HANDBOOK OF
TOXICOLOGY

Second Edition

ncasi

HANDBOOK OF
TOXICOLOGY

Second Edition

Edited by

Michael J. Derelanko, Ph.D., D.A.B.T., F.A.T.S.
Corporate Manager of Toxicology and Risk Assessment
Honeywell International Inc.
Morristown, New Jersey

Mannfred A. Hollinger, Ph.D.
Professor
Department of Medical Pharmacology and Toxicology
School of Medicine
University of California, Davis

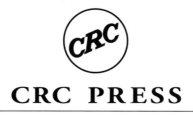

CRC PRESS

Boca Raton   London   New York   Washington, D.C.

Library of Congress Cataloging-in-Publication Data

Handbook of toxicology / Michael J. Derelanko, Mannfred A. Hollinger, editors.—2nd ed.
    p. cm.
    Updated and expanded ed. of: CRC handbook of toxicology. c1995.
    Includes bibliographical references and index.
    ISBN 0-8493-0370-2 (alk. paper)
    1. Toxicology—Handbooks, manuals, etc. I. Derelanko, Michael J. II. Hollinger,
Mannfred A. III. Derelanko, Michael J. CRC handbook of toxicology.

RA1215 .C73 2001
615.9—dc21   2001025086

Visit the CRC Press Web site at www.crcpress.com

© 2002 by CRC Press LLC

No claim to original U.S. Government works
International Standard Book Number 0-8493-0370-2
Library of Congress Card Number 2001025086
Printed in the United States of America 1 2 3 4 5 6 7 8 9 0
Printed on acid-free paper

Preface to the First Edition

Toxicologists working in the laboratory or office rely on a large information base to design, conduct, and interpret toxicology studies and to perform risk assessments. Diverse information such as normal hematology and clinical chemistry values, reproductive indices, physiological parameters, animal housing requirements, toxicity classifications, and regulatory requirements accumulated during the toxicologist's career are generally scattered in file cabinets and on office shelves. Although practicing toxicologists usually can locate information related to their own areas of expertise with minimal effort, obtaining reference information in less familiar areas of toxicology may require considerably more effort, possibly involving a trip to the library or a phone call to a colleague. A single basic reference source of toxicological information has not been previously available. We have attempted to fill this void with this publication.

Our goal was to produce a reference book containing practical reference information useful to practicing toxicologists in the chemical and pharmaceutical industries, contract laboratories, regulatory agencies, and academia. Contributors were asked to compile reference material for their own areas of expertise which would be of value to both experts and students. The task seemed easier in concept than it proved to be in reality. It quickly became evident that limits had to be placed on the amount and detail of information included to allow for publication in a reasonable time frame. Although information for most areas of toxicology is presented, coverage of some areas is clearly missing. We encourage and welcome constructive comments on improving the information provided as well as suggestions for additional material which could be included in possible future editions of this handbook.

We have designed the handbook to allow basic reference information to be located quickly. Each chapter begins with an outline of its contents. Where possible, text was purposely kept to a minimum. This book is intended only to be a basic reference source. The user requiring more detailed discussion should consult the sources cited. Much of the information provided has been previously published elsewhere. The editors and contributors cannot attest to the accuracy and completeness of such and, therefore, cannot assume any liability of any kind resulting from the use or reliance on the information presented in this handbook. Mention of vendors, trade names, or commercial products does not constitute endorsement or recommendation for use.

Preface to the Second Edition

It has been approximately 10 years since we began compiling information for the first edition of the CRC *Handbook of Toxicology*. In reviewing the material contained in the first edition it was apparent that information such as values for physiological parameters, substance toxicity, and information related to fundamental toxicology principles and practices remain virtually timeless. On the other hand, information on such topics as regulatory requirements and guidelines, contract laboratories, and contact information such as phone numbers and addresses clearly needed updating. Moreover, although information for most areas of toxicology was included in the first edition, coverage of some toxicology specialties was clearly missing.

In this respect, the *CRC Handbook of Toxicology, Second Edition* has been extensively updated and expanded. Nearly all of the original chapters from the first edition have been updated, with several receiving extensive revision. Additionally, coverage of inhalation toxicology, neurotoxicology, and histopathology has been expanded. Several new regulatory chapters dealing with pesticides, medical devices, consumer products, and worldwide notification of new chemicals have been added. Areas of toxicology missing from the first edition such as ecotoxicology and *in vitro* toxicology are now covered. Also included is a new chapter providing an extensive overview of the toxicology of metals.

Since the publication of the first edition, environmental and endocrine toxicology and children's health have become major issues that will clearly impact the field of toxicology in the future. To provide some basic information on these topics, two chapters on basic male and female endocrinology and toxicology have been included and tables have been added to the risk assessment chapter that provide information on differences in physiological and biochemical parameters between children and adults. When the first edition went to print, the Internet was in its infancy but has now become an important information-gathering tool for toxicologists. In the second edition, the authors were asked where possible to reference Web sites they consider sources of valuable information for their fields of expertise.

The *CRC Handbook of Toxicology* contains a considerable amount of reference information. However, because of the size of the handbook and the number of tables and figures it contains, some users of the first edition reported it was not always easy to identify and locate specific information quickly. As a search aid for the second edition, headings have been added at the top of each page identifying the chapter topics. Also we included pages at the end of some of the chapters to provide additional information closely related to the subject matter of the chapter. Constructive comments on how future editions of the *CRC Handbook of Toxicology* can be improved are welcome.

The number of chapters in the second edition has increased from the original 22 to 33 with over 200 new tables and figures added. It is said, "A picture is worth a thousand words." Thus, as in the first edition, text has been kept to a minimum where possible and practical reference information is provided in tables and figures that are useful to practicing toxicologists in the chemical and pharmaceutical industries, contract laboratories, regulatory agencies, and academia. As before, much of the information provided has been previously published elsewhere. Although considerable effort was made to obtain the information from reliable sources, the editors and contributors cannot attest to its accuracy and completeness and, therefore, cannot assume any liability of any kind resulting from the use or reliance on the information provided in this handbook. Mention of vendors, trade names, or commercial products does not constitute an endorsement or recommendation for use.

Michael J. Derelanko
Mannfred A. Hollinger

Editors

Michael J. Derelanko, Ph.D., D.A.B.T., F.A.T.S., is Corporate Manager of Toxicology and Risk Assessment at Honeywell International Inc., in Morristown, New Jersey. Dr. Derelanko received a B.S. degree from Saint Peter's College in 1973. He was a National Institutes of Health predoctoral trainee in the Albert S. Gordon Laboratory of Experimental Hematology at New York University, receiving M.S. and Ph.D. degrees. He received the 1976 New York University Gladys Mateyko Award for Excellence in Biology. Following a two-year postdoctoral fellowship in gastrointestinal pharmacology at Schering-Plough Corporation, he began his career in industrial toxicology in 1980 as a research toxicologist in the laboratories of Allied Chemical Corporation.

Dr. Derelanko is a Diplomate of the American Board of Toxicology and a Fellow of the Academy of Toxicological Sciences. He is a member of the Society of Toxicology, the Society for Experimental Biology and Medicine, and the honorary research society Sigma Xi. He has served on the content advisory committee of the New Jersey Liberty Science Center, has chaired or been a member of industrial and government toxicology advisory committees, is actively involved with the Chemical Industry Institute of Toxicology, and serves on the speaker's bureau of the New Jersey Association for Biomedical Research.

Dr. Derelanko has authored numerous papers in experimental hematology, gastrointestinal pharmacology, and toxicology. He has been actively involved in educating the public about toxicology, particularly at the middle school level. He has delivered invited lectures on this subject at national meetings. Dr. Derelanko's current research interests involve understanding the toxicity of aliphatic oximes. He is coeditor along with Dr. Mannfred A. Hollinger of the first edition of the *CRC Handbook of Toxicology* and author of CRC's *Toxicologist's Pocket Handbook*.

Mannfred A. Hollinger, Ph.D., is a Professor in the Department of Medical Pharmacology and Toxicology, School of Medicine, University of California, Davis. Dr. Hollinger is former editor of *Current Topics in Pulmonary Pharmacology and Toxicology, Focus on Pulmonary Pharmacology and Toxicology,* and *Yearbook of Pharmacology,* and assistant editor of *The Journal of Pharmacology and Experimental Therapeutics.* Dr. Hollinger serves on the editorial advisory board of *The Journal of Pharmacology and Experimental Therapeutics, Research Communications in Chemical Pathology and Pharmacology,* and *The Journal of The American College of Toxicology.* Dr. Hollinger is at present series editor of *Pharmacology and Toxicology: Basic and Clinical Aspects* for CRC Press. He is a member of the American Society of Pharmacology and Experimental Therapeutics and the Society of Toxicology.

Born in Chicago, he obtained his B.S. degree from North Park College in 1961 and his M.S. (1965) and Ph.D. (1967) degrees from Loyola University, Chicago. He was employed by Baxter Laboratories from 1961 to 1963. From 1967 to 1969, Dr. Hollinger was a postdoctoral research fellow in the Department of Pharmacology, Stanford University Medical School. Since coming to Davis in 1969, Dr. Hollinger has participated in several team-taught courses to undergraduate, graduate, and medical students.

While at Davis, Dr. Hollinger has published numerous research papers as well as a monograph on respiratory pharmacology and toxicology. He continues to serve as a referee for many of the principal pharmacology and toxicology journals. Dr. Hollinger was the recipient of a Burroughs-Wellcome Visiting Scientist Fellowship to Southampton, England in 1986 as well as a National Institutes of Health Fogarty Senior International Fellowship to Heidelberg, Germany in 1988. His current research interests deal with pulmonary fibrosis.

Contributors

Mohamed B. Abou-Donia, Ph.D.
Professor of Pharmacology and Neurobiology
Department of Pharmacology and Cancer
  Biology
Duke University Medical Center
Durham, North Carolina

Aqel W. Abu-Qare, Ph.D.
Research Associate
Department of Pharmacology and Cancer
  Biology
Duke University Medical Center
Durham, North Carolina

Carol S. Auletta, D.A.B.T., R.A.C., M.B.A.
Senior Director
Toxicology
Huntingdon Life Sciences
Princeton Research Center
East Millstone, New Jersey

William H. Baker, D.V.M., Dipl., A.C.V.P.
Associate Director of Pathology
Springborn Laboratories, Inc.
Spencerville, Ohio

Kimberly L. Bonnette, M.S., LATG
Manager of Acute Toxicology
Springborn Laboratories, Inc.
Spencerville, Ohio

G. Allen Burton, Jr., Ph.D.
Brage Golding Distinguished Professor of
  Research and Director
Institute for Environmental Quality
Wright State University
Dayton, Ohio

Rodger D. Curren, Ph.D.
President
Institute for In Vitro Sciences, Inc.
Gaithersburg, Maryland

Michael J. Derelanko, Ph.D., D.A.B.T., F.A.T.S.
Corporate Manager of Toxicology and Risk
  Assessment
Honeywell International Inc.
Morristown, New Jersey

Patrick J. Devine, Ph.D.
Research Associate
Department of Physiology
The University of Arizona
Tucson, Arizona

Jill Dolgin, Pharm.D.
Drug Information Product Manager
Product Information Department
SmithKline Beecham
Philadelphia, Pennsylvania

Brendan J. Dunn, M.S.
Manager, Toxicology and Risk Assessment
Honeywell International Inc.
Morristown, New Jersey

Donald J. Ecobichon, Ph.D.
Queen's University
Department of Pharmacology and Toxicology
Kingston, Ontario, Canada

Eman M. Elmasry, Ph.D.
Associate Professor
Faculty of Pharmacy
Zagazig University
Zagazig, Egypt

Henry C. Fogle, B.S., M.S.
Manager, International Regulatory Affairs
Honeywell International Inc.
Hopewell, Virginia

Ramadevi Gudi, Ph.D.
Study Director, Cytogenetics Studies
BioReliance Corp.
Rockville, Maryland

John W. Harbell, Ph.D.
Vice President and Chief Scientific Officer
Institute for In Vitro Sciences, Inc.
Gaithersburg, Maryland

Jane E. Harris, Ph.D.
Director of Toxicology
BASF Corp.
Princeton, New Jersey

Steven J. Hermansky, Pharm.D., Ph.D., D.A.B.T.
Associate Director
Product Safety and Toxicology
Schering-Plough HealthCare Products
Memphis, Tennessee

Kimiko Hirayama, Ph.D.
Professor
Kumamoto University College of Medical
    Science
Kumamoto, Japan

Richard M. Hoar, Ph.D.
Consultant in Developmental Toxicology
Williamstown, Massachusetts

David J. Hoffman, Ph.D.
Ecotoxicologist
Patuxent Wildlife Research Center
U.S. Geological Survey
Laurel, Maryland
and Adjunct Professor
University of Maryland

Gary M. Hoffman, B.A., D.A.B.T.
Study Director and Director of Inhalation
    Toxicology
Huntingdon Life Sciences
Princeton Research Center
East Millstone, New Jersey

Mannfred A. Hollinger, Ph.D.
Professor
Department of Medical Pharmacology and
    Toxicology
School of Medicine
University of California
Davis, California

Robert V. House, Ph.D.
Staff Scientist
Covance Laboratories, Inc.
Madison, Wisconsin

Patricia B. Hoyer, Ph.D.
Professor
Department of Physiology
The University of Arizona
Tucson, Arizona

David Jacobson-Kram, Ph.D., D.A.B.T.
Vice President
Toxicology and Laboratory Animal Health
BioReliance Corp.
Rockville, Maryland

Daniel R. Lavoie, M.S.
Aquatic Toxicologist
Institute for Environmental Quality
Wright State University
Dayton, Ohio

Barry S. Levine, D.Sc., D.A.B.T.
Director
Toxicology Research Laboratory
Associate Professor of Pharmacology
Department of Pharmacology
University of Illinois
Chicago, Illinois

Karen M. MacKenzie, Ph.D., D.A.B.T.
Consultant
Anderson, South Carolina

Rosemary C. Mandella, Ph.D., D.A.B.T.
Associate Director of Toxicology
Huntingdon Life Sciences
Princeton Research Center
East Millstone, New Jersey

Dennis J. Naas, B.S.
President, Owner
AccuTox Consulting Services, Ltd.
Midland, Michigan

Rajesh K. Naz, Ph.D.
Director
Division of Research
Department of Obstetrics and Gynecology
Medical College of Ohio
Toledo, Ohio

Paul E. Newton, Ph.D., D.A.B.T.
Senior Study Director and Director of
  Inhalation Toxicology
MPI Research, Inc.
Mattawan, Michigan

John C. Peckham, D.V.M., M.S., Ph.D.
Veterinary Pathologist
Experimental Pathology Laboratories, Inc.
Research Triangle Park, North Carolina

William J. Powers, Jr., Ph.D., D.A.B.T.
Vice President
Global Preclinical Development
Johnson & Johnson
Raritan, New Jersey

Barnett A. Rattner, Ph.D.
Ecotoxicologist
Patuxent Wildlife Research Center
U.S. Geological Survey
Laurel, Maryland
and Adjunct Professor
University of Maryland

Dawn D. Rodabaugh, B.S.
Assistant Toxicologist–Study Director
Springborn Laboratories, Inc.
Spencerville, Ohio

Richard H. C. San, Ph.D.
Scientific Director
Genetic Toxicology
BioReliance Corp.
Rockville, Maryland

Gene E. Schulze, Ph.D., D.A.B.T.
Associate Director
Department of Toxicology
Bristol-Myers Squibb Pharmaceutical Research
  Institute
Syracuse, New York

Joseph C. Siglin, Ph.D., D.A.B.T.
Director of Research
Springborn Laboratories, Inc.
Spencerville, Ohio

Suresh C. Sikka, Ph.D., H.C.L.D.
Associate Professor and Urology Research
  Director
Tulane University Health Sciences Center
New Orleans, Louisiana

Peter T. Thomas, Ph.D.
Director
Toxicology
Covance Laboratories, Inc.
Madison, Wisconsin

Valentine O. Wagner III, M.S.
Study Director
Bacterial Mutagenesis Studies
BioReliance Corp.
Rockville, Maryland

Christopher W. Wilson, B.S.
Assistant Toxicologist–Study Director
Springborn Laboratories, Inc.
Spencerville, Ohio

Akira Yasutake, Ph.D.
Chief in Biochemistry Section
National Institute for Minamata Disease
Kumamoto, Japan

Robert R. Young, M.S.
Director
Toxicology Operations
BioReliance Corp.
Rockville, Maryland

Acknowledgments

The editors and contributors thank the following individuals who helped with the preparation of the *CRC Handbook of Toxicology, Second Edition* by providing information, advice, constructive criticism, technical expertise, or secretarial skills: Dr. Bjorn Thorsrud, Dr. David Serota, Dr. David Dolan, Dr. George Rusch, Dr. Leigh Ann Naas, Dr. Hans Certa, Dr. George Dearlove, Dr. Gregory Kearns, Dr. Jill Merrill, Gary Roy, Donald Surprenant, Rita Levy, Renee Bolduc, Bob Nellis, Christy Calhoun, Michelle Delaurier, Ronald Brzozowski, Elise Larsen, Daniel Murray, Greg Mun, and Regina Carbon Tihan.

As the second edition of the handbook contains a significant amount of information from the first edition, the editors again acknowledge the following individuals for their help in the publication of the earlier handbook: Dr. David Serota, Dr. Kurt Weingand, Dr. Walter Loeb, Dr. George Rusch, Dr. Rosemary Mandella, Dr. C. Anita Bigger, Dr. Donald Putman, Renee Brown, Rita Levy, Cynthia Nofziger, Cathy Beck, Cindy Moore, Doris Bridgeman, Isabelle Baker, Antoinette Keesey, David Keesey, Robin Larkin, Donna Blaszcak, Diane Blansett, Ellen Whiting, Sharon Harris, Farrell Merriman, Gary Roy, Joseph Townsend, Pam Errico, Elizabeth Regan, Kristin Ballard, Kim Cayz, Michael Mercieca, Jane Clark, Hans Raabe, Betsy Schadly, Skip Wagner, Robert Young, Bernette Cockrell, Christine Holzer, Trina Rode, Carol Winiarski, Dolores Yili, Georgene Rutledge, Rusty Rush, Deborah Douds, Todd Merriman, and Gregory Kowalski.

The editors extend a special thanks to the authors and publishers who graciously allowed the reprinting of many of the tables and figures in the handbook.

Helpful Tips for Using This Handbook

The *CRC Handbook of Toxicology* has been designed to allow the working toxicologist to locate basic toxicological information quickly. Where possible, text has been kept to a minimum with most of the information provided in tables and figures. The information is organized into chapters dealing with various areas of toxicology. Each chapter begins with a detailed listing of all of the major topics, tables, and figures it contains. Headings are provided on the top of each page identifying the chapter topic to allow quick location of the subject matter. Because of the large and varied amount of information in the handbook, the user seeking a specific type of information may not always find reference to it in the index. It is recommended that a user seeking, for example, information on reproductive indices used in multigeneration studies use the page headings to locate the chapter on reproductive toxicology, turn to the first page of the chapter, and scan the contents listing. The user will quickly find that Table 11.13 provides the desired information. Similarly, cage requirements for rats can be quickly found in Table 1.16 of Chapter 1 by locating this chapter on laboratory animal management and scanning its contents listing. The user is cautioned that some information contained in the handbook may change over time, particularly as relates to regulatory requirements and guidelines, addresses, and phone numbers.

Table of Contents

Dedication

The second edition of the Handbook of Toxicology *is dedicated to toxicologists past, present, and future*

Dedication of the first edition

For MJD

To my wife, Patricia, and my sons, Michael and Robert, for their patience and understanding; to my parents, Anne and Frank, for their encouragement and support; to my mentors, Dr. Joseph LoBue, and the late Drs. Albert Gordon and Robert Kelly, for the example they set.

For MAH

To Georgia Lee Hollinger, Randolph Alan Hollinger, and Christopher Hastings Hollinger, for being special contributors in their own way.

1 Laboratory Animal Management

Joseph C. Siglin, Ph.D., D.A.B.T.
and William H. Baker, D.V.M., D.A.C.V.P.

CONTENTS

0-8493-0370-2/02/$0.00+$1.50
© 2002 by CRC Press LLC

SECTION 1. INTRODUCTION

The use of live animals continues to be an important and necessary component of research activities worldwide. To ensure the ethical and humane treatment of animals, scientists must possess a sound understanding of appropriate animal husbandry practices and must be knowledgeable of those variables which may impact and potentially confound experimental procedures and results.

The purpose of this chapter is to provide the scientist with a reference source covering many of the fundamental aspects of proper laboratory animal management for species commonly utilized in toxicological research. In keeping with the desired format of this book, the information provided herein is presented in concise fashion to allow a broad coverage of animal husbandry topics and related information. For more detailed information, the reader is referred to the reference materials identified in individual sections, and at the end of this chapter.

SECTION 2. ANIMAL HUSBANDRY

Animal husbandry may be simply defined as the methods used in the care and maintenance of animals. In a larger sense, however, animal husbandry encompasses all aspects of appropriate care, treatment, and management for a given species, including circadian rhythm, life span, environmental limits, breeding and reproductive patterns, nutritional and social requirements, and macro- and microenvironmental necessities. Of course, each species has its own unique peculiarities that are essential to its well-being. The scientist must be knowledgeable of these characteristics and of the various regulatory guidelines and policies that govern the use of animals in research.

SECTION 3. REGULATIONS AND GUIDELINES

Over the years, the United States and other countries have developed various federal mandates and statutes designed to protect animals from illicit commerce and use. The first such federal statute in the United States was the Pet Protection Act of 1966. This act became the forerunner of what is now called the Animal Welfare Act.

A. ANIMAL WELFARE ACT

The Animal Welfare Act (AWA)[1] refers to the Act of August 24, 1966 (P.L. 89-544), as amended by the Acts of December 24, 1970 (P.L. 91-579), April 22, 1976 (P.L. 94-279), December 23, 1985 (P.L. 99-198), and 1990 (P.L. 101-624). The various provisions of the AWA are designed to ensure that animals used in research, for exhibition, or as pets receive humane care and treatment. The AWA also regulates the transport, purchase, sale, housing, care, treatment, and handling of such animals. The standards set forth by the AWA are considered absolute minimal standards to which people who handle animals must adhere. According to the AWA, "animal" is defined as "any live or dead dog, cat, nonhuman primate, guinea pig, hamster, rabbit, or any other warm-blooded animal, which is being used or is intended for use for research, teaching, testing, experimentation, exhibition, or as a pet." The term dog means "all dogs including those used for hunting, security, or breeding purposes."

Regulatory authority under the AWA is implemented by the Animal and Plant Health Inspection Service (APHIS) of the U.S. Department of Agriculture. Rules and regulations pertaining to implementation of the law are provided in the Code of Federal Regulations (CFR), Title 9 (Animals and Animal Products), Subchapter A (Animal Welfare), Parts 1, 2, and 3. Copies of the regulations may be obtained on line searching for "Animal Welfare Act" or at www.nal.usda.gov/awia/legislat/usdaleg.htm. The relevant regulations and standards covered by the AWA are summarized below.

Subjects Addressed by the AWA

- Part 1: Definition of Terms
- Part 2: Regulations
  Subpart A: Licensing
  Subpart B: Registration
  Subpart C: Research Facilities
  Subpart D: Attending Veterinarian and Adequate Veterinary Care
  Subpart E: Identification of Animals
  Subpart F: Stolen Animals
  Subpart G: Records
  Subpart H: Compliance with Standards and Holding Period
  Subpart I: Miscellaneous
- Part 3: Standards
  Subparts A–F: Specifications for the Humane Handling, Care, Treatment and Transportation of Dogs and Cats, Guinea Pigs and Hamsters, Rabbits, Non-human Primates, Marine Mammals, and Other Warm-blooded Mammals

According to the AWA, "each dealer, exhibitor, operator of an auction sale, and intermediate handler must comply in all respects with the regulations set forth in Part 2 and the standards set forth in Part 3 for the humane handling, care, treatment, housing, and transportation of animals."

B. PUBLIC HEALTH SERVICE REGULATIONS

In 1973, a new policy applying to all Public Health Service (PHS) awardee institutions was drafted. The policy required that institutions conducting PHS-supported research comply with the AWA and the *Guide for the Care and Use of Laboratory Animals.*[2] Each institution is also required to provide the National Institutes of Health (NIH) with an assurance which gives a detailed plan for research, training, testing, education, experimentation, or demonstration purposes. In essence, the policy requires that institutions take responsibility for the quality of their animal research programs and the conduct of investigators and animal care personnel. In 1985, the Public Health Service Policy on Humane Care and Use of Laboratory Animals by awardee institutions was updated and the final version of the policy was made effective January 1, 1986. Subsequently, Congress enacted and later revised the *Health Research Extension Act* November 20, 1985 (P.L. 99-158) which added several key provisions to the PHS policy. Although the policy is not law, it has the same effect because an institution must comply in order to compete for funding for animal-related research from PHS and other funding sources. Key elements of the PHS policy include:

- Negotiation of Animal Welfare Assurances which include commitments by awardee institutions concerning animal care and use, training of staff, and occupational health programs for employees;
- Establishment of an Institutional Animal Care and Use Committee (IACUC) with defined responsibilities;
- Detailed requirements for the submission of applications for awards;
- Specific record keeping requirements to ensure clear accountability for the quality of the institutional program; and
- Specific reporting requirements which enable funding agencies and the NIH Office of Laboratory Animal Welfare (OLAW) to oversee the entire system.

Additional information concerning the PHS policy may be obtained from the Office of Laboratory Animal Welfare, National Institutes of Health, 6705 Rockledge, Pr, RKLI, Suite 1050, MSC 7982, Bethesda, MD 20892–7982.

Each institution subject to the PHS policy is expected to operate its research program in accordance with the U.S. Government Principles for the Utilization and Care of Vertebrate Animals Used in Research and Training. These principles are listed below.

U.S. Government Principles for the Utilization and Care of Vertebrate Animals Used in Research and Training

- The transportation, care, and use of animals should be in accordance with the Animal Welfare Act and other applicable federal laws, guidelines, and policies.
- Procedures involving animals should be designed and performed with due consideration of their relevance to human or animal health, the advancement of knowledge, or the good of society.
- The animals selected for a procedure should be of an appropriate species and quality and the minimum number required to obtain valid results. Methods such as mathematical models, computer simulation, and *in vitro* biological systems should be considered.
- Proper use of animals, including the avoidance or minimization of discomfort, distress, and pain when consistent with sound scientific practices, is imperative. Unless the contrary is established, investigators should consider that procedures that cause pain or distress in human beings may cause pain or distress in other animals.
- Procedures with animals that may cause more than momentary or slight pain or distress should be performed with appropriate sedation, analgesia, or anesthesia. Surgical or other painful procedures should not be performed on unanesthetized animals paralyzed by chemical agents.
- Animals that would otherwise suffer severe or chronic pain or distress that cannot be relieved should be painlessly killed at the end of the procedure or, if appropriate, during the procedure.

- The living conditions of animals should be appropriate for their species and contribute to their health and comfort. Normally, the housing, feeding, and care of all animals used for biomedical purposes must be directed by a veterinarian or other scientist trained and experienced in the proper care, handling, and use of the species being maintained or studied. In any case, veterinary care shall be provided as indicated.
- Investigators and other personnel shall be appropriately qualified and experienced for conducting procedures on living animals. Adequate arrangements shall be made for their in-service training, including the proper and humane care and use of laboratory animals.
- Where exceptions are required in relation to the provisions of these Principles, the decisions should not rest with the investigators directly concerned but should be made, with due regard to the second principle (see above), by an appropriate review group such as an institutional animal care and use committee. Such exceptions should not be made solely for the purposes of teaching or demonstration.

C. GUIDE FOR THE CARE AND USE OF LABORATORY ANIMALS

The *Guide for the Care and Use of Laboratory Animals*[2] was first published in 1963 under the title *Guide for Laboratory Animal Facilities and Care.* The *Guide* has been revised several times since 1963 with the latest edition prepared in 1996. The *Guide* provides information on common laboratory species housed under a variety of circumstances. Although the *Guide* is not intended to be an exhaustive review of all aspects of animal care and use, it does address a number of relevant issues, including physical construction of animal facilities, husbandry, veterinary care, sanitation, and qualifications and training of laboratory personnel. In the most recent version of the *Guide* (National Academy of Science ISBN-0-309-05377-3, Revised 1996), emphasis was placed on the establishment of an Animal Care and Use Committee to oversee animal care facilities and insure compliance with applicable federal, state, and local laws and regulations. Copies of the *Guide* may be obtained from the Institute of Laboratory Animal Resources, National Research Council, 2101 Constitution Ave., NW, Washington, D.C. 20418. www.nas.edu/cls/ilarhome.nsf. E-mail: ILAR@NAS.edu. FAX: 202-334-1687. Various topics covered by the *Guide* are listed below.

Topics Covered by the Guide for the Care and Use of Laboratory Animals[2]

- Institutional Policies
  Monitoring the Care and Use of Animals
  Veterinary Care
  Personnel Qualifications and Training
  Personal Hygiene
  Occupational Health
  Animal Experimentation Involving Hazardous Agents
  Special Considerations
- Laboratory Animal Husbandry
  Housing
  Animal Environment
  Food
  Bedding
  Water
  Sanitation
  Identification and Records
  Emergency, Weekend, and Holiday Care
- Veterinary Care
  Preventative Medicine

Surveillance, Diagnosis, Treatment, and Control of Disease
Anesthesia and Analgesia
Surgery and Postsurgical Care
Euthanasia
- Physical Plant
Physical Relationship of Animal Facilities to Laboratories
Functional Areas
Construction Guidelines
Aseptic Surgery
- Special Considerations
Genetics and Nomenclature
Facilities and Procedures for Animal Research with Hazardous Agents
Farm Animals

Appendices
A. Selected Bibliography
B. Professional and Certifying Laboratory Animal Science Organizations
C. Federal Laws Relevant to Animal Care and Use
D. Public Health Service Policy and Government Principles on Care and Use of Animals

SECTION 4. INSTITUTIONAL PROGRAMS

A. AAALAC

The American Association for Accreditation of Laboratory Animal Care (AAALAC) is a nonprofit corporation whose primary goal is to promote high-quality care and use of animals through a voluntary accreditation program. Institutions maintaining, using, importing, or breeding laboratory animals for scientific research are eligible to apply for AAALAC accreditation. The accreditation process involves inspection of the animal facilities and program by experts in laboratory animal science, who submit a comprehensive report for consideration by the Council on Accreditation. The Council reviews the report, using the *Guide for the Care and Use of Laboratory Animals* as a basis for determining whether full accreditation should be granted. If accreditation is granted, facilities are required to submit annual reports concerning the status of their animal facilities and animal program. Site reinspections are conducted by AAALAC representatives at intervals of 3 years or less to determine whether accreditation should be continued.

The specific standards which have been established by the AAALAC Board of Trustees for accreditation are listed below. AAALAC.org.

AAALAC Accreditation Standards

- Care and management of laboratory animals should be directed by qualified people.
- All animal care personnel should be qualified by training and experience in laboratory animal science.
- Physical facilities and husbandry methods for the animals should allow their maintenance in wellbeing and comfort.
- The NIH *Guide* is the basic guide to the establishment of specific standards for accreditation.
- The accreditable unit shall comply with all statutes and regulations including, but not limited to, the prevailing standards of sanitation, health, labor, and safety of the community and state of location.
- Membership in or affiliation with an organization dedicated to laboratory animal care and use is not required for accreditation.

Once a facility becomes fully accreditated, a certificate of accreditation is issued and the facility is identified on a list of accreditated facilities published in the Association's Activities Report. Full AAALAC accreditation is accepted as partial assurance by NIH that the animal facility and program are in compliance with PHS policy. Further information on AAALAC accreditation may be obtained from AAALAC, 11300 Rockville Pike, Suite 1211, Rockville, MD 20852. Telephone: (301) 231-5353. Fax: (301) 231-8282.

B. IACUC

The AWA, PHS policy, and *Guide for the Care and Use of Laboratory Animals* all require the establishment of an Institutional Animal Care and Use Committee (IACUC) that is responsible for monitoring the facility's animal care and use program. The AWA requires that the IACUC be appointed by the chief executive officer of the research facility and consist of a chairperson and at least two additional members as follows:

- A Doctor of Veterinary Medicine, with training or experience in laboratory animal science and medicine, who has direct or delegated program responsibility for activities involving the research facility; and
- An individual not affiliated in any way with the facility other than as a member of the committee, and not a member of the immediate family of a person who is affiliated with the facility. This individual should provide representation for general community interests in the proper care and treatment of animals.

The *Guide for the Care and Use of Laboratory Animals*[2] specifies an IACUC composition comparable to that required by the AWA, with the addition of "other members as required by institutional needs and by federal, state and local regulations and policies." The PHS policy is somewhat different in that it specifically requires that the IACUC be composed of at least five members, including a veterinarian with program responsibilities, a scientist experienced in laboratory animal research, a nonscientist, and an individual who has no other association with the institution besides membership in the IACUC (the specific role and background of the fifth member is not specified).

The AWA, PHS policy, and *Guide for the Care and Use of Laboratory Animals* all specify relatively similar functions for the IACUC, which include:

- Review, at least once every 6 months, the research facility's program for humane care and use of animals.
- Inspect, at least once every 6 months, all the animal facilities, including animal study areas and satellite facilities.
- Prepare and submit reports of IACUC evaluations to the institutional official.
- Review and, if warranted, investigate concerns involving the care and use of animals at the facility resulting from public complaints and from reports of noncompliance received from facility personnel or employees.
- Make recommendations to the institutional official regarding any aspect of the research facility's animal program, facilities, or personnel training.
- Review and approve, require modifications in (to secure approval), or withhold approval of those components of proposed activities related to the care and use of animals.
- Review and approve, require modifications in (to secure approval), or withhold approval of proposed significant changes regarding the care and use of animals in ongoing activities.

The IACUC may also suspend any activity involving animals which is deemed unacceptable. However, it is the intent of the guidelines above to avoid such situations through the implementation of sensible and ethical animal programs, training, and preliminary review of proposed animal activities by the IACUC.

Further information concerning IACUC authority and functions may be found in the AWA, 9 CFR, Subchapter A, Part 2, Subpart C, 2.3.1. In addition, an *Institutional Animal Care and Use Committee Guidebook,* prepared by the NIH Office of Laboratory Animal Welfare (OLAW), may be obtained from: Applied Research Ethics National Association, 132 Boylston Street, Boston, MA 02116, or from the Superintendent of Documents, U.S. Government Printing Office, Washington, D.C. 20402 ISBN-0-309-05377-3.

SECTION 5. PROFESSIONAL AND GOVERNMENTAL ORGANIZATIONS

Information concerning various professional and governmental organizations involved in laboratory animal science, animal welfare, or related activities is provided in the following sections.

A. AALAS

The American Association for Laboratory Animal Science (AALAS) is concerned with all aspects of laboratory animal care and use, and provides a means for collection and exchange of information on all phases of animal care and management. The association holds annual meetings and publishes a bimonthly journal, *Laboratory Animal Science.* The AALAS Animal Technician Certification Board provides for three levels of technical certification: Assistant Laboratory Animal Technician (ALAT), Laboratory Animal Technician (LAT), and Laboratory Animal Technologist (LATG). Additional information may be obtained from AALAS. Telephone: (901) 745-8620. Fax: (901) 753-0046. www.aalas.org

B. ACLAM

The American College of Laboratory Animal Medicine (ACLAM) was founded in 1957 to encourage education, training, and research; to establish standards of training and experience for qualification; and to certify, by examination, qualified laboratory animal specialists as diplomates. ACLAM meets biannually in conjunction with the American Veterinary Medical Association (AVMA) and the American Association for Laboratory Animal Science (AALAS). The College emphasizes and sponsors continuing education and autotutorial programs on the use, husbandry, and diseases of animals used in research. Additional information may be obtained through the ACLAM website at www.aclam.org/foundation_contacts.

C. ASLAP

The American Society of Laboratory Animal Practitioners (ASLAP) was organized to disseminate ideas, experiences, and knowledge among veterinarians involved in laboratory animal practice through education, training, and research. The Society, which was founded in 1966, is open to any graduate of a veterinary college accredited or recognized by the AVMA. ASLAP holds two educational meetings annually, one in conjunction with the AVMA annual meeting and one in conjunction with the AALAS annual meeting. Additional information may be obtained through the ASLAP Coordinator, 11300 Rockville Pike, Suite 1211, Rockville, MD 20852. Telephone: (301)231-6349. Fax: (231)231-6071. aslap@aaalac.org

D. AVMA

The American Veterinary Medical Association (AVMA) is the major national organization of veterinarians. The primary mission of the AVMA is the advancement of veterinary medical science, including its relationship to public health and agriculture. The AVMA is the major accrediting agency for colleges of veterinary medicine. The AVMA sponsors specialization in veterinary medicine through the recognition of specialty certifying organizations such as ACLAM. The AVMA Committee on Animal Technician Activities and Training accredits 2-year programs in animal technology throughout the United States. A summary of state laws and regulations relative to veterinarians and animal technicians is available from the AVMA, 1931 North Meacham Road, Suite 100, Schaumburg, IL 60173. Telephone: (847) 925-8070. Fax: (847) 925-1329.

E. ICLAS

The International Council for Laboratory Animal Science (ICLAS) is a nongovernmental organization that encourages international cooperation in laboratory animal science. ICLAS promotes the development of international standards for the care and use of laboratory animals, disseminates information concerning laboratory animals, sponsors scholarships for education, and supports programs that advance laboratory animal science in developing nations. ICLAS issues the *ICLAS Bulletin* every spring and autumn. Additional information may be obtained from www.iclas.org.

F. ILAR

The Institute of Laboratory Animal Resources (ILAR) was founded in 1952 under the auspices of the National Research Council. ILAR's mission is to provide expert counsel to the federal government, the biomedical research community, and the public on the scientific, technological, and ethical use of laboratory animals within the context of the interests and mission of the National Academy of Sciences. ILAR promotes the high-quality humane care of laboratory animals; the appropriate use of laboratory animals; and the exploration of alternatives in research, testing, and teaching. The most recent edition of the *Guide for the Care and Use of Laboratory Animals*[2] was prepared by ILAR for the National Institutes of Health. For more information, contact ILAR, National Academy of Sciences, 2101 Constitution Ave., NW, Washington, D.C. 20418. Telephone: (202) 334-2590. Fax: (202) 334-1687. ILAR@nas.edu.

G. SCAW

The Scientists' Center for Animal Welfare (SCAW) was founded in 1979 and consists of individuals and institutions concerned with various aspects of animal welfare. SCAW promotes the principle of humane animal care and treatment in all areas of animal science. Among other activities, SCAW develops educational materials and national guidelines on humane animal experimentation; monitors animal legislation issues; and conducts workshops and surveys. For more information, contact SCAW, 7833 Walker Drive, Suite 340, Greenbelt, MD 20770. Telephone: (301) 345-3500. www.scaw.com

H. NIH

The National Institutes of Health (NIH) is a federal agency that disburses funds for biomedical research and sets policy on laboratory animal welfare (PHS policy). Additional information may be obtained from: Office of Animal Care and Use, 9000 Rockville Pike, Bethesda, MD 20892. Telephone: (301) 496-5424.

I. DEA

The Drug Enforcement Administration (DEA) of the U.S. Department of Justice is the regulatory authority responsible for the enforcement of laws pertaining to controlled substances. Licenses to use controlled substances are obtained from this agency. Additional information may be obtained from: DEA, Registration Unit-ODRR, Washington, D.C. 20537. Telephone: (202) 307-7255.

J. FDA

The U.S. Food and Drug Administration (FDA) is the federal agency responsible for enforcing the FDA Good Laboratory Practice (GLP) regulations. Additional information may be obtained from: United States FDA, Parklawn Building, 5600 Fishers Lane, Rockville, MD 20857. Telephone: (301) 443-5006. 1-888-463-6332.

K. OLAW

The Office of Laboratory Animal Welfare (OLAW) of the NIH oversees compliance with the Public Health Service Policy on Humane Care and Use of Laboratory Animals. Additional information may be obtained from: OLAW, 9000 Rockville Pike, Building 31, Room 5B63, Bethesda, MD, 20892. Telephone: (301) 496-7005.

L. APHIS

The Animal, Plant and Health Inspection Service (APHIS) is the division of the U.S. Department of Agriculture that administers the federal Animal Welfare Act. Additional information may be obtained from: USDA, APHIS, 2568-A RIVA RD., ANNAPOLIS, MD 21401. Telephone: (410) 571-8692. aphis.web@usda.gov

M. AWI

The Animal Welfare Institute (AWI) is a national organization active in laboratory animal welfare issues. The AWI encourages lay persons to serve on IACUCs and has a number of publications pertinent to laboratory animal welfare. Additional information may be obtained from: AWI, P.O. Box 3650, Washington, D.C. 20007. Telephone: (202) 337-2332. FAX: (202) 338-9478. awi@animalwelfare.com

N. AWIC

The Animal Welfare Information Center (AWIC) is an information center of the National Agricultural Library established as result of the 1985 amendment to the Animal Welfare Act. Additional information may be obtained from: National Agricultural Library, Room 301, Beltsville, MD 20705. Telephone: (301) 504-6212.

O. CAAT

The Center for Alternatives to Animal Testing (CAAT) was established in 1981 to encourage and support the development of nonanimal testing methods. The center supports grants, sponsors symposia, and publishes a variety of materials related to animal testing and alternatives. Additional information may be obtained from: Johns Hopkins School of Hygiene and Public Health, Baltimore, MD 21202. Telephone: (410) 223-1612.

P. NABR

The National Association for Biomedical Research (NABR) is a nonprofit organization which was established in 1979 and merged with the National Society for Medical Research in 1985. Membership in NABR includes numerous institutions, universities, medical and veterinary schools; health agencies; academic and professional societies; and private and public research organizations.

NABR monitors legislation that could potentially impact the use of animals in research. Members of NABR may obtain copies of bills, summaries of bills, listings of current legislation, and related materials via the NABR computerized database. Additionally, a compilation of *State Laws Concerning the Use of Animals in Research* may be obtained through NABR.

NABR supports the responsible and ethical use of laboratory animals in research, education, and product safety testing. NABR recognizes that it may not be feasible to completely replace live animals in research because whole living organisms are an indispensable element of biomedical research and testing. Still, the Association believes that animal use should be minimized whenever possible; that pain and distress should be avoided and/or minimized; and that alternatives to live animals should continue to be developed and utilized, whenever feasible. Additional information may be obtained from: Ms. Frankie Trull, President, 818 Connecticut Ave., NW, Suite 200, Washington, D.C. 20006. Telephone: (202) 857-0540.

SECTION 6. ORGANIZATIONS THAT OPPOSE THE USE OF ANIMALS IN RESEARCH

A number of organizations strongly oppose the use of animals in research, or exhibit varying philosophies regarding this subject. There are, however, some deep divisions in the philosophies and strategies of these organizations. For example, animal welfare groups such as the humane societies tend to be most concerned with the proper care and treatment of animals, pet adoption, and humane euthanasia. On the other hand, "animal rights" groups are primarily concerned with establishing the "legal rights" of animals. These latter groups outwardly oppose the use of animals in research and the "exploitation" of animals for sport or food. The activities of these groups have challenged the research community to better inform and educate the public about the critical need for animals in research. Additional standing goals for scientists include:

- Reduction of the number of animals used through thoughtful selection of techniques and models.
- Relief of any unavoidable discomfort to animals.
- Improvement of animal facilities and assurance that personnel are fully informed and properly trained.
- Elimination or reduction of experimental procedures that cause pain or distress.
- Utilization of nonanimal alternatives whenever and wherever possible.

SECTION 7. ANIMAL PAIN

In accordance with the AWA, *Guide for the Care and Use of Laboratory Animals*, and Public Health Service Policy for the Humane Care and Use of Laboratory Animals, veterinarians and investigators must identify and eliminate sources of pain and distress, with the exception of those procedures that are essential to the research in question and approved by the IACUC. Although it is widely agreed that laboratory animals need not experience substantial pain or distress, there is a general lack of agreement on the specific meaning of such terms as comfort, wellbeing, discomfort, stress, fear, anxiety, pain, and distress. Nonetheless, provisional definitions for these terms have been developed[3] and are presented below.

- *Comfort:* A state of physiological, psychological, and behavioral equilibrium in which an animal is accustomed to its environment and engages in normal activities, such as feeding, drinking, grooming, social interaction, sleeping-waking cycles, and reproduction.
- *Wellbeing:* A positive mental state that reflects the level of welfare and comfort of an animal.

- *Discomfort:* A minimal change in an animal's adaptive level or baseline state as a result of changes in its environment or biological, physical, social, or psychotic alterations. Physiological or behavioral changes that indicate a state of stress might be observed, but are not marked enough to indicate distress.
- *Stress:* The effect produced by external (physical or environmental) events or internal (physiological or psychological) factors, referred to as stressors, which induce an alteration in an animal's biological equilibrium.
- *Anxiety and fear:* Emotional states that are traditionally associated with stress. They can be adaptive in that they inhibit an organism's actions that could lead to harm or cause it to act in ways allowing it to escape from potentially harmful situations.
- *Pain:* Results from potential or actual tissue damage. Pain can be considered a potent source of stress, that is, a stressor. It can also be considered a state of stress itself, however, and can lead to distress and maladaptive behaviors.
- *Distress:* An adverse state in which an animal is unable to adapt completely to stressors and the resulting stress and shows maladaptive behaviors. It can be evident in the presence of various experimental or environmental phenomena, such as abnormal feeding, absence or diminution of postprandial grooming, inappropriate social interaction with conspecifics or handlers, and inefficient reproduction.

With regard to the issues of animal discomfort and pain, researchers should consider the following questions before undertaking any live animal experiment:

- Will the procedure yield results that are beneficial to animal or human health and wellbeing?
- Has a literature search been performed to ensure that the proposed procedures do not unnecessarily duplicate previous experiments?
- Is the species and number of animals appropriate for the purpose of the experiment?
- Is the discomfort to the animals limited to that which is unavoidable in the conduct of the experiment?
- Have appropriate analgesic, anesthetic, and tranquilizing drugs been considered to minimize pain and discomfort?
- Has the method of euthanasia been considered?
- Are the individuals performing the experimental procedures and caring for the animals properly trained?

In general, procedures that cause minimal pain or discomfort to humans and place the animal in minimal distress are considered acceptable.

SECTION 8. ANIMAL MODELS AND ALTERNATIVES

Animal models may be broadly classified as experimental, negative, or spontaneous. An experimental model is one in which an experimentally induced condition mimics a human disease. A negative model, on the other hand, is one in which a particular condition cannot be produced, and is therefore studied to better understand the reason for the protective or resistant effect(s). A spontaneous model is one in which the animal naturally develops a disease or some other condition of interest.

In considering a particular animal model for an experiment, the investigator must first ensure that there are no acceptable nonanimal alternatives for the planned research. Once this has been clearly established and documented (e.g., by detailed literature search and review), special consideration must be given toward species availability, husbandry and technical expertise, space and caging requirements, special environmental requirements, genetic characteristics, nutritional requirements, microbial etiology and life span of the animal, and reproductive, anatomic, physiological, and behavioral characteristics of the species.

An alternative model is defined as any technique that reduces or eliminates the need for live animals and thereby prevents potential pain and distress in animals. Such alternative models include computer and mathematical simulations, microbiological systems, tissue/organ culture, epidemiological surveys, and plant analysis. A major drawback common to many of these alternative models is the lack of complex physiological interactions that occur in the whole animal. Nonetheless, the potential for reduction and replacement of live animals provides strong incentive for the continued development and validation of alternative models.

SECTION 9. ANIMAL FACILITY SAFETY

The Occupational Safety and Health Act (OSHA), which is administered by the U.S. Department of Labor, is not specifically directed at laboratories and research operations. However, the regulations apply to all work places and cover fire, electrical, and mechanical safety, and exposure to chemicals, radiation, and noise. In general, research laboratories have not been subjected to the frequent and rigorous OSHA inspections which are common to industries with intrinsically high accident rates. However, there now exist specific OSHA regulations concerning occupational exposures to toxic substances in research laboratories. These standards require that the laboratory develop a "Chemical Hygiene Program" designed to provide employee protection in the specific circumstances of the individual laboratory. In addition, there are requirements for training of employees, worker availability to reference materials concerning chemical hazards, and a provision for medical consultation and examination.

SECTION 10. ZOONOTIC DISEASES[4,10]

Zoonotic diseases are those which are transmissible from animals to humans under natural conditions. A few of the better known zoonotic diseases are described in the following sections.

A. HEPATITIS

Hepatitis A virus can infect chimpanzees, gorillas, patas monkeys, celebres, apes, woolly monkeys, and some tamarins. However, chimps recently introduced into captivity are the most common source of infection for humans. The incubation period for the virus may be 15–50 days, followed by abrupt onset of fever, anorexia, nausea, and jaundice. The severity of the disease is related to age, with fatality quite low among hospitalized patients. Lifelong immunity is conferred by development of an IgG immune response. Disease control measures involve quarantine, adequate protective clothing, sanitation, and personal hygiene. As an additional measure, the PHS recommends immunoprophylaxis (i.e., administration of immune serum globulin every 4 months) for personnel in close contact with newly imported chimps.

B. HERPESVIRUS B

Herpesvirus B, which is caused by *Herpesvirus simiae*, represents the most serious health hazard to humans from nonhuman primates. In the natural host of the virus, the *Macaca* spp, the disease is mild and similar to that of herpes simplex in humans, with the development of tongue and lip ulcers which heal in 7–14 days. In contrast, in infected humans, disease symptoms may be similar to polio, with rapid flaccid paralysis leading to death, or permanent paralysis in survivors. Transmission usually occurs through a bite from an infected animal, or by exposure of the broken skin or mucus membranes to infected saliva or infected tissues. Because of the potential danger to humans, all macaques should be viewed as potential carriers, and protective clothing should be worn at all times which protects the handler from bites and scratches. Although antiserum is available, its effectiveness is questionable.

Note: Herpes simplex in man can be transmitted to lower primates with generalized disease in owl monkeys, tree shrews, lemurs, marmosets, and tamaris.

C. RABIES

In the United States, the skunk and bat are the largest natural reservoirs of the rabies virus. The virus is transmitted through the saliva of infected animals via bites, scratches, abrasions, or across mucus membranes. In dogs, the virus is present in the saliva for 1–14 days before clinical symptoms manifest. In humans, the disease is almost always fatal, even when proper treatment is begun shortly after exposure. The most important disease control measure for domestic animals is vaccination. For humans, preexposure vaccination should be made available for all persons working with potentially infected animals.

D. LYMPHOCYTIC CHORIOMENINGITIS

Mice, hamsters, and humans serve as natural hosts for the virus causing lymphocytic choriomen-ingitis, and wild mice are a natural reservoir for the virus, which is the only latent virus in mice that naturally infects humans. The incidence of the disease may be 100% in wild populations, and may become 100% in breeding colonies if preventive measures are not instituted. However, only persistently infected mice and acutely infected hamsters are known to transmit the virus, which may be passed in the urine, feces, saliva, and nasal secretions of carrier animals. Lifelong infection with high concentrations in all organs is often observed in fetal and newborn infected mice. Hamsters, on the other hand, may remain infected for long periods, but eventually eliminate the virus. There are four different recognized forms of the disease in mice. In the cerebral form, death may occur with no previous symptoms on the fifth or sixth day after inoculation. In the visceral form, death may also occur after several days, but is often preceded by conjunctivitis and ruffled fur. In the late-onset form which occurs in neonatally infected mice, animals may seem healthy until 9–12 months of age when signs of chronic illness manifest, including ruffled fur, weight loss, and hunched posture. A form resulting in early death of neonatally exposed mice may also occur under poorly understood conditions. Infection of humans often results in mild influenza-like symptoms, and may or may not involve the central nervous system. Other than direct virus isolation, a rise in antibody titer serves as the most conclusive diagnosis of infection.

E. OTHER ZOONOSES

Other zoonoses are described briefly in Table 1.1.

TABLE 1.1
Other Zoonotic Diseases

Disease	Description
Monkey pox	Related to smallpox; clinical signs in humans include fever, headache, sore throat, and rash
Benign epidermal monkey pox (BEMP)	Primarily affects macaques and Leaf monkeys; circumscribed elevated lesions on eyelids, face, and elsewhere; in humans, disease regresses in 2–3 weeks
Yaba virus	Caused by a poxvirus transmitted via a mosquito vector; virus has been inoculated into humans, but natural transmission has not been recorded; infected animals develop benign histiocytomas that eventually regress

TABLE 1.1 *(Continued)*
Other Zoonotic Diseases

Disease	Description
Contagious ecthyma (ORF)	Caused by poxvirus of sheep and goats; characterized by epithelial proliferation and necrosis in the skin and mucus membranes of urogenital and gastrointestinal tracts; in humans, seen as painful nodules on hands which resolve in 1–2 mo
Yellow fever	Caused by an RNA flavivirus transmitted by mosquitos; classic lesion is massive hepatic midzonal necrosis; disease severity varies among species of nonhuman primates
Hentaviral Diseases (Korean hemorrhagic fever, epidemic hemorrhagic fever, Hentavirus pulmonary syndrome, nephropathia epidemica)	Caused by *Hantaan* virus carried by wild rodents worldwide, disease involves fever and renal and/or pulmonary involvement with headaches, diarrhea, nausea, vomiting, and possible hemorrhagic symptoms
Measles	Caused by a morbillivirus of the family *Paramyxoviridae*. Highly contagious disease with incubation time of 9–11 days; rash begins in oral cavity and spreads over face, neck, chest, and body; natural immunity develops after capture, but vaccination may be necessary for naive animals. Measles is not a natural disease of macaques, but is acquired through contact with humans.
Rickettsialpox	Caused by *Rickettsia akarii*; domestic mice are natural host, and vector is the mite, *Allodermanyssus sanguineus*; self-limiting disease in man characterized by fever, headache, myalgia, lymphadenopathy, leukopenia, eschar-like lesions, and generalized rash
Murine typhus	Caused by *Rickettsia typhi*: transmission to humans via rat fleas; clinical signs similar to those of rickettsialpox
Rocky Mountain Spotted Fever	Caused by *Rickettsia rickettssii*; transmitted by ticks (*Dermacentor spp.*) as vectors and reservoir hosts; mammalian hosts include wild rodents, lagamorphs, and dogs; disease in humans includes fever, headache, myalgia, and generalized hemorrhagic rash
Q fever	Caused by *Coxiella burnetti*; disease is widespread in sheep; dogs, cats, and chickens can become infected; organism is shad in urine, feces, milk, and placenta of asymptomatic ungulates; incubation is 2–3 wk and results in febrile systemic disease; most cases resolve in 2 wk
Psittacosis	Caused by *Chlamydia psittaci*; hosts include mice, guinea pigs, rabbits, cats, lambs, calves, birds, and frogs; disease includes conjunctivitis, pneumonitis, pericarditis, hepatitis, enteritis, urethritis, and arthritis; in humans, may be asymptomatic or present after 1–2 weeks of incubation, frequently with respiratory symptoms
Brucellosis	Caused in the laboratory by *Brucella canis*, due to use of random-source dogs; oral and transcutaneous routes of infection occur in the laboratory; brucellosis should be suspected when dog has history of abortion or infertility; source of infection is not known in most human cases. Other Brucella species may be contracted through the use of other species in the laboratory environment, i.e., goats, sheep, pigs, cattle
Leptospirosis	*Leptospira* spp. bacteria are found worldwide and divided into serovars based on DNA-relatedness; reservoirs are wild and domestic animals including rats, swine, cattle, and dogs; transmission primarily via contact with skin, especially if abraded, or mucous membranes with infected urine-contaminated materials; may be clinically inapparent or present with fever of sudden onset, headache, chills, severe myalgia, conjunctival suffusion or may present with a diphasic fever, meningitis, rash, hemolytic anemia, hemorrhage into skin and mucous membranes, hepatorenal failure, jaundice, mental confusion/depression, myocarditis, and pulmonary involvement.
Tuberculosis	Caused by *Mycobacterium* acid-fast bacilli; natural reservoirs are cattle, birds, and humans, with many other species susceptible: outbreaks occur in nonhuman primates, with Old World species more susceptible than New World monkeys and great apes; tuberculosis can occur in every organ system, although respiratory system is most familiar form

TABLE 1.1 *(Continued)*
Other Zoonotic Diseases

Disease	Description
Campylobacteriosis	Caused by *Campylobacter spp.* which has been isolated from dogs, cats, hamsters, ferrets, nonhuman primates, rabbits, swine, cattle, sheep, chickens, turkeys, and wild birds; disease in humans is self-limiting and usually brief; clinical symptoms include abdominal pain, fever, and diarrhea
Salmonella	Caused by over 1600 serotypes worldwide; two most common in laboratory colonies are *Salmonella typhimunum* and *Salmonella enteritidis*, due primarily to contaminated laboratory feed; acute gastroenteritis is most common presenting symptom; some cases proceed to septicemia after bacterial invasion of gut wall
Shigellosis	Caused by *Shigella spp.*, including *S. flexneri*, *S. sonnie*, and *S. dysenteriae*, all found in nonhuman primates; humans are main reservoir; nonhuman primates acquire disease after contact with infected primates or through contaminated facilities, food, or water; children may exhibit more severe disease with symptoms of dysentery with blood and mucus in feces
Streptobacillus moniliformis	Common in wild rodents, rare in laboratory rats, causes rat-bite fever (Haverhill Fever) in man, organism inhabits oropharynx of rat and is transmitted by bite
Yersinia	Species which are zoonotic in laboratory animals include *Y. pseudotuberculosis, Y. enterocolitica,* and *Y. pestis; Y. pseudotuberculosis* and *Y. enterocolitica* produce mesenteric lymphadenitis, septicemia, and appendicitis in humans; infection can occur through feces-contaminated food, or through direct contact with infected animals
Dermatophilosis	Caused by *Dermatophilus congolensis*; experimentally transmitted to mice, guinea pigs, and rabbits; produces circumscribed patches of alopecia in infected animals with exudative dermatitis; organism may persist in the fur and infect humans
Erysipeloid	Caused by *Erysipelothrix rhusiopathiae* in swine, lambs, calves, poultry, fish, and wild and laboratory mice: produces inflammatory lesions of the skin with occasional concurrent septicemia; pigs are the most common source in the laboratory
Listeriosis	Caused by *Listeria monocytogenes*; laboratory species most commonly affected are ruminants, guinea pigs, rabbits, and chinchillas; in normal hosts, disease may be expressed as pustular or papular cutaneous lesions or an acute, mild, febrile illness, sometimes with influenza-like symptoms; pregnant woman and fetuses are at risk with the potential for *in utero* infections and abortion
Pseudomonas	Opportunistic organism, especially for immunosuppressed animals; transmission from the caretakers or animals has been documented, but not the reverse
Dermatomycoses (ringworm)	Caused by three genera of fungi: *Microsporum, Trichophyton,* and *Epidermophyton*; frequently the animals are asymptomatic and not identified until caretaker develops the disease; transmission occurs by direct or indirect contact with infected animal; dermatomycosis is usually self-limiting in humans and presents as scaling, erythema, and occasional vesicles in the skin
Toxoplasmosis	Caused by *Toxoplasma gondii*; felines develop intestinal infection followed by shedding of oocysts resulting in transmission to humans; human infection is common, but clinical symptoms rare; congential infection can lead to systemic disease with neuropathological lesions
Amebiasis	Caused by *Entamoeba histolytica*; parasite is commonly found in feces of normal monkeys and apes, but may also cause severe clinical disease; most cases of human disease exhibit no clinical symptoms; mild diarrhea to acute bloody or mucoid dysentery with fever or chills may occur after invasion of colon wall
Balantidiasis	Caused by *Balantidium coli*: common in domestic swine and also found in humans, great apes, and several monkey species; most infections are asymptomatic
Giardiasis	Caused by *Giardia spp.*; found worldwide among all classes of vertebrates with no apparent host specificity; dogs and nonhuman primates may serve as reservoirs for human infection; in humans, infection often causes chronic or intermittent diarrhea, with light-colored, soft, and mucoid stools

TABLE 1.1 *(Continued)*
Other Zoonotic Diseases

Disease	Description
Pneumocystis pneumonia	Caused by *Pneumocystis carinii;* latent infections occur in rodents, lagomorphs, nonhuman primates, and domestic and zoo animals; zoonotic transmission has not been proven but may be possible; disease occurs in immunodeficient individuals or those with other debilities; frequently fatal and characterized by alveolitis as lungs fill with white foamy fluid containing parasites
Cyptosporidiosis	Caused by *Cryptospridium parvum*; affects epithelial cells of GI, biliary, and respiratory tract of humans, birds, fish, reptiles, rodents, cats, dogs, cattle, and sheep; diarrhea is major symptom in man, remitting in < 30 days in most immunologically competent people; may be fatal in immunodeficient persons

SECTION 11. RECOGNITION AND CONTROL OF DISEASE

Adequate veterinary care and daily observation of animals are essential for the recognition and control of disease. Diseases are transmitted by the following routes:

- *Vector*: A living carrier that transfers an infective agent from one host to another.
- *Fomite*: An inanimate object that is not intrinsically harmful, but is able to harbor pathogenic microorganisms.
- *Genes*: Inheritable abnormalities and mutations may result in disease states.

There are several procedures that can be instituted to control disease. Some routine procedures are listed below.

- Closely observe each animal at the time of receipt, and reject any animal(s) exhibiting abnormal physical, behavioral, or physiological conditions.
- Isolate and quarantine each new shipment of animals until their health status can be verified.
- Establish procedures that maintain barriers between animals and personnel (e.g., gloves, masks, and protective clothing); between animals and animals (e.g., changing gloves and disinfecting equipment between animals); and between animals and equipment (e.g., disinfect cleaning utensils and sanitize caging).
- Establish animal health and monitoring programs matched to the quality and types of animals and needs of the research laboratory.

Daily observation of animals allows early detection of signs of disease. While checking the general physical condition of each animal, the caretaker should also look for any signs of injury and/or abnormal physiological findings. Observations of any of the conditions listed in Table 1.2 should be

TABLE 1.2
Abnormal Conditions in Laboratory Animals

Abnormal physical conditions	Dehydrated, emaciated, listless, prostrate, dyspnea, alopecia, circling/head tilt, coughing, sneezing, discharges, scratching, unkempt, abscess/tumor(s), diarrhea, few or no feces, blood in feces, worms in feces, vomitus, bloody vomitus, worms in vomitus
Nonspecific signs of injury	Limping, paralysis, ataxia, dilated pupils, convulsions, fractures, hemorrhage, wounds, contusions
Abnormal physiological findings	Lack of urine, excess urination, few or no feces, anorexia, decreased water intake, excessive water intake

followed by diagnosis, prognosis, and treatment, after consultation with the attending veterinarian. If necessary, animals should be euthanized to control disease and alleviate pain and distress.

SECTION 12. ANIMAL NUTRITION

All animals require regular amounts of clean pure water and food. Fortunately, there are a variety of "complete balanced diets" available commercially for various laboratory species. These diets have been designed to provide the necessary fats, carbohydrates, proteins, fiber, vitamins, and minerals needed by the particular species. Researchers often select "certified" diets for use in their laboratories because these have been assayed for levels of various potential contaminants (e.g., aflatoxins and heavy metals; chlorinated hydrocarbons and polychlorinated biphenyls; and organophosphate pesticides). Similarly, in many laboratories, the water supplied to the animals is analyzed at regular intervals to ensure potability and absence of contaminants which may negatively impact animal health and research objectives. It is advisable that researchers closely review and retain all reports of food and water analyses. Some of the various types and sources of commercial laboratory diets are listed in Table 1.3. Various nutritional deficiencies which may affect laboratory animals are presented in Table 1.4.

TABLE 1.3
Types and Sources of Commercial Laboratory Diets

Source	Species	Diet Types
Purina Mills, Inc. 505 N. 4th St. Richmond, IN 47374 (765) 962-9561 www.labdiet.com	Rat/mouse/hamster	5001 Laboratory Rodent Diet; 5002 Certified Rodent Diet; 5008 Formulab Diet; 5010 Laboratory Autoclavable Rodent Diet; 5014 Certified Autoclavable Rodent Diet; 5L36 Certified Rodent Opti-Diet; 5P07 Prolab RMH 1000; 5P06 Prolab RMH 2000; 5P14 Prolab RMH 2500; 5R24 Autoclavable Prolab RMH 2500; 5P00 Prolab RMH 3000; 5P04 Autoclavable Prolab RMH 3500; 5053 Pico*Lab Rodent Diet 20; 5061 Pico-Vac Lab Rodent Diet; 5P75 and 5P76 Prolab Isopro RMH 3000
	Rat	5012 Rat Diet
	Mouse	5015 Mouse Diet; 5020 Mouse Diet 9F; 5021 Autoclavable Mouse Breeder Diet; 5058 PicoLab Rodent Diet 20; 5062 Pico-Vac Mouse Diet 20
	Rabbit	5304 Autoclavable Rabbit Diet; 5321 Laboratory Rabbit Diet; 5322 Certified Rabbit Diet; 5325 Certified High Fiber Rabbit Diet; 5326 Laboratory Rabbit Diet HF; 5P25 Prolab Hi-Fiber Rabbit; 5p26 Prolab Rabbit Diet
	Guinea Pig	5025 Guinea Pig Diet; 5026 Certified Guinea Pig Diet; 5L08 Guinea Pig Diet, Autoclavable 20; 5P18 Prolab Guinea Pig
	Mini-Pig	5080 Laboratory Mini-Pig Starter Diet; 5L80 Laboratory Mini-Pig HF Grower Diet; 5081 Laboratory Mini-Pig Grower Diet; 5082 Laboratory Mini-Pig Breeder Diet; 5084 Laboratory Porcine Grower Diet; 5P94 Prolab Mini-Pig Diet
	Dog	5006 Laboratory Canine Diet; 5007 Certified Laboratory Canine Diet; 5L18 Laboratory High Density Canine Diet; 5P40 Prolab Canine 1600; 5P41 Prolab Canine 2000
	Cat	5003 Laboratory Feline Diet
	Ferret	5280 Ferret Diet; 5L14 High Density Ferret Diet
	Avian	5065 Laboratory Chick Diet S-G; 5070 Laboratory Cage Layer Diet
Ruminant		5508 Rumilab Diet

TABLE 1.3 *(Continued)*
Types and Sources of Commercial Laboratory Diets

Source	Species	Diet Types
Primate		5037 & 5038 Monkey Diet Jumbo and Monkey Diet; 5040 New World Primate Diet; 5045 & 5047 High Protein Monkey Diet and Jumbo; 5048 Certified Primate Diet; 5049 & 5050 Laboratory Fiber-Plus Monkey Diet and Jumbo; 5052 Fiber-Balance Monkey Diet; 5K91 Certified Hi-Fiber Primate; 5P46 Prolab Primate 18
		*Pico diets are irradiated
Harlan Teklad	Rodents	2014 Protein Rodent Maintenance Diet (14%)
P.O. Box 44220		2014S Protein Rodent Maintenance Diet (14%) (Sterilizable)
Madison, WI 53744-4220		2016 Protein Rodent Diet (16%)
Toll Free: (800) 483-5523		2016S Protein Rodent Diet (16%) (Sterilizable)
Voice: (608) 277-2070		2018 Protein Rodent Diet (18%)
FAX: (608) 277-2066		2018S Protein Rodent Diet (18%) (Sterilizable)
www. Harlan.com/teklad/	Rabbits	2030 Rabbit Diet
global/index		2031 High Fiber Rabbit Diet
	Guinea Pig	2040 Guinea Pig Diet
		2041 High Fiber Guinea Pig Diet
	Primates	2050 Protein Primate Diet (20%)
		2055 Protein Primate Diet (25%)
		2021 Protein Dog Diet (21%)
		2025 Protein Dog Diet (25%)
		2027 Protein Dog Diet (27%)
	Cats	2060 Cat Diet

The above diets are standard diets. Harlan Teklad also provides services to custom design diets such as the examples listed below:

purified	mineral deficient
vitamin deficient	adjusted calories
adjusted protein	amino acid diet
adjusted carbohydrate	adjusted fat
essential fatty acid	atherogenic
deficient	basal mixes
rabbit diets with cholesterol	
isoflavone reduced	
basal mixes	

TABLE 1.4
Nutritional Deficiencies of Laboratory Animals

Nutritional Deficiency	Species Affected	Symptom(s)
Vitamin A	All species	Night blindness, dryness and thickness of cornea and conjunctiva, skin lesions
Vitamin C	Primates and guinea pigs	Scurvy conditions, breakdown of connective tissues
Vitamin D	All species	Lameness, enlargement of long bones with softening and deformation of all bones
Vitamin E	All species	Weak muscles, poor growth, low reproduction
Vitamin K	All species (the guinea pig *may* be an exception)	Slow blood clotting time

TABLE 1.4 *(Continued)*
Nutritional Deficiencies of Laboratory Animals

Nutritional Deficiency	Species Affected	Symptom(s)
Vitamin B_1	All species	Gastrointestinal, nervous, cardiovascular symptoms
Vitamin B_2	All species	Skin lesions or mucous membrane lesions, cardiac problems in dogs, collapse, comma
Nicotinic acid	All species	Skin, gastrointestinal, nervous symptoms, inflammation of the mouth in dogs
Vitamin B_6	All species	Convulsions, nausea, dermatitis, anemia
Biotin	Mice (raw egg whites or sulfur drugs can result in a deficiency for any mammal)	Skin lesions
Folic acid	All species	Anemia, diarrhea in primates
Choline	All species	Weight loss, reduced reproduction and lactation
Vitamin B_{12}	All species	Anemia
Calcium	All species	Lameness
Phosphorus	All species	Lameness
Magnesium	All species	Low blood pressure, nervous symptoms
Sodium	All species	Reduced growth, eye disturbances, low protein digestion
Chlorine	All species	Abnormal fluid and pH balances
Potassium	All species	Reduced appetite and growth
Iron	All species	Anemia
Copper	All species	Anemia, hair loss, dermatosis
Iodine	All species	Weak newborns, decreased basal metabolism rate
Cobalt	Guinea pig	Anemia

A. FOOD AND WATER REQUIREMENTS

Approximate daily food and water requirements for various species are presented in Table 1.5.

Most toxicology studies employ *ad libitum* feeding conditions in which animals are allowed to regulate their own dietary intake to meet energy requirements. However, the use of *ad libitum*

TABLE 1.5
Approximate Daily Food and Water Requirements for Various Species

Species	Daily Food Requirement	Daily Water Requirement
Mouse	3–6 g	3–7 ml
Rat	10–20 g	20–30 ml
Hamster	7–15 g	7–15 ml
Guinea pig	20–30 g[a]	12–15 ml/100 g
Rabbit	75–100 g	80–100 ml/kg
Cat	100–225 g	100–200 ml
Dog	250–1200 g	100–400 ml/day
Primate	40 g/kg[a]	350–1000 ml

[a] Like humans, guinea pigs and nonhuman primates require a continuous supply of vitamin C (ascorbic acid) in the diet.

feeding for long-term rodent bioassays has recently received increased attention since it appears that this practice impacts longevity, carcinogenesis, and overall animal health.

B. Fasting

Like humans, animals are often fasted in preparation for blood collection. Generally, fasting periods of 18–24 hours may be safely utilized for most species. However, for mice, fasting periods of 18–24 hours may lead to severe debility, dehydration, and even death. Therefore, it is recommended that fasting periods of no longer than 4–6 hours be used for this species.

SECTION 13. ANESTHESIA AND ANALGESIA*

A. General Considerations

As stated earlier, investigators using live animals must employ appropriate anesthetic, analgesic, and sedative agents when necessary to control pain and distress, unless use of such agents would interfere with the specific objectives of the research. If these agents are not used, both the Animal Welfare Act and *Guide for the Care and Use of Laboratory Animals* require that the procedures be directly supervised by the responsible investigator in accordance with all regulations and guidelines governing these situations. If pain-relieving procedures are not employed, the investigator must provide well-documented evidence demonstrating that the use of such agents would interfere with the results of the study.

B. Controlled Substances

To comply with these regulations, it is imperative that appropriate pain-relieving agents be available and that appropriate methods of administration and dosages be established. Because many pain-relieving agents are controlled substances, the use and handling of these agents are regulated by the Controlled Substances Act (84 Stat. 1242; 21 U.S.C. 801). This statute is specifically administered by the U.S. Drug Enforcement Agency (DEA). Among other requirements, users of controlled substances must ensure that drug supplies are adequately protected (stored in a secure cabinet or safe) and inventoried in accordance with the requirements of the statute.

C. Relevant Definitions

- *Analgesia:* The relief of pain without loss of consciousness.
- *Tranquilization:* A state of behavioral change in which the animal is relaxed, unconcerned by its surroundings, and often indifferent to minor pain.
- *Sedation:* Mild state of central nervous system (CNS) depression in which the animal is awake, but calm.
- *Local anesthesia:* Loss of sensation in a limited area.
- *Regional anesthesia:* Insensibility in a larger but still limited area.
- *Preanesthesia:* A state produced by the concomitant use of several drugs to decrease anxiety without producing excessive drowsiness, to facilitate smooth, rapid induction of general anesthesia without prolonging emergence, provide amnesia for the perioperative period while maintaining cooperation prior to loss of consciousness, relieve preoperative and postoperative pain, and minimize some of the undesirable effects of anesthesia, i.e., salivation, bradycardia, and postanesthetic vomiting.
- *General anesthesia:* A state of controlled and reversible unconsciousness characterized by lack of pain (analgesia), lack of memory (amnesia), and relatively depressed reflex responses without affecting the animal's vital systems, i.e., respiration and circulation.

* See Additional Related Information at the end of this chapter.

- *Surgical anesthesia:* Generally referred to as a surgical plane of anesthesia representing Stage III, plane 2 of the classical stages and planes of anesthesia; a medium depth of anesthesia suitable for most surgical procedures.

D. General Principles Regarding Anesthesia, Analgesia, and Tranquilization

The health of the animal should be carefully evaluated before instituting any anesthetic, analgesic, or tranquilizing procedure, and the specific drug(s) selected should provide the minimal level of CNS depression necessary. In addition, before undertaking any procedure, the investigator should closely consider the effect of the technique on experimental objectives, including potential drug interactions and interferences with test substance(s) (e.g., competing metabolic pathways, etc.).

E. Stages of Anesthesia

Indicators of anesthesia are commonly divided into four classic stages based on the depth of consciousness, presence or absence of reflex reactions, and degree of CNS and physiological depression. Stage I is characterized by disorientation, normal or panting respiration (20–30 breaths/min., unchanged heart rate, centrally positioned eyeball, normal pupil size, pupillary response to light, good muscle tone, and the presence of all reflexes. Stage II is marked by "excitement" with possible struggling, vocalization, paddling, chewing, or yawning; irregular respiration with possible holding of breath or hyperventilation; increased heart rate; centrally positioned eyeball or possible nystagmus (rapid involuntary oscillation of eyeball), possible dilation of pupils; pupillary response to light; good muscle tone; and presence of all reflexes with some possibly exaggerated. These first two stages represent presurgical anesthetic depths. Stage III anesthesia is subdivided into four different "planes" of progressively deeper unconsciousness. In plane 1 (light anesthesia), respiration is regular with a rate of 12–20 breaths/min.; pulse is strong (>90 beats per min., [bpm]); the animal may respond with movement, eyeballs may be centrally positioned or there may be nystagmus; pupil size is normal and responds to light; muscle tone is good and swallowing reflex is poor or absent and others present but diminished. In plane 2 (medium or surgical anesthesia), respiration may be shallow at 12–16 breaths/min.; heart rate >90 bpm; heart and respiration rates may increase in response to surgical activity; eyeballs may be ventrally rotated; pupil size moderately dilated; pupillary light response sluggish; muscle tone relaxed and patellar, ear flick, palpebral and corneal reflexes may be present, but others absent. In plane 3 (deep anesthesia), respiration is shallow at <12 breaths/min.; heart rate is 60–90 bpm with increased capillary refill time [CRT] and reduced strength of pulse; there is no response to surgical activity; eyeballs may be central or rotated ventrally; pupils are moderately dilated; pupillary light response if very sluggish; muscle tone greatly reduced and all reflexes are diminished or absent. In plane 4 (overdose), respiration is jerky; heart rate <60 bpm with prolonged CRT and pale mucous membranes; there is no response to surgical activity; eyeballs are centrally positioned; pupils are widely dilated; pupillary light response is absent; muscle tone is flaccid and there is no reflex activity. In Stage IV, the animal is moribund with loss of thoracic breathing, cardiovascular collapse, centrally positioned eyeballs; absence of pupillary light response flaccid muscle tone and absence of all reflexes.

The characteristics of the various stages and planes of anesthesia may vary with the anesthetic agent used, the species of animal, and the condition of individual animals with regard to study specific treatments prior to anesthesia.

F. Methods of Administration

Anesthetic agents are commonly administered by parenteral injection, inhalation, tracheal intubation, or topical application. For inhalant anesthetics, use of appropriate equipment (i.e., gas anesthesia machine) is highly recommended to help assure proper control of exposure. Masks or cones may be used with gas anesthesia machines to initially induce anesthesia, or to maintain animals at the desired level of anesthesia.

Injectable compounds may be administered by various routes (e.g., IV, IM, IP, or SC) for the purpose of preanesthesia, or to obtain a surgical level of anesthesia. However, in all cases, dosages and drugs must be calculated carefully and animals closely monitored throughout the anesthesia procedure. In larger species, tracheal intubation is often used for administration of inhalant anesthetics because this method allows for oxygen administration and forced ventilation, if necessary. When selecting an anesthetic agent and method of administration, the investigator must consider several factors, including the species, age, type and duration of surgery, available equipment, and personal knowledge. Of course, all procedures involving anesthesia and surgery must be supervised by a qualified veterinarian.

G. Commonly Used Anesthetic, Analgesic, and Tranquilizing Agents

Some of the more commonly used anesthetic, analgesic, and tranquilizing agents are briefly described below.

- *Atropine sulfate*: Anticholinergic agent often used as a preanesthetic to help decrease salivation, promote bronchodilation, prevent vagally induced bradycardia and reduced cardiac output, and reduce gastrointestinal activity.
- *Acepromazine maleate*: A phenothiazine sedative with antiemetic, antidysrhythmic, and antihistaminic properties.
- *Chlorpromazine hydrochloride*: This phenothiazine derivative potentiates barbiturate anesthesia.
- *Diazepam (Valium)*: Schedule IV drug with anticonvulsant and muscle relaxation properties.
- *Narcotic agents*: These agents produce hypnotic and analgesic effects, with resulting depression of cardiovascular and thermoregulatory systems (e.g., morphine, meperidine, etorphine (M99), and fentanyl).
- *Morphine*: May cause atropine-sensitive bradycardia and adverse gastrointestinal disturbance.
- *Meperdine (Demerol)*: Usually preferred over morphine because it produces fewer adverse side effects.
- *Fentanyl*: A potent short-acting narcotic used in Innovar-Vet (see below).
- *Etorphine Hydrochloride (M99)*: Commonly used to immobilize zoo animals and wild game.
- *Innovar-Vet*: Combination of narcotic analgesic fetanyl (0.4 mg/ml) and tranquilizer droperidol (20 mg/ml) which produces good analgesia and muscle relaxation.
- *Rompun (Xylazine)*: Non-narcotic sedative and analgesic muscle relaxant with a wide margin of safety.
- *Ketamine hydrochloride (Vetalar)(Ketaset)*: (Changed to a Schedule III drug by the DEA in August, 1999): Dissociative anesthetic agent that produces a state of chemical restraint and anesthesia. Reflexes remain intact. Excessive salivation may be controlled with atropine. Ketamine hydrochloride has a wide margin of safety and relatively short duration and recovery time, with minimal adverse side effects.
- *Medetomidine hydrochloride (Domitor)*: A synthetic α_2-adrenoreceptor agonist which produces sedation and analgesia for clinical and minor surgical procedures not requiring muscle relaxation. Domitor can be reversed with *Atipamezole hydrochloride (Antisedan)*.
- *Pentobarbital sodium (Nembutal)*: Long-acting barbiturate with a small margin of safety. Produces severe CNS depression and general anesthesia with increasing dose.

- *Thiamylal sodium (Surital)*: Short-acting barbiturate (approximately 15–30 minutes).
- *Chloralhydrate*: A hypnotic Schedule IV drug with a narrow margin of safety and weak analgesic properties.
- *Diethylether*: Inhalant anesthetic has so many shortcomings that it should not be used. Although it provides good analgesia and muscle relaxation, vapors irritate the respiratory mucosa and it is EXTREMELY FLAMMABLE AND EXPLOSIVE.
- *Halothane (Flurane)*: This highly volatile inhalant anesthetic produces reasonably good analgesia and muscle relaxation, but is a potent cardiovascular depressant. A vaporizer is essential to produce precise concentrations.
- *Methoxyflurane(Metafane)*: Nonexplosive inhalant anesthetic of relatively low volatility that produces good analgesia and muscle relaxation. Produces cardiovascular and respiratory depression.
- *Isoflurane (AErrane®)*: Nonflammable, nonexplosive general inhalation anesthetic agent. Produces profound respiratory depression. Increasing depth of anesthesia may increase hypotension and respiratory depression.
- *Nitrous oxide*: Potent inhalant anesthetic which is nonirritating, nonexplosive, and often used in conjunction with other agents.

Dosages and routes of administration of several commonly used anesthetic agents are presented in Table 1.6.

H. SPECIES PECULIARITIES AND CONTRAINDICATIONS

1. Mouse

- Use of chloroform in the mouse can cause renal tubular calcification and/or necrosis, especially in males. The DBA/2 mouse strain is particularly susceptible to these effects.

2. Rat

- Use of methoxyflurane is contraindicated in the Fischer 344 rat because this inhalant anesthetic may produce a diabetes-like syndrome in this strain.

3. Guinea Pig

- Intramuscular injection of Innovar-Vet should be avoided in guinea pigs because this can produce severe tissue necrosis.
- Repeated exposure to halothane in the guinea pig can produce hepatotoxicity. In addition, guinea pigs routinely hold their breath when first exposed to the irritating vapors (e.g., from halothane or chloroform). Thus, methoxyflurane is considered a safer alternative for this species.
- The larger cecum of the guinea pig can act as an anesthetic reservoir.

4. Rabbit

- A combination of 35 mg ketamine with 5 mg xylazine/kg given IM is a safe and effective method of anesthesia in the rabbit (20–75 minutes).
- The rabbit possesses a unique hypnotism/immobilization reflex.
- Like the guinea pig, the large cecum of the rabbit may act as an anesthetic reservoir.

5. Cat

- The use of morphine is contraindicated in the cat.

TABLE 1.6
Typical Routes and Dosages of Several Sedative, Analgesic, and Anesthetic Agents[a]

Agents	Dosage and Route in Species						
	Mouse	Rat	Hamster	Guinea Pig	Rabbit	Dog	Primate
Chlorpromazine (mg/kg)	3–35 (IM) 6 (IP)	1–20 (IM) 4–8 (IP)	0.05 (IM)	5–10 (IM)	10–25 (IM)	1–6 (IM) 0.5–8 (PO)	1–6 (IM)
Promazine (mg/kg)	0.5 (IM)	0.5–1 (IM)	0.5–1 (IM)	0.5–1 (IM)	1–2 (IM)	2–4 (IM)	2–4 (IM)
Acepromazine (mg/kg)	—	—	—	—	1 (IM)	0.5–1 (IM) 1–3 (PO)	0.5–1 (IM)
Meperidine (mg/kg)	60 (IM) 40 (IP)	44 (IM) 50 (IP) 25 (IV)	2 (IM)	1 (IP) 2 (IM)	10 (IV)	0.4–10 (IM)	3–11 (IM)
Innovar-Vet (ml/kg)	0.05 (IM)	0.13–0.16 (IM)	—	0.08–0.66 (IM)	0.2–0.3 (IM)	0.13–0.15 (IM)	0.05 (IM)
Ketamine (mg/kg)	25 (IV) 25–50 (IP) 22 (IM)	25 (IV) 50 (IP) 22 (IM)	40 (IM) 100(IP)	22–64 (IM)	22–44 (IM)	—	5–15 (IM)
Pentobarbital (mg/kg)	35 (IV) 40–70 (IP)	25 (IV) 40–50 (IP)	50–90 (IP)	24 (IV) 30 (IP)	25 (IV) 40 (IP)	30 (IV)	25–35 (IV)
Thiopental (mg/kg)	25–50 (IV)	40 (IM) 25–48 (IP)	—	55 (IM) 20 (IP)	25–50 (IV)	16 (IV)	25 (IV)

Note: See Chapter 22, Section 9 for additional information on anesthetics.

[a]Drugs and dosages presented are to serve only as a guideline. Selection and administration of specific agents and dosages should be supervised by a qualified veterinarian.

6. Primate

- Tranquilizers should never be used as the sole method of restraint for primates.
- The most commonly used immobilization agent for primates is 10–40 mg/kg ketamine given IM.
- For general surgical procedures, inhalation anesthesia is best, with 0.1 mg/kg atropine sulfate to control salivation.

SECTION 14. EUTHANASIA

Over the years, a number of acceptable and effective methods have been developed and utilized to induce euthanasia in various species. A detailed discussion of these and other euthanasia methods may be found in the 2000 Report of the AVMA Panel on Euthanasia.[5] The ultimate goal of euthanasia is to induce humane death, without causing unnecessary anxiety, pain, or distress to the animal. To achieve this, the euthanasia method must produce rapid CNS depression and insensitivity to pain to minimize potential stress and/or anxiety which might otherwise occur before unconsciousness. Thus, when employed in an appropriate manner, a good euthanasia method will induce CNS depression and rapid unconsciousness, followed by respiratory or cardiac arrest, and subsequent loss of brain function.

Unfortunately, there are a number of euthanasia techniques that, although generally recognized as humane, possess a high degree of intrinsic unpleasantness. Thus, researchers are challenged to select euthanasia techniques that (1) induce humane death without causing pain or distress to the animals, (2) do not negatively impact on experimental objectives and postmortem evaluations, and (3) do not produce an unnecessary level of unpleasantness for those involved. With regard to this latter consideration, it should be emphasized that some intrinsically unpleasant methods of euthanasia are nonetheless humane. Before using these "unpleasant methods," researchers are encouraged to educate personnel concerning the lack of an acceptable alternative method, and to have appropriate and detailed documentation supporting the need for the particular euthanasia method selected. Finally, it is imperative that individuals involved in performing any euthanasia procedure be properly trained and possess a demonstrated proficiency in the particular technique before undertaking the procedure with any animal.

A. MODES OF ACTION

Euthanasia agents produce death by three primary mechanisms: (1) direct or indirect hypoxia, (2) direct depression of neurons essential for life functions, or (3) physical disruption of brain activity via destruction of essential neuronal components. Agents that induce death by direct or indirect hypoxia should produce unconsciousness before loss of motor activity to ensure a painless and distress-free death. Agents that cause muscle paralysis without unconsciousness are therefore unacceptable as the sole method of euthanasia (e.g., curare, succinylcholine, etc.). Agents that produce unconsciousness and death by direct depression of neurons in the brain may produce an initial stage of "excitement" during which muscle contraction and vocalization may occur. These responses should not be regarded as indicators of distress because they do not seem to be purposeful. Death from these agents is attributable to direct depression of respiratory centers and/or cardiac arrest.

When properly implemented, physical disruption of brain activity (e.g., by concussion), direct destruction of the brain (e.g., by penetrating captive bolt), and electrical depolarization of neurons (e.g., by electrocution) are effective methods for the rapid induction of unconsciousness and death. However, these methods are often aesthetically objectionable for those involved. Exaggerated muscle activity may follow unconsciousness from these methods; however, the animal is not thought to experience pain or distress in the unconscious state.

B. Euthanasia Methods and Agents

The selection of a particular euthanasia method requires consideration of several factors, including the age and species to be euthanized; ability of the method/agent to induce unconsciousness and death without causing pain or distress; training and skill of personnel; reliability and irreversibility of the method; safety of personnel; and compatibility of the method with experimental objectives and endpoints. Euthanasia agents and methods which are currently considered acceptable or "conditionally acceptable" by the AVMA Panel are presented for several common laboratory species in Table 1.7. The characteristics and modes of action of these agents/methods are summarized in Table 1.8 and briefly described below.

TABLE 1.7
Acceptable and "Conditionally Acceptable" Methods for Euthanasia of Several Common Laboratory Species[5]

| | Agents/Methods[a] | |
Species	Acceptable	Conditionally Acceptable
Cats	Inhalant anesthetics, CO, CO_2, barbiturates	N_2, Ar
Dogs	Inhalant anesthetics, CO, CO_2, barbiturates	N_2, Ar, electrocution, penetrating captive bolt
Rabbits	Inhalant anesthetics, CO, CO_2, barbiturates	N_2, Ar, cervical dislocation, decapitation, penetrating captive bolt
Rodents and other small animals	Inhalant anesthetics, CO, CO_2, barbiturates	N_2, Ar, cervical dislocation, decapitation
Nonhuman primates	Barbiturates	Inhalant anesthetics, CO, CO_2, Ar

[a] See Table 1.8 for other conditions and requirements of "acceptable" and "conditionally acceptable" euthanasia methods.

1. Inhalant Agents

The suitability of a particular inhalant agent depends on whether the animal experiences distress before loss of consciousness. Additional considerations common to all inhalant agents are listed below.

- In general, unconsciousness is more rapid and euthanasia is more humane when the animal is rapidly exposed to a high concentration of the agent.
- Most inhalant agents are hazardous to humans. Therefore, appropriate safety precautions must be followed to ensure personnel safety.
- Compared to adult animals, neonates are often more resistant to the effects of inhalant agents due apparently to increased resistance to hypoxia.

Inhalant anesthetics, such as ether, halothane, methoxyflurane, isoflurane, and enflurane, have been used in overdose for euthanasia of smaller animals. Exposure is usually accomplished using a small chamber (e.g., a bell jar) containing cotton or gauze soaked with the inhalant anesthetic agent. The use of suspended wire flooring in the chamber allows equilibration of the chamber atmosphere, while avoiding direct contact by the animal with the irritating liquid anesthetic.

a. Advantages

- Inhalant anesthetics are useful for euthanasia of small animals in which venipuncture may be difficult.

TABLE 1.8
Summary of the Characteristics of Several Euthanasia Methods

Euthanasia Method	Classification	Mechanism of Action	Species	Effectiveness	Personnel Safety
Inhalant anesthetics	Acceptable	Hypoxia due to depression of vital centers	Small animals such as rats, mice, hamster, and guinea pigs via chamber administration	Moderately rapid onset of anesthesia; initial excitation may occur	Minimize exposure to personnel by scavenging or venting
Carbon dioxide	Acceptable	Hypoxia due to depression of vital centers	Small animals such as rats, mice, hamsters, and guinea pigs via chamber administration	Effective in adult animals; may be prolonged in immature and neonatal animals	Minimal hazard
Carbon monoxide	Acceptable	Hypoxia due to inhibition of O_2-carrying capacity of hemoglobin	Most small species including dogs, cats, and rodents	Effective and acceptable with proper equipment and operation	Extremely hazardous; difficult to detect
Barbiturates	Acceptable	Hypoxic due to depression of vital centers	Most species	Highly effective when administered appropriately	Safe, except human abuse potential of controlled substances(s)
Inert gasses (Ni, Ar)	Conditionally acceptable	Hypoxic hypoxemia	Cats, small dogs, rodents, rabbits, and other small species	Effective, but other methods are preferable; acceptable only if animal is heavily sedated or anesthetized	Safely used in ventilated area
Cervical dislocation	Conditionally acceptable	Hypoxia due to disruption of vital centers, direct depression of brain	Mice, rats <200 g, and rabbits <1 kg	Effective and irreversible; requires training, skill, and IACUC approval; aesthetically displeasing	Safe
Decapitation	Conditionally acceptable	Hypoxia due to disruption of vital centers, direct depression of brain	Rodents and small rabbits	Effective and irreversible; requires training, skill, and IACUC approval; aesthetically displeasing	Potential injury due to guillotine

- Halothane, enflurane, isoflurane, and methoxyflurane are nonflammable and nonexplosive under conditions of routine use.

b. *Disadvantages*
  - Struggling and anxiety may develop during induction due to irritating vapors.
  - Ether is extremely flammable and explosive.
  - Inhalant anesthetic vapors may be harmful to humans, particularly to the developing conceptus during the early stages of pregnancy.

c. *Recommendations*
  - Chamber administration of the inhalant anesthetics listed above is acceptable for euthanasia of small animals such as rats, mice, hamsters, and guinea pigs. However, if possible, use of ether should be avoided because it is extremely flammable and potentially explosive. In addition, appropriate safety precautions should be used with all inhalant anesthetic agents to avoid exposure of laboratory personnel.

2. Carbon Dioxide

Carbon dioxide (CO_2) is a nearly odorless, nonflammable, and nonexplosive gas that has been used extensively as an inhalant euthanasia agent for a number of species.

a. *Advantages*
  - CO_2 produces rapid depressant and anesthetic effects.
  - CO_2 may be obtained in compressed cylinders.
  - CO_2 is inexpensive, nonflammable, and nonexplosive; it does not pose a particular safety hazard to personnel under conditions of normal use.
  - CO_2 does not distort cellular architecture.

b. *Disadvantages*
  - There are no major disadvantages concerning the use of CO_2 as an euthanasia agent. However, it should be noted that because CO_2 is heavier than air, incomplete chamber filling may permit taller or climbing animals to avoid exposure. In most instances, prefilling the chamber with the desired CO_2 atmosphere will avoid this potentially stressful situation for the animal(s).

c. *Recommendations*
  - Chamber administration of CO_2 is an effective and often desirable method of euthanasia for small animals such as rats, mice, hamsters, and guinea pigs, provided that the chamber is not overcrowded. CO_2 is not recommended for larger animals such as rabbits, cats, and dogs, because these species may exhibit signs of distress before the onset of anesthesia and narcosis. CO_2 is best provided from pressurized tanks that allow precise regulation of CO_2 inflow. Effective exposure conditions for most smaller species are a CO_2 concentration of 70% (i.e., 70% CO_2 and 30% O_2), and a flow rate which displaces approximately 20% of the chamber volume per minute.

3. Carbon Monoxide

Carbon monoxide (CO) is a colorless, odorless gas that is flammable and potentially explosive at concentrations above 10%. In humans and animals, CO acts as a cumulative poison by combining with hemoglobin and blocking the uptake of oxygen by red blood cells, leading to fatal hypoxemia.

Although CO has been shown to induce unconsciousness in animals with minimal discernible discomfort, the many dangers associated with CO outweigh its routine use in most laboratory settings. Nonetheless, CO inhalation is an acceptable method for euthanasia of many species, including dogs and cats, provided that compressed CO is used and the following precautions are taken:

- Personnel must be thoroughly instructed in the use of CO and its associated hazards and limitations.
- The CO source and chamber must be in a well-ventilated area, preferably outdoors.
- The chamber must be well lit and have viewing ports that allow observation of the animals.
- The CO flow rate must be adequate to rapidly achieve a CO concentration of at least 6%.
- If the CO chamber is inside, CO monitors must be placed in the room to warn personnel of hazardous CO concentrations.

4. Inert Gases

Inert gases such as nitrogen and argon are colorless, odorless, nonflammable, and nonexplosive gases that have been used to induce euthanasia by hypoxemia. Although these gases are readily available and minimally hazardous to personnel, their use requires prior sedation or anesthesia of the animal to avoid discernible hypoxemia and ventilatory stimulation which commonly precede death and are obviously distressing. In addition, when preanesthesia is used, the time to death is often delayed. Consequently, inert gases should be used for euthanasia only when animals have been heavily sedated and chamber oxygen concentrations of less than 2% can be rapidly achieved.

5. Chloroform

Chloroform presents a significant hazard due to its known potent hepatotoxicity and suspected carcinogenicity in humans. Therefore, chloroform is not recommended for euthanasia.

6. Barbiturates and Barbiturate Combination Drugs

There are several commercially available euthanasia products that are formulated to include a barbituric acid derivative such as phenobarbital and local anesthetic agent(s). These products are often categorized as Schedule III drugs, making them somewhat easier to obtain and store compared with Schedule II drugs such as phenobarbital. These agents are acceptable and effective for euthanasia when properly used. Combination drugs containing neuromuscular blocking agents are not acceptable for euthanasia.

7. Chloral Hydrate

Chloral hydrate causes death by hypoxemia resulting from depression of the respiratory center. However, because this depression is slow, it may be preceded by aesthetically objectionable symptoms such as muscle spasms, gasping, and vocalization. Thus, chloral hydrate is not considered acceptable for euthanasia of dogs, cats, or other small animals.

8. T-61 Euthanasia Solution

T-61, an injectable nonbarbiturate, non-narcotic combination of three drugs, is no longer manufactured or commercially available in the United States.

9. Unacceptable Injectable Agents

The following injectable agents are considered unacceptable for euthanasia when used alone: strychnine, nicotine, caffeine, magnesium sulfate, potassium chloride, and all neuromuscular blocking agents.

10. Cervical Dislocation and Decapitation

Physical methods of euthanasia such as cervical dislocation and decapitation are considered by most to be aesthetically displeasing. However, when properly used by skilled personnel, these methods may cause less fear and anxiety, and may be more rapid, painless, and humane than other methods of euthanasia. In the laboratory, cervical dislocation and decapitation may be useful euthanasia techniques for small animals when other methods or agents may interfere with experimental objectives and results. However, before using these methods, it is imperative that personnel are properly trained and experienced, and that approval is obtained from the Institutional Animal Care and Use Committee.

a. Recommendations

Physical euthanasia methods such as cervical dislocation and decapitation are recommended only when scientifically justified and when other acceptable methods have been clearly ruled out. Use of these procedures must be preapproved by the Institutional Animal Care and Use Committee. Animals should be sedated or unconscious before using these techniques, if practical. When properly performed, cervical dislocation is considered humane for poultry, mice, rats weighing less than 200 g, and rabbits weighing less than 1 kg.

11. Verification of Death

Regardless of the specific euthanasia method used, it is imperative that death be verified by examining the animal for cessation of vital signs. Of course, the specific means for confirming death requires professional judgment and training.

SECTION 15. SOURCES OF LABORATORY ANIMALS

There are a number of reliable sources from which laboratory animals may be purchased. Company names, addresses, telephone numbers, and available species from several suppliers are presented in Table 1.9.

TABLE 1.9
Names, Addresses, and Phone Numbers of Several Animal Suppliers

Facility	Avian	Cats	Cattle	Chinchillas	Dogs	Gerbils	Guinea Pigs	Hamsters	Mice	Opossum	Primates	Rabbits	Rats	Sheep	Swine	Woodchucks	Contact Information
Ace Animals, Inc., PA							X		X				X				(610) 367-6047 netjunction.com/aceanimals
Alder Ridge Farms, Inc., PA					X												(717) 727-3458
Animal Biotech Industries, PA														X			(215) 766-7413 animalbiotech.com
Archer Farms, MD														X			(410) 879-4110
B&K Universal, Inc., CA					X		X	X	X		X		X				(510) 490-3036 bku.com
Barton's West End Facilites, NJ					X									X			(908) 637-4427
BIOQUAL, Inc., MD											X						(301) 251-0633
Butler Farms USA, Inc., NY					X				X								(315) 587-2295 infor@marfarms.com
Cedar River Laboratories, IA		X															(515) 228-2212
Charles River Laboratories, MA						X	X	X	X		X	X	X		X		(800) 522-7287 criver.com
CLEA Japan/Pegasus, NJ							X	X	X		X	X	X				(609) 737-3961 straube.com
Covance, PA					X		X	X	X		X	X			X		(717) 336-4921 covance.com
Crest Caviary, CA							X										(408) 728-5265
Cytogen Res & Dev, MA								X									(617) 325-7774
Davidson's Mill Breeding Laboratories, NJ							X					X					(732) 821-9094
Elm Hill Breeding Labs, Inc., MA							X	X	X			X					(978) 256-2545 elmhilllabs.com
Hare-Marland/Rabbits for Research, NJ												X					(973) 728-3745
Harlan Sprague Dawley, Inc., IN		X				X	X	X	X			X					(317) 894-7521 harlan.com
Hilltop Lab Animals, Inc., PA						X	X	X	X				X				(724) 887-8480 edmied@aol.com
HSD/Ridglan, IN					X												(317) 894-7521
INTEGRA Biosciences, Inc., MD								X	X								(301) 874-5790
Jackson Laboratory, ME									X								(800) 422-6423 micetech@jax.org
Kiser Lake Kennels		X			X												(937) 362-3193 kiserlakekennels.com
LABS of Virginia, SC										X	X						(803) 589-5190
Liberty Research, Inc., NY	X	X			X												(607) 565-8131
Lixit Animal Care Products, CA	X	X	X	X			X	X	X			X	X				(707) 252-1622

TABLE 1.9 (*Continued*)
Names, Addresses, and Phone Numbers of Several Animal Suppliers

Facility	Avian	Cats	Cattle	Chinchillas	Dogs	Gerbils	Guinea Pigs	Hamsters	Mice	Opossum	Primates	Rabbits	Rats	Sheep	Swine	Woodchucks	Contact Information
LSR Industries, WI												X					(414) 835-2742 calesser@execdc.com
Mallinckrodt Medical, Inc., MO							X		X			X	X				(314) 654-7908 mallinckrodt.com
Marshall Farms USA, Inc., NY					X												(315) 587-2295 marshallpet.com/index01
Moulton Chinchilla Ranch, MN				X													(507) 288-6334
Myrtle's Rabbitry, Inc., TN												X					(800) 424-9511
Northeastern Wildlife, NY										X						X	(607) 334-5809 whipplej@norwich.net
Osage Research Primates, MO											X						(573) 348-8002 geocities.com/ResearchTriangle/Lab/9341/index
Primate Products, FL											X						(305) 471-9557 hemi.com/~lspi
Robinson Services, Inc., NC												X					(910) 940-2550 keurob1@aol.com
Schroer Mfg. Co. (Shor-Line), MO		X			X												(816) 471-0488
Simonsen Laboratories, Inc., CA							X	X	X				X				(408) 847-2002 simlab.com
Sinclair Research Center, Inc., MO		X															(573) 446-6464 gbouchard@sockets.net
SINCONBREC USA, Inc., IL											X						(847) 734-1662
Taconic Farms, Inc., NY									X				X				(518) 537-6208 taconic.com
Thomas D. Morris, Inc., MD			X														(410) 356-6780
Three Springs Scientific, PA											X			X			(215) 257-6055
VWR Scientific Products, PA							X		X				X				(610) 431-1700 vwrsp.com
Western Oregon Rabbit Co., OR												X					(541) 929-2245
White Eagle Laboratories, Inc., PA	X	X															(215) 348-3868
Zivic-Miller Laboratories, Inc., PA													X				(724) 452-5200 zivic-miller.com

SECTION 16. SPECIES DATA

The following sections provide some general information concerning the husbandry and biology of several species commonly used in research.

A. MOUSE (*Mus musculus*)

1. Breeds and Strains

There are a variety of mouse breeds and strains which are available from commercial sources. Inbred strains are produced by 20 or more consecutive generations of brother × sister matings, with the primary objective of reducing genetic variability by increasing homozygosity at genetic loci. This results in a high degree of uniformity in the physical and physiological traits of the various inbred strains.

Outbred strains, on the other hand, are produced through the mating of totally unrelated individuals. This frequently results in the production of offspring that show more vigor than the parental animals in terms of growth, survival and fertility. The offspring of such matings (F1 hybrids) are heterozygous at all loci in which the parental animals differed. These F1 hybrids can be reproduced only from the designated parental strains.

Random breeding is a mating technique in which mating is undertaken with animals from the same stock, but without regard to genetic background. The primary purpose of this technique is to preserve genetic variability in the stock. Some of the more common mouse strains are listed and briefly described in Table 1.10.

TABLE 1.10
Common Strains of Laboratory Mice

Strain	Description
CD-1 Mice	Outbred albino strain descended from "Swiss" mice
CF-1 Mice	Outbred albino strain not descended from "Swiss" mice
Swiss-Webster Mice	Outbred albino strain from selective inbreeding of Swiss mice by Dr. Leslie Webster
SKH1 (Hairless) mice	Outbred strain that originated from an uncharacterized strain
BALB/c mice	Inbred albino strain developed originally by H.J. Bagg (Bagg albino)
C3H mice	Inbred agouti strain developed originally from "Bagg albino" female and DBA male
C57BL/6 mice	Inbred black strain developed originally by C.C. Little
DBA/2 mice	Inbred non-agouti, dilute brown strain developed originally by C.C. Little; oldest of all inbred mouse strains
FVB mice	Inbred albino strain derived originally from outbred Swiss colony
AKR mice	Inbred albino strain originally developed by Furth as a high leukemia strain
B6C3F1 mice	Hybrid agouti strain from female C57BL/6N × male C3H/He
DBF1 mice	Hybrid black strain from female C57BL/6N × male DBA/2N
CAF1 mice	Hybrid albino strain from female BALB/cAn × male A/HeN
CDF1 mice	Hybrid brown strain from female BALB/cAnN × male DBA/2N
CB6F1 mice	Hybrid black strain from female BALB/cAnN × male C57BL/6N
Nude CD-1 mice	Outbred hairless albino strain that is athymic and thus immunodeficient (unable to produce T-cells)
Nude BALB/cAnN mice	Inbred hairless albino strain that is athymic and thus immunodeficient (unable to produce T-cells)

Transgenic Lines (National Institute of Environmental Health Sciences is exploring the utility of genetically altered mice to study mechanisms of carcinogenesis, namely, the Tg.AC (carrier of an activated mouse H-*ras* oncogene) and the *p53±* (heterozygous for the wild-type tumor suppressor gene *Trp53*).

TABLE 1.10 (Continued)
Common Strains of Laboratory Mice

Strain	Description
Tg.AC mouse	Produced in FVB/N mice by pronuclear injection of a v-Ha-*ras* transgene linked to a fetal ζ-globulin promotor and an SV-40 polyadenylation/splice sequence. These mice respond as if genetically initiated, rapidly developing epidermal papillomas in response to topical tumor promotor or carcinogen treatment.
P53*def* mouse	This line has 1 functional wild-type *p53* allele and 1 inactivated allele, imparting sensitivity to the mutational and carcinogenic effects of genotoxic chemicals. The *p53* gene, often mutated or deleted in human and rodent tumors, is critical to cell cycle control and DNA repair.

2. Handling and Restraint

Handling and restraint of the mouse requires training and experience because of the mouse's small size and agile movement. The mouse is usually picked up by the tail, placed on a secure surface such as the forearm or table top, and then restrained by gently grasping the loose skin behind the neck and over the back, while maintaining a grip on the tail. The handler must use a firm but gentle grip to minimize twisting and movement of the animal that could potentially result in self-injury. Excessive pressure or force during handling and restraint could easily result in spinal separation or other injury to the mouse. Furthermore, extra care should be exercised when removing the mouse from a cage with a wire floor as the animal will forcefully grip the cage bottom to avoid removal.

3. Housing

Mice may be housed individually or with several animals per cage in plastic shoebox-type caging or suspended stainless steel caging. When housed in plastic shoeboxes, mice should be provided with some type of bedding material such as processed hardwood chips or ground corncobs. Fresh water may be provided using water bottles or via an automatic watering system. However, when using an automatic watering system, the line pressure must low enough to allow the animal to easily activate the sipper mechanism without receiving a frightening high-pressure "squirt" in the face. In addition, whenever possible, gang housing of adult males should be avoided because male mice will form a pecking order when placed together, and serious injury or death may result due to extensive fighting between cage mates. Minimum cage space requirements for mice are presented in Table 1.11.

TABLE 1.11
Minimum Cage Space Requirements for Mice[a]

Body Weight (g)	Floor Area/Mouse (sq. in.)	Cage Height (in.)
>10	6.0	5
10–15	8.0	5
15–25	12.0	5
>25	>15.0	5

[a] As per the *Guide for the Care and Use of Laboratory Animals*, 1996.

4. Environmental Conditions

Environmental conditions recommended for mice by the *Guide* are as follows:

Room temperature: 64–79°F, 18–26°C
Relative humidity: 30–70%
Room air changes: 10–15/hour

Environmental controls should be set toward the middle of the room temperature and relative humidity ranges to avoid extremes and large fluctuations in these environmental variables. The *Guide* does not specify any particular lighting cycle for mice; however, a 12 hour light/12 hour dark cycle is used routinely for this species.

5. Physical and Physiological Parameters

Physical and physiological parameters of laboratory mice are listed in Table 1.12.

TABLE 1.12
Physical and Physiological Parameters of Mice[4,6,7a]

Life span	1–2 yr
Male adult weight	20–35 g
Female adult weight	20–35 g
Birth weight	1.0–1.5 g
Adult food consumption	3–6 g/day
Adult water consumption	3–7 ml/day
Male breeding age/weight	6–8 wk/20–35 g
Female breeding age/weight	6–8 wk/20–30 g
Placentation	Discoidal endotheliochorial
Estrus cycle	4–5 days (polyestrous)
Gestation period	19–21 days
Weaning age/weight	21 days/8–12 g
Average litter size	10–12 pups
Mating system(s)	1:1 or 1 male to multiple females
Adult blood volume	6–7% of body weight
Maximum safe bleed	7–8 ml/kg
Red cell count	$7-12 \times 10^6/mm^3$
White cell count	$3-12 \times 10^3/mm^3$
Hemoglobin	13–17 g/dl
Hematocrit	40–54%
Mean corpuscular volume	43–54
Mean corpuscular hemoglobin	13–18
Mean corpuscular hemoglobin concentration	31–34
Platelet count	$1000-1600 \times 10^3/mm^3$
Heart rate	300–600 beats/min
Respiration rate	90–180 breaths/min
Rectal temperature	37.5°C
Urine pH	6.0–7.5
Urine volume	1–3 ml/day
Chromosome number	$2n = 40$

[a] See Chapters 2, 5, 11, 12, and 18 for more detailed information.

---

6. Identification, Bleeding, Anesthesia, and Euthanasia Methods for Mice

TABLE 1.13
Identification, Bleeding, Anesthesia, and Euthanasia Methods for Laboratory Mice

Identification methods
  Ear tags
  Ear punch, notch
  Tail tatoo identification number
  Subcutaneously implanted transponder
Bleeding methods
  Orbital sinus
  "Tail Nick"
  Via heart after euthanasia
Anesthesia methods
  Ketamine/xylazine, methoxyflurane, barbiturates, pentobarbital (5 mg/100 g IP)
Euthanasia methods
  Barbiturate overdose
  CO_2 inhalation
  Cervical dislocation

7. Diseases

Various diseases and adverse health conditions of laboratory mice are identified and briefly described in Table 1.14.

TABLE 1.14
Various Diseases and Adverse Health Conditions of Laboratory Mice[4,8,9]

Disease/Health Condition	Etiology, Clinical Signs, Symptoms, and/or Pathology
Tyzzer's	Caused by the bacterium *Clostridium piliforme,* an obligate intracellular organism that causes enterohepatic disease in many domestic and laboratory animal species; usually subclinical but immunosuppressant drugs may precipitate epidemics; signs include diarrhea, poor coat, and sudden death in young; focal necrosis in liver and inflammation of ileum may be seen at necropsy.
Murine respiratory mycoplasmosis (MRM)	Caused by bacterium *Mycoplasma pulmonis*; relatively common chronic disease characterized by inflammation of respiratory tract and middle ear; signs in mice include chattering and dyspnea; lesions include bronchitis, bronchopneumonia, rhinitis, and otitis media. Other mycoplasma organisms infect mice affecting the reproductive and central nervous systems.
Klebsiellsis	Caused by bacterium *Klebsiella pneumonia;* nonspecific signs include dyspnea, sneezing, cervical lymphadenopathy, inappetence, hunched posture, and rough coat; cervical, pharyngeal, renal, and hepatic abscesses; granulomatous pneumonia.
Staphylococcosis	Caused by bacterium *Staphylococcus aureus*; normal inhabitant of the skin; may cause skin and facial abscesses in nude mice.
Pseudotuberculosis	Caused by bacterium *Corynebacterium kutscheri*; infection usually inapparent but may cause nasal/ocular discharge, dyspnea, arthritis, or skin abscesses; focal caseous abscesses in liver, lungs, kidneys, and lymph nodes.
Helicobacter hepaticus	Causes chronic hepatitis and may be associated with increased incidence of hepatic neoplasms; mice may be infected with *H. bilis, H. muridarum, H. rappini,* and possibly others. H. muridarum may be associated with chronic gastritis and one or more of the above may be associated with chronic enterocolitis in immunodeficient mice.

TABLE 1.14 *(Continued)*
Various Diseases and Adverse Health Conditions of Laboratory Mice[4,8,9]

Disease/Health Condition	Etiology, Clinical Signs, Symptoms, and/or Pathology
Sendai virus	Caused by *Paramyxovirus*; clinically inapparent chronic infection or clinically apparent acute infection; variable signs may include chattering, mild respiratory distress, prolonged gestation, poor growth, and death in young; concurrent pulmonary infections may occur.
Pneumonia virus of the mouse (PVM)	Caused by *Pneumovirus*: common in laboratory rodents worldwide; subcinical in euthymic rodents.
K virus (Kilham virus of mice)	Caused by *Polyomavirus*; wild mice are natural host; natural infection is subclinical.
Epizootic diarrhea of infant mice (EDIM)	Caused by a rotavirus virus; mustard colored feces; rectal impaction follows intestinal inflammation.
Reovirus-3	Natural infections are usually subclinical and have little significance for most studies.
Murine hepatitis virus (MHV)	Caused by *Coronavirus* (25 different strains isolated); mice are natural host; clinically apparent infection in naive infant mice; diarrhea with high mortality may occur.
Mouse pox (ectromelia)	Caused by ectromelia virus; natural transmission due to direct contact and fomites; clinical manifestations may include variable mortality, facial edema, swelling of feet, and necrotic amputation of limbs or tail; necrosis of liver, spleen, and lymphoid tissue in acute disease.
Lymphocytic choriomeningitis	Caused by *Arenavirus*; may cause significant zoonotic infection in those working with transplantable rodent tumors and rodent cell lines; wild mice are principal reservoir; only infected mice and hamsters are known to transmit virus; natural infection of adult mice ranges from inapparent to severe disease with high mortality; clinical symptoms in humans are usually flu-like (see zoonoses).
Murine cytomegalovirus	Common subclinical infection of submaxillary salivary glands of wild mice; infrequent natural infections in laboratory mice; used as an animal model for human cytomegalovirus.
Mouse thymic virus	Natural infections are subclinical; wild and laboratory mice are hosts; prevalence in mouse stocks is unknown; characteristic lesion is lymphoid necrosis in thymus, nodes, and spleen.
Polyomavirus	Highly contagious but of limited significance as natural infection of mice; major importance is as model for viral carcinogenesis and cell transformation; prevalence is poorly understood.
Minute virus of mice (MVM)	Caused by *Parvovirus*: wild and laboratory mice are natural hosts; highly contagious but natural infections are inapparent and not known to produce disease.
Theiler's mouse encephalomyelitis	Caused by *Picornavirus*: laboratory mice and rats are natural hosts but infection is probably rare; predominant lesion is poliomyelitis.
Pneumocystis carinii	Caused by what molecular genetic data confirm to be a fungus. Not pathogenic for immunocompetent hosts; steroids, low-protein diets, and immunodeficent genotypes can precipitate expression of varying degrees of interstitial pneumonia.
Protozoan parasites	*Cryptosporidium muris, C. parvum*; *Eimeria spp.*; *Giardia muris* and *Spironucleus muris* can effect various levels of the gastrointestinal tract.
Fighting	Trauma due to fighting often results in morbidity and mortality in male mice housed together; fighting usually occurs at night; bite and scratch wounds often become infected; may be prevented by grouping males at weaning rather than later.
Hair chewing (barbering)	Alopecia in cage mates is most common in pigmented mice; early indication is loss of whiskers; alopecia of the muzzle, head, and trunk is common.
Ringtail	Condition of young rats and mice characterized by annular constriction and subsequent edema, necrosis, and sloughing of the tail; may be prevented by providing relative humidity $\geq 50\%$; much more common in rats than mice.

B. RAT (*Ratus norvegicus*)

1. Breeds and Strains

The laboratory rat is derived from the wild brown or "Norway" rat. Outbred strains include the Sprague-Dawley, Wistar, and Long-Evans rats. Inbred strains include the Fischer 344, Spontaneous Hypertensive, and Wistar Kyoto rat. Physiologically, the rat is similar to other single-stomached animals, except rats do not possess a gall bladder. Common breeds and strains of rats that are available from several commercial suppliers are presented in Table 1.15.

TABLE 1.15
Common Strains of Laboratory Rats

Strain	Description
Sprague-Dawley rats	Outbred albino strain originated by R.W. Dawley from a hybrid hooded male and female Wistar rat.
Wistar rats	Outbred albino strain originated at the Wistar Institute.
Long-Evans rats	Outbred white with black or occasional brown hood; originated by Drs. Long and Evans by cross of white Wistar females with wild gray male.
Zucker rats	Outbred obese strain with four principal coat colors (predominately brown; brown + white; predominately black; or black + white).
Fischer 344 (F-344) rats	Inbred albino strain originated from mating #344 of rats obtained from local breeder (Fischer).
Lewis rats	Inbred albino strain originally developed by Dr. Lewis from Wistar stock.
Wistar Kyoto (WKY) rats	Inbred albino strain originated from outbred Wistar stock from Kyoto School of Medicine.
Brown Norway rats	Inbred non-agouti brown strain originated from a brown mutation in a stock of rats trapped from the wild at the Wistar Institute in 1930.
Spontaneously hypertensive (SHR) rates	Inbred albino strain developed from Wistar Kyoto rats with spontaneous hypertension.

2. Handling and Restraint

Laboratory rats can be handled easily if they are treated kindly. Frequent handling usually makes the rat even more gentle and easy to handle. Rats may be picked up by gently grasping the animal around the torso. If necessary, rats may be picked up by grasping the base of the tail and then immediately transferring the animal to a more stable position. However, when using this technique, it is important to grasp near the base and not the tip of the tail because this could easily injure the animal.

3. Housing

The rat is a most adaptive creature; however, this does not preclude the need for appropriate housing and husbandry standards. Like mice, rats may be housed individually or with several animals per cage in plastic shoebox-type caging or suspended stainless steel caging. When housed in plastic shoeboxes, rats should be provided with some type of bedding material such as processed hardwood chips or ground corncobs. Fresh water may be provided using water bottles or via an automatic watering system. For newly weaned rats, it is advisable to gang house the animals for several days after receipt (e.g., 2–3/cage) to allow the animals to become accustomed to the food and water sources. This is particularly true if the animals are to be introduced to an automatic water system for the first time.

Each rat should be checked daily to ensure that an adequate supply of fresh food and water is available. In addition, the health of each animal should be verified at the time of receipt and on a daily basis thereafter by trained and qualified personnel. Minimum cage space requirements for the laboratory rat are presented in Table 1.16.

TABLE 1.16
Minimum Cage Space Requirements for Rats[a]

Body Weight (g)	Floor Area/Rat (sq. in.)	Cage Height (in.)
<100	17.0	7
100–200	23.0	7
200–300	29.0	7
300–400	40.0	7
400–500	60.0	7
>500	>70.0	7

[a] As per the *Guide for the Care and Use of Laboratory Animals*, 1996.

4. Environmental Conditions

Environmental conditions recommended for rats by the *Guide* are as follows:

Room temperature: 64–79°F, 18–26°C
Relative humidity: 30–70%
Room air changes: 10–15/hour

Environmental controls should be set toward the middle of the room temperature and relative humidity ranges to avoid extremes and possible large fluctuations in these variables. The *Guide* does not specify any particular lighting cycle for rats; however, a 12 hour light/12 hour dark cycle is routinely used for this species.

5. Physical and Physiological Parameters

Physical and physiological parameters for laboratory rats are listed in Table 1.17.

TABLE 1.17
Physical and Physiological Parameters of Rats[4,6,7a]

Life span	2–3 yr
Male adult weight	350–400 g
Female adult weight	180–200 g
Birth weight	5–6 g
Adult food consumption	10–20 g/day
Adult water consumption	20–30 ml/day
Male breeding age/weight	10–12 wk/300–350 g
Female breeding age/weight	8–10 wk/200–300 g
Placentation	Discoidal hemochorial
Estrus cycle	4–5 days (polyestrous)
Gestation	20–22 days
Weaning age/weight	21 days/35–45 g
Average litter size	10–12 pups
Mating system(s)	1:1 or 1 male to multiple females
Adult blood volume	6–7% of body weight
Maximum safe bleed	5–6 ml/kg

TABLE 1.17 *(Continued)*
Physical and Physiological Parameters of Rats[4,6,7a]

Red cell count	$6–10 \times 10^6/mm^3$
White Cell Count	$7–14 \times 10^3/mm^3$
Hemoglobin	11–18 g/dl
Hematocrit	34–48%
Mean corpuscular volume	50–65
Mean corpuscular hemoglobin	19–23
Mean corpuscular hemoglobin concentration	32–38
Platelet count	$800–1500 \times 10^3/mm^3$
Heart rate	250–500 beats/min
Respiration rate	80–150 breaths/min
Rectal temperature	37.5°C
Urine pH	6.0–7.5
Urine volume	10–15 ml/day
Chromosome number	$2n = 42$

[a] See chapters 2, 5, 10, 11, 12, and 18 for more detailed information.

6. Identification, Bleeding, Anesthesia, and Euthanasia Methods for Rats

TABLE 1.18
Identification, Bleeding, Anesthesia, and Euthanasia Methods for Laboratory Rats

Identification methods
    Ear tags
    Ear punch, notch
    Tail tatoo identification number
    Subcutaneously implanted transponder
Bleeding methods
    Orbital sinus
    Tail vein and artery
Anesthesia methods
    75 mg/kg ketamine and 5 mg/kg xylazine
    4–5 mg/100 g body weight sodium pentobarbital
Euthanasia methods
    CO_2 inhalation
    Sodium pentobarbital overdose

7. Diseases

Various diseases and adverse health conditions of laboratory rats are identified and briefly described in Table 1.19.

TABLE 1.19
Various Diseases and Adverse Health Conditions of Laboratory Rats[4,8,9]

Disease/Health Condition	Etiology, Clinical Signs, Symptoms, and/or Pathology
Mycoplasma pulmonis	Bacterial infection which is common in conventionally reared rats and mice; responsible for rhinitis, otitis, laryngitis, tracheitis, bronchiolitis, bronchopneumonia, and additionally perioophoritis and salphingitis. Other mycoplasma species have been isolated from rats but *M. pulmonis* is the only significant pathogen.

TABLE 1.19 *(Continued)*
Various Diseases and Adverse Health Conditions of Laboratory Rats[4,8,9]

Disease/Health Condition	Etiology, Clinical Signs, Symptoms, and/or Pathology
Klebsiellosis	Caused by bacterium *Klebsiella pneumonia*; rats with natural disease may have submaxillary, parotid, or inguinal lymph node abscesses.
Tyzzer's disease	Caused by bacterium *Clostridium piliforme*; may occur in mice, rats, gerbils, hamsters, guinea pigs, rabbits, cats, dogs, nonhuman primates, horses, and other species; has been reported in Europe, North America, and Asia; most outbreaks in laboratory rats and mice have occurred in conventional colonies; usually subclinical; signs may include diarrhea, poor coat, and sudden death in young; focal necrosis in liver and inflammation of ileum.
Bordetellosis	Caused by bacterium *Bordetella bronchiseptica* that is a common inhabitant of the respiratory tract of rats and mice; may cause pneumonia usually in association with a primary pathogen such as mycoplasma.
Pasteurellosis	Caused by bacterium *Pasteurella pneumotropica*, an opportunistic organism; associated with abortion and respiratory, ear, reproductive, mammary gland, conjunctival and skin lesions; usually a co-pathogen with respiratory pathogens such as Sendai virus and mycoplasma.
Sendai virus	Caused by *Paramyxovirus*; extremely contagious; clinically inapparent chronic infection or clinically apparent acute infection; variable signs may include chattering, mild respiratory distress, prolonged gestation, poor growth, and death in young; concurrent pulmonary infections may occur.
Sialodacryoadenitis (SDA)	Caused by *Coronavirus*; highly contagious; one of the most common viruses in laboratory rats; virus is present in tissues of infected rats for only about 7 days; suckling rats may have mild transient signs (e.g., conjunctivitis); alternatively, sudden high prevalence of overt disease may occur with signs such as cervical edema, sneezing, photophobia, nasal and ocular discharge, and corneal lesions; there is usually high morbidity and no mortality; histopathological changes in salivary and lacrimal glands are characteristic.
Rat parvoviruses	Rat Virus (RV), H-1 Virus, and Rat Parvovirus (RPV); all are common, but only RV is associated with natural disease. RV is usually subclinical, but can be associated with fetal resorption, neonatal cerebellar hypoplasia with ataxia, hepatitis, jaundice, steatorrhea, and hemorrhages in adults especially when immunosuppressed.
Pneumonia virus of mice	Caused by *Pneumovirus*; common infection in laboratory rodents worldwide; active infection lasts about 9 days; natural infections are subclinical in euthymic rodents.
Ringtail	Condition of young rats and mice characterized by annular constriction and subsequent edema, necrosis, and sloughing of the tail; much more common in rats; may be prevented by providing relative humidity $\geq 50\%$.

C. GUINEA PIG (*CAVIA PORCELLUS*)

1. Breeds and Strains

Compared with the variety of mouse and rat strains which are available commercially, relatively few strains of guinea pigs are produced commercially for research purposes. The most commonly used guinea pig strains are albino outbreds of the Dunkan-Hartley and Hartley varieties. These strains have short, smooth hair and characteristic nonpigmented eyes.

Hairless guinea pigs such as the IAF strain are available from Charles River Laboratories, Wilmington, MA. Although these guinea pigs are a bit more expensive than the standard Hartley guinea pig, the absence of hair and intact immune system of the hairless guinea pig makes it an attractive alternative for dermal studies, such as delayed contact hypersensitivity or photoirritation and photosensitization studies. Consequently, the hairless guinea pig seems to be gaining in popularity among scientists involved in dermatological research.

2.　Handling and Restraint

Although the guinea pig is probably the most nervous and panicky species used in research, it generally will not scratch or bite when picked up, provided it is well supported. It is advisable to approach and handle the guinea pig in a quiet and confident manner to avoid inducing any unnecessary stress in the animal. The guinea pig may be picked up easily by placing one hand firmly around the animal's thorax and the other hand beneath the body to support the animal's weight. The guinea pig will often wiggle and vocalize (whistle) when handled.

3.　Housing

Because guinea pigs cannot jump or climb very well, they may be housed in relatively shallow cages with solid bottoms or wire flooring. If solid-bottom caging is used, the animals should be provided with some type of bedding material, such as processed hardwood chips. If suspended stainless steel caging is used, the wire floor must not allow the animal's feet to extend between the grids or the animal may be injured accidentally. Water may be supplied to guinea pigs using water bottles or by an automatic watering system. Each guinea pig should be checked daily to ensure that it has an adequate supply of fresh, uncontaminated food and water. Like humans and nonhuman primates, guinea pigs require regular doses of vitamin C (ascorbic acid) to avoid developing scurvy. Fortunately, commercial diets are available that contain an adequate supplement of vitamin C for this species.

The health of each animal should be verified at the time of receipt and on a daily basis thereafter by trained and qualified personnel. Guinea pigs can be rather messy laboratory animals because they quickly foul their cages and seem to enjoy spilling their food and playing with their water sippers. Therefore, the condition of the cages and bedding should be monitored closely and cleaned regularly to provide a suitable habitat for the animals. Minimum cage space requirements for the guinea pig are as follows:

TABLE 1.20
Minimum Cage Space Requirements for Guinea Pigs[a]

Body Weight (g)	Floor Area/Guinea Pig (sq. in.)	Cage Height (in.)
≤350	60.0	7
>350	>101.0	7

[a] As per the *Guide for the Care and Use of Laboratory Animals*, 1996.

4.　Environmental Conditions

Environmental conditions for guinea pigs recommended by the *Guide* are as follows:

Room temperature: 64–79°F, 18–26°C
Relative humidity 30–70%
Room air changes: 10–15/hour

Environmental controls should be set toward the middle of the room temperature and relatively humidity ranges listed above to avoid extremes and large fluctuations in these environmental variables. The *Guide* does not specify any particular lighting cycle for guinea pigs; however, a 12 hour light/12 hour dark cycle is routinely used for this species.

5. Physical and Physiological Parameters

Physical and physiological parameters of guinea pigs are listed in Table 1.21.

TABLE 1.21
Physical and Physiological Parameters of Guinea Pigs[4,6,7a]

Life span	4–6 yr
Male adult weight	1,000–1,200 g
Female adult weight	850–900 g
Birth weight	90–120 g
Adult food consumption	20–30 g/day
Adult water consumption	12–15 ml/100 g
Dietary peculiarities	Vitamin C required to avoid scurvy
Male breeding age/weight	11–12 wk/600–700 g
Female breeding age/weight	7–8 wk/350–450 g
Placentation	Discoidal hemochorial
Estrus cycle	16–18 days
Gestation	65–70 days
Weaning age/weight	7–14 days/150–200 g
Litter size	2–5
Mating	1M:1F or 1M:10F
Adult blood volume	6–7% body weight
Maximum safe bleed	7–8 ml/kg
Red cell count	$4.5–7 \times 10^6/mm^3$
White cell count	$5–15 \times 10^3/mm^3$
Hemoglobin	11–17 g/dl
Hematocrit	39–47%
Platelet count	$250–750 \times 10^3/mm^3$
Heart rate	230–300 beats/min
Respiration rate	60–110 breaths/min
Rectal temperature	39.5°C
Urine pH	8.0–9.0
Urine volume	15–75 ml/day
Chromosome number	$2n = 64$

[a] See Chapters 5, 11, 12, and 18 for more detailed information.

---

6. Identification, Bleeding, Anesthesia, and Euthanasia Methods for Guinea Pigs

---

TABLE 1.22
Identification, Bleeding, Anesthesia, and Euthanasia Methods for Laboratory Guinea Pigs

Identification methods
    Ear tags
    Subcutaneously implanted transponder
Bleeding methods
    Cardiac puncture (only with prior anesthesia)
Anesthesia methods
    Ketamine, methoxyflurane, isoflurane, pentobarbital
Euthanasia methods
    CO_2 inhalation
    Sodium pentobarbital overdose

---

7. Diseases

Various diseases and adverse health conditions of guinea pigs are identified and briefly described in Table 1.23.

TABLE 1.23
Various Diseases and Adverse Health Conditions of Guinea Pigs[4,9]

Disease/Health Condition	Etiology, Clinical Signs, Symptoms, and/or Pathology
Antibiotic-induced toxicity	Guinea pigs and hamsters are highly susceptible to the toxic effects of many antibiotics; toxicity results from overgrowth of *Clostridium difficile* and subsequent elaboration of toxins; enterocolitis with diarrhea and death may occur in 3–7 days.
Conjunctivitis	Often caused by *Chlamydia psittaci; Salmonella spp., Streptococcus spp., Staphylococcus spp.,* and *Pasteurella multocida* may also be involved; clinical signs include conjunctival hyperemia and chemosis with purulent ocular exudate; may be treated with ophthalmic antibiotics.
Lymphadenitis (lumps)	Inflammation and enlargement of the cervical lymph nodes is common in guinea pigs; usually caused by *Streptococcus zooepidemicus*; clinical findings are large unilateral or bilateral swellings or abscesses in the ventral neck region; organisms may gain entry to lymphatics from abrasions of the oral mucosa, thus avoid abrasive materials in feed or litter; affected animals should be culled.
Metastatic calcification	Occurs most often in male guinea pigs >1 yr old, but is usually clinically inapparent; signs include stiff joints and high mortality; calcium deposits may be seen in the lungs, liver, heart, aorta, stomach, colon, kidneys, joints, and skeletal muscles at necropsy; may be due to diets low in magnesium and potassium.
Muscular dystrophy	Guinea pigs are extremely sensitive to vitamin E deficiency; clinical signs are stiffness, lameness, and refusal to move; microscopic lesions include coagulative necrosis, inflammation, and proliferation of skeletal muscle fibers.
Parasitic diseases	Several protozoa (*Toxoplasma gondii, Eimeria caviae, Encephalitozoon cuniculi*), nedatodes (*Paraspidodera uncinata*), and lice (*Gyropus ovalis, Gliricola porcelli*) may infect guinea pigs.
Pneumonia	May be caused in guinea pigs by several bacteria (e.g., *Bordetella bronchiseptica, Streptococcus zooepidemicus, Streptococcus pneumoniae, Klebsiella pneumoniae,* and *Patteurella pneumotropica*); clinical signs are respiratory distress; affected animals should be culled.
Pregnancy toxemia	Metabolic disorder caused by obesity and stress which might induce temporary anorexia during late pregnancy; clinical findings are anorexia, adipsia, muscle spasms, coma within 48 hr of onset, and death within 4–5 days; laboratory findings are aciduria, proteinuria, hyperlipemia, and fatty degeneration of parenchymatous organs.
Ringworm	Dermatomycotic infection usually caused in guinea pigs by *Trichophyton mentagophytes*; signs are alopecia (usually starting at head), characterized by crusty, flaking lesions of the skin; facial lesions are common and disease may spread over the posterior regions; contagious to man and other animals.
Scurvy	Caused by vitamin C deficiency; guinea pigs cannot synthesize or appreciably store vitamin C; clinical signs include unsteady gait, painful locomotion, hemorrhage of gums, swelling of joints, and emaciation; may be prevented by providing 15–25 mg of vitamin C per day; vitamin C is stable for 3 mo in commercial guinea pig diets that are properly stored after milling.
Slobbers	Actually represents several conditions characterized by wet, matted hair around the mouth, chin, and ventral neck; drooling occurs whenever mastication is impaired (e.g., from dental abnormalities such as malocclusion or mandibular deformity); incisor teeth may be clipped to improve occlusion; mandibular deformity may result from subacute scurvy, folate deficiency or excess dietary fluoride.

D. RABBIT (*ORYCTOLAGUS CUNICULUS*)

1. Breeds and Strains

There are more than 100 different breeds and varieties of rabbits recognized by the American Rabbit Breeders Association. However, relatively few breeds are used for research purposes. Two breeds which have been used quite extensively for research include the New Zealand White rabbit and the Dutch Belted rabbit.

The New Zealand White (NZW) rabbit is an albino breed with rather large ears and characteristic nonpigmented eyes. This breed commonly attains a mature body weight of approximately 4.5 kg (approximately 10 pounds). In contrast, the Dutch Belted rabbit is a nonalbino breed that is usually black with a white stripe on the face and around the thorax. This breed has a mature body weight which is substantially less than that of the NZW rabbit, in the range of 2 to 2.5 kg (approximately 4.5 to 5 pounds).

2. Handling and Restraint

As with all species, it is essential that personnel receive proper, supervised training in appropriate handling and restraint techniques before working with rabbits. The rabbit should NEVER BE PICKED UP BY THE EARS ALONE because this will undoubtedly result in injury to the animal, and possibly to the caretaker. If handled incorrectly, the rabbit usually becomes excited and kicks viciously with its powerful back legs while twisting and contorting its body. This often leads to spinal injury to the animal.

The best method for picking up the rabbit is to grasp the scruff of the neck with one hand, while supporting the rump of the animal with the other hand. A gentle but firm grip is necessary to control the animal and to reduce anxiety and fear which are associated with restraint and lifting of the animal. Because all rabbits resist restraint to some degree, handlers should wear long sleeves or other protective covering to avoid being scratched.

3. Housing

In the laboratory setting, rabbits are usually housed in individual, suspended stainless steel cages with wire or slatted metal flooring. Fresh water may be supplied by water bottles or via an automatic watering system. Commercial rabbit feed is usually supplied using "J-type" feeders in which the curved lower portion dwells inside the cage and the square "hopper" portion is attached to the outside of the cage. Because male rabbits commonly express urine outside their cages, it is desirable to use some type of feeder lid to avoid contamination of the food supply of animals on lower cage levels. Food may be provided *ad libitum,* or on a restricted daily basis (e.g., 30–60 g/kg per day for an adult rabbit). When fed *ad libitum,* rabbits (like some humans) often gorge themselves and eat more than is really needed. A large NZW rabbit can usually maintain its body weight while being fed no more than 110–150 g of pellets per day.

Rabbits produce two types of feces that are known as "day feces" and "night feces." The day feces are hard and round, whereas the night feces are soft and covered by gray mucus. The night feces are consumed by the rabbit directly from the anus in a practice known as "coprophagy." This provides the rabbit with some benefit in the way of increased digestibility of protein and vitamins. Because of this practice, overnight fasting of rabbits will rarely, if ever, result in complete emptying of the stomach. Use of cages with wire flooring does not in any way reduce or eliminate coprophagy.

As with all species, the health of each rabbit should be verified at the time of receipt and on a daily basis thereafter by trained and qualified personnel. The condition of the animals' cages should be closely monitored and cleaned regularly to provide a suitable habitat for the animals. Minimum cage space requirements for rabbits are presented in Table 1.24.

TABLE 1.24
Minimum Cage Space Requirements for Rabbits[a]

Body Weight (kg)	Floor Area/Rabbit (sq. ft.)	Cage Height (in.)
<2	1.5	14
2–4	3.0	14
4–5.4	4.0	14
>5.4	≥5.0	14

[a] As per the *Guide for the Care and Use of Laboratory Animals,* 1996.

4. Environmental Conditions

Environmental conditions recommended for rabbits by the *Guide* are as follows:

Room temperature: 61–72°F, 16–22°C
Relative humidity: 30–60%
Room air changes: 10–15/hour

Environmental controls should be set toward the middle of the room temperature and relative humidity ranges just described to avoid extremes and large fluctuations in these environmental variables. The *Guide* does not specify any particular lighting cycle for rabbits; however, a 12 hour light/12 hour dark cycle is routinely used for this species.

5. Physical and Physiological Parameters

Physical and physiological parameters for laboratory rabbits are listed in Table 1.25.

TABLE 1.25
Physical and Physiological Parameters of Rabbits[4,6,7a]

Life span	5–7 yr
Male adult weight	4.0–5.5 kg
Female adult weight	4.5–5.5 kg
Birth weight	90–110 g
Adult food consumption	75–100 g
Adult water consumption	80–100 ml/kg body weight
Dietary peculiarities	Pelleted diet
Male breeding age/weight	6–7 mo/3.5–4.0 kg
Female breeding age/weight	5–6 mo/4.0–4.5 kg
Placentation	Discoidal hemoendothelial
Estrus cycle	Polyestrous, induced
Gestation	30–32 days
Weaning age/weight	6–7 wk/1.0–1.5 kg
Litter size	4–12
Mating system(s)	1:1 or via artificial insemination
Adult blood volume	6% of body weight
Maximum safe bleed	6.5–7.5 ml/kg
Red cell count	$4.5–7.0 \times 10^6/mm^3$
White cell count	$5–12 \times 10^3/mm^3$
Hemoglobin	11–14 g/dl
Hematocrit	32–48%

TABLE 1.25 *(Continued)*
Physical and Physiological Parameters of Rabbits[4,6,7a]

Mean corpuscular volume	58–72
Mean corpuscular hemoglobin	18–24
Mean corpuscular hemoglobin concentration	30–35
Platelet count	$250–750 \times 10^3/mm^3$
Heart rate	250–300 beats/min
Respiration rate	35–55 breaths/min
Rectal temperature	39.5°C
Urine pH	8.2
Urine volume	50–130 ml/kg
Chromosome number	$2n = 44$

[a] See chapters 5, 11, 12, and 14 for more detailed information.

6. Identification, Bleeding, Anesthesia, and Euthanasia Methods for Rabbits

TABLE 1.26
Identification, Bleeding, Anesthesia, and
Euthanasia Methods for Laboratory Rabbits

Identification methods
  Ear studs/tags
  Ear tatoo
  Subcutaneously implanted transponder
Bleeding methods
  Marginal ear vein
  Jugular vein
  Cardiac puncture (only with prior anesthesia)
Anesthesia methods
  Halothane, pentobarbital, methoxyflurane, ketamine, xylazine
Euthanasia methods
  Barbiturate overdose (IV)
  Other chemical euthanasia solutions

7. Diseases

Various diseases and adverse health conditions of rabbits are identified and briefly described in Table 1.27.

TABLE 1.27
Various Diseases and Adverse Health Conditions of Rabbits[4,9]

Disease/Health Condition	Etiology, Clinical Signs, Symptoms and/or Pathology
Pasteurellosis	Common and highly contagious disease caused by *Pasteurella multocida*; may be transmitted by direct or indirect contact; some animals may be asymptomatic carriers; infection may manifest as rhinitis (snuffles), pneumonia, otitis media, conjunctivitis, abscesses, genital infections, or septicemia; best controlled by strict culling; rhinitis, abscesses, genital infection, and pneumonia due to *P. multocida* and other agents are described further below.

TABLE 1.27 *(Continued)*
Various Diseases and Adverse Health Conditions of Rabbits[4,9]

Disease/Health Condition	Etiology, Clinical Signs, Symptoms and/or Pathology
Rhinitis	*Pasteurella*—induced acute, subacute, or chronic inflammation of the air passages and lungs; serous exudate from nose and eyes may become purulent; fur on inside of front legs may become matted due to pawing at nose; infected animals usually sneeze and cough; infection may proceed to pneumonia.
Abscesses	*Pasteurella*—induced abscesses may be found in any part of the body or head; fight wounds may develop into abscesses; it is usually better to eliminate rather than treat affected rabbits.
Genital infections	Genital infections may be caused by *Pasteurella* or other organisms; the infections manifest as acute or subacute inflammation of the reproductive tract; occurs more often in does than bucks; females may exhibit yellowish gray vaginal discharge; best controlled by culling.
Pneumonia	*P. multocida* accounts for most cases, but other bacteria may be involved (e.g., *Klebsiella pneumoniae, Bordetella bronchiseptica*, and *pneumococci*); upper respiratory disease (snuffles) often precedes pneumonia; occurrence may be directly proportional to level of ammonia in rabbitry; affected animals usually die within 1 wk after signs appear.
Listeriosis	Sporadic septicemic disease caused by *Listeria monocytogenes* and characterized by sudden deaths, abortions, or both; clinical signs are nonspecific and may include anorexia. depression, and weight loss; seldom affects the CNS but may spread to the liver, spleen, and gravid uterus; multiple gray-white foci are commonly seen at necropsy.
Staphylococcosis	Caused by *Staphylococcus aureus*; manifests as fatal septicemia in young rabbits and suppurative inflammation in older rabbits involving almost any organ or tissue; infected rabbits may show no signs until resistance is decreased; abscesses develop in chronic infections; usually fever, depression, anorexia, and then death in acute septicemia.
Enterotoxemia	Explosive diarrheal disease of young rabbits (e.g., 4–8 wk of age) which occasionally affects adults; one recognized cause is *Clostridium spiroforme*; signs are lethargy, rough coat, greenish brown fecal staining, and death within 48 hr; necropsy shows fluid-distended intestine with petechiae on serosal surface.
Mucoid enteropathy	Diarrheal disease which may occur in rabbits of any age; exact etiology is unknown; clinical signs are mucoid feces, anorexia, lethargy, dehydration, rough coat, bloated abdomen, and perineal area covered with mucus and feces; impaction of cecum and gelatinous mucus in the colon are common necropsy findings.
Tyzzer's disease	Caused by *Bacillus piliformis*; produces severe diarrhea and death in young rabbits; characterized by profuse diarrhea, anorexia, dehydration, lethargy, and death in 1–3 days; bacterium may affect other species.
Hepatic coccidiosis	Caused by *Eimeria stiedae*; transmission is by ingestion of sporulated oocysts; severity of disease depends on the number of oocysts ingested; rabbits may fail to make normal gains, but infection is usually asymptomatic; small yellowish white nodules are found throughout the hepatic parenchyma at necropsy; microscopically, nodules are composed of hypertrophied bile ducts; oocysts may be demonstrated by fecal flotation and microscopic examination.
Intestinal coccidiosis	Caused by *E. magna, E. irresidua, E. media, E. perforans*, or other *Eimeria spp.*; like hepatic coccidiosis, transmission is by ingestion of sporulated oocysts; may occur in rabbits receiving the best of care; infections are usually mild with no clinical signs; intestines may become thickened and pale; oocysts may be demonstrated by fecal flotation and microscopic examination.
Ear mites	The ear mite, *Psoroptes cuniculi,* is a common parasite of rabbits; common signs are head shaking, ear flopping, and ear scratching; ears can be treated by removing exudate and applying miticide for dogs and cats, or light mineral oil alone; treatment should be repeated in 6–10 days and continued as necessary; ivermectin has been shown effective in treating ear mites.
Fur mites	Infestation is usually asymptomatic unless animals become debilitated; infestations are common by *Cheyletiella parasitovorax* and *Listrophorus gibbus*; occasional small scabs and sores may be seen on the necks of adult animals.
Encephalitozoonosis	Widespread protozoal infection of rabbits caused by *Encephalitozoon (Nosema) cuniculi*; occasionally infects mice, guinea pigs, rats, and dogs; usually no clinical signs are seen; pitting of the kidneys may be seen at necropsy; microscopic lesions consist of focal granulomas and pseudocysts in the brain and kidneys.

TABLE 1.27 *(Continued)*
Various Diseases and Adverse Health Conditions of Rabbits[4,9]

Disease/Health Condition	Etiology, Clinical Signs, Symptoms and/or Pathology
Pinworms	The rabbit pinworm, *Passalurus ambiguus*, is usually not clinically significantly; adult worm lives in cecum or anterior colon; not transmissible to man.
Pox Viruses Orthopox	Caused by Rabbitpox Virus which is closely related to vaccinia virus and the same as rabbit plaque or "pockless" rabbitpox; transmission is via direct contact (nasal secretions); clinical signs include fever, nasal and ocular discharge, enlarged lymph nodes, and typical pox lesions in the skin with associated high mortality; lesions include papules or nodules in the dermis (central necrosis with mononuclear cell infiltration), possible necrosis and hemorrhages in lung, spleen, lymph nodes, liver, testis, ovary and uterus.
Leporipox	Rabbit Myxoma Virus is world wide; transmission is mechanical via direct contact or arthropod vectors; rare in laboratory rabbits, endemic in the wild with 99% mortality in susceptible *Oryctolagus sp.*; lesions vary markedly due to virulence and resistance factors; clinical signs include dermal masses, gleatinous edema, especially around body orifices and face; lesions in the skin display proliferation of "myxoma cells" (undifferentiated stellate mesenchymal cells) in dermis with abundant mucinous matrix; epidermis may be hyperplastic to degenerate with numerous eosinophilic intracytoplasmic inclusions; hemorrhage or necrosis, as well as, myxoma cells may be seen in other organs.
	Rabbit Fibroma Virus (Shope Fibroma Virus) occurs under natural conditions in cottontail rabbit; has been experimentally induced *Oryctolagus sp.*; transmission is mechanical via arthropods; infection may be limited to subcutaneous rubbery masses that develop 3–5 days post exposure (PE), these masses display mesenchymal/fibroblastic proliferation in the superficial dermis with epithelial hyperplasia extending into the mass, at 10–15 days PE regression can be seen with infiltration of lymphocytes and plasma cells, and necrosis; lesions associated with a sub-type metastatic virus consist of subcutaneous fibromas at 3–6 days PE with systemic metastases, and reduced T and B-cell response in the spleen, death by PE day 10–14 from bronchopneumonia.
Papova Viruses (Papillomatosis)	Cottontail Rabbit Papilloma Virus (CRPV) is also called Rabbit or Shope Papilloma Virus; natural infection in wild rabbits, rare in domestic rabbits; infects skin, never the oral cavity; spread by direct contact and insects; lesions include long keratinized papillary projections (warts) that may persist for months; this lesion may progress to squamous cell carcinoma.
	Oral Papillomatosis Virus (OPV) infects nonkeratinized surfaces only; usually ventral aspects of tongue or, rarely, ventral oral cavity; never elsewhere on the body; growths are typically solitary and papillary that regress in weeks to 1–2 years; the CRPV and OPV are distinctly different viruses and do not cross react.
Viral hemorrhagic disease	Highly contagious acute infection primarily of domestic rabbits; causative agent is a calicivirus lactating and gestating females are most susceptible; rabbits are often found dead with no prior signs; clinical signs in protracted cases include dyspnea, congestion of eyelids, abdominal respiration, and tachycardia; death may be preceded by violent cage activity such as rapid turns and flips; bloody nasal discharge is sometimes seen; gross lesions are generally limited to congestion of the respiratory tract and liver; microscopically there may be marked focal coagulative hepatic necrosis; focal necrosis of the myocardium may also be seen.
Broken back	Fracture or dislocation of lumbar vertebrae is common; signs include posterior paresis or paralysis and urinary and fecal incontinence; this condition warrants immediate euthanasia
Cannibalism	Young does may kill and consume their young for any number of reasons; cannibalism of dead young is a natural nest-cleaning activity.
Dental malocclusion	Overgrowth of incisors can result in difficulty in eating and drinking; this can be corrected by cutting the teeth from time to time.
Hair chewing and hairballs	Hair may accumulate in the stomach due to grooming; excessive hair may produce blockage resulting in anorexia, weight loss, and death.
Ulcerative pododermatitis (sore hocks)	Commonly caused by body-weight pressure on wire-floored cages; factors such as accumulation of urine-soaked feces and the type of wire flooring can influence development; there is no effective treatment; affected animals should be culled.

E. DOG (*CANIS FAMILARIS*)

1. Breeds and Strains

A variety of breeds and strains of dogs are used for laboratory studies. For toxicology investigations, the pure-bred beagle is probably the most popular breed owing to its uniform and relatively small size, docile temperament, physiological similarities to humans, and ability to adapt well to cage life. Beagles and other pure-bred strains produced specifically for research purposes are available from a number of USDA licensed commercial suppliers (see Table 1.9). These "bred for research" dogs offer the additional advantages of known genetic pedigrees and documented health histories and therapeutic treatments.

2. Receipt

As with all species, the health of each dog should be verified at the time of receipt and on a daily basis thereafter by trained and qualified personnel. On receipt, each dog should be given a thorough physical examination by a qualified veterinarian. The extent of this examination may vary, but, as a minimum, it should include general physical appearance and behavior, assessment of heart and lung sounds, presence of external parasites, condition of gums and teeth, mobility, and presence of any abnormal secretions or signs of gastrointestinal disturbance. Additional evaluations should be undertaken as deemed appropriate by the veterinarian or required by laboratory standard operating procedures. These may include fecal flotation for internal parasites, hematology and clinical chemistry assessments, ophthalmological examinations, and ECG measurements.

Each dog must have a certificate of health that has been completed by a licensed veterinarian and states that the animal was determined to be in acceptable condition no longer than 10 days before shipping. The date of last access to feed and water must appear on the paperwork accompanying each dog and on the dog's transport cage. The paperwork must also provide a place to document that feed was offered at least every 24 hours for dogs 16 weeks of age or older, and at least every 12 hours for dogs less than 16 weeks of age. Potable water must be offered at least once every 12 hours to all dogs in transit.

3. Handling and Restraint

Compassionate treatment and common sense are the cornerstones of proper management of dogs and other laboratory species. Specifications for the humane handling, care, treatment, and transportation of dogs (and cats) may be found in Part 3, Subpart A of the Animal Welfare Act.[1] Other regulations concerning USDA licensing, registration, research facilities, veterinary care, animal identification, required records, and regulatory compliance may be found in Part 2, Subpart A of the Animal Welfare Act.

The dog may be handled and restrained in a safe manner, provided that personnel are properly trained and experienced in appropriate handling and restraint techniques. Smaller dogs such as the beagle may be lifted by extending one arm under the abdominal area in front of the hind legs and the other arm in front of the chest area. Like other species, dogs should be handled in a firm but gentle manner.

During experimental manipulation (e.g., dose administration, clinical and physical examinations, blood sampling, electrocardiograms, etc.), it is wise to employ a team of two individuals, one to provide restraint and reassurance to the dog while the other performs experimental procedures. For some experimental techniques, the dog may be placed in a suspended upright position using a body sling designed for this purpose. Alternatively, the dog may be placed and manually restrained on top of an examination table. Irrespective of the method used, the presence of a second individual is most helpful to provide reassurance to the animal during restraint.

Occasionally, even docile breeds such as the beagle may become aggressive and require muzzling and/or chemical restraint to protect laboratory personnel. Muzzles may be purchased for this purpose, or simply prepared by wrapping the animals snout with gauze. When aggressive animals are encountered, the investigator and facility veterinarian should attempt to determine the reason for the adverse behavior and take immediate action. If the animal is injured, it should be euthanized. If the aggressive behavior is a manifestation of experimental treatment, immediate steps should be taken to ensure the safety of laboratory personnel. Of course, these latter comments apply to all species used in laboratory research.

4. Housing

Although the dog is hardier than many laboratory species, it must still be provided with a safe and comfortable habitat which protects the animal from extreme temperatures and weather conditions that may be uncomfortable or hazardous to the animal.

Dogs may be housed in cages, pens, or runs, with one or more dogs per primary enclosure. However, if housed in group pens or runs, only compatible animals should be placed together. Primary enclosures must be designed and constructed in a suitable and structurally sound manner. The enclosures must be kept in good repair with surfaces that can be readily cleaned and sanitized. Floors must protect the animals feet and legs from injury. If mesh or slatted floors are used, the dog's feet must not be allowed to pass through the floor openings. Primary enclosures must be cleaned daily and sanitized a minimum of once every 2 weeks. Animals are not to be wetted or contaminated by water from other cages during the cleaning process.

All dogs must have easy and convenient access to fresh food and water. Food must be provided at least once each day, except as otherwise might be required to provide adequate veterinary care. The food must be uncontaminated, wholesome, palatable, and of sufficient quantity and nutritive value to maintain the normal condition and weight of the animal. If potable water is not continually available to the animal, it must be offered as often as necessary to ensure the health and well-being of the dog (i.e., not less than twice daily for at least 1 hour each time). Minimum cage space requirements for the dog are presented in Table 1.28.

TABLE 1.28
Minimum Cage Space Requirements for Dogs[a]

Body Weight (kg)[a]	Type of Housing[a]	Floor Area/Dog[b] (sq. ft.)	Cage Height[a] (in.)
<15	Pen/run	8.0	Not Applicable
15–30	Pen/run	12	Not Applicable
>30	Pen/run	24	Not Applicable
<15	Cage	8.0	32
15–30	Cage	12	36
>30	Cage	—[b]	—[b]

[a] As per the *Guide for the Care and Use of Laboratory Animals*, 1996.
[b] These guidelines may require modification based on the body conformation of individual animal and breed.

According to the *Guide*, some dogs, especially those toward the upper limit of each weight range, may require additional floor space or cage height to ensure compliance with the Animal Welfare Act. These regulations mandate that the height of each cage be sufficient to allow the dog to stand in a "comfortable position" and that the minimum square footage of floor space be equal to the "mathematical square of the sum of the length of the dog in inches, as measured from the tip of the nose to the base of the tail, plus 6 inches, expressed in square feet." As an example, the floor space calculation for a dog measuring 28 inches from the tip of the nose to the base of the tail would be:

$$\frac{(28 \text{ in.} + 6 \text{ in.})^2}{144 \text{ in. } (1 \text{ sq. ft.})} = 8.0 \text{ sq. ft.}$$

5. Environmental Conditions

Environmental conditions recommended for dogs by the *Guide* are as follows:

Room temperature: 64–84°F, 18–29°C
Relative humidity: 30–70%
Room air changes: 10–15/hour

Environmental controls should be set toward the middle of the room temperature and relatively humidity ranges stated above to avoid extremes and large fluctuations in these environmental variables. The *Guide* does not specify any particular lighting cycle for dogs; however, a 12 hour light/12 hour dark cycle is routinely used for this species.

6. Exercise

Dogs 12 weeks old or older which are housed separately from other dogs must be given an opportunity to exercise regularly if their cage size is less than two times the required size. Dogs which are gang housed in a pen that meets 100% of the required floor space (i.e., the sum of each dogs requirement) are not required to be provided with additional exercise. The specific exercise program must be approved by the attending veterinarian and IACUC. The program must be in the written form of a standard operating procedure and records documenting the regimen must be maintained for each dog. Each dog that is denied contact with another dog must have positive daily physical contact with an animal handler.

Exercise exemptions for health reasons deemed necessary by the veterinarian must be in written form and, unless the health condition is permanent, must be reviewed by the veterinarian every 30 days. The IACUC must also agree to the proposed exercise exemption and must review the proposal at least once each year. If the principle investigator determines that the exercise is detrimental to the research protocol for scientific reasons, exercise may be eliminated, provided that the IACUC approves of this action. In this case, the committee's approval must be in the IACUC-approved protocol.

7. Physical and Physiological Parameters

Physical and physiological parameters for dogs are listed in Table 1.29.

TABLE 1.29
Physical and Physiological Parameters of Dogs[4,7 a]

Life span	12–14 yr
Male adult weight	6–25 kg
Female adult weight	6–25 kg
Birth weight	300–500 g
Adult food consumption	250–1,200 g/day
Adult water consumption	100–400 ml/day
Breeding age (males)	9–12 mo
Breeding age (females)	10–12 mo
Estrus cycle	Biannual, monestrus
Gestation	56–58 days
Weaning age	6–8 wk
Litter size	4–8
Mating	Pairs, 1 male to multiple females

TABLE 1.29 *(Continued)*
Physical and Physiological Parameters of Dogs[4,7] [a]

Adult blood volume	8–9%, 75–110 ml/kg
Maximum safe bleed	8–10 ml/kg
Red cell count	$5.5–8.5 \times 10^6/mm^3$
White cell count	$6–14 \times 10^3/mm^3$
Hemoglobin	13–18 g/dl
Hematocrit	38–52%
Platelet count	$200–600 \times 10^3/mm^3$
Heart rate	80–140 beats/min
Respiration rate	10–30 breaths/min
Rectal temperature	38.5°C
Urine pH	7.0–7.8
Urine volume	25–45 ml/kg
Chromosome number	$2n = 78$

[a] See Chapters 5, 11, 12, and 18 for more detailed information.

8. Identification, Bleeding, Anesthesia, and Euthanasia Methods for Dogs

TABLE 1.30
Identification, Bleeding, Anesthesia, and Euthanasia Methods for Laboratory Dogs

Identification methods
    Chain collar with metal (numbered) tag
    Letter tattoo on ear or flank
    Cage card + individual animal records
    Subcutaneously implanted transponder
Bleeding methods
    Cephalic, saphenous, femoral, and jugular veins
Anesthesia methods
    Halothane, isoflurane, tranquilizers, narcotics, sodium pentobarbital
Euthanasia methods
    Overdose of anesthetic drugs or chemical euthanasia solutions (e.g., sodium pentobarbital)

9. Diseases

Various diseases and adverse health conditions of dogs are identified and briefly described in Table 1.31.

TABLE 1.31
Various Diseases and Adverse Health Conditions of Dogs[4,9]

Disease/Health Condition	Etiology, Clinical Signs, Symptoms and/or Pathology
Distemper (hardpad disease)	Caused by a paramyxovirus; highly contagious systemic disease characterized by diphasic fever, leukopenia, gastrointestinal and respiratory catarrh, and frequent pneumonic and neurological complications; suspected cause of multiple sclerosis in man; hyperkeratosis of footpads may occur; CNS signs include localized twitching, paresis, or paralysis, and convulsions with salivation and chewing movements; seizures may become more frequent and severe; atrophy of thymus is a consistent postmortem finding; prevention is available via vaccination.

TABLE 1.31 *(Continued)*
Various Diseases and Adverse Health Conditions of Dogs[4,9]

Disease/Health Condition	Etiology, Clinical Signs, Symptoms and/or Pathology
Parvovirus	An enteritis of acute onset and varying morbidity and mortality; dogs of all ages may be affected, but puppies seem to be more susceptible; older and immune-impaired dogs may also be more susceptible to the virus; virus produces two different disease forms (myocarditis and enteritis); intestinal crypts become infected resulting in collapse of villi and necrosis of crypt cells; clinical signs include anorexia, lethargy, and rapid dehydration; lymphopenia (but not leukopenia) is found in most affected dogs; death may follow due to dehydration, electrolyte imbalance, endotoxic shock, or secondary septicemia; small intestine is primarily affected in enteric form of disease; pulmonary edema is main finding in myocardial form; prevention is available via vaccination.
Hepatitis virus	Contagious disease with signs that vary from slight fever to severe depression, marked leukopenia, prolonged bleeding time, and death; caused by canine adenovirus-1; clinical signs include apathy, anorexia, thirst, conjunctivitis, ocular discharge, nasal discharge, and occasional abdominal pain; disseminated intravascular coagulation is common; liver, kidneys, spleen, and lungs are the main target organs; hepatic cell necrosis and "paint brush" hemorrhages of the gastrointestinal tract, lymph nodes, thymus, and pancreas are observed postmortem; 25% of recovered dogs develop bilateral corneal opacity; prevention is available via vaccination which is often given with distemper immunizations.
Canine herpesvirus	Fatal viral infection of puppies worldwide; transmission occurs between susceptible puppies and the infected dam; death usually occurs at 1–3 wk; characteristic lesions consist of disseminated focal necrosis and hemorrhages; no vaccine is available, however, subsequent litters receive maternal antibodies in the colostrum and disease does not develop.
Canine coronavirus	Highly contagious gastrointestinal disease of dogs characterized by emesis and diarrhea; signs are similar to parvovirus but usually milder; prevention is available via vaccination.
Parainfluenza virus	Virus is capable of causing disease by itself, but is probably more often involved as a primary infection followed by secondary invaders; clinical signs include fever, anorexia, serous nasal discharge, lacrimation, and coughing; histological lesions include bronchiolitis and alveolitis with marked congestion and hemorrhage; prevention is available via vaccination.
Brucellosis	Caused by *Brucella canis*; disease disseminates rapidly among dogs closely kenneled; both sexes seem to be equally susceptible; primary signs are abortion, stillbirths, and conception failures; infected dogs develop generalized lymphadenitis, epididymitis, periorchitis, and prostatitis; transmission is congenital, venereal, or by ingestion of contaminated materials; bacteremia may persist for up to 2 yr; attempts at immunization have not been uniformly successful.
Infectious tracheobronchitis (kennel cough)	Highly contagious but generally a mild and self-limiting disease that affects dogs of all ages and results from inflammation of the upper airways; may progress to fatal bronchopneumonia in puppies or chronic bronchitis in adult dogs; spreads rapidly among susceptible dogs; canine parainfluenza virus, canine distemper virus, canine adenovirus-2, or *Bordetella bronchiseptica* may act as primary pathogens; concurrent infections with several pathogens is common; prominent clinical sign is harsh dry cough which may be followed by retching and gagging; development of more severe signs indicates complicating systemic infection such as distemper or bronchopneumonia; dogs should be immunized against distemper, parainfluenza, and canine adenovirus-2.
Coccidiosis	Approximately 22 species of coccidia infect the intestinal tract of dogs; the most common coccidia of dogs are *Cystoisospora spp.*; common clinical signs in severe cases are diarrhea (sometimes bloody), weight loss, and dehydration; may be treated with coccidiostatic agents such as sulfadimethoxine or nitrofurazone.

TABLE 1.31 *(Continued)*
Various Diseases and Adverse Health Conditions of Dogs[4,9]

Disease/Health Condition	Etiology, Clinical Signs, Symptoms and/or Pathology
Giardiasis	Intestinal protozoan which causes acute enteritis; trophozoites of *Giardia canis* may be detected by direct saline smears of fecal samples; ova may be detected by fecal flotation.
Babesiosis	Caused by a protozoan, *B. canis*, transmitted by a variety of tick genuses. The organism parasitizes red blood cells leading to anemia, fever, lethargy, and poor appetite; in more severe cases, severe depression, drooling, vomiting, jaundice, hemoglobinuria (due to intravascular hemolysis), mucosal petechiae and congestion, ulcerative stomatitis, and angioneurotic edema of the head, legs, and body occur; disseminated intravascular coagulation is a consistent occurrence in severe *B. canis; B. gibsoni* is another agent of canine babesiosis, but is apparently restricted to Asia; extravascular hemolysis is the rule with *B. gibsoni* in which splenomegaly and death due to anemia are common.
Mange	Contagious skin disease caused by several species of mites; may be transmitted by larvae, nymphs, and fertilized females; signs include alopecia and pruritis with intense irritation; if untreated, infestation can lead to emaciation, debilitation, and even death; sarcoptic mites burrow in the skin and cause intense itching, scratching, chewing, and rubbing; this often leads to inflammation and secondary infections; skin becomes dry, thickened, wrinkled, and crusty; demodectic mites feed on cells of the hair follicles and are more likely to produce localized lesions.
Heartworm	Clinical or subclinical disease complex caused by the filarial worm *Dirofilaria immitis*; occurs frequently in mosquito-infected areas; duration and severity of infection determine the severity of clinical signs; common findings are coughing, decreased exercise tolerance, and weight loss; large numbers of worms in right atrium and vena cava can cause death; treatment is difficult; affected dogs are not suitable for research.
Roundworm	Roundworms are relatively common in dogs, especially puppies; *Toxocara canis* is the most important species because it is fatal in young pups and larvae may migrate in man; infected dogs fail to grow and exhibit dull coats and distended abdomens; signs in severe infestations include pneumonia, ascites, fatty degeneration of liver, and mucoid enteritis; worms may be vomited or voided in feces: animals may be treated with piperazine salts or broad-spectrum compounds such as dichlorvos, febantel, or ivermectin.
Stronglyoidosis	Small slender nematode (*Strongyloides stercoralis*) parasite that inhabits the small intestine of dogs; worms are practically transparent; infections are usually associated with warm, wet, crowded, unsanitary housing; presence of clinical signs indicates heavy infection; these include blood-streaked mucoid diarrhea, emaciation, and reduced growth; in advanced stages there is shallow rapid breathing and pyrexia (indicates grave prognosis); common postmortem findings are pneumonia with large areas of consolidation, marked enteritis with hemorrhage, mucosal exfoliation, and profuse mucus secretion.
Stomach worm	Stomach nematodes of dogs (*Physaloptera* spp) occur throughout the world; these parasites cause gastritis and duodenitis resulting in vomiting, anorexia, and dark feces; anemia and weight loss may develop in heavy infections; treatment with pyrantel and carbon disulfide is effective.
Hookworms	*Ancylostoma caninum* is the principal cause of canine hookworm disease; a characteristic change in young pups is acute normocytic, normochromic anemia followed by hypochromic, microcytic iron deficiency anemia; this is often fatal; anemia results from blood sucking and ulceration when *A. caninum* shift feeding sites; hydremia, emaciation, and weakness develop in chronic disease.
Whipworm	The whipworm (*Trichuris vulpis*) commonly inhabits the cecum in infected dogs; no signs are seen in light infestations; weight loss and diarrhea may become pronounced as the worm burden increases; fresh blood may accompany the feces and anemia occasionally follows.

TABLE 1.31 *(Continued)*
Various Diseases and Adverse Health Conditions of Dogs[4,9]

Disease/Health Condition	Etiology, Clinical Signs, Symptoms and/or Pathology
Cestode (tapeworm) infections	Adult cestodes such as *Dipylidium caninum* and *Taenia pisiformis* may inhabit the intestine of dogs, but rarely cause serious disease; if present, clinical signs may depend on the degree of infection, age, condition, and breed of host; clinical signs may vary from unthriftiness and malaise to colic and mild diarrhea.
Fleas	Ubiquitous blood-sucking ectoparasites, principally of dogs and cats; may cause pruritus and severe dermatological problems; act as intermediate hosts for the tapeworm *D. caninum*: adult fleas can jump long distances and attach to potential hosts; pruritus is usually the first sign of flea infestation in dogs.
Otitis externa	Acute or chronic inflammation of the epithelium of the external auditory meatus, sometimes involving the pinna; characterized by erythema, discharge, desquamation, and varying degrees of pain and pruritis; this is the most common disease of the ear canal of dogs.

REFERENCES

1. Code of Federal Regulations (CFR), Title 9; Subchapter A, Animal Welfare, Office of the Federal Register, Washington, 1985.
2. *Guide for the Care and Use of Laboratory Animals*, U.S. Department of Health and Human Services, Public Health Service, National Institutes of Health, NIH Publication No. 86–23, Revised 1996.
3. *Recognition and Alleviation of Pain and Distress in Laboratory Animals*, Institute of Laboratory Animal Resources, Commission on Life Sciences, National Research Council, National Academy Press, Washington, 1992, pp. 3–7.
4. Evans, I.E. and Maltby, C.J., *Technical Laboratory Animal Management*, MTM Associates, Manassas, VA, 1989.
5. Beaver, B.V. et al., Report of the AVMA Panel on Euthanasia, *J. Am. Vet. Med. Assoc.*, 218(5), 669–696, 2001.
6. Williams, C.S.F., *Practical Guide to Laboratory Animals*, C.V. Mosby, St. Louis, 1976.
7. *LAMA Lines*, Newsletter of the Laboratory Animal Management Association, 4, Sept./Oct., 1988.
8. *Infectious Diseases of Mice and Rats*, Institute of Laboratory Animal Resources, Commission on Life Sciences, National Research Council, National Academy Press, Washington, 1991.
9. *The Merck Veterinary Manual*, 7th ed., Merck & Co., Rahway, NJ, 1991.
10. Benenson, A.S., Ed., Control of Communicable Diseases Manual, 16th ed., American Public Health Association, Washington, 1995.

ADDITIONAL RELATED INFORMATION

TABLE 1.32
Guiding Principles in the Use of Animals in Toxicology

1. The use, care, and transportation of animals for training and for toxicological research and testing for the purpose of protecting human and animal health and the environment must comply with all applicable animal welfare laws.
2. When scientifically appropriate, alternative procedures that reduce the number of animals used, refine the use of whole animals, or replace whole animals (e.g., *in vitro* models, invertebrate organisms) should be considered.
3. For research requiring the use of animals, the species should be carefully selected and the number of animals kept to the minimum required to achieve scientifically valid results.
4. All reasonable steps should be taken to avoid or minimize discomfort, distress, or pain of animals.
5. Appropriate aseptic technique, anesthesia, and postoperative analgesia should be provided if a surgical procedure is required. Muscle relaxants or paralytics are not to be used in place of anesthetics.
6. Care and handling of all animals used for research purposes must be directed by veterinarians or other individuals trained and experienced in the proper care, handling, and use of the species being maintained or studied. Veterinary care is to be provided in a timely manner when needed.
7. Investigators and other personnel shall be qualified and trained appropriately for conducting procedures on living animals, including training in the proper and humane care and use of laboratory animals.
8. Protocols involving the use of animals are to be reviewed and approved by an institutional animal care and use committee before being initiated. The composition and function of the committee shall be in compliance with applicable animal welfare laws, regulations, guidelines, and policies.
9. Euthanasia shall be conducted according to the most current guidelines of the American Veterinary Medical Association (AVMA) Panel on Euthanasia or similar bodies in different countries.

From Society of Toxicology (1999). With permission.

TABLE 1.33
General Information Sources for the Care and Use of Research Animals

1. *Public Health Service Policy on Humane Care and Use of Laboratory Animals*. PHS (Public Health Service), 1996, U.S. Department of Health and Human Services, Washington, D.C. 22 pp. [PL 99-158. Health Research Extension Act, 1985].
2. The Animal Welfare Act of 1966 (P.L. 89-544) as amended by the Animal Welfare Act of 1970 (P.L. 91-579); 1976 Amendments to the Animal Welfare Act (P.L. 94-279); the Food Security Act of 1985 (P.L. 99-198), Subtitle F (Animal Welfare File Name: PL99198); and the Food and Agriculture Conservation and Trade Act of 1990 (P.L. 101-624), Section 2503, Protection of Pets (File Name: PL 101624). Rules and regulations pertaining to implementation are published in the Code of Federal Regulations, Title 9 (Animals and Animal Products), Chapter 1, Subchapter A (Animal Welfare). Available from Regulatory Enforcement and Animal Care, APHIS, USDA, Unit 85, 4700 River Road, Riverdale, MD 20737-1234, File Name 9CFR93. www.nal.usda.gov/awic/legislat/awicregs.html
3. *Guide for the Care and Use of Laboratory Animals*. Institute of Laboratory Animal Resources, Commission on Life Sciences, National Research Council, National Academy Press, Washington, D.C., 1996 or succeeding revised editions. www.nap.edu/readingroom/books/labrats
4. *International Guiding Principles for Biomedical Research Involving Animals*. Council for International Organizations of Medical Sciences (CIOMS), Geneva, 1985.
5. *Interdisciplinary Principles and Guidelines for the Use of Animals in Research, Testing, and Education*. Ad Hoc Animal Research Committee, New York Academy of Sciences, 1988.
6. *Recognition and Alleviation of Pain and Distress in Laboratory Animals. A report of the Institute of Laboratory Animal Resources Committee on Pain and Distress in Laboratory Animals.* NCR (National Research Council). Washington, D.C.: National Academy Press, 1992.
7. *Education and Training in the Care and Use of Laboratory Animals: A Guide for Developing Institutional Programs*. AVMA (American Veterinary Medical Association). Report of the AVMA panel on euthanasia. J. Am. Vet. Med. Assoc. 218(5), 669–696, 2001.
8. *Guide to the Care and Use of Experimental Animals*. CCAC (Canadian Council on Animal Care) Vol. 1, 2nd ed. Edited by E. D. Olfert, B. M. Cross, and A. A. McWilliam. Ontario, Canada: Canadian Council on Animal Care, 1993. 211 pp.

Compiled by the Society of Toxicology.

TABLE 1.34
Commonly Used Anesthetics

This table lists injectable anesthetics and preanesthetics used in various animal species. The medications are sometimes used in combination to produce anesthesia. These combinations are indicated by brackets where applicable. For example, atropine, morphine, and pentobarbital can be used in combination in dogs. Atropine and morphine are administered 30 minutes before pentobarbital to reduce paraympathetic secretions and to provide analgesia. The routes of exposure listed are those generally used. Other routes of administration may be used for some of the medications. The reader should consult the reference for information on alternate routes and dosage information.

Species	Anesthetic	Time[a] (min)	Route[b]	Dose (mg/kg)
Mouse	Amobarbital		IV	54
	Barbital		IV	234
	Chloral hydrate		IP	400
	α-Chloralose		IP	114
	Chlorobutanol (in 50% alcohol)		IP	175
	Droperidol(2%)-Fentanyl (0.04%)		IP	0.02–0.05[c]
	Etomidate		IP	22–25
	Hexobarbital		IV	47
	Ketamine		IV	50
	Ketamine		IP	100–200
	Ketamine		IM	400
	Pentobarbital		IV	35
	Phenobarbital		IV	134
	Probarbital		IP	75
	Secobarbital		IV	30
	Thiamylal		IV	25–50
	Thiopental		IV	25
	Tribromoethanol		IV	120
	Urethan		IP	1500
Rat	⎡ Acepromazine		IP	12 ⎤
	⎣ Ketamine		IP	120 ⎦
	Amobarbital		IV	55
	Barbital		IP	190
	Chloral hydrate		IP	300
	α-Chloralose		IP	55
	α-Chloralose		IV	100
	Diallybarbituric Acid		SC	60
	Droperidol(2%)-Fentanyl(0.04%)		IM	0.3[c]
	Droperidol(2%)-Fentanyl(0.04%)		IP	0.13[c]
	Hexobarbital		IP	75
	Inactin		IP	100
	Ketamine		IP	100
	Ketamine		IM	100
	Ketamine		IP	40–160
	Methohexital		IP	37.5
	Pentobarbital		IV	25
	⎡ Pentobarbital		IP	35 ⎤
	⎣ Chloral hydrate		IP	160 ⎦
	⎡ Pentobarbital		IP	10 ⎤
	⎣ Ketamine		IP	75 ⎦
	Phenobarbital		IP	40
	Phenobarbital		IV	100

TABLE 1.34 *(Continued)*
Commonly Used Anesthetics

Species	Anesthetic	Time[a] (min)	Route[b]	Dose (mg/kg)
	Probarbital		SC	225
	Secobarbital		IV	17.5
	Thiopental		IV	25
	Tiletamine-Zolazepam (1:1)		IM	20–30
	Tribromoethanol		IP	550
	Urethane		IP	780
	Urethane		SC	1,200
	Xylazine		IM	6
	Ketamine		IM	80
Guinea pig	Amobarbital		IV	50
	Chloral hydrate		IP	400
	Chlorobutanol (in 50% alcohol)		IP	175
	Droperidol(2%)-Fentanyl(0.04%)		IM	0.66–0.88[c]
	Droperidol(2%)-Fentanyl(0.04%)		IP	0.8
	Ketamine		IM	44–256
	Pentobarbital		IP	30
	Pentobarbital		IM	15–30
	Pentobarbital		IV	30
	Pentobarbital		IP	35
	Chloral hydrate		IP	160
	Phenobarbital		IP	100
	Secobarbital		IV	20
	Thiopental		IV	20
	Tribromoethanol		IV	100
	Urethane		IP	1,500
Rabbit	Amobarbital		IV	40
	Barbital		IV	175
	α-Chloralose		IV	120
	Chloral hydrate		IV	200
	Diallylbarbituric acid		IV	50
	Droperidol(2%)-Fentanyl(0.04%)		IM	0.22[c]
	Hexobarbital		IV	25
	Ketamine		IV	15–20
	Ketamine		IM	44
	Morphine	30	SC	10
	Chlorobutanol (in 50% alcohol)		PO	175
	Paraldehyde		IV	300
	Pentobarbital		IV	30
	Pentobarbital		IP	40
	Pentobarbital		IV	25–40
	Phenobarbital		IV	200
	Probarbital		IP	66
	Secobarbital		IV	22.5
	Thiamylal		IV,IP	45–50
	Thiopental		IV	20
	Tribromoethanol		IV	80
	Urethane		IV	1,000
	Urethane		IP	700
	Pentobarbital		IP	40
	Xylazine		IM	5

TABLE 1.34 *(Continued)*
Commonly Used Anesthetics

Species	Anesthetic	Time[a] (min)	Route[b]	Dose (mg/kg)
	Xylazine		IM	5
	Ketamine		IM	50
Cat	Amobarbital		IV	11
	Barbital		IV	200
	Chloral Hydrate		PO	250
	α-Chloralose		IV	75
	α-Chloralose		IV	50
	Urethane		IV	50
	α-Chloralose		IV	80
	Pentobarbital		IV	12
	α-Chloralose		IV	80
	Pentobarbital		IV	6
	Diallylbarbituric acid		IV	36
	Hexobarbital		IV	25
	Ketamine		IM	11–33
	Ketamine		IV	11–22
	Ketamine		IM	6.6–22
	Acepromazine		IV,IM	0.22–0.55
	Ketamine		IM	6.6–22
	Diazepam		IV,IM	0.33–1.1
	Ketamine	10–15	IM	10–15
	Pentobarbital		IV	30
	Ketamine		IM	6.6–22
	Xylazine		IM	0.44
	Pentobarbital		IP	20
	Barbital		IP	200
	Methohexital		IV	11
	Paraldehyde		IV	300
	Pentobarbital		IV	25
	Phenobarbital		IP	180
	Secobarbital		IV	25
	Thiamylal		IV	17.6
	Thiamylal		i.thoracic	25
	Thiopental		IV	28
	Tiletamine-Zolazepam (1:1)		IM	6–13
	Tribromoethanol		IV	100
	Urethane		IV	1250
	Urethane		IP	400
	α-Chloralose		IP	50
	Urethane		IP	280
	Diallylbarbituric acid		IP	70
	Urethane		IP	360
	Diallylbarbituric acid		IP	90
	Urethane		IP	250
	Pentobarbital		IP	30

TABLE 1.34 (Continued)
Commonly Used Anesthetics

Species	Anesthetic	Time[a] (min)	Route[b]	Dose (mg/kg)
Dog	Acepromazine	10–15	IM	0.55
	Ketamine	5	IM	11–22
	Thiamylal		IV	To effect
	Amobarbital		IV	50
	Barbital		IV	220
	Barbital		IV	250
	Thiopental		IV	15
	Barbital		IV	220
	Pentobarbital		IV	15
	Chloral hydrate		IV	125
	α-Chloralose		IV	100
	Dial-urethane		IV	10[c]
	Droperidol(2%)-Fentanyl(0.04%)		IM	0.05–0.15[c]
	Droperidol(2%)-Fentanyl(0.04%)		IV	0.03–0.09[c]
	Etomidate		IV	1.5–3
	α-Chloralose		IV	100
	α-Chloralose		IV	0. 17[d]
	Morphine		IM	2
	α-Chloralose		IV	100
	Morphine	30	SC	1
	α-Chloralose		IV	100
	Morphine	60	SC	1
	α-Chloralose		IV	80
	α-Chloralose		IV	50
	Thiopental		IV	15
	Morphine	30	SC	10
	Chlorobutonal (in 50% alcohol)		PO	225
	Morphine		SC	1
	Thiopental		IV	20
	Hexobarbital		IV	30
	Methohexital		IV	11
	Paraldehyde		IV	300
	Pentobarbital		IP	30
	Pentobarbital		IV	6[d]
	Pentobarbital		IV	10
	α-Chloralose		IV	80
	Morphine	30	SC	10
	Pentobarbital		IV	20
	Morphine	30	IM	2
	Pentobarbital		IV	15
	Morphine	60	IM	3
	Pentobarbital		IV	12

TABLE 1.34 *(Continued)*
Commonly Used Anesthetics

Species	Anesthetic	Time[a] (min)	Route[b]	Dose (mg/kg)
	Atropine	30	SC	1
	Morphine	30	SC	10
	Pentobarbital		IV	30
	Phenobarbital		IV	80
	Phenobarbital		IV	200
	Thiopental		IV	15
	Promazine	5	IV,IM	4.4
	Ketamine		IM	17.6
	Promazine	5	IV,IM	4.4
	Ketamine		IV	to effect
	Secobarbital		PO	40
	Thiamylal		IV	17.6
	Tiletamine-Zolazepam (1:1)		IM	6–13
	Thiopental		IV	25
	Tribromoethanol		IV	125
	Urethane		IV	1,000
	Urethane		IP	500
	α-Chloralose		IP	50
	Urethane		IV	480
	α-Chloralose		IV	48
	Morphine		IV	2
	Morphine	60	SC	2
	Urethane		IV	250
	α-Chloralose		IV	60
	Morphine	60	SC	3
	Urethane		IV	50
	α-Chloralose		IV	13
	Diallylbarbituric Acid		IV	8
	Morphine	30	SC	5
	Urethane		PO	1,500
	Xylazine	5	IV	1
	Ketamine		IV	10
Monkey	Amobarbital		IV	40
	Dial-Urethane		IV	0.7c
	Droperidol(2%)-Fentanyl(0.04%)		IM	0.11[c]
	Ketamine		IV	28–45
	Ketamine		IM	7–40
	Ketamine	10–15	IM	18
	Thiamylal		IV	15
	Pentobarbital		IV	20–33
	Pentobarbital		IP	30
	Pentobarbital		IV	25
	Phenobarbital		IP	100
	Secobarbital		IV	17.5
	Tiletamine-Zolazepam(1:1)		IM	3
	Thiamylal		IV	25

TABLE 1.34 *(Continued)*
Commonly Used Anesthetics

Species	Anesthetic	Time[a] (min)	Route[b]	Dose (mg/kg)
	Xylazine	10–15	IM	6
	Ketamine		IV	To effect
	Xylazine		IM	6
	Ketamine		IM	7–40

[a] The numbers refer to time elapsed (in minutes) before the injection of the following drug.

[b] Most common route of administration. IM = intramuscular; IP = intraperitoneal; IV= intravenous; PO = per os (orally).

[c] Dose is given as ml/kg.

[d] mg/kg/min infusion.

From Borchard, R.E., Barnes, C.D., and Eltherington, L.G., *Drug Dosage in Laboratory Animals. A Handbook,* 3rd ed., CRC Press, Boca Raton, FL, 1992. With permission.

TABLE 1.35
Advantages and Disadvantages for Anesthetic Agents and Adjuncts

Agent	Advantages	Disadvantages
1. Injection Anesthetics	Inexpensive, easy to use, rapid onset.	Constantly changing anesthetic state. Poor reproducibility.
α-Chloralose	Less reflex depression than barbiturates. Catecholamine release may support circulation.	Low water solubility. Inject warm or in a 10% solution with propylene glycol 200.
Dial (Ciba)[a]	More rapid onset and less toxic than urethane alone. Less reflex depression than with barbiturate alone.	Urethane toxicity limits use to acute experiment.
Droperidol-Fentanyl	IV use not generally required. Analgesic; can antagonize opioid component (fentanyl).	Cardiac and respiratory depression. Transient behavioral changes. Thermoregulatory upset; vomition, defecation.
Etomidate	Potent hypnotic, wide margin of safety, rapid induction.	Not analgesic in subanesthetic doses.
Ketamine	IV use not generally required. Large margin of safety; no cardiovascular nor respiratory depression. Analgesic.	Poor relaxation and poor recovery; convulsive, hallucinogenic. Retention of reflexes. Used in combination with phenothiazines, benzodiazepines, and xylazine to overcome disadvantages.
Methohexital	Very short duration (< 15 min, may be a disadvantage). Recovery from metabolism (use in low fat animal).	IV use required; short duration; violent recovery possible. Metabolism required; low margin of safety.
Pentobarbital	Rapid onset. High water solubility.	IV use required generally. Marked cardiovascular and reflex depression. Extravascular → severe inflammation, sloughing.
Thiamylal	Short duration (15–30 min). Recovery from redistribution (metabolism later). Good anesthesia and relaxation.	Longer duration in animals with low body fat. IV use generally required. Cardiovascular and respiratory depression; low margin of safety.

TABLE 1.35 *(Continued)*
Advantages and Disadvantages for Anesthetic Agents and Adjuncts

Agent	Advantages	Disadvantages
Thiopental	Short duration (15–30 min). Useful to include anesthesia prior to inhalation agents.	Solution rapidly decomposes. Fat solubility → remains in the body a long time.
Tiletamine-Zolazepam	Similar to ketamine-diazepam combinations.	
Urethane	Little reflex depression. High water solubility. Long duration.	Liver and bone marrow toxicity. Used only in acute experiments.
2. Inhalation Anesthetics	Constant and reproducible anesthesia; therefore, less data variability.	More skill required. Some need expensive equipment. Alveolar tension difficult to monitor in animal smaller than rat.
Cyclopropane	Rapid induction. Easy to measure—as difference from oxygen.	Explosive, circulatory adaptation. Tendency to laryngospasm.
Diethyl ether	Respiratory stimulation. Good muscle relaxation.	Slow induction and slow recovery. Explosive and stimulates secretions. Long duration in body fat. Circulatory adaptation occurs.
Floroxene	Cardiovascular stimulation. Little respiratory depression.	Irritating and explosive over 4%. Circulatory adaptation. Metabolized in the body.
Halothane	Rapid induction, rapid recovery. Non-explosive and potent.	Expensive. Cardiovascular depression and adaptation. Sensitization of myocardium to catecholamines. Poor analgesia; metabolized. Need precision vaporizers. Malignant hyperthermia implications.
Isoflurane	Low metabolism. Nonexplosive. No circulatory adaptation → "constant" anesthetic state. Rapid induction, rapid recovery.	Expensive. Cardiorespiratory depression. Need precision vaporizers.
Methoxyflurane	Potent and nonexplosive. Nonirritating to respiratory tract. Good analgesia (postanesthetic) and muscle relaxation. Precision vaporizers not needed.	Slow induction and slow recovery. Alveolar-arterial gradient. High fat solubility → long duration in body. High oxygen flows to vaporize. Highly metabolized. Ages rubber equipment.
Nitrous oxide	Not metabolized. Easily measured and used. Analgesic, additive to other anesthetics.	Only analgesia in safe concentrations. Need muscle relaxants to prevent movement. Hypoxia and diffusion hypoxia.
3. Adjuncts to Anesthesia	Facilitate induction and maintenance of anesthesia, improve safety.	Injectable drugs and not advised for acute experiments.
Atropine	Decreases respiratory secretion and vagal bradycardia.	Ganglionic blockade and CNS effects.
Benzodiazepine tranquilizers (Diazepam)	Used with several anesthetics, especially dissociative types (e.g., ketamine). Improves induction and recovery; better relaxation (allows intubation).	

TABLE 1.35 *(Continued)*
Advantages and Disadvantages for Anesthetic Agents and Adjuncts

Agent	Advantages	Disadvantages
Phenothiazine tranquilizers (Chlorpromazine)	Preanesthetic sedation. Reduces dose of anesthetic required.	Many pharmacological actions, especially cardiovascular depression. Prolonged recovery.
Curate	Immobility with minimal anesthesia or with nitrous oxide. "Ordinary doses" do not enter brain.	Release histamine. Need artificial ventilation. Must use analgesics.
Succinylcholine	Rapid onset and short duration. Can titrate IV. Immobility with minimal anesthesia.	Increased Serum K^+. Implicated in malignant hyperthermia. Other cholinergic actions. Must use analgesics.
Narcotics (morphine)	Analgesia and sedation facilitate anesthesia. Use as only anesthetic if support ventilation.	Release histamine. Respiratory depression causing delay in induction of inhalation anesthesia.
Xylazine	Preanesthetic sedation; reduces dose of anesthetic; analgesic. Emetic action (especially in cats; may be a disadvantage). Antagonized by α_2 blockers (e.g., yohimbine)	Cardiorespiratory depression; emesis; severe CNS depression.

[a] Contains: urethane, 400 mg/ml; diallybarbituric acid, 100 mg/ml.

From Borchard, R.E., Barnes, C.D., and Eltherington, L.G., *Drug Dosage in Laboratory Animals. A Handbook,* 3rd ed., CRC Press, Boca Raton, FL, 1992. With permission.

2 Acute, Subchronic, and Chronic Toxicology

Carol S. Auletta, D.A.B.T., R.A.C., M.B.A.

CONTENTS

SECTION 1. INTRODUCTION

This chapter presents information on designing and implementing acute, subchronic, and chronic toxicity studies and on interpreting results of these studies. Sample designs are provided to present an overview of typical studies of various duration in rodent and non-rodent species. A variety of government guidelines and regulations for study design have been published; several of these are summarized in tables presented in this chapter. Samples of much of the documentation necessary to implement a study in our laboratory, as well as checklists to confirm that all appropriate prestudy tasks have been performed, are presented for guidance in the type of information required to initiate a toxicity study. Tables presenting guidelines for many of the logistical and scientific decisions which must be made to select appropriate doses, dose volumes, dosing apparatus, and dose administration procedures summarize several formal and informal "rules" used in our and other laboratories. Formulas and sample calculations are provided for calculating doses, dietary concentrations, and test material requirements. Guidelines for types of clinical signs and their experimental significance, as well as historical control values for rodent body weight, food consumption, and survival in our laboratory, are provided for use in evaluating experimental results and interpreting the data. One particularly useful table summarizes the types of organ weight changes which would be expected as a result of food deprivation and resultant decreases in body weight gain; this is helpful in differentiating truly toxic effects from those which are secondary to decreases in weight gain associated with palatability problems or other causes.

It is important to remember that the information and guidelines provided are basic, general suggestions which will apply in many situations but which must be reviewed carefully to assure that they address specific needs. The toxicologist designing and interpreting a study will have information on scientific and regulatory concerns which may require modification of "standard" designs and procedures. It should also be noted that some of the information is specific to our laboratory and, although it should provide useful guidance, it may not be completely transferable to other situations.

SECTION 2. SAMPLE STUDY DESIGNS

The following tables illustrate sample study designs commonly used for toxicity studies. Studies in rodents and non-rodents are presented. Common species in these categories are:

Rodents: Commonly used are rats and mice. Studies conducted in rabbits, which are nonrodents, frequently follow similar designs.

Nonrodents: Commonly used are dogs and nonhuman primates.

TABLE 2.1
Experimental Design — Acute Toxicity Study (Rodent)

	No. of Animals			
	Initial		Necropsy, Day 15	
Doses (mg/kg)[a]	Males	Females	Males	Females
Limit Test (performed if material is expected to be nontoxic)				
[b]	5	5	A.S.	A.S.
ED$_{50}$ Test [performed if more than 50% of animals in limit test exhibit mortality (LD$_{50}$ study) or other effects (ED$_{50}$ study)]				
[c]	5	5	A.S.	A.S.
[c]	5	5	A.S.	A.S.

TABLE 2.1 *(Continued)*
Experimental Design — Acute Toxicity Study (Rodent)

Doses (mg/kg)[a]	No. of Animals			
	Initial		Necropsy, Day 15	
	Males	Females	Males	Females
c	5	5	A.S.	A.S.
c	5	5	A.S.	A.S.

[a] mg/kg = milligrams of test material per kilogram of body weight; A.S. = all survivors; complete postmortem evaluations are also performed on animals that are found dead or euthanatized in a moribund condition during the course of the study.

[b] Regulatory-specified limit dose (usually 2000 mg/kg orally and 2000 mg/kg dermally) or dose selected as a reasonable multiple (10–100×) of potential human exposure.

[c] Two to four doses lower than the limit dose are selected to produce a range of effects from a no-effect dose to one which produces slightly less-pronounced effects than the limit dose. (If a range of mortality is seen, these data can be used to calculate an LD_{50} value.) Doses may be administered concurrently (if adequate preliminary information is available to select appropriately) or stepwise, with new doses selected based on the results of preceding doses.

TABLE 2.2
Experimental Design — Acute Toxicity Study (Nonrodent)

Limit Test (performed if material is expected to be nontoxic)

Doses (mg/kg)	Number of Animals			
	Initial		Necropsy Day 15	
	Males	Females	Males	Females
a	2–3	2–3	A.S.	A.S.

Up and Down Test (performed if toxicity is expected)[b]

Dose Sequence	Dose Level (mg/kg)[c]		Number of Animals				
	Effect seen at preceding dose (severe toxicity)	No effect seen at preceding dose	Initial[d]	Pretest	Clinical Laboratory Studies[e] Termination	Necropsy	Microscopic Pathology
1st (a)	—	a	1	1	1	1	A.R.
2nd (b)	a ÷ m	a × m	1	1	1	1	A.R.
3rd (c)	b ÷ m	b × m	1	1	1	1	A.R.
4th (d)	c ÷ m	c × m	1	1	1	1	A.R.
5th (e)	d ÷ m	d × m	1	1	1	1	A.R.
6th (f)	e ÷ m	e × m	1	1	1	1	A.R.

[a] Regulatory-specified limit dose or dose selected as a reasonable multiple (10–100×) of potential human exposure.

[b] m = multiplier (generally between 1.5 and 3; usually 2); A.R. = as required Optional. These are sometimes performed to assess target organ toxicity.

[c] The initial dose (a) should he close to the estimated ED_{50}; if this estimate is poor, it would be best to err on the low side.

[d] Either sex may be used for the first dose (a). Subsequent animals will generally be of a different sex than the previous one. Attempts should be made to dose animals of both sexes at both toxic and nontoxic levels.

[e] Optional. These are frequently performed to assess target organ toxicity. Terminal studies are performed on all survivors 14 days after dosing; attempts are made to collect samples from moribund animals.

Adapted from Bruce, R.D., An up-and-down procedure for acute toxicity to testing, *Fund. Appl. Toxicol.*, 5, 151, 1985.[1]

TABLE 2.3
Experimental Design — Range-Finding Study (Rodent)[a]

Group	Dose (mg/kg/day or ppm)[b]	Initial		Week 2 or 4[c]					
				Clinical Laboratory Studies		Necropsy		Microscopic Pathology[a]	
		Males	Females	Males	Females	Males	Females	Males	Females
I	0[e]	5	5	5	5	A.S.	A.S.	5	5
II	*	5	5	5	5	A.S.	A.S.	A.R.	A.R.
III	*	5	5	5	5	A.S.	A.S.	A.R.	A.R.
IV	*	5	5	5	5	A.S.	A.S.	A.R.	A.R.
V	*	5	5	5	5	A.S.	A.S.	5	5

[a] A.S. = All survivors; complete postmortem evaluations are also performed on animals that are found dead or euthanatized in a moribund condition during the course of the study. A.R. = as required; examinations of tissues from animals at lower dose levels may be performed if indicated by findings in high-dose animals. mg/kg/day = milligrams of test material per kilogram of body weight per day; or ppm = parts per million (dietary concentration).

[b] Doses should be selected to produce a range of effects from a no-effect dose to one which produces clear toxicity. A minimum of three doses is recommended. More doses may be used to increase likelihood of achieving an appropriate range of effects.

[c] Two weeks is a common duration and is a recommended minimum. Four-week studies are frequently performed to provide additional information.

[d] Optional. Microscopic examination of tissues from control and high-dose animals may be performed to assess target organ toxicity.

[e] Control animals receive vehicle in the same volume as high-dose animals or receive untreated diet.

TABLE 2.4
Experimental Design — Range-Finding Study (Nonrodent)[a]

Group	Dose Level (mg/kg/day or ppm)[b]	Initial		Clinical Laboratory Studies Pretest and Week 2 or 4[c]		Necropsy Week 2 or 4[c]		Microscopic Pathology[d]	
		Males	Females	Male	Females	Male	Females	Male	Females
I	0[e]	1	1	1	1	A.S.	A.S.	1	1
II	*	1	1	1	1	A.S.	A.S.	1	1
III	*	1	1	1	1	A.S.	A.S.	1	1
IV	*	1	1	1	1	A.S.	A.S.	1	1
V	*	1	1	1	1	A.S.	A.S.	1	1

[a] A.S. = all survivors; complete postmortem evaluations are also performed on animals that are found dead or euthanatized in a moribund condition during the course of the study; mg/kg/day = milligrams of test material per kilogram of body weight per day; or ppm = parts per million (dietary concentration).

[b] Doses should be selected to produce a range of effects from a no-effect dose to one which produces clear toxicity. A minimum of three doses is recommended. More doses may be used to increase likelihood of achieving an appropriate range of effects.

[c] Two weeks is a common duration and is a recommended minimum. Four-week studies are frequently performed to provide additional information.

[d] Optional. Microscopic examination of tissues may be performed to assess target organ toxicity.

[e] Control animals receive empty capsules, vehicle in the same volume as high-dose animals, or untreated diet.

TABLE 2.5
Experimental Design — Subchronic Toxicity Study (Rodent): 4 Weeks

		Number of Animals							
				Week 4					
Group	Dose Level (mg/kg/day or ppm)[b]	Initial		Clinical Laboratory Studies		Necropsy		Microscopic Pathology	
		Males	Females	Males	Females	Males	Females	Males	Females
I (control)	0[c]	5	5	5	5	A.S.	A.S.	5	5
II (low)	*	5	5	5	5	A.S.	A.S.	A.R.	A.R.
III (mid)	*	5	5	5	5	A.S.	A.S.	A.R.	A.R.
IV (high)	*	5	5	5	5	A.S.	A.S.	5	5

[a] A.S. = all survivors; complete postmortem evaluations are also performed on animals that are found dead or euthanatized in a moribund condition during the course of the study. A.R. = as required: (1) target organs/tissues identified by Group IV evaluations; (2) macroscopic lesions; mg/kg/day = milligrams of test material per kilogram of body weight per day; or ppm = parts per million (dietary concentration).

[b] Doses should be selected to produce no effect at the low dose and clear toxicity (without significant mortality) at the high dose.

[c] Control animals receive vehicle in the same volume as high-dose animals or receive untreated diet.

TABLE 2.6
Experimental Design — Subchronic Toxicity Study (Rodent): 13 Weeks[a]

		Number of Animals							
				Month 3					
Group	Dose Level (mg/kg/day or ppm)[b]	Initial		Clinical Laboratory Studies		Necropsy		Microscopic Pathology	
		Males	Females	Males	Females	Males	Females	Males	Females
I (control)	0[d]	5–10	5–10	5–10	5–10	A.S.	A.S.	5–10	5–10
II (low)	*	5–10	5–10	5–10	5–10	A.S.	A.S.	A.R.	A.R.
III (mid)	*	5–10	5–10	5–10	5–10	A.S.	A.S.	A.R.	A.R.
IV (high)	*	5–10	5–10	5–10	5–10	A.S.	A.S.	5–10	5–10

[a] A.S. = all survivors; complete postmortem evaluations will also be performed on animals that are found dead or euthanatized in a moribund condition during the course of the study. A.R. = as required: 1) target organs/tissues identified by Group IV evaluations; 2) macroscopic lesions; mg/kg/day = milligrams of test material per kilogram of body weight per day; or ppm = parts per million (dietary concentration).

[b] Doses should be selected to produce no effect at the low dose and clear toxicity (without significant mortality) at the high dose.

[c] 5 or 10 animals per sex are used, depending on type of test material and government agency to which study will be submitted.

[d] Control animals receive vehicle in the same volume as high-dose animals or receive untreated diet.

TABLE 2.7
Experimental Design — Subchronic Toxicity Study (Nonrodent): 4 Weeks

		Number of Animals[a]							
		Initial		Clinical Laboratory Studies Pretest and Week 4		Necropsy Week 4		Microscopic Pathology	
Group	Dose Level (mg/kg/day or ppm)[b]	Males	Females	Males	Females	Males	Females	Males	Females
I (control)	0[c]	4	4	4	4	A.S.	A.S.	4	4
II (low)	*	4	4	4	4	A.S.	A.S.	4	4
III (mid)	*	4	4	4	4	A.S.	A.S.	4	4
IV (high)	*	4	4	4	4	A.S.	A.S.	4	4

[a] A.S. = all survivors; complete postmortem evaluations are also performed on animals that are found dead or euthanatized in a moribund condition during the course of the study; mg/kg/day = milligrams of test material per kilogram of body weight per day; or ppm = parts per million (dietary concentration).
[b] Doses should be selected to produce no effect at the low dose and clear toxicity (without mortality) at the high dose.
[c] Control animals receive empty capsules, vehicle in the same volume as high-dose animals, or untreated diet.

TABLE 2.8
Experimental Design — Subchronic Toxicity Study (Nonrodent): 13 Weeks

		Number of Animals[a]							
		Initial		Clinical Laboratory Studies Pretest and Month 3		Necropsy Month 3		Microscopic Pathology	
Group	Dose Level (mg/kg/day or ppm)[b]	Males	Females	Males	Females	Males	Females	Males	Females
I (control)	0[c]	4	4	4	4	A.S.	A.S.	4	4
II (low)	*	4	4	4	4	A.S.	A.S.	4	4
III (mid)	*	4	4	4	4	A.S.	A.S.	4	4
IV (high)	*	4	4	4	4	A.S.	A.S.	4	4

[a] A.S. = all survivors; complete postmortem evaluations are also performed on animals that are found dead or euthanatized in a moribund condition during the course of the study; mg/kg/day = milligrams of test material per kilogram of body weight per day; or ppm = parts per million (dietary concentration).
[b] Doses should be selected to produce no effect at the low dose and clear toxicity (without mortality) at the high dose.
[c] Control animals receive empty capsules, vehicle in the same volume as high-dose animals, or untreated diet.

TABLE 2.9
Experimental Design — Chronic Toxicity Study (Rodent): 6 Months

		Number of Animals[a]							
		Initial		Clinical Laboratory Studies[c] Months 3, 6		Necropsy Month 6		Microscopic Pathology	
Group	Dose Level[b] (mg/kg/day or ppm)	Males	Females	Males	Females	Males	Females	Males	Females
I (control)	0[d]	20	20	20	20	A.S.	A.S.	20	20
II (low)	*	20	20	20	20	A.S.	A.S.	A.R.	A.R.
III (mid)	*	20	20	20	20	A.S.	A.S.	A.R.	A.R.
IV (high)	*	20	20	20	20	A.S.	A.S.	20	20

[a] A.S. = all survivors; complete postmortem evaluations are also performed on animals that are found dead or euthanatized in a moribund condition during the course of the study; A.R. = as required: 1) target organs/tissues identified by Group IV evaluations, 2) all tissues from animals found dead or euthanatized in a moribund condition during the study; 3) gross lesions; mg/kg/day = milligrams of test material per kilogram of body weight per day; or ppm = parts per million (dietary concentration).

[b] Doses should be selected to produce no effect at the low dose and clear toxicity (without significant mortality) at the high dose.

[c] Hematology and clinical chemistry evaluations are performed (urinalysis is optional and is generally only performed when specific effects are anticipated).

[d] Control animals receive vehicle in the same volume as high-dose animals or receive untreated diet.

TABLE 2.10
Experimental Design — Chronic Toxicity Study (Nonrodent): 9 Months

		Number of Animals[a]							
		Initial		Clinical Laboratory Studies[c] Months 3, 6, 9		Necropsy Month 9		Microscopic Pathology	
Group	Dose Level (mg/kg/day or ppm)[b]	Males	Females	Males	Females	Males	Females	Males	Females
I (control)	0[d]	4	4	4	4	A.S.	A.S.	4	4
II (low)	*	4	4	4	4	A.S.	A.S.	4	4
III (mid)	*	4	4	4	4	A.S.	A.S.	4	4
IV (high)	*	4	4	4	4	A.S.	A.S.	4	4

[a] A.S. = all survivors; complete postmortem evaluations are also performed on animals that are found dead or euthanatized in a moribund condition during the course of the study; mg/kg/day = milligrams of test material per kilogram of body weight per day; or ppm = parts per million (dietary concentration).

[b] Doses should be selected to produce no effect at the low dose and clear toxicity (without mortality) at the high dose.

[c] Hematology and clinical chemistry evaluations are performed (urinalysis is optional and is generally only performed when specific effects are anticipated).

[d] Control animals receive empty capsules, vehicle in the same volume as high-dose animals, or untreated diet.

SECTION 3. REGULATORY GUIDELINES —
STUDY REQUIREMENTS

A. LIST OF GUIDELINES AND AGENCIES

1. Toxicology Testing

a. General (International) Harmonization

At the time of publication of this book (2001) efforts continue to establish guidelines that are accepted by regulatory agencies in all countries and by all regulatory agencies within each country. However, harmonized, universally accepted guidelines for acute, subchronic, and chronic toxicity testing have not yet been established. The most universally accepted guidelines are those published by the Organization for Economic Cooperation and Development (OECD) and accepted in many countries. These guidelines were developed for international use and were considered to be "adequate for the evaluation of most chemicals." Initial drafts were issued in 1979 by the lead countries (U.S.A. and U.K.) and they are reviewed and updated periodically.

OECD Guidelines for Acute Subchronic and Chronic Oral and Dermal Toxicity Studies are:

Duration	Guideline No.	Issue Date	Title
Acute	401	2/24/87	Acute Oral Toxicity
	402	2/24/87	Acute Dermal Toxicity
	420	7/17/92	Acute Oral Toxicity — Fixed Dose Method
	423	3/22/96	Acute Oral Toxicity — Acute Toxic Class Method
	425	9/21/98	Acute Oral Toxicity — Up-and-Down Procedure
Subchronic	407	7/27/95	Repeated Dose 28-Day Oral Toxicity study in Rodents
	408	9/21/98	Repeated Dose 90-day Oral Toxicity study in Rodents
	409	9/21/98	Repeated Dose 90-day Oral Toxicity study in Nonrodents
	410	5/12/81	Repeated Dose Dermal Toxicity: 21/28-Day Study
	411	5/12/81	Subchronic Dermal Toxicity: 90-Day Study
Chronic	452	5/12/81	Chronic Toxicity Studies
	453	5/12/81	Combined Chronic Toxicity/Carcinogenicity Studies

b. Pharmaceuticals

U.S.A.: The U.S. Food and Drug Administration (FDA) regulates approval of drugs. Although specific "Points to Consider" documents have been issued for some types of drugs, no detailed protocol requirements exist for acute, subchronic, and chronic toxicity evaluations.

Europe: European Community (EC). The Rules Governing Medicinal Products in the European Community — Volume III. Guidelines on the Quality, Safety and Efficacy or Medicinal Product for Human Use. January 1989.

Japan: JMHW (Japanese Ministry of Health and Welfare): Guidelines for Toxicity Studies of Drugs; Notification No. 88 of the Pharmaceutical Affairs Bureau, August 10, 1993.

c. Food Additives

FDA Bureau of Foods: Toxicological Principles for the Safety Assessment of Direct Food Additives and Color Additives Used in Food, 1982 (The "Redbook").

Draft revisions were published for comment in 1993 but are not yet finalized.

Guidelines, presented in Appendix II (Guidelines for Toxicological Testing), for Acute, Subchronic, and Chronic Oral Toxicity Studies are:

Pages	Guideline for:
1–7	Acute Oral LD_{50} Toxicity Studies
8–18	Short-Term Continuous Exposure Oral Toxicity Study [4 Weeks]
19–29	Subchronic Oral Toxicity Studies [90 Days]
30–41	Long-Term Toxicity in the Rodent
42–52	Long-Term Toxicity in the Dog

d. Agricultural and Industrial Chemicals

In August 1998, the United States Environmental Protection Agency developed a series of guidelines for the testing of pesticides and toxic substances. These were developed by the Office of Prevention, Pesticides and Toxic Substances (OPPTS) and are referred to as the OPPTS guidelines. They harmonize, update, and supersede previous guidelines developed specifically for agricultural chemicals (FIFRA, Federal Insecticide, Fungicide and Rodenticide Act) and industrial chemicals (TSCA, Toxic Substances Control Act).

Guidelines for Acute, Subchronic and Chronic Oral and Dermal Toxicity Studies are:

Duration	Guideline	Title
Acute	OPPTS 870.1100	Acute Oral Toxicity Study
	OPPTS 870.1200	Acute Dermal Toxicity Study
Subchronic	OPPTS 870.3100	90-Day Oral Toxicity in Rodents
	OPPTS 870.3150	90-Day Oral Toxicity in Nonrodents
	OPPTS 870.3200	21/28-Day Dermal Toxicity
	OPPTS 870.3250	90-Day Dermal Toxicity
Chronic	OPPTS 870.4100	Chronic Toxicity
	OPPTS 870.4300	Combined Chronic Toxicity/Carcinogenicity

Japan continues to have separate guidelines for agricultural and industrial chemicals:

Agricultural Chemicals

Japan: JMAFF (Japanese Ministry of Agriculture, Forestry and Fisheries) Guidance on Toxicology Study Data for Application of Agriculture Chemical Registration 59 Nohsan No. 4200, January 28, 1985.

Industrial Chemicals

Japan: MITI (Ministry of International Trade and Industry): The Law Concerning Examination and Regulation of Manufacture, etc. of Chemical Substances (Chemical Substances Control Law), enacted April 1, 1987.

2. Regulatory Guidelines — Good Laboratory Practices

a. International

OECD Principles of Good Laboratory Practices [ENV/MC/CHEM (98) 17].

b. Europe

European Economic Community (EEC) Good Laboratory Practice Regulations Council Directive 1999/11/EC.

c. U.S.A.

Food Additives and Pharmaceuticals: Part 58 of 21 CFR (FDA Good Laboratory Practice Regulations).

Agricultural Chemicals: Part 160 of 40 CFR (EPA/FIFRA Good Laboratory Practice Standards).

Industrial Chemicals: Part 792 of 40 CFR (EPA Good Laboratory Practices — TSCA).

d. Japan

Pharmaceuticals: Japanese Ministry of Health and Welfare (JMHW) Good Laboratory Regulations (Ordinance No. 21, 26 March 97).

Agricultural Chemicals: Japanese Ministry of Agriculture, Forestry and Fisheries (JMAFF) Good Laboratory Practice Regulations, Notification No. 6283).

Industrial Chemicals: Japanese Ministry of International Trade and Industry (MITI). Good Laboratory Practice Standards Applied to Industrial Chemicals. (Notification No. 85).

B. SUMMARY/COMPARISON TABLES

TABLE 2.11
Animal Requirements — Standard Study Guidelines

	Acute	Subchronic (2-, 3-, or 4-Week, 90-Day)		Chronic	
Species	Oral studies are most commonly performed in rodents (rats and/or mice); dermal studies are generally performed in rabbits and/or rats. If dogs are used, an "up-and-down" study (see Table 2) is usually performed	Oral Dermal	Rodent Nonrodent	Rat Dog Rat, rabbit[a]	Rodent Nonrodent	Rat Dog
Age/weight at initiation of treatment	"Adults" or "young adults" are usually specified	Oral	Rat	Before 6 wk (no more than 8 wk)	Rat	Before 6 wk (no more than 8 wk)
	Rats: 200–300 g		Dog	4–6 mo (no more than 9 mo)	Dog	4–6 mo (no more than 9 mo)
	Rabbits: 2–3 kg	Dermal	Rat, rabbit[a]	Adult: Rats: 200–300 g Rabbits: 2–3 kg		
No. of groups	Limit Test: one	At least four (control plus at least three dose levels)			At least four (control plus at least three dose levels)	
	Acute Toxicity: three or more (low-, medium-, and high-effect dose levels)[b]					

TABLE 2.11 *(Continued)*
Animal Requirements — Standard Study Guidelines

		Acute		Subchronic (2-, 3-, or 4-Week, 90-Day)			Chronic	
No of animals per group	5 per sex (some guidelines require both sexes for only one dose level)[b]	Rats	10/sex	Exceptions: 1 OECD: 5/sex for 2-, 3-, and 4-wk studies: 2 Redbook: 20/sex for 90-day studies	Rat	20/sex	Exception: JMHW: 10/sex	
		Dogs	4/sex	Exception: JMHW: 3/sex	Dog	4/sex	Exception: JMHW: 3/sex	

[a] Guinea pigs are also acceptable but are seldom used.
[b] Refinements using fewer animals for acute oral toxicity studies have been developed (OECD guidelines 420, 423, and 425).

TABLE 2.12
Body Weight and Food Consumption Intervals — Standard Study Guidelines

Study Type	Intervals	Exceptions
Body Weights		
Acute and subchronic	Pretest and weekly	
Chronic	Pretest, weekly through 13 wk, every 4 wk (or approximately monthly) thereafter	1. OECD: at approximately 3-mo intervals after 13 wk 2. Redbook: weekly for dogs
Food Consumption		
Subchronic	Pretest and weekly	
Chronic	Pretest, weekly through 13 wk, every 4 wk (or approximately monthly) thereafter	1. OECD: at approximately 3-mo intervals after 13 wk 2. Redbook: weekly for dogs 3. JMHW: weekly for dietary administration

TABLE 2.13
Ophthalmology Intervals — Standard Study Guidelines (Subchronic and Chronic Studies)[a]

	Duration					
	2–4 Weeks		3 Months		Chronic	
Guideline	Intervals	Groups	Intervals	Groups	Intervals	Groups
OECD	N.S.	N.S.	Pre & Term	C&H	N.S.	N.S.
EC	N.S.	N.S.	N.S.	N.S.	N.S.	N.S.
JMHW	R - Rx	All	R - Rx	All	R - Rx	All
	NR - Pre & Rx	All	NR - Pre & Rx	All	NR - Pre & Rx	All
Redbook	Pre & Term	C&H	Pre & Term	C&H	Pre, every 3 mo	C&H
OPPTS	Pre & Term	C&H	Pre & Term	C&H	Pre & Term	C&H

TABLE 2.13 *(Continued)*

Ophthalmology Intervals — Standard Study Guidelines (Subchronic and Chronic Studies)[a]

	Duration					
	2–4 Weeks		3 Months		Chronic	
Guideline	Intervals	Groups	Intervals	Groups	Intervals	Groups
JMAFF	Pre & Term	C&H	Pre & Term	C&H	Pre & Term	All
MITI	N.S.	N.S.	N.A.	N.A.	N.S.	N.S.

[a] N.S. = not specified; N.A. = not applicable (no guideline); R = rodent; NR = nonrodent; Pre = pretest (before initiation of dosing); Term = termination of dosing; C & H = at least control and high-dose groups; all groups if findings in high-dose group; Rx = at least once during treatment.

TABLE 2.14

Clinical Pathology Intervals — Standard Study Guidelines (Subchronic and Chronic Studies)[a]

	Duration								
	2–4 Weeks			3 Months			Chronic		
Guideline	Intervals	Animals	Studies	Intervals	Animals	Studies	Intervals	No. Animals (per sex/group)	Studies
OECD	Term	All	H,C	R: Term	All	H,C	3,6,12,18,24 mo (H,U)	R: 10	H,U,C
				NR: P,R,T	All	H,C,U	6,12,18,24 mo (C)	NR: all	
EC	R: Term NR: Pre & Term	All	H,C,U	R: Term NR: Pre & Term	All	H,C,U	R: Term NR: Pre & Term	All	H,C,U
JMHW	R: Term	All[b]	H,C,U	R: Term	All[b]	H,C,U	R: H,C: Term U: R	All[b]	H,C,U
	NR: Pre & Term	All	H,C,U	NR: P,R,T	All	H,C,U	NR: H,C: P,R,T U: Pre, R	All	
Redbook	Term	R: 5/sex N.R: all	H,C	Term	All	H,C	NR: Pre, every 3 mo; Term	R: 10 NR: all	H,C
OPPTS	Term	All	H,C	R: Term	All	H,C	Every 6 mo, Term (H,U)	R: 10	H,U,C
				NR:P,R,T			Pre, R, Term (C)	NR: all	
JMAFF	N.R.	N.R.	N.A.	R: Term NR: P,R,T	All	H,C,U[c]	Every 6 mo, Term	R: 10 NR: all	H,C,U
MITI	N.S.	N.S.	H,C	N.A.	N.A.	N.A.	N.S.	N.S.	H,C,U

[a] N.S. = not specified; N.A. = not applicable (no guideline); N.R. = not required; R = rodent (rabbits included for dermal studies,); NR = non-rodent; P or Pre = pretest (before initiation of dosing); T or term = termination of dosing; R = at least once during treatment; H = hematology; C = clinical chemistry; U = urinalysis.

[b] Urinalysis can be performed on a fixed number of animals per group.

[c] Urinalysis performed at termination only (if considered necessary).

[d] Differential counts should also be performed on animals in deteriorating health.

[e] Urinalysis on rodents only.

TABLE 2.15
Hematology Parameters of Subchronic and Chronic
Studies — Standard Study Guidelines

Hematology

All Guidelines

Erythrocyte count
Hematocrit
Hemoglobin concentration
Leukocyte count (total and differential)
Some measure of clotting function
Suggestions: Clotting time
                    Platelet count
                    Prothrombin time (PT)
                    Activated partial thromboplastin time (APTT)

Exceptions/Additions

OPPTS: MCV, MCH, MCHC
MHW: in addition, reticulocyte count, PT, APTT
JMAFF: specifies platelet count
MITI chronic studies: in addition, reticulocyte count; specifies platelet count
EC: Guidelines do not specify parameters.

TABLE 2.16
Clinical Chemistry Parameters of Subchronic and Chronic Studies —
Standard Study Guidelines

Parameter	Guidelines[a]					
	OECD	JMHW	RDBK	OPPTS	JMAFF	MITI
Alkaline phosphatase		×		×	×	×
Alanine aminotransferase (ALT)	×	×	×	×	×	×
Aspartate aminotransferase (AST)	×	×	×	×	×	×
γ-glutamyltransferase (GGT)	×			×	×		×
Glucose	×	×	×	×	×	×
Bilirubin: total	×	×	×	×[c]		
Creatinine	×	×	×	×		×
Urea (BUN)	×	×	×	×	×	×
Total protein	×	×	×	×	×	×
Albumin	×	×	×	×	×	
Albumin/globulin ratio		×				
Electrolytes (Na, K, Cl, Ca, P)	×	×	×	×	×	×
Cholesterol		×		×		×
Triglycerides		×		×		×
Ornithine decarboxylase (ODC)	[b]	[b]				[b]
Protein-electrophoretogram		×				
Lactate dehydrogenase						[c]
Creatine kinase						[c]
Phosphotipids						[c]
Uric acid						[c]

[a] EC guidelines do not specify parameters.

[b] Ornithine decarboxylase is a tissue enzyme; no acceptable analytical procedure for blood exists.

[c] Chronic studies only.

TABLE 2.17
Urinalysis Parameters of Subchronic and Chronic Studies — Standard Study Guidelines

Parameter	Guideline[a]				
	OECD	MHW	OPPTS	JMAFF	MITI (chronic)
Appearance	×		×	×	
Volume	×	×	×	×	×
Specific gravity	×	×	×	×	
Protein	×	×	×	×	×
Glucose	×	×	×	×	×
Ketones		×		×	×
Occult blood[b]	×	×	×	×	×
Sediment microscopy[b]		×	×	×	c
pH	×	×	×		×
Bilirubin		×	×		×
Urobilinogen		×			×
Electrolytes (Na, K, etc.)		×			

[a] EC guidelines do not specify parameters; other guidelines do not recommend routine urinalyses.
[b] Semiquantitative evaluation.
[c] When necessary.

TABLE 2.18
Organ Weight Requirements — Standard Study Guidelines

Organ to be Weighed	Guideline[a]					
	OECD	JMHW	RDBK	OPPTS	JMAFF	MITI
Adrenal glands	×	×	×	×	×	×
Kidneys	×	×	×	×	×	×
Liver	×	×	×	×	×	×
Testes	×	×	×	×	×	×
Epididymides	×					
Ovaries	×	×		×		×
Thyroid/ Parathyroids	NR	b	NR	NR	NR	
Brain	×	×		×	Chronic	Chronic
Heart	×	×		×		Chronic
Lungs		b				Chronic
Spleen	×	×		×		Chronic
Pituitary		×				Chronic
Salivary gland		b				
Seminal Vesicles		b				
Thymus	×	b		×		
Uterus	×	b		×		

[a] EC guidelines do not specify organs to be weighed. NR = non-rodent.
[b] Guidelines state that these organs are "often weighed."

TABLE 2.19
Microscopic Pathology Requirements of Subchronic and Chronic Studies (Rodents) — General — Standard Study Guidelines

Groups	Control and High-Dose All Tissues[a]	Intermediate Doses					
		Target Organs[b]	Lesions/Masses	Early Deaths[c]	Lungs[d]	Liver	Kidneys
OECD	×	×	×	C			
JMHW	×	×					
Redbook	×	×	×	×[e]	C	C	C
OPPTS	×	×	×	×[e]			
JMAFF	×	×	×	×	×	×	×
MITI	×	×					

Note: Nonrodents: most guidelines recommend examinations for all animals. Exception: OECD 90-day study: control and high-dose, all tissues; intermediate dose, target organs.

[a] Tissues listed in Tables 20 or 21. C = chronic studies only; SC = subchronic studies only.
[b] Target organs: organs for which possible test material-related effects are seen in high-dose animals.
[c] Animals found dead or euthanatized in moribund condition before study termination (all tissues).
[d] Examination recommended, primarily for evidence of infection.
[e] Not required for 21/28-day studies.
[f] Not required for dermal studies.

TABLE 2.20
Microscopic Pathology Requirements — Tissues Most Often Recommended for Subchronic Studies — Standard Study Guidelines

Tissues[a]	OECD		EC	JMHW	RDBK		JMAFF	OPPTS	MITI
	28 Day	90 Day			28 Day	90 Day			
Adrenal glands	×	×	×	×	R	×	×	×	×
Bone (sternum/femur/ vertebrae/rib)			S, F, or V	S, F		S	S, F	×	F+
Bone marrow (sternum/ femur/vertebrae/rib)	×	×	S, F, or V	S, F	R	S	S, F	×	F+
Brain (Medulla/pons, cerebrum, cerebellum)	×	×	×	×	R	×	×	×	+
Esophagus		×	×	×	×	×	×	×	
Heart	×	×	×	×	×	×	×	×	×
Kidney	×	×	×	×	×	×	*×	×	×
Large intestine (cecum, colon, rectum)	×	×	Colon	×	R	×	×	×	
Liver	×	×	×	×	×	×	*×	×	×
Lung (with mainstem bronchi)	×	×	×	×	×	×	×	×	+
Lymph node (representative)	×	×	×	×	R	×	×	×	
Ovaries	×	×	×	×	×	×	×	×	+
Pancreas		×	×	×	×	×	×	×	
Pituitary		×	×	×		×	×	×	
Prostate	×	+	×	×		×	×	+	
Salivary glands		+	×	×		×	×	×	

TABLE 2.20 *(Continued)*
Microscopic Pathology Requirements — Tissues Most Often Recommended for Subchronic Studies — Standard Study Guidelines

Tissues[a]	OECD 28 Day	OECD 90 Day	EC	JMHW	RDBK 28 Day	RDBK 90 Day	JMAFF	OPPTS	MITI
Small intestine (duodenum, ileum, jejunum)	×	×	×	×	R	×	×	×	
Spleen	×	×	×	×	×	×	×	×	×
Stomach	×	×	×	×	R	R	×	×	+
Testes (with epididymides)	×	×	×	×	×	×	×	×	+
Thymus	×	×	×	×		×	×	×	
Thyroid (with parathyroids)	×	×	×	×		×	×	×	+
Trachea	×	×	×	×		×	×	×	
Urinary bladder	×	×	×	×		×	×	×	+
Uterus	×	×	×	×	R	×	×	×	
Gross lesions/masses/ target organs	×	×	×	×	×	×	*×	×	×

[a] * = 21/28 day dermal studies; + = examination/preservation required only if indicated by signs of toxicity or target organ involvement (for, MITI, preservation suggested, examination not required); R = tissue required for rodents only.

TABLE 2.21
Microscopic Pathology Requirements — Tissues Occasionally Recommended for Subchronic Studies — Standard Study Guidelines

Tissue[a]	OECD 28 Day	OECD 90 Day	EC	JMHW	RDBK 90 Day	OPPTS	JMAFF	MITI
Aorta		×			×	×	×	
Eyes		+	×	×	×	+		+
Gallbladder (not present in rats)			×	×	×	×	×	
Lacrimal gland (rodent only)				×				
Larynx						×		
Mammary gland		♀+	×	×	×	♀	♀	
Muscle (skeletal, usually biceps femoris)		+			×		×	
Nasopharyngeal tissue						×		
Nerve (peripheral/sciatic)	×	×			×	×	×	
Seminal vesicles (not present in dogs)		+		×	×	×	×	
Skin		(×)		×		(×)	*×	
Spinal cord (no. of sections; total no. indicated)	3	3	×	×	2	+3	×	
Tongue				×				
Vagina				×				
Zymbal glands							+	

[a] ♀ from females only; * 21/28 day dermal studies + examination/preservation required only if indicated by signs of toxicity or target organ involvement (for MITI, preservation suggested examination not required); R = tissue required for rodents only; ( ) = dermal only.

TABLE 2.22
Microscopic Pathology Requirements — Standard Study Guidelines — Tissues Most Often Recommended for Chronic Studies

Tissues[a]	OECD	EC	JMHW	RDBK	OPPTS	JMAFF	MITI
Adrenal glands	×	×	×	×	×	×	×
Bone (sternum/femur/vertebrae)	S, F	S, F, or V	S, F	S	×	S, F	S, F, or V
Bone marrow (sternum/femur/vertebrae)	S	S, F, or V	S, F	S	×	S, F	S
Brain (medulla/pons, cerebrum, cerebellum)	×	×	×	×	×	×	×
Esophagus	×	×	×	×	×	×	×
Heart	×	×	×	×	×	×	×
Kidney	×	×	×	×	×	×	×
Large intestine (cecum, colon, rectum)	×	Colon	×	×	×	×	×
Liver	×	×	×	×	×	×	×
Lung (with mainstem bronchi)	×	×	×	×	×	×	×
Lymph node (representative)	×	×	×	×	×	×	×
Mammary gland	♀[a]	×	×	×	♀	♀	♀
Ovaries	×	×	×	×		×	×
Pancreas	×	×	×	×	×	×	×
Pituitary	×	×	×	×	×	×	×
Prostate	×	×	×	×	×	×	×
Salivary glands	×	×	×	×	×	×	×
Small intestine (duodenum, ileum, jejunum)	×	×	×	×	×	×	×
Spleen	×	×	×	×	×	×	×
Stomach	×	×	×	×	×	×	×
Testes (with epididymides)	×	×	×	×	×	×	×
Thymus	×	×	×	×	×	×	×
Thyroid (with parathyroids)	×	×	×	×	×	×	×
Trachea	×	×	×	×	×	×	×
Urinary bladder	×	×	×	×	×	×	×
Uterus	×	×	×	×	×	×	×
Gross lesions/masses/target organs	×	×	×	×	×	×	×

[a] ♀ from females.

TABLE 2.23
Microscopic Pathology Requirements — Tissues Occasionally Recommended for Chronic Studies — Standard Study Guidelines

Tissue	OECD	EC	JMHW	RDBK	JMAFF	OPPTS	MITI
Aorta	×			×	×	×	
Eyes	×	×	×	×		×	×
Gallbladder (not present in rats)		×	×	×	×	×	
Lacrimal gland (rodent only)			×				
Larynx						×	
Fallopian tubes				×			
Muscle (skeletal, usually biceps femoris)	×			×	×		
Nerve (peripheral/sciatic)	×			×	×	×	×

TABLE 2.23 *(Continued)*
Microscopic Pathology Requirements — Tissues Occasionally Recommended for Chronic Studies — Standard Study Guidelines

Tissue	OECD	EC	JMHW	RDBK	JMAFF	OPPTS	MITI
Nose						×	
Pharynx						×	
Seminal vesicles (not present in dogs)	×		×	×	×	×	×
Skin	×		×		×	×	×
Smooth muscle				×			
Spinal cord (number of sections; total number indicated)	3	×	×	2	×	3	×
Tongue			×				×
Vagina			×				

SECTION 4. STUDY IMPLEMENTATION

A. PROTOCOL COMPONENTS CHECKLIST

This is a form used in our laboratory to outline protocol components.

PROTOCOL & PRICE REQUEST

Sponsor: _____	Date of Contact: _____
Address: _____	Date Rec'd by B.D.: _____
_____	Contact Recipient: _____
Attention: _____	Program (Y/N): _____
_____	Information
Agent: _____	Requested: ❏ Protocol ❏ Cost
Industry: _____	❏ Brochures ❏ Other: _____

STUDY TYPE

ACUTE	TOXICITY	CARDIOVASCULAR
❏ Toxicity (LC_{50}/LD_{50})	❏ Range-Finding	❏ Range-Finding
❏ Irritation	❏ Oncogenicity	❏ Cardio Monitoring _____
❏ Dermal Sensitization *B/M&K*	❏ Toxicity/Oncogenicity	❏ Telemetry _____
	❏ _____	❏ _____

NEUROTOXICITY	REPRODUCTION	
❏ Range-Finding	❏ Range-Finding	❏ Two Generation
❏ Developmental	❏ Reproduction (Seg I)	❏ Male Fertility
❏ _____	❏ Developmental (Seg II)	❏ Dominant Lethal
	❏ Peri/Post (Seg III)	❏ _____

DURATION OF STUDY

❏ _____ Hours	❏ _____ Days	❏ _____ Weeks	❏ _____ Months	❏ _____ Years

SPECIES/STRAIN

❏ Rat/_____		Mouse/_____		❏ Monkey/__
❏ Dog	❏ Ferret	❏ Chicken	❏ Rabbit	❏ Guinea Pig	❏ Other/_____

ROUTE OF ADMINISTRATION

ORAL	INHALATION	DERMAL
❑ Diet ❑ Adj. ❑ Const.	❑ Head-Only	❑ Abraded #:_____
❑ Gavage ❑ Capsule	❑ Nose-Only	❑ Non-abraded #:_____
❑ Nasogastric	❑ Whole-Body	❑ Occluded ❑ Semi-Occluded
❑ _____	❑ _____	❑ _____

OCULAR	INJECTION/INFUSION	OTHER
❑ Washed #:_____	❑ SubQ ❑ IP ❑ IM ❑ IV	❑ Vaginal
❑ Unwashed #:_____	❑ Infusion (Continuous)	❑ Nasal
❑ _____	❑ Infusion (Intermittent)	❑ _____
	❑ _____	

FREQUENCY OF ADMINISTRATION

❑ Single	❑ Daily #:_____	❑ Weekly #:_____	❑ ____hr/_____days/week	❑ Other

REGULATORY GUIDELINE

❑ OPPTS	❑ FDA/Pharmacuetical	❑ OECD	❑ JMITI
	❑ JMAFF	❑ EEC	❑ WHO
❑ FDA/Red Book	❑ JMHW	❑ Non-Regulatory	❑ Other_____

EXPERIMENTAL DESIGN

Group	I		II		III		IV		V		VI	
	M	F	M	F	M	F	M	F	M	F	M	F
Dosage ❑ ppm ❑ mg/kg ❑ ml/kg ❑ mg/M³ ❑ ml(cc) ❑ _____												
NUMBER OF ANIMALS (MAIN STUDY)												
❑ Satellite/Recovery												
Ophthalmology												
❑ Intervals: Main Study												
Satellite/Recovery												
Hematology												
❑ Intervals: Main Study												
Satellite/Recovery												
❑ Standard Battery ❑ Additional (see attached)												
Clinical Chemistry												
❑ Intervals: Main Study												
Satellite/Recovery												
❑ Standard Battery ❑ Additional (see attached)												
Urinalysis												
❑ Intervals: Main Study												
Satellite/Recovery												
❑ Standard Battery ❑ Additional (see attached)												

Group		I		II		III		IV		V		VI	
		M	F	M	F	M	F	M	F	M	F	M	F
Toxico/Pharmacokinetics													
❏ Intervals:	Main Study												
❏ Timepoints:	Satellite/Recovery												
	❏ Plasma ❏ Serum ❏ In-House Analysis ❏ Shipped To Sponsor												
ECG													
❏ Intervals:	Main Study												
	Satellite/Recovery												
Blood Pressure													
❏ Intervals:	Main Study												
	Satellite/Recovery												
Necropsy													
❏ Interim Sacrifice													
❏ Terminal Sacrifice													
❏ Recovery Sacrifice													
❏ Organ Weights													
❏ Microscopic Examination													
Analytical													
❏ Dose Medium ❏ Product Chemistry ❏ RIA ❏ ADME													
Other													
❏ Special Stains ❏ Special Statistical Package Status Reports: ❏ Weekly ❏ Monthly ❏ Interim Only ❏ Term Only													

B. STUDY INITIATION CHECKLIST

The following checklist presents activities to be completed plus items to be addressed before initiation of the study.

1. PROTOCOL
   a. Finalized/scientific review and approval   _____
   b. IACUC review and approval   _____
   c. QA GLP review and approval   _____
   d. Distributed to appropriate personnel   _____

2. TEST ANIMALS
   a. Room assigned   _____
   b. Ordered   _____
   c. Received   _____
   d. Health examination completed (including prestudy EKG, ophthalmology, vaccinations,   _____
      vaccinations and TB testing as required)
   e. Assigned to groups; assignment reviewed and approved   _____

3. PRESTUDY CLINICAL PATHOLOGY (if required)
   a. Scheduled   _____
   b. Completed   _____
   c. Reviewed by Study Director (animal selection)   _____

4. STUDY SCHEDULE
    a. Completed   _____
    b. Distributed   _____

5. TEST MATERIAL
    a. Amount needed calculated/confirmed   _____
    b. Received   _____
    c. Storage:_____   _____
    d. Handling instructions (personnel protection)
       1) Technical material   _____
       2) Dosing solutions, treated feed, etc.   _____

6. PRESTUDY ANALYSIS OF DIETS/DOSE FORMULATIONS (if required)
    a. Method provided   _____
    b. Method validated   _____
    c. Scheduled   _____
    d. Completed   _____

7. DOSES, DOSE SOLUTIONS, DIET PREPARATION
    a. Doses/concentrations selected   _____
    b. Mixing instructions
       1) Developed/provided to appropriate personnel   _____
       2) Prestudy mix completed   _____
       3) Analysis required/completed   _____

		Required	Completed
Type:	Homogeneity	_____	_____
	Stability	_____	_____
	Concentration	_____	_____

8. WASTE DISPOSAL
    a. Technical material   _____
    b. Dosing solutions, treated feed, etc.   _____
    c. Procedures to minimize waste   _____

9. EXPECTED TOXICITY AND CLINICAL SIGNS

10. SUBCONTRACTORS (including pathology, clinical pathology, metabolism, microbiology)
    a. Required   _____
    b. QA notified   _____
       If required, list below subcontractor's name and address, work to be performed by the
       subcontractor, handling instructions, and the person responsible for shipment:

11. NECROPSY PROCEDURES (special instructions, e.g., photos of gross lesions, paired
    organs weighed together or separately, unusual fixative)

12. TOXICOKINETIC SAMPLES (blood, urine, etc.)
   a. Type _____
   b. Preservative/anticoagulant, etc. _____
   c. Storage/transfer instructions _____

13. REPORT SCHEDULE
   a. Status reports — frequency
      Weekly _____
      Monthly _____
   b. Special data handling/statistics _____
   c. Final draft — date required _____
   d. Histopathology — date required _____
   e. Final report — date required _____

C. GLP Protocol Review Checklist*

This is a checklist used by Huntingdon Life Sciences' Quality Assurance Unit to review protocols for GLP Compliance.

Sponsor, Study No._____

+ = Requirement Met
0 = Requirement Not Met
NA = Not Applicable

Date:_____

	Circle Agency	FDA	EPA	OECD	MHW	MAFF	MITI	NON
1.	A descriptive title and statement of purpose of the study.	—	—	—	—	—	—	—
2.	Identification of the test and control article by name and/or code number.	—	—	—	—	—	—	—
3.	The name and address of the test facility and the sponsor.	—	—	—	—	—	—	—
4a.	Proposed experimental start date.	NA	—	—	NA	—	—	—
4b.	Proposed termination date.	NA	—	—	NA	NA	—	—
4c.	Proposed duration of study.	NA	NA	NA	NA	—	—	NA
5.	Justification for selection of the test system.	NA	—	—	—	—	—	—
6.	Where applicable, the number, body weight range, sex, source of supply, species, strain, substrain and age of the test system.	—	—	—	—	—	—	—
7.	The procedure for unique ID of the test system.	—	—	NA	—	—	—	—
8.	A description of the experimental design, including the method for control of bias.	—	—	—	—	—	—	—
9.	A description and/or identification of the diet used in the study, to include statement of contaminants.	—	—	NA	—	—	—	—
10a.	Route of administration.	—	—	—	—	—	—	—
10b.	Reason for route.	NA	—	—	—	—	—	—
10c.	Reason for frequency and duration.	NA	NA	NA	—	—	—	NA
11.	Dose levels in appropriate units, and method and frequency of administration.	—	—	—	—	—	—	—
12.	Method degree of absorption is measured.	NA	NA	NA	—	—	—	—
13.	Type/frequency of test measurements.	—	—	—	—	—	—	—
14.	Records to be maintained.	—	—	—	—	—	—	—
15a.	Date sponsor approved, and dated study director signature.	—	—	—	—	NA	—	—
15b.	Signed by test facility management.	NA	NA	NA	—	—	—	NA
16.	Proposed statistical methods	—	—	NA	—	—	—	—

Circle Agency	FDA	EPA	OECD	MHW	MAFF	MITI	NON
17. Reference to OECD or other test guidelines.	NA	NA	__	NA	NA	NA	NA
18. Environmental conditions for the test system.	NA	NA	NA	__	__	__	NA
19. Test, control and reference substances or mixtures appropriately tested (or to be tested) for identity, strength, purity stability, uniformity and solubility.	__	__	__	__	__	__	__

D. Test and/or Control Material Handling Information

This is a form used in our laboratory to obtain information about materials to be tested.

STUDY NO(S):

TEST AND/OR CONTROL MATERIAL

HANDLING INFORMATION

_____   _____

_____   _____

_____   _____

This form is designed to specify test material handling and disposition instructions and to provide procedures (if known) in case of accidental exposure to the substance. As with all data, this information will be considered confidential and will be available only to persons involved with the study or studies using this substance. Please provide as complete information as possible for each category below and/or attach the information in your own form and return:

I.   IDENTIFICATION

Test Material (name or Code Number)_____

Batch or Lot Number:_____

Physical Description:_____

Purity:_____

Density (if known): _____

pH (if applicable): _____

Test Material is Soluble in (check one): ____Water; _____Acetone; _____Alcohol; _____Oil; _____Other (_____)

II. STORAGE INFORMATION - Material should be stored in:

_____Temperature-monitored room (60–85°F); _____Freezer; _____Refrigerator; _____Other (_____)

III. STABILITY

Length of time material is stable under conditions described above: _____

Expiration date: _____Indicated on label: YES/NO (circle one)

	Unknown	Less than 4 Hours	Up to 4 Hours	Up to 24 Hours	Other ( )
Stability in common vehicles:					
Water:	_____	_____	_____	_____	_____
Methylcellulose:	_____	_____	_____	_____	_____
Corn oil:	_____	_____	_____	_____	_____
Organic solvents (acetone, ethanol):	_____	_____	_____	_____	_____
Other (_____):	_____	_____	_____	_____	_____

If stability of neat material or of material in vehicle to be used in study is not known:

_____ Instructions for analysis will be provided.

_____ Samples are to be submitted to Sponsor for analysis.

_____ Analysis will not be required.

IV. HANDLING (EMPLOYEE SAFETY) INFORMATION

KNOWN HAZARDS: (If available, attach summary of pertinent results of any previous toxicity studies).

Approximate rodent oral LD_{50} = ____ mg/kg (if unavailable, enter NK, not known).

Is material a probable eye/skin irritant: YES/NO (circle one).

OTHER PERTINENT

INFORMATION:_____

PRECAUTIONS: Use of protective clothing (laboratory coats), latex gloves, safety glasses and dust mask is routine. Precautions in excess of the above should be specified: _____ Routine precautions adequate. Other:_____

IN CASE OF EMERGENCY RELATED TO THIS SUBSTANCE, CONTACT:

_____ of _____ at _____
(Person) (Company) (Phone Number)

V   DISPOSITION

All material will be returned to the Sponsor. Person and address to whom samples are to be returned:

Name: _____   Shipping Instructions: _____

Address: _____   _____

_____   _____

Note: Please enclose appropriate shipping labels for return.

V1.   SIGNATURE

Information submitted by: _____

Company: _____ Date: _____

E. FLOW CHART/TIME LINES FOR CONDUCT OF STUDY

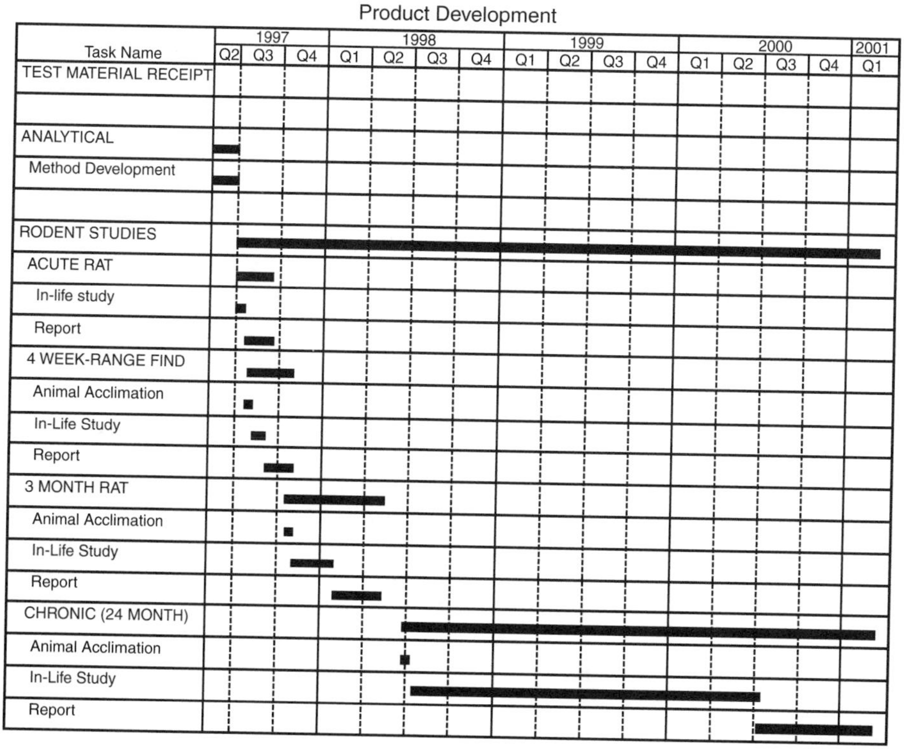

FIGURE 2.1 Flow chart/time line for rodent studies.

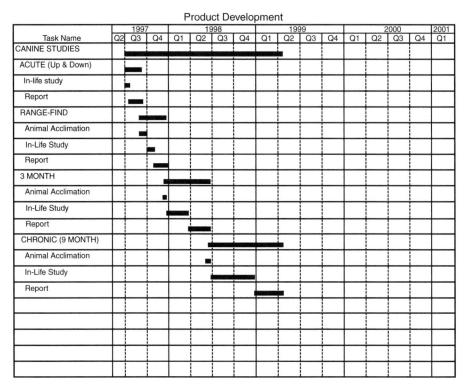

FIGURE 2.2 Flow chart/time line for nonrodent studies.

F. Sample Study Schedule

PROPOSED STUDY SCHEDULE

STUDY NUMBER:____ EXAMPLE ___   PAGE __1__OF __1__

PREPARED BY: _____ DATE: _____   APPROVED BY: _____ DATE: _____

VERIFIED BY: _____ DATE: _____   SCHEDULED BY: _____ DATE: _____

cc: _____

YEAR							O	YEAR	STUDY						O
2001	STUDY			B	F	F	B	2001				B	F	F	B
DATE	DAY	WK	EVALUATIONS	W	I	O	S	DATE	DAY	WK	EVALUATIONS	W	I	O	S
7/1								8/1	14			√		√	√
7/2								8/2	15	3			W		
7/3								8/3	16						
7/4								8/4	17						
7/5	−13	−1	Animal Receipt		N			8/5	18						
7/6	−12							8/6	19						
7/7	−11							8/7	20						
7/8	−10							8/8	21			√		√	√
7/9	−9							8/9	22	4			W		
7/10	−8							8/10	23						
7/11	−7		Vet. Examination	√			√	8/11	24						
7/12	−6	0			W			8/12	25						
7/13	−5							8/13	26						

7/14	−4							8/14	27						
7/15	−3		Ophthalmology					8/15	28				√	√	√
7/16	−2							8/16	29	5	Ophthalmology, Urine				
7/17	−1							8/17	30		Hematology, Necropsy				
7/18	0		Sort and Eartag	√		√	√	8/18							
7/19	1	1	Initiate treatment		W			8/19							
7/20	2							8/20							
7/21	3							8/21							
7/22	4							8/22							
7/23	5							8/23							
7/24	6							8/24							
7/25	7			√		√	√	8/25							
7/26	8	2			W			8/26							
7/27	9							8/27							
7/28	10							8/28							
7/29	11							8/29							
7/30	12							8/30							
7/31	13							8/31							

BW – BODY WEIGHT   GENERAL NOTES: _____

FI – FEEDER IN   _____

   W – WEIGHED FEEDER   _____

   N – NON-WEIGHED FEEDER   _____

FO – FEEDER OUT   _____

OBS – OBSERVATIONS   _____

G. Animal Selection — Randomization Procedures

Rodents are generally assigned to studies by use of computer programs which sort animals by weight and assign them to groups in a manner that results in similar mean weights.

The following procedures are used in our laboratory to assign small numbers of animals (usually dogs or monkeys) to groups:

1. Eliminate from selection any animals considered unsuitable on the basis of pretest examinations and evaluations.
2. List animals in ascending or descending order based on body weights.
3. Determine the number of blocks per sex and the number of animals per block by referring to the protocol. The number of blocks per sex is equal to the number of groups and the number of animals per block is equal to the number of animals per group. For example, if the study design calls for 4 groups of 5 animals per sex, then the number of blocks per sex equals 4 with 5 animals in a block.
4. Distribute the animals into the blocks so that the body weight means for each block are comparable.
5. Do not place littermates (dogs) in the same blocks.
6. Use a random numbers table to assign the blocks to study groups as follows:
   a. Assign a two-digit number to each block (00–99).
   b. When an assigned number is reached on the table, assign this block to Group I.
   c. Continue across the rows until the next assigned number is reached. If the block assigned to this number is a different sex than the first number found, assign this block as Group I. If it is the same sex as the first block assigned, assign this block to Group II.
   d. Continue in this manner until all the blocks are assigned to dose groups.

SECTION 5. DOSE/VEHICLE SELECTION
AND DOSE FORMULATION*

A. DEFINITIONS RELATIVE TO DOSES/DOSE SELECTION

1. Acute Studies

ED_{50}: The median effective dose, i.e., the dose for which half (50%) of the animals exhibit an effect (E) and half of the animals exhibit no effect.

The effect may be defined as a specific toxic event (e.g., tremors) and is sometimes defined as lethality (LD_{50}). Other subscripts may be used to designate the percentage of animals affected. For example, the ED_{10} and ED_{90} are the doses at which 10% or 90% of the animals, respectively, demonstrate the effect.

2. General Studies

Limit Dose: A dose which is considered high enough that if no mortality or significant toxicity is seen in animals receiving this dose, no higher doses are required.

Examples: Limit doses (EPA/OECD)

Acute Oral Toxicity	2,000 mg/kg
Acute Dermal Toxicity	2,000 mg/kg
21-Day Dermal Toxicity	1,000 mg/kg/day
Chronic Studies of Pesticides	1,000 mg/kg/day

Note: The "limit" dose of a non-nutritive material added to the diet is generally considered to be 5% (50,000 ppm).

3. Subchronic and Chronic Studies

ADI: Acceptable Daily Intake (established for food additives/residues and published by the EPA).

NOEL: No observed effect level. Dose at which no effect is seen.

NOAEL: No observed adverse effect level. Dose at which no adverse (toxic) effect is seen.

4. Chronic Studies

MTD: Maximum Tolerated Dose. Highest dose that can be tolerated without significant lethality from causes other than tumors. (A frequently cited criterion for EPA studies is that the MTD for chronic studies with pesticides is a dose which produces an approximate 10–15% decrement in body weight gain.)

HTD: Highest dose tested. Highest dose that can be expected to yield results relevant to humans. This is a proposed new dose which would be selected based on an evaluation of results of subchronic studies.

B. GEOMETRIC PROGRESSION TABLES FOR DOSE SELECTION

Table 2.24 is a series of approximately geometrically-spaced doses used frequently in our laboratory, primarily for acute toxicity studies.

---

* See Chapter 33, Section 4 for calculations, preparation, and properties of various types of substances commonly used in toxicology.

TABLE 2.24
Geometric Progressions

Interval	0.1 log	0.14 log		0.3 log
Multiples of	1.26	1.43		2
Doses		0.4 _or_	0.25	0.25
		0.6	0.35	0.5
	0.8	0.8	0.5	1.0
	1.0	1.2	0.7	2.0
	1.3	1.7	1.0	4.0
	1.6	2.5	1.4	8.0
	2.0	3.5	2.0	16.0
	2.5	5.0	2.8	
	3.2	7.1	4.0	
	4.0	10.0	5.6	
	5.0	14.2	8.0	
	6.3	20.0	11.2	
	8.0	28.4	16.0	
		40.3	22.4	

C. VEHICLES: GUIDELINES FOR DOSING

The following are commonly used vehicles which are generally regarded as nontoxic and nonirritating.

Oral
  Water
  Methylcellulose or carboxymethylcellulose (0.5 – 5% aqueous suspension)
  Oil (corn, peanut, sesame)
    Note: High volumes may be associated with soft stool
Dermal
  Physiological saline
  Water
  Ethanol
  Acetone
  Mineral oil
Parenteral
  Physiological saline (sterile)
  Water for injection (sterile)

D. Dose Volume and Needle Size Guidelines

TABLE 2.25
Suggested Dose Volumes (mL/kg) for Test Material Administration

Species	GAVAGE Ideal	GAVAGE Limit	DERMAL Ideal	DERMAL Limit	IV Ideal	IV Limit	IP Ideal	IP Limit	SC Ideal	SC Limit	IM Ideal	IM Limit	NASAL[a] Ideal	NASAL[a] Limit
							ROUTE							
Mouse	10	20–50	—	—	5	15–25	5–10	30–50	1–5	10–20	0.1	0.5–1	—	—
Rat	10	20–50	2	6	1–5	10–20	5–10	10–20	1	10–20	0.1–1	1–10	0.1	0.2
Rabbit	10	10–20	2	8	1–3	5–10	—	—	1–2.5	5–10	0.1–0.5	1	0.2	1
Dog	10	10–20	—	—	1	5–10	3	5	0.5	1–2	0.1–0.2	1	0.2	2
Monkey	10	10	—	—	1	5–10	3	5	0.5	1–2	0.1–0.5	1	0.2	1

[a] Nasal doses (ml/Animal, 1/2 doses per nostril) based on experience in our laboratory.

Adapted from *SYNAPSE*, American Society of Laboratory Animal Practitioners, Vol. 24, March 1991.[2] Some adaptations have been made based on experience in our laboratory.

TABLE 2.26
Suggested Dosing Apparatus/Needle Sizes (Gauge) for Test Material Administration[a]

Species	Gavage Recommended	IV Ideal	IV Range	IP Ideal	IP Range	SC Ideal	SC Range	IM Ideal	IM Range
					Route				
Mouse	Premature infant feeding tube cut to 70 mm, marked at 38 mm	25 or 27	25–30	25 or 27	22–30	25 or 27	22–30	25 or 27	22–30
Rat	3-inch ball-tipped intubation needle	25	25–30	25	22–30	25	25–30	25	22–30
Rabbit	No. 18 French catheter, cut to 15 inches, marked at 12 inches	21	21–22	21	18–23	25	22–25	25	22–30
Dog	Kaslow stomach tube 12Fr ≥ 24 inches; Davol 32Fr intubation tube	21	21–22	—	—	22	20–23	21 or 25	20–25
Monkey	No. 8 French tube (nasogastric gavage)	25	25–30	—	—	22	22–25	25	22–25

[a] Recommended gavage equipment and ideal needle sizes are those used in our laboratory. Suggested ranges of needle sizes are from: *Laboratory Manual for Basic Biomethodology of Laboratory Animals*, MTM Associates, Inc.[3]

E. Dermal Exposure Methods

Procedures used in our laboratory are:

Dose site:
- An area on the back is used.
- Hair is removed from the application site before administration of test material.
- Care must be taken to avoid damaging the skin during clipping. Animals with damaged skin should not be used.
- The site is reclipped as necessary throughout the study.
- The maximum exposure site consists of an area of skin from the scapulae to the wings of the ilium extending to the lateral midline on either side.
- This area represents approximately 10% of the body surface.
- If no covering (occlusion) will be used, it is preferable to use a smaller area in the scapular area to prevent/minimize ingestion of test material.

Application procedures:
- *Open, nonoccluded:* The test material is spread evenly over the dose site with a glass rod or gloved fingers. Animals (rabbits and rats) are generally fitted with polyethylene collars to prevent ingestion.
- *Occlusive covering:* The test material is applied and covered with an impervious material designed to hold the material in place and prevent ingestion and evaporation.

Rabbits:
   Preparation of covering:
      1. Cut 4-1/2 inch wide 8-ply gauze to a length of approximately 18 inches.
      2. Cut polyethylene sheeting to a size of approximately 10×24 inches.
      3. Fold both edges of the polyethylene lengthwise toward the middle. Tape the ends of the polyethylene to hold the folded edges.
      4. Cut 2- or 3-inch-wide athletic tape (e.g., Zonas®) to a length of approximately 21 inches.
   Application:
      1. Apply the test material as described previously.
      2. Wrap the gauze around the animal's midsection.
      3. Cover the gauze with the polyethylene sheeting.
      4. Wrap each end of the polyethylene with athletic tape, making contact with the animal's skin. Also place a piece of athletic tape over the middle of the polyethylene sheeting.

Rats:
   Preparation of covering:
      1. Cut 2- or 3-inch wide elastic adhesive bandages (e.g., Elastoplast®) to a length of approximately 14 inches. Adjust length as needed depending on the size of the animal.
      2. Cut polyethylene sheeting to an approximate size of 3×4 inches.
      3. Place the 3×4-inch square of polyethylene on the adhesive side of the elastic bandage approximately 1/2 inch from one end of the bandage.
   Application:
      1. Apply the test material as described previously.
      2. Place a gauze patch of appropriate size over the dose site.
      3. Place the end of the bandage containing the polyethylene square over the patch and wrap the bandage around the animal so that the edges of the bandage come in contact with the animal's skin. Apply the bandage in a manner that prevents the animal from disturbing the dose site but does not cause undue stress.

Semiocclusive covering:
   The test material is applied beneath a gauze wrapping designed to hold the material in place and prevent ingestion without completely occluding the dose site.
   Procedures used in our laboratory are:

Rabbits:
   Preparation of covering:
      1. Cut 4-1/2-inch wide 8-ply gauze or a suitable substitute to a length of approximately 18 inches.
      2. Cut 2-inch wide athletic tape (e.g., Zonas®) to a length of approximately 21 inches.
   Application:
      1. Apply test material as described previously.

2. Wrap the gauze around the animal to cover the dose site.
3. Place one piece of athletic tape over each edge of the gauze (upper and lower) to secure it. The tape must come in contact with the animal's skin to secure the bandage.

Removal of coverings:

If necessary, cut the bandages using bandage scissors (generally used for rabbits). Carefully remove the bandage and any underlying gauze. Remove any excess test material from the dose site by wiping gently with gauze (dry or moistened with warm water).

F. BODY WEIGHT/SURFACE AREA CONVERSION TABLES

TABLE 2.27
Body Weight: Surface Area Conversion Table

Species	Representative Body Weight to Surface Area[a]		
	Body Weight (kg)	Surface Area (m²)	Conversion Factor (km)
Mouse	0.02	0.0066	3
Rat	0.15	0.025	5.9
Monkey	3	0.24	12
Dog	8	0.4	20
Human			
Child	20	0.8	25
Adult	60	1.6	37

[a] Example: To express a mg/kg dose in any given species as the equivalent mg/m² dose, multiply the dose by the appropriate *km*. In human adults, 100 mg/kg is equivalent to 100 mg/kg × 37 kg/m² = 3700 mg/m².

Adapted from Freireich, E.J. et al., Quantitative comparison of toxicity of anti-cancer agents in mouse, rat, dog, monkey and man, *Cancer Chemother. Rep.*, 50; 219, 1966.

TABLE 2.28
Equivalent Surface Area Dosage Conversion Factors[a]

		TO				
		Mouse (20 g)	Rat (150 g)	Monkey (3 kg)	Dog (8 kg)	Human (60 kg)
	Mouse	1	1/2	1/4	1/6	1/12
F	Rat	2	1	1/2	1/3	1/6
R	Monkey	4	2	1	3/5	1/3
O	Dog	6	4	3/2	1	1/2
M	Man	12	7	3	2	1

Example: To convert a dose of 50 mg/kg in the mouse to an equivalent dose in the monkey, assuming equivalency on the basis of mg/m²; multiply 50 mg/kg × 1/4 = 13 mg/kg.

[a] This table gives approximate factors for converting doses expressed in terms of mg/kg from one species to an equivalent surface area dose expressed as mg/kg in the other species tabulated.

Adapted from Freireich, E.J. et al., Quantitative comparison of toxicity of anti-cancer agents in mouse, rat, dog, monkey and man, *Cancer Chemother. Rep.*, 50, 219, 1966.

G. Dose Calculations — Oral, Dermal, or Parenteral Administration

Abbreviations: ml = milliliter; mg = milligram; g = gram (equal to 1000 mg); kg = kilogram (equal to 1000 g); b.w. = body weight (generally expressed in kilograms).

1. Dose Volume

To calculate dose volume when dose and concentration are known:

$$\text{Dose volume (ml / kg b.w.)} = \frac{\text{dose (mg / kg b.w.)}}{\text{concentration (mg / ml)}}$$

Example: To determine the dose volume needed to administer 200 mg of test material per kilogram of body weight of a dose solution containing 20 mg of test material per milliliter:

$$\frac{\text{dose: 200 mg / kg b.w.}}{\text{concentration: 20 mg / ml}} = \text{dose volume: 10 ml / kg b.w.}$$

2. Concentration of Dosing Mixture

To calculate dose concentration when dose and desired dose volume are known:

$$\text{Concentration (mg / ml)} = \frac{\text{dose (mg / kg b.w.)}}{\text{dose volume (ml / kg b.w.)}}$$

Example: To determine the concentration of dose solution needed to administer 200 mg of a test material per kilogram of body weight at a dose volume of 10 ml/kg of body weight:

$$\frac{\text{dose: 200 mg / kg}}{\text{dose volume: 10 ml / kg}} = \text{concentration: 20 mg / ml}$$

3. Individual Animal Doses

    A. Solids

        To calculate the weight of a solid material to be administered to an animal (used for oral administration in capsules, dermal dosing of neat powders): Dose for animal (mg) = dose (mg/kg b.w.) × animal's body weight (kg).

        Example: To administer a dose of 25 mg/kg b.w. to a dog weighing 9.4 kg: 25 mg/kg b.w. × 9.4 kg b.w. = 235 mg.

    B. Liquids

        To calculate the dose volume to be administered to an individual animal: Dose volume for animal (ml) = dose volume (ml/kg b.w.) × animal's body weight (kg).

        Example: To administer a dose of 6 ml of test material per kilogram of body weight to a rat weighing 325 g:

            Convert body weight to kilograms: 325 grams × 0.001 kg/g = 0.325 kg

            Calculate dose: 6 ml/kg b.w. × 0.325 kg b.w. = 1.95 ml

4. Adjustment for Active Ingredient

If doses are to be administered as doses of pure material or active ingredient, the dose must be adjusted as follows: Desired dose of active ingredient × (100%/% active ingredient) = calculated total dose.

Example: To administer a dose of 10 mg/kg b.w. of active ingredient of a test material which is 85% active.

$$10 \, mg \, / \, kg \times \frac{100}{85} = 11.76 \, mg \, / \, kg \, (dose \, to \, be \, administered)$$

5. Dose Solution Conversions

To convert percent to milligrams per milliliter: Concentration in % × 10 = concentration in mg/ml.
Rationale: A 100% mixture contains 1g (or 1000 mg)/ml. Therefore:

$$100\% = 1000 \, mg/ml$$
$$10\% = 100 \, mg/ml$$
$$1\% = 10 \, mg/ml$$

Example: To determine the concentration in milligrams per milliliter of a 30% w/v (weight/volume) solution:

$$30\% \, w/v \times 100 = 300 \, mg/ml$$

H. CALCULATIONS FOR DIETARY AND DRINKING WATER ADMINISTRATION

Abbreviations: t.m. = test material; mg = milligram; g = gram (equal to 1000 mg); kg = kilogram (equal to 1000 g); b.w. = body weight (generally expressed in kilograms); f.c. = food consumption.

1. Calculation of Concentration — General

- Conversions
  Concentrations are usually expressed as ppm (parts per million) or %. Conversion: % × 10,000 = ppm.
  For solids (dietary administration)
      1 ppm = 1 mg of test material per kg of mixture
      1% = 10,000 mg of test material per kg of mixture
  For liquids (drinking water administration)
      1 ppm = 1 mg of test material per liter of mixture
      1% = 10,000 mg of test material per liter of mixture
- Calculation of amount of test material needed
  To calculate the amount of test material needed when desired concentration and total amount of diet are known:
  Desired concentration (ppm) × required amount of diet (kg) = amount of test material needed (mg).
  Example: To prepare 20 kg of a diet containing 6 ppm of test material:

$$6 \, ppm = 6 \, mg/kg$$
$$6 \, mg/kg \times 20 \, kg = 120 \, mg$$

Therefore, mix 120 mg of test material in 20 kg of diet.

- Adjustment for active ingredient
  If doses are to be administered as doses of pure material or active ingredient, the concentration must be adjusted as follows: Desired concentration of active ingredient × (100%/% active ingredient) = calculated concentration.
  Example: To prepare 20 kg of diet containing 6 ppm of active ingredient of a test material which is 80% active:

$$6 \text{ ppm} = \text{mg/kg} \times 100/80 = 7.5 \text{ mg/kg}$$
$$7.5 \text{ mg/kg} \times 20 \text{ kg} = 150 \text{ mg}$$

  Therefore, mix 150 mg of test material in 20 kg of diet.
- Adjustment for high test material concentrations
  When high concentrations of test material are used, displacement of diet must be considered and an appropriate adjustment made. This is usually done when the amount of test material to be added is 5 g or more. The correction is made by subtraction of an equivalent weight of diet rounded to the nearest 10 g as shown below:

Test Material (g)	Feed Displaced (g)
5.0–15.0	10
15.1–25.0	20
25.1–35.0	30
35.1–45.0	40
45.1–55.0	50

  Example: To prepare 60 kg of a diet containing 30 g of test material (concentration of 500 ppm):

  30 g of test material displaces 30 g of feed
  60 kg of diet = 60,000 g of diet
  60,000 g of diet – 30 g of test material = 59,970 g of feed

  Therefore, mix 30 g of test material with 59,970 g of feed.

2. Adjustment of Concentration for Body Weight

Dietary concentrations are often adjusted to administer a specified amount of test material per unit of body weight each day, e.g., mg/kg b.w./day. Each time the diet is prepared, adjustments are made based on body weight and food consumption data from the preceding interval(s) and the new concentration is calculated as follows:

- Calculation of dietary concentration
  Dietary concentration (mg test material/kg diet) = desired dose (mg/kg b.w./day) ÷ predicted food consumption (g diet/kg b.w./day) × 1000 (g/kg).
  In our laboratory, predictions are made as follows:
- Predicted food consumption
  The preceding interval's food consumption (expressed as grams of food consumed per animal per day) and a predicted body weight are used as follows: Predicted food consumption (g diet/kg b.w./day) = previous food consumption (g diet/day) ÷ predicted body weight (kg).

- Predicted body weight is calculated as follows: Predicted body weight (kg) = current weight (kg) × 1.33 − previous weight (kg) × 0.33.

  Example: To calculate the dietary concentration needed to administer 100 mg of test material per kg b.w. per day during Week 3 to a group of rats which had a mean body weight of 200 g at the end of Week 1 and 249 g at the end of Week 2 and a mean food consumption value of 120 g of food per animal during a 6-day measurement period (20 g per animal per day) during Week 2.

  1. Calculate predicted body weight:

     To predict the Week 3 weight of a group of rats which had mean weights of 200 g at the end of Week 1 and 249 g at the end of Week 2:

     This week's (Week 2) weight × 1.33   249 × 1.33 = 331 g
     Last week's (Week 2) weight × 0.33   200 × 0.33 = 66 g

     Predicted Week 3 weight: 331 − 66 = 265 g

  2. Calculate predicted food consumption:

     $$\frac{\text{Previous week's f.c.: 20 g / day}}{\text{Predicted b.w.: 265 g}} = 75.5 \text{ g diet / kg b.w. / day}$$

  3. Calculate dietary concentration:

     100 mg t.m./kg b.w./day (dose) ÷ 75.5 g diet/kg b.w./day (predicted f.c.) × 1000
     = 1324.5 g t.m./kg diet

     Check: Based on prediction, rat consumes 75.5 g/kg b.w./day of diet containing 1324.5 mg/kg of test material. 1324.5 mg test material/kg of diet × 0.0755 kg of diet = 100 mg test material/kg b.w./day.

3. Test Material Intake

To calculate actual test material intake (dose): Dose (mg of t.m./kg b.w./day) × dietary concentration (mg t.m./g of diet) × diet consumed (g diet/kg b.w./day).

Example: To determine the dose of test material received by a rat which consumed 120 g of diet/kg b.w./day of a diet containing 800 ppm of test material.

- 800 ppm = 800 mg t.m./kg of diet = 0.8 mg t.m./g of diet
- 0.8 mg t.m./g of diet × 120 g of diet/kg b.w./day = 96 mg t.m./kg b.w./day

4. Approximate Conversion Factors (ppm to mg/kg/day)

When diets of a constant concentration are administered throughout a study, the actual test material intake per unit of body weight decreases as the animal grows older. Approximate conversion factors, assuming normal food consumption, to convert ppm in diet to mg test material/kg b.w./day are in Table 2.29.

TABLE 2.29
Conversion Factors (ppm to mg/kg)[a]

Species	Age	Conversion Factor (Divide ppm by)
Mice	Young (1–12 wk of study)	5
	Older (13–78 wk of study)	6–7
Rats	Young (1–12 wk of study)	10
	Older (13–104 wk of study)	20
Dogs		40

[a] *Example*: To estimate the approximate test material intake of rats receiving a 1000 ppm dietary concentration during a 4-week study: 1000 ppm ÷ 10 = 100 mg/kg b.w./day.

I. Calculation of Test Material Requirements

1. Amount of Material Needed for Capsule Administration or Dermal Administration of Neat Material

Sum of doses (mg/kg b.w./day) × number of animals per group × b.w. (kg)[a] × number of days.
[a] Guidelines: Average Body Weight (kg).

Duration of Study	Rat Sprague-Dawley	F344	Mouse CD-1	B6C3F1	Rabbit NZW
<4 wk	0.300	0.200	0.030	0.025	3
<12 wk	0.400	0.250	0.035	0.030	4
>12 wk	0.500	0.350	0.040	0.035	4

	Nonhuman Primate Cynomolgus	Rhesus	Dog
<12 wk	3	4	10
>12 wk	4	6	12

Notes: This is an approximate minimal amount. A safety factor of 20–50% is usually added to allow for remixes, etc. Adjustment for active ingredient should be made if required.

Example: To calculate the amount of material needed for a 4-week study in dogs with doses of 10, 30, and 100 mg/kg b.w./day and a group size of 4 dogs/sex.

- Sum of doses (10 + 30 + 100) = 140 mg/kg/day
- 140 mg/kg/day × 8 dogs × 10 kg × 30 days = 336,000 mg (336 g) with safety factor (additional 50%) request approximately 500 g.

2. Amount of Material Needed for Administration in a Solution or Suspension

1. Calculate amount of solution to be prepared at each interval (i.e., each mix): Dose (ml/kg b.w./ day) × b.w. × number of animals × number of days = ml/interval.

Example: To calculate the volume to be prepared to administer 10 ml/kg b.w./day to rats for a 6-month study in 20 rats per sex per group with dose solutions prepared weekly.

$$10 \text{ ml/kg b.w./day} \times 0.500 \text{ kg per rats} \times 40 \text{ rats} \times 8 \text{ days} = 1600 \text{ ml}$$

2. Calculate amount of material to be used for each mix: Sum of concentrations (mg/ml) × volume (ml) = amount needed (mg).

   Example: To calculate test material needs when 1600 ml of dose solution per week per dose level are mixed and dose concentrations are 20, 40, and 80 mg/ml:
   - Sum of concentrations: 20 + 40 + 80 = 140 mg/ml
   - 140 mg/ml × 1600 ml/wk = 224,000 mg (224 g) per week.

3. Calculate amount of test material needed for entire study: mg or g/interval × number of intervals = mg or g needed.

   Example: To calculate the total amount of material needed for the examples presented above: 224 g/week × 27 weeks (one additional week added for pretest mix) = 5824 g, with safety factor (additional 20%), request approximately 7000 g.

3. Amount of Material Needed for Dietary Administration

1. Calculate the amount of dietary mixture to be prepared at each interval (i.e., each mix): Amount of feed per animal per interval × number of feeders to be prepared. The amount of feed depends on size of feeders. In our laboratory, the following are used: mice, 64 g/wk; rats, 275 g/wk; dogs, 3.5 kg/wk (400 g/day).

   In our laboratory, we prepare 5–10% more feeders than needed for rodents (minimum of two extra feeders per group) and one extra feeder per dog per week.

   Example: To calculate the amount of diet to be mixed each week for a group of 10 rats per sex:

$$275 \text{ g of feed/rat/wk} \times 20 \text{ rats} = 5500 \text{ g}$$
$$\text{plus } 10\% \text{ (two additional feeders)} = \underline{550 \text{ g}}$$
$$\text{Total} = 6000 \text{ g}$$

A safety factor of 500 to 1000 additional grams may be added here.

2. Calculate the amount of test material to be used for each batch of diet to be mixed: Sum of concentrations (mg t.m./kg diet) × batch size (kg) = mg of t.m. needed per batch.

   a. For studies with the same concentration throughout the study: Sum of concentrations = sum of dose levels.

      Example: To calculate the amount of material needed per week to administer dietary concentrations of 100, 200, and 400 ppm to groups of 10 rats per sex
      - Sum of concentrations (100 + 200 + 400) = 700 ppm (mg t.m./kg diet)
      - 700 mg t.m./kg diet × 6 kg diet = 4200 mg (4.2 g)

   b. For studies with adjustment of concentration based on body weights and food consumption:

$$\text{Sum of concentrations} = \frac{\text{Sum of dose levels (mg / kg / day)}}{\text{Predicted feed consumed (g / kg b.w. / day)} \times 1000}$$

The following numbers, based on historical control data, are used in our laboratory for estimating the predicted feed consumed.

Duration of Study	Amount of Feed Consumed (g feed/kg b.w./day)	
(wk)	Rat	Mouse
4	100	250
12	80	215
26	70	190
>26	50	165

Example: To calculate the amount of material needed per week to administer doses of 50, 250, and 1250 mg/kg b.w./day to groups of 10 rats per sex for 4 weeks.

- Sum of concentrations (50, 250, and 1250) = 1550 mg/kg b.w./day

- $$\frac{1550 \text{ mg / kg b.w. / day}}{100 \text{ g / kg b.w. / day} \times 1000} = 0.1155 \text{ mg / kg diet}$$

- 0.1155 mg t.m./kg diet × 6 kg diet = 693 mg

3. Calculate amount of test material needed for entire study: mg or g/interval × number of intervals = mg or g needed.

  Example a: To calculate the total amount of test material needed for a 13-week study in which dietary concentrations of 100, 200, and 400 ppm are administered to groups of 10 rats per sex.

  4.2 g/week × 14 weeks (one additional week added for pretest mix) = 58.8 g, with safety factor (additional 20–25%), request approximately 70–75 g.

  Example b: To calculate the total amount of test material needed for a 4-week study in which dietary doses of 50, 250, and 1250 mg/kg b.w./day are administered to groups of 10 rats/sex.

  693 mg/wk × 5 wk (one additional week added for pretest mix) = 3465 mg (3.465 g) with safety factor (additional 50%), request approximately 5 g.

4. Examples of Calculation Sheets Used In Our Laboratory

1. Test material calculations for a constant concentration dietary study.

  The study has four groups with 50 rats/sex/group. The dose levels are 0, 30, 100, and 300 ppm.

Test Material Calculation Sheet: Constant Concentration Diet

Duration:	105 wk	Sponsor code:	_____
Test material:	_____	Study No.:	_____
Percent active:	100	AICF = 100% active:	1

Batch size calculation

Groups	No. of Feeders/Group*	kg (Feed)/Animal/wk	Calculated Batch Size
I–IV	110	× 0.275	30.25 kg
	Mixed Batch Size: 31.5 kg/group/wk		

Test material/batch calculations

Group	Dose Level (ppm)	(mg/kg)	×	AICF	×	Mixed Batch Size (kg)	=	Test Material per Batch
II	30	30	×	1	×	31.5 ÷ 1000	=	0.945 g/wk
III	100	100	×	1	×	31.5 ÷ 1000	=	3.15 g/wk
IV	300	300	×	1	×	31.5 ÷ 1000	=	9.45 g/wk
						Total	=	13.545 g/wk

Total test material requirements

Total per Batch	×	No. of Mixes	×	Safety Factor	=	Test Material Required
13.545 g	×	106	×	1.2 ÷ 1000	=	1.7 kg

AICF = active ingredient correction factor.

*Includes extra feeders

2. Test material calculations for an adjusted concentration dietary study. The study has four groups with 50 rats/sex/group. The dose levels are 0, 30, 100, and 300 mg/kg/day.

Test Material Calculation Sheet: Adjusted Concentration Diet Calculations

Test Material: _____   Sponsor code: _____
Percent active: 98%   Study No: _____
AICF = 100/% active: 1.02   Study duration: 105 Weeks
Batch Size Calculations

Group & Sex	No. of Feeders/ Sex/Group*		kg (Feed Presented) Animal/Wk		Calculated Batch Size	Mixed Batch Size
I–IV ♂	55	×	0.275	=	15.1 kg	16.5 kg
I–IV ♀	55	×	0.275	=	15.1 kg	16.5 kg

Amount of Test Material Required for Study Completion

$$\frac{\text{Sum of the dose level (mg/kg/day)}}{1000 \times \text{amount consumed/animal/day (g/kg/day)}} \times \frac{\text{Combined mixed batch size}}{\text{(male + female) in kilograms}} \times \frac{\text{No. of}}{\text{Wk}}$$

$$\times \text{AICF} \times \frac{\text{Safety}}{\text{Factor}} = \frac{\text{Test Material}}{\text{Required}}$$

$$\frac{430}{1000 \times 50} \times 33 \times 106 \times 1.02 \times 1.2 = 37 \text{ kg}$$

AICF = active ingredient correction factor.

* Includes extra feeders.

3. Test material calculations for an oral intubation study. The study has four groups with 10 dogs/sex/group. The dose levels are 0, 30, 100, and 300 mg/kg/day, and the dose volume is 5 ml/kg. The test material is prepared on a weekly basis.

Test Material Calculation

Study duration: 13 wk   Sponsor code: _____
Test Material: _____   Study No.:   _____
Percent active: 100   AICF = 100% active: 1
Batch Size Calculations

Group & Sex	b.w. (kg)		Dose Volume (ml/kg)		No. of Animals per Group		No. of Doses		Batch Size		Mixed Batch Size (ml)
II–IV	12	×	5	×	20	×	7	=	8400	=	10,080

Test material/batch calculations

Group	Dose Level (mg/kg day)		Dose Volume (ml/kg)		Conc. (mg/ml)		Batch (ml)		AICF		Test Material (g)
II	30	÷	5	=	6	×	10,080	×	1 ÷ 1000	=	60.48
III	100	÷	5	=	20	×	10,080	×	1 ÷ 1000	=	201.60
IV	300	÷	5	=	60	×	10,080	×	1 ÷ 1000	=	604.80
							Total per batch			=	866.88

Total test material requirements

Total per Batch (kg)		No. of Mixes		Safety Factor		Test Material Required (kg)
0.867	×	14	×	1.2	=	15

AICF = active ingredient correction factor.

J. PROCEDURES FOR PREPARATION OF DOSE SOLUTIONS/SUSPENSIONS AND TEST DIETS

The following are samples of standard procedures used in our laboratory. Individual procedures are developed as needed, based on the properties of the test material. Preliminary analyses are performed to confirm adequacy of preparation procedure.

1. Preparation of Dose Solutions/Suspensions

Materials: Test material
             Vehicle
Equipment: Balances
             Beakers (or volumetric flasks)
             Weighing spatulas
             Glassine weigh paper of weigh boats
             Sonicator (if needed)
             Stir plates and stir bars (if needed)
             Calculation sheet

Procedure (Sample) for Suspension Preparation

1. Remove vehicle (methylcellulose) from refrigerator 1 hour before mixing.
2. Using a weigh boat or weigh paper, weigh out the specified amount of test material (as per the current calculation sheet). Carefully transfer the test material into a 50-ml beaker.
3. Add approximately 2 ml of vehicle (methylcellulose) to the beaker, and begin stirring until a paste is formed. Continue adding vehicle (methylcellulose) to the beaker until reaching 3/4 of the total volume, rinsing off the spatula at this time.
4. Repeat steps 1 and 2 for each concentration to be prepared.

5. Place the beakers in a sonicator for approximately 15 minutes.
6. Remove the beakers from the sonicator and Q.S. each suspension with methylcellulose. Add a stir bar to the beakers, and allow the suspensions to stir on the stir plates for approximately 30 minutes.
7. Transfer to appropriately labeled storage containers.

2. Preparation of Test Diets

Materials: Test material
             Certified rodent diet No. 5002 meal
Equipment: Balances
             Scales
             Mixers: mortar/pestle, Hobart mixer, Twinshell mixer
             Weigh boats or glassine weigh paper
             Weighing spatulas
             Appropriately labeled test material transfer containers
             Appropriately labeled diet storage buckets
             Calculation sheet

Handling Precaution (Specified as Necessary):

Respirator type: Disposable dust/mist facemask
Gloves/hand protection: Natural rubber or latex
Eye protection: Safety glasses with sideshields
Foot protection: Disposable shoe covers
Head protection: Bouffant cap
Outer clothing: White Tyvek suit or gray lab coat

Procedure (Sample)

1. Weigh out the specified amount of test material using a weigh boat or weigh paper and transfer to appropriate container.
2. Weigh out the specified amount of diet into diet storage bucket.
3. Prepare an initial premix as follows: Place approximately 10 g of untreated feed from the diet storage bucket into a mortar. Pour the test material into the layer of feed in the mortar. Rinse the test material container with several grams of untreated feed (from the diet bucket), add this rinse to the mortar. Pestle mixture until homogeneous.
4. Prepare an additional premix as follows: Place approximately 2 kg of untreated feed (from the diet bucket) into the bowl of the Hobart mixer. Pour the initial premix (from the mortar) into the Hobart mixer bowl. Rinse the mortar and pestle with several grams of untreated diet (from the bucket) to incorporate any residual test material, and add this rinse to the bowl of the Hobart mixer. Pour an additional 2.0 kg of diet (from the diet bucket) into the bowl of the Hobart mixer. Using the paddle blade, run the Hobart mixer on speed 1 for approximately 10 minutes.
5. Complete mix as follows: Pour approximately half the diet remaining in the bucket into a Twinshell mixer. Add the premix from the Hobart mixer and rinse the Hobart bowl with several grams of untreated diet (from the diet bucket); add this rinse to the Twinshell. Pour remaining diet into the Twinshell mixer and run the mixer for approximately 15 minutes. On completion, empty the mix into the appropriate dose group bucket (lined

with a plastic bag). Attach the dose group identification tag to the bucket. Repeat for each concentration.

K. ANALYSES OF DOSING SOLUTIONS/SUSPENSIONS AND DIETS

The following are recommended procedures.

1. Method Validation

Analytical methods are developed and/or validated in the testing facility's laboratory. The designated vehicle (or diet) is mixed with the test material at concentrations over the range expected to be administered during the study. Mixtures are assayed according to the proposed method. The data obtained are evaluated for reproducibility of results. Means and standard deviations are computed for multiple extractions and injections of the low- and high-concentration mixtures. Modifications are made as necessary until acceptable results are obtained.

2. Homogeneity Analyses

Before initiation of the study, batches of the low- and high-concentration mixtures are prepared. Three samples each from the top, middle, and bottom portion of each mix are taken for analysis. If the data demonstrate that the mean of the values for the three levels are within ±10% (solutions) or ±15% (diets) of each other and of the nominal (desired) concentration, the batch is considered homogeneous.

3. Stability Analyses

Stability of the test material in the mixture under storage conditions to be used for the study are determined for at least 2 weeks. Duplicate samples of the low- and high-concentration mixtures are assayed 4, 7, and 14 days after preparation (samples for homogeneity assays, evaluated on the day of preparation, are used to establish concentration at time of preparation). If the data indicate the test material is unstable at room temperature, frozen or refrigerated storage stability is evaluated.

4. Confirmation of Concentrations During Study

Solutions/suspensions or diets for all dose levels are assayed weekly for the first 4 weeks (one sample per concentration is taken and two subsamples are analyzed). Subsequent assays are performed at monthly intervals for the remainder of the study. The concentration determined in the batch must be within ±10% (solutions) or ±15% (diets) of each other before the mixtures are acceptable. If mixtures are not within the acceptable range, new mixtures are prepared and analyzed.

5. Summary

The number of analyses performed is as follows:

Homogeneity Analyses
9 samples per concentration × 2 concentrations = 18
1 control sample (vehicle)   =   1
                                                       Total = 19

Stability Analyses
2 samples per concentration × 2 concentrations × 3 intervals = 12
1 control sample × 3 intervals   =   3
                                                                       Total = 15

Confirmation of Concentration

	4-Wk Study	24-Mo Study
Two samples per concentration × concentrations × 4–27 intervals	= 24	162
1 control sample × 4–27 intervals	= 4	27
Total	= 28	189

SECTION 6. EXPERIMENTAL EVALUATIONS

A. CLINICAL SIGNS OF TOXICITY

TABLE 2.30
Clinical Signs of Toxicity

Clinical Observation	Observed Signs	Organs, Tissues, or Systems Most Likely To Be Involved
I. Respiratory: blockage in the nostrils, changes in rate and depth of breathing, changes in color of body surfaces	A. Dyspnea: difficult or labored breathing, essentially gasping for air, respiration rate usually slow	
	1. Abdominal breathing: breathing by diaphragm, greater deflection of abdomen upon inspiration	CNS respiratory center, paralysis of costal muscles, cholinergic inhibition
	2. Gasping: deep labored inspiration, accompanied by a wheezing sound	CNS respiratory center, pulmonary edema, secretion accumulation in airways (increase cholinergic)
	B. Apnea: a transient cessation of breathing following a forced respiration	CNS respiratory center, pulmonary cardiac insufficiency
	C. Cyanosis: bluish appearance of tail, mouth, foot pads	Pulmonary-cardiac insufficiency, pulmonary edema
	D. Tachypnea: quick and usually shallow respiration	Stimulation of respiratory center, pulmonary-cardiac insufficiency
	E. Nostril discharges: red or colorless	Pulmonary edema, hemorrhage
II. Motor activities: changes in frequency and nature of movements	A. Decrease or increase in spontaneous motor activities, curiosity, preening, or locomotions	Somatomotor, CNS
	B. Somnolence: animal appears drowsy, but can be aroused by prodding and resumes normal activities	CNS sleep center
	C. Loss of righting reflex: loss of reflex to maintain normal upright posture when placed on the back	CNS, sensory, neuromuscular
	D. Anesthesia: loss of righting reflex and pain response (animal will not respond to tail and toe pinch)	CNS, sensory
	E. Catalepsy: animal tends to remain in any position in which it is placed	CNS, sensory, neuromuscular, autonomic
	F. Ataxia: inability to control and coordinate movement while animal is walking with no spasticity, epraxia, paresis, or rigidity	CNS, sensory, autonomic

TABLE 2.30 *(Continued)*
Clinical Signs of Toxicity

Clinical Observation	Observed Signs	Organs, Tissues, or Systems Most Likely To Be Involved
	G. Unusual locomotion: spastic, toe walking, pedaling, hopping, and low body posture	CNS, sensory, neuromuscular
	H. Prostration: immobile and rests on belly	CNS, sensory, neuromuscular
	I. Tremors: involving trembling and quivering of the limbs or entire body	Neuromuscular, CNS
	J. Fasciculation: involving movements of muscles, seen on the back, shoulders, hind limbs, and digits of the paws	Neuromuscular, CNS, autonomic
III. Convulsion (seizure): marked involuntary contraction or seizures of contraction of voluntary muscle	A. Clonic convulsion: convulsive alternating contraction and relaxation of muscles	CNS, respiratory failure, neuromuscular, autonomic
	B. Tonic convulsion: persistent contraction of muscles, attended by rigid extension of hind limbs	
	C. Tonic-clonic convulsion: both types may appear consecutively	
	D. Asphyxial convulsion: usually of clonic type, but accompanied by gasping and cyanosis	
	E. Opisthotonos: tetanic spasm in which the back is arched and the head is pulled towards the dorsal position	
IV. Reflexes	A. Corneal (eyelid closure): touching of the cornea causes eyelids to close	Sensory, neuromuscular
	B. Pinnal: twitch of external ear elicited by light stroking of inside surface of ear	Sensory, neuromuscular, autonomic
	C. Righting	CNS, sensory, neuromuscular
	D. Myotact: ability of animal to retract its hind limb when limb is pulled down over the edge of a surface	Sensory, neuromuscular
	E. Light (pupillary): constriction of pupil in the presence of light	Sensory, neuromuscular, autonomic
	F. Startle reflex: response to external stimuli such as touch, noise	Sensory, neuromuscular
V. Ocular signs	A. Lacrimation: excessive tearing, clear or colored	Autonomic
	B. Miosis: constriction of pupil regardless of the presence or absence of light	Autonomic
	C. Mydriasis: dilation of pupils regardless of the presence or absence of light	Autonomic
	D. Exophthalmos: abnormal protrusion of eye from orbit	Autonomic

TABLE 2.30 *(Continued)*
Clinical Signs of Toxicity

Clinical Observation	Observed Signs	Organs, Tissues, or Systems Most Likely To Be Involved
	E. Ptosis: dropping of upper eyelids, not reversed by prodding animal	Autonomic
	F. Chromodacryorrhea (red lacrimation)	Autonomic, hemorrhage, infection
	G. Relaxation of nictitating membrane	Autonomic
	H. Corneal opacity, iritis, conjunctivitis	Irritation of the eye
VI. Cardiovascular signs	A. Bradycardia: decreased heart rate	Autonomic, pulmonary-cardiac insufficiency
	B. Tachycardia: increased heart rate	Autonomic, pulmonary-cardiac insufficiency
	C. Vasodilation: redness of skin, tall, tongue, ear, foot pad, conjunctivae, and warm body	Autonomic, CNS, increased cardiac output, hot environment
	D. Vasoconstriction: blanching or whitening of skin, cold body	Autonomic, CNS, cold environment, cardiac output decrease
	E. Arrhythmia: abnormal cardiac rhythm	CNS, autonomic, cardiacpulmonary insufficiency, myocardial infarction
VII. Salivation	A. Excessive secretion of saliva: hair around mouth becomes wet	Autonomic
VIII. Piloerection	A. Contraction of erectile tissue of hair follicles resulting in rough hair	Autonomic
IX. Analgesia	A. Decrease in reaction to induced pain (e.g., hot plate)	Sensory, CNS
X. Muscle tone	A. Hypotonia: generalized decrease in muscle tone	Autonomic
	B. Hypertonia: generalized increase in muscle tension	Autonomic
XI. Gastrointestinal signs: dropping (feces)	A. Solid, dried, and scant	Autonomic, constipation, GI motility
	B. Loss of fluid, watery stool	Autonomic, diarrhea, GI motility
Emesis	A. Vomiting and retching	Sensory, CNS, autonomic (in rat, emesis is absent)
Diuresis	A. Red urine (Hematuria)	Damage in kidney
	B. Involuntary urination	Autonomic, sensory
XII. Skin	A. Edema: swelling of tissue filled with fluid	Irritation, renal failure, tissue damage, long term immobility
	B. Erythema: redness of skin	Irritation, inflammation, sensitization

From Chan, P.K. and Hayes, A.W., Principles and methods for acute toxicity and eye irritancy, in *Principles and Methods of Toxicology,* 2nd ed., Raven Press, New York, 1989.[5] With permission.

TABLE 2.31
Autonomic Signs

Sympathomimetic	Piloerection
	Partial mydriasis
Sympathetic block	Ptosis
	Diagnostic if associated with sedation
Parasympathomimetic	Salivation (examined by holding blotting paper)

TABLE 2.31 *(Continued)*
Autonomic Signs

	Miosis
	Diarrhea
	Chromodacryorrhea in rats
Parasympathomimetic block	Mydriasis (maximal)
	Excessive dryness of mouth (detect with blotting paper)

From Chan, P.K. and Hayes, A.W., Principles and methods for acute toxicity and eye irritancy, in *Principles and Methods of Toxicology*, 2nd ed., Raven Press, New York, 1989.[5] With permission.

TABLE 2.32
Toxic Signs of Acetylcholinesterase Inhibition

Muscarinic Effects[a]	Nicotinic Effects[b]	CNS Effects[c]
Bronchoconstriction	Muscular twitching	Giddiness
Increased bronchosecretion	Fasciculation	Anxiety
Nausea and vomiting (absent	Cramping	Insomnia
in rats)	Muscular weakness	Nightmares
Diarrhea		Headache
Bradycardia		Apathy
Hypotension		Depression
Miosis		Drowsiness
Urinary incontinence		Confusion
		Ataxia
		Coma
		Depressed reflex
		Seizure
		Respiratory depression

[a] Blocked by atropine.

[b] Not blocked by atropine.

[c] Atropine might block early signs.

From Chan, P.K. and Hayes, A.W., Principles and methods for acute toxicity and eye irritancy, in *Principles and Methods* of *Toxicology*, 2nd ed., Raven Press, New York, 1989.[5] With permission.

B. FORMULAS/METHODS FOR CALCULATING ED_{50}

1. Standard Acute Toxicity Study

The following methods are generally used for calculating ED_{50} (LD_{50}) values for acute toxicity studies in rodents: Finney (1971);[6] Litchfield and Wilcoxon (1949);[7] Miller and Tainter (1944).[8]

2. Up-and-Down Study

The following is used for the up-and-down toxicity study (Bruce[1]). The ED_{50} is computed by following the procedure on pages 386–388 of *Introduction to Statistical Analysis,* Dixon, W.J. and Massay, F.J., 3rd ed., McGraw-Hill, New York, 1969, (presented below with permission). Note that in applying the formula, X_f should be the logarithm of the final dose and d is the logarithm of m. The result of applying the formula is the logarithm of the ED_{50}. The antilogarithm of this result is the ED_{50}.

STATISTICAL ANALYSIS FOR N SMALL

In analyses of measured response the usual t test and analysis-of-variance procedures are widely used for (1) comparing mean response between two or more groups and (2) separating the components of variation due to the design variables of an experiment by the use of factorial designs, Latin squares, and so on. The same analyses are desirable when the basic measurement is an all-or-none response. Such comparisons or analyses can more easily be made from shorter series of trials.

The method given in Sec. 19.3 provides estimates of μ and σ for a long series of trials, and a satisfactory estimate of μ can be obtained by that method for series of as few as 10 or 15 trials when the starting level is not too far from the mean. However, even shorter series are desirable when the elapsed time for observing the response is long or when several series are to be tested concurrently, with each series at some different level of an associated variable. For very short series the estimate of μ is somewhat dependent on the starting level, and if a predetermined number of tests are performed the standard error of the mean will also depend on the starting level.

This section presents a modified up-and-down estimate of μ which is almost independent of the choice of starting level and has a smaller and uniform standard error. This is accomplished by allowing the sample size to vary slightly, depending on the outcome of the first few trials, and by using the list of estimates provided in Table 19-3 for each particular sequence of results.

The trials are performed in the same up-and-down manner described in the first sections of this chapter, except that the testing continues for a total number of tests N' performed in each series, which is determined by choosing a "nominal" sample size N. This nominal N is the total number of trials reduced by one less than the number of like responses at the beginning of the series.

EXAMPLE 19-3. A test-series shown in Fig. 19-4 with the outcome $\bigcirc$, X, X, $\bigcirc$, X, $\bigcirc$ has $N' = 6$. Since the response changed after the first trial, N is also 6. For the series $\bigcirc$, $\bigcirc$, $\bigcirc$, X, X, $\bigcirc$, X, $\bigcirc$, where there are three like responses at the beginning, we have $N' = 8$ and $N = 6$.

We obtain several estimates of P_{10} with equal standard errors by continuing testing in each series so that each series is of the same nominal sample size. If, for example, we wish the standard error of P_{10} to be .56σ, we see from Table 19-3 that a nominal sample of size 6 is required. Thus four additional observations will be needed after the first reversal of response. For example, a sequence starting $\bigcirc$, X, or $\bigcirc$, $\bigcirc$, X, or $\bigcirc$, $\bigcirc$, $\bigcirc$, X, and so on, or X, $\bigcirc$, or X, X, $\bigcirc$, and so on would be followed by four more observations.

The resulting configuration of responses and nonresponses for each series is referred to in Table 19-3, and we compute

$$X_i + kd$$

where X_i = the last dose administered; k = the tabular value; d = the interval between dose levels.

Table 19-3 lists all solutions for all N' and for $N \leq 6$. If the series begins with more than four like responses, that is, $N' - N > 3$, the entry in the final column of Table 19-3 may be used (except for five tabular entries where an additional increment in the third decimal place is indicated). The estimate for Example 19-3 is $P_{10} = 0.602 + (.831 \times .301) = 852$.

For N greater than 6, P_{10} may be estimated by computing for the last N trials the mean of the test levels corrected by a factor which is dependent on the constants A and C of Table 19-4. The estimate is

$$\frac{\Sigma X_i}{N} + \frac{d}{N}(A+C)$$

where the X_i's are the test levels and A and C are obtained from Table 19-4. In Table 19-4 n_0 refers to the number of $\bigcirc$'s and n_x to the number of X's in the final N trials. The standard error of this estimated mean is approximately $\sigma\sqrt{2/N}$. The additional adjustment C, which improves this estimate, particularly for the smaller sample sizes, is based on the initial trials. This adjustment has little effect except in a few cases with small probability of occurrence, that is, where there are great differences of the number of X's and $\bigcirc$'s in the final N trials and where the series starts with a compensating run of $\bigcirc$'s or X's, respectively. If the use of this adjustment has any appreciable effect on the estimate it is advisable to investigate the possible disagreement of the experimental situation with the assumptions of this model; for example, the assumption that the interval may be very much smaller than σ or that the sampling is not all from the same population.

Log dose	Results of tests
1.204	×
.903	○ × ×
.602	○ ○
.301	
0	

FIGURE 19-4
Results of six tests in an up-down experiment.

TABLE 19-3

Values of k for estimating P_{50} from up-and-down sequence of trials of nominal length N. The estimate of P_{50} is $X_f + kd$, where X_f is the final test level and d is the interval between dose levels. If the table is entered from the foot, the sign of k is to be reversed.

Sample Size N	Second part of series	k For Test Series Whose First Part Is ○	○○	○○○	○○○○	Second part of series	Standard Error of P_{50}
2	×	−.500	−.388	−.378	−.377	○	.55σ
3	× ○	.842	.890	.894	.894	○ ×	.76σ
	× ×	−.178	.000	.026	.028	○ ○	
4	× ○ ○	.299	.314	.315	.315	○ × ×	.67σ
	× ○ ×	−.500	−.439	−.432	−.432	○ × ○	
	× × ○	1.000	1.122	1.139	1.140	○ ○ ×	
	× × ×	.194	.449	.500	.506	○ ○ ○	
5	× ○ ○○	−.157	−.154	−.154	−.154	○× × ×	.61σ
	× ○ ○ ×	−.878	−.861	−.860	−.860	○ × × ○	
	× ○ × ○	.701	.737	.741	.741	○ × ○ ×	
	× ○ × ×	.084	.169	.181	.182	○ × ○ ○	
	× × ○ ○	.305	.372	.380	.381	○ ○ × ×	
	× × ○ ×	−.305	−.169	−.144	−.142	○ ○ × ○	
	× × × ○	1.288	1.500	1.544	1.549	○ ○ ○ ×	
	× × × ×	.555	.897	.985	1.000^{+1}	○ ○ ○ ○	
6	× ○ ○ ○ ○	−.547	−.547	−.547	−.547	○ × × × ×	.36σ
	× ○ ○ ○ ×	−1.250	−1.247	−1.246	−1.246	○ × × ×○	
	× ○ ○ × ○	.372	.380	.381	.381	○ × ×○ ×	
	× ○ ○ × ×	−.169	−.144	−.142	−.142	○ × × ○ ○	
	× ○ × ○ ○	.022	.039	.040	.040	○ × ○ × ×	
	× ○ × ○ ×	−.500	−.458	−.453	−.453	○ × ○ × ○	
	× ○ × × ○	1.169	1.237	1.247	1.248	○ × ○ ○ ×	
	× ○ × × ×	.611	.732	.756	.758	○ × ○ ○ ○	
	× × ○ ○ ○	−.296	−.266	−.263	−.263	○ ○ × × ×	
	× × ○ ○ ×	−.831	−.763	−.753	−.752	○ ○ × ×○	
	× × ○ × ○	.831	.935	.952	.954	○ ○ × ○ ×	
	× × ○ × ×	.296	.463	.500	$.504^{+1}$	○ ○ × ○ ○	
	× × × ○ ○	.500	.648	.678	.681	○ ○ ○ × ×	
	× × × ○ ×	−.043	.187	.244	$.252^{+1}$	○ ○ ○ × ○	
	× × × × ○	1.603	1.917	2.000	2.014^{+1}	○ ○ ○ ○ ×	
	× × × × ×	.893	1.329	1.465	1.496^{+1}	○ ○ ○ ○ ○	
		×	××	×××	××××	Second part of series	
		$-k$ For Series Whose First Part Is					

The estimates are given in Table 19-3 for each possible configuration of responses, with the assumption that the proportion of successes is given by a normal cumulative distribution. For estimates as given in Table 19-3 it is assumed that $d = \sigma$. Fortunately, estimates for this design with $N \geq 3$ prove to have standard errors which depend very little on the actual value of σ and, in addition, are almost independent of the starting level and of μ. This is approximately true even when the spacing d differs from σ.

TABLE **19-4**

Values of A and C for approximate estimate of P^{50} for $N > 6$. The estimate is $\Sigma N_x \cdot d(A + C)/N$, where the X_x's are the test levels of the final N trials with $n_\bigcirc$ nonresponses and n_x responses and d is the interval between dose levels. $C = 0$ for a series whose first part is a single $\bigcirc$ or $\times$.

$n_\bigcirc - n_x$	A	$\bigcirc\bigcirc$	$\bigcirc\bigcirc\bigcirc$	$\bigcirc\bigcirc\bigcirc\bigcirc$	$\bigcirc\bigcirc\bigcirc\bigcirc\bigcirc$
		C For Test Series Whose First Part Is			
5	10.8	0	0	0	0
4	7.72	0	0	0	0
3	5.22	.03	.03	.03	.03
2	3.20	.10	.10	.10	.10
1	1.53	.16	.17	.17	.17
0	0	.44	.48	.48	.48
−1	−1.55	.55	.65	.65	.65
−2	−3.30	1.14	1.36	1.38	1.38
−3	−5.22	1.77	2.16	2.22	2.22
−4	−7.55	2.48	3.36	3.52	3.56
−5	−10.3	3.5	4.8	5.2	5.3
$n_x - n_\bigcirc$	−A	$\times\times$	$\times\times\times$	$\times\times\times\times$	$\times\times\times\times\times$
		−C For Test Series Whose First Part Is			

C. HISTORICAL CONTROL DATA — RODENT BODY WEIGHTS AND FOOD CONSUMPTION

The following are representative mean values from several chronic studies conducted in our laboratory. (Age at week − 1 is approximately 5 weeks.)

TABLE 2.33
Body Weight and Food Consumption — CD-1 Mice

Week	Males Body Weight (g)	Males Food Consumption (g/kg/day)	Females Body Weight (g)	Females Food Consumption (g/kg/day)
−1	23.64	—	19.24	—
0	27.46	235.55	21.62	293.20
1	28.82	212.60	22.66	267.00
2	30.00	198.36	24.24	262.42
3	31.02	196.14	24.80	273.80
4	31.92	196.60	25.92	252.74
5	32.46	182.76	26.32	269.70
6	33.36	181.46	27.06	245.48

TABLE 2.33 *(Continued)*
Body Weight and Food Consumption — CD-1 Mice

	Males		Females	
Week	Body Weight (g)	Food Consumption (g/kg/day)	Body Weight (g)	Food Consumption (g/kg/day)
7	34.44	170.20	27.80	247.56
8	34.40	180.72	27.96	240.86
9	34.88	169.70	28.50	222.38
10	35.08	166.00	28.90	216.24
11	35.36	166.90	29.26	211.50
12	36.14	153.94	29.34	209.74
13–14	36.30	166.34	29.80	218.14
17–18	37.62	146.16	30.98	209.00
21–22	38.00	152.86	31.54	204.54
25–26	38.24	153.40	32.28	190.88
27–30	38.40	149.40	32.30	190.95
31–34	39.40	134.50	33.12	177.30
35–38	39.66	135.48	33.48	166.90
39–42	40.26	136.42	33.28	180.42
43–46	40.03	131.80	34.10	165.70
47–50	40.40	126.46	34.34	156.52
51–54	39.90	128.72	35.10	149.16
55–58	40.16	135.80	34.46	173.96
59–62	39.80	137.88	35.20	158.84
63–66	40.46	133.70	34.76	172.72
67–70	40.24	133.18	34.78	161.12
71–74	39.88	142.22	35.14	167.62
75–79	40.56	142.66	35.48	171.02

TABLE 2.34
Body Weight and Food Consumption — Sprague-Dawley Rats

	Males		Females	
Week	Body Weight (g)	Food Consumption (g/kg/day)	Body Weight (g)	Food Consumption (g/kg/day)
−1	132.46	—	103.82	—
0	188.64	146.00	139.14	122.30
1	236.12	115.98	161.56	122.58
2	286.94	101.12	182.80	111.00
3	327.78	90.28	203.46	104.30
4	362.78	82.02	222.10	94.04
5	393.70	75.12	232.70	87.44
6	417.26	68.98	243.04	84.82
7	432.70	63.32	250.68	77.12
8	446.16	62.08	255.40	76.44
9	457.80	58.44	261.36	73.40
10	475.74	60.96	268.62	75.84
11	481.42	57.14	274.52	73.34
12	497.12	59.78	278.24	73.26
13	508.12	56.14	282.46	70.68

TABLE 2.34 *(Continued)*
Body Weight and Food Consumption — Sprague-Dawley Rats

Week	Males Body Weight (g)	Males Food Consumption (g/kg/day)	Females Body Weight (g)	Females Food Consumption (g/kg/day)
17–18	549.84	50.30	299.70	67.42
21–22	577.62	47.62	311.82	63.30
25–26	603.22	45.04	327.22	62.18
29–30	616.76	44.36	334.22	61.84
33–34	635.46	43.94	348.96	61.74
37–38	651.96	42.60	363.38	58.44
41–42	660.34	41.12	374.96	56.40
45–46	678.16	40.12	389.65	52.63
49–50	695.72	39.24	409.40	52.34
53–54	703.72	39.20	412.76	51.28
57–58	720.88	37.70	430.90	49.16
61–62	728.74	37.56	441.18	48.82
65–66	735.76	38.00	455.06	48.26
69–70	735.04	38.46	460.24	48.24
72–74	737.54	37.80	465.70	47.78
77–78	736.58	39.34	467.70	46.78
81–82	738.04	38.48	471.72	47.74
85–86	733.70	39.22	473.98	47.38
89–90	725.80	38.52	479.42	47.82
93–94	723.62	37.92	490.06	45.68
97–98	721.50	37.48	494.10	45.04
101–102	703.84	35.60	498.56	44.10

TABLE 2.35
Body Weight and Food Consumption — Fischer 344 Rats

Week	Males Body Weight (g)	Males Food Consumption (g/kg/day)	Females Body Weight (g)	Females Food Consumption (g/kg/day)
−1	86.03	—	68.43	—
0	118.27	137.73	89.90	146.93
1	151.50	112.73	108.07	124.63
2	183.60	99.33	123.70	107.00
3	211.07	85.73	135.70	96.43
4	228.17	77.73	142.80	90.93
5	244.10	75.07	150.60	89.03
6	256.27	67.13	155.77	80.47
7	263.53	63.07	162.07	72.73
8	275.23	60.40	164.40	69.67
9	281.90	56.17	166.47	68.20
10	290.47	54.20	170.20	66.27
11	296.60	55.63	172.23	67.40
12	300.23	54.40	173.07	69.10
13	301.10	54.25	174.75	64.10
16	319.07	51.10	181.53	65.63

TABLE 2.35 *(Continued)*
Body Weight and Food Consumption — Fischer 344 Rats

Week	Males		Females	
	Body Weight (g)	Food Consumption (g/kg/day)	Body Weight (g)	Food Consumption (g/kg/day)
20	331.67	48.17	186.87	62.63
24	343.40	47.97	193.67	62.07
28–30	355.70	46.67	201.90	59.87
32–34	366.23	45.33	206.70	60.00
36–38	374.67	44.23	211.37	61.10
40–42	382.90	44.07	215.40	58.27
44–46	384.13	42.63	218.90	56.00
48–50	385.90	38.17	223.53	57.07
52–54	396.23	44.17	228.47	57.37
56–59	400.87	43.57	236.17	55.23
60–62	401.90	40.97	241.47	50.63
64–66	404.87	43.77	246.37	53.43
68–70	406.57	44.37	253.80	54.60
72–74	410.20	43.67	259.53	54.57
76–78	404.93	46.00	265.07	54.77
80–82	394.77	43.60	262.80	51.50
84–86	393.60	43.37	264.47	50.37
88–90	397.07	43.73	270.70	51.50
92–94	391.43	42.93	275.13	50.83
96–98	388.77	42.47	277.17	49.63
100–102	388.03	43.33	277.70	51.57

D. Effect of Decreased Body Weights on Organ Weights of Rats

TABLE 2.36
Effect of Decreased Body Weights on Relative Organ Weights[a] of Rats[b]

Decrease	No Change	Increase
Liver (?)	Heart	Adrenal glands (?)
	Kidneys	Brain
	Prostate	Epididymides
	Spleen	Pituitary
	Ovaries	Testes
		Thyroid (?)
		Uterus

[a] Relative weights = organ/body weight ratios (?)
? = Differences slight or inconsistent.
[b] For absolute weights, all except thyroids decrease.
Summary of results reported in: Schwartz, E. R. et al.,[10] Scharer, K.[11]

E. Rodent Survival Rates

TABLE 2.37
Monthly Survival Rates of Untreated CD-1 Mice in Chronic Toxicity Studies Conducted Between 1985 and 1992

Month of Study	Males Mean % Survival	±SD	No. of Studies	Females Mean % Survival	±SD	No. of Studies
1	99.7	0.7	21	99.9	0.4	20
2	99.6	0.8	21	99.7	0.7	20
3	99.2	1.3	21	99.5	0.9	20
4	98.7	1.5	21	99.4	0.9	20
5	98.1	1.6	21	99.4	0.9	20
6	97.8	1.5	21	99.0	1.5	20
7	97.4	1.6	21	98.4	1.9	20
8	96.6	2.2	21	98.1	1.9	20
9	95.7	2.6	21	97.5	2.0	20
10	94.8	3.2	21	96.9	2.0	20
11	93.4	3.2	21	96.0	2.3	20
12	92.6	3.7	21	95.1	3.4	20
13	89.5	7.0	21	92.9	4.3	20
14	86.7	7.5	21	90.0	4.3	20
15	83.1	7.5	21	87.3	4.3	20
16	76.8	9.0	21	81.9	6.3	20
17	69.4	10.6	21	76.0	7.8	20
18	59.7	12.9	21	67.0	10.4	20

TABLE 2.38
Eighteen-Month Survival Rates of Untreated CD-1 Mice in Chronic Toxicity Studies Between 1985 and 1992

Study Code	Route of Administration	Termination Date	Supplier[a]	Survivorship[b] Male Incidence	%	Female Incidence	%
A	Diet	3/87	CR-K	26/48	54	27/49	55
B	Diet	6/87	CR-K	30/50	60	32/50	64
C	Diet	1/88	CR-K	38/65	58	46/65	71
D	Diet	3/88	CR-K	27/50	54	33/50	66
E	Diet	4/88	CR-K	46/69	67	56/69	81
F	Gavage	11/88	CR-K	38/66	58	33/67	49
G	Diet	1/89	CR-K	24/47	51	26/47	55
H	Diet	8/89	CR-K	33/49	67	27/46	59
I	Diet	1/90	CR-K	32/50	64	28/45	62
J	Diet	3/90	CR-K	30/48	63	—	—
K	Gavage	4/90	CR-K	25/59	43	42/59	71
M	Diet	7/90	CR-K	35/51	68	39/50	78
N	Diet	12/90	CR-K	25/50	50	31/49	63
O	IM	1/91	CR-K	19/48	40	25/49	51

TABLE 2.38 *(Continued)*
Eighteen-Month Survival Rates of Untreated CD-1 Mice in Chronic Toxicity Studies Between 1985 and 1992

Study Code	Route of Administration	Termination Date	Supplier[a]	Survivorship[b]			
				Male		Female	
				Incidence	%	Incidence	%
P	Diet	8/91	CR-P	37/50	74	36/50	72
Q	Diet	9/91	CR-P	46/50	92	42/50	84
R	Diet	4/92	CR-K	24/50	48	34/49	69
S	Diet	5/92	CR-K	32/50	64	30/50	60
T	Diet	6/92	CR-K	26/60	43	49/60	82
U	Diet	9/92	CR-K	28/50	56	38/48	79
V	Diet	11/92	CR-K	39/48	81	33/49	67

[a] Supplier: CR-K, Charles Rive-Kingston, NY, CR-P, Charles River-Portage, MI.
[b] Animals killed accidentally were excluded from calculations of survivorship.

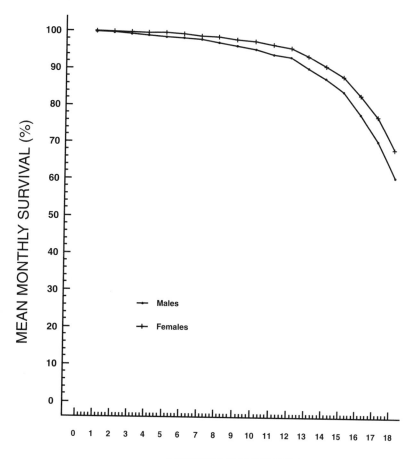

FIGURE 2.3 Mean monthly survival — mice.

TABLE 2.39
Monthly Survival Rates of Untreated Sprague-Dawley
Rats in Chronic Toxicity Studies Conducted Between
1984 and 1992

Month of Study	Males			Females		
	Mean % Survival	±SD	No. of Studies	Mean % Survival	±SD	No. of Studies
1	99.8	0.6	19	99.8	0.6	19
2	99.4	1.0	19	99.8	0.6	19
3	99.1	1.3	19	99.7	1.0	19
4	98.9	1.4	19	99.5	1.1	19
5	98.6	1.9	19	99.4	1.1	19
6	98.1	2.1	19	99.1	1.4	19
7	97.7	2.1	19	99.1	1.4	19
8	97.2	2.1	19	98.8	1.4	19
9	96.9	2.1	19	98.2	1.9	19
10	96.5	2.0	19	97.8	2.1	19
11	95.3	2.6	19	97.1	2.7	19
12	94.5	3.2	19	96.2	3.0	19
13	93.2	4.3	19	94.9	3.2	19
14	91.9	4.0	19	93.5	3.7	19
15	89.9	5.1	19	91.2	4.4	19
16	86.4	6.5	19	88.8	5.0	19
17	82.9	7.6	19	84.5	6.3	19
18	78.5	8.7	19	80.6	7.7	19
19	72.0	9.9	19	74.4	7.9	19
20	66.4	9.7	19	68.9	9.7	19
21	57.8	9.0	18	61.7	11.2	19
22	50.3	9.9	18	56.5	12.2	19
23	43.0	10.6	18	49.7	12.7	19
24	34.7	8.9	18	42.3	12.2	19

TABLE 2.40
Twenty-Four-Month Survival Rates of Untreated Sprague-Dawley Rats in
Chronic Toxicity Studies Conducted Between 1984 and 1992

Study Code	Route of Administration	Termination Date	Supplier[a]	Survivorship[b]			
				Male		Female	
				Incidence	%	Incidence	%
DD	Diet	7/86	CR-P	27/55	49	22/55	40
EE	Diet	7/86	CR-P	20/70	29	31/70	44
FF	Diet	10/86	CR-K	20/55	36	25/55	45
GG	Diet	12/87	CR-P	20/63	32	31/63	49
HH	Diet	1/88	CR-K	21/50	42	21/50	42
II	Diet	3/88	CR-K	15/50	30	24/50	48
JJ	Diet	5/88	CR-P	27/60	45	28/50	56
KK	Gavage	11/88	CR-K	20/60	33	19/60	32
LL	Diet	4/89	CR-K	21/55	38	24/54	44
MM	Gavage	10/89	CR-K	17/60	28	14/60	23

TABLE 2.40 *(Continued)*
Twenty-Four-Month Survival Rates of Untreated Sprague-Dawley Rats in Chronic Toxicity Studies Conducted Between 1984 and 1992

Study Code	Route of Administration	Termination Date	Supplier[a]	Male Incidence	%	Female Incidence	%
NN	Diet	11/89	CR-K	22/52	42	23/50	46
OO	Diet	7/90	CR-K	20/52	38	19/54	35
PP	Diet	8/90	CR-K	17/53	32	21/52	40
QQ	IntraMuscular	12/91	CR-K	—	—	41/50	82
RR	Diet	5/92	CR-K	21/50	42	21/50	42
SS	Diet	4/92	CR-K	7/46	15	16/50	32
TT	Diet	10/92	CR-K	26/58	45	22/60	37
UU	Diet	11/92	CR-K	13/60	22	21/60	35
VV	Diet	12/92	CR-K	13/49	27	17/50	34

[a] Supplier: CR-K, Charles River-Kingston, NY; CR-P, Charles River-Portage, MI.
[b] Animals killed accidentally were excluded from calculations of survivorship.

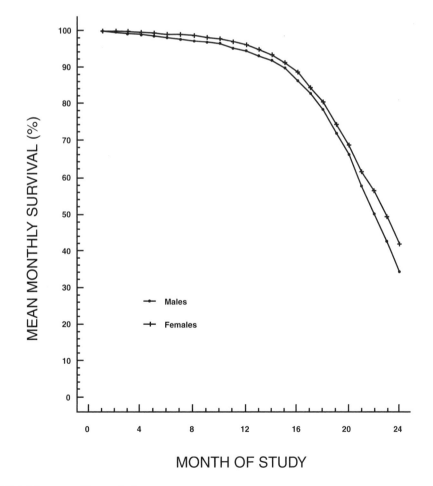

FIGURE 2.4 Mean monthly survival — rats.

REFERENCES

1. Bruce, R.D., An up-and-down procedure for acute toxicity testing, *Fund Appl. Toxicol.,* 5, 151, 1985.
2. *SYNAPSE,* American Society of Laboratory Animal Practitioners, Vol. 24, 1991.
3. *Laboratory Manual For Basic Biomethodology of Laboratory Animals,* MTM Associates, Inc.
4. Freireich, E.J. et al., Quantitative comparison of toxicity of anti-cancer agents in mouse, rat, dog, monkey and man, *Cancer Chemother. Rep.,* 50, 219, 1966.
5. Chan, P.K. and Hayes, A.W., Principles and methods for acute toxicity and eye irritancy, in *Principles and Methods of Toxicology,* 2nd ed., Hayes, A.W., Ed., Raven Press, New York, 1989.
6. Finney, D.J., *Probit Analysis,* 3rd ed., Cambridge University Press, London, 1971.
7. Litchfield, J.T. and Wilcoxon, F., A simplified method for evaluating dose-effect experiments, *J. Pharmacol. Erp. Ther.,* 96, 99, 1949.
8. Miller, L.C. and Tainter, M.L., Estimation of the ED_{50} and its error by means of logarithmic-probit graph paper, *Proc. Soc. Exp. Biol. Med.,* 57, 261, 1944.
9. Dixon, W.J. and Massay, M.J., Eds., *Introduction to Statistical Analysis,* 3rd ed., McGraw-Hill, New York, 1969.
10. Schwartz, E., Tomaben, J.A., and Boxill, G.C., The effects of food restriction on hematology, clinical chemistry and pathology in the albino rat, *Toxicol. Appl. Parmacol.,* 25, 515, 1973.
11. Scharer, K., The effect of underfeeding on organ weights of rats. How to interpret organ weight changes in cases of marked growth retardation in toxicity tests, *Toxicol.,* 7, 45, 1977.

3 Dermal Irritation and Sensitization

Kimberly L. Bonnette, M.S., L.A.T.G.,
Dawn D. Rodabaugh, B.S., and
Christopher W. Wilson, B.S.

CONTENTS

0-8493-0370-2/02/$0.00+$1.50
© 2002 by CRC Press LLC

SECTION 1. COMPARISON OF MAJOR STUDY DESIGNS

TABLE 3.1
Comparison of Dermal Irritation Study Designs[1-5]

Category	EPA-OPPTS (870.2500)
Number of animals	At least three healthy adults
Species	Albino rabbit recommended
Preliminary screens	May not test if: pH $\leq$ 2, $\geq$ 11.5, dermal LD_{50} < 200 mg/kg, dermal limit test at 2000 mg/kg did not produce irritation, a validated and accepted *in vitro* test demonstrates corrosive properties, or corrosive potential is predicted from structure–activity relationships.
Control group	None required
Preparation of skin	Clip or shave $\approx$ 24 hr before test
	Use only healthy, intact skin
Application site	Dorsal area of trunk
Application area	$\approx$ 6 cm^2
Patch types	Gauze patch held loosely in contact with skin using nonirritating tape
Occlusion	Semiocclusive dressing
Preparation of test substance	Solids: pulverized if necessary, moistened sufficiently with water or suitable vehicle to ensure good skin contact
	Liquids: generally used undiluted
Dose level	Solids: 0.5 g
	Liquids: 0.5 ml
Exposure interval	4 h (3 min, 1 h if corrosion is anticipated)
No. of applications	One
Test substance residue removal	Water or another appropriate solvent
Observation intervals	30–60 min, 24, 48, and 72 h after patch removal
Minimum observation period	72 h
Maximum observation period	14 days

Category	Japanese-MAFF (Current)	Japanese-MAFF (Draft)
Number of animals	At least six young adults	At least three young adults
Species	Albino rabbit	White rabbit
Preliminary screens	May not test if: pH $\leq$ 2, $\geq$ 11.5	May not test if: pH $\leq$ 2, $\geq$ 11.5
Control group	None required	None required
Preparation of skin	Clip or shave $\approx$ 24 hr before test	Clip $\approx$ 24 hr before test
		Use only healthy, intact skin
Application site	Dorsal area of trunk	Dorsal area of trunk
Application area	$\approx$ 6 cm^2	$\approx$ 6 cm^2
Patch types	Gauze patch held loosely in contact with skin using nonirritating tape	Gauze patch held in contact with skin using nonirritating tape
Occlusion	Semiocclusive dressing preferred; occlusive may be appropriate	Semiocclusive dressing preferred; occlusive may be appropriate
Preparation of test substance	Solids: Pulverized if necessary, moistened sufficiently with water or suitable vehicle	Solids: crushed if necessary, moistened thoroughly with water or suitable vehicle to ensure good skin contact
	Liquids: Generally used undiluted	Liquids: Applied undiluted
Dose level	Solids: 0.5 g	Solids: 0.5 g
	Liquids: 0.5 ml	Liquids: 0.5 ml

TABLE 3.1 *(Continued)*
Comparison of Dermal Irritation Study Designs[1-5]

Category	Japanese-MAFF (Current)	Japanese-MAFF (Draft)
Exposure interval	4 h	4 h (3 min, 1 h, 4 h to the first animal if severe potential irritation/corrosion is anticipated)
No. of applications	One	One
Test substance residue removal	Water or another appropriate solvent	Water or another appropriate solvent
Observation intervals	30–60 min, 24, 48, and 72 h after patch removal	30 or 60 min, 24, 48, and 72 h after patch removal
Minimum observation period	72 h	72 h
Maximum observation period	14 days	14 days

Category	European-OECD	European-EEC
Number of animals	Generally three healthy adults, one animal may sometimes be used	At least three healthy adults, one animal may sometimes be used
Species	Albino rabbit recommended	Albino rabbit recommended
Preliminary screens	Do not test if: pH ≤ 2, ≥ 11.5, material is highly toxic by dermal route, dermal limit test at 2000 mg/kg did not produce irritation, *in vitro* test indicate corrosive properties	Do not test if: pH ≤ 2, ≥ 11.5, material is highly toxic by dermal route, dermal limit test at 2000 mg/kg did not produce irritation, *in vitro* test indicate corrosive properties
Control group	None required	None required
Preparation of skin	Closely clip ≈ 24 h before test; use only healthy, intact skin	Clip or shave ≈ 24 h before test; use only healthy, intact skin
Application site	Dorsal area of trunk	Dorsal area of trunk
Application area	≈ 6 cm^2	≈ 6 cm^2
Patch types	Gauze patch held loosely in contact with skin using nonirritating tape	Gauze patch held loosely in contact with skin using nonirritating tape
Occlusion	Semiocclusive	Semi-occlusive or occlusive
Preparation of test substance	Solids: Pulverized if necessary, moistened with smallest amount of water or suitable vehicle to ensure good skin contact	Solids: Pulverized if necessary, moistened sufficiently with water or suitable vehicle to ensure good skin contact
	Liquids: Applied undiluted	Liquids: Applied undiluted
Dose level	Solids: 0.5 g	Solids: 0.5 g
	Liquids: 0.5 ml	Liquids: 0.5 ml
Exposure interval	4 h, may be reduced to 1 h or 3 min	4 h, may be reduced to 1 h or 3 min
No. of applications	One	One
Test substance residue removal	Water or another appropriate solvent	Water or another appropriate solvent
Observation intervals	60 min, 24, 48, and 72 h after patch removal	60 min, 24, 48, and 72 h after patch removal
Minimum observation period	72 h	72 h
Maximum observation period	Not indicated	14 days

TABLE 3.2
Comparison of Sensitization Study Designs.[6–11]

Category	EPA OPPTS 870.2600	Japanese-MHW
Acceptable test methods	Buehler Test,[a] Guinea Pig Maximization Test (GPMT),[a] Open Epicutaneous Test, Mauer Optimization Test, Split Adjuvant Technique, Freund's Complete Adjuvant Test, Draize Sensitization Test	Adjuvant and Patch Test; Buehler Test;[a] Draize Test; Freund's Complete Adjuvant Test; Maximization Test;[a] Open Optimization Test; Split Adjuvant Test
Species	Guinea pig	Guinea pig
Number and sex	Dependent on method used	Dependent on method used
Control animals	Periodic (every 6 months) use of a positive control substance with an acceptable level of reliability for the test system selected is recommended; irritation controls may or may not be used	Positive controls are required; preferred substances include p-phenylenediamine, 1-chloro-2,4-dinitrobenzene, neomycin sulfate, and nickel sulfate
Dose level	Dependent on method used	Dependent on method used
Preparation of skin	Clipping, shaving, or depilation depending on method used	Dependent on method used
Observation of animals	Skin reactions are to be graded and recorded after the challenge exposure at the time specified by the methodology selected (usually 24, 48, and 72 h)	Skin reactions are to be noted at 24, 48, or 72 h after challenge exposure
Body weights	Initial and terminal body weights required	Initial and terminal body weights required

Category	Japanese-MAFF (current)	Japanese-MAFF (draft)
Acceptable test methods	Draize Test, Freund's Complete Adjuvant Test, Mauer Optimization Test, Buehler Test,[a] Open Epicutaneous Test, Guinea Pig Maximization Test,[a] Split Adjuvant Technique	Buehler Test,[a] Guinea Pig Maximization Test,[a] other methods may be used provided that they are well validated and scientific justification is given
Species	Guinea pig	Guinea pig
Number and sex	Dependent on method used	Dependent on method used
Control animals	Use of a positive control substance for the reliability of the test system selected is recommended	Positive control are required to evaluate the responsivity of the test system
Dose level	Dependent on method used	Dependent on method used
Preparation of skin	Dependent on method used	Dependent on method used
Observation of animals	Dependent on method used	Skin reactions are to be graded and recorded after the challenge exposure at the time specified by the methodology selected (usually 24, 48, and 72 h)
Body weights	Initial and terminal body weights required	Initial and terminal body weights required

Category	European-OECD	European-EEC
Acceptable test methods	Buehler Test,[a] Guinea Pig Maximization Test,[a] other methods may be used provided that they are well validated and scientific justification is given	Buehler Test,[a] Guinea Pig Maximization Test,[a] other methods may be used provided that they are well validated and scientific justification is given
Species	Guinea pig	Guinea pig
Number and sex	Dependent on method used	Dependent on method used

TABLE 3.2 *(Continued)*
Comparison of Sensitization Study Designs.[6-11]

Category	European—OECD	European—EEC
Control animals	Mild-to-moderate positive controls are required every 6 months (response of at least 30% in an adjuvant test and 15% in a nonadjuvant test should be expected); preferred substances are hexylcinnamicaldehyde, mercaptobenzothiazol, and benzocaine; others are accepted with justification	Mild-to-moderate positive controls are required every 6 months (response of at least 30% in an adjuvant test and 15% in a nonadjuvant test should be expected); preferred substances are phenylenediamine, 2,4-dinitrochlorobenzene, potassium dichromate, neomycin sulfate, and nickel sulfate, or others that are known sensitizing substances from the literature
Dose level	Dependent on method used	Dependent on method used
Preparation of skin	Clipping, shaving, or depilation depending on method used	Clipping, shaving, or depilation dependent on method used
Observation of animals	24 and 48 h after patch removal at challenge	All skin reactions from induction and challenge procedures should be recorded and reported
Body weights	Initial and terminal body weights required	Initial and terminal body weights required

[a] These test methods are the most widely used.

SECTION 2. COMPARISON OF REGULATORY GUIDELINES

TABLE 3.3
Quick Reference Chart for Common U.S. Test Guidelines[1-15]

Regulatory Group Dermal	Reference	Specific Section for Dermal Irritation	Specific Section for Dermal Sensitization
U.S. Environmental Protection Agency (EPA)	Health Effects Test Guidelines, August 1998	OPPTS 870.2500	OPPTS 870.2600
U.S. Consumer Product Safety Commission (CPSC)	Subchapter C—Federal Hazardous Substances Act Regulations, 16 CFR Part 1500, January 1993 (FHSA)	Section 1500.41	Section 1500.3
U.S. Department of Transportation (DOT)	49 CFR, Part 173, October 1998 (DOT)	Sections 173.136, 173.137	Not specified
U.S. Food and Drug Administration (FDA)	Toxicological Principles for the Safety Assessment of Direct Food Additives and Color Additives Used in Food, Redbook II, 1993 (FDA)	Not specified	Not specified
U.S. Pharmacopeia (USP)	The U.S. Pharmacopeia, USP24 and The National Formulary, NF 19, January 1, 2000 (USP)	Chapter 88	Not Specified

TABLE 3.4
Quick Reference Chart for Common Foreign Test Guidelines[2,4,5,7,8,10,11,16]

| | | Specific Section for | |
| | | Dermal | Dermal |
Regulatory Group	Reference	Irritation	Sensitization
Government of Canada, Environment Canada, and Health and Welfare Canada (CEPA)	Canadian Environmental Protection Act, Guidelines for the Notification and Testing of New Substances: Chemicals and Polymers, March 1993	Section 5.1	Section 5.1
European Organization for Economic Cooperation and Development (OECD)	Guidelines for Testing of Chemicals, Section 4, Health Effects, July 1992	Subsection 404	Subsection 406
European Economic Community (EEC)	Part B: Methods for the Determination of Toxicity, December 1992	No. L 383 A/124, B.4	No. L 383 A/131, B.6
Japanese Ministry of Forestry and Fisheries (MAFF)	Agricultural Chemicals Laws and Regulations, Testing Guidelines for Toxicology Studies, January 1985	pp. 25–26	pp. 27–29
Japanese Ministry of Forestry and Fisheries (MAFF)	Guidelines on the Compiling of the Results on Toxicity (draft) December 1987	pp. 9–11	pp. 16–19
Japanese Ministry of Health and Welfare (MHW)	1990 Guidelines for Toxicity Studies of Drugs Manual, September 1989	Not specified	Chap. 7, pp. 75–80

TABLE 3.5
Quick Reference Chart for Miscellaneous Test Guidelines[17–23]

Regulatory Group	Reference	Study Type
International Maritime Organization (IMO)	International Maritime Dangerous Goods Code	Dermal corrosion
Occupational Safety and Health Administration (OSHA)	OSHA's Hazard Communication Standard, 29 CFR 1900.1200, Appendix A, August 1987	Dermal irritation and sensitization
American Society for Testing and Materials (ASTM)	Annual Book of ASTM Standards, F719 (13.01), E993 (11.04), F720 (13.01)	Dermal irritation and sensitization
The Cosmetic, Toiletry and Fragrance Association, Inc. (CTFA)	CTFA Safety Testing Guidelines, Sections II and IV	Dermal irritation and sensitization

TABLE 3.6
Comparison of Excerpts from Selected Dermal Irritation Test Guidelines

EPA OPPTS 870.2500

(a) *Scope* — (1) Applicability. This guideline is intended to meet testing requirements of both the Federal Insecticide, Fungicide, and Rodenticide Act (FIFRA) (7 USC 136, *et seq.*) and the Toxic Substances Control Act (TSCA) (15 USC 2601).

(2) *Background.* The source of materials used in developing this harmonized OPPTS test guideline are 40 CFR 798.4470 Primary Dermal Irritation; OPP 81-5 Primary Dermal irritation (Pesticide Assessment Guidelines, Subdivision F — Hazard Evaluation; Human and Domestic Animals); EPA report 540/09-82-025, 1982; and OECD 404 Acute Dermal Irritation/Corrosion.

(b) *Purpose.* Determination of the irritant and/or corrosive effects on skin of mammals is useful in the assessment and evaluation of the toxic characteristics of a substance where exposure by the dermal route is likely. Information derived from this test serves to indicate the existence of possible hazards likely to arise from exposure of the skin to the substance.

(c) *Definitions.* The definitions in section 3 of TSCA and in 40 CFR Part 792 — Good Laboratory Practice Standards (GLP) apply to this test guideline. The following definitions also apply to this test guideline.

"Dermal corrosion" is the production of irreversible tissue damage in the skin following the application of a test substance.

"Dermal irritation" is the production of reversible inflammatory changes in the skin following the application of a test substance.

"Pharmacological effect" means any chemically induced physiological changes in the test animal.

"Target Organ" means any organ of a test animal showing evidence of an effect of chemical treatment.

(d) *Principle of the test methods.* (1) The substance to be tested is applied in a single dose to the skin of several experimental animals, each animal serving as its own control [except when severe irritation/corrosion is suspected and the stepwise procedure is used (see paragraph (f)(1)(iii))]. The degree of irritation is read and scored at specified intervals and is further described to provide a complete evaluation of the effects. The duration of the study should be sufficient to permit a full evaluation of the reversibility or irreversibility of the effects observed but need not exceed 14 days.

(2) When testing solids (which may be pulverized if considered necessary), the test substance should be moistened sufficiently with water or, where necessary, a suitable vehicle, to ensure good contact with the skin. When vehicles are used, the influence of the vehicle on irritation of skin by the test substance should be taken into account. Liquid test substances are generally used undiluted.

(e) *Initial considerations.* (1) Strongly acidic or alkaline substances, for example, with a demonstrated pH of 2 or less, or 11.5 or greater, need not be tested for primary dermal irritation, owing to their predictable corrosive properties.

(2) It is unnecessary to test materials which have been shown to be highly toxic (LD_{50} less than 200 mg/kg) by the dermal route or have been shown not to produce irritation of the skin at the limit test dose level of 2000 mg/kg body weight.

(3) It may not be necessary to test *in vivo* materials for which corrosive properties are predicted on the basis of results from well validated and accepted *in vitro* tests. If an *in vitro* test is performed before the *in vivo* test, a description or reference to the test, including details of the procedure, must be given together with results obtained with the test and reference substances.

(4) It may not be necessary to test materials for which corrosive potential is predicted from structure-activity relationships.

(f) *Test procedures* — (1) Animal selection — (i) *Species and strain.* The albino rabbit is recommended as the preferred species. If another mammalian species is used, the tester should provide justification/reasoning for its selection.

(ii) *Number of animals.* At least three healthy adult animals (either sex) should be used unless justification/reasoning for using fewer animals is provided. It is recommended that a stepwise procedure be used to expose one animal, followed by additional animals to clarify equivocal responses.

(iii) *Stepwise exposure of animals.* A single rabbit may be used if it is suspected that the test material might produce severe irritation/corrosion. Three test patches are applied concurrently or sequentially to the animal. The first patch is removed after 3 min. If no serious skin reaction is observed, the second patch is removed after 1 h. If observations indicate that exposure can be continued humanely, the third patch is removed after 4 h and the responses graded. If a corrosive effect is observed after an exposure of up to 4 h, then further animal testing is not required. If no corrosive effect is observed in one animal after a 4-h exposure, the test is completed using two additional animals, each with one patch only, for an exposure period of 4 h. If it is expected that the test substance will not produce severe irritancy or corrosion, the test may be started using three animals, each receiving one patch for an exposure period of 4 h.

TABLE 3.6 *(Continued)*
Comparison of Excerpts from Selected Dermal Irritation Test Guidelines

(2) *Control animals.* Separate animals are not recommended for an untreated control group. Adjacent areas of untreated skin of each animal may serve as a control for the test.

(3) *Dose level.* A dose of 0.5 ml of liquid or 500 mg of solid or semisolid is applied to the test site.

(4) *Preparation of test area.* Approximately 24 h before the test, fur should be removed from the test area by clipping or shaving from the dorsal area of the trunk of the animals. Care should be taken to avoid abrading the skin. Only animals with healthy intact skin should be used.

(5) *Application of the test substance.* (i) The recommended exposure duration is normally 4 h unless corrosion is observed [see paragraph (f)(1)(ii)]. Longer exposure may be indicated under certain conditions (e.g., expected pattern of human use and exposure). At the end of the exposure period, residual test substance should generally be removed, where practicable, using water or an appropriate solvent, without altering the existing response or the integrity of the epidermis.

(ii) When vehicles are used, the influence of the vehicle on irritation of skin by the test substance should be taken into account. If a vehicle is used, it should not alter the absorption, distribution, metabolism, retention or the chemical properties of the test substance nor should it enhance, reduce, or alter its toxic characteristics. Although water or saline is the preferred agent to be used for moistening dry test materials, other agents may be used providing the use is justified. Acceptable alternatives include: gum arabic, ethanol and water, carboxymethyl cellulose, polyethylene glycol, glycerol, vegetable oil, and mineral oil.

(iii) The test substance should be applied to a small area (approximately 6 cm^2) of skin and covered with a gauze patch, which is held in place with nonirritating tape. In the case of liquids or some pastes, it may be necessary to apply the test substance to the gauze patch and apply that to the skin. The patch should be loosely held in contact with the skin by means of a suitable semiocclusive dressing for the duration of the exposure period. Access by the animal to the patch and resultant ingestion/inhalation of the test substance should be prevented.

6. *Observation period.* The duration of the observation period need not be rigidly fixed. It should be sufficient to fully evaluate the reversibility or irreversibility of the effects observed. It need not exceed 14 days after application.

7. *Clinical examination and scoring.* (i) After removal of the patch, animals should be examined for signs of erythema and edema and the responses scored within 30–60 min, and at 24, 48, and 72 h after patch removal.

(ii) Dermal irritation should be scored and recorded according to the grades provided in the guidelines. Further observations may be needed, as necessary, to establish reversibility. In addition to the observation of irritation, any lesions and other toxic effects should be fully described.

(g) *Data and reporting* — (1) Data summary. Data should be summarized in tabular form, showing for each individual animal the irritation scores for erythema and edema at 30 to 60 min, and 24, 48, 72 h after patch removal, any other dermal lesions, a description of the degree and nature of the irritation, corrosion and reversibility, and any other toxic effects observed.

(2) *Evaluation of results.* The dermal irritation scores should be evaluated in conjunction with the nature and reversibility or otherwise of the responses observed. The individual scores do not represent an absolute standard for the irritant properties of a material. They should be viewed as reference values which are only meaningful when supported by a full description and evaluation of the observations.

(3) *Test report.* In addition to the reporting recommendations as specified under 40 CFR part 792, subpart J, the following specific information should be reported:

(i) Species, strain, sex, age, and source of test animal.

(ii) Rationale for selection of species (if species is other than the species preferred or required by the OPP toxicology data requirements for pesticide registration).

(iii) Tabulation of erythema and edema data and any other dermal lesions/responses for each individual animal at each observation time point (e.g., 30–60 min and 24, 48, 72 h until end of test/reversibility).

(iv) Description of any lesions observed.

(v) Narrative description of the degree and nature of irritation or corrosion observed.

(vi) Description of any systemic effects observed.

(vii) Description of any pretest conditioning, including diet, quarantine, and treatment of disease.

(viii) Description of caging conditions including number (and any change in number) of animals per cage, bedding material, ambient temperature and humidity, photoperiod, and identification of diet of test animal.

(ix) Manufacturer, source, purity, and lot number of test substance.

(x) Physical nature and, where appropriate, concentration and pH value for the test substance.

TABLE 3.6 *(Continued)*
Comparison of Excerpts from Selected Dermal Irritation Test Guidelines

(xi) Identification and composition of any vehicles (e.g., diluents, suspending agents, and emulsifiers) or other materials used in administering the test substance.

(xii) A list of references cited in the body of the report, i.e., references to any published literature used in developing the test protocol, performing the testing, making and interpreting observations, and compiling and evaluating the results.

Japanese-MAFF (Current)

1. *Purpose.* The purpose of this study is to obtain the data which will make the basis to establish safe handling procedures in use.

2. *Test Substance.* The end-use product should be used. However, strongly acidic or alkaline substances (approximately pH 2 or less or pH 11.5 or greater) might not be tested.

3. *Test Animals.* At least six of young adult albino rabbits should be used.

4. *Exposure Conditions.*

(1) Approximately 24 hours before the test, fur should be removed from the dorsal area of the trunk of the test animals by clipping or shaving.

(2) When testing solids (which may be pulverized if considered necessary), the test substance should be moistened sufficiently with water or, where necessary, a suitable vehicle, to ensure good contact with the skin. When vehicles are used, the influence of the vehicle should be taken into account. Liquid test substances are generally used undiluted.

(3) A dose of 0.5 ml of liquid or 0.5 g of solid or paste is applied to the test site.

(4) The test substance should be applied to a small area (approximately 6 cm^2) of skin and covered with a gauze patch, which is held in place with non-irritating tape. In the case of liquids or some pastes, it may be necessary to apply the test substance to the gauze patch and then apply that to the skin. The patch should be loosely held in contact with the skin by means of a suitable semi-occlusive dressing for the duration of the exposure period. (However, the use of occlusive dressing maybe considered appropriate in some cases.)

(5) Exposure duration is for four hours. At the end of the exposure period, residual test substance should generally be removed by using water or an appropriate solvent.

5. *Clinical Examination and Scoring.* After removal of the patch, animals should be examined for signs of erythema and edema and the responses scored within 30 minutes or 60 min, and then at 24, 48 and 72 h after patch removal. Dermal irritation is scored and recorded according to the grades in Table 3.8. Further observations may be needed, as necessary, to establish reversibility. It need not normally exceed 14 days after application. In addition to the observation of irritation, any lesions and other toxic effects should be fully described.

Japanese-MAFF (Draft)

1. *Objective*

This test seeks to provide information on potential skin irritation or corrosion forming a basis for establishing the safe method of handling the agrochemical during use.

2. *Test substance*

The preparation. However this test should not be undertaken with strongly acidic or alkaline materials (generally those up to pH 2 and from pH 11.5) as these may be expected to be corrosive.

3. *Test animal species and age*

Young adult white rabbits are used. Three or more are used.

4. *Method of administration*

(1) About 24 h before the test, the hair in the dorsal region of the trunk of the test animals is clipped short. Care is taken not to damage the skin and only animals with healthy, undamaged skin are used.

(2) If the test substance is a solid, it is moistened thoroughly with water or a suitable vehicle to ensure good contact with the skin. If necessary it may also be crushed. Care must also be taken that the vehicle used has no effects on the test. Test substances in liquid form are applied undiluted.

(3) 0.5 ml of liquid test substance and 0.5 g of solid or paste test substances are applied to the test site.

TABLE 3.6 *(Continued)*
Comparison of Excerpts from Selected Dermal Irritation Test Guidelines

(4) The test substance is applied to a small area of skin (about 6 cm²), covered with a gauze patch and secured with nonirritant tape. For liquid or paste materials, a method may also be adopted in which the test substance is applied to the gauze patch and the gauze patch applied to the skin. Contact between the patch and skin is maintained with a suitable semiocclusive dressing during the exposure period (an occlusive dressing may be used in some cases). Untreated skin of the animal is taken as the control.

(5) The exposure period is normally 4 hours. Test substance remaining at the end of the period of application is removed with water or a suitable vehicle.

5. *Points to note regarding administration*

(1) If severe potential irritation/corrosion is suspected

(1) If the test substance is suspected of being severely irritating or corrosive, a test is conducted in one animal.

1) If the test substance is suspected of being corrosive, three test patches are applied simultaneously to one animal. The first patch is removed after three min. If no strong skin reaction is observed, the second patch is removed after one hour. If it is judged in terms of the humane treatment of the animal at this stage that the exposure can be extended to 4 h, the third patch is removed after 4 h and the reactions are graded. If a strong irritant reaction is observed after 3-min or 1-h exposure, the remaining patches are removed and the test stopped immediately. The three patches may also be applied successively to different sites on the same animal for examination.

2) If severe irritation is suspected with the test substance, one patch is applied to one animal for 4 h.

3) If no severe irritation or corrosion is observed after a 4-h exposure, two more animals are tested with one patch each for 4 h.

(2) If it is anticipated that severe irritation/corrosion will not occur with the test substance, the test is started using three animals and one patch is applied to each for 4 h.

6. *General condition and scoring*

The animals are examined and scored for signs of erythema and edema 30 or 60 minutes, and 24, 48, and 72 h after removal of the patch.

Skin irritation is scored and recorded in accordance with the evaluation scores given in the appendix. If necessary, subsequent examinations are given to demonstrate reversibility. There is generally no need to go beyond 14 days. In addition to examining for irritation, any serious injury or other toxic actions are recorded thoroughly.

European-OECD

Introduction

1. OECD Guidelines for Testing of Chemicals are periodically reviewed in light of scientific progress. In the review, special attention is given to possible improvements in relation to animal welfare. This updated version of the original guideline 404 (adopted in 1981) is the outcome of a meeting of OECD experts held in Paris in May 1991.

2. The main differences between this and the original version of the guidelines are (a) the inclusion of data from *in vitro* tests in the information on which a decision not to proceed to an *in vivo* test can be based; and (b) the possibility to use one animal in a first step of the *in vivo* procedure allowing certain chemicals to be exempted from further testing.

3. Definitions used are set out in the Annex.

Initial Considerations

4. In the interests of animal welfare, it is important that the unnecessary use of animals is avoided, and that any testing which is likely to produce severe responses in animals is minimized. Consequently, test substances meeting any of the following criteria should not be tested in animals for dermal irritation/corrosion:

(i) Materials that have predictable corrosive potential based on structure-activity relationships and/or physicochemical properties such as strong acidity or alkalinity, e.g., when the material to be applied has a pH of 2 or less or 11.5 or greater (alkaline or acidic reserve (1) should also be taken into account);

(ii) materials which have been shown to be highly toxic by the dermal route;

(iii) materials which, in an acute dermal toxicity test (2), have been shown not to produce irritation of the skin at the limit test dose level of 2000 mg/kg body weight.

In addition, it may not be necessary to test *in vivo* materials for which corrosive properties are predicted on the basis of results from *in vitro* tests (3).

TABLE 3.6 *(Continued)*
Comparison of Excerpts from Selected Dermal Irritation Test Guidelines

Principle of the In Vivo Test

5. The substance to be tested is applied in a single dose to the skin of one or more experimental animals, untreated skin areas of the test animal(s) serving as control. The degree of irritation is read and scored at specified intervals and is further described in order to provide a complete evaluation of the effects. The duration of the study should be sufficient to evaluate fully the reversibility of the effects observed. Animals showing severe distress and/or pain at any stage of the test must be humanely killed.

Description of the In Vivo Method

Selection of Animal Species

6. Several mammalian species may be used. The albino rabbit is the preferred species.

Number and Sex of Animals

7. Three healthy adult animals are required for the complete test. Male and/or female animals can be used. Additional animals may be used to clarify equivocal responses. Sometimes the test can be performed with one animal only.

Housing and Feeding Conditions

8. Animals should be individually housed. The temperature of the experimental animal room should be 20°C (± 3°C) for rabbits, 22°C (± 3°C) for rodents and the relative humidity 30–70%. Where the lighting is artificial, the sequence should be 12 h light, 12 h dark. Conventional laboratory diets are suitable for feeding and an unrestricted supply of drinking water should be available.

Preparation of the Animals

9. Approximately 24 h before the test, fur should be removed by close-clipping the dorsal area of the trunk of the animals. Care should be taken to avoid abrading the skin and only animals with healthy intact skin should be used.

10. Some strains of rabbit have dense patches of hair which are more prominent at certain times of the year. Such areas of dense hair growth should not be used as patch sites.

Procedure
Application of the Test Substance

11. The test substance should be applied to a small area (approximately 6 cm²) of skin and covered with a gauze patch, which is held in place with non-irritating tape. In the case of liquids or some pastes, it may be necessary to apply the test substance to the gauze patch and then apply that to the skin. The patch should be loosely held in contact with the skin by means of a suitable semi-occlusive dressing for the duration of the exposure period. Access by the animal to the patch and resultant ingestion/inhalation of the test substance should be prevented.

12. Liquid test substances are generally used undiluted. When testing solids (which may be pulverized if considered necessary), the test substance should be moistened with the smallest amount of water, or where necessary a suitable vehicle, needed to ensure good contact with the skin. When vehicles are used, the influence of the vehicle on irritation of the skin by the test substance should be taken into account.

13. At the end of the exposure period, normally 4 h, residual test substance should be removed, where practicable, using water or an appropriate solvent without altering the existing response or the integrity of the epidermis.

Dose Level

14. A dose of 0.5 ml of liquid or 0.5 g of solid or semi-solid is applied to the test site.

Exposure of One Animal

15. If it is suspected that the test substance might produce severe irritancy/corrosion, a single animal test should be employed. When it is suspected that the substance may cause corrosion, three test patches are applied simultaneously to the animal. The first patch is removed after three minutes. If no serious skin reaction is observed, the second patch is removed after one hour. If the observations at this stage indicate that the exposure can humanely be allowed to extend to four hours, the third patch is removed after four hours and the responses are graded. If a corrosive effect is observed after either three minutes or one hour exposure, the test is immediately terminated by removal of the remaining patches. Alternatively, three patches may be applied sequentially. When it is suspected that the substance may cause severe irritancy, a single patch should be applied to the animals for four hours.

TABLE 3.6 *(Continued)*
Comparison of Excerpts from Selected Dermal Irritation Test Guidelines

Exposure of a Further Two Animals

16. If neither a corrosive effect nor a severe irritant effect is observed after a four hour exposure, the test should be completed using two additional animals, each with one patch only, for an exposure period of four hours.

Exposure of Three Animals

17. If it is expected that the test substance will not produce severe irritancy or corrosion, the test may be started using three animals, each receiving one patch for an exposure period of four hours.

Observation Period

18. The duration of the observation period should not be fixed rigidly but should be sufficient to evaluate fully the reversibility of the effects observed.

Clinical Observations and Grading of Skin Reactions

19. Animals should be examined for signs of erythema and oedema and the responses scored at 60 min, and then at 24, 48, and 72 h after patch removal. Dermal irritation is scored and recorded according to the grades in the table below. Further observations may be needed to establish reversibility. In addition to the observation of irritation, all lesions and other toxic effects should be recorded and fully described.

Data and Reporting
Data

20. Data should be summarized in tabular form, showing for each individual animal the irritation scores for erythema and oedema at 60 minutes, 24, 48, and 72 hours after patch removal, all lesions, a description of the degree and nature of irritation, corrosion or reversibility, and any other toxic effects observed.

Test Report

21. The test report must include the following information:
Test substance:
- physical nature and, where relevant, physicochemical properties;
- identification data.

Vehicle:
- justification for choice of vehicle.

Test animals:
- species/strain used;
- number, age and sex of animals;
- source, housing conditions, diet, etc.;
- individual weights of animals at the start and at the conclusion of the test.

Test conditions:
- technique of patch site preparation;
- details of patch materials used and patching technique;
- details of test substance preparation, application and removal.

Results:
- tabulation of irritation response data for each individual animal for each observation time period (e.g., 60 min, 24, 48, and 72 h after patch removal);
- description of all lesions observed;
- narrative description of the degree and nature of irritation observed, and any histopathological findings;
- description of any other toxic effects in addition to dermal irritation/corrosion.

Discussion of the results:

If an *in vitro* test is performed before the *in vivo* test, the description or reference of the test, including details of the procedure, must be given together with results obtained with the test and reference substances.

TABLE 3.6 *(Continued)*
Comparison of Excerpts from Selected Dermal Irritation Test Guidelines

European-EEC

1.4 Principle of the Test Method

Initial Considerations

Careful consideration needs to be given to all the available information on a substance to minimize the testing of substances under conditions that are likely to produce severe reactions. The following information may be useful when considering whether a complete test, a single-animal study, or no further testing is appropriate.

i) Physiochemical properties and chemical reactivity. Strongly acidic or alkaline substances (demonstrated pH of 2 or less or 11.5 or greater, for example) may not require testing for primary dermal irritation if corrosive properties can be expected. Alkaline or acidic reserve should also be taken into account.

ii) If convincing evidence of severe effects in well validated *in vitro* tests is available, a complete test may not be required.

iii) Results from acute toxicity studies. If an acute toxicity test by the dermal route has been conducted with the substance at the limit test dose level (2,000 mg/kg body weight), and no skin irritation was observed, further testing for skin irritation may be unnecessary. In addition, testing of materials which have been shown to be highly toxic by the dermal route is unnecessary.

The substance to be tested is applied in a single dose to the skin of several experimental animals, each animal serving as its own control. The degree of irritation is read and graded after a specific interval, and is further described to provide a complete evaluation of the effects. The duration of the observations should be sufficient to evaluate fully the reversibility of the effects observed.

Animals showing severe and enduring signs of distress and pain may need to be humanely killed.

1.6 Description of the Test Method

1.6.1. Preparations

Approximately 24 hours before testing, fur should be removed, by clipping or shaving, from the dorsal area of the trunk of the animal.

When clipping or shaving the fur, care should be taken to avoid abrading the skin. Only animals with healthy intact skin should be used.

Some strains of rabbit have dense islets of hair which are more prominent at certain times of the year. Test substances should not be applied to these zones of dense hair growth.

When testing solids (which may be pulverized if considered necessary) the test substance should be moistened sufficiently with water or, where necessary, a suitable vehicle, to ensure good contact with the skin. When vehicles are used, the influence of the vehicle on irritation of skin by the test substance should be taken into account. Liquid test substances are generally used undiluted.

1.6.2. Test Conditions

1.6.2.1. Experimental Animals

Although several mammalian species may be used, the albino rabbit is the preferred species.

1.6.2.2. Number of Animals

If it is suspected from *in vitro* screening results or other considerations that the substance might produce necrosis (i.e., be corrosive) a single-animal test should be considered. If the results of this test do not indicate corrosivity, the test should be completed using at least two additional animals.

For the complete test, at least three healthy adult animals are used. Separate animals are not required for an untreated control group. Additional animals may be required to clarify equivocal responses.

1.6.2.3. Dose Level

Unless there are contra-indications 0.5 ml of liquid or 0.5 g of solid or semi-solid is applied to the test site. Adjacent areas of untreated skin of each animal serve as controls for the test.

1.6.2.4. Observation Period

The duration of the observation period should not be fixed rigidly. It should be sufficient to evaluate fully the reversibility or irreversibility of the effects observed, but need not normally exceed 14 days after application.

TABLE 3.6 *(Continued)*
Comparison of Excerpts from Selected Dermal Irritation Test Guidelines

1.6.3. Procedure

Animals should be caged individually. The test substance should be applied to a small area (approximately 6 cm^2) of skin and covered with a gauze patch, which is held in place with non-irritating tape. In the case of liquids or some pastes it may be necessary to apply the test substance to the gauze patch and then apply that to the skin. The patch should be loosely held in contact with the skin by means of a suitable occlusive or semi-occlusive dressing for the duration of the exposure period. Access by the animal to the patch and resultant ingestion/inhalation of the test substance should be prevented.

At the end of the exposure period, residual test substance should be removed, where practicable, using water or an appropriate solvent, without altering the existing response or the integrity of the epidermis.

Exposure duration normally is four hours.

If it is suspected that the substance might produce necrosis (i.e., be corrosive), the duration of exposure should be reduced (e.g., to one hour or three minutes). Such testing may also employ a single animal in the first instance and, if not precluded by the acute dermal toxicity of the test compound, three patches may be applied simultaneously to this animal. The first patch is removed after three minutes. If no serious skin reaction is observed, the second patch is removed after one hour. If the observations at this stage indicate that a four-hour exposure is necessary and can be humanely conducted, the third patch is removed after four hours and the responses are graded. In this case (i.e. when a four-hour exposure has been possible), the test should then be completed using at least two additional animals, unless it is not considered humane to do so (e.g., if necrosis is observed following the four hour exposure).

If a serious skin reaction (e.g., necrosis) is observed at either three minutes or one hour, the test is immediately terminated.

Longer exposures may be indicated under certain conditions, e.g., expected pattern of human use and exposure.

1.6.3.1. Observation and Grading

Animals should be observed for signs of erythema and oedema and the response graded at 60 minutes, and then at 24, 48, and 72 hours after patch removal. Dermal irritation is graded and recorded according to the system in Table 3.8. Further observations may be needed if reversibility has not been fully established within 72 hours. In addition to the observation of irritation, any serious lesions such as corrosion (irreversible destruction of skin tissue) and other toxic effects should be fully described.

Techniques such as histopathological examination or measurement of skin-fold thickness may be used to clarify doubtful reactions or responses masked by staining of the skin by test substance.

2. Data

Data should be summarized in tabular form, showing for each individual animal the irritation gradings for erythema and oedema throughout the observation period. Any serious lesions, a description of the degree and nature of irritation, reversibility or corrosion and any other toxic effect observed should be recorded.

3. Reporting
3.1 Test Report

The test report shall, if possible, include the following information:

- species, strain, source, environmental conditions, diet, etc.;
- test conditions (including the relevant physicochemical properties of the chemical, the technique of skin preparation and cleansing, and the type of dressing: occlusive or semi-occlusive);
- tabulation of irritation response data for each individual animal for each observation time period (e.g., 1, 24, 48, and 72 hours, etc., after patch removal);
- description of any serious lesions observed, including corrosivity;
- description of the degree and nature of irritation observed and any histopathological findings;
- description of any toxic effects other than dermal irritation,
- discussion of the results;
- interpretation of the results.

TABLE 3.7
Comparison of Excerpts from Selected Sensitization Test Guidelines[6-11]

EPA OPPTS 870.2600

This guideline is one of a series of test guidelines that have been developed by the Office of Prevention, Pesticides and Toxic Substances, United States Environmental Protection Agency for use in the testing of pesticides and toxic substances, and the development of test data that must be submitted to the agency for review under Federal regulations.

The Office of Prevention, Pesticides and Toxic Substances (OPPTS) has developed this guideline through a process of harmonization that blended the testing guidance and requirements that existed in the Office of Pollution Prevention and Toxics (OPPT) and appeared in Title 40, Chapter I, Subchapter R of the code of Federal Regulations (CFR), the Office of Pesticide Programs (OPP) which appeared in publications of the National Technical Information Service (NTIS), and the guidelines published by the Organization for Economic Cooperation and Development (OECD).

The purpose of harmonizing these guidelines into a single set of OPPTS guidelines is to minimize variations among the testing procedures that must be performed to meet the data requirements of the U.S. Environmental Protection Agency under the Toxic Substance Control Act (15 U.S.C. 2601) and the Federal Insecticide, Fungicide and Rodenticide Act (7 U.S.C. 136, *et seq.*).

(a) Scope. (1) Applicability. This guideline is intended to meet testing requirements of both the Federal Insecticide, Fungicide, and Rodenticide Act (FIFRA) (7 USC 136, *et seq.*) and the Toxic Substances Control Act (TSCA) (15 USC 2601).

(2) Background. The source materials used in developing this harmonized OPPTS test guideline are the OPPT 40 CFR 798.4100 Dermal Sensitization; OPP 81-6 Dermal Sensitization (Pesticide Assessment Guidelines, Subdivision F-Hazard Evaluation; Human and Domestic Animals); EPA report 540/09-82-025, 1982; and OECD 406 Skin Sensitization.

(b) Purpose. In the assessment and evaluation of the toxic characteristics of the substance, determination of its potential to provoke skin sensitization reactions is important. Information derived from test for skin sensitization serves to identify the possible hazard to a population repeatedly exposed to the test substance. While the desirability of skin sensitization testing is recognized, there are some real differences of opinion about the best method to use. The test selected should be a reliable screening procedure which should not fail to identify substances with significant allergenic potential, while at the same time avoiding false negative results.

(c) Definitions. (1) "Challenge exposure" is an experimental exposure of a previously treated subject to a test substance following an induction period, to determine if the subject will react in a hypersensitive manner.

(2) "Induction exposure" is an experimental exposure of a subject to a test substance with the intention of inducing a hypersensitive state.

(3) "Induction period" is a period of at least 1 week following an induction exposure during which a hypersensitive state is developed.

(4) "Skin sensitization" ("allergic contact dermatitis") is an immunologically mediated cutaneous reaction to a substance. In the human, the responses may be characterized by pruritis, erythema, edema, papules, vesicles, bullae, or a combination of these. In other species, the reactions may differ and only erythema and edema may be seen.

(d) Principle of the test method. Following initial exposure(s) to a test substance, the animals are subsequently subjected, after a period of not less that 1 week, to a challenge exposure with the test substance to establish whether a hypersensitive state has been induced. Sensitization is determined by examining the reaction to the challenge exposure and comparing this reaction to that of the initial induction exposure. The test animals are initially exposed to the test substance by intradermal and/or epidermal application (induction exposure). Following a rest period of 10 to 14 days (the induction periods), during which an immune response may develop, the animals are exposed to a challenge dose. The extent and degree of skin reaction to the challenge exposure is compared with that demonstrated by control animals that undergo sham treatment during induction and then receive the challenge exposure.

(e) Test procedures. (1) Any of the following seven test methods is considered to be acceptable. It is realized, however, that the methods differ in their probability and degree of reaction to sensitizing substances.

(i) Buehler test;
(ii) Guinea pig maximization test;
(iii) Open epicutaneous;
(iv) Mauer optimization test;
(v) Split adjuvant technique;
(vi) Freund's complete adjuvant test;
(vii) Draize sensitization test;

TABLE 3.7 *(Continued)*
Comparison of Excerpts from Selected Sensitization Test Guidelines[6–11]

(2) The GPMT of Magnusson and Kligman, which uses adjuvant, and nonadjuvant Buehler test are given preference over other methods. Although strong preference is given to either the Buehler test or the GPMT, it is recognized that other tests may give useful results. If other tests are used, the tester should provide justification/reasoning for their use, methods and protocols must be provided, and each test should include a positive and a negative control group.

(f) *Screening tests.* The mouse ear swelling test (MEST) or the local (auricular) lymph node assay (LLNA) in the mouse may be used as screening tests to detect moderate to strong sensitizers. If a positive result is seen in either assay, the test substance may be designated a potential sensitizer, and it may not be necessary to conduct a further test in guinea pigs. If the LLNA or MEST does not indicate sensitization, the test substance should not be designated a nonsensitizer without confirmation in an accepted test with guinea pigs.

(g) *Animal selection.* (1) Species and strain. The young adult guinea pig is the preferred species. Commonly used laboratory strains should be employed. If other species are used, the tester should provide justification/reasoning for their selection.

(2) *Housing and feeding.* The temperature of the experimental animal room should be $20\pm3°C$ with the relative humidity 30–70%. Where the lighting is artificial, the sequence should be 12 h light/12 h dark. Conventional laboratory diets may be used with an unlimited supply of drinking water. It is essential that guinea pigs receive an adequate amount of ascorbic acid.

(3) *Number and sex.* The number and sex will depend on the method used. If females are used, they should be nulliparous and not pregnant.

(4) *Control animals.* (i) The sensitivity and reliability of the experimental technique used should be assessed every 6 months in naive animals by the use of positive control substance known to have mild-to-moderate skin-sensitizing properties. In a properly conducted test, a response of at least 30% in an adjuvant test and at least 15% in a nonadjuvant test should be expected for mild-to-moderate sensitizes. Preferred substances are hexylcinnamicaldhyde (CAS No. 101-86-0), mercaptobenzothiazole (CAS No. 149-30-4), benzocaine (CAS No. 94-09-7), dinitro-chloro-benzene (CAS No. 97-00-7), or DER 331 epoxy resin. There may be circumstances where, given adequate justification, other control substances meeting the above criteria may be used.

(ii) Depending upon the test selected, animals may be used as their own controls, but usually there will be a separate group of sham-treated animals that are exposed to the test substance only after the induction period, whose reactions are compared to those of the animals that have received both induction and challenge exposures. Control groups which provide the best design should be used. Some cases may best be served by both naive and vehicle control groups.

(5) (i) The dose level will depend upon the method selected.

(6) (i) Skin reactions should be graded and recorded after the challenge exposures at the time specified by the methodology selected. This is usually at 24 and 48 h. Additional notations should be made as necessary to fully describe unusual responses.

(ii) Regardless of method selected, initial and terminal body weights are to be recorded.

(7) *Procedures.* (i) The procedures to be used are those described by the methodology chosen.

(h) *Data and reporting.* Data should be summarized in tabular form, showing for each individual animal the skin reaction, results of the induction exposure, and the challenge exposure at times indicated by the method chosen. As a minimum, the erythema and edema should be graded and any unusual findings should be recorded.

(1) Evaluation of the results. The evaluation of results will provide information on the proportion of each group that became sensitized and the extent (slight, moderate, severe) of the sensitization reaction in each individual animal.

(2) *Test report.* In addition to the information required by 40 CFR part 158 (for pesticides) and 40 CFR part 792 subpart J (for toxic substances), the test report shall include the following information:

(i) A description of the methods used and the commonly accepted name;

(ii) Information on positive control study, including:

    (A) Positive control used;

    (B) Method used; and

    (C) Time conducted.

(iii) The number, species, strain, age, source, and sex of the test animals;

(iv) Individual weights of the animals at the start of the test and at the conclusion of the test;

(v) A brief description of the grading system; and

(vi) Each reading made on each individual animal.

(vii) The chemical identification and relevant physicochemical properties of the test substance.

TABLE 3.7 *(Continued)*
Comparison of Excerpts from Selected Sensitization Test Guidelines[6-11]

(viii) The vehicles used for induction and challenge, and justification for their use, if other than water or physiological saline. Any material that might reasonably be expected to react with or enhance or retard absorption of the test substance should be reported.

(ix) The total amount of test substance applied for induction and challenge, and the technique of application in each case.

(x) Description of any pretest conditioning, including diet, quarantine, and treatment of disease.

(xi) Description of caging conditions including number (and any change in number) of animals per cage, bedding material, ambient temperature and humidity, photoperiod, and identification of diet of test animal.

(xii) Histopathological findings, if any.

(xiii) Discussion of results.

(xiv) Manufacturer, source, purity, and lot number of test substance.

(xv) Physical nature and, where appropriate, concentration and pH value for the test substance.

(xvi) A list of references cited in the body of the report, i.e., references to any published literature used in developing the test protocol, performing the testing, making and interpreting observations, and compiling and evaluating the results.

Japanese-MHW

2. Selection of Test Methods

These test methods are given as examples because they have been adopted in most laboratories, and because that they all represent well established assay techniques with a high degree of reproducibility. Generally, original reports pertaining to the individual test methods are cited herein, although some of these tests are in use with modifications. Testing procedure need not be limited to those cited herein, and in cases where any other test method is employed, justification of its application should be stated along with citation of the appropriate literature.

(a) Adjuvant and patch test

The test comprises intradermal injections of FCA and abrasion of the skin, topical application of the test substance onto the scratched region, and covering of the test site with an occlusive patch for sensitization. The topical challenge is made without a covering. The test is used for such test substances which are not injectable intradermally.

(b) Buehler test

This test also employs topical application of the test substance. The test site is covered with an occlusive patch and a wrapping and the topical challenge is carried out with a wrap, as during induction, to enhance penetration and prevent evaporation of the test substance.

(c) Draize test

The test method was the first predictive sensitization assay accepted by regulatory agencies. It is characterized by the intradermal introduction of a dilution of the test substance for sensitization, and a challenge by subsequent intradermal injection.

(d) Freund's complete adjuvant test

The test comprises intradermal injections of the test substance incorporated in a 1:1 mixture of FCA and distilled water.

(e) Maximization test

The maximization test, as described in the Guidelines, combines FCA, sodium lauryl sulfate, intradermal injection and occlusive topical application of the test substance during the sensitization period.

(f) Open epicutaneous test

This test closely simulates the conditions of drug use in humans by utilizing repeated topical application of the test substance.

(g) Optimization test

The optimization test is analogous to Draize test but involves the use of FCA for sensitization and an intradermal challenge with covering of the test site.

(h) Split adjuvant test

The test utilizes skin damage caused by the application of dry ice onto a shaved area of skin, and FCA as an adjuvant. The test substance is applied topically with a dressing.

TABLE 3.7 *(Continued)*
Comparison of Excerpts from Selected Sensitization Test Guidelines[6–11]

Whichever test method is selected, it is impracticable to accomplish a perfect prediction of the sensitizing potential of a substance in humans based solely on results of the test, but the test results may provide important information valid for the extrapolation of data to the conditions of human use.

In the current Guidelines, the spirit of concern for research animals is incorporated. Test methods, for example, are roughly divided into two groups: those involving the use of an adjuvant and those which do not, so as to systematically minimize the types of tests to be adopted. Thus, scientific considerations have been made for the reduction of the number of animals used in tests. They are, in brief, 1) reduction of the number of animals used in tests, 2) limitation of types of testing methods and delineation of test methods that may be selected, 3) classification of the test methods according to assay sensitivity, and so forth.

3. Selection of Test Animals

Primarily, animals highly susceptible to the sensitizing action of the test substance are to be selected as a test system. In all the test methods mentioned above, regardless, the animal species used is the guinea pig. Young, healthy adult albino guinea pigs (usually between 1 and 3 months of age) weighing not more than 500 g at the start of the test are used as a rule. They may be male or female, or of both sexes, and, in the case of females, the animals should be nonpregnant and nulliparous.

This animal species is selected primarily for the reasons that guinea pigs are known to elicit, if at all, reactions similar to those that occur in man and that a substantial amount of background laboratory data has been accumulated for this species.

4. Number of Animals

An extreme reduction in the number of animals used in tests may render statistical data analysis meaningless. Only the minimum number of animals required for test groups (groups subject to sensitization with the test substance) and control groups (positive control and control groups) are stated in these Guidelines. If any influence of the minimized number of animals on test results is anticipated, the number should be increased appropriately. The above stated minimum number of animals (5/group) may suffice only for such circumstances where the response is either obviously negative or strongly positive. It follows that, otherwise, each test group need consist of at least 10 animals and each control group of at least 5 animals.

5. Positive Controls

Positive controls are required as references for comparative assessments of the responsiveness of animals used and of the sensitizing potency of the drug substance being tested. Compounds currently in use for this purpose include: *p*-phenylenediamine (CAS No. 106-50-3), 1-chloro-2,4-dinitrobenzene (CAS No. 97-00-7), neomycin sulfate (CAS No. 1405-10-3) and nickel sulfate (CAS No. 7786-81-4), but any other suitable sensitizers documented in the biomedical literature may also be used.

6. Test Methods

Detailed accounts are given of the maximization test (Magnusson and Kligman) and the adjuvant and patch test, under Description of the Test Procedure in the Guidelines, while the other six test methods are only cited. All the test methods mentioned in the Guidelines may be regarded as essentially equivalent and none given a preference to others. That is, any of the test methods mentioned above may be adopted.

The maximization test and adjuvant and patch test are selected as examples to be detailed on the rationale that those involving the use of Freund's complete adjuvant are likely to be superior in assay sensitivity to those not using it.

It is most desirable to conduct the testing stepwise in evaluating a substance for skin sensitizing potential. In the first step, one of the five tests incorporating the use of the adjuvant is to be performed to ascertain if the property of the test substance is to be further assessed by comparison with a known sensitizing substance or by conducting a test not involving the use of an adjuvant so as to permit evaluation of the intensity of sensitization by the test substance.

All these tests are designed to determine the potential of test substances to induce hypersensitivity by, in general, exposure (sensitization) of experimental animals to the test substance and a challenge exposure (elicitation) after a subsequent rest period of about 2 weeks. Test results are for sensitizing potential interpreted by comparing cutaneous responses of experimental animals with those of controls. Each of the test methods described has advantages and drawbacks and, therefore, it is most desirable that the tests by performed properly by personnel well versed in these aspects.

TABLE 3.7 *(Continued)*
Comparison of Excerpts from Selected Sensitization Test Guidelines[6–11]

In preparing animals for tests, they should be randomly allocated to experimental groups. Test sites on the skin must be clipped free of hair or shaven prior to administration of the test substance.

Study conditions must be carefully set up since test results may vary with the conditions.

7. Dose Levels

In case where graded dose levels appropriate to the assay are employed, the physicochemical properties of the test substance, such as the solubility at test concentrations and the tolerated local or systemic dose need be taken into account. The concentrations of the test substance for sensitizing and challenge chosen for the assay may be justified whenever deemed necessary.

8. Observation Parameters

Body weights of animals must be recorded at least at the initiation and at the completion of testing. All animals should be observed for any signs of skin irritation during the sensitization period. Skin reactions are to be noted at 24, 48, or 72 hours after challenge exposure, and interpreted for sensitizing activity of the test substance. The reactions must be rated as specified for each test. All observed cutaneous reactions and any adverse findings noted must be recorded.

9. Reporting of Test Results

It is advisable that test results be summarized by tabulation or other means in such a way that the skin reactions of individual animals at respective periods of observation can be clearly recognized.

In reporting the test results, data concerning the following parameters must be included:
1) Strain of guinea pigs used.
2) Number, age in weeks, and sex(es) of animals used.
3) Individual animal body weights at the start and at the completion of test.
4) All reactions observed in animals, along with details of reactions if any scoring system or classification scheme is employed.
5) Evaluation of test results, and comments.

10. Evaluation of Test Results

The skin sensitizing potential of the test substance should be evaluated according to the reactions observed in animals in the test group and in each control group. Interpretation of the test results must be based on evaluation of the potential of the test substance to sensitize the skin. Basically, it is to be made according to the evaluation criteria specified in the literature reporting the test method.

In cases where the incidence of a positive skin reaction is to be assessed, it is advisable that increased numbers of animals be used in test and control groups, and that data obtained be processed by an appropriate statistical procedure.

What should be noted here is that the tests mentioned herein, unfortunately, are not necessarily adequate as assays for predicting the sensitizing potential of the test substance in humans. To evaluate the sensitizing activity of the material, therefore, the material is first to be subjected to any one of the test methods involving the use of an adjuvant and determined thereby as to whether it has sensitizing activity or not. If the material has proven to be positive, then it should be further assessed, preferably by a test method not involving the use of an adjuvant in order to make practical risk assessment and classification of the test substance.

Japanese-MAFF (Current)

1. Purpose

The purpose of this study is to obtain the data which will make the basis to establish safe handling procedures in use.

2. Test Substance

The end-use product should be used. However, strongly acidic or alkaline substance (approximately pH 2 or pH 11.5 or greater) might not be tested.

3. Test Animals

At least one mammalian species should be used. The young adult guinea pig is the preferred species.

TABLE 3.7 *(Continued)*
Comparison of Excerpts from Selected Sensitization Test Guidelines[6–11]

4. Test Methods

Any of the following seven test methods is considered to be acceptable. Use of a positive control substance for the reliability for the test system selected is recommended.

Draize Test

Freund's Complete Adjuvant Test

Mauer Optimisation Test

Buehler Test

Open Epicutaneous Test

Guinea Pig Maximization Test

Split Adjuvant Technique

Japanese-MAFF (draft)

1. Objective

This test seeks to provide information on potential skin sensitization forming a basis for establishing the safe method of handling the agrochemical during use.

2. Test substances

Basic compound and preparation

3. Test animal species, age, and sex

Young adult guinea pigs are used. Females are nulliparous, nonpregnant animals.

4. Test methods

The test methods which are undertaken with a relatively high frequency are the guinea pig maximization test (GPM method) and the Buehler test (Buehler method). However, if information about sensitization is available, the test method therein may be substituted.

A positive control group is also provided in order to evaluate the responsivity of the test system.

5. Test procedures

Both the GPM method and the Buehler method are described in detail in the guidelines.

(1) *Number of animals.* This is dependent on the method used.

(2) *Dose settings.* The maximum concentration of the test substance used in exposure for sensitization is one to which there is satisfactory resistance systemically but producing mild to moderate skin irritation. The maximum concentration of test substance used for challenge exposure is the highest at which no irritation is shown. Two or three animals are used to determine the appropriate concentration of the test substance.

(3) *Sensitization.* Procedures are dependent on the method used.

(6) *Examination.* About 21 h after removing the patches, the challenged area is shaved if necessary. Three hours later (about 48 h after the start of application of the challenging patches), the skin is examined for any reaction which is then recorded in accordance with the grades shown in the table. Skin reactions are observed and recorded again 24 h after the first examination.

Table: Evaluation criteria for challenge patch test reaction

No visible change	0
Diffuse or patchy erythema	1
Moderate and chronic erythema	2
Marked erythema and oedema	3

(8) Examination of general condition. All skin reactions and all abnormal findings which occur as a result of sensitization and challenge are recorded.

European-OECD

Introduction

2. Currently, quantitative structure–activity relationships and *in vitro* models are not yet sufficiently developed to play a significant role in the assessment of the skin-sensitization potential of substances which therefore must continue to be based on *in vitro* models.

TABLE 3.7 *(Continued)*
Comparison of Excerpts from Selected Sensitization Test Guidelines[6–11]

3. The guinea pig has been the animal of choice for predictive sensitization tests for several decades. Two types of tests have been developed: adjuvant tests in which sensitization is potentiated by injection of Freund's complete adjuvant (FCA), and nonadjuvant tests. In the original guideline 406, four adjuvant test and three nonadjuvant tests were considered to be acceptable. In this updated version, the guinea pig maximization test (GPMT) of Magnusson and Kligman which uses adjuvant and the nonadjuvant Buehler test are given preference over other methods and the procedures are presented in detail. It is recognized, however, that there may be circumstances where other methods may be used to provide the necessary information on sensitization potential.

4. The immune system of the mouse has been investigated more extensively than that of the guinea pig. Recently, mouse models for assessing sensitization potential have been developed that offer the advantages of having an end point which is measured objectively, being of short duration, and treating a minimal number of animals. The mouse ear swelling test (MEST) and the local lymph node assay (LLNA) appear to be promising. Both assays have undergone validation in several laboratories and it has been shown that they are able to detect reliably moderate to strong sensitizes. The LLNA or the MEST can be used as a first stage in the assessment of skin sensitization potential. If a positive result is seen in either assay, a test substance may be designated as a potential sensitizer, and it may not be necessary to conduct a further guinea pig test. However, if a negative result is seen in the LLNA or MEST, a guinea pig test (preferably a GPMT or Buehler test) must be conducted using the procedure described in this guideline.

5. Definitions:

"Skin sensitization" (allergic contact dermatitis): An immunologically mediated cutaneous reaction to a substance. In the human, pruritis, erythema, edema, papules, vesicles, bullae, or a combination of these may characterize the responses. In other species the reactions may differ and only erythema and edema may be seen.

"Induction exposure" An experimental exposure of a subject to a test substance with the intention of inducing a hypersensitive state.

"Induction period" A period of at least 1 week following an induction exposure during which a hypersensitive state may develop.

"Challenge exposure" An experimental exposure of a previously treated subject to a test substance following an induction period, to determine if the subject reacts in a hypersensitive manner.

General Principle of Sensitization Tests in Guinea Pigs

6. The test animals are initially exposed to the test substance by intradermal injection and/or epidermal application (induction exposure). Following a rest period of 10 to 14 days (induction period), during which an immune response may develop, the animals are exposed to a challenge dose. The extent and degree of skin reaction to the challenge exposure in the test animals is compared with that demonstrated by control animals which undergo sham treatment during induction and receive the challenge exposure.

Elements Common to Sensitization Tests in Guinea Pigs

Sex of Animals

7. Male and/or female healthy young adult animals can be used. If females are used they should be nulliparous and nonpregnant.

Housing and Feeding Conditions

8. The temperature of the experimental animal room should be 20°C (± 3°C) and the relative humidity 30–70%. Where the lighting is artificial, the sequence should be 12 h light, 12 h dark. For feeding, conventional laboratory diets may be used with an unlimited supply of drinking water. It is essential that guinea pigs receive an adequate amount of ascorbic acid.

Preparation of the Animals

9. Animals are acclimatized to the laboratory conditions for at least 5 days prior to the test. Before the test, animals are randomized and assigned to the treatment groups. Removal of hair is by clipping, shaving or possibly by chemical depilation, depending on the test method used. Care should be taken to avoid abrading the skin. The animals are weighed before the test commences and at the end of the test.

Reliability Check

10. The sensitivity and reliability of the experimental technique used should be assessed every six months by use of substances which are known to have mild-to-moderate skin sensitization properties.

TABLE 3.7 *(Continued)*
Comparison of Excerpts from Selected Sensitization Test Guidelines[6-11]

11. In a properly conducted test, a response of at least 30% in an adjuvant test and at least 15% in a non-adjuvant test should be expected for mild/moderate sensitisers. Preferred substances are hexyl cinnamic aldehyde (CAS No. 101-86-0), mercaptobenzothiazole (CAS No. 149-30-4) and benzocaine (CAS No. 94-09-7). There may be circumstances where, given adequate justification, other control substances meeting the above criteria may be used.

Removal of the Test Substance

12. If removal of the test substance is considered necessary, this should be achieved using water or an appropriate solvent without altering the existing response or the integrity of the epidermis.

Description of the Guinea Pig Methods

13.-36. Both the guinea pig maximization test and the Buehler test methods are described in the guideline.

Data and Reporting

Data

37. Data should be summarized in tabular form, showing for each animal the skin reactions at each observation.

Test Report

38. The test report must include the following information:

Test substance:

— physical nature and, where relevant, physicochemical properties

— identification data

Vehicle:

— justification of choice of vehicle

Test animals:

— strain of guinea pig used

— number, age, and sex of animals

— source, housing conditions, diet, etc.

— individual weights of animals at the start and at the conclusion of the test

Test conditions

— technique of patch site preparation

— details of patch materials used and patching technique

— result of pilot study with conclusion on induction and challenge concentrations to be used in the test

— details of test substance preparation, application, and removal

— vehicle and test substance concentrations used for induction and challenge exposures and the total amount of substance applied for induction and challenge.

Reliability check:

— a summary of the results of the latest reliability check including information on substance, concentration, and vehicle used.

Results:

— on each animal including grading system

— narrative description of the nature and degree of effects observed

— any histopathological findings

Discussion of results

— If a screening assay is performed before the guinea pig test, the description or reference of the test, including details of the procedure, must be given together with results obtained with the test and reference substances.

European-EEC

Method

1.1 Introduction

Remarks:

The sensitivity and ability of tests to detect potential human skin sensitizers are considered important in a classification system for toxicity relevant to public health. There is no single test method which will adequately identify all substances with a potential for sensitizing human skin and which is relevant for all substances.

TABLE 3.7 *(Continued)*
Comparison of Excerpts from Selected Sensitization Test Guidelines[6–11]

Factors such as the physical characteristics of a substance, including its ability to penetrate the skin, must be considered in the selection of a test.

Tests using guinea pigs can be subdivided into the adjuvant-type tests, in which an allergic state is potentiated by dissolving or suspending the test substance in Freunds Complete Adjuvant (FCA), and the non-adjuvant tests.

Adjuvant-type tests are likely to be more accurate in predicting a probable skin sensitizing effect of a substance in humans than those methods not employing Freunds Complete Adjuvant and are thus the preferred methods.

The Guinea Pig Maximization Test (GPMT) is a widely used adjuvant-type test. Although several other methods can be used to detect the potential of a substance to provoke skin sensitization reaction, the GPMT is considered to be the preferred adjuvant technique.

With many chemical classes, non-adjuvant tests (the preferred one being the Buehler test) are considered to be less sensitive.

In certain cases there may be good reasons for choosing the Buehler test involving topical application rather than the intradermal injection used in the Guinea Pig Maximization Test. Scientific justification should be given when the Buehler test is used.

The Guinea Pig Maximization Test (GPMT) and the Buehler test are described in this method. Other methods may be used provided that they are well-validated and scientific justification is given.

Regardless of the methods used, the sensitivity of the strain of guinea pig being used for skin sensitization testing must be checked at regular intervals (six months) using a known mild to moderate sensitizer and a satisfactory number of positive responses obtained.

1.3. Reference Substances
The following substances, diluted as necessary, are recommended, as well as any other sensitizing substance known either from the literature or which belongs to the group of the substance being tested.
- *p*-phenylenediamine
  CAS No. 106-50-3
- 2,4-dinitrochlorobenzene
  CAS No. 97-00-7
- potassium dichromate
  CAS No. 7778-50-9
- neomycin sulphate
  CAS No. 1405-10-3
- nickel sulphate
  CAS No. 7786-81-4

1.4. Principle of the Test Methods
Following initial exposure to a test substance (the 'induction' period) the animals are subjected approximately two weeks after the last induction exposure to a 'challenge' exposure to the test substance in order to establish if a hypersensitive state has been induced. Sensitization is determined by examining the skin reaction to the challenge exposure.

1.5 Quality Criteria
None.
1.6 Description of the Test Method
The guinea pig maximization test (GPMT) and the Buehler test are described in the guideline.

2. Data (GPMT and Buehler test)
Data should be summarized in tabular form, showing for each animal the skin reactions at each observation.

3. Reporting (GPMT and Buehler test)
3.1 Test Report (GPMT and Buehler test)
The test report shall, if possible, include the following information:
— strain of guinea pig used
— test conditions, vehicle and test substance concentrations used for induction and challenges
— number, age, and sex of animals

TABLE 3.7 *(Continued)*
Comparison of Excerpts from Selected Sensitization Test Guidelines[6-11]

— individual weights of animals at the start and at the conclusion of the test
— discussion of the results
— interpretation of the results

3.2 Evaluation and Interpretation (GPMT and Buehler test)

There are limitations in the extent to which the results of animal and *in vitro* tests can be extrapolated directly to humans and this must be borne in mind when tests are evaluated and interpreted. When available, evidence of adverse effects in humans may be of relevance in determining the potential effects of chemical substances on the human population.

SECTION 3. MATERIALS AND PROCEDURES FOR PERFORMING DERMAL IRRITATION STUDIES[24-33]

A. THE OCCLUDED DERMAL IRRITATION TEST IN RABBITS

1. Materials

a. Gauze Dressing

Type: Ace-Tex Corporation nonsterilized
Thickness: 4-ply gauze dressing
Size: 1 × 1 inch

b. Tape — Nonirritating

Type: Blenderm® . . . (Medical-Surgical Division/3M, St. Paul, MN)
Size: 1 inch wide

c. Occlusive Materials

Type: Impervious material (e.g., plastic wrap)

d. Binding Materials

Elastic wrap
Type: Rubber elastic bandage: Ace® Bandage or Coban® (Medical-Surgical Division/3M, St. Paul, MN), or Expandover® (Sherwood Medical, St. Louis, MO)
Size: Adequate wrapping of the entire test site

e. Securing Materials

Type: Zonas® (Johnson & Johnson Medical Inc., Arlington, TX) porous athletic tape
Size: 2 inches wide

f. Elizabethan or similar Collars: Optional.

g. Animal Species

New Zealand white rabbits.

2. Procedures

The hair is removed from a sufficient area on the rabbit's back on the day before dosing. Care should be taken to avoid abrading the skin during the clipping procedure. On the day of dosing, the test site (approximately 1 × 1 inch square of intact skin) should be designated and the gauze patch (1 × 1 inch) should be secured to the animal on at least two cut edges of the gauze patch, using the nonirritating Blenderm tape. The test substance, either 0.5 ml or 0.5 g, should be administered under the gauze dressing and the remaining cut edges secured to the animal's back with nonirritating tape.

Liquids are administered as received, powders should be moistened with a suitable vehicle before application (e.g., distilled water). If the test article is a solid or powder that does not work well as a paste (e.g., does not spread well), 0.5 g of the test article will be applied to an approximate 1 × 1 in. 4-ply gauze patch and will be moistened with the appropriate amount of distilled water or suitable vehicle (generally 0.5 ml) and the gauze patch applied to the test site. An impervious sheet of material (e.g., plastic wrap) is then wrapped around the trunk of the animal. The elastic wrap is then wrapped around the animal's torso and is secured in place using the Zonas athletic tape. The Zonas is wrapped around the outermost portion of the elastic wrap at the cranial and caudal ends. An Elizabethan or similar collar may then be placed around the animal's neck. After the designated time of exposure (i.e., 4 or 24 hours), the tape, elastic wrap, impervious wrap, and gauze patch are removed and the test site is delineated using an indelible marker. The test site should then be rinsed with a suitable vehicle (e.g., distilled water). At the appropriate grading intervals (e.g., 1, 24, 48, and 72 hours after patch removal), the animals should be examined and scored for signs of erythema and edema according to the Draize dermal grading system. Grading of the test sites may be continued after the 72-hour scoring interval if irritation persists (e.g., day 7, day 10, day 14).

B. The Semioccluded Dermal Irritation Test in Rabbits

1. Materials

a. Gauze Dressing
Type: Ace-Tex Corporation nonsterilized
Thickness: 4-ply gauze dressing
Size: 1 × 1 inch

b. Tape — Nonirritating
Type: Blenderm®
Size: 1 inch wide

c. Binding Materials
Elastic wrap
Type: Rubber elastic bandage : Ace® Bandage, Coban®, or Expandovert®
Size: Adequate wrapping of the entire test site

d. Securing-Materials
Type: Zonas® porous athletic tape
Size: 2 inches wide

e. Elizabethan or similar collars: Optional.

f. Animal Species
New Zealand White Rabbit

2. Procedures

The hair is removed from a sufficient area on the rabbit's back on the day before dosing. Care should be taken to avoid abrading the skin during the clipping procedure. On the day of dosing, the test site (approximately 1 × 1 inch square of intact skin) should be designated and the gauze patch (1 × 1 inch) should be secured to the animal on at least two cut edges of the gauze patch using the nonirritating Blenderm tape. The test substance, either 0.5 ml or 0.5 g, should be administered under the gauze dressing and the remaining cut edges secured to the animal's back with nonirritating tape. Liquids are administered as received. Powders should be moistened with a suitable vehicle prior to application (e.g., distilled water). If the test article is a solid or powder that does not work well as a paste (e.g., does not spread well), 0.5 g of the test article will be applied to an approximate 1 × 1 inch 4-ply gauze patch and will be moistened with the appropriate amount of distilled water or suitable vehicle (generally 0.5 ml) and the gauze patch applied to the test site. The elastic wrap is then wrapped around the animal's torso and secured in place using the Zonas athletic tape. The Zonas tape is wrapped around the outermost portion of the elastic wrap at the cranial and caudal ends. An Elizabethan or similar collar may then be placed around the animal's neck. After the designated exposure time (i.e., 4 or 24 h), the tape, elastic wrap, and gauze patch are removed and the test site is delineated using an indelible marker. The test site should then be rinsed with a suitable vehicle (e.g., distilled water). At the appropriate grading intervals (e.g., 1, 24, 48, and 72 h after patch removal), the animals should be examined and scored for signs of erythema and edema according to the Draize dermal grading system. Grading of the test sites may be continued after the 72-h scoring interval if irritation persists (e.g., day 7, day 10, day 14).

C. THE NONOCCLUDED DERMAL IRRITATION TEST IN RABBITS

1. Materials

a. Elizabethan or similar collars or restrainer

b. Animal Species
New Zealand White Rabbit

2. Procedures

The hair is removed from a sufficient area on the rabbit's back on the day before dosing. Care should be taken to avoid abrading the skin during the clipping procedure. On the day of dosing, the test site (approximately 1 × 1 inch square of intact skin) should be designated and the test substance (0.5 ml or 0.5 g) should be administered to that area. Liquids are administered as received, powders should be moistened with a suitable vehicle before application (e.g., distilled water). The animal should then be placed in a restraining device or an Elizabethan or similar collar should be applied. After the designated exposure time (i.e., 4 or 24 hours), the test site should be delineated with an indelible marker and rinsed with a suitable vehicle (e.g., distilled water). At the appropriate grading intervals (e.g., 1, 24, 48, and 72 hours following patch removal), the animals should be examined and scored for signs of erythema and edema according to the Draize dermal grading system. Grading of the test sites may be continued after the 72-hour scoring interval if irritation persists.

D. THE CORROSIVITY TEST IN RABBITS

1. Materials

a. Gauze Dressing
Type: Ace-Tex Corporation nonsterilized
Thickness: 4-ply gauze dressing.
Size: 1 × 1 inch

b. Tape-Nonirritating
Type: Blenderm®
Size: 1 inch wide

c. Binding Materials
Elastic wrap
Type: Rubber elastic bandage: Ace® Bandage or Coban®

d.   Securing Materials
Type: Zonas® porous athletic tape
Size: 2 inches wide

e.   Elizabethan or similar collars: Optional.

f.   Animal Species
New Zealand White Rabbit

2.   Procedures

The hair is removed from a sufficient area on the rabbit's back on the day before dosing. Care should be taken to avoid abrading the skin during the clipping procedure. On the day of dosing, each test site (approximately 1 × 1 inch square of intact skin) should be selected based on the number of exposure periods required (i.e., 3 minutes, 1 hour, and/or 4 hours). The 1 × 1 inch gauze dressing should be secured to the animal's back at the designated exposure site on at least two cut edges of the gauze patch using the nonirritating Blenderm tape. The test substance, either 0.5 ml or 0.5 g, should be administered under the gauze dressing at each exposure site and the remaining cut edges secured to the animal's back. Liquids and powders should be administered as received. If the test article is a solid or powder that does not work well as a paste (e.g., does not spread well), 0.5 g of the test article will be applied to an approximate 1 × 1 inch 4-ply gauze patch and will be moistened with the appropriate amount of distilled water or suitable vehicle (generally 0.5 ml) and the gauze patch applied to the test site. The elastic wrap is then wrapped around the animal's torso and secured in place using the Zonas athletic tape. The Zonas is wrapped around the outer most portion of the elastic wrap at the cranial and caudal ends. If more than one exposure interval is utilized, the elastic wrap overlying the gauze dressings may be delineated using an indelible marker. This should aid in the unwrapping process. An Elizabethan or similar collar may then be applied to the animal. After the designated exposure interval (i.e., 3 min, 1 h, and/or 4 h), a window can be cut into the elastic wrap overlying the gauze patch for the appropriate test site and the gauze patch removed. The test site should be delineated with an indelible marker and then rinsed with a suitable vehicle (e.g., distilled water). If more than one exposure interval is utilized, the cut out window of the elastic wrap should be secured to the animal with additional Blenderm tape. This will help prevent possible disruption of the remaining site(s). These steps are repeated until the last exposure interval is completed, at which time the entire elastic wrap is removed. At the appropriate grading intervals (e.g., after patch removal and at 24, 48, and 72 h after patch application), the animals should be examined and scored for signs of erythema and edema according to the Draize dermal grading system. Grading of the test sites may be continued after the 72-h scoring interval if irritation persists.

E.   THE PHOTOIRRITATION TEST IN RABBITS

1.   Materials

a.   UVA Bulbs
Eight (nonoccluded procedure) or four (occluded procedure) Sylvania (Osram Sylvania, Danvers, MD) F-40/350 BL blacklight flourescent or equivalent.

b.   UVA/UVB Photometer
IL 1350 radiometer/photometer.

c.   Irradiation Deflector
Aluminum foil.

d.   Materials for Nonocclusive Procedure

Rabbit stocks or other restraining device

e.   Materials for Occlusive Procedure

1. Occlusive Materials
   Type: Impervious material: plastic wrap or other suitable plastic wrap
2. Binding Materials
   Type: Rubber elastic bandage: Ace® bandage, or Coban®, or Expandover®
   Size: Adequate wrapping of the entire test site
3. Securing Materials
   Type: Zonas® porous athletic tape
   Size: 2 inches wide
4. Tape — Nonirritating
   Type: Blenderm®
   Size: 1 inch wide
5. Gauze Dressing
   Type: Ace-Tex Corporation nonsterilized
   Thickness: 4-ply gauze dressing
   Size 1 × 1 in. square

f.   Animal Species

New Zealand White Rabbit

2.   Procedures

a.   Preliminary Procedures

The photoirritation study is conducted using three or six adult New Zealand White rabbits per group. Animals of either sex should be utilized for the test and positive control (if utilized) groups. On the day before dose administration, the animals selected for study should have the fur clipped for the dorsal area of the trunk of each animal using a small animal clipper. Care should be taken to avoid abrading the skin during the clipping procedure.

b.   Nonoccluded Procedure

On the following day (day 0), the test article (or positive control material, e.g., Oxsoralen Lotion, 1% 8-MOP from CN Pharmaceuticals, Inc., Cosa Mesa, CA, if used) will be applied initially to one small area of intact skin on the right side of each animal as follows: a 0.025 ml dose of the test article (or positive control material, if used) will be applied to one approximate 2.5 cm × 2.5 cm test site on the animals. The test sites will be delineated with a marker. The test sites will remain unoccluded. Immediately after application, the animals will be placed in stocks. Animals will remain in stocks until the completion of the UVA light exposure period and completion of the left site dose period. Approximately 2 h after test article application, excess test article may be removed using dry gauze to have adequate UVA light exposure. The test site may be re-delineated, if needed. Each animal will be wrapped with aluminum foil. An approximate 2.5 × 2.5 cm square section will be cut in the aluminum foil to expose the test site on the right side. Treatment sites on the right side will then be exposed to a target dose of 5 or 10 J/cm². UVA light (320 to 400 nm) will be emitted from a bank of eight Sylvania F-40/350 BL blacklight fluorescent tubes. The peak emission of the light source will be 360 nm. After the completion of the UVA light exposure period, the foil will be removed. Any residual test article (from right test sites) will be removed with gauze moistened in deionized water (or appropriate solvent) followed by dry gauze. Animals will be removed from the stocks and the test article (or positive control material) will be applied to an area of intact skin approximate 2.5 × 2.5 cm on the left side of each animal. The test sites will be delineated with a marker. The test site will remain unoccluded. The animals will be returned to the stocks until the completion of the exposure period. Approximately 2 h after test article application on the second test site (on the left side), any residual test article (from the left test site) will be removed with gauze moistened in deionized water (or appropriate solvent) followed by dry gauze. The test sites may be re-delineated, if needed. The animals will be returned to their cages.

c.   Occluded Procedure

On the day of dose administration (day 0), the test article (or positive control material, if utilized) will be applied to two small areas of intact skin of each animal as follows: 0.5 ml or 0.5 g aliquots of the test substance should be applied to two separate areas of intact skin, one on the left side and one on the right side of each test animal. The test substance is held in contact with the skin using an approximately 1 × 1 in. square gauze patch secured to the animal with a nonirritating tape. An impervious plastic wrap is placed over the trunk of the animal and further wrapped with an elastic wrap. The elastic wrap is then secured to the animal using the athletic tape. Animals will be placed in stocks following dosing and will remain in stocks until completion of UVA light exposure period. Approximately 2 h after chamber application, the elastic wrap, plastic wrap, and gauze patch located on the right side of each animal will be removed. Excess test article may be removed using dry gauze to have adequate UVA light exposure. The test site may be re-delineated (if needed). The patch on the left side of the animal will remain undisturbed. Each animal will be wrapped with aluminum foil. An approximate 2.5 × 2.5 cm square section will be cut in the aluminum foil to expose each test site on the right side. Treatment sites on the right side will then be exposed to a target dose of 5 or 10 J/cm^2. UVA light (320 to 400 nm) will be emitted from a bank of four or eight Sylvania F-40/350 BL blacklight fluorescent tubes. The peak emission of the light source will be 360 nm. After the completion of the UVA light exposure period, the foil and chamber (from the left side) will be removed. Any residual test article (from all sites) will be removed with gauze moistened in deionized water (or appropriate solvent) followed by dry gauze. Animals will be returned to their cages.

F.   The Photoirritation Test in Guinea Pigs

1.   Materials

a.   UVA Bulbs

Eight Sylvania (Osram Sylvania, Danvers, MD) F-40/350 BL blacklight flourescent or equivalent.

b.   UVA/UVB Photometer

IL 1350 radiometer/photometer.

c.   Irradiation Deflector

Aluminum foil.

d.   Materials for Nonocclusive Procedure

Type: Buehler restainer or similar device
Type: Dental dam

e.   Materials for Occlusive Procedure

   1.   Occlusive Materials
       Type: 25 mm Hilltop® Chamber
   2.   Binding Materials
       Type: Buehler restainer or similar device
       Type: Dental dam

f.   Animal Species

Hartley-derived albino guinea pig

2.   Procedures

a.   Preliminary Procedures

The photoirritation study is conducted using six adult Hartley-derived albino guinea pigs per group. Animals of either sex should be utilized for the test and positive control (if utilized) groups. On the day before dose administration, the animals selected for study should have the fur clipped for the dorsal area of the trunk of each animal using a small animal clipper. Care should be taken to avoid abrading the skin during the clipping procedure.

b.   Nonoccluded Procedure

On the following day (day 0), immediately prior to application, the animals will be placed in individual restrainers. The dental dam will be pulled taut over the back and secured to the bottom of the restrainer. An approximate 2.5×2.5 cm window will be cut into the right side of the dental dam to ensure that the test sites remain unoccluded. The restrainers will be adjusted as necessary to minimize any discomfort of the animals. Animals will remain in restrainers until the completion of the UVA light exposure period and completion of the left site dose period.

The test article (or positive control material, e.g., Oxsoralen Lotion 1% 8-MOP from CN Pharmaceuticals, Cosa, CA, if used) will be applied initially to one small area of intact skin on the right side of each appropriate animal as follows: a 0.025 ml dose of the test article (or positive control material, if used) will be applied to one approximate 2.5×2.5 cm test site on the animals. The test sites will then be delineated with a marker. The test sites will remain unoccluded. Approximately 2 h after test article application, excess test article may be removed using dry gauze in order to have adequate UVA light exposure. The test sites may be re-delineated, if needed. The back of each animal will be covered with aluminum foil. An approximate 2.5×2.5 cm square section will be cut in the aluminum foil to expose each test site on the right side. Treatment sites on the right side will then be exposed to a target dose of 10 J/cm^2. UVA light (320 to 400 nm) will be emitted from a bank of eight Sylvania F-40/350 BL blacklight fluorescent tubes. The peak emission of the light source will be 360 nm. After the completion of the UVA light exposure period, the foil will be removed. Any residual test article (from right test sites) will be removed with gauze moistened in deionized water (or appropriate solvent) followed by dry gauze. Animals will remain in restrainers and an approximate 2.5×2.5 cm window will be cut in the dental dam on the left side. The test article (or positive control material, if used) will be applied to an area of intact skin on the left side of each animal. The test material will be applied to an approximate 2.5×2.5 cm test site on the left side of the animals. The test site will remain unoccluded. Approximately 2 h after test article application on the second test site (on the left side), the remaining dental dam will be removed. Any residual test article (from the left test site) will be removed with gauze moistened in deionized water (or appropriate solvent) followed by dry gauze. The test sites may be re-delineated, if needed. The animals will be returned to their cages.

c.   Occluded Procedure

On the day of dose administration (day 0), the test article will be applied to two small areas of intact skin on the left and right side of each appropriate animal as follows: a 0.3 ml or 0.3 g (or maximum dose, powders to be moistened with the appropriate vehicle) dose of the test article (or positive control material as described previously, if used) will be applied to two 25 mm Hilltop chambers just prior to applying the chambers to the back. The Hilltop chambers will be applied to the back as quickly as possible. The test sites will be delineated with a marker. Immediately following application, the animals will be placed in individual restrainers and the chamber will be held at the designated site using rubber dental dam. The dental dam will be pulled taut over the back and secured to the bottom of the restrainer. The restrainers will be adjusted as necessary to minimize any discomfort of the animals. Animals will remain in restrainers until the completion of the UVA light exposure period. Approximately 2 h after chamber application, an approximate 2.5 × 2.5 cm square will be cut into the dental dam and the chamber located on the right side of each animal will be removed. Excess test article may be removed using dry gauze to have adequate UVA light exposure. The test site may be re-delineated (if needed). The chamber on the left side of the animal will remain undisturbed. The back of each animal will be covered with aluminum foil. An approximate 2.5 × 2.5 cm square section will be cut in the aluminum foil to expose each test site on the right side. Treatment sites on the right side will then be exposed to a target dose of 10 J/cm². UVA light (320 to 400 nm) will be emitted from a bank of eight Sylvania F-40/350 BL blacklight fluorescent tubes. The peak emission of the light source will be 360 nm. After the completion of the UVA light exposure period, the foil, the remaining dental dam, and chamber (from the left side) will be removed. Any residual test article (from all sites) will be removed with gauze moistened in deionized water (or appropriate solvent) followed by dry gauze.

SECTION 4. MATERIALS AND PROCEDURES FOR PERFORMING DERMAL SENSITIZATION STUDIES[33–50]

A. THE MODIFIED BUEHLER SENSITIZATION TEST IN GUINEA PIGS

1. Materials

a. Occlusive Materials

Type: 25 mm Hilltop® chamber (Hilltop Research, Inc., Cincinnati, OH), 2 × 2 cm Webril® patch; (Professional Medical Products, Greenwood, SC)

b. Binding Materials

Elastic wrap
Type: Expandover®, Coban®

c. Securing Materials

Type: Conform® (Kendall Health Care Products Co. Mansfield, MA)
Size: 1 inch wide

d. Depilatory Materials

Neet® (Reckitt & Coleman Inc., Wayne, NJ) hair remover cream

e. Animal Species

Hartley albino guinea pig

2. Procedures

A topical range-finding irritation screen should generally be performed before initiating the sensitization study. Four graded levels (generally 25% w/v, 50% w/v, 75% w/v, and 100%) are used for this procedure. Optimally, the topical range-finding study should produce no systemic toxicity and a spectrum of dermal responses that includes grades 0 ±, 1 and 2 unless the test substance is not dermally irritating at 100%.

Based on the range-finding results, the test substance concentration used for induction should produce no systemic toxicity and a mild to moderate dermal response (grades ±, 1 or 2) unless the test substance is not dermally irritating at 100%.

The test substance concentration used for challenge/rechallenge should produce no systemic toxicity and dermal responses generally consisting of grades 0 to ± unless the test substance is not dermally irritating at 100%.

3. Topical Range-Finding Study

On the day before dose administration, four topical range-finding guinea pigs should be weighed and the hair removed from the right and left side of the animals with a small animal clipper. Care should be taken to avoid abrading the skin during clipping procedures. On the following day, up to four closed patches/chambers at four different concentrations of test substance can be applied to the clipped area of each animal (one patch/chamber for each level of test substance). For liquids, gels, and pastes, a dose of 0.3 or 0.4 ml should be placed on a 25 mm Hilltop Chamber or Webril patch. For solids and powders, the maximum volume of solid/powder that can be contained in a 25 mm Hilltop Chamber (with cotton pad removed) should be utilized. Before chamber application, the test substance should be moistened with a suitable vehicle (e.g., distilled water). The patches/chambers should then be applied to the clipped surface as quickly as possible. The trunk of the animal should be wrapped with elastic wrap which is secured with adhesive tape (if necessary) to prevent removal of the patch/chamber and the animal returned to its cage. Approximately 6 hours after patch/chamber application, the elastic wrap, tape, and patches/chambers should be removed. The test substance should be removed with a suitable vehicle (e.g., distilled water). The test sites of the topical range-finding animals should be graded for irritation at approximately 24 and 48 hours after patch/chamber application using the Buehler dermal grading system.

4. Induction

On the day before the first induction dose administration (day −1), all sensitization study animals should be weighed. The hair should then be removed from the left side of the test animals with a small animal clipper. Care should be taken to avoid abrading the skin during clipping procedures. On the following day (day 0), patches/chambers containing the test substance should be applied to the clipped area of 10 to 20 test animals. For liquids, gels, and pastes, a dose of 0.3 ml or 0.4 ml should be placed on a 25 mm Hilltop Chamber or Webril patch. For solids and powders, the maximum volume of solid/powder that can be contained in a 25-mm Hilltop Chamber (with cotton pad removed) should be utilized. Before chamber application, the test substance should be moistened with a suitable vehicle (e.g., distilled water). The patch/chamber should then be applied to the clipped surface as quickly as possible. The trunk of each animal should be wrapped with elastic wrap which is secured with adhesive tape (if necessary) to prevent removal of the patch/chamber and the animal returned to its cage. Approximately 6 hours after dosing, the elastic wrap, tape, and patch/chamber will be removed. The test substance should be removed with a suitable vehicle (e.g., distilled water). The induction clipping, patch application, and grading procedure should be repeated on study day 7 (± 1 day) and study day 14 (± 1 day) so that a total of three consecutive induction exposures should be administered to the test animals. Test sites should be graded for dermal irritation at approximately 24 and 48 h after patch application using the Buehler dermal grading system. The application site may be moved if irritation persists from a previous induction exposure but will remain on the left side of the animal. If a positive control group is necessary, 2, 4-dinitrochlorobenzene (DNCB) and α-hexylcinnamaldehyde is an acceptable positive control substance and a positive control group consisting of 10 DNCB or HCA test animals and 10 DNCB or HCA control animals may be used. The DNCB or HCA test and DNCB or HCA control animals should be treated in the same manner as the sensitization study test and challenge control animals throughout the study. The DNCB concentrations standardly used for induction and challenge are 0.1 to 0.5% w/v and 0.05 to 0.1% w/v, respectively. The HCA concentrations standardly used for induction and challenge are 3.0 to 5.0% and 1.0 to 2.5%, respectively. A response of at least 15% in a nonadjuvant test should be expected for a mild to moderate sensitizer.

5. Challenge

On the day before challenge dose administration, the hair should be removed from the right side of the test and challenge control animals with a small animal clipper. Care will be taken to avoid abrading the skin during clipping procedures. On the next day (day 28 ± 1 day), patches/chambers containing the test substance should be applied to a naive site within the clipped area of the test and challenge control animals. For liquids, gels, and pastes, a dose of 0.3 ml or 0.4 ml should be placed on a 25 mm Hilltop Chamber or Webril patch. For solids and powders, the maximum volume of solid/powder that can be contained in a 25 mm Hilltop Chamber (with cotton pad removed) should be used. Before chamber application, the test substance should be moistened with an appropriate vehicle (e.g., distilled water). The patch/chamber should then be applied to the clipped surface as quickly as possible. The trunk of each animal should be wrapped with elastic wrap which is secured with adhesive tape (if necessary) to prevent removal of the patch/chamber and the animal returned to its cage. Approximately 6 h after dosing, the elastic wrap, tape, and patch/chamber should be removed. The test substance should then be removed with a suitable vehicle (e.g., distilled water).

Approximately 20 hours after patch/chamber removal, the test sites may be depilated (optional) as follows:

1. Neet Hair Remover cream should be placed on the test sites and surrounding areas and left on for no more than 15 minutes.
2. The depilatory should then be thoroughly removed with a stream of warm water. The animals should be dried with a towel and returned to their cages.

Note: The depilatory process has an advantage of being able to view test sites without hair, however, from time to time suspected test article/depilatory reactions may be observed producing unanticipated dermal responses in the test and control animals.

Test sites should be graded for dermal irritation at approximately 24 and 48 hours after patch removal using the Buehler dermal grading system.

6. Rechallenge

If a rechallenge phase is required, the procedure should be performed on day 35 (± 1 day). The animal's haircoat should again be clipped on the right side of the animal on the day before dosing. The exposure period, dosing, wrapping, and depilation procedures should be the same as used in the challenge procedure except that the 10 to 20 test and 10 naive rechallenge control animals and a naive skin site is utilized.

B. THE STANDARD BUEHLER SENSITIZATION TEST IN GUINEA PIGS

1. Materials

a. Occlusive Materials
Type: 25 mm Hilltop® Chamber, 2 × 2 cm Webril® Patch

b. Binding Materials
Elastic wrap
Type: Expandover®, Coban®

c. Securing Materials
Type: Conform®
Size: 1 inch wide

d. Depilatory Materials
Neet®Hair Remover Cream

e. Animal Species
Hartley albino guinea pig

2. Procedures

A topical range-finding irritation screen generally should be performed before initiating the sensitization study. Four graded levels (generally 25% w/v, 50% w/v, 75% w/v, and 100%) are utilized for this procedure. Optimally, the topical range-finding study should produce no systemic toxicity and a spectrum of dermal responses that includes grades 0, ±, 1, and 2 unless the test substance is not dermally irritating at 100%.

Based on the range-finding results, the test substance concentration used for induction should produce no systemic toxicity and a mild to moderate dermal response (grades ±, 1 or 2) unless the test substance is not dermally irritating at 100%.

The test substance concentration used for challenge/rechallenge should produce no systemic toxicity and dermal responses generally consisting of grades 0 to ± unless the test substance is not dermally irritating at 100%.

3. Topical Range-Finding Study

On the day before dose administration, four topical range-finding guinea pigs should be weighed and the hair removed from the right and left side of the animals with a small animal clipper. Care should be taken to avoid abrading the skin during clipping procedures. On the next day, up to four closed patches/chambers at four different concentrations of test substance can be applied to the clipped area of each animal (one patch/chamber for each level of test substance). For liquids, gels, and pastes, a dose of 0.3 ml or 0.4 ml will be placed on a 25-mm Hilltop Chamber or Webril patch. For solids and powders, the maximum volume of solid/powder that can be contained in a 25-mm Hilltop Chamber (with cotton pad removed) should be utilized. Before chamber application, the test substance should be moistened with a suitable vehicle (e.g., distilled water). The patches/chambers should then be applied to the clipped surface as quickly as possible. The trunk of the animal should be wrapped with elastic wrap which is secured with adhesive tape (if necessary) to prevent removal of the patch/chamber and the animal returned to its cage. Approximately 6 h after patch/chamber application, the elastic wrap, tape, and patches/chambers should be removed. The test substance should be removed with a suitable vehicle (e.g., distilled water). The test sites of the topical range-finding animals should be graded for irritation at approximately 24 and 48 h after patch/chamber application using the Buehler dermal grading system.

4. Induction

On the day before the first induction dose administration (day −1), all sensitization study animals should be weighed. The hair should then be removed from the left side of the test animals with a small animal clipper. Care will be taken to avoid abrading the skin during clipping procedures. On the next day (day 0), patches/chambers containing the test substance should be applied to the clipped area of 10 to 20 test animals. For liquids, gels, and pastes, a dose of 0.3 ml or 0.4 ml should be placed on a 25 mm Hilltop Chamber or Webril patch. For solids and powders, the maximum volume of solid/powder that can be contained in a 25 mm Hilltop Chamber (with cotton pad removed) should be used. Before chamber application, the test substance should be moistened with a suitable vehicle (e.g., distilled water). The patch/chamber should then be applied to the clipped surface as quickly as possible. The trunk of each animal should be wrapped with elastic wrap which is secured with adhesive tape (if necessary) to prevent removal of the patch/chamber and the animal returned to its cage. Approximately 6 h after dosing, the elastic wrap, tape, and patch/chamber will be removed. The test substance should be removed with a suitable vehicle (e.g., distilled water). The induction clipping, patch application, and grading procedure should be repeated three times a week (i.e., Monday-Wednesday-Friday) for 3 consecutive weeks so that a total of nine consecutive induction exposures are administered to the test animals. Test sites should be graded for dermal irritation at approximately 24 and 48 h after patch application using the Buehler dermal grading system. The application site may be moved if irritation persists from a previous induction exposure but will remain on the left side of the animal. If a positive control group is necessary, DNCB or HCA is an acceptable positive control substance, and a positive control group consisting of 10 DNCB or HCA test animals and 10 DNCB or HCA control animals may be used. The DNCB or HCA test and DNCB or HCA control animals should be treated in the same manner as the sensitization study test and challenge control animals throughout the study. The DNCB concentrations standardly used for induction and challenge are 0.1 to 0.5% w/v and 0.05 to 0.1% w/v, respectively. The HCA concentrations standardly used for induction and challenge are 3.0 to 5.0% and 1.0 to 2.5%, respectively. A response of at least 15% in a nonadjuvant test should be expected for a mild to moderate sensitizer.

5. Challenge

On the day before challenge dose administration, the hair should be removed from the right side of the test and challenge control animals with a small animal clipper. Care will be taken to avoid abrading of the skin during clipping procedures. On the next day (day 32 ± 1 day), patches/ chambers containing the test substance should be applied to a naive site within the clipped area of the test and challenge control animals. For liquids, gels, and pastes, a dose of 0.3 ml or 0.4 ml should be placed on a 25 mm Hilltop Chamber or Webril patch. For solids and powders, the maximum volume of solid/powder that can be contained in a 25 mm Hilltop Chamber (with cotton pad removed) should be utilized. Before chamber application, the test substance should be moistened with an appropriate vehicle (e.g., distilled water). The patch/chamber should then be applied to the clipped surface as quickly as possible. The trunk of each animal should be wrapped with elastic wrap which is secured with adhesive tape (if necessary) to prevent removal of the patch/chamber and the animal returned to its cage. Approximately 6 h after dosing, the elastic wrap, tape, and patch/chamber should be removed. The test substance should then be removed with a suitable vehicle (e.g., distilled water).

Approximately 20 h after patch/chamber removal, the test sites may be depilated (optional) as follows:

1. Neet Hair Remover cream should be placed on the test sites and surrounding areas and left on for no more than 15 min.
2. The depilatory should then be removed thoroughly with a stream of warm water. The animals should then be dried with a towel and returned to their cages.

Note: The depilatory process has an advantage of being able to view test sites without hair, however, from time to time, suspected test article/depilatory reactions may be observed producing unanticipated dermal responses in the test and control animals.

Test sites should be graded for dermal irritation at approximately 24 and 48 h after patch removal using the Buehler dermal grading system.

6. Rechallenge

If a rechallenge phase is required, the procedure should be performed on day 39 (± 1 day). The animal's haircoat should again be clipped on the right side of the animal on the day before dosing. The exposure period, dosing, wrapping, and depilation procedures should be the same as used in the challenge procedure except that the 10 to 20 test and 10 naive rechallenge control animals and a naive skin site is utilized.

C. THE GUINEA PIG MAXIMIZATION TEST

1. Materials

a. Injection Materials

Monoject® (Sherwood Medical, St. Louis, MO) or equivalent 1 cc Tuberculin syringe with 25 to 27 gauge–⅝-inch needle

b.   Occlusive Materials
Type: 2 × 2 cm Webril® patch, 2 × 4 cm Modified Webril® Patch, 25 mm Hilltop® Chamber

c.   Binding Materials
Elastic wrap
Type: Coban®

d.   Securing Materials
Type: Conform® Zones® Athletic Tape
Size: 1-in. wide

e.   Animal Species
Hartley albino guinea pig

2.   Procedures

For the topical screen, four graded levels (generally 25% w/v, 50% w/v, 75% w/v, and 100%) are used for this procedure. Optimally, the topical range-finding study should produce no systemic toxicity and a spectrum of dermal responses that includes grades 0, ±, 1 and 2 unless the test substance is not dermally irritating at 100%.

For the intradermal screen, four graded levels (generally 0.1% w/v, 1.0% w/v, 3.0% w/v, and 5.0% w/v) are used for this procedure. Optimally, the intradermal range-finding study should produce no systemic toxicity and only localized reactions at the injection site (responses that do not notably extend beyond the site of injection).

Based on this information, the test substance concentration used for intradermal induction should produce no systemic toxicity and only localized reactions at the injection site (responses that do not notably extend beyond the site of injection). For the topical induction, the test substance concentration used should produce a mild to moderate dermal response (grades ±, 1 or 2) unless the test substance is not dermally irritating at 100%.

The test substance concentration used for challenge/rechallenge should produce no systemic toxicity and dermal responses generally consisting of grades 0 to ± unless the test substance is not dermally irritating at 100%.

3.   Topical Range-Finding Study

On the day before dose administration, four topical range-finding guinea pigs should be weighed and the hair removed from the right and left side of the animals with a small animal clipper. Care should be taken to avoid abrading the skin during clipping procedures. On the next day, up to four closed patches/chambers at four different concentrations of test substance can be applied to the clipped area of each animal (one patch/chamber for each level of test substance). For liquids, gels and pastes, a dose of 0.3 ml or 0.4 ml should be placed on a 25 mm Hilltop Chamber or Webril patch. For solids and powders, the maximum volume of solid/powder that can be contained in a 25 mm Hilltop Chamber (with cotton pad removed) should be used. Before chamber application, the test substance should be moistened with a suitable vehicle (e.g., distilled water). The patches/chambers should then be applied to the clipped surface as quickly as possible. The trunk of the animal should be wrapped with elastic wrap which is secured with adhesive tape (if necessary) to prevent removal of the patch/chamber. Approximately 24 h after patch/chamber application, the elastic wrap, tape, and patches/chambers should be removed. The test substance should be removed with a suitable vehicle (e.g., distilled water). The test sites of the topical range-finding animals should be graded for irritation at approximately 24 and 48 h after patch/chamber removal using the Buehler dermal grading system.

4. Intradermal Range-Finding Study

On the day before dose administration, four intradermal range-finding guinea pigs should be weighed and the hair removed from the right and left side of the animals with a small animal clipper. Care should be taken to avoid abrading the skin during clipping procedures. On the next day, up to four intradermal injections at four different concentrations of test substance can be injected into the clipped area of each animal (one injection for each level of test substance). A dose of 0.1 ml should be injected for each concentration using a syringe attached to a hypodermic needle.

The test sites of the intradermal range-finding animals should be graded for irritation at approximately 24 and 48 h after intradermal injections using the Buehler dermal grading system.

5. Induction

On the day before intradermal dosing (day − 1), all sensitization study animals should be weighed. The hair should then be removed from the scapular area of 10 to 20 test and 10 challenge control animals with a small animal clipper. Care should be taken to avoid abrading the skin during clipping procedures. On the next day (day 0), three pairs of intradermal injections should be made in the clipped area of all sensitization study animals. The injections should be kept within an approximate 2 × 4 cm area with one row of three injections on each side of the back bone as indicated below:

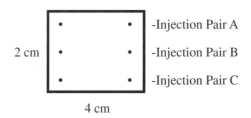

$$2 \text{ cm} \qquad \qquad 4 \text{ cm}$$

-Injection Pair A

-Injection Pair B

-Injection Pair C

Injections for the test animals should be as indicated: 1) Injection Pair A , 0.1 ml of a 1:1 v/v Freund's Complete Adjuvant in sterile water emulsion (FCA emulsion); 2) Injection Pair B, 0.1 ml of the test substance preparation; 3) Injection Pair C, 0.1 ml of the test substance in the FCA emulsion.

Injections for the challenge control animals should be as indicated: 1) Injection Pair A, 0.1 ml of the FCA emulsion; 2) Injection Pair B, 0.1 ml of the vehicle; 3) Injection Pair C, 0.1 ml of the vehicle/ FCA emulsion.

On the day before topical induction, the hair should be clipped from the scapular area of the test and challenge control animals using a small animal clipper. Care should be taken to avoid abrading the skin during the clipping procedures. A 10% w/w sodium lauryl sulfate preparation in petrolatum should then be applied to the 2 × 4 cm intradermal injection area so that the injection area is sufficiently covered with the preparation (0.5 ml). On the next day (day 7 ± 1 day), any residual sodium lauryl sulfate preparation should be removed with a dry gauze, and the test animals should receive a topical dose of the test substance. The challenge control animals should receive a topical dose of the vehicle. Each animal's dose first should be applied to a modified Webril patch and the patch applied over the intradermal injection sites as quickly as possible. For liquids, gels, and pastes, a dose of 0.8 ml should be placed on the modified Webril patch. For solids and powders, the maximum volume of solid/powder that can be maintained on the modified Webril patch should be used. Before solid/powder application, the test substance should be moistened with a suitable vehicle (e.g., distilled water). The trunk of each animal should then be wrapped with elastic wrap which is secured with adhesive tape (if necessary) to prevent removal of the patch and the animal returned to its cage. Approximately 48 h after dosing, the elastic wrap, tape, and patch should be removed. The test substance should be removed with a suitable vehicle (e.g., distilled water).

If a positive control group is necessary, DNCB or HCA are acceptable positive control substances, and a positive control group consisting of 10 DNCB or HCA test animals and 10 DNCB or HCA control animals may be used. The DNCB or HCA test and control animals should be treated in the same manner as the sensitization study test and control animals throughout the study. The DNCB concentrations standardly used for induction and challenge are 0.1 to 0.5% w/v and 0.05 to 0.1% w/v, respectively. The HCA concentrations standardly used for induction and challenge are 3.0 to 5.0% w/v and 0.5 to 1.0% w/v, respectively. A response of at least 30% in an adjuvant test should be expected for a mild to moderate sensitizer.

6. Challenge

On the day before challenge dose administration, all test and challenge control animals should be weighed. The hair should then be removed from the right side of the test and challenge control animals with a small animal clipper. Care should be taken to avoid abrading of the skin during clipping procedures. On the next day (day 21 ± 1 day), the test and challenge control animals should receive a topical dose of the test substance. For liquids, gels, and pastes, a dose of 0.3 ml or 0.4 ml should be placed on a 25 mm Hilltop Chamber or Webril patch. For solids and powders, the maximum volume of solid/powder that can be contained in a 25 mm Hilltop Chamber (with cotton pad removed) should be used. The weight of the solid/powder placed in the chamber should be recorded. Before chamber application, the test substance should be moistened with a suitable vehicle (e.g., distilled water). The patch/chamber should then be applied to the clipped surface as quickly as possible. The trunk of each animal should be wrapped with elastic wrap which is secured with adhesive tape (if necessary) to prevent removal of the patch/chamber and the animal returned to its cage. Approximately 24 h after dosing, the elastic wrap, tape, and patch/chamber should be removed. The test substance should be removed with a suitable vehicle (e.g., distilled water). The test sites should be graded for dermal irritation at approximately 24 and 48 hours after patch removal using the Buehler dermal grading system.

7. Rechallenge

If a rechallenge phase is required, the rechallenge procedure should be performed on day 28 (±1 day). The animal's haircoat should be clipped on the left side of the animal on the day before dosing. The exposure period, dosing, and the wrapping procedures are the same as used in the challenge procedure except that 10 naive rechallenge control animals and a naive skin site are utilized.

D. The Murine Local Lymph Node Assay

1. Materials

a. *Dosing Materials*

1. Calibrated pipette or syringe
2. 1-cc disposable syringe, 25 to 27 gauge needle

b. *Lymph Node Collection/Cell Suspension Materials*

1. Tissue culture dish (e.g., 60 mm)
2. Tissue culture tube (e.g., 12 × 75 mm)
3. Centrifuge tube (e.g., 15 ml)
4. Nylon or stainless steel screen, ~100 to 200 μm mesh opening, ~85 μm thick

5. Pasteur pipet
6. Forceps
7. Scintillation cocktail (e.g., Ecovolume®)

c. Animal Species
Female CBA mice.

2. Procedures

The test material is applied directly to the ears for assessing the contact hypersensitization. These procedures evaluate the ability of the test article to cause lymphocyte proliferation as determined by incorporation of 3H-thymidine by lymphocytes within the appropriate draining lymph nodes of topically treated mice, which is then compared to appropriate control mice. Generally, no range-finding animals are utilized unless there is a concern for dermal trauma (corrosion/severe irritation) or systemic toxicity. Instead, at least three consecutive concentrations from the following range are utilized: 100, 50, 25, 10, 5, 2.5, 1, 0.5, 0.25, and 0.1% (w/v). The selection is made to provide the highest possible test concentration, which is generally limited by compatibility with the vehicle chosen and the suitability of the resulting preparation for unoccluded dermal application. The following vehicles are recommended, in order of preference: acetone–olive oil (4:1), acetone, dimethylformamide, methyl ethyl ketone, propylene glycol, and dimethysulfoxide. Aqueous vehicles are not normally recommended because of insufficient absorption during the dosing procedure; however, aqueous-organic mixtures such as 3:1 acetone–water or 80% ethanol have been used successfully. Materals for positive control include 2,4-dinitrochlorobenzene (DNCB), α-hexylcin-namaldehyde (HCA), 2-mercaptobenzothiazole, and benzocaine. A threefold or greater increase in proliferative activity of the test animals compared with concurrent vehicle treated control animals is the criterion for a classification of skin-sensitizing activity.

3. Topical Induction

On day 0, 5 females per test article concentration and control group (and positive control test and control group, if utilized) will be weighed and 25 µl of test article will be applied to the dorsal surface of the left and right ear. Care will be taken to ensure that the test article will not run off of the ear during application. Approximately 24 h later (day 1) and 48 h later (day 2), each animal will receive additional applications as described previously. The animals will then be rested for 2 days. The vehicle control animals (and positive control animals, if used) are treated the same as above.

4. Injection of 3H-thymidine for Lymphocyte Incorporation

On day 5 (approximately 72 h after the final application), the five females per group will receive an intravenous injection of 3H-thymidine for lymphocyte incorporation. The injection will consist of 0.250 ml of phosphate-buffered saline (PBS) containing 20 µCi of 3H-thymidine (specific activity of 5.0 or 6.7 Ci/mmol). An animal will be excluded from the study if the full 0.250 ml of 3H-thymidine/PBS is not properly injected intravenously.

5. Lymph Node Collection

Approximately 5 h after the 3H-thymidine injections, the animals will be euthanized with carbon dioxide and the appropriate draining (auricular) lymph nodes will be removed and pooled for each individual animal. Care will be taken to assure that the lymph nodes are removed intact and placed in a capped tissue culture tube (e.g. 12×75 mm) containing 4 ml of PBS.

6. Cell Suspension

The lymph nodes will be transferred to a tissue culture dish (e.g., 60 mm) by pouring the PBS tube containing the lymph nodes. The lymph nodes will be mechanically passed through a nylon or stainless steel screen. A pasteur pipet and a small pair of forceps will be used to rinse the screen with PBS into the tissue culture dish, which will then be rinsed with the PBS back into the culture tube to allow the capsule debris to settle to the bottom. The PBS will then be carefully drawn off with a pasteur pipet and will be placed in a centrifuge tube containing 6 ml of PBS (approximately 10 ml total tube volume). The cell suspensions will then be centrifuged and then resuspended in 20 ml of PBS and a second wash will be performed. After completion of the second wash, the cells will be suspended in 3 ml of 5% trichloroacetic acid (w/v TCA in deionized water) and left at approximately 4°C for approximately 18 h.

7. Scintillation Counting

The cell suspensions will be centrifuged and resuspended in 1 ml of 5% TCA. The individual cell suspensions will be transferred into the appropriate scintillation vials containing 10 ml of scintillation cocktail along with an additional 1 ml of TCA, which has been used to rinse the bottom portion of the tube. The TCA and scintillation fluid will be thoroughly mixed by gently swirling the contents of the vial until the solution becomes clear. The sample will then be counted and recorded in disintergrations per minute (DPM).

E. THE PHOTOSENSITIZATION TEST IN MICE

1. Materials

a. UVA Bulbs

Four Sylvania® F-40/350 BL blacklight fluorescent or equivalent.

b. UVB Bulbs

Phillips® (Phillips Lighting Co. Somerset, NJ) F-40 UVB fluorescent sunlamps or equivalent.

c. UVA/UVB Photometer

IL 1350 radiometer/photometer.

d. Dyer® (Dyer Company, Lancaster, PA) Micrometer

Model D-1000.

e. Irradiation Deflector

3-mm thick sheet of plate glass (large enough to cover UVA-exposed animals).

f. Micropipettor

Eppendorf® (Brinkman Instruments, Inc., Westbury, NY) 1 to 50 µL micropipetter.

g. Animal Species

BALB/c mice.

2. Procedures

A preliminary irritation screen should generally be included in this test to observe the degree of primary irritation the test substance may produce. Twenty female mice, separated into 4 dose groups (5 mice/ group), are used for this procedure. Up to four different concentrations of the test substance can be utilized. Each mouse should be placed in a restrainer and two measurements of ear thickness should be performed using an engineer's micrometer. Two different concentrations may be utilized on each mouse, one concentration for each ear. Eight microliters of the test substance should be used for animals in groups 3 and 4 and 8 µl of the vehicle for groups 1 and 2. The appropriate material should be applied to both sides of the ear. After a 60-min waiting period, the ears should be wiped with gauze moistened with an appropriate vehicle (e.g., distilled water). Mice from groups 2 and 4 should then be exposed to 10 J/cm^2 UVA and 25 to 60 mJ/cm^2 UVB. Mice in groups 1 and 3 are not irradiated. At approximately 3, 24, and 48 h postirradiation, the mice should be placed back into the restraining device and ear measurements should once again be performed and recorded.

3. Induction

An induction phase of the photosensitization study should be initiated with an intraperitoneal injection of cyclophosphamide (CP). A dose of 200 mg/kg CP in sterile phosphate-buffered saline at a dose volume of 10 ml/kg should be injected approximately 3 days before the first induction. Because the CP injections may induce toxicity and/or mortality, additional mice should be used for this procedure to allow for a sufficient number of animals on study. On day 0, the backs of all mice should be clipped using a small animal clipper and appropriately sized clipper blade. Standard study designs are set up with four groups of five female mice each. The first two groups are designated as test substance groups with the remaining two groups set up as vehicle control and ultraviolet control groups, respectively. The mice designated for groups 1, 2, and 4 are induced on days 0, 1, and 2. Group 3 animals are not treated during the induction phase. Mice in groups 1 and 2 should receive 50 µl of the appropriate test substance gently rubbed into the skin on the dorsal back of each animal on each of the induction days. Mice in group 4 should receive 50 µl of the designated vehicle in the same manner. Each mouse is then placed in an individual compartment of an irradiation box with a wire lid restraining device. Approximately 60 min after application of the appropriate material, the treated area of each animal should be gently wiped against the grain of hair growth with a gauze patch moistened with an appropriate vehicle. After the wiping procedure, animals from group 2 should be returned to their respective cages and should not receive irradiation. Mice in groups 1 and 4 should be exposed to 10 J/cm^2 UVA and 25 mJ/cm^2 UVB from a distance of approximately 20 ± 1.0 cm. For the UVA exposure, a 3-mm-thick sheet of plate glass should be placed over the UVA radiometer detector during irradiation measurements to filter out any UVB wavelengths that may be emitted. The mice from groups 1 and 4 are then exposed to UVA light (320 to 400 nm) emitted from a bank of four Sylvania F-40/350 BL blacklight fluorescent tubes. The bank of lights are positioned approximately 20 ± 1.0 cm above the irradiation boxes containing the mice for a target dose of 10 J/cm^2. A peak emission of the UVA lights should be at 360 nm. For the UVB exposure, the mice should be positioned under a bank of eight Phillips F40 UVB fluorescent sunlamps for an exposure of 25 mJ/cm^2 UVB light. It is preferable to rotate the animals' positions for each induction exposure so that no one group is irradiated in the same location.

4. Challenge

A challenge phase of the photosensitization study should be performed 7 days after the first induction phase. Before challenge, each mouse should have the ear thickness measured on both ears using an engineer's micrometer (Model D-1000). Measurements should be read and recorded as millimeters $\times 10^{-2}$. These measurements should take place while the animal is in a restraining device. While the animal is still restrained, 8 µl of the test substance will be administered to each side of one ear. The vehicle is then applied to both sides of the opposite ear. After approximately 60 min, the ears should be wiped with the appropriate vehicle and the animals in groups 1, 3, and 4 exposed to 10 J/cm^2 UVA and 25 mJ/cm^2 UVB as indicated previously. The group 2 mice should not be irradiated. Ear thickness measurements as described previously should be performed at approximately 24 and 48 h after the challenge procedure.

5. Rechallenge

If a rechallenge phase is required, the procedure should be performed 7 days after the challenge exposure. The exposure period, irradiation, and ear measurement procedures should be the same as used in the challenge procedure.

F. THE PHOTOSENSITIZATION TEST IN GUINEA PIGS

1. Materials

a. UVA Bulbs
Four Sylvania® F-40/350 BL blacklight fluorescent or equivalent.

b. UVA/UVB Photometer
IL 1350 radiometer/photometer.

c. Irradiation Deflector
Aluminum foil.

d. Patching Materials
Webril® patch 2 × 2 cm or 25 mm Hilltop® Chamber; rubber dental dam; Blenderm® tape.

e. Animal Species
Hartley albino guinea pig.

2. Procedures

Unless the irritation potential of the test substance is known, the study should begin with a topical range-finding study. The range-finding study should include eight Hartley-derived albino guinea pigs (4 males and 4 females). Up to four graded concentrations of the test substance may be used in this procedure. On the day before dose administration, the eight guinea pigs should be weighed and the hair removed from the left and right side of each animal using a small animal clipper. Care should be taken to avoid abrading the skin during the clipping procedure. On the day of dose administration, a 0.3 ml or 0.4-ml dose of the appropriate concentration of the test substance should be administered to a 25 mm Hilltop Chamber or Webril patch and the patch immediately placed on the right or left side of the guinea pig (one patch on either side of the back bone). Four patches (two patches per concentration) may be applied. Immediately after application, the animals should be placed in a Buehler restrainer and the patches occluded using rubber dental dam. The dental dam should be pulled taut over the back of the animal and fastened to the bottom of the restrainer. After an exposure period of 2 hours, a 2 × 2 cm square should be cut into the dental dam and the patch removed from the right side of each animal. The patch on the left side of the animal should remain intact. The back of each animal should then be covered with aluminum foil. An approximately 2 × 2 cm square section should be cut in the aluminum foil on each animal to expose the test site on the right side. The treated sites on the right side of the animal should then be exposed to UVA light (320 to 400 nm) at a target dose of 10 J/cm^2. Any heavy residual test substance is removed with dry gauze before irradiation to fully expose the test site. After the exposure, the foil, dental dam, and remaining patches from the left side should be removed and any residual test substance removed with an appropriate vehicle. The dermal test sites should be graded at approximately 24 and 48 h after the initiation of the UVA light exposure.

3. Induction

The induction phase of the study is initiated by weighing the animals and clipping the hair from the scapular area of the 10 test and 10 challenge control animals. Care is taken to avoid abrading the skin during the clipping procedure. On the day of dose administration (day 0), four 0.1-ml intradermal injections of a 1:1 v/v Freund's Complete Adjuvant in sterile water emulsion are administered to the previously prepared animals. The injections should be made on each side of the back bone. The center portion of the skin between the injection sites is then tape-stripped using an adhesive tape to remove the outer layers of the epidermis. A single 25 mm Hilltop® Chamber or Webril patch containing 0.3 ml or 0.4 ml of the test substance for the test animals and 0.3 ml or 0.4 ml of vehicle for the challenge control animals should be applied immediately to the center of the tape-stripped area. A piece of rubber dental dam should be placed over the application site and secured to the bottom of the restrainer to provide an occlusive binding. After approximately 2 hours of exposure a 2×2 cm square will be cut in the rubber dam and the patch removed. Aluminum foil is then placed over the entire back of each guinea pig and an approximately 2×2 cm square window over the test area is cut to allow exposure to the UVA treatment. Any heavy residual test substance is removed with dry gauze before irradiation to fully expose the test site. The test sites should then be exposed to UVA light (320 to 400 nm) at a target dose of 10 J/cm². After the completion of the exposure period, the aluminum foil and dental dam should be removed and the test substances removed with an appropriate vehicle. The induction procedure should be repeated three times a week (e.g., Monday-Wednesday-Friday) for 2 consecutive weeks for a total of six induction exposures. If a positive control group is necessary, Musk Ambrette is an acceptable positive control substance, and a positive control group consisting of 10 Musk Ambrette test animals and 10 Musk Ambrette control animals should be treated in the same manner as the photosensitization study test and challenge control animals throughout the study. The Musk Ambrette concentrations standardly used for induction and challenge are 15% w/v and 0.5% w/v, respectively.

4. Challenge

A challenge procedure should be performed on study day 25 ($\pm$ 1 day). On the day before challenge dose administration, the test and challenge control animals should be weighed and the hair removed from the left and right side of the animal using a small animal clipper. On the next day, a 0.3 ml or 0.4 ml volume of the test substance should be applied to each of 2 25 mm Hilltop Chamber or Webril patches. One patch will be applied to each side of each animal. Immediately after the patching procedure, the animals should once again be placed into restrainers and the test sites immediately occluded with a piece of rubber dental dam. After approximately 2 h of exposure, a 2×2 cm square should be cut into the dental dam and the patch from the right side of each animal removed. Aluminum foil should then be placed over the back of each animal and a 2×2 cm square window cut in the foil to allow the test area to be exposed to the UVA light. Any heavy residual test substance is removed with dry gauze before irradiation to fully expose the test site. The test sites on the right side should then be exposed to UVA light (320 to 400 nm) at a target dose of 10 J/cm². After the target exposure, the foil, dental dam, and patches should be removed and any residual test substance removed with an appropriate vehicle. The test sites should be graded at approximately 24 and 48 h after the initiation of the UVA exposure using a Draize grading system.

5. Rechallenge

If the results of the challenge phase are not conclusive, a rechallenge procedure can be performed on study day 32 ($\pm$ 1 day). The rechallenge phase should be similar in design to the challenge phase except that 10 naive rechallenge control animals and a naive skin site should be utilized for this phase.

SECTION 5. COMPARISON OF SCORING SYSTEMS

TABLE 3.8
Draize Dermal Irritation Scoring System[24]

Erythema and Eschar Formation	Value	Edema Formation	Value
No erythema	0	No edema	0
Very slight erythema (barely perceptible)	1	Very slight edema (barely perceptible)	1
Well-defined erythema	2	Slight edema (edges of area well defined by definite raising)	2
Moderate to severe erythema	3	Moderate edema (raised approximately 1 mm)	3
Severe erythema (beet-redness) to slight, eschar formation (injuries in depth)	4	Severe edema (raised more than 1 mm and extending beyond the area of exposure)	4

TABLE 3.9
Human Patch Test Dermal Irritation Scoring System[51]

Skin Reaction	Value
No sign of inflammation; normal skin	0
Glazed appearance of the sites, or barely perceptible erythema	± (0.5)
Slight erythema	1
Moderate erythema, possible with barely perceptible edema at the margin; papules may be present	2
Moderate erythema, with generalized edema	3
Severe erythema with severe edema, with or without vesicles	4
Severe reaction spread beyond the area of the patch	5

TABLE 3.10
Chamber Scarification Dermal Irritation Scoring System[51]

Skin Reaction	Value
Scratch marks barely visible	0
Erythema confined to scratches perceptible erythema	1
Broader bands of increased erythema, with or without rows of vesicles, pustules, or erosions	2
Severe erythema with partial confluency, with or without other lesions	3
Confluent, severe erythema sometimes associated with edema, necrosis, or bullae	4

TABLE 3.11
Magnusson Sensitization Scoring System[38]

Skin Reaction	Value
No reaction	0
Scattered reaction	1
Moderate and diffuse reaction	2
Intense reddening and swelling	3

TABLE 3.12
Split Adjuvant Sensitization Scoring System[52]

Skin Reaction	Value
Normal skin	0
Very faint, nonconfluent pink	±
Faint pink	+
Pale pink to pink, slight edema	+ +
Pink, moderate edema	+ + +
Pink and thickened	+ + + +
Bright pink, markedly thickened	+ + + + +

TABLE 3.13
Buehler Sensitization Scoring System[34]

Skin Reaction	Value
No reaction	0
Very faint erythema, usually confluent	±(0.5)
Faint erythema, usually confluent	1
Moderate erythema	2
Strong erythema, with or without edema	3

TABLE 3.14
Contact Photosensitization Scoring System[48]

Skin Reaction	Value
No erythema	0
Minimal but definite erythera confluent	1
Moderate erythema	2
Considerable erythema	3
Maximal erythema	4

TABLE 3.15
Human Patch Test Sensitization Scoring System[53]

Skin Reaction	Value
Doubtful reaction; faint erythema only	? or + ?
Weak positive reaction; erythema, infiltration, discrete papules	+
Strong positive reaction: erythema, infiltration, papules, vesicles	+ +
Extreme positive reaction; intense erythema, infiltration and coalescing vesicles	+ + +
Negative reaction	–
Irritant reaction of different types	IR
Not tested	NT

SECTION 6. COMPARISON OF CLASSIFICATION SYSTEMS

TABLE 3.16
Environmental Protection Agency (EPA) Method of Calculating the Primary Irritation Index (PII) for Dermal Irritation Studies[54,55]

Option 1

Separately add up each animal's erythema and edema scores for the 1-, 24-, 48-, and 72-h scoring intervals. Add all six values together and divide by the (number of test sites × 4 scoring intervals).

Option 2

Add the 1-, 24-, 48-, and 72-h erythema and edema scores for all animals and divide by the (number of test sites × 4 scoring intervals).

TABLE 3.17
Federal Hazardous Substances Act (CPSC-FHSA) Method of Calculating the Primary Irritation Index (PII) for Dermal Irritation Studies[56]

Option 1

Separately add up each animal's intact and abraded erythema and edema scores for the 25- and 72-hr scoring intervals. Add all six values together and divide by the (number of test sites × 2 scoring intervals).

Option 2

Add the 25- and 72-h erythema and edema scores for all animals (intact and abraded sites) and divide by the (number of test sites × 2 scoring intervals).

TABLE 3.18
European Economic Community's (EEC) Method of Calculating the Primary Irritation Index (PII) for Dermal Irritation Studies[5]

For six animals

1. *Erythema:* Add all 24-, 48-, and 72-h erythema scores for each animal together and divide by the (number of test sites × 3 scoring intervals).
2. *Edema:* Add all 24-, 48-, and 72-h edema scores for each animal together and divide by the (number of test sites × 3 scoring intervals),

For three animals

1. *Erythema:* Add all 24-, 48-, and 72-h erythema scores of each animal individually and divide by the number of scoring intervals.
2. *Edema:* Add all 24-, 48-, and 72-h edema scores of each animal individually and divide by the number of scoring intervals.

TABLE 3.19
Environmental Protection Agency (EPA)
Dermal Classification System[57]

Primary Irritation Index	Irritation Rating
0.00	Nonirritant
0.01–1.99	Slight irritant
2.00–5.00	Moderate irritant
5.01–8.00	Severe irritant

TABLE 3.20
Environmental Protection Agency (EPA) Standard Evaluation Procedure Dermal Classification System[58]

Mean Score (Primary Irritation Index)	Response Category
0–0.4	Negligible
0.5–1.9	Slight
2–4.9	Moderate
5–8.0	Strong (primary irritant)

TABLE 3.21
Federal Fungicide, Insecticide, and Rodenticide Act (EPA-FIFRA) Dermal Classification System[59]

Toxicity Category	Warning Label
I	Corrosive. Causes eye and skin damage (or irritation). Do not get in eyes, on skin, or on clothing. Wear goggles or face shield and gloves when handling. Harmful or fatal if swallowed. (Appropriate first aid statement required.)
II	Severe Irritation at 72 h. Causes eye (and skin) irritation. Do not get on skin or on clothing. Harmful if swallowed. (Appropriate first aid statement required.)
III	Moderate Irritation at 72 h. Avoid contact with skin, eyes, or clothing. In case of contact immediately flush eyes or skin with plenty of water. Get medical attention if irritation persists.
IV	Mild or slight irritation at 72 h. (No precautionary statements required.)

TABLE 3.22
European Economic Community (EEC) Dermal Classification System[60]

Mean Erythema Score	Irritation Rating
0.00–1.99	Nonirritant
≥ 2.00	Irritant

Mean Edema Score	Irritation Rating
0.00–1.99	Nonirritant
≥ 2.00	Irritant

TABLE 3.23
Federal Hazardous Substances Act (CPSC-FHSA) Dermal Classification System[56]

Primary Irritation Score	Irritation Rating
0.00–4.99	Nonirritant
≥ 5.00	Irritant

TABLE 3.24
Draize Dermal Classification System[51]

Primary Irritation Index	Irritation Rating
< 2	Mildly irritating
2–5	Moderately irritating
> 5	Severely irritating

TABLE 3.25
Department of Transportation (DOT), Occupational Safety and Health Administration (OSHA), and International Maritime Organization (IMO) Packing Group Classification System[14,17,61]

Packing Group	Definition
I	Materials that cause full-thickness destruction of intact skin tissue within an observation period of up to 60 min starting after the exposure time of 3 min or less.
II	Materials other than those meeting Packing Group I criteria that cause full-thickness destruction of intact skin tissue within an observation period of up to 14 days starting after the exposure time of more than 3 min but not more than 60 min.
III	Materials, other than those meeting Packing Group I or II criteria — 1. That cause full-thickness destruction of intact skin tissue within an observation period of up to 14 days starting after the exposure time of more than 60 min but not more than 4 h; or 2. That do not cause full-thickness tissue destruction of intact skin tissue but exhibit a corrosion rate on steel or aluminum surfaces exceeding 6.25 mm (0.25 in.)/year at a test temperature of 55°C (130°F).

TABLE 3.26
Maximization Sensitization Classification System[38]

Sensitization Rate, %	Grade	Classification
0	—	Nonsensitizer
> 0–8	I	Weak sensitizer
9–28	II	Mild sensitizer
29–64	III	Moderate sensitizer
65–80	IV	Strong sensitizer
81–100	V	Extreme sensitizer

TABLE 3.27
Optimization Sensitization Classification System[51]

Intradermal Positive Animals %	Epidermal Positive Animals %	Classification
s, > 75	And/or s, > 50	Strong sensitizer
s, 50–75	And/or s, 30–50	Moderate sensitizer
s, 30–50	n.s., 0–30	Weak sensitizer
n.s., 0–30	n.s., 0	No sensitizer

s, significant; n.s., not significant (using Fisher's Exact Test).

SECTION 7. MATERIALS THAT PRODUCE DERMAL IRRITATION AND/OR SENSITIZATION

TABLE 3.28
Common Materials Used as Positive Controls[10,11,25,27,29–32,44,46,47,50]

Material	CAS No.	Suggested Concentrations	Category
Sodium lauryl sulfate	151-21-3	1.0%	Irritant
Hexyl cinnamic aldehyde	101-86-0	—	Mild to moderate sensitizer
Mercaptobenzothiazole	149-30-4	—	Mild to moderate sensitizer
Benzocaine	94-09-7	—	Mild to moderate sensitizer
p-Phenylenediamine	106-50-3	—	Sensitizer
2,4-Dinitrochlorobenzene (DNCB)	97-00-7	Induction: 0.1 to 0.5%, 0.25% w/v in echanol/acetone Challenge: 0.1 to 0.3%, w/v in ethanol/acetone	Sensitizer
Potassium dichromate	7778-50-9	—	Sensitizer
Neomycin sulfate	1405-10-3	—	Sensitizer
Nickel sulfate	7786-81-4	—	Sensitizer
8-Methoxypsoralen (Oxsoralen Lotion®)	298-81-7	1.0%	Photoirritant
5-Methoxypsoralen (Bergapten)	298-81-7	1.0%	Photoirritant
2,4-Dinitro-3-methyl-6-tertiary-butyl-anisole (musk ambrette)	83-66-9	Induction: 10.0% w/v in ethanol/acetone Challenge: 0.5% w/v in ethanol/acetone	Photosensitizer
2-Chloro- 10-[3-dimethylaminopropyl] phenothiazine hydrochloride (chloropromazine)	50-53-3	Induction: 1.0% w/v in methanol Challenge: 0.1% w/v in methanol	Photosensitizer
3,3,4,5-Tetrachlorosalicylandide (TCSA)	1154-59-2	Induction: 1.0% w/v in acetone Challenge: 1.0% w/v in acetone	Photosensitizer (in mice and guinea pigs), possible sensitizer in guinea pigs

TABLE 3.29
Materials Categorized by Their Ability to Produce Dermal Irritation or Sensitization[45,49,53,62,63]

Material	Irritants	Sensitizer	Photoirritant	Photosensitizer
Clothing and Textiles				
Dyes				
Aminoazotoluene		√		
Anthraquinones dyes (Disperse blue 35)		√	√	
Azo dyes		√		
Chromium dyes		√		
Disperse yellow 39 (methene dye)		√		
Naphthol AS (azo dye)	√			
p-Phenylenediamine (PPD)		√		
Resins				
Dimethyl oldihydroxyethylene		√		
Dimethyl olethylene urea		√		
Dimethyl urea (urea formaldehyde)		√		
Formaldehyde		√		

TABLE 3.29 *(Continued)*
Materials Categorized by Their Ability to Produce Dermal Irritation or Sensitization[45,49,53,62,63]

Material	Irritants	Sensitizer	Photoirritant	Photosensitizer
Melamine formaldehyde		√		
Adhesives				
Dodecyl mercaptan	√	√		
p-tertiary-butylphenol formaldehyde (PTBP resin)		√		
Rubber boots				
Isopropylaminodiphenylamine (IPPD)		√		
Mercaptobenzothiazole (MBT)		√		
Fiberglass	√			
Cosmetics				
Aldehyde citronellal		√		
Aluminum palls (in deodorants)	√			
Ammonium persulfate		√		
Balsam Peru		√		√
Benzoyl salicylate		√		
Celaltronium chloride		√		
Chloro-3,5-xylenol 4-(chloroxylenol)	√	√		
Cinnamic acid		√		
Cinnamic aldehyde		√		
di-tert-butyl hydrogunone		√		
dl-α–tocopherol		√		
Henna		√		
Lanolin		√		
Lemongrass oil		√		
Perfume		√		
Propellants in deodorant		√		
Sorbitan monostearate	√	√		
Sorbitan monoleate	√	√		
Triethanolamine	√			
Zerconium		√		
Foods				
Artichoke		√		
Asparagus		√		
Carrot		√		√
Cheese		√		
Chives		√		
Cucumber		√		
Endive		√		
Fish		√		
Flour		√		
Garlic		√		
Horseradish		√		
Leek		√		
Lemon peel		√		
Lettuce		√		
Meats		√		

TABLE 3.29 *(Continued)*
Materials Categorized by Their Ability to Produce Dermal Irritation or Sensitization[45,49,53,62,63]

Material	Irritants	Sensitizer	Photoirritant	Photosensitizer
Onion		✓		
Poultry skin and flesh		✓		
Shellfish		✓		
Wheat flour		✓		
Vanilla		✓		
Food Additives				
4-Hydroxybenzoic acid		✓		
Ammonium and potassium persulfates		✓		
Butylated hydroxyanisole		✓		
Butylated hydroxytoluene		✓		
Dodecyl gallate	✓			
Ethoxyquin				✓
Hydroquinone		✓		✓
Monosodium glutamate		✓		
Octyl gallate	✓			
Propyl gallate		✓		
Sodium benzoate		✓		
Sorbic acid		✓		
Sulfur dioxide		✓		
Medicants				
Ampicillin		✓		
Antihistamines		✓		
Benadryl		✓		
Benzoic acid		✓		
Benzophenone		✓		
Benzoyl peroxide		✓		
Coumarin	✓			✓
Dimercaprol		✓		
Estrogen cream		✓		
Fluorouracil		✓		✓
Gentian violet		✓		
Hydrocortisone		✓		✓
Mafenide acetate		✓		✓
Monoamyl amine		✓		
Neomycin sulfate		✓		
Oxyphenbutazone		✓		
p-Chlorobenzenesulfonylglycolic acid nitrile		✓		
Penicillin		✓		
Pristinamycin		✓		
Promethazene hydrochloride				✓
Quinoderm		✓		
Retinoic acid		✓		
Salicylic acid		✓		
Streptomycin		✓		
Sulisobenzone		✓		✓
Sulfonamides		✓		
Tetracycline (also phototoxic)		✓		

TABLE 3.29 *(Continued)*
Materials Categorized by Their Ability to Produce Dermal Irritation or Sensitization[45,49,53,62,63]

Material	Irritants	Sensitizer	Photoirritant	Photosensitizer
		Metals		
Arsenic	√			
Beryllium salts		√		
Cadmium sulfide				√
Chromate		√		
Nickel		√		
Selenium	√			
		Pesticides		
Dichlorphene	√			
Dinitrochlorobenzene		√		
Dinobuton	√			
Diothiocarbarnates		√		
Lindane		√		
Malathion		√		
Maneb		√		
Omite	√			
Randox		√		
Zineb		√		
		Plants		
Angelica	√			
Anise	√			
Boneset		√		
Burdock		√		
Caraway	√			
Celeriac	√			
Celery	√			
Chamomile		√		
Cocklebur		√		
Coriander	√			
Cow parsley	√			
Daffodil, narcissus		√		
Dill	√			
Fennel	√			
Feverfew		√		
Giant hogweed	√			
Hogweed, cow parsnip	√			
Ivy		√		
Marshelder		√		
Masterwort	√			
Poison ivy and oak		√		
Poverty weed		√		
Primula		√		
Pyrethrum, tansy		√		
Ragweed		√		
Ragweed of florists and species (alantolactone and parthenium)		√		
Sage brush/wormwood		√		

TABLE 3.29 *(Continued)*
**Materials Categorized by Their Ability to Produce Dermal Irritation or
Sensitization**[45,49,53,62,63]

Material	Irritants	Sensitizer	Photoirritant	Photosensitizer
Sneezeweed (alantolactone and parthenium)		✓		
Tansy		✓		
Tulip		✓		
Fruits and Vegetables				
Artichoke		✓		
Brussels sprouts, cabbage		✓		
Carrot	✓	✓		
Celery		✓		
Chicory, endive		✓		
Chive, leek, onion, garlic		✓		
Horseradish		✓		
Lettuce		✓		
Orange, lemon, lime		✓		✓
Parsley	✓	✓		
Parsnip	✓	✓		
Pineapple		✓		
Woods				
Abura	✓			
African blackwood	✓			
African mahogany	✓			
American mahogany	✓			
Australian blackwood	✓			
Ayan	✓			
Camphor	✓	✓		
Cassia oil		✓		
Ceylon satinwood	✓			
Cocobolo	✓			
Cocus	✓			
Common alder	✓			
Douglas fir	✓			
English elm	✓			
Gaboon	✓			
Grevillea	✓			
lpe	✓			
Iroko	✓			
Limba	✓			
Louro	✓			
Macassar ebony	✓			
Makore	✓			
Mansonia	✓			
Opepe	✓			
Peroba rosa	✓			
Pine oil	✓			
Ramin	✓			
Teak	✓			
Toporite	✓			
Western red cedar	✓			

TABLE 3.29 *(Continued)*
Materials Categorized by Their Ability to Produce Dermal Irritation or Sensitization[45,49,53,62,63]

Material	Irritants	Sensitizer	Photoirritant	Photosensitizer
White peroba	√			
White poplar	√			
West Indian satinwood	√			
Yew	√			
Plastics				
Acrylamide		√		
Acrylonitrile		√		
Cyanoacrylic acids and esters	√			
Diacrylates (delayed)	√			
Methacrylonitrile (poison)		√		
Methyl, ethyl, and *n*-butyl methacrylates		√		
Epoxy Resin Systems				
Allyl resin — diallylglycol carbonate	√			
Diallylphthalate	√			
Dimethylaniline (poison)	√			
Diphenylmethane diisocyanate	√			
Epoxy monomer		√		
Hardener		√		
Hexamethylene diisocyanate	√			
Maleic acid anhydride	√			
Napththalene diisocyanate		√		
Naphthoquinone (poison)	√			
Peroxides (catalyst)	√			
Phthalic acid anhydride	√			
p-tert-Butyl phenol formaldehyde (PTBP)		√		
Reactive diluent		√		
Toluene diisocyanate	√			
Hardeners				
Isophoronediamine		√		
N-Aminoethylpiperazine		√		
Polyether alcohol		√		
Polyurethane laquar	√			
Triethylamine	√			
Cellulose Polymers				
Cellophane		√		
Celluloid		√		
Cellulose nitrate		√		
Collodion		√		
Gun cotton		√		
Pyroxylin		√		
Rayon		√		
Regenerated cellulose		√		
Cellulose Acetate				
Antioxidant: *p-tert*-butyl phenol		√		
Colors: azo dyes solvent yellow 3, solvent red 26, pigment red 481		√		

TABLE 3.29 *(Continued)*
Materials Categorized by Their Ability to Produce Dermal Irritation or Sensitization[45,49,53,62,63]

Material	Irritants	Sensitizer	Photoirritant	Photosensitizer
Components: plastizer, triphenyl phosphate		√		
Polish turpentine		√		
Solvent: ethylene glycol monomethyl ether acetate		√		
Ultraviolet light stabilizer: resorcinol monobenzoate		√		
		Preservatives and Antibacterials		
Preparations Containing Lanolins (l)/Parabins (P)/Chlorocresol (c)				
Adcortyl cream (p)		√		
Betnovate cream (c)		√		
Betnovate lotion (p)		√		
Cortenema (p)		√		
Dermovate cream (c)		√		
Efcortelan cream (c)		√		
Efcortelan lotion (p)		√		
Hydrocortistab eye ointment (1)		√		
Hydromycin-Dornluent ear/eye (1)		√		
Medrone acne lotion (p)		√		
Medrone cream (p)		√		
Motivate cream (c)		√		
Myciguent ointment (1)		√		
Myciguent opthalmic ointment (1)		√		
Neo-Cortef eye and ear ointment (1)		√		
Neo-Cortef ointment (p)		√		
Neo-Cortef lotion (p)		√		
Neo-Medione acne lotion (p)		√		
Nerisone cream (p)		√		
Nystadermal cream (p)		√		
Nystadermal gel (c)		√		
Propaderm cream (c)		√		
Propaderm lotion (c)		√		
Remiderm cream (p)		√		
Schericur ointment (l)		√		
Synolar creams except for Synalar Forti cream (p)		√		
Synolar combination creams (p)		√		
Synolar ointments (l)		√		
Topilar ointment (l)		√		
Topisone (l)		√		
Triadcortyl cream (p)		√		
Ultradil cream plain (p)		√		
Ultradil ointment plain (l)		√		
Ultralanum cream plain (l)		√		
Ultralanum lotion (p)		√		
Ultralanum ointment (l)		√		
Ultralanum ointment plain (l)		√		

Phenolic Compounds
Hexachlorophane   √

TABLE 3.29 *(Continued)*
Materials Categorized by Their Ability to Produce Dermal Irritation or Sensitization[45,49,53,62,63]

Material	Irritants	Sensitizer	Photoirritant	Photosensitizer
Mercury				
Ammoniated mercury		√		
Mercuric chloride	√	√		
Mercurochrome	√			
Mercury fulminate (mercuric cyanate)	√			
Merthiolate	√			
Phenylmercuric acetate	√	?		
Phenylmercuric borate		√		
Phenylmercuric nitrate		√		
Phenylmercuric proprimate		√		
Quaternary Ammonium Compounds				
Benzalkonium chloride	√			
Bronopol	√			
Cetalkonium chloride		√		
Cetrimide		√		
Chlorhexidine		√		
Chloroacetamide		√		
Ethylene oxide	√			

Rubber/Latex Components

Material	Irritants	Sensitizer	Photoirritant	Photosensitizer
Thiurams				
Dipentamethylenethiuram disulfide		√		
Tetraethylthiuram disulfide		√		
Tetramethylthiuram disulfide		√		
Tetramethylthiuram monosulfide		√		
Mercapto Group				
Cyclohexylbenzothiazylsulfenamide		√		
Dibenzothiazyldisulfide		√		
Mercaptobenzothiazole		√		
Morpholinylmercaptobenzothiazole		√		
PPD Group				
Diaminodiphenylmethane		√		
Diphenyl-PPD		√		
Isopropylphenyl-PPD (isopropylamino diphenylamine)		√		
Phenylcyclohexyl-PPD		√		
Naphthyl Group				
Phenyl-β–naphthylamine		√		
sym-Di-β–napthyl-PPD		√		
Carbamates				
Zinc diethyldithiocarbamate		√		
Zinc dibutyldithiocarbamate		√		
Miscellaneous				
Dioxydiphenyl		√		
Diphenylguanidine		√		
Dithiodimorpholine		√		

TABLE 3.29 *(Continued)*
Materials Categorized by Their Ability to Produce Dermal Irritation or Sensitization[45,49,53,62,63]

Material	Irritants	Sensitizer	Photoirritant	Photosensitizer
Miscellaneous Compounds				
Acetaldehyde (10%)		√		
Acetyl-1,1,2,3,3,6-hexamethylindan				√
Acetylacetone (slightly)		√		
Acridine				√
Acriflavine				√
Alcohol, anhydrous		√		
Allyl butyrate (4%)	√			
Allyl cinnamate (0.1%)	√			
Allyl cyclohexylacetate	√			
Allyl epoxypropoxybenzene		√		
Allyl phenylacetate	√	√		
Aminobenzoic acid derivatives			√	
Aminobenzoic acid p⁻				√
Aminophenol o⁻ and p⁻		√		
Aminosalicylic acid p⁻				√
Aminothiazole		√		
Aminodarone			√	
Ammonia		√		
Amyl dimethylamino benzoate, mixed *ortho* and *para* isomers			√	
Amyl dimethyl PABA				√
Amyl nitrite	√			
Amyl phenylacetate	√			
Anthracene-acridine			√	
Atranorin				√
Benzaldehyde		√		
Benzydamine hydrochloride				√
Bergamot oil				√
Bergapten (5-methoxypsoralen)			√	
Bromomethyl-4-nitrobenzene		√		
Buclosamide				√
Butylphenol		√		
Cadmium chloride				√
Cadmium sulfate				√
Caraway oil				√
Carbimazole				√
Carotene β-				√
Cephalosporins		√		
Cetyl alcohol		√		
Chlor-2-phenylphenol				√
Chloramine-T		√		
Chlormercaptodicarboximide				√
Chloro-6-fluorobenzaldehyde-α-chlorooxime2–		√		
Chlorodiazepoxide			√	
Chlorothalonil	√			
Chlorothiazides			√	√
Chlorpromazine				√

TABLE 3.29 *(Continued)*
**Materials Categorized by Their Ability to Produce Dermal Irritation or
Sensitization**[45,49,53,62,63]

Material	Irritants	Sensitizer	Photoirritant	Photosensitizer
Cinoxate				√
Cinnamon bark oil Ceylon				√
Citral		√		
Clobetasol-17-proprionate		√		
Coal tar			√	√
Cobalt chlorate				√
Cobaltous chloride		√		
Cobaltous chlorate				√
Cobaltous nitrate				√
Cobaltous sulfate				√
Cocamide DEA	√			
Cocamphocarboxyglycinate		√		
Coniferyl benzoate		√		
Cu(II)-acetyl acetonate		√		
Cumin oil				√
Cyanamide		√		
Dacarbazine			√	
Decylaminoethanethiol 2-n⁻		√		
Deneclocycline			√	
Dexpanthenol	√			
Diamine N⁻		√		
Diaminodiphenylmethane		√		√
Dibucain hydrochloride				√
Dichloro-2-phenylphenol				√
Dichloroquinoline		√		
Dicyclohexylcarbodiimide		√		
Diethazine				√
Diethylaminopropylamine		√		
Diethyl fumarate		√		
Diethylstilbestrol				√
Digalloyl trioleate				√
Diglycidyl ether		√		
Dihydrocoumarin		√		
Dimethoxane				√
Dimethyl antranilate				√
Dimethyl sulfoxide		√		
Dioctyl-p-phenylenediamine		√		
Diphenhydramine hydrochloride				√
Diphenylcyclopropenone		√		
Diphenyl-p-phenylenediamine		√		
Dipyrone		√		
Docusate sodium	√			
Erythrosine				√
Ethacridine lactate monohydrate				√
Ethyl aminobenzoate		√		√
Ethyl ether	√			
Ethylparaben		√		
Fig leaf absolute				√
Furocoumarins			√	

TABLE 3.29 *(Continued)*
Materials Categorized by Their Ability to Produce Dermal Irritation or Sensitization[45,49,53,62,63]

Material	Irritants	Sensitizer	Photoirritant	Photosensitizer
Geraniol		√		
Geranyl formate	√			
Ginger oil				√
Griseofulvin			√	√
Gylceryl *p*-aminobenzoate				√
Halogenated Phenols				
Bithionol				√
Bromochlorosalicylanilide (Multifungin)				√
Chlorophenylphenol				√
Dibromosalicylanilide (DBS)				√
Fentichlor				√
Hexachlorophene Buclosamide (Jadit)				√
Tetrachlorosalicylanilide 3, 3′, 4′, 5 (TCSA)				√
Tribomosalicylanilide (TBSA)				√
Trichlorcarbanilide (TCCA)				√
Hexanediol diacrylate	√			√
Hexantriol		√		
Hydratropic aldehyde	√			
Iothion		√		
Isoamyl alcohol		√		
Isocamphyl cyclohexanol	√			
Isopropyl alcohol		√		
Isostearoamphopropionate		√		
Ketoprofen				√
Kynuremic acid			√	
Lauroamphocarboxyglycinate		√		
Lauroamphoglycinate		√		
Lauroamphopropionate		√		
Lauryl isoquinolinium bromide	√			
Lavender oil				√
Mannide monooleate	√			
Mechlorethamine hydrochloride (nitrogen mustard)		√		
Menthol 1-		√		
Mepazine				√
Metamizole		√		
Methoxyethylepoxypropoxybenzene		√		
Methylanisalacetone α-	√			
Methylcoumarin 6–				√
Methylcoumarin 7–				√
Methylene blue				√
Methylisothiazolinone		√		
Methylparaben		√		
Methyl salicylate		√		
Minoxidil				√
Musk ambrette	√			
Musk xylol				√
Mycanodin				√
Neosilversalvarsan		√		

TABLE 3.29 *(Continued)*
Materials Categorized by Their Ability to Produce Dermal Irritation or Sensitization[45,49,53,62,63]

Material	Irritants	Sensitizer	Photoirritant	Photosensitizer
Neroli oil				✓
Neutral Red		✓	✓	
Nicotinyl alcohol		✓		
Nitrofuroxime		✓		
Nitrose dimethyl aniline		✓		
Nonoxynol-9	✓			
Oak moss				✓
Octoxynol-9	✓			
Oleamide		✓		
Oxybenzone				✓
Padimate A or Escalol 506 (amyl p-dimethylaminobenzoate)			✓	
Papain		✓		
PBA-1				✓
Pelargonic acid	✓			
Pentadecylcatechol 3–		✓		
Pentamethyl-4,6-dinitroindane 1, 1, 3, 3, 5–	✓			✓
Pentanol		✓		
Pentylidenecyclohexanone		✓		
Perphenazine				✓
Petitgrain oil Paraguay				✓
Phenanthrene				✓
Phenol		✓		
Phenothiazine				✓
Phenylacetaldehyde		✓		
Phenylbenzimidazol sulfate 2–				✓
Phenyl butazone		✓		
Phenyl gylcidyl ether				✓
Phenylphenol				✓
Phosphorus sesquisulfide		✓		
Picryl chloride		✓		
Pigment orange 5				✓
Pigment orange red 49, calcium lake				✓
Pinus pumilio oil	✓			
Pitch			✓	✓
Platinum salts		✓		
Polysorbate 20	✓			
Polysorbate 60		✓		
Polysorbate 80	✓			
Primin		✓		
Prochlorperazine			✓	
Promazine				✓
Propionaldehyde		✓		
Propyl alcohol n–		✓		
Propylphenbutazone		✓		
Psoralens			✓	
Pyridine				✓
Pyridoxine hydrochloride		✓		
Pyrilamine maleate				✓

TABLE 3.29 *(Continued)*
Materials Categorized by Their Ability to Produce Dermal Irritation or Sensitization[45,49,53,62,63]

Material	Irritants	Sensitizer	Photoirritant	Photosensitizer
Quinine				✓
Quinine hydrochloride				✓
Quinine sulfate				✓
Quinoline methanol			✓	
Rhodamine B				✓
Ricinoleic acid	✓			
Rose Bengal				✓
Rue oil				✓
Silver bromide				✓
Silver fulminate	✓			
Silver nitrate				✓
Sodium hypochlorite	✓			
Sodium monoglyceride sulfide	✓			
Sodium monoglyceride sulfonate	✓			
Sodium octoxynol-2 ethane sulfonate	✓			
Sodium oleyl laurate	✓			
Sodium stearate	✓			
Sodium sulfide	✓	✓		
Sodium thiosulfate	✓			
Sorbitan laurate	✓	✓		
Squaric acid-diethylester		✓		
Stearalkonium chloride	✓			
Stearoamphoglycinate		✓		
Stearyl alcohol		✓		
Stictic acid				✓
Stilbene triazine				✓
Sulbentine				✓
Sulfadiazine				✓
Sulfamerazine				✓
Sulfamethazine				✓
Sulfanilamide			✓	✓
Sulfathiazole				✓
Sulfur		✓		
Sulisobenzone				✓
Thioridazine				✓
Thiourea				✓
Thurfyl nicotinate		✓		
Toluidine red				✓
Tribomsalan				✓
Tributyltin oxide	✓			
Trichlorosalicylanilide 3',4',5–				✓
Triclocarban				✓
Triethylenemelamine				✓
Trimeprazine				✓
Trinitrobenzene sym–		✓		
Tropicamide		✓		
Turkey-red oil	✓			
Umbelliferone				✓
Undecylenic aldehyde digeranyl acetal	✓			

TABLE 3.29 *(Continued)*
Materials Categorized by Their Ability to Produce Dermal Irritation or Sensitization[45,49,53,62,63]

Material	Irritants	Sensitizer	Photoirritant	Photosensitizer
Valeraldehyde		√		
Vetiverol	√			
Vinyl pyridine 4–		√		
Xanthotoxin (8-methoxypsoralen)			√	
Zinc pyrithione				√

TABLE 3.30
Dermal Irritants and Sensitizers Listed by Occupation[45,49,53,62,63]

Occupation	Irritant	Sensitizer
Agricultural workers	Artificial fertilizers Disinfectants and cleansers for milking machines Petrol and diesel oil	Rubber (clothing and milking equipment) Oats Barley Animal feed (antibiotics, preservatives, additives, and cobalt) Veterinary medicaments Cement Plants Pesticides Wood Preservatives
Artists and sculptors	Solvents Clay Plaster	Turpentine Pigments (cobalt, nickel, and chromium) Azo dyes Anthraquinone dyes Aminoazotoluene Colophony Epoxy resin
Automobile and aircraft mechanics	Solvents Cutting oils Paints Hand cleansers	Chromate (primers, passivators, anticorrosives, welding fumes, oils) Nickel Cobalt Rubber Epoxy resins Dimethacrylate resins Dipentene in thinners
Bakers and confectioners	Flour Detergents	Flavors and spices (cinnamon, eugenol, vanilla, cardamom) Orange Lemon Lime Pineapple Essential oils Dyes Ammonium persulfate Benzoyl peroxide (improvers in flour)
Bartenders	Detergents Citrus fruit	Orange Lemon

TABLE 3.30 *(Continued)*
Dermal Irritants and Sensitizers Listed by Occupation[45,49,53,62,63]

Occupation	Irritant	Sensitizer
	Wet work	Lime
		Flavors
		ortho-Phenylphenol (in some detergents)
Bookbinders	Solvents	Glues
	Glues	Resins
		Leather
Butchers	Detergents	Meat (contact urticaria)
	Meat	Teak (knife handles)
	Offal	Nickel
		Sawdust
Cabinetmakers, French polishers, carpenters	Detergents	Stains (including dichromate)
	Solvents	Glues (urea, phenol, PTBP-formaldehyde resins)
	Thinners for cleaning metal (as a cause of koilonychia, Ancona- Alayon, 1975)	Woods
		Turpentine
	Wood and wood preservatives	Varnishes
		Colophony
Cablejointers	Solvents	Epoxy resin
		Fluxes (aminoethylethanolamine)
Cleaners	Detergents	Rubber gloves
	Solvents	Chromates (bleaches in some countries)
	Wet work	
Coal miners	Dust (coal, stone)	Rubber boots
	Cement	Masks
	Wet conditions	
Construction workers	Cement	Chromate
		Cobalt
		Gloves (rubber, leather)
		Resins (epoxy and formaldehyde)
		Woods
Cooks and catering	Detergents	Foods (contact urticaria)
	Food juices	Onion
	Wet work	Garlic
	Parsley	Lettuce
	Parsnip	Carrots
	Carrots	Celery
		Parsley
		Parsnip
		Brussels sprouts
		Cabbage
		Spices
		Flavors
		Rubber gloves
		Sodium metabisulfite
		Lauryl
		Octyl gallate
		Formaldehyde (deodorizing solution, fishmongers)

TABLE 3.30 *(Continued)*
Dermal Irritants and Sensitizers Listed by Occupation[45,49,53,62,63]

Occupation	Irritant	Sensitizer
Dentists and dental technicians	Detergents Hand cleaners Wet work	Local anesthetics (amethocaine, procaine) Methacrylates Eugenol (eugenol and colophony gingivectomy dressing) Mercury Disinfectants Rubber Dental impression material (Impregum and Scutan: the sensitizers are the catalysts methyldichlorobenzene sulfonate and methyl-*p*-toluoylsulfonate
Dry cleaners	Solvents	Rubber gloves
Electricians	Soldering fluxes	Fluxes (colophony, hydrazine) Insulating tape (colophony) Resins (epoxy and formaldehyde) Rubber
Electroplaters	Acids Alkalis	Nickel Chromium Other metals Rubber gloves
Embalmers and morticians	Disinfectants Detergents	Formaldehyde
Floor layers	Solvents	Cement Resins (epoxy and formaldehyde) Woods Varnish Linoleum (colophony)
Florists	Manure Fertilizers Pesticides Wet work	Plants (alantolactone and parthenium) Pesticides (DNCB, dichlorphene, lindane) Rubber gloves
Foundry workers	Cleansers	Phenol and urea formaldehyde (resin-coated sand) Colophony (nitrogen-free sand) Gloves (rubber, chromium)
Funeral directors		Floral tributes (alantolactone and parthenium)
Garage workers	Petroleum products Diesel fuel Cleansers Detergents Solvents	Rubber gloves Chromate Epoxy resin Antifreeze (MBT)
Gardeners	Artificial fertilizers	Pesticides Plants/flowers Rubber gloves Boots
Hairdressers	Shampoos Perming solutions Bleaching solutions	Dyes (*p*-phenylenediamine, *p*-toluoylenediamine, *o*-nitro-*p*-phenylenediamine, *p*-aminiphenol, henna)

TABLE 3.30 *(Continued)*
Dermal Irritants and Sensitizers Listed by Occupation[45,49,53,62,63]

Occupation	Irritant	Sensitizer
	Wet work	Persulfates
		Rubber gloves
		Lanolin
		Perfumes
		Lemongrass oil
		Formaldehyde (shampoos)
		Resorcinol
		Pyrogallol
		Nickel
Hospital workers	Detergents	Rubber gloves
	Disinfectants	Disinfectants
	Foods	Flowers
	Wet work	Foods
		Polishes
		Hand creams
Housework	Detergents	Rubber gloves
	Cleaners	Foods (onions, garlic, citrus fruit; contact
	Foods	urticaria)
	Disinfectants	Spices
	Wet work	Flavors
		Hand creams
		Nickel
		Chromate (bleaches)
		Flowers
		Polishes
Jeweler	Detergents	Epoxy resin
	Solvents	Metals (nickel, chromium)
		Sawdust (used for drying jewelry)
Metal workers	Cutting and drilling oils	Chromates
	Solvents	Additives in cutting oils (antibacterials and
	Hand cleansers	antioxidants)
Nurses	Disinfectants	Rubber gloves
	Detergents	Formaldehyde
	Wet work	Glutaraldehyde
		Dettol
		Disinfectants
		Medicaments (including antibiotics,
		antihistamines, hydrocortisone, retinoic
		acid, chlorpromazine)
		Flowers
Office workers	Photocopying (ammonia)	Rubber (finger stalls)
		Nickel (clips, photocopying solutions)
		Copy papers
		Carbon papers
		Correction paper fluids
Painters	Solvents	Turpentine
	Thinners	Dipentene
	Wallpaper adhesives	Cobalt (driers, colors)

TABLE 3.30 *(Continued)*
Dermal Irritants and Sensitizers Listed by Occupation[45,49,53,62,63]

Occupation	Irritant	Sensitizer
	Hand cleansers	Chromate (colors)
		Wallpaper adhesives (formaldehyde, chloroacetamide, and fungicides)
		Paints (preservatives, e.g., mercurials)
Photograph developers (X-ray technicians)	Wet work	Rubber gloves
	Solvents	p-Aminophenol (Metol)
		Color developers
		Hydroquinone
		Phenindone
		Sodium metabisulfite
		EDTA
		Glutaraldehyde
		Pyrogallol
		Amidol
		Ethylenediamine
		Resorcinol
		Triazine
		Salicylaldoxime
Plastic industry	Solvents	Monomers
	Acids	Hardeners (isophoronediamine, polyether alcohol)
	Styrene	
	Oxidizing agents	Additives
	Hardeners (Polyurethane lacquer, triethylamine)	Cellulose polymers
		Cellulose acetate
		Epoxy resin systems
Plating industry	Acids	Nickel
	Alkalis	Chromate
	Solvents	Cobalt
		Mercury
Plumbers	Wet work	Chromate (cement)
	Cleaners	Rubber (gloves, packing)
Printers	Solvents	Chromate
		UV-cured inks
		Colophony (paper)
		Turpentine
		Rubber gloves
		Rubber blanket in offset printing
		Formaldehyde (gum arabic)
Radio and television workers	Fluxes	Resins (epoxy)
		Fluxes (colophony and hydrazine)
		Chromate
Rubber workers	Solvents	Rubber chemicals
	Talc	Dyes
	Zinc stearate	Colophony
Secretaries		Carbon paper
		Photocopy paper (azo compound, thiourea-photosensitizer)
		Correcting paper
		Rubber (fingerstall and rubber bands)

TABLE 3.30 *(Continued)*
Dermal Irritants and Sensitizers Listed by Occupation[45,49,53,62,63]

Occupation	Irritant	Sensitizer
Shoemakers and cobblers	Solvents	Glues (PTBP resin, colophony)
		Leather
		Rubber
		Turpentine
Tannery workers	Acids	Tanning agents (chromium, vegetable tans,
	Alkalis	glutaraldehyde, formaldehyde)
	Reducing and oxidizing agents	Rubber (gloves and boots)
	Wet work	Fungicides
		Dyes
Textile workers	Fibers	Formaldehyde resins
	Bleaching agents	Dyes
	Solvents	Chromate (mordant)
		Nickel
Veterinarians (and	Disinfectants	Rubber gloves
slaughterhouse workers)	Wet work	Medicaments used to treat animals and
	Entrails	which contaminate their fur
	Animal secretions	Medicaments
		Tuberculin
		Benethamate
		Benzylpenicillin
		Spiramycin
		Tylosin
		Penethamete
		Neomycin in a calf drench
		Mercaptobenzothiazole in a medication
		Benzisothiazolone fungicide
		Topical pesticides; malathion
		Contact urticaria from animal tissues
		Cow hair and dander in bacon factories,
		workers eviscerating or cleaning the guts
		develop an eczema of the fingers, known
		as "gut" or "fat" eczema; its cause is
		unknown
Woodworkers	Woods	Lichens (atranorin)
		Glues
		Varnishes
		Colophony
		Turpentine
		Balsams

SECTION 8. GLOSSARY OF COMMON TERMINOLOGY[64–68]

Acanthosis Hypertrophy of the stratum spinosum and granulosum.

Blanching To take color from, to bleach. Characterized by a white or pale discoloration of the exposure area due to decreased blood flow to the skin (ischemia).

Challenge exposure A dermal exposure to a test substance after one or more previous induction exposures, to determine whether the subject will react in a hypersensitive manner.

Concomitant sensitization When an individual is sensitized to different substances in different products at the same time.

Contact dermatitis A delayed type of induced sensitivity (allergy) of the skin with varying degrees of erythema, edema, and vesiculation, resulting from cutaneous contact with a specific allergen.

Contact urticaria Wheal-and-flare response generally elicited within 30 to 60 minutes after cutaneous exposure to a test substance. May be IgE mediated or nonimmunologically mediated.

Corrosion Direct chemical action on normal living skin that results in its disintegration or irreversible alteration at the site of contact. Corrosion is generally manifested by ulceration and necrosis with subsequent scar tissue formation.

Cross-sensitization An individual that is sensitized to a primary allergen acquires sensitivity to a chemically related molecule, which is called a secondary allergen.

Cumulative irritation Irritation resulting from repeated exposures to materials at the same skin site.

Dermatitis Inflammation of the skin.

Desquamation The shedding of the cuticle in scales or the outer layer of any surface. To shred, peel, or scale off, as the casting off of the epidermis in scales or shreds, or the shedding of the outer layer of any surface.

Diagnostic patch testing Utilized to confirm the existence of allergic contact dermatitis. A concentration of the test substance that is known to be nonirritating is applied to the skin in a suitable vehicle.

Eczema Inflammatory condition in which the skin becomes red and small vesicles, crusts, and scales develop.

Edema An excessive accumulation of serous fluid or water in cells, tissues, or serous cavities.

Erythema An inflammatory redness of the skin, as caused by chemical poisoning or sunburn, usually a result of congestion of the capillaries.

Eschar A dry scab, thick coagulated crust or slough formed on the skin as a result of a thermal burn or by the action of a corrosive or caustic substance.

Exfoliation To remove in flakes, scales or to peel. To cast off in scales, flakes, or the like. To come off or separate, as scales, flakes, sheets, or layers. Detachment and shedding of superficial cells of an epithelium or from any tissue surface. Scaling or desquamation of the horny layer of epidermis, which varies in amount from minute quantities to shedding the entire integument.

False cross-sensitivity Occurs when the same antigen is present in different products (e.g., eugenol in perfumes, soft drinks, and underarm deodorants).

Fissuring Characterized by a crack or cleft in the skin.

Hyperkeratosis Hypertrophy and thickening of the stratum corneum.

Index of sensitivity The prevalence of sensitivity to a substance in a given population at a given time.

Induction exposure An experimental exposure to a test substance with the intention of inducing a hypersensitive state.

Induction period A period of at least 1 week after a dermal exposure during which a hypersensitive state is developed.

Irritant A substance that causes inflammation and other evidence of irritation, particularly of the skin, on first contact or exposure; a reaction of irritation not dependent on a mechanism of sensitization.

Latent sensitization Subsequent exposure of the skin of a sensitized individual to a lower concentration of a sensitizer can elicit a more intense response than the initial exposure. This response may take hours or even days to develop, and hence it is delayed.

Necrosis Pathologic death of one or more cells, or of a portion of tissue or organ, resulting from irreversible damage.

Nonocclusive Site of application of test substance to the skin is not covered with any material and movement of the air to the site is not restricted.

Occlusive A bandage or dressing that covers the skin and excludes it from air. Prevents loss of a test substance by evaporation.

Photoallergy An increased reactivity of the skin to UV and/or visible radiation produced by a chemical agent on a immunologic basis. Previous allergy sensitized by exposure to the chemical agent and appropriate radiation necessary. The main role of light in photoallergy seems to be in the conversion of the hapten to a complete allergen.

Photoirritation Irritation resulting from light-induced molecular changes in the structure of chemicals applied to the skin.

Photosensitization The processes whereby foreign substances, either absorbed locally into the skin or systemically, may be subjected to photochemical reactions within the skin, leading to either chemically induced photosensitivity reactions or altering the "normal" pathologic effects of light. UV-A is usually responsible for most photosensitivity reactions.

Semiocclusive Site of application of test substance is covered; however, movement of air through covering is only partially restricted.

Sensitization (allergic contact dermatitis) An immunologically mediated cutaneous reaction to a substance.

Sensitizing potential The relative capacity of a given agent to induce sensitization in a group of humans or animals.

Superficial sloughing Characterized by dead tissue separated from a living structure. Any outer layer or covering that is shed. Necrosed tissue separated from the living structure.

Ulceration The development of an inflammatory, often suppurating lesion, on the skin or an internal mucous surface of the body caused by superficial loss of tissue, resulting in necrosis of the tissue.

REFERENCES

1. U.S. Environmental Protection Agency, Health Effects Guidelines, OPPTS 870.2500, Acute Dermal Irritation, August, 1998.
2. Japan Agricultural Chemicals Laws and Regulations, Testing Guidelines for Toxicology Studies, 25, 1985.
3. Japan Ministry of Agriculture, Forestry and Fisheries, Agricultural Chemicals Inspection Station, Guidelines on the Compiling of Test Results on Toxicity, Skin Irritation Test, 9–11, December, 1998 (Draft Proposal).
4. Organization for Economic Co-operation and Development, OECD Guidelines for Testing of Chemicals, Section 4: Health Effects, Subsection 404: Acute Dermal Irritation/Corrosion, 1, 1992.
5. The Commission of the European Communities, Official Journal of the European Communities, Part B: Methods for the Determination of Toxicity, No. L 383 A/124, B.4. Acute Toxicity (Skin Irritation), 1992.
6. U.S. Environmental Protection Agency, Federal Insecticide, Fungicide, Rodenticide Act, Pesticide Assessment Guidelines, Subdivision F, Hazard Evaluation: Human and Domestic Animals, Series 81-6: Dermal Sensitization Study, 59, 1984.
7. Japan New Drugs Division Pharmaceutical Affairs Bureau, Ministry of Health and Welfare, 1990 Guidelines for Toxicity Studies of Drugs Manual, 1991, Chap. 7.
8. Japan Agricultural Chemicals Laws and Regulations, Testing Guidelines for Toxicology Studies, 27, 1985.
9. Japan Ministry of Agriculture, Forestry and Fisheries, Agricultural Chemicals Inspection Station, Guidelines on the Compiling of Test Results on Toxicity, Skin Sensitization Test, 16–19, December, 1998 (Draft Proposal).

10. Organization for Economic Co-operation and Development, OECD Guidelines for Testing of Chemicals, Section 4: Health Effects, Subsection 406: Skin Sensitization, 1, 1992.
11. The Commission of the European Communities, Official Journal of the European Communities, Part B: Methods for the Determination of Toxicity, No. L 383 A/131, B.6: Skin Sensitization, 1992.
12. U.S. Consumer Products Safety Commission, 16 CFR Chapter II, Subchapter C: Federal Hazardous Substances Act Regulation, Part 1500, Subsection 1500.41: Method of Testing Primary Irritant Substances, 401, 1993.
13. U.S. Consumer Products Safety Commission, 16 CFR Chapter II, Subchapter C: Federal Hazardous Substances Act Regulation, Part 1500, Subsection 1500.3: Definitions, 382, 1993.
14. U.S. Research and Special Programs Administration, Department of Transportation, 49 CFR, Part 173. 136 and 173. 137, 1998.
15. U.S. Pharmacopeia, National Formulary, USP 24 NF 19 Biological Reactivity Test, IN-VIVO, 1832, 2000, Chap. 88.
16. Canadian Environmental Protection Act, Guidelines for the Notification and Testing of New Substances: Chemicals and Polymers, Section 5.1: Test Procedures and Practices, 50, 1993.
17. International Maritime Dangerous Goods Code, Class 8 Corrosives, International Maritime Organization, London, 1994.
18. Occupational Safety and Health Administration, Labor, 29 CFR Chapter XVII, Part 1910, Appendix A to Section 1900.1200: Health Hazard Definitions (Mandatory), 364, 1991.
19. American Society for Testing and Materials, *1991 Annual Book of ASTM Standards,* F719–81 (1986), 13.01: Practice for Testing Biomaterials in Rabbits for Primary Skin Irritation, 976, 1991.
20. American Society for Testing and Materials, *1991 Annual Book of ASTM Standards,* F720–81 (1986), 13.01, Practice for Testing Guinea Pigs for Contact Allergens: Guinea Pig Maximization Test, 976, 1991.
21. American Society for Testing and Materials, *1991 Annual Book of ASTM Standards, E* 993–88, 11.01, Test Method for Evaluation of Delayed Contact Hypersensitivity, 964, 1991.
22. The Cosmetic, Toiletry and Fragrance Association, Inc., *CTFA* Safety Testing Guidelines, Section II: Guidelines for Evaluating Primary Skin Irritation Potential, 2, 1991.
23. The Cosmetic, Toiletry and Fragrance Association, Inc., *CTFA Safety Testing Guidelines,* Section IV, Guidelines for Evaluating Contact Sensitization Potential, 7, 1991.
24. Draize, J. H., *Appraisal of the Safety of Chemicals in Foods, Drugs and Cosmetics,* The Association of Food and Drug Officials of the United States, 49, 1959.
25. Springborn Laboratories, Inc., Protocol for a Primary Irritation Study in Rabbits, EPA/PSI 1 — 10/2000, Spencerville, OH, 2000.
26. Springborn Laboratories, Inc., Protocol for a Dermal Corrosivity Study in Rabbits, DOT/COR-1 — 5/2000, Spencerville, OH, 2000.
27. Hakim, R.E., Freeman, R.G., Griffin, A.C., and Knox, J.M., Experimental toxicologic studies on 8-methoxypsoralen in animals exposed to the long ultraviolet, *J. Pharmacol. Exp. Ther.,* 131:394, 1961.
28. OECD Guidelines for the Testing of Chemicals, Acute Dermal Photoirritation Screening Test, February, 1995 (Draft Proposal).
29. Springborn Laboratories, Inc., Protocol for a Photoirritation Study in Rabbits with Non-Occlusive Conditions, SLI No. OECD/PHIRBU-1-8/2000, Spencerville, OH, 2000.
30. Springborn Laboratories, Inc., Protocol for a Photoirritation Study in Rabbits with Occlusive Conditions, SLI No. OECD/PHIRBO-1-8/2000, Spencerville, OH, 2000.
31. Springborn Laboratories, Inc., Protocol for a Photoirritation Study in Guinea Pigs with Non-Occlusive Conditions, SLI No. OECD/PHIGPU-1-8/2000, Spencerville, OH, 2000.
32. Springborn Laboratories, Inc., Protocol for a Photoirritation Study in Guinea Pigs with Occlusive Conditions, SLI No. OECD/PHIGPO-1-8/2000, Spencerville, OH, 2000.
33. Gad, S.C. and Chengelis, C.P., Photosensitization and phototoxicity, *Acute Toxicol. Testing,* 117, 1990.
34. Buehler, E.V. and Griffin, F., Experimental skin sensitization in the guinea pig and man, *Animal Models Dermatol.,* 55, 1975.
35. Springborn Laboratories, Inc., Protocol for a Dermal Sensitization Study in Guinea Pigs — Modified Buehler Design, EPA/MB-1–10/2000, Spencerville, OH, 2000.
36. Buehler, E.V., Delayed contact hypersensitivity in the guinea pig, *Arch. Dermatol,* 91, 171, 1965.
37. Springborn Laboratories, Inc., Protocal for a Dermal Sensitization Study in Guinea Pigs — Standard Buehler Design, EPA/MB-1–10/2000, Spencerville, OH, 2000.

38. Magnusson, B. and Kligman, A., *Allergic Contact Dermatitis in the Guinea Pigs,* C.C. Thomas, Springfield, IL, 1970.
39. Springborn Laboratories, Inc., Protocol for a Dermal Sensitization Study in Guinea Pigs — Maximization Design, EPA/MAX-1-10/2000 Spencerville, OH, 2000.
40. Gerberick, G.F., Kimber, I., and Basketter, D., The local lymph node assay ICCVAM test method submission, April, 1998, in *The Murine Local Lymph Node Assay: A Test Method for Assessing the Allergic Contact Dermatitis Potential of Chemicals/Compounds,* NIH Publication No. 99-4494, February 1999.
41. Kimber, I., Hilton, J., Dearman, R., Gerberick, G.F., Ryan, C., Basketter, D.A., Lea, L., House, R.V., Ladics, G.S., Loveless, S.E., and Hastings, K.L., Assessment of the skin sensitization potential of topical medicaments using the local lymph node assay: an interlaboratory evaluation, *J. Toxicol. Environ. Health,* A, 52, 563–579, 1998.
42. Loveless, S.E., Ladics, G.S., Gerberick, B.F., Ryan, C.A., Basketter, D.A., Scholes, E.W., House, R.V., Hilton, J., Dearman, R.J., and Kimber, I., Further evaluation of the local lymph node assay in the final phase of an international collaborative trial, *Toxicol.,* 108, 141–152, 1996.
43. Dearman, R.J., Hilton, J., Evans, P., Harvey, P., Basketter, D.A., and Kimber, I., Temporal stability of local lymph nodes assay response to hexylcinnamic aldehyde, *J. Appl. Toxicol.,* 18, 281–284, 1998.
44. Siglin, J.C., Jenkins, P.K., Smith, P.S., Ryan, C.A., and Gerberick, G.F., *Evaluation of a New Murine Model for the Predictive Assessment of Contact Photoallergy (CPA),* American College of Toxicology Annual Meeting, Savannah, GA, 1991.
45. Gerberick, G.F. and Ryan, C.A., A predictive mouse ear-swelling model for investigating topical phototoxicity, *Fd. Chem. Toxicol.,* 27, 813, 1989.
46. Springborn Laboratories, Inc., Protocol for a Photoallergy Study in Mice, FDA/PHS-2-2/94, Spencerville, OH, 1994.
47. Ichikawa, H., Armstrong, R.B., and Harber, L.C., Photoallergic contact dermatitis in guinea pigs: Improved induction technique using Freund's complete adjuvant, *J. Invest. Dermatol.,* 76, 498, 1981.
48. Harber, L.C., Shalita, A.R., and Armstrong, R.B., Immunologically mediated contact photosensitivity in guinea pigs, in *Dermatotoxicology,* 2nd ed., Marzulli, F.N. and Maibach, H.I., Eds., Hemisphere Publishing, Washington, 1983.
49. Maurer, T., Predictive animal test methods for allergenicity, in *Contact and Photocontact Allergens, a Manual of Predictive Test Methods,* Vol. 3, Calnan, C.D. and Maibach, H.I., Eds., Marcel Dekker, New York, 1983.
50. Springborn Laboratories, Inc., Protocol for a Photosensitization Study in Guinea Pigs, FDA/PHS OECD-1-1/2000 Spencerville, OH, 2000.
51. Patrick, E. and Maibach, H.I., Dermatotoxicology, in *Principles and Methods* of *Toxicology,* 2nd ed., Hayes, A.W., Ed., Raven Press, New York, 1989.
52. Klecak, G., Identification of contact allergies: predictive tests in animals, in *Dermatotoxicology,* 2nd ed., Marzulli, F.N. and Maibach, H.I., Eds., Hemisphere Publishing, Washington, 1983.
53. Fischer, T. and Maibach, H.I., Patch testing in allergic contact dermatitis, in *Exogenous Dermatoses: Environmental Dermatitis,* Menné, T. and Maibach, H.I., Eds., CRC Press, Boca Raton, FL, 1991.
54. U.S. Environmental Protection Agency, *Federal Insecticide, Fungicide, Rodenticide Act, Pesticide Assessment Guidelines,* Subdivision F, Hazard Evaluation: Human and Domestic Animals, Series 81-5 Dermal Irritation, 55e, 1984.
55. U.S. Environmental Protection Agency, *Toxic Substances Control Act, Test Guidelines,* 40 CFR Part 798, Subpart E — Specific Organ/Tissue Toxicity, Section 798.4470 Primary Dermal Irritation, 491, 1992.
56. U.S. Consumer Products Safety Commission, 16 CFR Chapter II, Subchapter C: Federal Hazardous Substances Act Regulation, Part 1500, Subsection 1500.3: Definitions, 381, 1993.
57. U.S. Environmental Protection Agency, *Federal Insecticide, Fungicide, Rodenticide Act, Pesticide Assessment Guidelines,* Subdivision F: Hazard Evaluation: Humans and Domestic Animals — Addendum 3 on Data Reporting, 1988.
58. U.S. Environmental Protection Agency, *Federal Insecticide, Fungicide, Rodenticide Act, Pesticide Assessment Guidelines,* Hazard Evaluation Division, Standard Evaluation Procedure, Guidance for Evaluation of Dermal Irritation Testing, 1, 1984.
59. U.S. Environmental Protection Agency, *Toxic Substances Control Act, Test Guidelines,* 40 CFR Chap. 1 (7-1-93), Part 156: Labeling Requirements for Pesticides and Devices, Section 156.10, 75, 1993.

60. The Commission of the European Communities, Official Journal of the European Communities, Annex VI, General Classification and Labelling Requirements for Dangerous Substances, No. L 257/11, 1983.

61. U.S. Occupational Safety and Health Administration, Labor, 29 CFR Chapter XVII, Part 1910, Appendix A to Section 1900.1200 — Health Hazard Definitions (Mandatory), 364, 1991.

62. DeGroot, A.C., *Patch Testing, Test Concentrations and Vehicles for 2800 Allergens,* Elsevier Science, Amsterdam, 1986.

63. Cronin, E., *Contact Dermatitis,* Churchill Livingstone, New York, 1980.

64. *Casarett and Doull's Toxicology, The Basic Science of Poisons,* 4th ed., Klaassen, C.D., Amdur, M.O., and Doull, J., Eds., Pergamon Press, New York, 1991.

65. Marzulli, F.N. and Maibach, H.I., Eds., *Dermatotoxicology,* 2nd ed., Hemisphere Publishing, Washington, 1977.

66. *Stedman's Medical Dictionary,* 25th ed., Williams & Wilkins, Baltimore, 1990.

67. *The American Heritage Dictionary of the English Language,* New College Edition, Morris, W., Ed., Houghton Mifflin, Boston, 1978.

68. U.S. Environmental Protection Agency, *Federal Insecticide, Fungicide, Rodenticide Act, Pesticide Assessment Guidelines,* Hazard Evaluation Division, Standard Evaluation Procedure, Guidance for Evaluation of Dermal Sensitization, 1, 1984.

ADDITIONAL RELATED INFORMATION

TABLE 3.31
Relative Ranking of the Skin Permeability in Different Animal Species

Ranking	Animal Species	Thickness of Stratum Corneum	Epidermis (μm)	Whole Skin (mm)
Most permeable	Mouse	5.8	12.6	0.84
	Guinea pig			
	Goat			
	Rabbit			
	Horse			
	Cat			
	Dog			
	Monkey			
	Pig	26.4	65.8	3.43
	Human	16.8	46.9	2.97
Least permeable	Chimpanzee			

From Leung, H-W. and Paustenbach, D.J., Percutaneous toxicity, in: *General and Applied Toxicology,* Ballantyne, B., Marrs, T.C., and Syversen, T., Eds., Groves's Dictionaries, New York, 1999, chap. 29, pp. 577–586. With permission. © Nature Publishing Group Reference.

TABLE 3.32
In Vivo **Human Percutaneous Absorption Rates of Some Neat Chemical Liquids**

Chemical	Percutaneous Absorption Rate (mg cm^{-2} h^{-1})
Aniline	0.2–0.7
Benzene	0.24–0.4
2-Butoxyethanol	0.05–0.68
2-(2-Butoxyethoxy) ethanol	0.035
Carbon disulfide	9.7
Dimethylformamide	9.4
Ethylbenzene	22–33
2-Ethoxyethanol	0.796
2-(2-Ethoxyethoxy) ethanol	0.125
Methanol	11.5
2-Methoxyethanol	2.82
Methyl *n*-butyl ketone	0.25–0.48
Nitrobenzene	2
Styrene	9–15
Toluene	14–23
Xylenes (mixed)	4.5–9.6
m-Xylene	0.12–0.15

From Leung, H-W. and Paustenbach, D.J., Percutaneous toxicity, in *General and Applied Toxicology,* Ballantyne, B., Marrs, T.C., and Syversen, T., Eds., Groves's Dictionaries, New York, 1999, chap. 29, pp. 577–586. With permission. © Nature Publishing Group Reference.

TABLE 3.33

In Vitro **Human Percutaneous Permeability Coefficients of Aqueous Solutions of Some Industrial Chemicals**

Organic Chemical	K_p (cm h^{-1})	Organic Chemical	K_p (cm h^{-1})	Inorganic Chemical	K_p (cm h^{-1})
2-Amino-4-nitrophenol	0.00066	2-Ethoxyethanol	0.0003	Cobalt chloride	0.0004
4-Amino-2-nitrophenol	0.0028	*p*-Ethylphenol	0.035	Mercuric chloride	0.00093
Benzene	0.11	Heptanol	0.038	Nickel chloride	0.0001
p-Bromophenol	0.036	Hexanol	0.028	Nickel sulfate	<0.000009
Butane-2,3-diol	<0.00005	Methanol	0.0016	Silver nitrate	<0.00035
n-Butanol	0.0025	Methyl hydroxybenzoate	0.0091		
Butan-2-one	0.0045	β–Naphthol	0.028		
Chlorocresol	0.055	3-Nitrophenol	0.0056		
o-Chlorophenol	0.033	4-Nitrophenol	0.0056		
p-Chlorophenol	0.036	Nitrosodiethanol amine	0.0000055		
Chloroxylenol	0.059	Nonanol	0.06		
m-Cresol	0.015	Octanol	0.061		
o-Cresol	0.016	Pentanol	0.006		
p-Cresol	0.018	Phenol	0.0082		
Decanol	0.08	Propanol	0.0017		
2,4-Dichlorophenol	0.06	Resorcinol	0.00024		
Diethanolamine	0.000034	Thymol	0.053		
Diethyl ether	0.016	Toluene	1.01		
1,4-Dioxane	0.00043	2,4,6-Trichlorophenol	0.059		
Ethanol	0.0008	3,4-Xylenol	0.036		
Ethanolamine	0.000043				

Note: Values obtained from viable excised human skin using a temperature-controlled skin penetration chamber.

From Leung, H-W. and Paustenbach, D.J., Percutaneous toxicity, in *General and Applied Toxicology,* Ballantyne, B., Marrs, T.C., and Syversen, T., Eds., Groves's Dictionaries, New York, 1999, chap. 29, pp. 577–586. With permission. © Nature Publishing Group Reference.

4 Ocular Toxicology

Brendan J. Dunn, M.S.

CONTENTS

0-8493-0370-2/02/$0.00+$1.50
© 2002 by CRC Press LLC

SECTION 1. ANATOMY OF THE EYE

Ocular tissues are described which generally show toxicological effects resulting from either topical exposure or systemic administration of chemical substances. The descriptions provided below are for the human eye, unless otherwise noted. Figures 4.1 through 4.3 show anatomical structures of the human eye in sagittal section; whereas, Figure 4.4 depicts the basic structures of the rabbit eye in sagittal section.

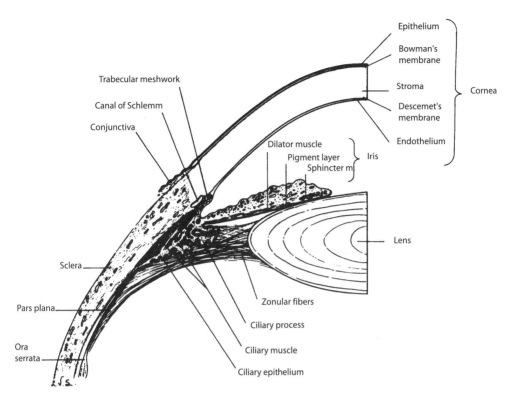

FIGURE 4.1 Sagittal section of the anterior chamber angle of the human eye showing the structure associated with the ciliary body, iris, cornea, and lens. (From Vaughan, D., Asbury, T., and Riordan-Eva, P., *General Ophthalmology*, 13th ed., Appleton & Lange, East Norwalk, CT, 1992. With permission.)

A. The Eyeball

The outer protective tissues of the eye are composed of the cornea, the conjunctiva, and the sclera.

1. Cornea: an avascular, transparent tissue that is composed of five layers:
   - Epithelium (approximately 10% of total thickness)
   - Bowman's layer or membrane
   - Stroma (approximately 90% of total thickness)
   - Descemet's membrane
   - Endothelium (one cell layer thick)
2. Conjunctiva: a thin vascularized, transparent layer of mucous membrane that covers the posterior surface of the eyelids (palpebral conjunctiva) and the anterior surface of the sclera (bulbar conjunctiva). The conjunctiva is squamous, nonkeratinized epithelium that contains numerous mucous-secreting cells.
3. Nictitating membrane: in the rabbit, a prominent cartilaginous flap of tissue covered by a layer of squamous epithelium that is attached in the medial canthus of the eye and moves laterally or diagonally across the eye behind the external eyelids.
4. Sclera: the fibrous white, dense, protective coating of the eye that is continuous with the cornea anteriorly and with the dural sheath of the optic nerve posteriorly.
   a. Lamina cribrosa: a few strands of modified scleral tissue that passes over the optic disk.
   b. Episclera: the outer layer of the sclera composed of thin, fine elastic tissue.
   c. Lamina fusca: the brownish inner scleral layer continuous with the sclera; related to the optic nerve at the choroid.

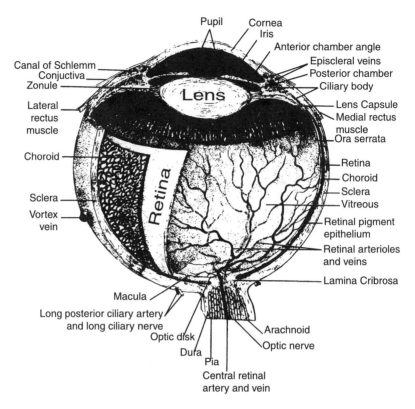

FIGURE 4.2 Sagittal section of the human eye showing internal structures. (From *The Anatomy of the Eye,* from original drawing by Paul Peck. Copyright, Lederle Laboratories Division of American Cyanamid Company, Wayne, NJ. All rights reserved. Reprinted with permission.)

B. THE UVEAL TRACT

The middle vascular layer of the eye is composed of the iris, the ciliary body, and the choroid.

1. Iris: a highly vascularized anterior extension of the ciliary body located in front of the lens. It forms the posterior wall of the anterior chamber and the anterior wall of the posterior chamber. Within the stroma of the iris are the sphincter and dilator muscles that determine the size of the medially located round aperture, the pupil. There are two pigmented layers on the posterior surface of the iris (except in albinos).
2. Ciliary body: the vascularized tissue extending forward from the anterior end of the choroid to the root of the iris. The ciliary muscle within this tissue is composed of longitudinal, circular, and radial fibers. The action of the ciliary muscle alters the tension on the capsule of the lens, giving the lens a variable focus for both near and distant objects in the visual field.
3. Choroid: the heavily vascularized posterior segment of the uveal tract located between the retina and sclera. It is composed of three layers of choroidal blood vessels: large, medium, and small. Anteriorly it joins the ciliary body and posteriorly it attaches to the margins of the optic nerve.

C. THE LENS

A biconvex, avascular, colorless, and almost completely transparent structure suspended behind the iris by the zonule, which connects to the ciliary body. The zonule, or suspensory ligament of the

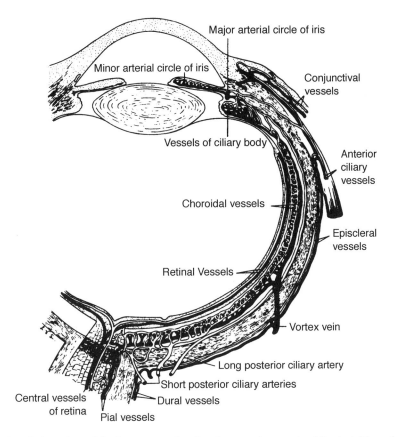

FIGURE 4.3 Saggital section of the human eye showing the vascular supply. All arterial branches originate with the ophthalmic artery. (From Vaughan, D., Asbury, T., and Riordan-Eva, P., *General Ophthalmology,* 13th ed., Appleton & Lange, East Norwalk, CT, 1992. With permission.)

lens, is composed of numerous fibrils arising from the ciliary body and inserting into the equator of the lens. The aqueous is anterior to the lens and the vitreous is posterior to it. The lens is encapsulated by a semipermeable membrane, the lens capsule.

D. THE AQUEOUS

A slightly alkaline liquid, composed mainly of water, that is secreted by the ciliary process and fills the anterior and posterior chambers of the eye. The aqueous passes through the pupil from the posterior chamber into the anterior chamber. In the anterior chamber, it flows toward the filtering trabecular meshwork at the periphery and into the canal of Schlemm.

E. THE VITREOUS

A clear avascular gelatinous body that fills the space bounded by the lens, retina, and optic disk. It comprises two-thirds of the volume and weight of the eye. It helps to maintain the shape and transparency of the eye.

F. THE RETINA

The innermost posterior coat of the eye composed of 10 histologically distinct layers of highly organized, delicate nerve tissue. The inner surface is in contact with the vitreous and the outer surface is related to the choroid. The layers of the retina are: 1) internal limiting membrane, 2) a

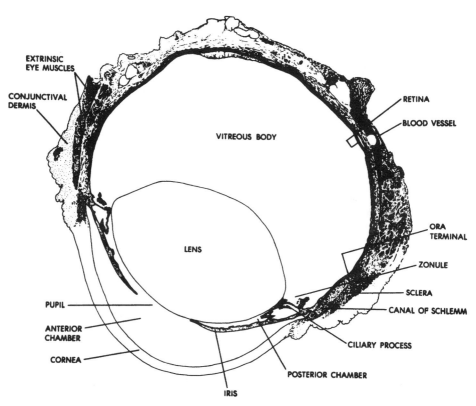

FIGURE 4.4 Sagittal section of the rabbit eye showing the basic structures. (From McLaughlin, C.A. and Chiasson, R.B., *Laboratory Anatomy of* the *Rabbit,* 3rd ed., Wm. C. Brown Communications, Dubuque, IA, 1990. All rights reserved. Reprinted with permission.)

layer of nerve fibers, 3) a ganglion cell layer, 4) inner plexiform layer, 5) inner nuclear layer, 6) outer plexiform layer, 7) outer nuclear layer, 8) external limiting membrane, 9) layer of rods and cones, and 10) pigment epithelium. Anteriorly, it extends almost as far as the ciliary body, ending in a ragged edge called the ora serrata. At the ora serrata, the nerve tissue of the retina ends, but a thin pigment layer of the retina continues further anteriorly to relate to the posterior surfaces of the ciliary processes and the iris. In the center of the posterior segment of the retina is the macula lutea, an oval yellowish spot with a depressed center called the fovea centralis. The optic disk (the visible portion of the optic nerve) is located about 3 mm to the medial side of the macula.

G. THE OPTIC NERVE

A nerve fiber tract whose fibers are derived from the ganglion cells of the retina. The optic nerve emerges from the posterior surface of the eyeball through a short, circular opening in the sclera located about 1 mm below and 3 mm nasal to the posterior pole of the eye. From the orbit the optic nerve travels through the bony optic foramen into the cranial cavity where it joins the opposite optic nerve, forming the optic chiasm.

SECTION 2. COMPARATIVE ANATOMY AND PHYSIOLOGY OF THE EYE

A. ANATOMICAL COMPARISONS

TABLE 4.1
Corneal Thickness and Area

Species	Thickness (mm)	Area (%)[a]	Ref.
Human	0.51–0.54	7	1, 2
Rhesus monkey	0.52	—	3
Rabbit	0.37–0.4	25	1, 3
Mouse	0.1	50	1
Rat	0.15	50	1
Cat	0.62	—	3
Dog	0.55	—	3

[a] Percentage of the total area of the globe.

TABLE 4.2
Comparison of the Type of Retinal Vasculature of Various Species

Species pig	Holangiotic	Merangiotic	Paurangiotic	Anangiotic
Dog	×			
Cat	×			
Human	×			
Primate	×			
Rabbit		×		
Rat	×			
Mouse	×			
Gerbil	×			
Cattle	×			
Horse			×	
Guinea pig				×
Chinchilla				×
Degu				×
Bird				×

Note: Holangiotic: The retinal blood supply is from a central retinal or cilioretinal arteries and extends over the entire retina. Merangiotic: A portion of the retina is supplied by retinal vessels. Paurangiotic: Retinal vessels are small and extend only a very short distance from the optic nerve. Anangiotic: The retina is without vessels. From David W. Hobson, *Dermal and Ocular Toxicology, Fundamentals and Methods,* CRC Press, Boca Raton, FL, 1991. With permission.

TABLE 4.3
Percentage of Optic Nerve Fibers Decussating at the Optic Chiasm

Species	Decussation (%)
Human	50
Primate	50

TABLE 4.3 *(Continued)*
Percentage of Optic Nerve Fibers
Decussating at the Optic Chiasm

Species	Decussation (%)
Dog	75
Cat	65–70
Horse	81
Cow	83
Pig	88
Bird	100

From David W. Hobson, *Dermal and Ocular Toxicology, Fundamentals and Methods,* CRC Press, Boca Raton, FL, 1991. With permission.

TABLE 4.4
Comparison of the Tapetum in the Cat, Dog, and Ferret

Parameter	Dog	Cat	Ferret
Number of central cell layers	9	16–20	7–10
Thickness of central tapetum	26–33 μm	61–67 μm	23–24 μm
Presence of microtubule-like structure in tapetal rod	Present	Absent	Present
Presence of electron-dense cores in tapetal rod	Absent	Present	Absent
Presence of electron-dense cores in tapetal rods after prolonged glutaraldehyde fixation	Absent	Present	Absent
Retention of tapetal color after prolonged glutaraldehyde fixation	Lost	Retained	Lost
Tapetal zinc concentration	26,000 ppm	1497 ppm	22,500 ppm
Tapetal cysteine concentration	241 μmol/g	0	216 μmol/g

Modified from Wen, G.Y., Sturman, J.A., and Shek, J.W., *Lab. Anim. Sci.*, 35, 200, 1985, in David W. Hobson, *Dermal and Ocular Toxicology, Fundamentals and Methods,* CRC Press, Boca Raton, FL, 1991. With permission.

B. PHYSIOLOGICAL COMPARISONS

TABLE 4.5
Concentrations of the Principal Components of the Aqueous Humor as Compared with Plasma of Various Species

Substance and Units	Aqueous	Plasma	Species	Ref.
Ascorbate				
μmol/ml	1.18	0.02	Monkey	4
	0.96	0.02	Rabbit	5
	1.06	0.04	Human	6
mg/dl	20.0		Horse	7
	5.5	—	Dog	7
	1.0	—	Cat	7
	21.0	—	Cow	7
Bicarbonate				
μmol/ml	22.5	18.8	Monkey	4
	27.7	24.0	Rabbit	5
	20.2	27.5	Human	6

TABLE 4.5 *(Continued)*
Concentrations of the Principal Components of the Aqueous Humor as Compared with Plasma of Various Species

Substance and Units	Aqueous	Plasma	Species	Ref.
mm/g H$_2$O	Ratio of aqueous/plasma	0.82	Horse	7
	Ratio of aqueous/plasma	1.13	Dog	7
	30.4	25.3	Cat	8
	36.0	—	Cow	8
Calcium				
μmol/ml	2.5	4.9	Monkey	9
	1.7	2.6	Rabbit	8
	—	—	Human	
mEq/L	3.0	5.5	Horse	7
	2.9	5.24	Dog	8
	2.7	4.8	Cat	8
	—	—	Cow	7
Chloride				
μmol/ml	—	—	Monkey	
	105.1	111.8	Rabbit	10
	131.0	107.0	Human	6
mEq/L	12.1	10.1	Horse	7
	Ratio of aqueous/plasma	1.07	Dog	7
	—	—	Cat	
	Ratio of aqueous/plasma	1.15	Cow	8
Glucose				
μmol/ml	3.0	4.1	monkey	5
	4.9	5.3	Rabbit	10
	2.8	5.9	Human	6
mg/dl	98	91	Horse	7
	51	70	Dog	7
	45	56	Cat	7
	33	57	Cow	7
Hyaluronate				
μmol/ml	—	—	Monkey	
	—	—	Rabbit	
	1.1	—	Human	11
	—	—	Horse	
	—	—	Dog	
	—	—	Cat	
	4.4	—	Cow	11
Lactate				
μmol/ml	4.3	3.0	Monkey	4
	9.3	10.3	Rabbit	10
	4.5	1.9	Human	6
	—	—	Horse	
	—	—	Dog	
			Cat	
	—	—	Cow	
Oxygen				
mm Hg	—	—	Monkey	
	30	77	Rabbit	12
	53	—	Human	13
	—	—	Horse	

TABLE 4.5 *(Continued)*
Concentrations of the Principal Components of the Aqueous Humor as Compared with Plasma of Various Species

Substance and Units	Aqueous	Plasma	Species	Ref.
	45	—	Dog	8
	—	—	Cat	
	—	—	Cow	
Phosphate				
µmol/ml	0.14	0.68	Monkey	5
	0.89	1.49	Rabbit	10
	0.62	1.11	Human	14
	0.33	0.31	Horse	15
	0.53	1.26	Dog	7
	0.48	1.87	Cat	7
	—	—	Cow	
Potassium				
µmol/ml	3.9	4.0	monkey	4
	5.1	5.6	Rabbit	10
	—	—	Human	
mEq/AL	5.1	5.5	Horse	15
	5.0	4.4	Dog	8
	4.4	4.0	Cat	8
	7.1	4.7	Cow	8
Protein				
mg/100ml	33.3	—	Monkey	4
	25.9	—	Rabbit	16
	23.7	—	Human	16
	20.0	730	Horse	15
	38.0	650	Dog	17
	15–55	780	Cat	17
	17.0	750	Cow	15
Sodium				
µmol/ml	152	148	Monkey	4
	143	146	Rabbit	10
	—	—	Human	
	117.4	143.5	Horse	15
	149.4	154	Dog	8
	158.5	163.6	Cat	8
	149.5	143	Cow	7
Urea				
µmol/ml	6.1	7.3	Monkey	4
	7.0	9.1	Rabbit	8
	—	—	Human	
mg/dl	28	27	Horse	15
	Ratio of aqueous/plasma	0.70	Dog	7
	Ratio of aqueous/plasma	0.73	Cat	7
	—	12	Cow	7
Creatinine				
µmol/ml	0.04	0.03	Monkey	4
	0.11	—	Rabbit	18
	—	—	Human	
	0.18	0.18	Horse	15
	—	—	Dog	

TABLE 4.5 *(Continued)*
Concentrations of the Principal Components of the Aqueous Humor as Compared with Plasma of Various Species

Substance and Units	Aqueous	Plasma	Species	Ref.
	—	—	Cat	
	—	—	Cow	

Modified from Schmidt, G.M. and Coulter, D.B., *Veterinary Ophthalmology*, Gelatt, K.N., Ed., Lea & Febiger, Philadelphia, 129, 1981, in David W. Hobson, *Dermal and Ocular Toxicology, Fundamentals and Methods,* CRC Press, Boca Raton, FL, 1991. With permission.

TABLE 4.6
Concentration of the Various Components of the Vitreous[7,19]

Constituent	Cattle	Rabbit	Pig	Human	Horse
Inorganic Constituents (mmol/kg H_2O)					
Sodium	130.5	133.9–152.2	142	137	118–153
Potassium	7.7	5.1–10.2	5.0	3.8	4.9–7.3
Calcium	3.9	1.5	5.7		4.9–7.3
Magnesium	0.8	—	2.6		—
Chloride	115.6	104.3	118	112.8	112–120
Water and Organic Constituents (mg/100 ml H_2O)					
Creatinine	1.0	—	0.5	—	—
Water	99%	99%	99%	99%	99%
Glucose	55–62	55–80	—	30–70	57–100
Lactic acid	14.8	65		70	17.5

Modified from Nordman, J., *Biologie et Chirurgie du Corps Vitre*, Brini, A., Ed., Masson et Cie, Paris, 1968, in David W. Hobson, *Dermal and Ocular Toxicology, Fundamentals and Methods,* CRC Press, Boca Raton, FL, 1991. With permission.

TABLE 4.7
Concentration of Mucopolysaccharide and Collagen of the Vitreous in Various Species

Species	Mucopolysaccharide (µg/ml)	Collagen (µg/ml)
Rabbit	31	104
Guinea pig	37	134
Human	240	286
Owl monkey	423	25
Steer	710	57

Modified from Gloor, B.P., *Adler's: Physiology of the Eye,* 8th ed., Moses, R.A. and Hart, W.H., Eds., C.V. Mosby, St. Louis, 246, 1987, in David W. Hobson, *Dermal and Ocular Toxicology, Fundamentals and Methods,* CRC Press, Boca Raton, FL, 1991. With permission.

TABLE 4.8
Distribution of the Anterior Uveal Adrenergic Receptors in Various Species

	Dilator	Sphincter	Ciliary Muscle
Cat	Mainly alpha, some beta	Mainly beta, some alpha	Mainly beta, some alpha
Rabbit	Mainly alpha, few beta	Mainly beta, few alpha	Mainly alpha, few beta
Monkey	Mainly alpha, very few beta	Mainly alpha, perhaps beta	Exclusively beta, no alpha
Man	Mainly alpha, very few beta	Alpha and beta in equal amounts	Mainly beta, very few or no alpha

Modified from Van Alpen, G.W., *Invest. Ophthalmol. Visual Sci.,* 15, 502, 1976, from David W. Hobson, *Dermal and Ocular Toxicology, Fundamentals and Methods,* CRC Press, Boca Raton, FL, 1991. With permission.

SECTION 3. REGULATORY GUIDELINES

A. CONTACT LENS MATERIALS

At a minimum, the following toxicology test procedures are recommended for contact lens materials by the Premarket Notification [510(k)] Guidance Document for Daily Contact Lenses. This guidance document was last revised May 1994 by the Contact Lens Branch, Division of Ophthalmic Devices, Center for Devices and Radiological Health, Food and Drug Administration (FDA). The toxicology studies are generally consistent with the applicable studies recommended for evaluating plastic polymers in the Tripartite Biocompatibility Guidance for Medical Devices, which categorizes contact lenses as Externally Communicating Devices: Intact Natural Channels. The Tripartite Guidance has been harmonized with the International Standards Series ISO 10993, Biological Evaluation of Medical Devices.

1. Systemic Injection Test (USP/NF)*

This test assesses the potential of leachable chemical constituents from a contact lens material to produce an acute systemic toxicity in mice. Extracts of the lens material are prepared in two types of solvents (polar and non-polar), injected into mice, and the mice observed for acute systemic toxicity.

2. Eye Irritation Test (USP/NF)*

This test evaluates the potential for ocular irritation resulting from residual chemical leachables in contact lens materials. The effects are assessed *in vivo* using rabbits.

3. *In Vitro* Cytotoxicity Test (USP/NF)*

This test evaluates the potential for cytotoxicity resulting from residual chemical leachables in contact with lens materials. The effects are assessed *in vitro* using cytotoxicity studies (e.g., tissue culture–agar overlay method or a suitable validated alternative).

Additional Recommended Testing. The following tests are not required if the applicant provides appropriate documentation demonstrating that either of the following criteria have been met:

- The recommended lens care regimen has been approved for use with the specific lens material group; or

---

* United States Pharmacopeia (USP) 24/National Formulary (NF) 19, 2000 (or current update).

- The plastic lens carries no charge or the same electric charge as the preservative system used in the approved care regimen.

However, the following tests are required if:

- A lens material is manufactured using a new monomer not previously used in a currently marketed hydrophilic or hydrophobic lens; or
- A UV-absorber is incorporated into the material, unless a scientific justification is provided to the contrary (e.g., use of a UV-absorber that has been previously cleared by the manufacturer for use in contact lenses of the same generic class; i.e., hydrophilic or hydrophobic materials), and will be incorporated into the lens by a method that has been approved in a PMA or cleared in a substantial equivalence [section 513(I)(1)(A)] premarket notification [510 (k)] for the manufacturer.

a. Sensitization Tests

i. *Preservative Uptake and Release.* Contact lens polymers may absorb or adsorb preservative materials that could possess irritating or sensitizing properties that are potentially irritating to some users. A quantitative analysis of preservative uptake per lens, the amount released, and the time course of release is conducted. Results taken from these test data are used to predict the potential for a preservative-related toxicity, as well as the potential for inducing a sensitivity/allergic response associated with the lens group.

ii. *Skin Sensitization (Guinea Pig Maximization Test)*.* This test grades or ranks chemical constituents on a scale of I through V as to their potential for inducing a sensitivity response in the guinea pig model. The grade or ranking is based on the number of animals sensitized, and the results are classified on an ascending scale from a weak (grade I) to an extreme sensitizing agent (grade V).

b. Three Week Ocular Irritation Test in Rabbits

This *in vivo* test of the contact lenses in rabbits is used as a biocompatibility test as well as a toxicity test of the lens material. The test assesses the effects of the ocular environment on the lens material, as well as the effects of the lens material on the ocular tissues.

B. Contact Lens Care Products (i.e., Solutions, Tablets)

The following *in vitro* and *in vivo* tests for contact lens care products are recommended by the Premarket Notification [510(k)] Guidance Document for Contact Lens Care Products, which was last revised in May, 1997 by the Center for Devices and Radiological Health, FDA.

1. *In Vitro* Cytotoxicity Test (USP/NF)

This test evaluates the potential for toxicity of residual chemicals leaching from the lens into the lens care products [i.e., solution(s)/solubilized tablets]. In addition, this test may be used to detect potential toxic carryover from uptake/release of the solution by the lens. The tissue culture-agar diffusion test, direct contact test, and/or elution test, or suitable validated alternative method may be used.

---

* Magnusson, B. and Kligman, A.M., The identification of contact allergens by animal assay. The Guinea Pig Maximization Test, *J. Invest. Dermatol.*, 52(3), 268–276, 1969.

2. Acute Ocular Irritation Test

This test evaluates the potential for ocular irritation resulting from residual chemical leachables from the finished device that may be extracted in the lens care products (i.e., solution(s)/solubilized tablets). This method is also used to detect the potential for ocular irritation due to carryover from uptake/release of the solution by the lens and from direct instillation of an in-eye solution. This test should not be needed in cases where formulations contain known ocular irritants. In such cases, an appropriate warning should be required on the label for products known to cause ocular irritation (i.e., daily cleaners/periodic cleaners) in lieu of performing the test.

3. Acute Oral Toxicity Study

This study assesses the potential of the contact lens care product (i.e., solution(s)/solubilized tablets) to produce a toxic response as a result of deliberate or accidental ingestion of the product by adults or children. These data are used to determine the need for additional warnings or precautions in the labeling of the product for the purpose of consumer protection. For rodent testing, the maximum volume of an aqueous solution generally should not exceed 2 ml/100 g of body weight. This single large dose is referred to as the maximum tolerable dose (MTD). Should signs of toxicity be demonstrated at the MTD, further testing consistent with accepted toxicological practices is recommended to complete a risk/benefit assessment of the product.

Additional Recommended Testing. The following tests are recommended if a manufacturer is using a new preservative or an active ingredient/chemical component not previously used in a currently marketed contact lens care product:

1. *Skin Sensitization (Guinea Pig Maximization Test):* described previously.
2. *In Vivo Ocular Biocompatibility Test (ISO 9394-1998):* This ISO test method, entitled "Optics and optical instruments — Determination of biological compatibility of contact lens material — Testing of the contact lens system by ocular study with rabbit eyes," should be acceptable in its entirety to address preclinical ocular biocompatibility of contact lens products.

C. Plastic Ophthalmic Containers

In the Premarket Notification [510(k)] Guidance Document for Contact Lens Care Products (revised May 1997), the Center for Devices and Radiological Health of the FDA recommends the following *in vitro* and *in vivo* tests that are consistent with the procedures listed in the USP 24/NF19, Containers for Ophthalmics — Plastics (Biological Test Procedures):

1. Systemic Injection Test
2. Acute Ocular Irritation Test
3. *In Vitro* Cytotoxicity Test

These tests (described previously) indirectly or directly assess the potential toxicity of constituent(s) that may leach from the container for a prolonged period of time.

D. Ophthalmic Therapeutic Formulations

Nonclinical study protocols, based on guidelines set forth by Goldenthal[21] and Hackett,[26] have been developed to assess acute and systemic toxicity of ophthalmic formulations. The toxicity data developed from the following preclinical study designs are used to establish an adequate safety profile and assess risk.

1. One Day Acute Topical Ocular Irritation Test

This test is used for formulation ingredients that have not been previously used by the topical ocular route and that have been placed in Category 1 by FDA ophthalmic panel(s), e.g., a single-application diagnostic drug used for producing mydriasis or a single-application topical anesthetic for producing corneal anesthesia. The test is designed to determine the ocular toxicity potential in the event accidental or intentional drug misuse occurs.

- Dosing should be according to the anticipated clinical regimen. However, the dosing frequency may be adjusted or exaggerated to enhance the chance of observing toxicity for the purpose of predicting human risk. Typically, formulation ingredients are instilled at 0.03 to 0.05 ml every 30 min for 6 consecutive h, using at least 6 eyes (rabbit).
- When possible, use of multiples of the active ingredients is essential.
- If available, use of a marketed product (control) is included for comparison.

2. Subchronic (1 to 3 months) and Chronic (≥ 1 year) Topical Ocular Irritation with Systemic Toxicological Evaluations

These tests are intended for drugs that require multiple dose therapy. Therefore, testing requirements are more extensive for development of an adequate safety profile. The extent of testing depends on the intended use of the drug. For example, drugs administered intermittently (up to several times/day for treatment periods of 2 weeks to 3 months) for external eye disease (i.e., anti-inflammatory and antimicrobial drugs) require less comprehensive testing than drugs intended for chronic administration (daily for years or for remaining lifetime) for diseases such as glaucoma.

- If the ingredients have adequate published safety data or a FDA panel has placed them into Category 1 by another route of administration, then hematology, clinical chemistry, urinalysis, and histopathology may not be required. But, if the ingredients have not been evaluated by any other route, have not been given a safe and effective rating by the FDA, or there are no published toxicology data, then systemic toxicity is monitored by including hematology, clinical chemistry, urinalysis, and histopathology of tissues, including the eyes.
- The dosing regimen (rabbit and/or dog/monkey) should be similar to that which is used clinically.
- When possible, use of multiples of the active ingredients is essential.
- If available, use of a marketed product (control) is included for comparison.

E. CHEMICAL SUBSTANCES (LIQUIDS, SOLIDS, AEROSOLS, AND LIQUIDS UNDER PRESSURE)

1. IRLG Guidelines

Eye irritation testing guidelines were developed by the Interagency Regulatory Liaison Group (IRLG), five federal agencies (Consumer Product Safety Commission, Occupational Safety and Health Administration, Food and Drug Administration, Environmental Protection Agency, and Food Safety and Quality Service of the Department of Agriculture) (Fed. Reg. 1977, 1979). Standardized guidelines for eye irritation (Fed. Reg. 1981)[22] are summarized below.

a. General Considerations
  1. *Good laboratory practices.* Studies should be conducted according to good laboratory practice regulations (21 CFR, Part 58).
  2. *Test substance.* As far as is practical, composition of the test substance should be known and should include the names and quantities of all major components, known

contaminants and impurities, and the percentages of unknown materials. The lot of the substance should be stored under conditions that maintain its stability, strength, quality, and purity from the date of its production until the tests are complete.

3. *Animals.* Healthy animals, without eye defects or irritation and not subjected to any previous experimental procedures, must be used. The test animal shall be characterized as to species, strain, sex, weight, and/or age. Each animal must be assigned an appropriate identification number. Recommendations in DHEW publication (NIH) 74-23, entitled "Guide for the Care and Use of Laboratory Animals," should be followed for the care, maintenance, and housing of animals.

4. *Documentation.* Color photographic documentation may be used to verify gross and microscopic findings.

b. Specific Considerations

1. *Test preparation.* Testing should be performed on young, adult, albino rabbits (male or female) weighing approximately 2.0 to 3.0 kg. Other species may also be tested for comparative purposes. For a valid eye irritation test, at least six rabbits must survive the test for each test substance. A trial test on three rabbits is suggested. If the substance produces corrosion, severe irritation, or no irritation, no further testing is necessary. However, if equivocal responses occur, testing in at least three additional animals should be performed. If the test substance is intended for use in or around the eye, testing on at least six animals should be performed.

2. *Test procedure.* Both eyes of each animal in the test groups must be examined by appropriate means within 24 hours before substance administration. For most purposes, anesthetics should not be used; however, if the test substance is likely to cause significant pain, local anesthetics may be used before instillation of the test substance for humane reasons. In such cases, anesthetics should be used only once, just before instillation of the test substance; the eye used as the control in each rabbit should also be anesthetized. The test substance is placed in one eye of each animal by gently pulling the lower lid away from the globe (conjunctival cul-de-sac) to form a cup into which the test substance is dropped. The lids are then gently held together for 1 second and the animal is released. The other eye, remaining untreated, serves as a control. Vehicle controls are not included. If a vehicle is suspected of causing irritation, additional studies should be conducted using the vehicle as the test substance. For testing liquids, 0.1 ml is used. For solid, paste, or particulate substances (flake, granule, powder, or other particulate form), the amount used must have a volume of 0.1 ml, or a weight of not more than 100 mg. For aerosol products, the eye should be held open and the substance administered in a single, short burst for about 1 second at a distance of about 4 inches directly in front of the eye. The dose should be approximated by weighing the aerosol can before and after each treatment for liquids. After the 24-hour examination, the eyes may be washed, if desired. Tap water or isotonic saline solution of sodium chloride (USP or equivalent) should be used for all washings.

3. *Observations.* The eyes should be examined 24, 48, and 72 hours after treatment. At the option of the investigator, the eyes may also be examined at 1 hour and at 7, 14, and 21 days. In addition to the required observations of the cornea, iris, and conjunctivae, serious lesions such as pannus, phlyctena, and rupture of the globe should be reported. The grades of ocular reaction (see Section 4.B) must be recorded at each examination. Evaluation of reactions can be facilitated by using a binocular loupe, hand slit lamp, or other appropriate means. After the recording of observations at 24 hours, the eyes of any or all rabbits may be examined further after applying fluorescein stain. An animal has exhibited a positive reaction if the test substance has produced one or more of the following signs at any observation:

    a. Ulceration of the cornea (other than a fine stippling).

    b. Inflammation of the iris (other than slight deepening of the rugae or light hyperemia of the circumcorneal blood vessels).

    c. An obvious swelling in the conjunctivae (excluding the cornea and iris) with partial eversion of the eyelids or a diffuse crimson color with individual vessels not easily discernible.

4. *Evaluation.* The test result is considered positive if four or more animals in either test group exhibit a positive reaction. If only one animal exhibits a positive reaction, the test result is regarded as negative. If two or three animals exhibit a positive reaction, the investigator may designate the substance an irritant. When two or three animals exhibit a positive reaction and the investigator does not designate the substance an irritant, the test shall be repeated with a different group of six animals. The second test result is considered positive if three or more of the animals exhibit a positive reaction. Opacity grades 2–4 and/or perforation of the cornea are considered to be corrosive effects or when opacities persist to 21 days. If only one or two animals in the second test exhibit a positive reaction, the test should be repeated with a different group of six animals. When a third test is needed, the substance will be regarded as an irritant if any animal exhibits a positive response.

c. Data Reporting

1. *Identification.* Each test report should be signed by the persons responsible for the test, identify the laboratory where the test was performed by name and address, and give inclusive dates of the test.

2. *Body of report.* The test report must include all information necessary to provide a complete and accurate description and evaluation of the test procedures and results in the following sections:

    a. Summary and conclusions.

    b. Materials, including the identification of the test substance (chemical name, molecular structure, and a qualitative and quantitative determination of its chemical composition), manufacturer and lot number of the substance tested, and specific identification of diluents, suspending agents, emulsifiers, or other materials used in administering the test substance. Specific animal data are to be included in the report. This includes species and strain, source of supply of the animals, description of any pretest acclimation, and number, age, and condition of animals of each sex in each test group.

    c. Methods, such as deviation from guidelines, specifications of test methods, data on dosage administration, and data on observation methods.

    d. Results, such as tabulation of individual animal data must accompany each report in sufficient detail to permit independent evaluation of results, including summaries and tables that show relation of effects to time of dosing, etc.

2. OECD Guidelines

The Organization for Economic Cooperation and Development (OECD) Guideline for "Acute Eye Irritation/Corrosion," No. 405 (Adopted: 24 February 1987).[23]

a. Introductory Information

i. Prerequisites

- Solid or liquid test substance
- Chemical identification of test substance
- Purity (impurities) of test substance
- Solubility characteristics

- pH and buffer capacity (where appropriate)
- Melting point/boiling point

ii.   Standard Document

There are no relevant international standards.

b.   Method

i.   Introduction, Purpose, Scope, Relevance Application and Limits of Test

In the assessment and evaluation of the toxic characteristics of a substance, determination of the irritant and/or corrosive effects on eyes of mammals is an important initial step. Information derived from this test serves to indicate the possible existence of hazards likely to arise from exposure of the eyes and associated mucous membranes to the test substance.

ii.   Definitions

Eye irritation is the production of reversible changes in the eye after the application of a test substance to the anterior surface of the eye.

Eye corrosion is the production of irreversible tissue damage in the eye after application of a test substance to the anterior surface of the eye.

iii.   Principle of the Test Method

The substance to be tested is applied in a single dose to one of the eyes in each of several experimental animals; the untreated eye is used to provide control information. The degree of irritation/corrosion is evaluated and scored at specific intervals and is further described to provide a complete evaluation of the effects. The duration of the study should be sufficient to evaluate fully the reversibility or irreversibility of the effects observed.

Animals showing severe and enduring signs of distress and pain may need to be humanely killed.

iv.   Initial Considerations

All the available information on a substance must be considered carefully to minimize the testing of substances under conditions that are likely to produce severe reactions. The following information may be useful in this regard.

1. *Physical-chemical properties and chemical reactivity.* Strongly acidic or alkaline substances, for example, which can be expected to result in a pH in the eye of 2 or less, or 11.5 or greater, need not be tested because of their probable corrosive properties. Buffer capacity also should be considered.
2. *Results from skin irritation studies.* Materials that have demonstrated definite corrosive or severe skin irritancy in a dermal study need not be tested further for eye irritancy, presuming that such substances will produce similarly severe effects on the eyes.
3. *Results from well-validated alternative studies.* Materials that have demonstrated potential corrosive or severe irritancy need not be tested further for eye irritation, presuming that such substances will produce similarly severe effects on the eyes in a test using this guideline.

c.   Description of the Test Procedure

i.   Preparations

Both eyes of each experimental animal provisionally selected for testing should be examined within 24 hours before testing starts. Animals showing eye irritation, ocular defects, or preexisting corneal injury should not be used.

ii.   Experimental Animals

Selection of Species. A variety of experimental animals have been used, but it is recommended that testing should be performed using healthy adult albino rabbits.

A Single-Animal Test. A single-animal test should be considered if marked effects are anticipated. If the results of this test in one rabbit suggest that the substance is severely irritant
(reversible effect) or corrosive (irreversible effect) to the eye using the procedure described,
further testing for ocular irritancy in subsequent animals may not need to be conducted.
Occasionally, further testing in additional animals may be appropriate to investigate specific aspects.

Number of Animals. In cases other than a single-animal test, at least three animals should be
used. Additional animals may be required to clarify equivocal responses.

Housing and Feeding Conditions. Animals should be housed individually. The room temperatures for experimental animals should be 22°C (±3°C) for rodents and 20°C (±3°C) for
rabbits; the relative humidity should be 30 to 70%. Where the lighting is artificial, the
sequence should be 12 h light/12 h dark. Conventional laboratory diets are suitable for
feeding, and an unrestricted supply of drinking water should be available.

iii.   Test Conditions

Dose Level

1. *Testing of Solids and Liquids.* For testing liquids, a dose of 0.1 ml is used. Pump sprays
   should not be used, but the liquid should be expelled instead and 0.1 ml collected and
   instilled in the eye as described for liquids. In testing solids, pastes, and particulate
   substances, the amount used should have a volume of 0.1 ml, or a weight of not more
   than 100 mg (the weight must always be recorded). If the test material is solid or granular
   it should be ground to a fine dust. The volume of particulates should be measured after
   gently compacting them, e.g., by tapping the measuring container.

   Testing of Aerosols. To test a substance contained in a pressurized aerosol container, the
   eye should be held open and the test substance administered in a single burst of about
   1 second from a distance of 10 cm directly in front of the eye. Care should be taken not
   to damage the eye. In appropriate cases, aerosols may be tested in the manner already
   described for pump sprays.

   An estimate of the dose may be made by simulating the test as follows: the substance
   is sprayed through a window, the size of a rabbit eye, placed directly before a weighing
   paper. The weight increase of the weighing paper is considered to approximate the amount
   sprayed into a rabbit eye. For volatile substances the dose may be estimated by weighing
   the container before and after use.

2. *Observation Period.* The duration of the observation period should not be fixed rigidly
   but should be sufficient to evaluate fully the reversibility or irreversibility of the effects
   observed. It usually should not exceed 21 days after instillation.

d.   Procedure

i.   Application

The test substance should be placed in the conjunctival sac of one eye of each animal after gently
pulling the lower lid away from the eyeball. The lids are then gently held together for about 1
second to prevent loss of the material. The other eye, which remains untreated, serves as a control.

ii.   Local Anesthetics

If it is thought that the substance might cause unreasonable pain, a local anesthetic may be used
before instillation of the test substance. The type and concentration of the local anesthetic should
be selected carefully to ensure that no significant differences in reaction to the test substance will
result from its use. The control eye should be similarly anesthetized.

iii.   Irrigation

The eyes of the test animals should not be washed out for 24 hours after instillation of the test
substance. At 24 hours a washout may be used if considered appropriate.

For some substances shown to be irritating by this test, additional tests using rabbits with eyes washed soon after instillation of the substance may be indicated. In these cases it is recommended that three rabbits be used. Half a minute after instillation the eyes of the rabbits are washed for half a minute using a volume and velocity of flow that will not cause injury.

iv.   Clinical Observations and Scoring

The eyes should be examined at 1, 24, 48, and 72 hours. If there is no evidence of irritation at 72 hours the study may be ended. Extended observation may be necessary if there is persistent corneal involvement or other ocular irritation to determine the progress of the lesions and their reversibility or irreversibility. In addition to the observations of the conjunctivae, cornea, iris, and any other lesions which are noted should be recorded and reported. The grades of ocular reaction (see Section 4.B) should be recorded at each examination.

Examination of reactions can be facilitated by use of a binocular loupe, hand slit lamp, biomicroscope, or other suitable devices. After recording the observations at 24 hours, the eyes of any or all rabbits may be examined further using fluorescein.

The grading of ocular responses is subject to various interpretations. To promote harmonization and to assist testing laboratories and those involved in making and interpreting the observations, an illustrated guide in grading eye irritation should be used.

e.   Data and Reporting

i.   Treatment of Results

Data may be summarized in tabular form, showing for each individual animal the irritation scores at the designated observation time, a description of the degree and nature of irritation, the presence of serious lesions, and any effects other than ocular that were observed.

ii.   Evaluation of the Results

The ocular irritation scores should be evaluated in conjunction with the nature and reversibility or otherwise of the responses observed. The individual scores do not represent an absolute standard for the irritant properties of a material. They should be viewed as reference values and are only meaningful when supported by a full description and evaluation of the observations.

iii.   Test Reports

The test report should include the following information:

- Species/strain used
- Physical nature and, where applicable, concentration and pH value for the test substance
- Tabulation of irritant/corrosive response data for each animal at each observation time (e.g., 1, 24, 48, and 72 hours)
- Description of any serious lesions observed
- Narrative describing the degree and nature of irritation or corrosion observed
- Description of the method used to score the irritation at 1, 24, 48, and 72 hours (e.g., hand slit lamp, biomicroscope, fluorescein); and
- Description of any nonocular topical effects noted.

iv.   Interpretation of the Results

Extrapolation of the results of eye irritation studies in animals to man is valid only to a limited degree. The albino rabbit is more sensitive than man to ocular irritants or corrosives in most cases. Similar results in tests on other animal species can give more weight to extrapolation from animal studies to man.

Care should be taken in the interpretation of data to exclude irritation resulting from secondary infection.

f.   Literature Cited by the OECD

1. WHO Publication: Environmental Health Criteria 6, *Principles and Methods for Evaluating the Toxicity of Chemicals.* World Health Organization, Geneva, 1978.

2. U.S. National Academy of Sciences, Committee for the Revision of NAS Publication 1138, *Principles and Procedures for Evaluating the Toxicity of Household Substances,* Washington, 1977.

3. Draize, J.H., Woodward, G., and Calvery, H.O., *J. Pharmacol. Exp. Ther.,* 82, 377–390, 1944.

4. Draize, J.H., *Appraisal of the Safety of Chemicals in Foods, Drugs, and Cosmetics — Dermal Toxicity,* Association of Food and Drug Officials of the United States, Topeka, KS, 1965, pp. 49–52.

5. Draize, J.H., *The Appraisal of Chemicals in Foods, Drugs and Cosmetics,* Association of Food and Drug Officials of the U.S., Austin, TX, 1965, pp. 36–45.

6. U.S. Federal Hazardous Substances Act Regulations, Title 16, Code of Federal Regulations, 38 FR 27012, September 27, 1973; 38 FR, 30105, November 1, 1973.

7. Loomis, T.A., *Essentials of Toxicology,* 2nd ed., Lea & Febiger, Philadelphia, 1974, pp. 207–213.

3. OPPTS 870.2400 Acute Eye Irritation

The Office of Prevention, Pesticides and Toxic Substances (OPPTS) developed this guideline through a process of harmonization that blended the testing guidance and requirements of the Office of Pollution Prevention and Toxics (OPPT), the Office of Pesticide Programs (OPP), and the Organization for Economic Cooperation and Development (OECD).

a.   Scope

1. Applicability. This guideline is intended to meet testing requirements of both the Federal Insecticide, Fungicide, and Rodenticide Act (FIFRA) (7 USC 136, et seq.) and the U.S. Environmental Protection Agency under the Toxic Substances Control Act (15 USC 2601).

2. Background. The source materials used in developing this harmonized OPPTS test guideline are OPPTS 798.4500 Primary Eye Irritation; OPP 81-4 Acute Eye Irritation — Rabbit (Pesticide Assessment Guidelines, Subdivision F — Hazard Evaluation; Human and Domestic Animals); EPA report 540/09-82-025, 1982; and OECD 405 Acute Eye Irritation/Corrosion.

b.   Purpose

1. In the assessment and evaluation of the toxic characteristics of a substance, determination of the irritant and/or corrosion effects on eyes of mammals is an important initial step. Information derived from this test serves to indicate the existence of possible hazards likely to arise from exposure of the eyes and associated mucous membranes to the test substance.

2. Data on primary eye irritation are required by 40 CFR 158.340 to support the registration of each manufacturing-use product and end-use product. (See §158.50 to determine whether these data must be submitted and which purity/grade of the test substance should be tested.)

c.   Definitions

The definitions in section 3 of TSCA and in 40 CFR Part 792 — Good Laboratory Practice Standards (GLP) apply to this test guideline. The following definitions also apply to this guideline.

Eye corrosion is the production of irreversible tissue damage in the eye following application of a test substance to the anterior surface of the eye.

Eye irritation is the production of reversible changes in the eye following the application of a test substance to the anterior surface of the eye.

d. Principle of the Test Method

The substance to be tested is applied in a single dose to one of the eyes in each of several experimental animals; the untreated eye is used to provide control information. The degree of irritation/corrosion is evaluated and scored at specified intervals and is fully described to provide a complete evaluation of the effects. The duration of the study should be sufficient to permit a full evaluation of the reversibility or irreversibility of the effects observed. The period of observation should be at least 72 h, but need not exceed 21 days. Animals showing severe and enduring signs of distress and pain may need to be killed in a humane fashion.

e. Initial considerations

1. Strongly acidic or alkaline substances, for example, with a demonstrated pH of 2 or less or 11.5 or greater, need not be tested owing to their predictable corrosive properties. Buffer capacity should be taken into account.
2. Materials that have demonstrated definite corrosion or severe irritation in a dermal study need not be further tested for eye irritation. It may be presumed that such substances will produce similarly severe effects in the eyes.
3. Results from well-validated and accepted *in vitro* test systems may serve to identify corrosives or irritants such that the test material need not be tested *in vivo*.

f. Test procedures

1. *Animal selection*
   a. *Species and strain.* A variety of experimental animals have been used, but it is recommended that testing should be performed using healthy adult albino rabbits. Commonly used laboratory strains should be used. If another mammalian species is used, the tester should provide justification/reasoning for its selection.
   b. *Number of animals.* A single animal should be considered if marked effects are anticipated. If the results of this test in one animal suggest the test substance to be a severe irritant (reversible effect) or corrosive (irreversible effect) to the eye using the procedure described, further tests may not need to be performed. In cases other than a single animal test, at least three animals should be used. Occasionally, further testing in additional animals may be appropriate to clarify equivocal responses.
2. *Dose level.* For testing liquids, a dose of 0.1 ml is recommended. In testing solids, pastes, and particulate substances, the amount used should have a volume of 0.1 ml, or a weight of not more than 100 mg (the weight must always be recorded). If the test material is solid or granular, it should be ground to a fine dust. The volume of particulates should be measured after gently compacting them (e.g., by tapping the measuring container). To test a substance contained in a pressurized aerosol container, the eye should be held open and the test substance administered in a single burst of about 1 s duration from a distance of 10 cm directly in front of the eye. The dose may be estimated by weighing the container before and after use. Care should be taken not to damage the eye. Pump sprays should not be used, but instead the liquid should be expelled and 0.1 ml collected and instilled into the eye as described for liquids. For volatile substances, the dose may be estimated by weighing the container before and after use.
3. *Examination of eyes prior to test.* Both eyes of each experimental animal provisionally selected for testing should be examined within 24 h before testing starts by the same

procedure to be used during the test examination. Animals showing eye irritation, ocular defects, or preexisting corneal injury should not be used.

4. *Application of test substance*

   a. The test substance should be placed in the conjunctival sac of the eye of each animal after gently pulling the lower lid away from the eyeball. The lids are then gently held together for about 1 s to limit loss of the material. The other eye, which remains untreated, serves as a control. If it is thought that the substance may cause extreme pain, local anesthetic may be used prior to instillation of the test substance. The type and concentration of the local anesthetic should be carefully selected to ensure that no significant differences in reaction to the test substance will result from its use. The control eye should be similarly anesthetized.

   b. The eyes of the test animals should not be washed out for 24 h following instillation of the test substance. At 24 h, a washout may be used if considered appropriate. This is to show whether washing with water palliates or exacerbates irritation.

   c. For some substances shown to be irritating by this test, additional testing using animals with eyes washed soon after instillation of the substance may be indicated. Half a minute after instillation, the eyes of the animals are washed with water for 30 s, using a volume and velocity of flow that will not cause injury.

5. *Observation period.* The duration of the observation period is at least 72 h, and should not be fixed rigidly, but should be sufficient to evaluate fully the reversibility or irreversibility of the effects observed. The observation period normally need not exceed 21 days after instillation.

6. *Clinical examination and scoring*

   a. The eyes should be examined at 1, 24, 48, and 72 h. If there is no evidence of irritation at 72 h, the study may be ended. Extended observation (e.g., at 7 and 21 days) may be necessary if there is persistent corneal involvement or other ocular irritation to determine the progress of the lesions and their reversibility or irreversibility. In addition to the observations of the cornea, iris, and conjunctivae, any other lesions that are noted should be recorded and reported. The grades for ocular reactions (using the grading system in Section 4.B) should be recorded at each examination.

   b. Examination of reactions can be facilitated by use of a binocular loupe, hand slit-lamp, biomicroscope, or other suitable device. After recording the observations at 24 h, the eyes of any or all rabbits may be further examined with the aid of fluorescein.

   c. The grading of ocular responses is subject to various interpretations. To promote harmonization and to assist testing laboratories and those involved in making and interpreting the observations, an illustrated guide in grading eye irritation should be used.

g. *Data and reporting*

1. *Data summary.* Data should be summarized in tabular form, showing for each individual animal the irritation scores at observation time up until reversal (nonpositive grades) or 21 days, when the test is concluded; a description of the degree and nature of irritation, the presence of serious lesions, and any effects other than ocular that were observed should be provided.

2. *Evaluation of the results.* The ocular irritation scores should be evaluated in conjunction with the nature and reversibility or otherwise of the responses observed. The individual scores do not represent an absolute standard for the irritant properties of a material. They should be viewed as reference values and are only meaningful when supported by a full description and evaluation of the observations.

3. *Test report.* In addition to the reporting requirements as specified under 40 CFR part 792, subpart J, the following specific information should be reported:
   a. Species, strain, sex, age, and source of test animal;
   b. Rationale for selection of species (if species is other than the species preferred);
   c. Tabulation of irritant/corrosive response data for each individual animal at each observation time point (e.g., 1, 24, 48, and 72 h until reversibility of lesions or termination of the test);
   d. Description of any lesions observed;
   e. Narrative description of the degree and nature of irritation or corrosion observed;
   f. Description of the method used to score the irritation at 1, 24, 48, and 72 h (e.g., hand slip-lamp, biomicroscope, fluorescein stain);
   g. Description of any nonocular effects noted;
   h. Description of any pretest conditioning, including diet, quarantine, and treatment of disease;
   i. Description of caging conditions including number (and any change in number) of animals per cage, bedding material, ambient temperature and humidity, photoperiod, and identification of diet of test animals;
   j. Manufacture, source, purity, and lot number of test substance;
   k. Physical nature and, where appropriate, concentration and pH value for the test substance;
   l. Identification, composition, and characteristics of any vehicles (e.g., diluents, suspending agents, emulsifiers, and anesthetics) or other materials used in administering the test substance;
   m. A list of references cited in the body of the report, i.e., references to any published literature used in developing the test protocol, performing the testing, making and interpreting observations, and compiling and evaluating the results.

h. References

The following references should be consulted for additional background information on this guideline:

1. Buehler, E.V. and Newmann, E.A., A comparison of eye irritation in monkeys and rabbits, *Toxicol. Appl. Pharmacol.,* 6, 701–710, 1964.
2. Draize, J.H., *Dermal Toxicity. Appraisal of the Safety of Chemicals in Foods, Drugs and Cosmetics*, The Association of Food and Drug Officials of the U.S., 1959, 3rd printing, 1975, pp. 49–52.
3. Draize, J.H. et al., Methods for the study of irritation and toxicity of substances applied topically to the skin and mucous membranes, *J. Pharmacol. Experimental Therapeautics,* 83, 377–390, 1944.
4. Kay, J.H. and Calandra, J.C., Interpretation of eye irritation tests, *J. Soc. Cosmetic Chem.,* 13, 281–289, 1962.
5. Loomis, T.A., *Essentials of Toxicology*, 3rd ed., Lea & Febiger, Philadelphia, 1978, pp. 226–232.
6. National Academy of Sciences, *Principles and Procedures for Evaluating the Toxicity of Household Substances*, A report prepared by the Committee for the revision of NAS Publication 1138, under the auspices of the Committee on Toxicology, National Research Council, National Academy of Sciences, Washington, 1977.
7. World Health Organization, *Part I. Environmental Health Criteria 6. Principles and Methods for Evaluating the Toxicity of Chemicals.* World Health Organization, Geneva, 1978.

SECTION 4. OCULAR SCORING CRITERIA

A. SCALE OF WEIGHTED SCORES FOR GRADING THE SEVERITY OF OCULAR LESIONS DEVELOPED BY DRAIZE ET AL.

In 1944, Draize et al.[24] described an eye irritancy grading system for evaluating drugs and other materials intended for use in or around the eye. Numerical scores were assigned for reactions of cornea, iris, and conjunctivae. The total ocular irritation score was calculated by a formula that gave the greatest weight to corneal changes (total maximum = 80). A total maximum score = 10 for the iris, and 20 for the conjunctiva.

1. Cornea
   A. Opacity-Degree of Density (area which is most dense is taken for reading)
      Scattered or diffuse area — details of iris clearly visible..1
      Easily discernible translucent areas, details of iris clearly visible 2
      Opalescent areas, no details of iris visible, size of pupil barely discernible..............3
      Opaque, iris invisible 4
   B. Area of Cornea Involved
      One quarter (or less) but not zero..1
      Greater than one quarter — less than one half 2
      Greater than one half — less than three quarters 3
      Greater than three quarters — up to whole area...4
      Score equals A × B × 5   Total maximum = 80
2. Iris
   A. Values
      Folds above normal, congestion, swelling, circumcorneal injection (any one or all of these or combination of any thereof), iris still reacting to light (sluggish reaction is positive) 1
      No reaction to light, hemorrhage; gross destruction (any one or all of these) 2
      Score equals A × 5   Total possible maximum = 10
3. Conjunctivae
   A. Redness (refers to palpebral conjunctivae only)
      Vessels definitely injected above normal...1
      More diffuse, deeper crimson red, individual vessels not easily discernible 2
      Diffuse beefy red..3
   B. Chemosis
      Any swelling above normal (includes nictitating membrane) 1
      Obvious swelling with partial eversion of the lids..2
      Swelling with lids about half closed 3
      Swelling with lids about half closed to completely closed.......................................4
   C. Discharge
      Any amount different from normal (does not include small amounts observed in inner canthus of normal animals)...1
      Discharge with moistening of the lids and hairs just adjacent to the lids.................2
      Discharge with moistening of the lids and considerable area around the eye 3
      Score (A + B + C) × 2   Total maximum = 20

Note: The maximum total score is the sum of all scores obtained for the cornea, iris, and conjunctivae.

B. Grades for Ocular Lesions

The following standardized grading system is used in testing guidelines of several U.S. federal agencies (Consumer Product Safety Commission, Occupational Safety and Health Administration, Food and Drug Administration, Environmental Protection Agency, and Food Safety and Quality Service of the Department of Agriculture) and the Organization for Economic Cooperation and Development (OECD) member countries.

Cornea

Opacity: degree of density (area most dense taken for reading)
No ulceration or opacity 0
Scattered or diffuse areas of opacity (other than slight dulling of normal luster,
  details of iris clearly visible) ....1[a]
Easily discernible translucent areas, details of iris slightly obscured 2
Nacreous areas, no details of iris visible, size of pupil barely discernible..................3
Opaque cornea, iris not discernible through the opacity 4

Iris

Normal..0
Markedly deepened rugae, congestion, swelling, moderate circumcorneal hyperemia, or
  injection, any of these or any combination thereof, iris still reacting to light (sluggish
  reaction is positive) ....1[a]
No reaction to light, hemorrhage, gross destruction (any or all of these) 2

Conjunctivae

Redness (refers to palpebral and bulbar conjunctivae excluding cornea and iris)
Blood vessels normal 0
Some blood vessels definitely hyperemic (injected)...1
Diffuse, crimson color, individual vessels not easily discernible................................2[a]
Diffuse beefy red...3

Chemosis: lids and/or nictitating membranes
No swelling 0
Any swelling above normal (includes nictitating membranes)......................................1
Obvious swelling with partial eversion of lids..2[a]
Swelling with lids about half closed 3
Swelling with lids more than half closed...4

[a] Readings at these numerical values or greater indicate positive responses.

C. Representative Illustrations of Draize Eye Irritation Scores

Color Figures 4.1 through 4.6* are intended to illustrate the subjective grades for corneal, conjunctival, and iridial manifestations of ocular irritation. Each plate is reproduced directly from the *Consumer Product Safety Commission's Illustrated Guide for Grading Eye Irritation Caused by Hazardous Substances* (*CPSC, 1972*). Color figures are grouped together in a separate section.

* Color Figures follow page 232.

D. Scoring Criteria for Ocular Effects Observed in Slit Lamp Microscopy

Location of Observations	Grades
Corneal Observations	
Intensity	
Only epithelial edema (with only slight stromal edema or without stromal edema)	1
Corneal thickness 1.5 × normal	2
Corneal thickness 2 × normal	3
Cornea entirely opaque so that corneal thickness cannot be determined	4
Area involved	
≤ 25% of total corneal surface	1
> 25% but ≤ 50%	2
> 50% but ≤ 75%	3
> 75%	4
Fluorescein staining	
≤ 25% of total corneal surface	1
> 25% but ≤ 50%	2
> 50% but ≤ 75%	3
> 75%	4
Neovascularization and pigment migration	
≤ 25% of total corneal surface	1
> 25% but ≤ 50%	2
> 50% but ≤ 75%	3
> 75%	4
Perforation	4
Maximal corneal score	20
Iridal Observations	
Iritis is quantitated by the cells and flare in the anterior chamber, iris, hyperemia, and capillary light reflex	
Cells in aqueous chamber	
A few	1
A moderate number	2
Many	3
Aqueous flare (Tyndall effect)	
Slight	1
Moderate	2
Marked	3
Iris hyperemia	
Slight	1
Moderate	2
Marked	3
Pupillary reflex	
Sluggish	1
Absent	2
Maximal iridal score	11
Conjunctival Observations	
Hyperemia	
Slight	1
Moderate	2
Marked	3
Chemosis	
Slight	1

Location of Observations	Grades
Moderate	2
Marked	3
Fluorescein staining	
Slight	1
Moderate	2
Marked	3
Ulceration	
Slight	1
Moderate	2
Marked	3
Scarring	
Slight	1
Moderate	2
Marked	3
Maximal conjunctival score	15

From Chan, P-K. and Hayes, A.W., in *Toxicology of the Eye, Ear, and Other Special Senses,* Hayes, A.W., Ed., Raven Press, New York, 1985. With permission.

E. Ocular Scoring System for Rabbits Based on Slit Lamp Examination

From *Dermatotoxicology,* 4th ed., pp. 780–785, Marzulli, F.N. and Maibach, H.I., Eds., Hemisphere, New York, 1991. Reproduced with permission. All rights reserved.[26]

1. Conjunctiva

Conjunctival changes can be divided clinically into congestion, swelling (chemosis), and discharge. Generally, the sequence of events for these changes is congestion, discharge, and swelling.

a. Conjunctival Congestion

0 = Normal. May seem blanched to reddish pink without perilimbal injection (except at 12 and 6 o'clock positions) with vessels of the palpebral and bulbar conjunctivae easily observed.

+1 = A flushed, reddish color predominantly confined to the palpebral conjunctiva with some perilimbal injection but primarily confined to the lower and upper parts of the eye from the 4, 7, 11, and 1 o'clock positions.

+2 = Bright red color of the palpebral conjunctiva with accompanying perilimbal injection covering at least 75% of the circumference of the perilimbal region.

+3 = Dark, beefy red color with congestion of both the bulbar and the palpebral conjunctivae along with pronounced perilimbal injection and the presence of petechia on the conjunctiva. The petechiae generally predominate along the nictitating membrane and the upper palpebral conjunctiva.

b. Conjunctival Swelling

There are five divisions from 0 to +4.

0 = Normal or no swelling of the conjunctival tissue.

+1 = Swelling above normal without eversion of the lids (can be ascertained easily by noting that the upper and lower eyelids are positioned as in the normal eye); swelling generally starts in the lower cul-de-sac near the inner canthus, which requires slit lamp examination.

+2 = Swelling with misalignment of the normal approximation of the lower and upper eyelids; primarily confined to the upper eyelid so that in the initial stages the misapproximation of the eyelids begins by partial eversion of the upper eyelid. In this stage, swelling is confined generally to the upper eyelid, although it exists in the lower cul-de-sac (observed best with the slit lamp).

+3 = Swelling definite with partial eversion of the upper and lower eyelids essentially equivalent. This can be easily ascertained by looking at the animal head-on and noticing the positioning of the eyelids; if the eye margins do not meet, eversion has occurred.

+4 = Eversion of the upper eyelid is pronounced with less pronounced eversion of the lower eyelid. It is difficult to retract the lids and observe the perilimbal region.

c. Conjunctival Discharge

Discharge is defined as a whitish-gray precipitate, which should not be confused with the small amount of clear, inspissated, mucoid material that can be formed in the medial canthus of a substantial number of rabbit eyes. This material can be removed with a cotton swab before the animals are used.

0 = Normal. No discharge.

+1 = Discharge above normal and present on the inner portion of the eye but not on the lids or hairs of the eyelids. The small amount that is in the inner and outer canthus can be ignored if it has not been removed before starting the study.

+2 = Discharge is abundant, easily observed, and has collected on the lids and around the hairs of the eyelids.

+3 = Discharge has been flowing over the eyelids, wetting the hairs substantially on the skin around the eye.

d. Aqueous Flare

The intensity of the Tyndall phenomenon is scored by comparing the normal Tyndall effect observed when the slit lamp beam passes through the lens with that seen in the anterior chamber. The presence of aqueous flare is presumptive evidence of breakdown of the blood-aqueous barrier

0 = Absence of visible light beam in the anterior chamber (no Tyndall effect).

+1 = The Tyndall effect is barely discernible. The intensity of the light beam in the anterior chamber is less than the intensity of the slit beam as it passes through the lens.

+2 = The Tyndall beam in the anterior chamber is easily discernible and is equal in intensity to the slit beam as it passes through the lens.

+3 = The Tyndall beam in the anterior chamber is easily discernible; its intensity is greater than the intensity of the slit beam as it passes through the lens.

2. Light Reflex

The pupillary diameter of the iris is controlled by the radial and sphincter muscles. Contraction of the radial muscle due to adrenergic stimulation results in mydriasis, whereas contraction of the sphincter muscle due to cholinergic stimulation results in miosis. Because an ophthalmic drug can exert potential effects on these neural pathways, it is important to assess the light reflex of an animal as part of the ophthalmic examination. Using full illumination with the slit lamp, the following scale is used:

0 = Normal pupillary response.

1 = Sluggish pupillary response.

2 = Maximally impaired (i.e., fixed) pupillary response.

3. Iris Involvement

In the following definitions the primary, secondary, and tertiary vessels are used as an aid to determine a subjective ocular score for iris involvement. The assumption is made that the greater the hyperemia of the vessels and the more the secondary and tertiary vessels are involved, the greater the intensity of iris involvement. The scores range from 0 to +4.

0 = Normal iris without any hyperemia of the iris vessels. Occasionally around the 12 to 1 o'clock position near the pupillary border and the 6 and 7 o'clock position near the pupillary border there is a small area around 1 to 3 mm in diameter in which both the secondary and tertiary vessels are slightly hyperemic.

+1 = Minimal injection of secondary vessels but not tertiary. Generally, it is uniform, but may be of greater intensity at the 1 or 6 o'clock position. If it is confined to the 1 or 6 o'clock position, the tertiary vessels must be substantially hyperemic.

+2 = Minimal injection of tertiary vessels and minimal to moderate injection of the secondary vessels.

+3 = Moderate injection of the secondary and tertiary vessels with slight swelling of the iris stroma. This gives the iris surface a slightly rugose appearance, which is usually most prominent near the 3 and 9 o'clock positions.

+4 = Marked injection of the secondary and tertiary vessels with marked swelling of the iris stroma. The iris seems rugose; may be accompanied by hemorrhage (hyphema) in the anterior chamber.

4. Cornea

The scoring scheme measures the severity of corneal cloudiness and the area of the cornea involved. Severity of corneal cloudiness is graded as follows:

0 = Normal cornea. Appears with the slit lamp adjusted to a narrow slit image as having a bright gray line on the epithelial surface and a bright gray line on the endothelial surface with a marble-like gray appearance of the stroma.

+1 = Some loss of transparency. Only the anterior half of the stroma is involved as observed with an optical section of the slit lamp. The underlying structures are clearly visible with diffuse illumination, although some cloudiness can be readily apparent with diffuse illumination.

+2 = Moderate loss of transparency. In addition to involving the anterior stroma, the cloudiness extends all the way to the endothelium. The stroma has lost its marble-like appearance and is homogeneously white. With diffuse illumination, underlying structures are clearly visible.

+3 = Involvement of the entire thickness of the stroma. With optical section, the endothelial surface is still visible. However, with diffuse illumination the underlying structures are just barely visible (to the extent that the observer is still able to grade flare and iritis, observe for pupillary response, and note lenticular changes).

+4 = Involvement of the entire thickness of the stroma. With the optical section, cannot clearly visualize the endothelium. With diffuse illumination, the underlying structures cannot be seen. Cloudiness removes the capability for judging and grading flare, iritis, lenticular changes, and pupillary response.

The surface area of the cornea relative to the area of cloudiness is divided into five grades from 0 to +4.

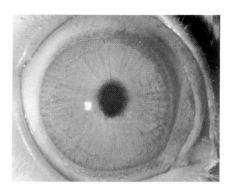

Normal Eye

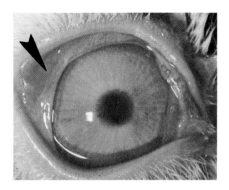

1 Redness

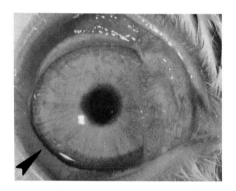

2 Redness

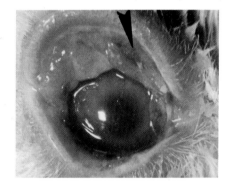

3 Redness

Chapter 4, Color Figure 1 The four photographs demonstrate the grades for conjunctival redness. Conjunctival redness is typically not homogeneous; therefore, only the most severely affected area of the conjunctiva should be graded, as shown by the arrows in the photographs.

Chapter 4, Color Figures 1-6 Reproduced from *Illustrated Guide for Grading Eye Irritation Caused by Hazardous Substances*, Consumer Product Safety Commission, Washington, D.C., 1972.

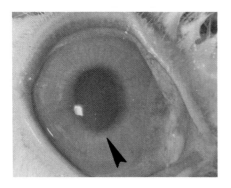

1 Opacity

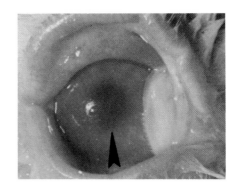

2 Opacity

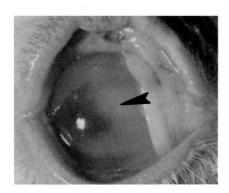

3 Opacity

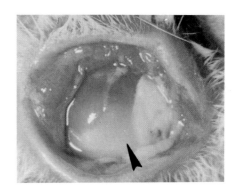

4 Opacity

Chapter 4, Color Figure 2 These four photographs demonstrate the four grades for corneal opacity. Because a corneal lesion is not distributed homogeneously, the most severely affected part of the cornea (see arrows) is graded.

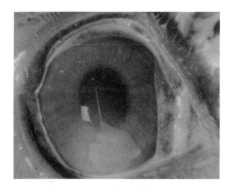

1 Opacity

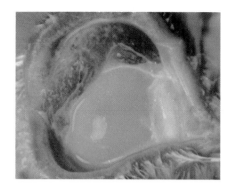

2 Opacity

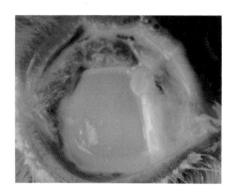

3 Opacity

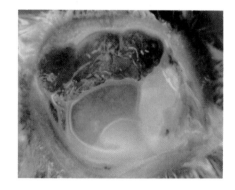

4 Opacity

Chapter 4, Color Figure 3 The eyes are stained with fluorescein and photographed under UV light. Fluorescein-stained areas demarcate corneal epithelial erosion, not opacity. Therefore, the areas stained with fluorescein do not necessarily correspond to the grades for opacity.

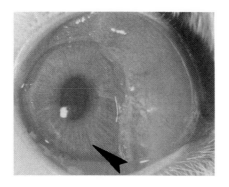

1 Iritis

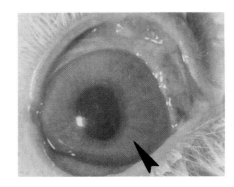

1 Iritis

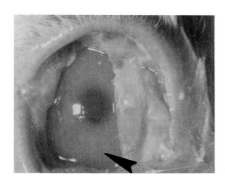

2 Iritis

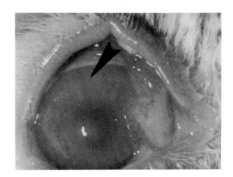

2 Iritis

Chapter 4, Color Figure 4 The two grades for iritis are demonstrated in these photographs. Grade 1 is a deepening of iridial rugae, or injection (hyperemia) of iridial vessels. The upper left photograph clearly shows injection of the secondary vessels of the iris, but this finding is more difficult to perceive in the upper right photograph due to loss of corneal clarity. Grade 2 iritis involves no reaction to light, hemorrhage, and/or destruction of the iris. Since this is almost invariably accompanied by significant corneal opacity, it may be difficult to observe. The two lower photographs demonstrate hemorrhage of the iris.

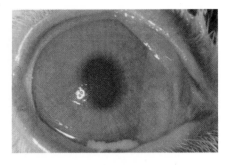

1 Chemosis

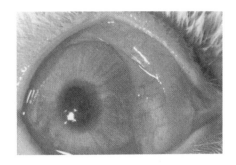

2 Chemosis

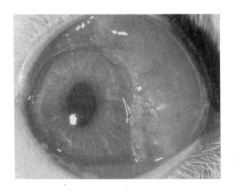

3 Chemosis

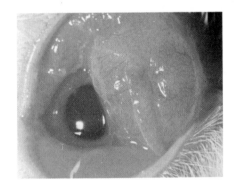

4 Chemosis

Chapter 4, Color Figure 5 These photographs are intended to indicate the degree of difference between each conjunctival chemosis grade. They may not accurately represent chemosis because the eyes have been held open to show other aspects of irritation.

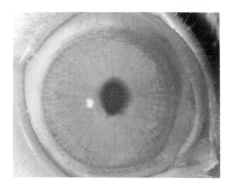

Normal Eye

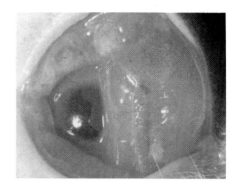

1 Hour

2-3 Redness	> 2 Opacity
1 Iritis	4 Chemosis

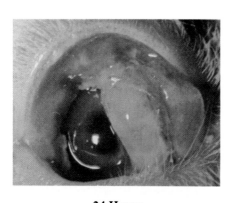

24 Hours

3 Redness	1 Opacity
2 Iritis	> 3 Chemosis

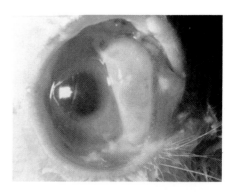

48 Hours

3 Redness	> 1 Opacity
2 Iritis	3 Chemosis

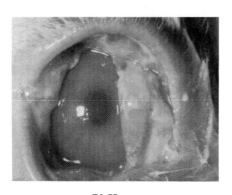

72 Hours

3 Redness	> 1 Opacity
2 Iritis	> 2 Chemosis

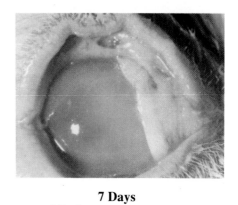

7 Days

3 Redness	4 Opacity
2 Iritis	2 Chemosis

Chapter 4, Color Figure 6 A time sequence of the same eye is shown from before administration of an irritant to seven days after exposure.

0 = Normal cornea with no area of cloudiness.
+1 = 1 to 25% area of stromal cloudiness.
+2 = 25 to 50% area of stromal cloudiness.
+3 = 51 to 75% area of stromal cloudiness.
+4 = 76 to 100% area of stromal cloudiness.

Pannus is vascularization or the penetration of new blood vessels into the corneal stroma. The vessels are derived from the limbal vascular loops. Pannus is divided into three grades.

0 = No pannus.
+1 = Vascularization is present but vessels have not invaded the entire corneal circumference. Where localized vessel invasion has occurred, vessels have not penetrated beyond 2 mm.
+2 = Vessels have invaded 2 mm or more around the entire corneal circumference.

The use of fluorescein is a valuable aid in defining epithelial damage. For fluorescein staining, the area can be judged on a 0 to +4 scale.

0 = Absence of fluorescein staining.
+1 = Slight fluorescein staining confined to a small focus. With diffuse illumination the underlying structures are easily visible. (The outline of the pupillary margin is as if there were no fluorescein staining).
+2 = Moderate fluorescein staining confined to a small focus. With diffuse illumination the underlying structures are clearly visible, although there is some loss of detail.
+3 = Marked fluorescein staining. Staining may involve a larger portion of the cornea. With diffuse illumination, underlying structures are barely visible but are not completely obliterated.
+4 = Extreme fluorescein staining. With diffuse illumination, the underlying structures cannot be observed.

Interpretation is facilitated by rinsing the eye with an isotonic irrigating solution to remove excess and nonabsorbed fluorescein.

Slit lamps are equipped with cobalt blue filters, which can be placed in front of the light from the slit illuminator to excite fluorescence of the fluorescein. Photographs using fluorescein staining require the use of this filter, and fluorescence will be enhanced by a yellow filter placed in front of the objectives of the corneal microscope.

5. Lens

The crystalline lens is readily observed with the aid of the slit lamp biomicroscope, and the location of lenticular opacity can be discerned readily by direct and retroillumination. The location of lenticular opacities can be divided arbitrarily into the following lenticular regions beginning with the anterior capsule: anterior capsular, anterior subcapsular, anterior cortical, posterior cortical, posterior subcapsular, posterior capsular. The lens should be evaluated routinely during ocular evaluations and graded as either N (normal) or A (abnormal). The presence of lenticular opacities should be described and the location noted as defined above.

SECTION 5. CLASSIFICATION SCHEMES

A. CLASSIFICATION OF COMPOUNDS BASED ON EYE IRRITATION PROPERTIES

This classification scheme developed by Kay and Calandra[27] utilizes the Draize scoring system to rate the irritating potential of substances.

1. STEP 1

Using the Draize eye irritation scoring system, find the maximum mean total score for all three tissues (cornea, iris, and conjunctivae) occurring within the first 96 h after instillation for which the incidence of this score plus or minus 5 points is at least 40%.

2. Step 2

Choose an initial or "tentative rating" on the basis of the score found in Step 1 as follows:

Score from Step 1	Tentative Eye Irritation Rating	Symbol
0.0–0.5 points	Nonirritating	N
0.5–2.5 points	Practically nonirritating	PN
2.5–15 points	Minimally irritating	M_1
15–25 points	Mildly irritating	M_2
25–50 points	Moderately irritating	M_3
50–80 points	Severely irritating	S
80–100 points	Extremely irritating	E
100–110 points	Maximally irritating	M_x
For borderline scores, choose the higher rating		

3. Step 3

Tentative Rating	Requirement for Maintenance
N	$MTS_{24} = 0$; for $MTS_{24} > 0$, raise one level
PN	As for N
M_1	$MTS_{48} = 0$; for $MTS_{48} > 0$, raise one level
M_2	$MTS_{96} = 0$; for $MTS_{96} > 0$, raise one level
M_3	1. $MTS \leq 20$; for $MTS_f > 20$, raise one level
	2. $ITS_f = 10$ (60%); if not true then no rabbit may show ITS_f 30; otherwise raise one level
S	1. As for M_3 except use $MTS_f \leq 40$
	2. As for M_3 except use $ITS_f \leq 30$ (60%) and 60 for high
E	1. As for M_3 except use $MTS_f \leq 80$
	2. As for M_3 except use $ITS_f \leq 60$ (60%) and 100 for high
M_x	1. $MTS_f > 80$ (60%); for $MTS_f \leq 80$, lower one level
	2. $ITS_f > 60$ (60%); otherwise lower one level

Symbols: MTS = mean total score; ITS = individual rabbit total score. Subscripts denote scoring interval: 24, 48, or 96 hr; f = final score (7 days).

Two requirements must be met before a tentative rating may become final. First, the mean total score for the 7-day scoring interval may not exceed 20 points if the rating is to be maintained. Second, individual total scores for at least 60% of the rabbits should be 10 points or less and in no case may any individual rabbit's total score exceed 30. If either or both of these requirements are not met, then the "tentative rating" must be raised one level and the higher level becomes the "final rating."

B. NATIONAL ACADEMY OF SCIENCES (NAS) METHOD BASED ON SEVERITY AND PERSISTENCE[28]

This descriptive scale, adapted from work conducted by Green et al.,[29] attaches significance to the persistence and reversibility of responses. It is based on the most severe response observed in a group of animals rather than the average response.

1. Inconsequential or Complete Lack of Irritation

Exposure of the eye to a material under the specified conditions causes no significant ocular changes. No staining with fluorescein can be observed. Any changes that occur clear within 24 h and are no greater than those caused by isotonic saline under the same conditions.

2. Moderate Irritation

Exposure of the eye to the material under the specified conditions causes minor, superficial, and transient changes of the cornea, iris, or conjunctiva as determined by external or slit lamp examination with fluorescein staining. The appearance at the 24-hour or subsequent grading interval of any of the following changes is sufficient to characterize a response as moderate irritation: opacity of the cornea (other than a slight dulling of the normal luster), hyperemia of the iris, or swelling of the conjunctiva. Any changes that are seen clear up within 7 days.

3. Substantial Irritation

Exposure of the eye to the material under the specified conditions causes significant injury to the eye, such as loss of the corneal epithelium, corneal opacity, iritis (other than a slight injection), conjunctivitis, pannus, or bullae. The effects clear up within 21 days.

4. Severe Irritation or Corrosion

Exposure of the eye to the material under the specified conditions results in the same types of injury as in the previous category and in significant necrosis or other injuries that adversely affect the visual process. Injuries persist for 21 days or more.

C. Modified NAS Method Developed by Alliedsignal, Inc.[30]

This classification scheme helps distinguish mildly irritating substances from moderately irritating substances, as well as identifying strongly and severely irritating substances. It is based on the most severe ocular response observed in a group of animals, rather than the average response, and on the persistence of the response.

1. Nonirritation

Exposure of the eye to the material under the specified conditions causes no ocular changes. No tissue staining with fluorescein is observed. Slight conjunctival injection (grade 1, some vessels definitely injected) that does not clear within 24 h is not considered a significant change. This level of change is inconsequential as far as representing physical damage to the eye and can be seen to occur naturally for unexplained reasons in otherwise normal rabbits.

2. Mild Irritation

Exposure of the eye to the material under the specified conditions causes minor and/or transient changes as determined by external or slit lamp examination or fluorescein staining. No opacity, ulceration, or fluorescein staining of the cornea (except for staining that is characteristic of normal epithelial desquamation) are observed at any grading interval. The appearance of any of the following changes is sufficient to characterize a response as mild irritation:

- Grade 1 hyperemia of the iris that is observed at 1 hour, but resolves by 24 h.
- Grade 2 conjunctival hyperemia (redness) that is observed at 1, 24, and/or 48 h, but resolves by 72 h.

- Grade 2 conjunctival chemosis (swelling) that is observed at 1 hour, but diminishes to grade 1 or 0 by 24 h; or Grade 1 conjunctival chemosis that is observed at 1 and/or 24 and/or 48 h, but resolves by 72 h.

3. Moderate Irritation

Exposure of the eye to the material under the specified conditions causes major ocular changes as determined by external or slit lamp examination or fluorescein staining. The appearance of any of the following changes is sufficient to characterize a response as moderate irritation:

- Opacity of the cornea (other than slight dulling of the normal luster) is observed at any observation period, but resolves by day 7.
- Ulceration of the cornea (absence of a confluent patch of corneal epithelium) is observed at any observation period, but resolves by day 7.
- Fluorescein staining of the cornea (greater than that which is characteristic of normal epithelial desquamation) is observed at 1, 2, 3, and/or 4 days, but no staining is found by day 7.
- Grade 1 or 2 hyperemia of the iris (circumcorneal injection, congestion) is observed and persists to 24 h or longer, but resolves by day 7.
- Grade 2 conjunctival hyperemia is observed and persists to at least 72 h, but resolves by day 7; or Grade 3 conjunctival hyperemia is observed at any observation period, but resolves by day 7.
- Grade 1 or greater conjunctival chemosis is observed and persists to 72 h or longer, but resolves by day 7.

4. Strong Irritation (Clearing within 21 Days)

Exposure of the eye to the material under the specified conditions results in the type of injury described in the former category, but the effects (possibly including pannus or bullae) heal or clear within 21 days.

5. Severe Irritation (Persisting for 21 Days) or Corrosion

Exposure of the eye to the material under the specified conditions results in the type of injury described in the two former categories, but causes significant tissue destruction (necrosis) or injuries that probably adversely affect the visual process. The effects of the injuries persist for at least 21 days.

D. CATEGORIZATION OF SUBSTANCES USING THE SLIT LAMP BIOMICROSCOPE AND FLUORESCEIN

Site	"Accept"	"Accept with Caution"	"Probably Injurious to Human Eyes"
Conjunctiva	Hyperemia without chemosis	Chemosis, less than 1 mm at the limbus	Chemosis, greater than 1 mm at the limbus
Cornea	Staining, corneal stippling[a] without confluence at 24 h	Confluence[b] of staining at 24 to 48 h	Staining with infiltration or edema
Anterior chamber	0	0	Flare[c] (visibility of slit beam; rubeosis of iris)

[a] Corneal stippling: multiple discrete punctate irregularities in the corneal epithelial layer which retain fluorescein.

[b] Confluence: uniform zones for fluorescein retention larger than 1 mm in diameter.

[c] Flare: Tyndall effect in a beam traversing the aqueous humor.

From Beckley, J.H. et al.[31] Source: Environmental Protection Agency, 1988. Guidance for Evaluation of Eye Irritation Testing, Hazard Evaluation Division, Standard Evaluation Procedures, EPA-540/09-88-105, Washington.[32]

E. CATEGORIZATION AND LABELING OF PESTICIDES[33]

Label Statements Regarding Eye Irritation Hazards Due to Pesticides.

Toxicity Category	Signal Word	Skull and Crossbones and "Poison" Required	Precautionary Statement	Practical Treatment
I. Corrosive (irreversible destruction of ocular tissue), corneal involvement, or irritation persisting for more than 21 days.	Danger	No	Corrosive.[a] Causes irreversible eye damage. Harmful if swallowed. Do not get in eyes or on clothing. Wear (goggles, face shield, or safety glasses)[b]. Wash thoroughly with soap and water after handling. Remove contaminated clothing and wash before reuse.	*If in eyes:* Flush with plenty of water. Get medical attention. *If swallowed:* drink promptly a large quantity of milk, egg whites, gelatin solution, or, if these are not available, drink large quantities of water. Avoid alcohol. *Note to physician:* Probable mucosal damage may contraindicate the use of gastric lavage.
II. Corneal involvement or irritation clearing in 21 days or less.	Warning	No	Causes substantial but temporary eye injury. Do not get into eyes or on clothing. Wear (goggles, face shield, or safety glasses).[b] Harmful if swallowed. Wash thoroughly with soap and water after handling. Remove contaminated clothing and wash before reuse.	Same as above; omit *note to physician* statement.
III. Corneal involvement or irritation clearing in 7 days or less.	Caution	No	Causes (moderate) eye injury (irritation). Avoid contact with eyes or clothing. Wash thoroughly with soap and water after handling.	*If in eyes:* Flush with plenty of water. Get medical attention if irritation persists.
IV. Minimal effects clearing in less than 24 h.	Caution	No	None required.	None required.

[a] The term "corrosive" may be omitted if the product is not actually corrosive.

[b] Choose appropriate form of eye protection. Recommendation for goggles or face shield is more appropriate for industrial, commercial, or nondomestic uses. Safety glasses may be recommended for domestic or residential use.

F. CONSUMER PRODUCT SAFETY COMMISSION, FEDERAL HAZARDOUS SUBSTANCES ACT (FHSA) REGULATIONS FOR CLASSIFYING AN EYE IRRITANT (16 CFR 1500.42)

Ocular reactions to a test substance are examined and scored in six test rabbits. An animal is considered as exhibiting a *positive reaction* if the test substance produces any of the following ocular tissue responses 24, 48, or 72 h after instillation:

Ocular Tissue	Positive Response
Cornea	Ulceration of the cornea (other than a fine stippling) or opacity (other than slight dulling of normal luster)
Iris	Inflammation (other than a slight deepening of the folds or rugae, or a slight circumcorneal injection of the blood vessels)
Conjunctivae	An obvious swelling with partial eversion of the lids or diffuse crimson-red with individual vessels not easily discernible

Classification of a test substance is based on the number of animals exhibiting a positive reaction.

Test Group Result (n = 6)	FHSA Classification
4–6 animals exhibit a positive reaction	Eye Irritant
2–3 animals exhibit a positive reaction	Inconclusive[a]
0–1 animals exhibit a positive reaction	Nonirritant

[a] If two to three animals exhibit a positive reaction, the test is repeated using six new animals. If three or more animals in the second test exhibit a positive reaction, the test substance is classified as an "eye irritant." If one to two animals in the second test exhibit a positive reaction, a third test is conducted using new animals. If one or more animals in the third test exhibit a positive reaction, the test substance is classified as an "eye irritant."

SECTION 6. SPECIALIZED TECHNIQUES USED TO EXAMINE THE EYE FOR TOXIC EFFECTS

Technique	Description	Refs.
Slit lamp biomicroscopy	Used as a visual aid to evaluate the external features of the eye and the anterior portion of the globe (conjunctiva, cornea, iris, lens, anterior portion of the vitreous)	25, 26, 34, 35
Direct ophthalmoscopy	Used as a monocular visual aid to evaluate the ocular media and fundus	36
Pachymetry	Used to measure the degree of corneal swelling	37–41
Electroretinography	Used to determine diffuse retinal damage and to evaluate the functional integrity of the retina when fundoscopic viewing is impaired due to lens opacification (the technique measures the normal change in electrical potential of the eye caused by a diffuse flash of light)	36
Specular microscopy	Used to evaluate the integrity of the corneal endothelium	42
Scheimpflug photography	Used to analyze and document changes in lens transparency (cataract development)	43
Tonometry	Used to measure intraocular pressure of the eye (both contact and noncontact techniques are available)	44–47

SECTION 7. PROPOSED TIER APPROACHES TO EYE IRRITATION TESTING

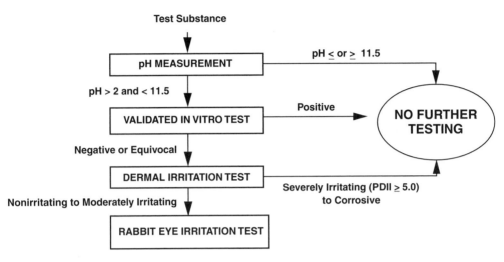

FIGURE 4.5 Schematic screening procedure to assess a test substance's irritation potential before conducting an eye irritation test.

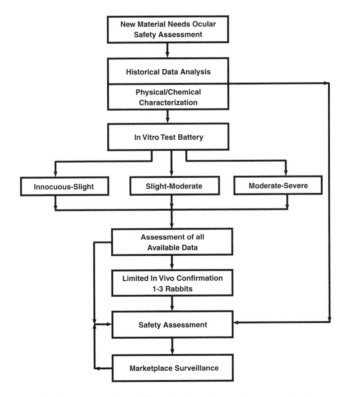

FIGURE 4.6 Diagrammatical representation of how *in vitro* alternatives may be incorporated into the ocular saftey assessment process. Initially, all previous testing data and physical chemical characterstics are evaluated. If necessary, the materials are then evaluated in a battery of *in vitro* assays. After the *in vitro* testing, all data are assessed again. Then either a saftey assessment would be made or an *in vivo* test would be performed in a limited number of animals before making the final saftey assessment. (From Hobson, D.W., *Dermal and Ocular Toxicology, Fundamentals and Methods,* CRC Press, Boca Raton, FL, 1991. With permission.)

SECTION 8. OCULAR ADVERSE EFFECTS
OF CHEMICAL SUBSTANCES

Tables 4.9 through 4.20 present lists of chemicals that are capable of producing certain ocular adverse effects. The tables were developed from information found in Grant's *Toxicology of the Eye,*[49] an excellent reference on chemicals, drugs, plants, toxins, and venoms, and their effects on the eyes or vision.

TABLE 4.9
Possible Adverse Corneal Effects

Chemical/Drug	Adverse Effects
Beryllium poisoning Calcium hydroxide burn Phenylmercuric nitrate Polyethylene sulfonic acid Vitamin D poisoning	Corneal calcification (band keratopathy)
Allyl alcohol Diethylamine Diethyl diglycolate Diisopropylamine Dimethylamine Dimethylaminopropylamine Dimethyl diglycolate Ethylenediamine N-Ethylmorpholine N-Ethylpiperidine N-Methylmorpholine Morpholine tert-Octylamine Tetramethylbutanediamine Tetramethylethylenediamine Triethylenediamine	Corneal epithelial edema (painless) with delayed onset of haloes from local action
Allyl alcohol p-Anisyl chloride Butyl amine Cardiac glycosides Colchicine Diazomethane Dichlorobutenes Diethylamine Digitalis glycosides Diisopropylamine Dimethylaminopropylamine Dimethylphosphorochloridothionate Dimethyl sulfate Diphenylcyanoarsine Diving mask defogger Dyes (cationic) Emetine Erythrophleine Ethylene oxide Ethylenimine Euphorbias Fish (decomposing) Formaldehyde	Corneal epithelial injury (painful) with delayed onset from local action

TABLE 4.9 *(Continued)*
Possible Adverse Corneal Effects

Chemical/Drug	Adverse Effects
Hydrogen sulfide	
Hypochlorite-ammonia mixtures	
Ipecac	
Manchineel	
Methyl bromide	
Methyl chloroacrylate	
Methyl dichloropropionate	
Methyl fluorolsulfate	
Methyl silicate	
Mustard gas	
Mustard oil	
Nitrosomethyl urethane	
Osmic acid	
Oxalyl chloride	
Podophyllum	
Poison ivy	
Squill	
Sulfur	
Surfactants	
Triacetoxyanthracene	
Trimethyl siloxane	
Vinblastine	
Amiodarone	Corneal epithelial deposits from systemic drugs (humans)
Amodiaquine	
Bismuth subnitrate	
Chloroquine	
Chlorpromazine	
Clofazimine	
Fluphenazine	
Gold	
Hydroxychloroquine	
Isotretinoin	
Mepacrine	
Monobenzone	
Perhexiline	
Tilorone	
Triparanol	
BA 6650	Corneal opacities from systemic drugs (animals)
Carbutamide	
Chlorpropamide	
1,2-Dibromoethane	
1,2-Dichloroethane	
Dichloronitroaniline	
Dimethylhydrazine	
Epinephrine	
Iminodipropionitrile	
Isoretinoin	
Phthalofyne	
Practolol	
Tobutamide	
Aniline	Corneal scarring, late (humans)
Hydroquinone	
Mustard gas	

TABLE 4.10
Possible Adverse Corneal and Conjunctival Effects

Chemical/Drug	Adverse Effects
Acetone	Burns (humans)
Alcohol	
Ammonia	
Benzalkonium chloride	
Benzene	
Brake fluid	
Brilliant green	
Calcium hydroxide	
Castor beans (ricin)	
a-Chloroacetophenone	
o-Chlorobenzylidene malononitrile	
Chlorobromomethane	
Chlorobutanol	
2-Chloroethanol	
Chloroform	
Chrysarobin (chrysophanic acid)	
Clove oil	
Croton oil	
Crystal violet	
2-Cyanoacrylic acid esters	
Cytarabine	
Dibenzoxazepine	
Dibutyl phthalate	
Dieffenbachia juice	
Digitoxin	
Digoxin	
Dimethyl phthalate	
Dimethyl sulfate	
Emetine hydrochloride	
Euphorbia latex	
Formaldehyde	
Gentian violet	
Hydrochloric acid	
Hydrogen peroxide	
Hydrogen sulfide	
Hydroquinone-benzoquinone	
Iodine vapor	
Isopropyl alcohol	
Lewisite	
Mustard gas	
Mustard oil	
Nitrogen mustards	
Osmium tetroxide	
Podophyllum	
Potassium permanganate	
Propylene imine	
Silver nitrate	
Spitting Cobra venom	
Soap	
Sodium hydroxide	
Styrene	

TABLE 4.10 *(Continued)*
Possible Adverse Corneal and Conjunctival Effects

Chemical/Drug	Adverse Effects
Sulfur dioxide	
Trichloroacetic acid	
Trichloroethylene	
Urea	
Vinblastine	
Zinc chloride	

TABLE 4.11
Possible Adverse Conjunctival Effects

Chemical/Drug	Adverse Effects
Allyl cyanide (rats)	Inflammation from systemic substances
Aminosalicylic acid	
Arsenic (inorganic)	
Arsphenamine	
Barbiturates	
Bromide	
Chloral hydrate	
Chlorambucil	
Chlorpropamide	
Cyclophosphamide	
Cytarabine	
Dixyrazine	
Ethylphenylhydratoin	
Gold	
Hexachlorobenzene	
Hypericum	
Isotretinoin	
Lantana (animals)	
Methotrexate	
Methyldopa	
Noramidopyrine	
Novobiocin	
Oxprenolol	
Penicillamine	
Phenazone	
Phenolphthalein	
Phenazopyridine (dogs)	
Phensuximide	
Phenylbutazone	
Phenytoin	
Phthalofyne	
Practolol	
Sulfadiazine	
Sulfamerazine	
Sulfarsphenamine	
Sulfathiozole	

TABLE 4.12
Possible Adverse Lens Effects

Chemical/Drug	Adverse Effects
Acetaminophen (A)	Opacity (cataract) from systemic administration or exposure
Alloxan (A)	
Allyl cyanide (A)	
Aminotriazole (A)	
Arabinose (A)	
5-Aziridino-2, 4-dinitrobenzamide (A)	
Bis-(phenylisopropyl)-piperidine & UVA (H)	
Bleomycin (A)	
Boron hydride disulfide (A)	
Bromodeoxuridine (reversible) (A)	
Busulfan (A)(H)	
Carbutamide (A)	
Chlorphentermine (A)	
Chlorophenylalanine (A)	
Chlorpropamide (A)	
Clomiphene (A)	
Cobalt chloride (A)	
Corticosteroids (H)	
Decahydronaphthalene (A)	
Diazacholesterol (A)	
Diazoxide (reversible) (A)	
Dichlorisone (H)	
Dichloroacetate (reversible) (A)	
Diethylaminoethoxyandrostenone (A)	
4-(*p*-Dimethylaminostyryl)quinoline (A)	
Dimethylnitroquinoline (A)	
Dimethyl terephthalate (A)	
Dinitrocresol (A,H)	
Dinitrophenol (A,H)	
Diquat (A)	
Disophenol (A)	
Dithizone (A)	
Epinephrine (A)	
Galactose (A,H)	
Hematoporphyrin (A)	
Hygromycin B (A)	
ICI 33828 (A)	
Iodoacetate (A)	
Methoxsalen and UVA (A)	
Methyl dichlorisone (H)	
Mimosine (A)	
Miotics (H)	
Mirex (A)	
Mitotane (H)	
Nafoxidine (A)	
Naphthalene (A)	
2-Naphthol (A)	
1,2-Naphthoquinone (A)	
Nitrogen mustard (A)	
Nitroquinolones (A)	

TABLE 4.12 *(Continued)*
Possible Adverse Lens Effects

Chemical/Drug	Adverse Effects
Opiates (A)	
Petroleum fraction (A)	
Phenelzine and serotonin (A)	
3-(2-Phenyl)-hydrazopropionitrile (A)	
2-(4-Phenyl-l-piperazinylmethyl)-cyclohexanone (A)	
(4′-Pyridyl)l-piperazine derivatives (A)	
Pyrithione (A)	
Selenium (A)	
SQ 11290 (A)	
Streptomycin (A)	
Streptozotocin (A)	
Sulfaethoxypyridazine (A)	
Tetrahydronaphthalene (A)	
Thallium (A)	
Tolbutamide (A)	
Tretamine (A)	
Triaziquone (A)	
Trinitrotoluene (H)	
Triparanol (A,H)	
Verapamil (A)	
Xylose (A)	
Amiodarone (H)	Lens deposits or discoloration
Chlorpromazine (A) (H)	
Copper (H)	
Fluphenazine (H)	
Iprindole (A)	
Iron (H)	
Mercury (H)	
Phenylmercuric salts (H)	
Silver (H)	

Note: A = animals; H = humans.

TABLE 4.13
Possible Adverse Eyelid Effects

Chemical/Drug	Adverse Effects
Amphetamine	Lid retraction
Cocaine	
Levodopa	
Methoxamine	
Phenylephrine	
Barbiturates	Ptosis of eyelids (topical or systemic substances)
Botulism	
Bretylium	
Chloral hydrate	
Chloralose	

TABLE 4.13 *(Continued)*
Possible Adverse Eyelid Effects

Chemical/Drug	Adverse Effects
Conhydrine	
Coniine	
Corticosteroids	
Curare	
Gelsemium sepervirens	
Guanethidine	
Levodopa	
Mephenesin	
Methylpentynol	
Pelletierine	
Penicillamine	
Phenoxybenzamine	
Primidone	
Reserpine	
Snake venoms	
Spider venoms	
Sulfonal	
Tetraethylammonium	
Thallium	
Trichloroethylene decomposition	
Trimethadione	
Vincristine	

TABLE 4.14
Possible Adverse Retinal Effects

Chemical/Drug	Adverse Effects
Acridine (A)	Retinal edema from systemic administration
Ammi majus seeds (H)	
Chloramphenicol (H)	
Cobalt (A)	
Cyanide (A)	
Dithizone (A)	
Ergotamine (H)	
Ethyl hydrocuprein (H)	
Fluoride (A)	
Glue sniffing (H)	
Glutamate (A)	
Helichrysum (A)	
Iminodipropionitrile (A)	
Iodate (A) (H)	
Iodoquinol (H)	
Methanol (H)	
Naphthalene (A)	
Optochin (H)	
Phosphorus (A)	
Quinine (H)	
Pyrithione (A)	

TABLE 4.14 *(Continued)*
Possible Adverse Retinal Effects

Chemical/Drug	Adverse Effects
Radiopaque media (H)	
Streptomycin (A)	
Triaziquone (A)	
Acetylphenylhydrazine (H)	Retinal hemorrhages from systemic administration
Alloxan (A)	
Arsphenamine (H)	
Aspirin (H)	
Benzene (H)	
Bicycloheptadiene dibromide (H)	
Carbenoxolone (H)	
Carbon disulfide (H)	
Carbon monoxide (H)	
Chloramphenicol (H)	
Dapsone (H)	
Desoxycortone acetate (A)	
Dextran (A)	
Dicumarol (H)	
Diodone (H)	
Diquat (A)	
Dithizone (A)	
Epinephrine (A)	
Ethambutol (H)	
Hexachlorophene (H)	
Iodoform (H)	
Isotretinoin (H)	
Lead (H)	
Licorice (H)	
Methaqualone (H)	
Methyl bromide (H)	
Miotane (H)	
Naphthalene (A)	
2-(2-Naphthyloxy) ethanol (A)	
Phenprocoumon (H)	
Phenylbutazone (H)	
Phosphorus (A)	
Potato leaf smoking (H)	
Pyrithione (A)	
Radiopaque media (H)	
Snake venoms (H)	
Sulfanilamide (H)	
Sulfathiozole (H)	
Trichloroethylene decomposition (H)	
Triethyl tin (H)	
Vitamin A (H)	
Warfarin (H)	
Amiodarone (A) (H)	Retinal lipidosis (phospholipidosis) from systemic administration
AY 9944 (A)	
Chlorcyclizine (A)	
1-Chloroamitriptyline (A)	
Chloroquine (A)	

TABLE 4.14 *(Continued)*
Possible Adverse Retinal Effects

Chemical/Drug	Adverse Effects
Clomipramine (A)	
Diethylaminoethoxyhexestrol (A)	
Dithiozone (A)	
Imipramine (A)	
Iprindole (A)	
Perhexilene (A)	
Triparanol (A)	
Ammeline (A)	Retinal photoreceptor damage by systemic administration
Ammi majus seeds (A)	
Aramite (A)	
Benzoic acid (A)	
Bracken fern (A)	
Bromoacetate (A)	
Cardiac glycosides (H)	
Colchicine (A)	
Diaminodiphenylmethane (A)	
Digitalis (H)	
Digitoxin (H)	
Ethylenimine	
Ethylhydrocupreine (A)	
Fluorescein (with light) (A)	
Fluoride (A)	
Furmethonol (H)	
Halothane (A)	
Helichrysum (A)	
Hematoporphyrin (with light) (A)	
Hexachlorophene (A)	
Iodate (A)	
Iodoacetate (A)	
Methylazoxymethanol acetate (A)	
N-Methyl-N-nitrosourea (A)	
2-Naphthol (A)	
P-1727 (A)	
Quinine (A) (H)	
Quinoline (A)	
Sodium azide (A)	
Stypandra imbricata (A)	
Sucrose (A)	
Urethane (A)	
Aspidium (A)	Retinal vessel narrowing from systemic administration
Diaminodiphenoxypentane (A)	
Ergotamine (H)	
Ethylenimine (A)	
Ethylhydroxycupreine (H)	
Eucupine (H)	
Iron (H)	
Lead (A)	
Oxygen (A) (H)	
P-1727 (A)	
Quinine (H)	

TABLE 4.14 *(Continued)*
Possible Adverse Retinal Effects

Chemical/Drug	Adverse Effects
Ammi majus seeds (A)	Retinal ganglion cell damage by systemic administration
Arsanilic acid (A) (H)	
Aspidium (A)	
Carbon dioxide (H)	
Carbon disulfide (A)	
Chloramphenicol (H)	
Cinchona derivatives (A)	
Cysteine (A)	
Ergot (A)	
Ethylhydrocupreine (A) (H)	
Glutamate (A)	
Locoweed (A)	
Methanol (H)	
Quinine (A) (H)	
Quinoline (A)	
Swainsona plants (A)	
Tellurium (A)	
Thallium (H)	
Vincristine (H)	
Alloxan (A)	Retinal pigment epithelial changes from systemic administration
Aminophenoxyalkanes (A)	
Ammeline (A)	
Ammi majus seeds (A)	
Amopyroquin (A)	
Aspartate (A)	
Bilirubin (A)	
Bromoacetate (A)	
Cephaloridine (A)	
Chloroquine (A) (H)	
Cobalt (A)	
Colchicine (A)	
Deferoxamine (H)	
Diaminodiphenoxyheptane (A)	
Diaminodiphenoxypentane (A)	
Diaminodiphenylmethane (A)	
Dibutyl oxalate (A)	
Dihydro-dihydroxynaphthalene (A)	
Dithizone (A)	
Epinephrine (A)	
Ethambutol (high dose) (H)	
Ethylenimine (A)	
Ethylhydrocupreine (H)	
Fluoride (A)	
Glutamate (A)	
Hydroxychloroquine (H)	
Iminodipropionitrile (A)	
Iodate (A) (H)	
Iodoacetate (A)	
Isopropylhydroxybenzylpyrazolopyrimidine (A)	
Lead (A)	

TABLE 4.14 *(Continued)*
Possible Adverse Retinal Effects

Chemical/Drug	Adverse Effects
Mesidine (A)	
N-Methyl-N-nitrosourea (A)	
Naphthalene (A)	
Naphthoquinone (A)	
Naphthyl benzoate (A)	
Nitrofurazone (A)	
Ouabain (A)	
Oxygen (A) (H)	
Penicillamine (H)	
Pheniprazine (A)	
Phenylhydrazine (A)	
Phlorizin (A)	
Phosphorus (A)	
Piperidychlorophenothiazine (A) (H)	
Quinine (H)	
Quinoline (A)	
Sodium azide (A)	
Sparsomycin (H)	
Tetrahydronaphthalene (A)	
Thioridazine (A) (H)	
Toxotoxin (A)	
Trenimon (A)	
Triaziquone (A)	
Trifluoromethylphenylisopropylamine (A)	
Urethane (A)	
Vinblastine (A)	
Vincristine (A)	
Vitamin A (A)	
Acetazolamide (H)	Electroretinogram altered by systemic administration
Aldrin (A)	
4-Aminobutyric acid (A)	
Aminophoxyalkanes (A)	
Ammeline (A)	
Ammonium poisoning (A)	
Amodiaquine (H)	
Amyl acetate (A)	
Aramite (A)	
Aspartate (A)	
Barbiturates (A)	
Befunolol (A)	
Carbaryl (A)	
Carbon disulfide (A)	
Carbon monoxide (A)	
Cardiac glycosides (A)	
Chloramphenicol (H)	
Deferoxamine (H)	
2-Deoxyglucose (A)	
Desipramine (A)	
Diaminodiphenoxypentane (A)	
Digitalis (H)	

TABLE 4.14 *(Continued)*
Possible Adverse Retinal Effects

Chemical/Drug	Adverse Effects
Digoxin (A) (H)	
Dithizone (A)	
Epinephrine (A)	
Ethambutol (A)	
Fluoride (A)	
Formaldehyde (A)	
Glucose 6-phosphate (A)	
Glutamate (A)	
Halothane (H)	
Hydroxychloroquine (A) (H)	
Iminodipropionitrile (A)	
Iodate (A)	
Iodoacetate (A)	
Methanol (H)	
Mitomycin C (A)	
Nitrofurazone (A)	
Ouabain (A)	
Oxygen (A) (H)	
Oxypertine (A)	
Piperidylchlorophenothiazine (A)	
Quinine (A) (H)	
Rifampin (A)	
Sodium azide (A)	
Styrene (A)	
Sucrose (A)	
Thallium (A)	
Trimethadione (A) (H)	
Urethane (A)	
Vincristine (H)	
Vitamin A (A)	
Amoproxan	Central (or cecocentral) scotomas from systemic administration
Caramiphene	(humans)
Carbon disulfide	
Chloramphenicol	
Chloroquine	
Chlorpropamide	
Clomiphene	
Digitalis	
Diogitoxin	
Digoxin	
Dinitrobenzene	
Dinitrochlorobenzene	
Dinitrotoluene	
Disulfiram	
Ergotamine	
Emetine	
Ethambutol	
Ethchlorvynol	
Ethyl alcohol	
Ethylene glycol	

TABLE 4.14 *(Continued)*
Possible Adverse Retinal Effects

Chemical/Drug	Adverse Effects
Flumequine	
Ibuprofen	
Iodate	
Iodoform	
Isoniazid	
Lead	
Methanol	
Methyl bromide	
Minoxidil	
Octamoxin	
Pheniprazine	
Plasmocid	
Streptomycin	
Sulfonamides	
Tetraethyl lead	
Thallium	
Thiacetazone	
Tobacco smoking	
Trichloroethylene decomposition	
Wasp sting	
Amodiaquine	Peripheral visual field constriction from systemic administration
Arsacetin	(humans)
Arsanilic acid	
Bee sting	
Botulism toxin	
Carbon dioxide	
Carbon monoxide	
Chloramphenicol	
Cortex granati	
Dionitrochlorobenzene	
Emetine	
Ethambutol	
Ethylhydrocupreine	
Ethylmercuritoluenesulfonanilide	
Eucupine	
Iodate	
Methylmercury compounds	
Methanol	
Naphthalene	
Orsudan	
Oxygen	
Pheniprazine	
Piperidylchlorophenothiazine	
Quinine	
Trichloroethylene decomposition	
Tryparsamide	

Note: A = animals; H = humans.

TABLE 4.15
Possible Adverse Optic Nerve Effects

Chemical/Drug	Adverse Effects
Acetarsone (H)	Optic nerve atrophy from systemic administration
Acetylarsone (H)	
Antimony potassium tartrate (H)	
Arsacetin (H)	
Arsanilic acid (A) (H)	
Aspidium (A) (H)	
Bee sting	
Brayera (H)	
Broxyquinoline (H)	
Carbon dioxide (H)	
Carbon disulfide (H)	
Caster beans (H)	
Chloramphenicol (H)	
Clioquinol (H)	
Cortex granati (H)	
Dapsone (H)	
Dinitrobenzene (H)	
Dinitrochlorobenzene (H)	
Ethambutol (H)	
Ethyl hydrocuprein (H)	
Ethylmercuritoluenesulfonanilide (H)	
Eucupine (H)	
Finger cherries (H)	
Formic acid (A)	
Halquinols (H)	
Hexachlorophene (A) (H)	
Hexamethonium (H)	
Iodoform (H)	
Iodoquinol (H)	
Isoniazid (H)	
Lead (H)	
Methanol (A) (H)	
Octamoxin (H)	
Pheniprazine (H)	
Plasmocid (H)	
Quinine (H)	
Solvent sniffing (H)	
Thallium (H)	
Trichloroethylene decomposition (H)	
Triethyl tin (H)	
Tryparsamide (H)	
Vincristine (H)	
Acetarsone (H)	Optic neuropathy from systemic administration
Acetylarsan (H)	
Acrylamide (A)	
Antirabies vaccine (H)	
Arsacetin (H)	
Arsanilic acid (A) (H)	
Aspidium (H)	
Bee sting (H)	
Botulism (H)	

TABLE 4.15 *(Continued)*
Possible Adverse Optic Nerve Effects

Chemical/Drug	Adverse Effects
Carbon disulfide (H)	
Cassava (H)	
Chloramphenicol (H)	
Clioquinol (A) (H)	
Cyanoacetic acid (A)	
Deferoxamine (H)	
Dinitrobenzene (H)	
Dinitrochlorobenzene (H)	
Dinitrotoluene (H)	
Disulfiram (H)	
Ethambutol (A) (H)	
Ethchlorvynol (H)	
Ethylene glycol (H)	
Filicin (A)	
Glutamate (A)	
Helichrysum (A)	
Hexachlorophene (H)	
Iminodipropionitrile (A)	
Indarsol (A)	
Iodoform (H)	
Isoniazid (H)	
Lead (A) (H)	
Methanol (H)	
Octamoxin (H)	
Penicillamine (H)	
Perhexiline maleate (H)	
Phosphorus (H)	
Plasmocid (H)	
Sodium azide (A)	
Streptomycin (H)	
Stypandra imbricata (A)	
Sulfonamides (H)	
Tellurium (A)	
Thallium (H)	
Tolbutamide (H)	
Trichloroethylene decomposition (H)	
Triethyl tin (A)	
Trinitrotoluene (H)	
Tryparsamide (H)	
Vincristine (H)	
Antimony potassium tartrate (H)	Papilledema (swelling of the optic disc) from systemic
Arsphenamine (H)	administration
Aspirin (H)	
Bee sting (H)	
Carbenoxolone (H)	
Cephaloridine (H)	
Chlorambucil (H)	
Chloramphenicol (H)	
Chlordecone (H)	
Cisplatin (H)	
Contraceptive hormones (H)	
Corticosteroids (H)	

TABLE 4.15 *(Continued)*
Possible Adverse Optic Nerve Effects

Chemical/Drug	Adverse Effects
p-Dichlorobenzene (A)	
Dynamite (H)	
Ergotamine (H)	
Ethylene glycol (H)	
Helichrysum (A)	
Hexachlorophene (A) (H)	
Isoniazid (H)	
Isotretinoin (H)	
Ketoprofen (H)	
Lead (H)	
Levothyroxine (H)	
Minocycline (H)	
Minoxidil (H)	
Mitotane (H)	
Nalidixic acid (H)	
Nitrofurantoin (H)	
DL-Penicillamine (H)	
Penicillin (H)	
Perhexilene maleate (H)	
m-Phenylenediamine (H)	
p-Phenylenediamine (H)	
Phosphorus (H)	
Sulfonamides (H)	
Tetracycline (H)	
Triethyl tin (H)	
Vitamin A (H)	
Aspidium	Retrobulbar neuritis from systemic administration
Carbon disulfide	
Cassava	
Chloramphenicol	
Deferoxamine	
Dinitrobenzene	
Dinitrochlorobenzene	
Dinitrotoluene	
Disulfiram	
Ethambutol	
Iodoform	
Isoniazid	
Lead	
Octamoxin	
m- or *p*-Phenylenediamine	
Thallium	
Tolbutamide	
Trichloroethylene decomposition	
Trinitrotoluene	
Chloramphenicol (A)	Optic chiasm injury by systemic administration
Cyanide (A)	
Chloramphenicol (A)	
Cyanide (A)	
Ethambutol (A) (H)	
Helichrysum (A)	

TABLE 4.15 *(Continued)*
Possible Adverse Optic Nerve Effects

Chemical/Drug	Adverse Effects
Hexachlorophene (H)	
Stypandra imbricata (A)	
Tellurium (A)	
Triethyl tin (A)	
Vincristine (H)	

Note: A = animals, H = humans.

TABLE 4.16
Possible Adverse Extraocular Muscle Effects

Chemical/Drug	Adverse Effects
Alcuronium	Weakness or paralysis from systemic administration
Amanita phalloides	
Amitriptyline	
Anesthesia, spinal	
Antirabies vaccine	
Arsphenamine	
Barbiturates	
Botulinus toxin	
Carbamazepine	
Curare	
Diazinon	
Ethyl alcohol	
Ethylene glycol	
Furmethonol	
Gelsemium sempervirens	
Hexachlorophene	
Isopentaquine	
Lead	
Minocycline	
Nalidixic acid	
Pamaquine	
Penicillamine	
Pentaquine	
Piperazine	
Plasmocid	
Primidone	
Scorpion venom	
Snake venoms	
Streptomycin	
Sulfonal	
Thallium	
Trichloroethylene decomposition	
Triethyl tin	
Vincristine	
Vitamin A	

TABLE 4.17
Possible Adverse Effects on Intraocular Pressure

Chemical/Drug	Adverse Effects
Acetazolamide (A) (H)	Reduction of intraocular pressure by systemic administration
Alcohol (H)	
Alcuronium (H)	
Aminophylline (H)	
Ascorbic acid (H)	
BA 6650 (A)	
Bromocriptine (H)	
Calcium chloride (A)	
Cardiac glycosides (H)	
Catha edulis (H)	
Chlorpromazine (H)	
Chlorthalidone (H)	
Cholera toxin (H)	
Contraceptive hormones (H)	
Dextran A (H)	
Dibenamine (H)	
Dichlorphenamide (H)	
Digitoxin (H)	
Digoxin (H)	
Dihydroergotoxine (H)	
Ethoxolamide (H)	
Glucose (H)	
Glycerine (H)	
Iodate (A)	
Iodoacetate (A)	
Isosorbide (H)	
Lanatoside C (A)	
Mannitol (H)	
Meprobamate (H)	
Mercaptomerin (A)	
Mercuderamide (A)	
Methazolamide (H)	
Methyldopa (H)	
Nialamide (A)	
Nitroglycerin (H)	
Ouabain (A)	
Pargyline (H)	
Phentolamine (H)	
Propranolol (H)	
Propylene glycol (H)	
Quinine (H)	
Sodium ascorbate (H)	
Sodium chloride (H)	
Sodium lactate (H)	
Sorbitol (H)	
Thiopental (H)	
Timolol (H)	
Trometamol (H)	
Urea (H)	

Note: A = animals; H = humans.

TABLE 4.18
Possible Adverse Effects on Vision

Chemical/Drug	Adverse Effects
Barbiturates	Cortical blindness (humans)
Carbon monoxide	
Diatrizoate	
Lead	
Lomotil	
Methadone	
Methylergonovine	
Methylmercury compounds	
Vincristine	
Acetyl digitoxin	Color vision alterations from systemic administration
Aconite	
Amodiaquine	
Barbiturates	
Cannabis	
Carbon dioxide	
Carbon disulfide	
Chloramphenicol	
Chlorothiazide	
Contraceptive hormones	
Digitalis	
Digoxin	
Dihydrostreptomycin	
Diphenhydramine theoclate	
Ethambutol	
Furmethonol	
Herbatox	
Ibuprofen	
Lead	
Lysergide	
Nalidixic acid	
Pentylenetetrazole	
Salicylate	
Carbon dioxide	Altered dark adaption from systemic administration (humans)
Carbon disulfide	
Carbon monoxide	
Deferoxamine	
Digitalis	
Digitoxin	
Halothane	
Indomethacin	
Piperidylchlorophenothiazine	
Acetazolamide	Acute transient myopia from systemic administration without cyclotonia
Aminophenazone	or miosis (humans)
Arsphenamine	
Bendrofluazide	
Chlorothiazide	
Chlorthalidone	
Clofenamide	

TABLE 4.18 *(Continued)*
Possible Adverse Effects on Vision

Chemical/Drug	Adverse Effects
Dichlorphenamide	
Ethoxolamide	
Hydrochlorothiazide	
Isotretinoin	
Neoarsphenamine	
Phenformin	
Polythiazide	
Prochlorperazine	
Promethazine	
Quinine	
Spironolactone	
Sulfonamides	
Tetracycline	
Trichlormethiazide	

TABLE 4.19
Possible Adverse Irritating Effects

Chemical/Drug	Adverse Effects
Acrolein	Lacrimation from direct exposures
Allyl propyl disulfide	
Bromoacetone	
Bromoacetophenone	
Bromobenzylcyanide	
Bromomethyl ethyl ketone	
Bromotoluene	
Bromoxylene	
Chloroacetone	
Chloroacetophenone	
Chlorobenzylidene malononitrile	
Chlorosulfonic acid esters	
Cyanic acid	
Cyanogen chloride	
Dibenzoxazepine	
Dibromomethyl ether	
Dichloroformoxime	
Dichloronitroethane	
Diphenylchlorarsine	
Ethylarsine dichloride	
Ethyl benzene	
Ethyl bromoacetate	
Ethyl ioodoacetate	
Hexafluoroisopropanol	
Iodotoluene	
Lewisite	
Methyl arsine dichloride	

TABLE 4.19 *(Continued)*
Possible Adverse Irritating Effects

Chemical/Drug	Adverse Effects
Methyl iodoacetate	
Methyl vinyl ketone	
Nitrobenzyl chloride	
Nitroethylene	
Onion vapor	
Pelargonic acide morpholide	
Phenylcarbylamine chloride	
Trichloroacetronitrile	
Trichloromethane sulfonyl chloride	
Trichloromethanethiol	
Trichloropyrimidine	
Xylyl bromides	
Xylyl chlorides	
Arsenic, inorganic (H)	Lacrimation with burning or itching sensation from systemic
Bethanechol (H)	administration
Bismuth subnitrate (A)	
Chloral hydrate (H)	
Cyclohexanol (A)(H)	
Diazoxide (H)	
Dichlorophenoxy acetic acid (A)	
Dimercaprol (H)	
Dimidium bromide (A)(H)	
Diphenylarsenic acid (H)	
Emetine (H)	
Fish (Ciquatera) poisoning (H)	
Herion (H)	
Hexachloronaphthalene (A)	
Hydralazine (H)	
Iodide (H)	
Mercury (acrodynia)(H)	
Methotrexate (H)	
Morphine withdrawal (H)	
Nicothiazone (H)	
Nitrofurantoin (H)	
Pentazocine withdrawal (H)	
Phthalofyne (A)(H)	
Practolol (H)	
Pyrithione (A)	
Reserpine (H)	
Scorpion venom (H)	
Sulfathiazole (H)	
Tegafur (H)	
Thiacetazone (H)	
Triethyl tin (H)	
Zoxazolamine (H)	

Note: A = animals; H = humans.

TABLE 4.20
Possible Ocular Teratogenesis

Chemical/Drug	Adverse Effects
Alloxan (A)	Abnormalities of the eyes
Aspidium (A)	
Azathioprine (A)	
Busulfan (H)	
Butylated hydroxytoluene (A)	
Caffeine (A)	
Carbutamide (A)	
Chlorambucil (A) (H)	
Clomiphene (A)	
Colchicine (A)	
Cyclizine (A)	
Cyclophosphamide (A)	
2,4-Dichlorophenyl-*p*-nitrophenyl ether (A)	
Felicin (A)	
Heptachlor (A)	
Idoxuridine (A)	
Isotretinoin (A)	
Lysergide (A) (H)	
1-Methyl-3-nitro-1-nitroguanidine (A)	
2-Naphthol (A)	
Nickel carbonyl (A)	
Quinine (A) (H)	
Salicylate (A)	
Thalidomide (A) (H)	
Trimethadione (H)	
Trypan blue (A)	
Urethane (A)	
Veratrum californicum (A)	
Vidarabine (A)	
Vinblastine sulfate (A)	
Vitamin A (A)	
Warfarin (H)	

Note: A = animals, H = humans.

SECTION 9. GLOSSARY OF TERMS RELATING TO THE EYE

Accommodation The adjustment of the eye for seeing at different distances, accomplished by changing the shape of the lens through action of the ciliary muscle, thus focusing a clear image on the retina.

Aniridia Congenital absence of the iris.

Anophthalmos Absence of a true eyeball.

Anterior chamber The aqueous-containing cavity of the eye, bounded by the cornea anteriorly, the chamber angle structures peripherally, and the iris and lens posteriorly.

Aphakia Absence of the lens.

Biomicroscopy Examination of the eye using a biomicroscope (slit lamp).

Blepharitis Inflammation of the eyelids.

Blepharoptosis Drooping of an upper eyelid due to paralysis.

Blepharospasm Involuntary spasm of the lids.

Bulla A large bleb or blister filled with lymph or serum.

Bullous Characterized by bullae.

Canal of Schlemm A circular modified venous structure in the anterior chamber angle.

Canthus The angle of either end of the eyelid aperture; specified as outer (temporal) and inner (nasal).

Cataract An opacity of the lens or its capsule.

Chemosis Intense edema of the conjunctiva. The conjunctiva is a loose fibrovascular connective tissue which is relatively rich in lymphatics and responds to noxious stimuli by swelling to the point of prolapse between the lids.

Choroid The vascular middle coat between the retina and sclera.

Ciliary body Portion of the uveal tract between the iris and the choroid consisting of ciliary processes and the ciliary muscle.

Cones Retinal receptor cells concerned with visual acuity and color discrimation.

Conjunctiva Mucous membrane that lines the posterior aspect of the eyelids (palpebral conjunctiva) and the anterior sclera (bulbar conjunctiva).

Conjunctivitis Inflammation of the conjunctiva.

Cornea Transparent portion of the outer coat of the eyeball forming the anterior wall of the anterior chamber.

Corneal perforation A hole made through the cornea, resulting from the destruction of corneal tissue (secondary infectious agent(s) may or may not play a contributing role).

Corneal vascularization The development of blood vessels in the cornea. If there is sufficient tissue necrosis, then vascularization accompanies wound healing. Uncomplicated healing of corneal wounds occurs without vascularization.

Cycloplegic A drug that causes paralysis of the ciliary muscle, thus preventing accommodation.

Dacryocystitis Infection of the lacrimal sac.

Ectropion Turning out of the eyelid.

Edema The presence of an abnormally large amount of fluid in the intercellular tissue spaces (e.g., edema of the cornea is manifested as increased thickness).

Endophthalmitis Inflammation of one or more of the intraocular cavities and adjacent structures.

Enophthalmos Abnormal retrodisplacement of the eyeball.

Entropion A turning inward of the eyelid.

Enucleation Complete surgical removal of the eyeball.

Exophthalmos Abnormal protrusion of the eyeball.

Exudate Material, such as fluid, cells, or cellular debris, which has escaped from blood vessels and has deposited in tissues or on tissue surfaces, usually as a result of inflammation. An exudate, in contrast to a transudate, is characterized by a high content of protein, cells, or solid material derived from cells.

Fibrosis The formation of fibrous connective tissue.

Flare (aqueous flare) The scattering of light as it passes through a medium that contains particles. It is analogous to the Tyndall effect, and is seen when a thin beam of high intensity light is passed into the anterior chamber (of the eye) containing cellular material or increased amounts of protein.

Fluorescein (fluorescein sodium) A fluorescent dye, the simplest of the fluorane dyes and the mother substance of eosin, which is commonly used intravenously to determine the state of adequacy of circulation in the retina and to a lesser degree the choriod and iris. Another important use is to detect epithelial lesions of the cornea and conjunctiva. Peak excitation occurs with light at a wavelength between 485 and 500 nm and peak emission occurs between 520 and 530 nm.

Fornix The junction of the palpebral and bulbar conjunctiva.

Fovea Depression in the macula adapted for most acute vision.

Fundus The posterior portion of the eye visible through an ophthalmoscope.

Gonioscope An optical instrument used for examination of the anterior chamber angle.

Granulation The formation of fibrovascular tissue in wounds or ulcers.

Hemorrhage An escape of blood from the vessels; bleeding.

Hyperemia Excess of blood in a part due to local or general relaxation of the arterioles. Blood vessels become congested and give the area involved a reddish or red-blue color.

Hyphema Hemorrhage within the anterior chamber of the eye.

Hypopyon An accumulation of pus in the anterior chamber of the eye.

Hypotony Abnormally soft eye from any cause.

Injection Congestion of blood vessels.

Iris The circular pigmented membrane behind the cornea and immediately in front of the lens; the most anterior portion of the vascular tunic of the eye. It is composed of the dilator and sphincter muscles and the two-layered posterior epithelium, and mesodermal components that form the iris stroma.

Iritis Inflammation of the iris, manifested by vascular congestion (hyperemia). An outpouring of serum proteins into the aqueous (flare) may accompany the inflammatory reaction.

Keratitis Inflammation of the cornea.

Keratoconus Cone-shaped deformity of the cornea.

Keratocyte One of the connective tissue cells found between the layers of fibrous tissue in the corneal stroma.

Keratometer An instrument for measuring the curvature of the cornea, used in fitting contact lenses.

Lens A transparent biconvex structure suspended in the eyeball between the aqueous and the vitreous. Its function is to bring rays of light to a focus on the retina. Accommodation is produced by variations in the magnitude of this effect.

Lens remnants Those portions of the lens capsule and variable amounts of cortex and nucleus remaining after discontinuity of the lens capsule. Such remnants are usually opaque and may also be called cataractous lens remnants.

Limbal Of or pertaining to the limbus.

Limbus Zone of merger between cornea and sclera. In the normal eye, the cornea is transparent, the limbus semitransparent, and the sclera opaque. The limbus may vary from 1 to 3 mm in width.

Macula lutea The small avascular area of the retina surrounding the fovea, often having yellow pigment.

Megalocornea Abnormally large cornea (> 13 mm in diameter).

Microphthalmos Abnormal smallness of the eyeball.

Miotic A drug causing pupillary constriction.

Mydriatic A drug causing pupillary dilation.

Necrosis Death of tissue, usually as individual cells, groups of cells, or in a small localized area.

Nystagmus An involuntary, rapid movement of the eyeball that may be horizontal, vertical, rotatory, or mixed.

Ophthalmoscope An instrument with a special illumination system for viewing the inner eye, particularly the retina and associated structures.

Optic atrophy Optic nerve degeneration.

Optic disk Ophthalmoscopically visible portion of the optic nerve.

Optic nerve The nerve that carries visual impulses from the retina to the brain.

Palpebral Pertaining to the eyelid.

Panophthalmitis Inflammation of the entire eyeball.

Pannus Vascularization and connective tissue deposition beneath the epithelium of the cornea.

Papilledema Swelling of the optic disk.

Phlyctenule Localized lymphocytic infiltration of the conjunctiva.

Photophobia Abnormal sensitivity to light.

Posterior chamber Space filled with aqueous anterior to the lens and posterior to the iris.

Proptosis A forward displacement of the eyeball.

Pterygium A triangular growth of tissue that extends from the conjunctiva over the cornea.

Ptosis Drooping of the upper eyelid.

Pupil The round opening at the center of the iris which allows transmission of light to the posterior of the eyeball.

Pupillary light reflex The abrupt narrowing of pupillary aperture occurring when light is cast into the eye. The neuromotor reflex is mediated through the brain stem and involves both eyes.

Retina The innermost or nervous tunic of the eye which is derived from the optic cup (the outer layer develops into the pigmented monolayer of epithelium and the inner layer develops into the complex sensory layer).

Retinal detachment The condition in which the inner sensory layer of the retina separates from the outer layer of retinal pigment epithelium.

Retrocorneal fibrous membrane Formation of fibrous tissue on the posterior surface of the cornea; this tissue may replace the corneal endothelium.

Rods Retinal receptor cells concerned with peripheral vision under decreased illumination.

Schlemm's canal A narrow channel in the anterior chamber angle that drains aqueous to the aqueous veins.

Sclera The white tough covering of the eye that, with the cornea, forms the external protective coat of the eye.

Slit lamp A biomicroscope especially adapted to examine the eye.

Symblepharon Adhesions between the bulbar and palpebral conjunctiva.

Synechia Adhesion of the iris to the cornea (anterior synechia) or to the lens (posterior synechia).

Tonometer An instrument for measuring intraocular pressure.

Ulcer A lesion resulting from the loss of substance on a cutaneous or mucosal surface. It may lead to gradual disintegration and necrosis of the tissues.

Ulceration The formation or development of an ulcer.

Uvea (uveal tract) The iris, ciliary body, and choroid considered together.

Uveitis Inflammation of one or all portions of the uvea.

Vascular congestion Excessive or abnormal accumulation of blood in a tissue caused by dilatation of its blood vessels.

Vascularization The process of becoming vascular, or the development of vessels in a tissue.

Vitreous Transparent, colorless mass of soft, gelatinous material filling the space in the eyeball posterior to the lens and anterior to the retina.

Zonule A system of fine fibers which extends from the ciliary processes to the equator of the lens and which holds the lens in place.

REFERENCES

1. Beckley, J.H., Comparative eye testing: man vs. animal, *Toxicol. Appl. Pharmacol.,* 7, 93, 1965.
2. Maurice, D.M. and Giardini, A.A., A simple optical apparatus for measuring the corneal thickness, and the average thickness of the human cornea, *Br. J. Opthalmol.,* 48, 61, 1951.
3. Marzulli, F.N. and Simon, M.E., Eye irritation from topically applied drugs and cosmetics: preclinical studies, *Am. J. Optom.,* 48, 61, 1971.
4. Gaasterland, D.E., Barranger, J.A., Rapoport, S.I., Girton, M.E., and Doppman, J.L., Long-term ocular effects of osmotic modification of the blood-brain barrier in monkeys. I. Clinical examinations; aqueous ascorbate and protein, *Invest. Ophthalmol. Visual, Sci.,* 24(2), 153, 1983.

5. Kinsey, V.E., Comparative chemistry of aqueous humor in posterior and anterior chambers of rabbit eye, *Arch. Ophthalmol.*, 50, 401, 1953.
6. DeBarnadinis, E. et al., The chemical composition of the human aqueous humor in normal and pathological conditions, *Exp. Eye Res.*, 4, 179, 1965.
7. Graymore, C.N., *Biochemistry of the Eye*, Academic Press, New York, 1970.
8. Davson, H. and Graham, L.T., Comparative aspects of the intraocular fluids, in *The Eye*, vol. 5, Davson, H., Ed., Academic Press, New York, 1974.
9. Bito, L., Intraocular fluid dynamics. I. Steady-state concentration gradients of magnesium, potassium and calcium in relation to the sites and mechanisms of ocular cation transport processes, *Exp. Eye Res.*, 10, 102, 1970.
10. Kinsey, V.E. and Reddy, D.V.N., *The Rabbit in Eye Research*, Prince, J.H., Ed., Charles C Thomas, Springfield, IL, 1964.
11. laurent, V.B.G., Hyaluronate in aqueous humour, *Exp. Eye Res.*, 33, 147, 1981.
12. Wegener, J.K. and Moller, P.M., Oxygen tension in the anterior chamber of the rabbit eye, *Acta Ophthalmol.*, 49, 577, 1971.
13. Kleifeld, O. and Neumann, H.G., Der sauerstaffgehalt des menschlichen kammerwassers, *Klin. Monatsbl. Augenheilkd.*, 35, 224, 1959.
14. Walker, A.M., Comparison of the chemical composition of aqueous humor, cerebrospinal fluid, lymph and blood from frogs, higher animals and man. Reducing substances, inorganic phosphate, uric acid, urea., *J. Biol. Chem.*, 101, 269, 1933.
15. Duke-Elder, Sir S., *Physiology of the Eye*, vol. 4 of *System of Ophthalmology*, C.V. Mosby, St. Louis, 1968.
16. Dernouchamps, J.P., The proteins of the aqueous humour, *Doc. Ophthalmol.*, 53, 193, 1982.
17. Blogg, J.R. and Coles, E.H., *Vet. Bull.*, 40, 347, 1970.
18. Furuichi, C., The influence of various experimental injuries on creatine, creatinene metabolism of aqueous fluid of the rabbit's eye, *Acta Soc. Ophthalmol.*, 65, 561, 1961.
19. McLaughlin, P.S. and McLaughlin, B.G., Chemical analysis of bovine and porcine vitreous humors: correlation of normal values with serum chemical values and changes with time and temperature, *Am. J. Vet. Res.*, 48, 467, 1987.
20. Nordmann, J., *Biologie et Chirurgie due Corps Vitre*, Brini, A., Ed., Masson & Cis, Paris, 1968.
21. Goldenthal, E.I., Current views on safety evaluation of drugs, *FDA Papers*, 2, 13, 1968.
22. Federal Register, Interagency Regulatory Liaison Group recommended guideline for acute eye irritation testing, National Technological Information Service PB82-117557, 1981.
23. Organization for Economic Cooperation and Development, Acute eye irritation and corrosion, Publication 405, OECD Publications and Information Center, Washington, 1987.
24. Draize, J.H., Woodard, G., and Calvery, H.O., Methods for the study of irritation and toxicity of substances applied topically to the skin and mucous membranes, *J. Pharmacol., Exp. Ther.*, 82, 377, 1944.
25. Baldwin, H.A., McDonald, T.O., and Beasley, C.H., Slit-lamp examination of experimental animal eyes. II. Grading scales and photographic evaluation of induced pathological conditions, *J. Soc. Cosmet. Chem.*, 24, 181, 1973.
26. Hackett, R.B. and McDonald, T.O., Eye irritation, in *Dermatotoxicology*, 4th ed., Marzulli, F.N. and Maibach, H.I., Eds., Hemisphere, New York, 1991.
27. Kay, J.H. and Calandra, J.C., Interpretation of eye irritation tests, *J. Soc. Cosmet. Chem.*, 13, 281, 1962.
28. Committee for the revision of NAS Publication 1138, *Principles and Procedures for Evaluating the Toxicity of Household Substances*, National Academy of Sciences, Washington, 1977.
29. Green, W.R. et al., *A Systematic Comparison of Chemically Induced Eye Injury in the Albino Rabbit and Rhesus Monkey*, The Soap and Detergent Association, New York, 1978, 407.
30. Dunn, B., Toxicology of the eye, in *CRC Handbook of Toxicology*, Derelanko, M.J. and Hollinger, M.A., Eds, CRC Press, Boca Raton, FL, 1995, 186.
31. Beckley, J.H., Russell, T.J., and Rubin, L.F., Use of the Rhesus monkey for predicting human response to eye irritants, *Toxicol. Appl. Pharmacol.*, 15, 1, 1969.
32. Environmental Protection Agency, Guidance for evaluation of eye irritation testing, Hazard Evaluation Division Standard Evaluation Procedures, EPA-540/09-88-105, Washington, 1988.
33. Camp, D.D., *Federal Register*, 49, 188, 1984.

34. McDonald, T.O., Baldwin, H.A., and Beasley, C.H., Slit-lamp examination of experimental animal eyes. I. Techniques of illumination and the normal animal eye, *J. Soc. Cosmet. Chem.,* 24, 163, 1973.

35. McDonald, T.O., Kasten, K., Hervey, R., Gregg, S., Borgmann, A.R., and Murchison, T., Acute ocular toxicity of ethylene oxide, ethylene glycol, and ethylene chlorohydrin, *Bull. Parenter. Drug Assoc.,* 27, 153, 1973.

36. Chang, D.F., Ophthalmic examination, in *General Ophthalmology,* 12th ed., Vaughan, D., Asbury, T., Tabbara, K., Eds., Appleton & Lange, Norwalk, CT, San Mateo, CA, 1989.

37. Mishima, S., Corneal thickness, *Survey Ophthalmol.,* 13, 57, 1968.

38. Mishima, S. and Hedbys, B.O., Measurements of corneal thickness with the Haag-Streit pachometer, *Arch. Ophthalmol.,* 80, 710, 1968.

39. Jacobs, G.A. and Martens, M.A., An objective method for the evaluation of eye irritation *in vivo, Fd. Chem. Toxicol.,* 27, 255, 1989.

40. Morgan, R.L., Sorenson, S.S., and Castles, T.R., Prediction of ocular irritation by corneal pachymetry, *Food Chem. Toxicol.,* 25, 609, 1987.

41. Kennah, H.E., Hignet, S., Laux, P.E., Dorko, J.D., and Barrow, C.S., An objective procedure for quantitating eye irritation based on changes of corneal thickness, *Fundam. Appl. Toxicol.,* 12, 258, 1989.

42. Leibowitz, H.M. and Laing, R.A., Specular microscopy, in *Corneal Disorders: Clinical Diagnosis and Management,* Leibowitz, H. M., Ed., W.B. Saunders, Philadelphia, 1984.

43. Scheimpflug, T., Der photoperspektograph und seine Anweedung, *Photor. Korr.,* 43, 516, 1906.

44. Forbes, M., Pico, G. Jr., and Grolman, B., A noncontact applanation tonometer, *Arch. Ophthal.,* 91, 134, 1974.

45. Callaway, S., Gazzard, M.F., Price Thomas, D., and Swanston, D.W., The calibration and evaluation of a handheld tonometer as a means of measuring the intraocular pressure in the conscious rabbit, *Exp. Eye Res.,* 15, 383, 1973.

46. Pollack, I.P., Viernstein, L.J., and Radius, R.L., An instrument for constant-pressure tonography, *Exp. Eye Res.,* 29, 579, 1979.

47. Hilton, G.F. and Shaffer, R.N., Electronic applanation tonometry, *Am. J. Ophthalmol.,* 62, 838, 1966.

48. Reinhardt, C.A., Pelli, D.A., and Zbinden, G., Interpretation of cell toxicity data for the estimation of potential irritation, *Food Chem. Toxicol.,* 23, 247, 1985.

49. Grant, W.M., *Toxicology of the Eye,* 3rd ed., Charles C Thomas, Springfield, IL, 1986.

5 Fundamental Inhalation Toxicology

Paul E. Newton, Ph.D., D.A.B.T.

CONTENTS

SECTION 1. INTRODUCTION

Potential exposure to toxic materials is greater via inhalation than any other route of exposure. The potential is greatest through the lung because more air is inhaled each day than water or food is ingested. The surface area of the lung far exceeds the surface area of the skin and gastrointestinal tract. Some inhalation exposures may be intentional, as with inhaled drugs. However, most exposures are unintentional via environmental pollutants in the industrial setting or ambient air. Inhalation toxicity studies determine the health effects of these materials through exposure to animals, which then allows for human risk assessment. Inhalation studies involve all the standard types of toxicity studies and their various endpoints including acute, subchronic, chronic, oncogenicity, reproductive, developmental, neurotoxicity, as well as *in vitro* exposures. The following tables and graphs are a compilation that has proved to be useful in the conduct of inhalation studies and the extrapolation of effects among different species. The compilation includes data on respiratory tract anatomy, pulmonary function, bronchoalveolar lavage, metabolism, pulmonary deposition and clearance, pulmonary toxicity, and data associated with exposure chambers and the generation and monitoring of exposure atmospheres.

SECTION 2. RESPIRATORY TRACT ANATOMY

TABLE 5.1

Comparative Lung Biology: Morphologic Features of Pleura, Interlobular and Segmental Septa, and Distal Airways

	Human	Macaque Monkey	Dog, Cat	Ferret	Mouse, Rat, Gerbil Hamster, Guinea Pig, Rabbit	Horse, Sheep	Ox, Pig
Pleura	Thick	Thin	Thin	Thin	Thin	Thick	Thick
Interlobular and segmental connective tissue	Extensive, interlobular partially surrounds many lobules	Little	Little, if any	Little	Little, if any	Extensive[a] interlobular partially surrounds many lobules	Extensive, interlobular surrounds many lobules completely

TABLE 5.1 *(Continued)*
Comparative Lung Biology: Morphologic Features of Pleura, Interlobular and Segmental Septa, and Distal Airways

	Human	Macaque Monkey	Dog, Cat	Ferret	Mouse, Rat, Gerbil Hamster, Guinea Pig, Rabbit	Horse, Sheep	Ox, Pig
Nonrespiratory bronchiole (nonalveolarized)	Several generations	Fewer generations, commonly only one	Fewer generations	Several generations	Several generations	Several generations	Several generations
	TB ends in respiratory bronchioles	TB ends in respiratory bronchioles	TB ends in respiratory bronchioles	TB ends in respiratory bronchioles	TB ends in alveolar ducts or very short respiratory bronchioles	TB ends in alveolar ducts or very short respiratory bronchioles	TB ends in alveolar ducts or very short respiratory bronchioles
Respiratory bronchiole (alveolarized)	Several generations	Several generations	Several generations	Several generations	Absent or a single short generation	Absent or a single short generation	Absent or a single short generation

Note: TB = terminal nonrespiratory bronchiole.

[a] The interlobular connective tissue of the sheep appears extensive and lobules appear completely separated in gross preparations, but not in LM, SEM, or HRCT.

From Tyler, W.S. and Julian, M.D., in *Treatise on Pulmonary Toxicology*, vol. 1, *Comparative Biology of the Normal Lung*, CRC Press, Boca Raton, FL, 1992. With permission.

TABLE 5.2
Interspecies Comparison of Nasal Cavity Characteristics

	Sprague-Dawley Rat	Guinea Pig	Beagle Dog	Rhesus Monkey	Man
Body weight	250 g	600 g	10 kg	7 kg	~70 kg
Naris cross-section	0.7 mm^2	2.5 mm^2	16.7 mm^2	22.9 mm^2	140 mm^2
Bend in naris	40°	40°	30°	30°	
Length	23 cm	3.4 cm	10 cm	5.3 cm	7–8 cm
Greatest vertical diameter	9.6 mm	12.8 mm	23 mm	27 mm	40–45 mm
Surface area (both sides of nasal cavity)	10.4 cm^2	27.4 cm^2	220.7 cm^2	61.6 cm^2	181 cm^2
Volume (both sides)	0.4 cm^3	0.9 cm^3	20 cm^3	8 cm^3	16–19 cm^3 (does not include sinuses)
Bend in nasopharynx	15°	30°	30°	80°	~90°
Turbinate complexity	Complex scroll	Complex scroll	Very complex membranous	Simple scroll	Simple scroll

From Schreider, J.P., in *Nasal Tumors in Animals and Man*, vol. III, *Experimental Nasal Carcinogenesis*, CRC Press, Boca Raton, FL, 1983.[26] With permission.

TABLE 5.3

Comparative Anatomy of the Lung Parenchyma and Air-Blood Tissue Barrier[a]

Species	N	Body Weight (g)	Lung Volume (ml)	Alveolar Surface Area (Both lungs), cm²	Capillary Surface Area (Both lungs), cm²	Capillary Volume (Both lungs), ml	Tissue (μm)
Shrew (*Surcus etrascus*)	4	2.6 ± 0.2	0.10 ± 0.01	170 ± 10	130 ± 15	0.0118 ± 0.002	0.27 ± 0.02
White mouse (*Mus musculus*)	5	23 ± 2	0.74 ± 0.07	680 ± 85	590 ± 60	0.084 ± 0.009	0.32 ± 0.01
Waltzing mouse (*Mus wagneri*)	5	13 ± 1	0.58 ± 0.06	630 ± 40	540 ± 30	0.065 ± 0.008	0.26 ± 0.002
Syrian golden hamster (*Mesocricetus auratus*)	4	118 ± 7	2.81 ± 0.24	2,760 ± 250	2,410 ± 190	0.294 ± 0.011	0.39 ± 0.10
White rat (*Rattus rattus*)	8	140 ± 7	6.34 ± 0.25	3,880 ± 190	4,070 ± 200	0.480 ± 0.022	0.37 ± 0.02
White rat (Sprague-Dawley)	6	360 ± 4	10.82 ± 0.38	4,865 ± 380	4,270 ± 385	0.63 ± 0.07	0.40 ± 0.02
White rat (Fischer-344)							
Male: 5 mo	4	289 ± 13	8.60 ± 0.31	3,915 ± 390	3,830 ± 395	0.65 ± 0.06	0.38 ± 0.03
Female: 5 mo	4	182 ± 5	7.48 ± 0.10	3,420 ± 125	3,260 ± 185	0.46 ± 0.10	0.34 ± 0.01
Male: 26 mo	4	391 ± 11	12.67 ± 0.74	4,630 ± 440	4,490 ± 485	0.67 ± 0.10	0.37 ± 0.01
Female: 26 mo	4	298 ± 7	9.39 ± 0.40	4,020 ± 25	3,570 ± 165	0.34 ± 0.05	0.37 ± 0.01
Guinea pig (*Cavia porcellus*)	15	429 ± 11	13.04 ± 3.03	9,100 ± 280	7,400 ± 230	1.50 ± 0.08	0.42 ± 0.01
Rabbit (*Oryctolagus cuniculus*)	6	3,560	79.2	58,600 ± 12,400	47,000 ± 8,800	7.15 ± 1.88	0.50 ± 0.04
Dwarf mongoose (*Helogalepervula*)	3	52,800 ± 9,800	30.6 ± 5.6	16,100 ± 2,600	14,600 ± 3,400	2.06 ± 0.52	0.39 ± 0.02
Genet cat (Genetta ligrino)	2	137,200 ± 4,300	99.0 ± 12.2	56,300 ± 6,400	42,300 ± 1,600	5.04 ± 0.63	0.51 ± 0.02
Dog (*Canis familiaris*)	3	5,400	284.2	182,000 ± 135,000	141,000 ± 111,000	26.0 ± 24.9	0.43 ± 0.02
Dog (*C. familiaris*)	8	11,200 ± 400	736 ± 25	407,000 ± 39,000	329,000 ± 16,000	50.2 ± 5.0	0.46 ± 0.01
Dog (*C. familiaris*)	4	16,000 ± 3,000	1,322 ± 64	510,000 ± 10,000	570,000 ± 20,000	92 ± 5	0.45 ± 0.01
Dog (*C. familiaris*)	6	22,800 ± 600	1,501 ± 74	897,000 ± 69,000	718,000 ± 69,000	71.8 ± 4.5	0.48 ± 0.01

Species	n						
Dog (*C. familiaris*)	5	46,100	2,888	1,769,000 ± 456,000	1,319,000 ± 375,000	234 ± 69	0.53 ± 0.08
Camel (*Camelus dromedarus*)	2	231,700 ± 2,700	15,900 ± 1,400	4,305,000 ± 584,000	2,726,000 ± 292,000	378 ± 100	0.60 ± 0.06
Giraffe (*Giraffa camelopordalis*)	1	383,000	21,000	6,361,000	5,516,000	965	0.60
Suni (*Nesotragus moschatus*)	2	3,300 ± 300	209.4 ± 0.6	96,900 ± 5,500	81,300 ± 13,000	12.4 ± 0.7	0.56 ± 0.09
Dik-dik (*Madogua kirkii*)	2	4,200 ± 100	313.4 ± 1.2	146,000 ± 700	130,000 ± 6550	22.6 ± 3.3	0.43 ± 0.02
Wildebeest (*Connochaetes tauriras*)	1	102,000	7,678	3,908,000	2,813,000	472	0.37
Waterbuck (*Kobus defasso*)	2	109,800 ± 16,300	7,835 ± 1,550	3,829,000 ± 950,000	3,378,000 ± 460,000	584 ± 98	0.46 ± 0.04
African goat (*Capra hircus*)	2	20,900 ± 1,000	1,370 ± 15	449,000 ± 12,000	439,000 ± 12,000	101 ± 8	0.54 ± 0.03
African sheep (*Ovis aries*)	2	21,800 ± 200	17,055 ± 435	671,000 ± 71,000	645,000 ± 139,000	146 ± 35	0.53 ± 0.05
Zebu cattle (*Bos indicus*)	4	192,500 ± 24,000	10,145 ± 1,960	3,850,000 ± 420,000	3,795,000 ± 392,000	700 ± 124	0.50 ± 0.04
Swiss cow (*B. taurus*)	1	700,000	22,450	12,830,000	11,380,000	2,770	0.51
Horse (*Equis cabalbus*)	2	510,000 ± 0	37,650 ± 1,050	24,560,000 ± 124,000	16,630,000 ± 1,080,000	2,800 ± 300	0.60 ± 0.02
Monkey (*Macaca irus*)	6	3,710	184.2	133,000 ± 12,700	116,000 ± 15,400	15.5 ± 2.7	0.50 ± 0.03
Baboon (*Papio papio*)	5	29,000 ± 3,000	2,393 ± 100	496,000 ± 77,000	386,000 ± 95,000	44 ± 17	0.67 ± 0.06
Man (*Homo sapiens*)	8	74,000 ± 4,000	4,341 ± 285	1,430,000 ± 120,000	1,260,000 ± 120,000	213 ± 31	0.62 ± 0.04

[a] All values are mean ± SEM.

From Pinkerton, R.E., Gehr, P., and Crapo, J.D., in *Treatise on Pulmonary Toxicology*, vol. 1, *Comparative Biology of the Normal Lung*, CRC Press, Boca Raton, FL. 1991.[3] With permission.

TABLE 5.4
Allometry of Pulmonary Structural Variables

Taxon	Intercept	Slope	N	M_b Range
V_L, ml; Lung Volume				
Mammals	56.7	1.02	21	0.01–2.000
Mammals	40.0	1.021	13	0.003–3.71
Mammals	46.0	1.059	33	0.003–700
Mammals	47.5	1.060	47	0.003–700
Canids	54.9	1.15	4	4.6–27.6
Dog (*Canis familiaris*)	52.8	1.07	1	2.65–57
Bats	96.4	1.07	5	0.005–0.173
S(A), m², Alveolar Surface Area				
Mammals	1.87	0.888	13	0.003–3.71
Mammals	3.34	0.949	33	0.003–700
Mammals	3.36	0.935	47	0.003–700
Canids	1.12	1.38	4	4.6–27.6
Dog (*C. familiaris*)	3.12	1.05	1	2.65–57
Bats[b]	5.18	1.01	5	0.005–0.173
S(c), m²; Pulmonary Capillary Surface Area				
Mammals	2.73	0.952	33	0.003–700
Mammals	2.72	0.941	47	0.003–700
Canids	1.14	1.25	4	4.6–27.6
Dog (*C. familiaris*)	2.53	1.05	1	2.65–57
V(c), ml; Pulmonary Capillary Volume				
Mammals	3.20	1.000	33	0.003–700
Mammals	3.63	1.009	47	0.003–700
Canids	1.92	1.23	4	4.6–27.6
Dog (*C. familiaris*)	3.28	1.12	1	2.65–57
Bats	3.73	0.954	5	0.005–0.173
τ_{ht} μm; Harmonic Mean Thickness of Alveolar Membrane				
Mammals	0.416	0.050	33	0.003–700
Mammals	0.413	0.053	47	0.003–700
Canids	0.476	0.000	4	4.6–27.6
Dog (*C. familiaris*)	0.39	0.80	1	2.65–57
Bats	0.249	0.021	5	0.005–0.173

Note: Allometry of pulmonary structural variables that contribute to gas conductance of the lung and morphometric estimates of pulmonary diffusing capacity (DL_0). Variables are related to body mass (M_b, in kg) by the function: $Y = a \cdot M_b^b$, where Y is the variable. a is the intercept of the log-transformed linear regression, and b is the slope of the log-transformed linear regression. N is the number of species. In some cases, regression equations were calculated from data given in the reference. Units have been converted for equivalence, where necessary.

From Jones, J.H. and Longworth, K.E., in *Treatise on Pulmonary Toxicology*, vol. 1, *Comparative Biology of the Normal Lung,* CRC Press, Boca Raton, FL, 1992.[6] With permission.

TABLE 5.5
Total Tissue Volumes, Surface Areas, and Mean Tissue Thickness in the Alveolar Region of Normal Mammalian Lungs[†]

	Fischer-344 Rat ($n = 4$)	Sprague-Dawley Rat ($n = 8$)	Dog ($n = 4$)	Baboon ($n = 5$)	Human ($n = 8$)
Body weight, kg	0.29 ± 0.01^a	0.36 ± 0.01	16 ± 3	29 ± 3	74 ± 4
Lung volume, ml	8.6 ± 0.31^a	10.55 ± 0.37^a	1322 ± 64	2393 ± 100	4341 ± 284
Total volumes, cm³/both lungs					
Air	5.978 ± 0.197	7.216 ± 0.278^a	914 ± 52	1851 ± 24	3422 ± 223
Capillary lumen	0.649 ± 0.057^a	0.659 ± 0.055^a	92 ± 5^b	44 ± 17^b	169 ± 24
Tissue	0.428 ± 0.046^a	0.671 ± 0.041^a	78 ± 4^b	68 ± 9^b	314 ± 41
Type I epithelium	0.082 ± 0.006^a	0.144 ± 0.010^a	16.5 ± 1.9^b	14.4 ± 2.3^b	32.5 ± 3.9
Type II epithelium	0.037 ± 0.009^a	0.053 ± 0.009^a	5.6 ± 0.5^b	3.5 ± 0.8^b	32.1 ± 5.0
Cellular interstitium	0.068 ± 0.005^a	0.079 ± 0.015^a	12.9 ± 0.7^b	9.4 ± 1.6^b	54.0 ± 7.0
Noncellular interstitium	0.128 ± 0.016^a	0.214 ± 0.016^a	22.8 ± 0.7^b	24.6 ± 3.7^b	98.3 ± 12.4
Endothelium	0.094 ± 0.009^a	0.156 ± 0.007^a	17.6 ± 1.6	13.4 ± 2.6	42.6 ± 5.4
Macrophages	0.019 ± 0.007^a	0.025 ± 0.006^a	2.5 ± 1.1^b	2.4 ± 1.1^b	54.7 ± 15.7
Surface area, m² both lungs[‡]					
Alveolar epithelium					
Type I	0.391 ± 0.39^a	0.387 ± 0.025^a	51.0 ± 1.0^b	47.7 ± 7.7^b	89.0 ± 8.0
Type II	0.015 ± 0.005^a	0.015 ± 0.002^a	1.0 ± 0.2	1.9 ± 0.3	7.0 ± 1.0
Capillary endothelium	0.383 ± 0.39^a	0.452 ± 0.035^a	57.0 ± 2.0	38.6 ± 9.5	91.0 ± 9.0
Arithmetic mean, tissue thickness, μm					
Epithelium					
Type I	0.212 ± 0.008^b	0.384 ± 0.038^a	0.327 ± 0.043^{ab}	0.308 ± 0.021^{ab}	0.361 ± 0.024^a
Type II	2.758 ± 0.424^{ab}	3.653 ± 0.266^a	4.138 ± 0.340^{ac}	1.839 ± 0.141^b	5.019 ± 0.551^c
Interstitium	0.500 ± 0.028^a	0.693 ± 0.058^a	0.658 ± 0.033^a	0.847 ± 0.140^a	1.634 ± 0.164
Endothelium	0.246 ± 0.011^a	0.358 ± 0.031^a	0.308 ± 0.019^a	0.361 ± 0.038^{ab}	0.474 ± 0.052^b

[†] All data are mean ± SEM. For comparisons between species all data connected by the same letter subscript are not statistically different from each other.

[‡] Type I surface area (SA) is the SA of basement membrane under type I cells: type II SA is the air surface of type II cells excluding the extra SA contributed by microvilli; endothelial SA is the luminal surface of the endothelial cells.

From Pinkerton, K.E., Gehr, P., and Crapo, J.D., in *Treatise on Pulmonary Toxicology,* vol. 1, *Comparative Biology of the Normal Lung,* CRC Press, Boca Raton, FL, 1992.[3] With permission.

TABLE 5.6
Tracheobronchial and URT Liquid Lining Layer Thicknesses

Species	Location	Thickness[a] (μm)	Comments
Cat	Trachea	≤20, usually <10	Not uniform "in some areas not detected"
Guinea pig	Trachea	~10	"Constantly biophasic"
	Intrapulmonary	0.0	Liquid lining never extended beyond ciliary tips
Human	Bronchi (main stem)	8.3^b	Combination of airway and vascular fixation,
	Bronchi (segmental)	6.9^b	lobes were surgical resections in
	Bronchioles	1.8^b	nonsmokers
Rabbit	Bronchi (1–3 mm)[c]	5 or more[b]	
	Bronchioles (0.5–1.0 mm)[c]	1–4[b]	Mucous blanket observed

TABLE 5.6 *(Continued)*
Tracheobronchial and URT Liquid Lining Layer Thicknesses

Species	Location	Thickness[a] (μm)	Comments
	Bronchioles (<0.5 mm)[c]	0.3–0.5[b]	
	Terminal bronchioles	<0.1[b]	
Rat	Nose	≤15	Observed a continuous blanket
	Trachea large bronchi	5–10	"Distribution was focal"
	Trachea	3–15, generally 8–12[b]	Mucous blanket observed
	Lobar bronchi	Few tenths-8, generally 2–5[b]	
	Trachea	6.1[b]	
	Bronchi	3[b]	Combination of airway and vascular fixation
	Bronchioles	2[b]	
	Terminal bronchioles	0.0	No epiphase or mucus observed
	Trachea, major bronchi, peripheral airways		"Well defined streams up to 500 mm wide." "Mucus was transported as discrete particles" as small as 0.5 mm in diameter. A continuous mucous blanket was not observed.

[a] Unless specified, values apply only to the epiphase above cilia lips.
[b] Thickness of epiphase plus hypophase.
[c] Diameter range of airways.

From Miller, F.J., Overton, J.H., Kimbell, J.S., and Russel, M.L., in *Toxicology of the Lung,* Raven Press, New York, 1993.[9] With permission.

TABLE 5.7
Alveolar Region Tissue and Blood Compartment Dimensions of Normal Mammalian Lungs

	Fischer-344 Rat (*n* = 4)	Sprague-Dawley Rat (*n* = 8)	Dog (*n* = 4)	Baboon (*n* = 5)	Human (*n* = 8)
Body weight (kg)	0.29 ± 0.01[a]	0.36 ± 0.01	16 ± 3	29 ± 3	79 ± 4
Lung volume (ml)	8.6 ± 0.31	10.55 ± 0.37	1,322 ± 64	2,393 ± 100	4,341 ± 284
Total volumes (cm³ both lungs)					
Air	5.978 ± 0.197	7.216 ± 0.278	914 ± 52	1,851 ± 24	3,422 ± 223
Capillary lumen	0.649 ± 0.057	0.659 ± 0.055	92 ± 5	44 ± 17	169 ± 24
Tissue	0.428 ± 0.046	0.671 ± 0.041	78 ± 4	68 ± 9	314 ± 41
Type I epithelium	0.082 ± 0.006	0.144 ± 0.010	16.5 ± 1.9	14.4 ± 2.3	32.5 ± 3.9
Type II epithelium	0.037 ± 0.009	0.053 ± 0.009	5.6 ± 0.5	3.5 ± 0.8	32.1 ± 5.0
Cellular interstitium	0.068 ± 0.005	0.079 ± 0.015	12.9 ± 0.7	9.4 ± 1.6	54.0 ± 7.0
Noncellular interstitium	0.128 ± 0.016	0.214 ± 0.016	22.8 ± 0.7	24.6 ± 3.7	98.3 ± 12.4
Endotheliurn	0.094 ± 0.009	0.156 ± 0.007	17.6 ± 1.6	134 ± 2.6	42.6 ± 5.4
Macrophages	0.019 ± 0.007	0.025 ± 0.006	2.5 ± 1.1	2.4 ± 1.1	54.7 ± 15.7
Surface area (m²/both lungs)					
Alveolar epithelium					
Type I	0.391 ± 0.039	0.387 ± 0.025	51.0 ± 1.0	47.7 ± 7.7	89.0 ± 8.0
Type II	0.015 ± 0.005	0.015 ± 0.002	1.0 ± 0.2	1.9 ± 0.3	7.0 ± 1.0
Capillary endothelium	0.383 ± 0.039	0.452 ± 0.035	57.0 ± 2.0	38.6 ± 9.5	91.0 ± 9.0
Tissue component of diffusion capacity (ml O_2 min^{-1} mm Hg^{-1})	3.43 ± 0.17	3.55 ± 0.33	399 ± 12	23.1 ± 5.2	436 ± 53.6

TABLE 5.7 *(Continued)*
Alveolar Region Tissue and Blood Compartment Dimensions of Normal Mammalian Lungs

	Fischer-344 Rat (*n* = 4)	Sprague-Dawley Rat (*n* = 8)	Dog (*n* = 4)	Baboon (*n* = 5)	Human (*n* = 8)
Tissue thickness (μm)					
Harmonic mean (air/plasma)	0.379 ± 0.030	0.405 ± 0.017	0.450 ± 0.007	0.674 ± 0.055	0.745 ± 0.059
Arithmetic mean					
Epithelium					
Type I	0.212 ± 0.008	0.384 ± 0.038	0.327 ± 0.043	0.308 ± 0.021	0.361 ± 0.024
Type II	2.578 ± 0.424	3.653 ± 0.266	4.138 ± 0.340	1.839 ± 0.141	5.019 ± 0.551
Interstitium	0.500 ± 0.028	0.693 ± 0.058	0.658 ± 0.033	0.847 ± 0.140	1.634 ± 0.164
Endothelium	0.246 ± 0.011	0.358 ± 0.031	0.308 ± 0.019	0.361 ± 0.038	0.474 ± 0.052

[a] All data are mean ±SEM.

Source: Crapo, J.D. et al., 1983.[10]

From Miller, F.J., Overton, J.H., Kimbell, J.S., and Russel, M.L., in *Toxicology of the Lung,* Raven Press, New York, 1993.[9] With permission.

TABLE 5.8
Anatomical Data: Trachea of Various Species

Species	Length (cm)	Internal Diameter (mm)	Goblet Cells per cm	Glands
Dog	10	15	350	+ + +
Baboon	3.5	5	600	+ + +
Pig	13	10	150	+ + +
Macaca	6	7	300	+ +
Mouse	2	2	—	±
Rabbit	6.5	10	150	−
Guinea pig	3.3	4	600	−
Hamster	1.5	2	6	−
Sheep	24	26	300	+ + +
Cat (SPF)	7	7	600	+ + + +
Squirrel monkey	2.5	3	150	+
Rat	3.2	3	8	±
Man	11.0	20	200[a]	+ + +[a]

[a] Varies considerably.

From Phalen, R.F., *Inhalation Studies: Foundations and Techniques,* CRC Press, Boca Raton. FL, 1984.[11] With permission.

TABLE 5.9
Dimensions of the Cross Sections of the Nasal
Cast of the Rat

Section No.	Distance from Anterior End of Nose (mm)	Perimeter (mm)	Area (mm²)
1	0	8.3	1.4
2	1	5.6	1.3
3	2	11.9	2.0
4	3	21.7	3.5
5	4	23.4	3.8
6	5	27.3	4.5
7	5.5	35.0	7.6
8	7	38.3	9.9
9	8	44.0	9.3
10	10	73.9	13.2
11	12	63.5	10.3
12	14	54.4	10.3
13	16	48.3	8.1
14	17	67.6	16.7
14[a]	17	57.8	13.0
15	18	58.4	21.7
16	19	104.1	25.8
16[a]	19	47.5	14.0
17	20	97.8	17.0
17[a]	20	9.0	5.0
18	21	44.5	12.5
18[a]	21	9.0	5.0
19	22	30.9	7.7
19[a]	22	8.5	4.2
20	23	17.4	5.9
20[a]	23	8.9	4.9
21	25	7.5	3.6
22	32	7.9	3.7
23	35	8.6	2.8
24	37	7.7	2.2
25	40	8.4	3.4
26	41	8.7	3.4
27	42	23.7	15.8
28	43	24.2	14.9
29	44	9.2	3.2
30	44.5	12.8	3.2
31	45	7.6	1.8
32	45.5	7.4	1.9
33	46	7.8	3.1
34	47	6.5	3.0
35	52	7.1	3.8

[a] Main airway alone. Does not include separate pockets.

From *Toxicology of the Nasal Passages,* J.P. Schreider, Hemisphere Publishing, Taylor & Francis, Washington, D.C., 1986, p. 10.[12] Reproduced with permission. All rights reserved.

TABLE 5.10
Dimensions of the Cross Sections of the Nasal Cast of the Guinea Pig

Section No.	Distance from Anterior End of Nose (mm)	Perimeter (mm)	Area (mm^2)
1	0	18.0	5.0
2	1	14.0	4.4
3	2	15.3	4.9
4	2.5	12.4	3.6
5	3	13.9	4.2
6	3.5	18.5	5.4
7	4	32.9	13.0
8	5.0	19.8	13.4
9	8	66.4	20.4
10	11	88.0	21.5
11	16	91.5	28.5
12	18	91.2	31.1
13	20	82.0	36.2
14	22	62.7	30.1
15	24	75.1	38.1
16	26	109.4	44.4
16[a]	26	94.3	39.2
17	28	153.5	58.1
17[a]	28	14.9	11.2
18	31	184.6	73.4
18[a]	31	14.5	10.8
19	34	14.2	13.3
19[a]	34	8.2	11.7
20	39	13.9	13.7
21	45	13.2	31.2
22	50	12.0	8.1
23	55	8.0	4.1
24	56	18.9	8.8
25	57	20.7	12.7
26	59	8.9	2.8
27	62	9.1	5.1
28	70	8.6	5.7

[a] Main airway alone. Does not include side pockets.

From *Toxicology of the Nasal Passages,* J.P. Schreider, Hemisphere Publishing, Taylor & Francis, Washington, D.C., 1986, p. 11.[12]

TABLE 5.11
Dimensions of the Cross Sections of the Nasal Cast of the Beagle

Section No.	Distance from Anterior End of Nose (mm)	Perimeter (mm)	Area (mm²)
1	0	44.0	33.3
2	5	50.3	42.3
3	10	72.5	44.8
4	15	66.5	32.0
5	20	63.8	37.6
6	25	70.1	49.6
7	30	106.3	75.9
8	35	143.4	95.5
9	40	294.8	155.0
10	43	503.0	205.8
11	50	674.3	228.4
11[a]	50	665.6	227.3
12	55	470.6	267.3
13	60	333.9	312.5
14	65	318.8	240.9
14[a]	65	64.3	91.2
15	70	424.1	277.5
15[a]	70	55.1	68.0
16	75	266.8	289.5
16[a]	75	109.1	143.8
17	80	200.9	272.5
17[a]	60	54.5	113.9
18	90	121.5	138.3
18[a]	90	52.6	105.3
19	100	44.4	95.2
19[a]	100	35.6	92.6
20	120	39.3	88.8
21	150	64.0	139.1
22	160	184.5	1022.5
23	170	131.0	871.3
24	180	210.0	1055.4
25	185	250.9	933.6
25[a]	185	53.1	89.1
26	190	50.8	112.6
27	195	50.6	175.4
28	205	57.5	251.3
29	275	57.0	237.1

[a] Main airway alone. Does not include separate pockets.

From *Toxicology of the Nasal Passages,* J.P. Schreider, Hemisphere Publishing, Taylor & Francis, Washington, D.C., 1986, p. 11.[12]

TABLE 5.12
Dimensions of the Cross Sections of the Nasal
Cast of the Rhesus Monkey

Section No.	Distance from Anterior End of Nose (mm)	Perimeter (mm)	Area (mm^2)
1	0	45.8	55.6
2	3	43.3	51.0
3	8	62.3	61.0
4	13	73.8	86.2
5	18	95.6	105.6
6	23	119.3	161.1
7	25	121.0	155.0
8	28	169.1	180.8
9	33	192.9	165.6
10	38	211.8	165.3
11	40	171.8	164.1
12	43	143.4	161.7
13	48	116.1	152.6
14	53	58.5	91.5
15	58	45.0	53.2
16	63	37.9	38.0
17	68	24.0	18.8
18	73	29.0	27.3
19	78	37.9	66.0
20	80	66.5	224.9
21	83	73.6	253.1
22	88	90.5	263.0
22[a]	88	75.4	256.4
23	90	118.8	257.3
24	93	34.1	43.8
25	95	27.6	15.8
26	98	29.5	18.2
27	103	35.0	72.0
28	105	33.3	75.4
29	110	27.9	56.1

[a] Main airway alone. Does not include separate pockets.

From *Toxicology of the Nasal Passages,* J.P. Schreider, Hemisphere Publishing, Taylor & Francis, Washington, D.C., 1986, p. 13.[12]

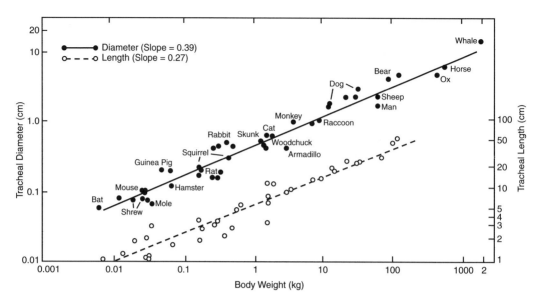

FIGURE 5.1 Relationship between body mass and the logarithms of tracheal diameter and length for a variety of species. From Tenney, S.M. and Bartlett, D., *Respir. Physiol.,* 3, 130, 1967.[4] With permission.

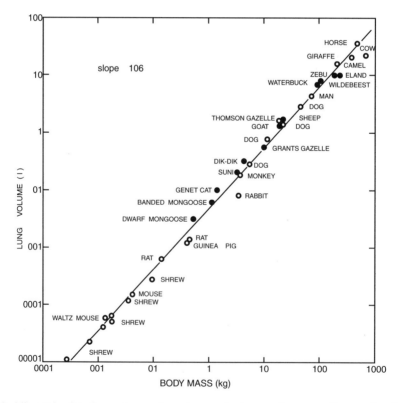

FIGURE 5.2 Allometric plot of mean lung volume to mean body mass for mammalian species. Closed circles are African species and open circles are other species. From Gehr et al., *J. Respir. Physiol.,* 44, 61, 1981.[5] With permission.

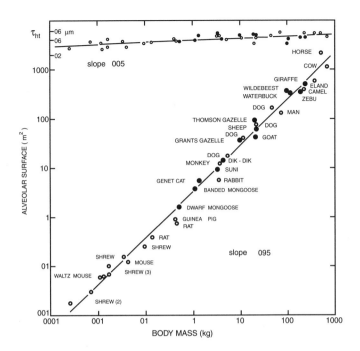

FIGURE 5.3 Allometric plot of alveolar surface area and harmonic mean tissue thickness (T_{ht}) to body mass for mammalian species. From Gehr et al., *J. Respir. Physiol.*, 44, 61, 1981.[5] With permission.

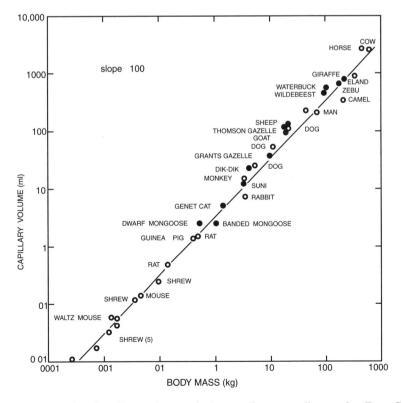

FIGURE 5.4 Allometric plot of capillary volume to body mass for mammalian species. From Gehr et al., *J. Respir. Physiol.*, 44, 61, 1981.[5] With permission.

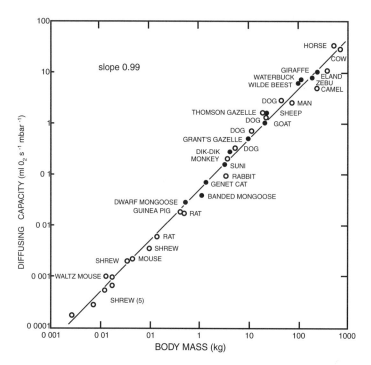

FIGURE 5.5 Allometric plot of pulmonary diffusing capacity to body mass for mammalian species. From Gehr et al., *J. Respir. Physiol.*, 44, 61, 1981.[5] With permission.

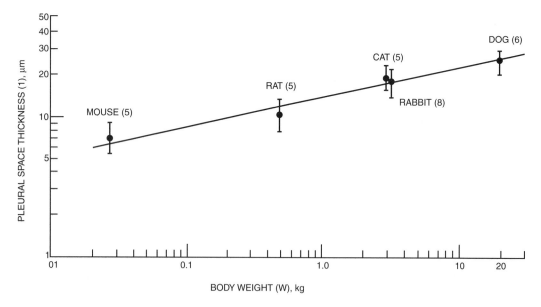

FIGURE 5.6 Pleural space thickness (t) vs. body weight (W) measured using light microscopy in five mammalian species. The power curve fit to the data was $t = 13.1\ W^{0.2}$. From Li-Fook et al., *J. Appl. Physiol.*, 59, 603, 1985.[7] With permission.

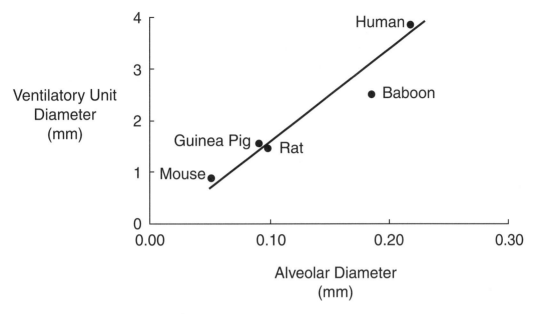

FIGURE 5.7 Mean alveolar diameter vs. mean ventilatory unit diameter. The alveolar diameters and corresponding ventilatory unit diameters from the lung of different species are shown. The lungs were preserved by vascular perfusion fixation at a lung volume near functional residual capacity. A remarkable similarity in lung structure across species is demonstrated by the fact that the ratio of ventilatory unit diameter to alveolar diameter is constant over the large range of lung sizes examined. The ventilatory unit averaged 17.5 alveolar diameters in size. From Pinkerton et al., *J. Appl. Physiol.,* 1993.[8] With permission

SECTION 3. CELLS IN THE RESPIRATORY TRACT

TABLE 5.13
Comparison of Abundance and Percentage of Cell Types in Tracheas of Seven Mammalian Species

Species	N	Total Nuclei	Percentage						
			Basal Cells	Ciliated Cells	Clara Cells	Mucous Goblet Cells	Serous Cells	Other Cells	Unidentified
Sheep	5	414.3[a] ± 33.2	28.5	30.6	0	5.1	0	35.9	0
Bonnet monkey	3	266.0 ± 12.0	31	41	0	8	0	16	4
Rhesus monkey	5	181.4 ± 50.7	42.0	32.9	0	16.8	0	4.3	4.0
Cat	3	273.0 ± 15.0	37.3	36.1	0	20.2	0	5.4	1.1
Rabbit	3	210.9 ± 29.7	28.2	43.00	17.6	1.3	0	0	9.4
Rat	3	147.9 ± 3.1	13.4	40.6	0	0.5	39.2	0	6.2
Hamster	3	151.4 ± 11.2	5.6	47.5	41.4	0	0	0	5.3

[a] Mean ±SD, number of nuclei per millimeter.

Source: Plopper, C.G., Mariassy, A.T., Wilson, D.W., Alley, J.L., Nishio, S.J., and Nettesheim, P., *Exp. Lung Res.,* 5, 281, 1983.[13]

From St. George, J.A., Harkema, J.R., Hyde, D.M., and Plopper, C.G., in *Toxicology of the Lung,* Raven Press, New York, 1993.[14] With permission.

TABLE 5.14
Density of Cells in the Bronchiolar
Epithelium of Adults

| | Cell Density/mm^{2a} | |
Species	All Cell Types	Noncillated Cells
Cat	19,532 ± 383	19,532 ± 383
Rat	18,813 ± 2,722	14,030 ± 3,373
Rabbit	15,073 ± 706	9,261 ± 434
Hamster	14,238 ± 2,794	8,489 ± 2,407
Mouse	9,759 ± 1,700	8,732 ± 2,200
Bonnet monkey	9,565 ± 304	8,800 ± 280

[a] Mean ±SD.

From St. George, J.A., Harkema, J.R., Hyde, D.M., and Plopper, C.G., in *Toxicology of the Lung*, Raven Press, New York, 1993.[14] With permission.

TABLE 5.15
Height μm of the Airway Epithelium in Adult Mammals from Various Reports

	Trachea		Bronchi					
	N	(Generation 0)	N	(Generation 1–2)	N	(Generation 4–6)	N	(Generation 7–11)
Primates								
Human	3	50–100; 43 ± 2	5	50–; 39–	—	—	—	—
Bonnet monkey	3	20 ± 7	3	21 ± 6	—	—	—	—
(*M. radiata*)								
Rhesus monkey	5	28 ± 5	5	19 ± 1	5	17 ± 1	5	13 ± 1
(*M. mullata*)								
Carnivores								
Dog	5	26 ± 4	—	20–50	—	—	—	—
Cat	5	20–24; 24±	—	—	—	—	—	—
Ferret	4	—	—	—	—	—	—	—
Perissodactyla								
Horse	3	48 ± 3	—	—	—	—	—	—
Artiodactyla								
Cow	5	60 ± 3	—	—	—	—	—	—
Sheep	5	41–57; 59 ± 7[a]	6	40 ± 3	8	32 ± 4[a]	6	30 ± 5[a]
Pig	5	46 ± 5	3	35–50	—	—	—	—
Rodentia								
Guinea pig	5	30 ± 3	—	15–30	—	—	—	—
Hamster	3	20 ± 0; 8–14	—	151 ± 11	5	20–	—	—
Rat	3	24 ± 1	20	13–	6	13–	—	—
Mouse	6	11–14	—	—	3	8–16	—	—
Lagomorpha								
Rabbit	—	21 ± 1	4	22 ± 3	6	9 ± 2	5	9 ± 1

[a] Insufflation fixed, epon-embedded Trachea (±SD).

From Mariassy, A.T., in *Treatise on Pulmonary Toxicology,* vol. 1, *Comparative Biology of the Normal Lung,* CRC Press, Boca Raton, FL, 1992.[15] With permission.

TABLE 5.16
Population Densities (% Cells) of the Tracheal Surface Epithelium in Adult Mammals and Juvenile Birds

	N	Cells/mm Basal Lamina	Basal	Ciliated	Mucous (Goblet)	Serous	Other[a]	Clara	Brush	Unidentified
							Epithelial Cells			
Primates										
Human	3	303 ± 20	33	49	9	0	9	0	—	—
Bonnet monkey (*Macaca radiata*)	3	266 ± 12	31	41	0	0	16 SMGC[b]	0	<1	4
Rhesus monkey (*Macaca mullata*)	5	181 ± 51	42	33	17	0	4 SMGC	0	<1	4
Carnivores										
Dog	5	—	—	—	—	—	—	—	—	—
Cat	5	273 ± 15	37	36	20	0	5	0	<1	1
Ferret	4	183–	25	54	22	0	—	0	Rare	—
Perissodactyla										
Horse	3	307 ± 23	31	46	5	0	18	0	—	—
Artiodactyla										
Cow	5	323 ± 24	31	42	4	0	23	0	<1	—
Sheep	5	414 ± 33	29	31	5	0	36 M3[c]	0	<1	0
Pig	5	303 ± 17	31	43	3	0	23	0	<1	—
Rodentia										
Guinea pig	5	307 ± 5	34	32	5	0	29	0	<0	—
Hamster	3	151 ± 11	6	48	0	0	0	41	<1	5
Rat	3	148 ± 3	13	41	1	39	0	0	1	6
Rat	5	168 ± 12	21	32	2	42	1	0	>1	1
Rat	—	142–	27	33	<1	27	13	0	—	—
Mouse	6	215–	10	39	<1	0	1	49	<1	—
Lagomorpha										
Rabbit	—	211 ± 30	28	43	1	0	0	18	Rare	9
Avia										
Goose	—	213–	33	50	12	<0.01	0	0	0	5

Note: ±S.D.

a Nonciliated cells, mostly eccrine.
b Small mucous granule cell.
c Mucous cell.

From Mariassy, A.T., in *Treatise on Pulmonary Toxicology*, vol. 1, *Comparative Biology of the Normal Lung*, CRC Press, Boca Raton, FL, 1992.[15] With permission.

TABLE 5.17
Population Densities (% Cells) of the Bronchial Surface Epithelium in Adult Mammals (Mainstem, Primary Bronchi)

	N	Cells/mm Basal Lamina	Basal	Ciliated	Mucous (Goblet)	Serous	Other[a]	Clara	Brush	Unidentified
Primates										
Human	5	—	6 ± 1	56 ± 10	26 ± 5	Scarce	31 ± 2	0	—	—
Bonnet monkey (*Macaca radial*)	3	210 ± 16	35	33	10	0	15 SMGC[b]	0	—	6
Rhesus monkey (*Macaca mullata*)	5	175 ± 46	32	44	15	0	5 SMGC	0	—	3
Carnivores										
Dog	—	—	—	—	—	—	—	—	—	—
Cat	—	—	—	—	—	—	—	—	—	—
Ferret	3	—	—	—	50/mm	—	20/mm	0	—	—
Perissodlactyla										
Horse	—	—	—	—	—	—	—	—	—	—
Artiodactyla										
Cow	—	—	—	—	—	—	—	—	—	—
Sheep	6	285 ± 24	18	48	4	0	30 M3[c]	0	<1	0
Pig	—	—	—	—	—	—	—	—	—	—
Rodentia										
Guinea pig	—	—	—	—	—	—	—	—	—	—
Hamster	6	—	22	49	4	0.2	8	15	Rare	1
Rat	20	126–	27	35	<1	21	16	0	—	—
Mouse	3	215–	4	47	1	0	2	46	<1	0
Lagomorpha										
Rabbit	4	194 ± 17	27	43	1	0	7	22	<1	—

Note: ±S.D.

[a] Nonciliated, mostly eccrine.
[b] Small mucous granule cell.
[c] Mucous cell.

From Mariassy, A.T., in *Treatise on Pulmonary Toxicology*, vol. 1, *Comparative Biology of the Normal Lung*., CRC Press, Boca Raton, FL, 1992.[15] With permission.

TABLE 5.18
Population Densities (% Cells) of the Bronchial Surface Epithelium in Adult Mammals (Lobar Bronchi, Generations 2–6)

	N	Cells/mm Basal Lamina	Epithelial Cells							
			Basal	Ciliated	Mucous (Goblet)	Serous	Other[a]	Clara	Brush	Unidentified
Primates										
Human	—	—	—	—	—	—	—	—	—	—
Bonnet monkey (*Macaca radiata*)	—	—	—	—	—	—	—	—	—	—
Rhesus monkey (*Macaca muilata*)	5	184 ± 49	32	47	15	0	5 SMGC[b]	0	—	2
Carnivores										
Dog	—	—	—	—	—	—	—	—	—	—
Cat	—	—	—	—	—	—	—	—	—	—
Ferret	—	—	—	—	—	—	—	—	—	—
Perissodactyla										
Horse	—	—	—	—	—	—	—	—	—	—
Artiodactyla										
Cow	—	—	—	—	—	—	—	—	—	—
Sheep	8	248 ± 23	19	39	12	0	30 M3[c]	0	<1	0
Pig	—	—	—	—	—	—	—	—	—	—
Rodentia										
Guinea pig	—	—	—	—	—	—	—	—	—	—
Hamster	5	179–	18	35	27	0	12	7	<1	1
Rat	6	116–	14	53	<1	20	12	0	Infrequent	
Mouse	3	199–	1	36	0	0	2	61	<1	<1
Lagomorpha										
Rabbit	6	114 ± 12	2	49	0	0	7	41	<1	—

Note: ±SD.

[a] Nonciliated, mostly eccrine.
[b] Small mucous granule cell.
[c] Mucous cell.

From Mariassy, A.T., in *Treatise on Pulmonary Toxicology*, vol. 1, *Comparative Biology of the Normal Lung*, CRC Press, Boca Raton, FL, 1992.[15] With permission.

TABLE 5.19
Population Densities (% Cells) of the Bronchial Surface Epithelium in Adult Mammals (Segmental Bronchi, Generations 7–11)

	N	Cells/mm Basal Lamina	Basal	Ciliated	Mucous (Goblet)	Serous	Other[a]	Clara	Brush	Unidentified
Primates										
Human	—	—	—	—	—	—	—	—	—	—
Bonnet monkey (*Macaca radiata*)	—	—	—	—	—	—	—	—	—	—
Rhesus monkey (*Macaca muilata*)	5	158 ± 15	29	49	14	0	3 SMGC[b]	0	—	2
Carnivores										
Dog	—	—	—	—	—	—	—	—	—	—
Cat	—	—	—	—	—	—	—	—	—	—
Ferret	—	—	—	—	—	—	—	—	—	—
Perissodactyla										
Horse	—	—	—	—	—	—	—	—	—	—
Artiodactyla										
Cow	—	—	—	—	—	—	—	—	—	—
Sheep	8	223 ± 17	18	43	8	0	31 M3[c]	0	<1	0
Pig	—	—	—	—	—	—	—	—	—	—
Rodentia										
Guinea pig	—	—	—	—	—	—	—	—	—	—
Hamster	—	—	—	—	—	—	—	—	—	—
Rat	—	—	—	—	—	—	—	—	—	—
Mouse	—	—	—	—	—	—	—	—	—	—
Lagomorpha										
Rabbit	5	147 ± 18	0	49	0	0	4	47	—	0

Note: ±SD.

a Nonciliated, mostly eccrine.
b Small mucous granule cell.
c Mucous cell.

From Mariassy, A.T., in *Treatise on Pulmonary Toxicology*, vol. 1, *Comparative Biology of the Normal Lung*, CRC Press, Boca Raton, FL, 1992.[15] With permission.

TABLE 5.20
Comparison of Species Differences in Microenvironment of Bronchiolar Cells: Centriacinar Organization and Tracheobronchial Distribution

| | Transitional or Respiratory Bronchiole | | Nonciliated Bronchiolar Cells Found in | |
Species	Extensive	Minimal	Trachea	Lobar Bronchus
Mouse		+	>50%	>60%
Hamster		+	>40%	>15%
Rat		+	0	0
Guinea pig		+	0	0
Rabbit		+	>15%	>25%
Dog	+		0	0
Cat	+		0	0
Ferret	+		0	0
Macaque monkey	+		0	0
Sheep	+	+	0	0
Pig		+	0	0
Horse		+	0	0
Cow		+	0	0
Human			0	0

From Plopper, C.G. and Hyde, D.M., in *Treatise on Pulmonary Toxicology,* vol. 1, *Comparative Biology of the Normal Lung,* CRC Press, Boca Raton, FL, 1992.[16] With permission.

TABLE 5.21
Comparison of Species Differences in Cellular Composition of Centriacinar Bronchiolar Epithelium

| | Cell Types in Terminal Bronchiole | | | | Cell Types in Respiratory Bronchiole | | | |
Species	Clara	Ciliated	Goblet	Basal	Clara	Ciliated	Goblet	Basal
Mouse	>50%	<50%	–	–	N/A	N/A	N/A	N/A
Hamster	>50%	<50%	–	–	N/A	N/A	N/A	N/A
Rat	>50%	<50%	–	–	N/A	N/A	N/A	N/A
Guinea pig	>50%	<50%	–	–	N/A	N/A	N/A	N/A
Rabbit	>50%	<50%	–	–	N/A	N/A	N/A	N/A
Dog	>95%	<5%	–	–	>95%	<5%	–	–
Cat	>95%	<5%	–	–	>95%	<5%	–	–
Macaque monkey	–	~50%	~20%	~10%	>90%	<10%	+	+
Sheep	>60%	<40%	–	–	N/A	N/A	N/A	N/A
Pig	+	+	–	–	N/A	N/A	N/A	N/A
Horse	>50%	>50%	–	–	N/A	N/A	N/A	N/A
Cow	>50%	<50%	–	–	N/A	N/A	N/A	N/A
Human	–	+	+	+	+	+	+	+

Note: N/A, not applicable; –, not present; +, present in variable amounts.

From Plopper, C.G., and Hyde, D.M., in *Treatise on Pulmonary Toxicology,* vol. 1, *Comparative Biology of the Normal Lung,* CRC Press, Boca Raton, FL, 1992.[16] With permission.

TABLE 5.22
Comparison of Numerical Density of Bronchiolar Epithelium and Density and Percentage of Clara Cells in Bronchiolar Epithelial Population of Adults

		Clara Cells	
Species	Bronchiolar Epithelium Density[a] (No./mm²)	Density[a] (No./mm²)	% of Population
Rat	17,070 ± 791	4,336 ± 201	25.4
Rabbit	15,073 ± 706	9,261 ± 434	61.4
Cat	19,532 ± 383	19,532 ± 383	100
Bonnet monkey	9,565 ± 304	8,800 ± 280	92

[a] Mean ±SD.

From Plopper, C.G. and Hyde, D.M., in *Treatise on Pulmonary Toxicology,* vol. 1, *Comparative Biology of the Normal Lung,* CRC Press, Boca Raton, FL, 1992.[16] With permission.

TABLE 5.23
Comparison of Relative Proportions (Percentages)[a] of Cellular Components in Clara Cells

Species	Nucleus	Agranular Endoplasmic Reticulum	Secretory Granules	Cytoplasmic Glycogen	Mitochondria	Large Mitochondria	Lateral Cytoplasmic Extensions
Mouse	21.8 ± 6.5	54.8 ± 7.5	+	0	34.7 ± 6.4	+	+
Hamster	25.2 ± 6.1	79.3 ± 7.6	+	0	10.7 ± 4.4	−	+
Rat	28.5 ± 10.4	66.2 ± 9.4	+	0.1 ± 0.4	16.3 ± 6.0	+	+
Guinea pig	28.6 ± 8.9	58.3 ± 9.0	+	0 ± 8.5	25.1	+	+
Rabbit	23.8 ± 8.8	61.6 ± 5.4	+	7.0 ± 5.4	19.1 ± 7.6	+	+
Dog	23.4 ± 11.4	24.7 ± 8.6	+	57.1 ± 13.7	8.0 ± 6.7	−	+
Cat	26.7 ± 9.2	10.7 ± 6.7	−	61.3 ± 10.1	19.5 ± 9.6	+	+
Macaque monkey	28.6 ± 4.4	5.2 ± 3.3	+	0	14.1 ± 2.8	−	+
Sheep	26.6 ± 10.3	64.6 ± 18.3	+	6.8 ± 12.1	13.8 ± 8.8	−	+
Pig	?	?	+	?	?	+	+
Horse	8.6 ± 4.1	70.6 ± 4.5	+	0	10.6 ± 4.4	−	+
Cow	27.7 ± 10.1	21.9 ± 10.1	+	62.3 ± 11.5	12.0 ± 7.5	−	+
Human	41.9 ± 10.0	3.1 ± 3.5	+	4.6 ± 5.8	15.3 ± 6.6	−	+

[a] As percent of cytoplasmic volume; mean ±SD; + = as present; − = not present.

From Plopper, C.G. and Hyde, D.M., in *Treatise on Pulmonary Toxicology,* vol. 1, *Comparative Biology of the Normal Lung,* CRC Press, Boca Raton, FL, 1992.[16] With permission.

TABLE 5.24
Characteristics of Cells from the Alveolar Region of Normal Mammalian Lungs[†]

	Fischer-344 Rat	Sprague-Dawley Rat	Dog	Baboon	Human
Total number of cells/lung, 10^9	0.67 ± 0.02^a	0.89 ± 0.04^a	114 ± 13^b	99 ± 9^b	230 ± 25
Total lung cells, %					
Alveolar type I	8.1 ± 0.3^a	8.9 ± 0.9^a	12.5 ± 1.7^b	11.8 ± 0.6^b	8.3 ± 0.6^a
Alveolar type II	12.1 ± 0.7^a	14.2 ± 0.7^{ab}	11.8 ± 0.6^a	7.7 ± 1.0	15.9 ± 0.8^b
Endothelial	51.1 ± 1.7^a	42.2 ± 1.1^a	45.7 ± 0.8^a	36.3 ± 2.4	30.2 ± 2.4
Interstitial	24.4 ± 0.7^a	27.7 ± 1.8^a	26.6 ± 0.7^a	41.8 ± 2.7	36.1 ± 1.0
Macrophage	4.3 ± 1.0^a	3.0 ± 0.3^a	3.4 ± 0.6^a	2.3 ± 0.7^a	9.4 ± 2.2
Alveolar surface covered, %					
Alveolar type I	96.4 ± 0.5^a	96.2 ± 0.5^a	97.3 ± 0.4^a	96.0 ± 0.6^a	92.9 ± 1.0
Alveolar type II	3.6 ± 0.3^a	3.8 ± 0.5^a	2.7 ± 1.0^a	4.0 ± 0.6^a	7.1 ± 1.0^a
Average cell volume, μm^3					
Alveolar type I	1530 ± 121^a	2042 ± 374^a	1196 ± 88^a	1224 ± 136^a	1764 ± 155
Alveolar type II	455 ± 108^a	443 ± 80^a	428 ± 37^a	539 ± 184^a	889 ± 101
Endothelial	275 ± 25^a	387 ± 30^a	343 ± 19^a	365 ± 61^a	632 ± 64
Interstitial	427 ± 55^a	331 ± 67^{ab}	440 ± 47^a	227 ± 30^b	637 ± 26
Macrophage	639 ± 131^a	1058 ± 257^a	654 ± 116^a	1059 ± 287^a	2492 ± 167
Average cell surface area, μm^2					
Alveolar type I	7287 ± 755^b	5320 ± 694^{ab}	3794 ± 487^a	4004 ± 383^a	5098 ± 659^a
Alveolar type II	185 ± 56^{ab}	123 ± 20^a	107 ± 15^a	285 ± 85^b	183 ± 14^{ab}
Endothelial	1121 ± 95^a	1105 ± 72^a	1137 ± 127^a	1040 ± 209^a	1353 ± 67^a

[†] All data are mean ±SEM. For comparisons between species, letter subscripts (a, b) indicate those values that are not different from other values having the same letter subscript.

Note: Modified from Crapo et al. (1983).[10]

From Pinkerton, K.E., Gehr, P., and Crapo, J.D., in *Treatise on Pulmonary Toxicology,* vol. 1, *Comparative Biology of the Normal Lung,* CRC Press, Boca Raton, FL, 1992.[3] With permission.

TABLE 5.25
Summary of Experimentally Determined Turnover Times for Selected Cells of Respiratory Tracts of Rats and Mice

	Turnover time (days)	
Tissue	Rat	Mouse
Tracheal epithelium	7–48	2–20
Bronchial epithelium	8–27	2–21
Bronchiolar epithelium	—	10–59
Alveolar epithelium	29	28–35
Alveolar macrophage	8–35	6–21

From Snipes, M.B., *Crit. Rev. Toxicol.,* 20, 174, 1989.[18] With permission.

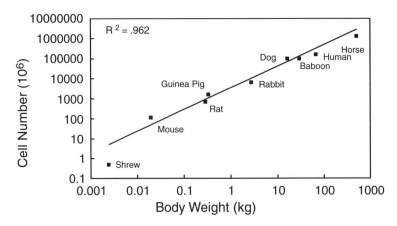

FIGURE 5.8 Allometric relationship for alveolar cells. On a log/log scale, the total number of alveolar cells within a species increases proportionally with body weight. For total number of lung cells, the slope is near 1 (0.95 ± 0.05) and statistically significant (*P* < .0001). A similar relationship holds for epithelial type I, epithelial type II, and interstitial and endothelial cells. A larger lung is therefore composed of more cells, not necessarily larger cells. From Stone et al., *Am. J. Respir. Cell. Mol. Biol.,* 6, 235, 1992.[17] With permission.

SECTION 4. PULMONARY FUNCTION

TABLE 5.26
Allometry of Pulmonary Diffusing Capacity

Taxon	Method	Intercept	Slope	N	M_b Range
DL_{co} ml [STPD] CO · min⁻¹ · torr⁻¹; Pulmonary Diffusing Capacity for CO (Physiologic)					
Mammals	—	0.22	1.14	—	—
Mammals	—	0.614	0.985		0.025–500
Canids	sb	0.592	1.275	4	4.6–27.6
Laboratory mammals	sb	0.4680	0.74	4	0.040–3.50
Dog (*Canis familiaris*)	sb	1.67	0.79	1	7.3–63
Rabbit (*Oryctolagus cuniculus*)	sb	0.4074	0.92	1	1.30–3.50
Guinea pig (*Cavia porcellus*)	sb	0.4571	0.74	1	0.250–1.000
Rat (*Rattus norvegicus*)	sb	0.4467	0.75	1	0.050–0.400
Hamster (*Mesocricetus auratus*)	sb	0.7943	0.91	1	0.040–0.120
Mouse (*Mus musculus*)	rb	0.00106	0.971	1	0.020–0.039
Mammals		0.16	1.18	—	—
Mammals		3.92	0.991	33	0.003–700
Mammals		6.49	0.962	47	0.003–700
Canids		1.92	1.25	4	4.6–27.6
Dog (*C. familiaris*)		6.56	1.00	1	2.65–57
Bats		6.25	0.932	5	0.005–0.173

Note: Allometry of pulmonary diffusing capacity for carbon monoxide (DL_{co}, physiologic) and oxygen (DL_{O2}, morphometric); both are in ml [STPD] · min⁻¹ · torr⁻¹. DL is related to body mass (M_b in kg) by the function: $D_L = a \cdot M_b^b$, where *a* is the intercept of the log-transformed linear regression, and *b* is the slope of the log-transformed linear regression. Method indicates if DL_{co} was determined by the single-breath (sb) or rebreathing (rb) technique. *N* is the number of species. In some cases, regression equations were calculated from data given in the reference. Units have been converted for equivalence, where necessary.

From Jones, J.H. and Longworth, K.E., in *Treatise on Pulmonary Toxicology,* vol. 1, *Comparative Biology of the Normal Lung,* CRC Press, Boca Raton, FL, 1992.[6] With permission.

TABLE 5.27
Allometry of O_2 Consumption and Flux

Taxon	Status	Intercept	Slope	N	M_b Range
Mammals + 7 birds	Basal	10.2	0.734	19	0.016–3.833
Mammals	Rest	10.7	0.739	10	0.173–679
Mammals	Rest	11.6	0.76	—	—
Mammals	Std	9.8	0.756	12	0.021–600
Small mammals	Std	9.13	0.727	56	0.003–3.71
Fossorial mammals	Basal	5.62	0.557	16	0.021–0.63
Monotremes	Rest	4.72	0.79	6	0.73–4.9
Dasyurid marsupials	Basal	6.75	0.74	12	0.008–5.05
Marsupials	Std	6.94	0.737	8	0.014–32.49
Marsupials	Rest	14.4	0.74	29	0.01–5.1
Insectivores (>25 g)	Rest	21.4	0.73	12	0.03–0.89
Chiropterans	Rest	18.8	0.73	17	0.005–0.59
Edentates	Rest	14.6	0.77	12	1.6–4.7
Lagomorphs	Rest	23.7	0.72	11	0.07–5.9
Rodents	Rest	24.9	0.69	133	0.007–0.96
Higher primates	Rest	37.6	0.73	10	0.23–71
Carnivores	Rest	30.0	0.73	24	0.17–26
Artiodactyls and perissodactyls	Rest	34.6	0.73	19	13–665
Mammals	Max	100	0.845	45	0.007–677
Mammals	Max	107	0.854	19	0.020–469
Mammals	Max	128	0.856	33	0.007–469
Mammals	Max	115	0.809	22	0.007–263
Canids	Max	219	0.905	4	4.6–27.6
Mammals	Max	54.0	0.678	14	0.003–2.54
Mammals	Max	67.5	0.73	4	0.033–0.841

Note: Allometry of oxygen consumption and flux through the respiratory system (V_{O2} ml [STPD] $O_2 \cdot min^{-1}$) under resting (rest), basal (basal), standard (std), and maximal (max) conditions. V_{O2} is related to body mass (M_b in kg) by the function. $V_{O2} = a \cdot M_b^b$, where a is the intercept of the log-transformed linear regression, and b is the slope of the log-transformed linear regression. N is the number of species. In some cases, regression equations were calculated from data given in the reference. Units have been converted for equivalence, where necessary.

From Jones, J.H. and Longworth, K.E., in *Treatise on Pulmonary Toxicology,* vol. 1, *Comparative Biology of the Normal Lung,* CRC Press, Boca Raton, FL, 1992.[6] With permission.

TABLE 5.28
Allometry of Blood Variables

Taxon	Intercept	Slope	N	M_b Range
Blood Volume ($cm^3 \cdot kg^{-1}$)				
Eutherians	65.6	1.02	—	—
Mammals	76	1.0	97	$0.01–10^3$
Hematocrit (%)				
Mammals	45.8	–0.01	123	—
Oxygen Half-Saturation Pressure (P_{90}, torr)				
Eutherians and marsupials	39.4	–0.03	89	
Marsupials	32.1	–0.074	7	—
Small mammals	50.3	–0.054	17	0.021–6.35
Bohr Effect (Δlog P_{90}/ΔpH)				
Mammals (hemoglobin solution)	0.76	–0.0596	10	0.03–3140
Erythrocyte Carbonic Anhydrase (U/μl erythrocyte* or U/100 μg hemoglobin)**				
Mammals*	1.146	–0.107	15	0.006–601
Mammals**	0.695	–0.107	13	0.025–4000

Note: Variables are related to body mass (M_b, in kg) by the function: $Y = a \cdot M_b^b$ where Y is the variable, a is the intercept of the log-transformed linear regression, and b is the slope of the log-transformed linear regression. N is the number of species. In some cases, regression equations were calculated from data given in the reference. Units have been converted for equivalence, where necessary.

From Jones, J.H. and Longworth, K.E., in *Treatise on Pulmonary Toxicology,* vol. 1, *Comparative Biology of the Normal Lung,* CRC Press, Boca Raton, FL, 1992.[6] With permission.

TABLE 5.29
Values of Standard (Basal) Oxygen Consumption for Representative Mammalian Species of Different Body Mass

Species	M_b (kg)	V_{O2} std (ml [STPD]$O_2 \cdot S^{-1}$ kg^{-1})
Horse (*Equus caballus*)	703	0.040
Ox (*Bos taurus*)	700	0.031
Pig (*Sus scrofa*)	122	0.048
Human (*Homo sapiens*)	71.5	0.058
Sheep (*Ovis aries*)	51.5	0.071
Goat (*Capra hircus*)	36	0.054
Dog (*Canis familiaris*)	13.2	0.026
Rabbit (*Oryctolagus cuniculus*)	4	0.183
Rhesus monkey (*Macaca mulatta*)	3.2	0.034
Cat (*Felis catus*)	3	0.122
Guinea pig (*Cavia porcellus*)	0.900	0.230
Rat (*Rattus norvegicus*)	0.375	0.247
Hamster (*Mesocricetus auratus*)	0.115	0.278
Gerbil (*Meriones unguiculatus*)	0.090	0.389
Mouse (*Mus musculus*)	0.030	0.528

From Jones, J.H. and Longworth, K.E., in *Treatise On Pulmonary Toxicology,* vol. 1, *Comparative Biology of the Normal Lung,* CRC Press, Boca Raton, FL, 1992.[6] With permission.

TABLE 5.30
Allometric Equations for Respiratory Variables in
Mammals ($Y = aM^b$; M = mass in kg)

Variable (Y)	Coefficient (a)	Exponent(b)
Tidal volume (ml)	7.69	1.04
Dead space volume (ml)	2.8	0.96
	—	1.05
Lung volume	—	1.02
Total lung capacity (ml)	53.5	1.06
Vital capacity (ml)	56.7	1.03
Functional residual cap (ml)	24.1	1.13
Wet lung wt (g)	11.3	0.99
	7.72	1.03
Lung compliance (ml/cm H_2O)	2.10	1.08
Inflationary	1.94	1.08
Deflationary PoMax[a]20	3.09	1.15
Deflationary PoMax[a]8	2.2	1.09
Chest wall compliance	4.52	0.86
Inflationary	5.59	1.2
Deflationary PoMax 20	4.61	1.07
Deflationary PoMax 8	4.9	1.16
Respiratory system comp.	1.56	1.04
Inflationary	1.34	1.1
Deflationary PoMax 20	1.8	1.11
Deflationary PoMax 8	1.56	1.06
Ventilation (ml/min)	379	0.8
Oxygen consumption (V_{O2})(ml/min)	11.6	0.76
Oxygen consumption (V_{O2}) (ml/s)	0.188	0.75
V_{O2} Max (ml/s)	1.92	0.809
V_t/T_t(inspiratory flow)(ml/s)	13.5	0.74
Resistance (raw) (cm H_2O/L/s)	24.4	−0.70
Resistance (raw) (cm H_2O/ml/s)	0.078	−0.819
Reciprocal time const. (s^{-1})	8.97	−0.298
Upper airway R (cm H_2O/ml/s)	0.056	−0.702
Rec. time const. law + uaw[b]	5.272	−0.326
Frequency (min^{-1})	53.5	−0.26
	—	0.28

[a] PoMax = maximum airway pressure.

[b] law = lower airways; uaw = upper airways.

From Boggs, D.F., in *Treatise on Pulmonary Toxicology*, vol. 1, *Comparative Biology of the Normal Lung*, CRC Press, Boca Raton, FL, 1992.[19]
With permission.

TABLE 5.31
Maximal Oxygen Consumption for Mammals

Species	M_b (kg)	V_{O2max} (ml [STPD] $O_2 \cdot s^{-1} \cdot kg^{-1}$)
Horse, thoroughbred (*Equus caballus*)	466	2.76
Horse, standardbred (*E. caballus*)	453	2.23
Ox, steer (*Bos taurus*)	449	0.85
Eland (*Taurotragus oryx*)	240	0.60
Zebu ox (*Bos indicus*)	232	0.49
Pony (*E. caballus*)	171	1.48
Hereford calf (*B. taurus*)	141	0.61
Waterbuck (*Kobus deffassa*)	109.8	0.79
Pony (*E. caballus*)	105.0	1.61
Wildebeest (*Connochaetes taurinus*)	102.0	0.73
Human, untrained (*Homo sapiens*)	69.8	0.81
Human, trained (*H. sapiens*)	63.9	1.18
Goat (*Capra hircus*)	30.0	0.95
Lion (*Panthera leo*)	30.0	1.00
Dog (*Canis familiaris*)	28.0	2.29
Wolf (*Canio lupus*)	27.6	2.60
Dog (*C. familiaris*)	25.3	2.67
African sheep (*Ovis aries*)	21.8	0.78
Dog (*C. familiaris*)	21.0	2.64
African goat (*Capra hircus*)	20.9	0.87
Pig (*Sus scrofa*)	18.5	1.56
Coyote (*Canis latrans*)	12.4	3.10
Grant's gazelle (*Gazella granti*)	10.1	0.89
Red fox (*Vulpes vulpes*)	4.61	2.89
Blue fox (*Alopex lagopus*)	4.40	3.62
Dik-dik (*Madoqua kirkii*)	4.2	0.91
Spring hares (*Pedetes capensis*)	3.00	1.62
Genet cat (*Genetta tirina*)	1.4	1.8
Banded mongoose (*Mungos mungo*)	1.14	1.9
Rat kangaroo (*Bettongia penicillata*)	1.10	2.95
Guinea pig (*Cavia porcellus*)	0.841	1.12
Dwarf mongoose (*Helogale pervula*)	0.58	2.1
White rat (*Rattus norvegicus*)	0.376	1.51
White rat, untrained (*R. norvegicus*)	—	1.21
White rat, trained (*R. norvegicus*)	—	1.56
White rat (*R. norvegicus*)	0.205	1.61
Hamster (*Mesocricetus auratus*)	0.100	1.97
Chipmunk (*Tamias striatus*)	0.0902	3.97
Merriam's chipmunk (*Eutamias merriami*)	0.075	1.96
Lemming (*Dicrostonyx groenlandicus*)	0.061	2.05
Mouse (*Mus musculus*)	0.033	2.89
Deer mouse (*Peromyscus maniculatus*)	—	2.95
European woodmouse (*Apodemus sylvaticus*)	0.020	4.4
Pygmy mouse (*Baiomys taylori*)	0.0072	4.36

Note: Values of maximal oxygen consumption for mammals of different body mass measured with animals running on a motorized treadmill.

From Jones, J.H. and Longworth, K.E., in *Treatise on Pulmonary Toxicology*, vol. 1, *Comparative Biology of the Normal Lung*, CRC Press, Boca Raton, FL, 1992.[6] With permission.

TABLE 5.32
Blood Respiratory Variables

Species	M_b (kg)	$[Hb]$ (g·dl^{-1})	HCT (%)	O_2 capacity (ml [STPD] O_2·dl^{-1})	P_{50} (torr)	Bohr Effect ($\Delta\log P_{50}/\Delta pH$)	Haldane Effect (ml [STPD] CO_2 dl^{-1})	Temperature Coefficient ($\Delta\log P_{50}/\Delta T$)
African elephant (*Loxodonia africana a.*)	2000	15.3	42.7	20.5	23.2	−0.351	5.5	0.023
Asian elephant (*Elephas maximus*)	1400	14.9	42	20.0	25.2	−0.351	5.5	0.023
White rhinoceros (*Cerathotherium sinum*)					20	−0.62		
Ox (*Bos taurus*)		11.5	40		31.5	−0.49		
Horse (*Equus caballus*)		11.1	33.4		25.1	−0.45		
Camel (*Camelus dromedarus*)		9.41	22.1	12.6	25.9			
Tapir (*Tapirus terrestris*)					26.5	−0.58		
Man (*Homo sapiens*)	67.0		44.8		24	−0.47	8.4	0.024
Bladdernose seal (*Cystophora cristata*)	50	26.4	63	36	28.3	−0.66		
Pronghorn antelope (*Antilocapra americana*)	38.4	16.8	42.7	22.5	24.4	−0.55		
Orangutan, juvenile (*Pongo pygmaeus*)	34.6	12.9	40.9	17.4	32.0	−0.49		
Sheep (*Ovis aries*)	33.0		35.0		26.7			
Chimpanzee (*Pan troglodytes*)	30.4	13.5	41.2	17.3	35.7	−0.462	4.7	
Pig (*Sus scrofa*)	30				29.3	−0.441		0.016
Goat (*Capra hircus*)	25.0		34.0		29.3	−0.48		
Dog (*Canis familiaris*)	20.0		40.0		29.0	−0.48		0.022
Gorilla, juvenile (*Gorilla gorillo*)	16.5	12.3	42.0	16.4	25.4	−0.48		
Kangaroo (*Macropus giganteus*)	15	18.6	53.0	24.9	27.5	−0.54		
Wallaby (*Macropus eugenii*)					32			
Baboons (*Papio anubis*)	10.36	11.7	37.1	15.4	37.2	−0.550	4.7	
Pigtail monkey (*Macaca nemestrina*)	9.50	12.6	42.0	16.6	36.7	−0.520	4.5	
Tasmanian devil (*Sarcophilus harrisii*)	8	20.1	47.0	26.9	41.2	−0.47		
Woodchuck (*Marmot monax*)	4.45	13.5	39.4		27.8	−0.72		
Rhesus monkey (*Macaca mulatta*)	3.94	12.9	41.5	16.9	35.2	−0.518	4.4	
Armadillo (*Dasypus novemcinctus*)	3.9	11.1	31	14.8	23.3	−0.55		
Pangolin (*Manis pentadactyla*)	3.6		36.5		25	−0.51		
Opossum (*Didelphis virginianis*)	3.40		31.5		38.7	−0.49		
Rabbit (*Oryctolagus cuniculus*)	3.10		35.0		30.0	−0.43		

TABLE 5.32 (*Continued*)
Blood Respiratory Variables

Species	M_b (kg)	[Hb] (g · dl⁻¹)	HCT (%)	O₂ capacity (ml [STPD] O₂ · dl⁻¹)	P_{50} (torr)	Bohr Effect (Δlog P_{50}/ΔpH)	Haldane Effect (ml [STPD] CO₂ dl⁻¹)	Temperature Coefficient (Δlog P_{50}/ΔT)
Cat (*Felis domesticus*)	2.64		42		35.0	−0.50		0.014
Echidna (*Tachyglossus setosus*)	2.1	17.6	48	21.9	21.3	−0.49		0.014
Platypus (*Ornithorynchus anatinus*)	1.8	18.3	52	22.7	27.2	−0.56		
Prairie dog (*Cynomys ludociciana*)	1.28	15.1	47.3		22			
Muskrat (*Ondatra zibethica*)	0.97	13.3	36.2		26.1	−0.66		
Squirrel monkey (*Saimiri sciureus*)	0.95	14.3	42.0	17.7	35.5	−0.542	4.5	0.017
Hedgehog (*Erinaceus europaeus*)	0.820		47.0	19.0	36	−0.49		
Guinea pig (*Cavia porcellus*)	0.669		41.1		26.7	−0.48		
Ground squirrel (*Spermophilus beecheyi*)	0.598	15.1	48.7		26			
White rat (*Rattus norvegicus*)	0.555		41.9		36.0	−0.52		
Guinea pig (*Cavia porcellus*)	0.291	12.6			25.3			
Mole rat (*Spaiax ehrenbergi*)	0.196	15.0	45.6		29.5	−0.53		
Bat (*Rousettus aegyptiacus*)	0.146	20.0	55		30.8	−0.55		
Golden hamster (*Mesocricetus auratus*)	0.135		42.4		26.0	−0.44		
Pocket gopher (*Thomomys bottae*)	0.135	17.1	46		33.3	−0.61		
Naked mole rat (*Heterocephalus glaber*)	0.106	13.6	46		23.3	−0.43		
Gerbil (*Meriones unguiculatus*)	0.078		31.2		28.5	−0.51		
Mouse (*Mus musculus*)	0.029		36.4		34.7	−0.50		
Bat (*Pipistrellus pipistrellus*)	0.005	24.4	61.5		36.6	−0.47		
Mole (*Talpa europa*)			47.2	22.4	24	−0.47		
Shrew (*Crocidura russula*)			35.5	21.7	37	−0.63		

Note: Body mass is M_b; hemoglobin concentration, [Hbl]; hematocrit, Hct; O₂ carrying capacity of the blood, O₂ capacity; oxygen half-saturation pressure, P_{50}, and oxygen equilibrium curve, temperature coefficient.

From Jones, J.H. and Longworth, K.E., in *Treatise on Pulmonary Toxicology*, vol. 1, *Comparative Biology of the Normal Lung*, CRC Press, Boca Raton, FL, 1992.[6] With permission.

TABLE 5.33
Normal Values of Blood Gases and Blood Buffering

Species	Body Weight (kg)	T_B (°C)	Pa_{CO_2} (torr)	pHa	Pa_{O_2} (torr)	HCO_3^- (mEq/L)	$\dfrac{\Delta \log Pa_{CO_2}}{\Delta pH}$
Mice	0.028	37.5	20.1			12.3	−1.75
Gerbil	0.078	36.4	31.2			19.0	−1.45
Hamster	0.135	35.8	45.1			27.5	−1.53
Rat	0.555	37.6	40.7	7.426	83.5	24.9	−1.48
Rat	0.531		33.1	7.425	87.1		
Rat	0.297		39.8	7.467	91	28.7	
Guinea pig	0.669	37.8	40.2	7.395	90	23.5	−1.43
Cat	2.64	38.8	29.4	7.384	102	18	−1.39
Cat		38.9	32.5	7.426	108	21	
Rabbit	3.1	38.8	32.8	7.388	86	21	
Porcupine	5.87	37.8	34.6	7.383	95	23	−1.35
Coatimundi	6	37.6	23.4	7.411	99	15	
Baboon	8–11		37.6	7.388	106		
Mini-pig	11–19		47	7.432	94.3	30.5	
Dog	20	38.3	41.6	7.386	93	23.2	−1.53
Goat	25	39	41.0	7.40	94.6	25.7	−1.30
Sheep	33	39	40.9	7.44	96	27.6	−1.35
Sheep	32–37	40	40.2	7.46	107		
Calf	45–73		38.7	7.340	85.7	20.6	
Calf			47.3	7.41	92	29	
Man	67	37	40.5	7.38	93	23.3	−1.55
Pony	176–204	38	39.6	7.429	90	25.6	
Horse	387–543			7.408		25.8	
Burrowers and Hibernators							
Pocket gopher			45	7.381		28.1	−2.67
Syrian hamster	0.142		52.3	7.419	70.9		
Hamster (*Cricetus*)		37	45.3	7.40		28.2	
Ground squirrels (13-lined)		38	55.9	7.44		36.8	
			47.7	7.4	65		
			52.4	7.418	75.3	33	
Echidna	3.4		53	7.429	60.5	33	
Woodchuck	4.5	37.3	48	7.357	72	25.7	−1.29

From Boggs, D.F., in *Treatise on Pulmonary Toxicology*, vol. 1, *Comparative Biology of the Normal Lung*, CRC Press, Boca Raton, FL, 1992.[19] With permission.

TABLE 5.34
Body Weight and Lung Volumes in Fischer-344 Rats at Various Ages[a]

Parameter	3 Months	18 Months	27 Months
Body weight (g)	222 ± 61	334 ± 106	332 ± 71
Total lung capacity (TLC) (ml)	11.9 ± 1.7	13.9 ± 2.2	14.4 ± 1.9
TLC/body weight (ml/kg)	56 ± 8	42 ± 7	43 ± 6
Vital capacity (ml)	11.0 ± 1.8	13.4 ± 2.3	13.4 ± 1.7
Functional residual capacity (ml)	2.1 ± 0.3	1.7 ± 0.3	2.7 ± 0.4
Residual volume (RV) (ml)	1.0 ± 0.3	0.6 ± 0.2	1.1 ± 0.5
RV/TLC, (ml/ml)	0.08 ± 0.03	0.04 ± 0.01	0.07 ± 0.03

[a] Values are means ±SD.

Adapted from Mauderly (1982).[20] From Sahebjami, H., in *Treatise on Pulmonary Toxicology*, vol. 1, *Comparative Biology of the Normal Lung*, CRC Press, Boca Raton, FL, 1992.[21] With permission.

TABLE 3.35
Body Weight and Lung Volumes in Adult and Older Hamsters[a]

Parameter	15 Weeks	65 Weeks	P Value
Body weight (g)	126 ± 12	125 ± 7	>0.20
Total lung capacity (ml)	9.6 ± 1.3	11.1 ± 1.0	<0.02
Vital capacity (ml)	6.9 ± 1.0	7.8 ± 0.9	<0.10
Functional residual capacity (ml)	3.5 ± 0.5	4.3 ± 0.3	<0.05
Residual volume (RV) (ml)	2.7 ± 0.60	3.3 ± 0.3	<0.05
RV/TLC (%)	28 ± 5	30 ± 5	>0.20

[a] Values are means ±SD.

Adapted from Mauderly (1979).[22] From Sahebjami, H., in *Treatise on Pulmonary Toxicology,* vol. II, *Comparative Biology of the Normal Lung,* CRC Press, Boca Raton, FL, 1992.[21] With permission.

TABLE 5.36
Ventilatory Parameters in Fischer-344 Rats of Various Ages[a]

Parameter	3 months	18 months	27 months
Respiratory frequency (breath/min)	48 ± 6	54 ± 7	54 ± 6
Tidal volume (ml)	1.1 ± 0.3	1.5 ± 0.3	1.5 ± 0.3
Minute ventilation ($\dot{V_e}$) (ml/min)	54 ± 14	82 ± 23	82 ± 18
$\dot{V_e}$, body weight (ml/min/kg)	254 ± 48	251 ± 45	252 ± 52

[a] Values are means ±SD.

Adapted from Mauderly (1982).[20] From Sahebjami, H., in *Treatise on Pulmonary Toxicology,* vol. 1, *Comparative Biology of the Normal Lung,* CRC Press, Boca Raton, FL, 1992.[21] With permission.

TABLE 5.37
Ventilatory Parameters in Hamsters at Various Ages[a]

Parameter	15 weeks	65 weeks
Respiratory frequency (breath/min)	24 ± 2.7	25 ± 3.9
Tidal volume (ml)	1.2 ± 0.2	1.1 ± 0.2
Minute volume (ml/min)	27.8 ± 3.3	28.1 ± 4.0

[a] Values are means ±SD.

Adapted from Mauderly (1979).[22] From Sahebjami, H., in *Treatise on Pulmonary Toxicology,* vol. 1, *Comparative Biology of the Normal Lung,* CRC Press, Boca Raton, FL, 1992.[21] With permission.

TABLE 5.38
The Lung Volumes (% TLC)[a] at Transpulmonary Pressures of 10 (V_{10})
and 5 cm H_2O (V_5) for Various Young Adult Mammals

Species	(% TLC) V_{10}	V_5	Conditions
Sci whale	68	45	Excised, room temperature, peak P_L = 25 cm H_2O
Horse	86	66	*In vivo,* anesthetized, body temperature, peak P_L = 30 cm H_2O
Humans	63	53	*In vivo,* body temperature, sitting, peak P_L = 35 cm H_2O
Sheep	78	66	*In vivo,* anesthetized, body temperature, peak P_L = 30 cm H_2O
Goat	81	51	Excised, room temperature, peak P_L = 35 cm H_2O
Dog	77	61	*In vivo,* anesthetized, body temperature, peak P_L = 30 cm H_2O
Monkey	93	82	*In vivo,* anesthetized, body temperature, peak P_L = 30 cm H_2O
Cat	93	71	Excised, room temperature, peak P_L = 23 cm H_2O
Rabbit	84	70	Excised, room temperature, peak P_L = 30 cm H_2O
Guinea pig	79	56	*In vivo,* anesthetized, body temperature, peak P_L = 28 cm H_2O
Rat	80	52	*In vivo,* anesthetized, body temperature, peak P_L = 25 cm H_2O
Hamster	84	64	*In vivo,* anesthetized, body temperature, peak P_L = 25 cm H_2O
White mouse	81	61	*In vivo,* anesthetized, body temperature, peak P_L = 38 cm H_2O

[a] TLC = total lung capacity.

From Lai, Y-L, in *Treatise on Pulmonary Toxicology,* vol. 1, *Comparative Biology of the Normal Lung,* CRC Press, Boca Raton, FL, 1992.[23] With permission.

TABLE 5.39
Morphometric Values in Sprague-Dawley Rats of
Various Ages[a]

Parameter	4 Months	8 Months	18 Months
V_L body weight (ml/kg)[b]	21.7 ± 1.0	30.9 ± 1.5	38.4 ± 2.8
Lm (μm)[b]	54 ± 2	71 ± 2	87 ± 7
ISA (cm²)	5.571 ± 445[c]	7.979 ± 318	8.733 ± 721

[a] Values are means ±SEM. V_L postfixation lung volume; Lm. mean chord length; ISA, internal surface area.

[b] Significantly different among groups.

[c] Significantly different compared with other groups.

Adapted from Johanson and Pierce (1973).[24] From Sahebjami, H., in *Treatise on Pulmonary Toxicology,* vol. 1, *Comparative Biology of the Normal Lung,* CRC Press, Boca Raton, FL, 1992.[21] With permission. All rights reserved.

SECTION 5. BRONCHOALVEOLAR LAVAGE FLUID (BALF)

TABLE 5.40
Normal Cytology of BALF (% of Total Cells)[a]

Animal	Macrophages	Neutro	EOS	Lymph
Rat, mouse, rabbit, Syrian hamster	95	<1	<1	<1
Guinea pig	90	—	10	—
Rabbit	95	<1	<1	4
Dog	85	5	5	5
Sheep	70	5	5	15
Horse	83	5	< 1	10
Monkey	89	—	—	10
Human (nonsmoker)	88	<1	<1	10

[a] Abbreviations: BALF = bronchoalveolar lavage fluid; Neutro = neutrophil; EOS = eosinophils; Lymph = lymphocytes.

From *Concepts in Inhalation Toxicology,* R.F. Henderson, Hemisphere Publishing, Taylor & Francis, Washington, D.C., 1989, p. 422.[25] Reproduced with permission. All rights reserved.

TABLE 5.41
Normal Biochemical Content of BALF, $\bar{X}$(SE)[a]

Animal	n	LDH (mIU/ml)	Alkaline Phosphatase (mIU/ml)	Acid Phosphatase (mIU/ml)	β-Glucuronidase (mIU/ml)	Protein (mg/ml)
Rat	240–280	109 (2)	53 (1)	2.4 (0.1)	0.34 (0.02)	0.39 (0.02)
Mouse	45–95	233 (13)	2.5 (0.2)	7.5 (0.8)	0.53 (0.08)	0.82 (0.07)
Guinea pig	6	69 (26)	5.7 (1.6)	2.5 (0.2)	0.65 (0.12)	0.13 (0.03)
Syrian hamster	6	72 (7)	3.6 (1.0)	2.0 (0.1)	0.57 (0.09)	0.37 (0.03)
Rabbit	6	27 (6)	8.5 (4.4)	5.3 (0.5)	0.37 (0.02)	0.44 (0.10)
Dog	4–12	134 (25)	22 (5)	1.4 (0.1)	0.30 (0.04)	0.35 (0.18)
Chimpanzee	5	51 (12)	53 (3)	—	—	0.01 (9.01)

[a] Values are normalized per milliliter of lung volume washed.

From *Concepts in Inhalation Toxicology,* R.F. Henderson, Hemisphere Publishing, Taylor & Francis, Washington, D.C., 1989, p. 423.[25] Reproduced with permission. All rights reserved

TABLE 5.42
Relative Proportions of Immunocompetent Cell Populations Obtained by Bronchoalveolar Lavage

Species	Bronchoalveolar Cells (%)			Lymphocyte (%)	
	Macrophages	Lymphocytes	Granulocytes	T	B
Human	78–91	9–20	1–3	47	15–17
Monkey	90–91	3–6	3–6	62	4
Dog	59–75	22–39	0–9	—	—
Swine	60–70	30–33	0–6	—	—
Guinea pig	50–80	12–50	2–19	68–76	10–20
Rabbit	84–98	2–16	0	—	—
Hamster	89	3	10	—	—
Mouse	45–96	3–39	1–6	—	—
Rat	93	2	5	50	12

Adapted from McDermott et al., *Int. Rev. Exp. Pathol.,* 23, 47, 1982.[26] From Murray, M.J. and Driscoll, K.E., in *Treatise on Pulmonary Toxicology,* vol. 1, *Comparative Biology of the Normal Lung,* CRC Press, Boca Raton, FL, 1992.[27] With permission.

TABLE 5.43
Lymphocyte Subpopulations Observed in Bronchoalveolar Lavage Fluid of Lung Tissue

Species: Source[a]	T Lymphocytes (%)				B Lymphocytes (%)
	Total	Helper	Suppressor	Helper/Suppressor	
Human					
BALF	73	46	25	1.8	NR
	72	46	28	1.7	9
	63	45	25	1.9	5.3
	66	48	27	1.8	NR
Tissue	40	NR[b]	NR	—	10
Rat					
BALF	32	29	NR	—	NR
	50	31	25	1.2	12.3
Tissue	90	50	40	1.2	10
	62	29	NR	—	15
	51	26	24	1.1	25
	44	16	19	0.8	10
	59	28	36	0.8	12
Mouse					
Tissue	38	13	6	2.2	23

[a] BALF = bronchoalveolar lavage fluid. Tissue lymphocyte populations were obtained by enzyme digestions and/or mechanical disruption techniques.

[b] NR = not reported.

From Murray, M.J. and Driscoll, K.E., in *Treatise on Pulmonary Toxicology,* vol. 1, *Comparative Biology of the Normal Lung,* CRC Press, Boca Raton, FL, 1992.[27] With permission.

SECTION 6. PULMONARY DEPOSITION AND CLEARANCE

TABLE 5.44
Lung and Alveolar Macrophage (AM) Parameters as They May Relate to *In Vivo* Particle Uptake

	Mouse	Hamster	Rat	Guinea Pig	Rabbit	Dog	Human
Average body weight (g)	42	122	380	430	2600	16,000	74,000
Lung volume (ml)	1.45	3.9	10.9	13	112	1320	4340
Lung surface area (m²)	0.125	0.28	0.66	0.91	3.3	52	143
Alveolar diameter (μm)	47	60	70	65	88	126	219
Calculated no. of alveoli (millions)[a]	18	25	43	69	135	1040	950
Lavagable no. of AM animal (millions)	0.36	2.0	1.6	1.4	12	3876	6500
	0.38	4.2	3.0	3.4	17		
	0.53	5.1	3.8	4.7	28		
	0.73	5.8	7.6		43		
	1.36	6.3	8.3		49		
Average	0.67	4.7	4.9	3.2	30	3876	6500
Calculated AMs alveolus	0.037	0.19	0.11	0.046	0.22	3.7	6.8
Area patrolled by each AM (μm²)	190,000	60,000	140,000	280,000	110,000	13,400	22,000
In vivo gold colloid uptake by AM, $T_{1/2}$ (h)	7.1	0.8	4.2			3.2	Corr. coeff. with area = r² = 0.99

[a] Number of alveoli = alveolar surface area/π (alveolar diameter).[2]

From Valberg, P.A. and Blanchard, J.D., in *Treatise on Pulmonary Toxicology,* vol. 1, *Comparative Biology of the Normal Lung,* CRC Press, Boca Raton, FL, 1992.[29] With permission.

TABLE 5.45
Tracheal Mucociliary Clearance

Species	Mucous Velocity[a] (mm/min)
Mouse	+
Rat	1.9 ± 0.7
	5.1 ± 3.0
	5.9 ± 2.5
Ferret	+
	18.2 ± 5.1
	10.7 ± 3.7
Guinea pig	2.7 ± 1.4
Rabbit	3.2 ± 1.1
	+
Chicken	*
Cat	2.5 ± 0.8
Dog	21.6 ± 5.0
	9.8 ± 2.1
	19.2 ± 1.6
	7.5 ± 3.7

TABLE 5.45 *(Continued)*
Tracheal Mucociliary Clearance

Species	Mucous Velocity[a] (mm/min)
	14.5 ± 6.3
Baboon	+
Sheep	17.3 ± 6.2
	10.5 ± 2.9
Pig	*
Cow	*
Donkey	14.7 ± 3.8
Horse	16.6 ± 2.4
	17.8 ± 5.1
Human	3.6 ± 1.5
	5.5 ± 0.4
	5.1 ± 2.9
	11.5 ± 4.7
	10.1 ± 3.5
	21.5 ± 5.5
	15.5 ± 1.7

Note: *, transport studied but no velocity given; +, inhalation study, clearance measured but no tracheal velocities given.

[a] Mean ±SD.

From Wolff, R.K., in *Treatise on Pulmonary Toxicology,* vol. 1, *Comparative Biology of the Normal Lung,* CRC Press, Boca Raton, FL, 1992.[31] With permission.

TABLE 5.46
Nasal Mucociliary Clearance

Species	Velocity[a] (mm/min)
Rat	2.3 ± 0.8
Dog	3.7 ± 0.9
Man	5.2 ± 2.3
	5.5 ± 3.2
	5.3 (0.5–23.6)
	8.4 ± 4.8
	6.8 ± 5.1
	7 ± 4

[a] Mean ±SD.

From Wolff, R.K., in *Treatise on Pulmonary Toxicology,* vol. 1, *Comparative Biology of the Normal Lung,* CRC Press, Boca Raton, FL, 1992.[31] With permission.

TABLE 5.47

Comparative Pulmonary Clearance Data for Relatively Insoluble Particles Inhaled by Laboratory Animals and Humans

Species	Aerosol Matrix	Particle Size μm	Measure	P_1	T_1	P_2	T_2	Study Duration (days)
Mouse	FAP	0.7	AMAD	0.93	34	0.07	146	850
	FAP	1.5	AMAD	0.93	35	0.07	171	850
	FAP	2.8	AMAD	0.93	36	0.07	201	850
	Ru Oxide	0.38	CMD	0.88	28	0.12	230	490
	Pu Oxide	0.2	CMD	0.86	20	0.14	460	525
Rat	Diesel soot	0.12	MMAD	0.37	6	0.63	80	330
	FAP	1.2	CMD	0.62	20	0.38	180	492
	FAP	0.7	AMAD	0.91	34	0.09	173	850
	FAP	1.5	AMAD	0.91	35	0.09	210	850
	FAP	2.8	AMAD	0.91	36	0.09	258	850
	Latex	3.0	CMD	0.39	18	0.61	63	190
	Pu Oxide	<1.0	CMD	0.20	20	0.80	180	350
	Pu Oxide	2.5	AMAD	0.75	30	0.25	250	800
	U_3O_8	~1–2	CMD	0.67	20	0.33	500	768
Guinea pig	FAP	2.0	AMAD	0.22	29	0.78	385	1100
	Diesel soot	0.12	MMAD			1.00	>2000	432
	Latex	3.0	CMD			1.00	83	190
Dog	Coal dust	2.4	MMAD			1.00	1000	160
	Coal dust	1.9	MMAD			1.00	~700	301–392
	Ce Oxide	0.09–1.4	MMD			1.00	>570	140
	FAP	2.1–2.3	AMAD	0.09	13	0.91	440	181
	FAP	0.7	AMAD	0.15	20	0.85	257	850
	FAP	1.5	AMAD	0.15	21	0.85	341	850
	FAP	2.8	AMAD	0.15	21	0.85	485	850
	Nb Oxide	1.6–2.5	AMAD			1.00	>300	128
	Pu Oxide	1–5	CMD			1.00	1500	280
	Pu Oxide	4.3	MMD			1.00	300	300
	Pu Oxide	1.1–4.9	MMAD		~1		400	468
	Pu Oxide	0.1–0.65	CMD	0.10	200	0.90	1000	~4000
	Pu Oxide	0.72	AMAD	0.10	3.9	0.90	680	730
	Pu Oxide	1.4	AMAD	0.32	87	0.68	1400	730
	Pu Oxide	2.8	AMAD	0.22	32	0.78	1800	730
	Tantalum	4.0	AMAD	0.40	1.9	0.60	860	155
	U_3O_8	0.3	CMD	0.47	4.5	0.53	120	127
	Zr Oxide	2.0	AMAD			1.0	340	128
Monkey	Pu Oxide	2.06	CMAD			1.0	500–900	200
	Pu Oxide	1.6	AMAD			1.0	770–1100	990
Human	FAP	1	CMD	0.14	40	0.86	350	372–533
	FAP	4	CMD	0.27	50	0.73	670	372–533
	Latex	3.6	CMD	0.27	30	0.73	296	~480
	Latex	5	CMD	0.42	0.5	0.58	150–300	160
	Pu Oxide	0.3	MMD			1.00	240	300
	Graphite and PuO$_2$	6	AMAD			1.00	240–290	566
	Pu Oxide	<4–5	CMD			1.00	1000	427

TABLE 5.47 *(Continued)*

Comparative Pulmonary Clearance Data for Relatively Insoluble Particles Inhaled by Laboratory Animals and Humans

Species	Aerosol Matrix	Particle Size		Pulmonary Burden[a]				Study Duration (days)
		μm	Measure	P_1	T_1	P_2	T_2	
	Th Oxide	<4–5	CMD			1.00	300–400	427
	Teflon	4.1	CMD	0.30	4.5–45	0.60	200–2500	300
	Zr Oxide	2.0	AMAD			1.00	224	261

Note: FAP = fused aluminosilicate particles; AMAD = activity median aerodynamic diameter; MMAD = mass median aerodynamic diameter; CMD = count median diameter; MMD = mass median diameter. Some aerosols were monodisperse, most were polydisperse, with geometric standard deviation in the range of 1.5 to 4. Clearance halftimes are approximations for biological clearance, the net result of dissolution-absorption processes and physical clearance processes. In some examples, the original data were subjected to a computer curve-fit procedure to derive the values for P and T.

[a] Pulmonary burden $P_1 e_1^{(\ln 2)t/\tau} + P_2 e_2^{(\ln 2)t/\tau}$, where P_1 and P_2 equal fractions of the initial pulmonary deposition, T_1 and T_2 equal retention half-times in days, and t equals days after exposure.

From Snipes, M.B., *Critical Reviews on Toxicology,* 20, 174, 1989.[18] With permission.

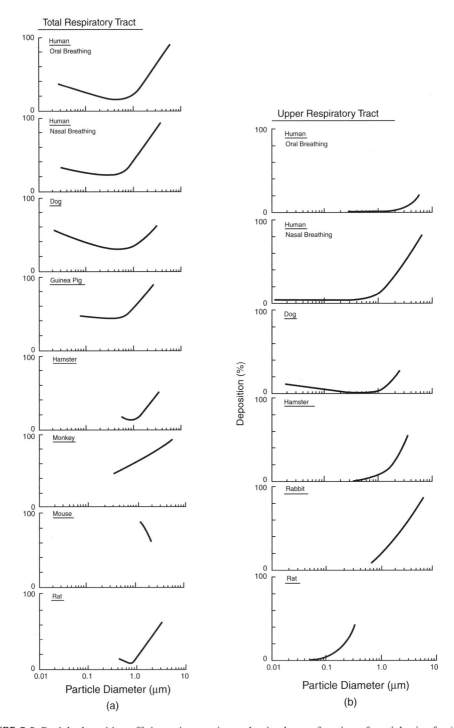

FIGURE 5.9 Particle deposition efficiency in experimental animals as a function of particle size for (a) total respiratory tract, (b) upper respiratory tract, (c) tracheobronchial tree, and (d) pulmonary region. Each curve represents an eye fit through mean values (or centers of ranges) of the data. Similar curves for humans are shown for comparison. Particle diameters are aerodynamic for those ≥0.5 μm and diffusion equivalent for those <0.5 μm. From *Concepts in Inhalation Toxicology,* Schlesinger, R.B., Hemisphere Publishing, Taylor & Francis, Washington, D.C., 1989, p. 208.[22] Reproduced with permission. All rights reserved.

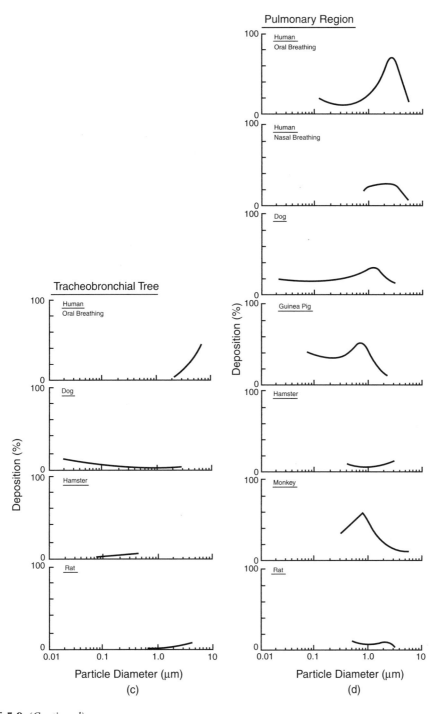

FIGURE 5.9 *(Continued)*

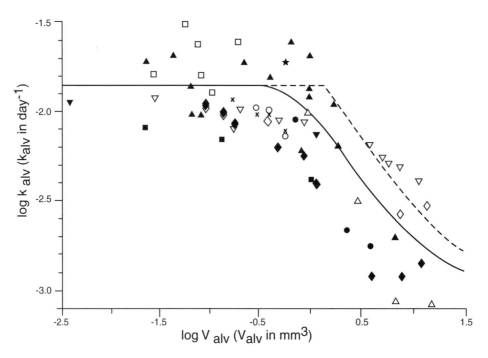

FIGURE 5.10 Alveolar clearance rate (k_{alv}) as a function of total particle volume in the lung, with data from different investigators using different insoluble particles. From Stöber et al., in *Toxicology of the Lung,* Raven Press, New York, 1993.[30] With permission.

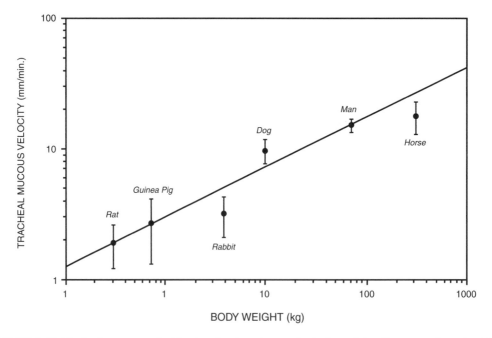

FIGURE 5.11 Tracheal mucous velocities in a log-log plot vs. the body weight of a range of species. The same techniques of intratracheal instillation of ^{99m}Tc-MAA were used in all cases. The function TMV = 3.0 $(BW)^{0.39}$ defines the relation between tracheal mucous velocity and body weight, with a correlation of 0.94. From Wolff, R.K., in *Treatise on Pulmonary Toxicology,* vol. 1, *Comparative Biology of the Normal Lung,* CRC Press, Boca Raton, FL, 1992.[31] With permission.

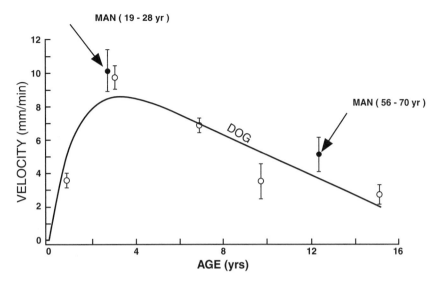

FIGURE 5.12 Tracheal mucous velocity (mean ±SE) is shown for beagle dogs (□) vs. age. The fitted function that describes this relation is $V(t) = 11[1 - \exp(-0.9t)] - 0.6t$. The available data for humans (●) are also shown after transforming for age. From Wolff, R.K., in *Treatise on Pulmonary Toxicology*, vol. 1, *Comparative Biology of The Normal Lung*, CRC Press, Boca Raton, FL, 1992.[3] With permission.

SECTION 7. PULMONARY TOXICITY

TABLE 5.48
Slopes of Ventilatory Responses to Carbon Dioxide

Species	Slope
Rat (Sprague-Dawley)	6.6
Rat (Wistar)	6.4
Rabbit	23.0
Cat	12.8
Porcupine	33.0
Woodchuck	12.0
Coatimundi	23.0
Baboon	34
Dog	38.3
Dog	13.4
Goat	32.7
Human	28
Pony	38
Weddell seal	16.7
Harbor seal	7.7
Harbor seal	23.12
Hooded seal	6.52
Harp seal	11.1

From Boggs, D.F., in *Treatise on Pulmonary Toxicology*, vol. 1, *Comparative Biology of the Normal Lung*, CRC Press, Boca Raton, FL, 1992.[19] With permission.

TABLE 5.49
Species Comparison of Lung Function Response After Exposure to Air Pollutants

Toxicant	Species	mg/m³	Time	f	V_T	V_g	R	C
Ozone	GP	2.1	2 h	↑	↓	–	↑	NR
	Rabbit	23.5	~35 h	↑	↓	↑	↑	↓
	Rat	0.7	2 h	↑	↓	–	–	–
	Dog	~2.0	2 h	↑	↓	–	↑	NR	↓
	Cat	0.5	4.6 h	Fix	Fix	Fix	↑	↓
Sulfur dioxide	GP	0.84	1 h	↑	↓	NR	↑	↓
	Monkey	13.4	78 wk	–	–	–	–	–
	Dog	13.4	225 day	–	–	–	↑	↓
	Sheep	13.1	4 h	–	–	–	–	–
	Mouse	44.5	10 min	↓	NR	NR	NR	NR
	Ferret	1308	12 wk	↓	–	–	–	–
	Cat	52.4	30 min	Fix	Fix	Fix	↑	↓
Sulfuric Acid	GP	0.7	1 h	–	–	–	↑	↓
	Rat	6.4	14 wk	–	–	–	–	–
	Dog	5.0	4 h	–	–	–	–	–
	Monkey	4.8	78 wk	↑	–	–	–	–
	Donkey	1.5	1 h	NR	NR	NR	–	–
	Rabbit	0.3	1 yr	NR	NR	NR	–	NR
Nitrogen dioxide	Rat	3.8	2 yr	↑	↑	–	–	–
	Monkey	9.4	90 day	↑	↑	–	–	–
	GP	9.8	4 h	↑	↓	–	–	–
	Rabbit	15.0	12 wk	NR	NR	NR	↑	NR
	Cat	19.2	12 mo	NR	NR	NR	↑	↓
	Sheep	28	4 h	NR	NR	NR	↑	
	Hamster	38.4	14 mo	NR	NR	NR	↑	–
	Dog	69.5	4 h	↑	↓	NR	NR	NR
Formaldehyde	GP	4.7	8 h	↓	↑	NR	↑	NR
	Rat	38.9	10 min	↓	↓	↓	NR	NR
	Mice	6.0	10 min	↓	↑	↓	NR	NR

Note: f, Frequency of breathing: V_T, tidal volume; V_E, minute ventilation; R, resistance; C, compliance; GP, guinea pig; ↑, increase; ↓, decrease; –, no change observed; NR, not reported; Fix, mechanically ventilated.

From Costa, D.L., Tepper, J.S., and Raub, J.A., in *Treatise on Pulmonary Toxicology,* vol. 1, *Comparative Biology of the Normal Lung,* CRC Press, Boca Raton, FL, 1992.[35] With permission.

TABLE 5.50
Lung Dysfunction After Toxicant Exposure

Toxicant	Species	Functional Variable[a]
SO_2 + ZnO	G. pig	↓ LV, ↓ DL_{co}
$(NH_4)_2SO_4$	G. pig	↑ LV, ↓ N_2 slope
Coal dust	Rat	↓ LV, ↑ FEF
Diesel exhaust	Rat	↑ LV, ↑ FEF
Diesel exhaust	Rat	DL_{co}, ↓ C_{rs}, ↑/↓ N_2 slope
O_3	Rat	–VP, ↑ R_{sw}
O_3	Rat	↑ VP
O_3	Rat	↑ LV, –C_{rs}, –N_2 slope, – DL_{co}
O_3	Rat	↑ LV, ↑ VP, ↓ Pa_{O_2}
O_3	Rat	↑ LV, ↑ VP, ↓ FEF, – DL_{co}

TABLE 5.50 *(Continued)*
Lung Dysfunction After Toxicant Exposure

Toxicant	Species	Functional Variable[a]
Acrolein	Rat	↑ LV, ↑/↓ C_{rs}, ↓ N_2 slope, DL_{co}, ↑ ↓ FEF
MIC	Rat	↓ PK flow
		↓ FEF 50, 25, +10
SiO_2	Rat	↓ LV, ↓ C_{rs}, ↓ N_2 slope, ↓ DL_{co}, ↓ FEF
Cl_2	Rat	↑ LV, ↑ C_{rs}, –N_2 slope, – DL_{co}, –FEF
MIC	Rat	↓ DL_{co}, ↓ C_{rs}, ↓ N_2 slope
Cd	Rat	↓ LV, ↓ C_{rs},/↓ N_2 slope, ↓ DL_{co}, ↑ ↓ FEF
O_2	Rat	↑/↓ LV, ↓ C_{rs}, ↓ DL_{co}, ↓ FEF
Oil fog	Rat	↓ LV, DL_{co}, –C_{rs}, –N_2 slope
Volcanic ash/SO_2	Rat	–LV, – DL_{co}, –C_{rs}, –N_2 slope
SiO_2	Rat	↓ LV, ↓ DL_{co}
NO_2	Mouse	–LV, DL_{co}, ↓ C_{rs},/↑ N_2 slope
O_3	Rabbit	↑ LV, ↓ FEF
O_3, SO_2 olefin	Hamster	–LV, ↓ N_2 slope, ↑ DL_{co}

[a] Functional variables; LV, lung volume; DL_{co}, diffusion capacity for carbon monoxide; FEF, forced expiratory flow; C_{rs}, respiratory system compliance; R_{sw}, airway resistance; VP, volume-pressure curve; ↑ = increase; ↓ = decrease, – no change.

From Costa, D.L., Tepper, J.S., and Raub, J.B., in *Treatise on Pulmonary Toxicology,* vol 1, *Comparative Biology of the Normal Lung,* CRC Press, Boca Raton, FL, 1992.[35] With permission.

TABLE 5.51
Agents Causing Lung Tumors in Laboratory Animals After Inhalation Exposure

Organic chemicals
  Gases
    Bis(chloromethyl)ether
    Bromoethane (ethyl bromide)
    1,3-Butadiene
    1,2-Dibromo-3-chloropropane
    1,2-Dibromoethane
    Dimethyl sulfate
    1,2-Epoxybutane
    Ethylene oxide
    Methylene chloride
    3-Nitro-3-hexene
    1,2-Propylene oxide
    Tetrachloroethylene
    Tetranitromethane
    Urethan
    Vinyl chloride
  Particles
    Benzo(a)pyrene
    Polyurethan dust
  Inorganic compounds
    Metallic
      Antimony compounds
      Beryllium compounds
      Cadmium chloride
      Chromium dioxide
      Nickel compounds

TABLE 5.51 *(Continued)*
Agents Causing Lung Tumors in Laboratory Animals After Inhalation Exposure

Titanium compounds
Nonmetallic
  Asbestos fibers
  Zeolite fibers
  Ceramic aluminosilicate fibers
  Kelvar aramid fibers
  Silica
  Oil shale dust
  Quartz
  Volcanic ash
Radionuclides
  Alpha-emitting radionuclide particles
  Beta-emitting radionuclide particles
  Radon and its decay products
Complex mixture
  Cigarette smoke
  Diesel engine exhaust
  Gasoline engine exhaust
  Coal tar aerosols
  Artificial smog

From Hahn, F.F., in *Toxicology of the Lung,* Raven Press, New York, 1993.[36] With permission.

TABLE 5.52
Carcinogenic Agents Causally Associated with Human Lung or Pleural Cancer

Industrial processes
  Aluminum production
  Coal gasification
  Coke production
  Hematite mining, underground with exposure to radon
  Iron and steel founding
  Painter, occupational exposure
  Rubber industry
Chemicals and groups of chemicals for which exposure has been primarily occupational
  Asbestos
  Bis(chloromethyl)ether
  Chromium compounds, hexavalent
  Coal tars
  Coal tar pitches
  Mustard gas
  Nickel and nickel compounds
  Soots
  Talc containing asbestiform fibers
  Vinyl chloride
Environmental agents and cultural risk factors
  Erionite
  Radon and its decay products
  Tobacco smoke

Based on database of IARC Monographs Program. From Hahn, F.F., in *Toxicology of the Lung,* Raven Press, New York, 1993.[36] With permission.

TABLE 5.53
Effects of Inhaled Toxicants on Mucociliary Clearance

Toxicant	Exposure Concentration	Exposure Duration	Animal Species	Region Examined[a]	Response[b]
Ozone (O₃)	0.5 ppm	2 h	Sheep	T	NE
	1 ppm	2 h	Sheep	T	↓
	0.4–1.2 ppm	4 h	Rat	B	↓ at _0.8 ppm
	0.1–0.6 ppm	2 h	Rabbit	B	↓ at 0.6 ppm
	0.62–1.25 ppm	4 h	Mouse	B	NE
	0.25, 0.6 ppm	2 h/day, 14 days	Rabbit	B	NE
	0.2, 0.4 ppm	2 h (with exercise)	Human	B	↑
Nitrogen dioxide(NO₂)	7.5, 15 ppm	2 h	Sheep	T	↓ at 15 ppm
	0.3–10 ppm	2 h	Rabbit	B	NE
	6 ppm	7 days/wk 6 wk	Rat	T	↓
	0.3, 1 ppm	2 h/day, 14 days	Rabbit	B	NE
Sulfur dioxide (SO₂)	1, 5, 25 ppm	6 h	Human	N	↓ at 5, 25 ppm
	5 ppm	3 h	Human	B	NE
	5 ppm	2 h (with exercise)	Human	B	↑
	20 ppm	4 h	Rat	B	↓
	1 ppm	1 yr	Dog	T	↓
Formaldehyde (HCHO)	20 ppm	4 h	Rat	PB	↓ at _6 ppm
	0.5, 15 ppm	6 h/days, 5 days/wk, 3 wk	Rat	N	↑
Carbon particles	50 mg/m³	Few minutes	Human	TB	NE
Diesel exhaust particles	0.4–0.5 mg/m³	0.5 h	Sheep	T	↓
	17 mg/m³	4 h	Rat	T	NE
	2 mg/m³	7 h/day, 5 days/wk, 6 mo	Rat	B	NE
	0.35–7 mg/m³	7 h/day, 5 days/wk, 30 mo	Rat	T	NE
Sulfuric acid (H₂SO₄)	0.4–0.5 mg/m³	0.5 h	Sheep	T	NE
	14 mg/m³ (0.1 μm)[c]	0.3 h	Sheep	T	NE
	4 mg/m³ (0.1 μm)	4 h	Sheep	T	NE
	1, 5 mg/m³ (0.3 μm)	1 h	Dog	T	NE
	0.2–1.4 mg/m³ (0.4 μm)	1 h	Donkey	T, B	NE on T, ↓ B persistent in 2 of 4 animals

TABLE 5.53 *(Continued)*
Effects of Inhaled Toxicants on Mucociliary Clearance

Toxicant	Exposure Concentration	Exposure Duration	Animal Species	Region Examined[a]	Response[b]
	0.1–10 mg/m^3 (0.5 μm)	1 h	Human	T, B	NE on T, ↑↓ B (depending on concentration)
	0.5, 1 mg/m^3 (0.9 μm)	1 h	Dog	T	→
	3.6 mg/m^3 (1 μm)	4 h	Rat	B	NE
	1.5 mg/m^3 (0.6 μm)	4 h	Mouse	B	NE
	15 mg/m^3 (3.2 μm)	4 h	Mouse	B	→
	0.1–2.2 mg/m^3 (0.3 μm)	1 h	Rabbit	B	↑ at low concentration
				B	↓ at high concentration
	0.25 mg/m^3 (0.3 μm)	1 h/day, 5 days/wk, 1 yr	Rabbit	B	→
	0.25–0.5 mg/m^3 (0.3 μm)	1 h/day, 5 days/wk, 4 wk	Rabbit	B	↑
	0.1 mg/m^3 (0.5 μm)	1 h/day, 5 days/wk, 6 mo	Donkey	B	→
Ammonium bisulfate (NH$_4$HSO$_2$)	0.6–1.7 mg/m^3 (0.4 μm)	1 h	Rabbit	B	↓ only at 1.7 mg/m^3
	1 mg/m^3 (0.1 μm)	4 h	Sheep	T	NE
Ammonium sulfate [(NH$_4$)$_2$SO$_2$]	2 mg/m^3 (0.4 μm)	1 h	Rabbit	B	NE
	0.3–3 mg/m^3 (0.4 μm)	1 h	Donkey	T, B	NE
	3.6 mg/m^3 (0.4 μm)	4 h	Rat	B	NE
	1.1 mg/m^3 (0.1 μm)	4 h	Sheep	T	NE

[a] N = nasal passages; B = bronchial tree; T = trachea.
[b] NNE = no effect; ↑ = acceleration of clearance or mucus transport rate or time; ↓ = retardation of clearance or mucus transport rate or time. Median particle size.

From Schlesinger, R.B., *Crit. Rev. Toxicol.*, 20, 297, 1990.[37] With permission.

TABLE 5.54
Effects of Inhaled Toxicants on Clearance from the Respiratory Region of the Lungs

Toxicant	Exposure Concentration	Exposure Duration	Animal Species	Response[a]
Ozone (O$_3$)	0.1–1.2 ppm	2 h	Rabbit	↑ at 0.1 ppm, ↓ at 1.2 ppm
	0.1, 0.6 ppm	2 h/day, 14 days	Rabbit	↑
	0.4–1 ppm	4 h	Rat	↑ at 0.8, 1 ppm
	0.5 ppm	16 h/day, 2 or 5 mo	Rabbit	NE
Nitrogen dioxide (NO$_2$)	0.3–10 ppm	2 h	Rabbit	↑
	0.3, 1 ppm	2 h/day, 14 days	Rabbit	↑
	1, 10 ppm	2 h/day, 14 days	Rabbit	↑
	30, 60 ppm	5 h/day, 5 days/wk, 2 wk	Mouse	↓ at 60 ppm
	3–24 ppm	7 h/day, 5 days/wk, 2–3 wk	Rat	↑ at low conc. × time values; ↓ at high conc. × time values
Formaldehyde (HCHO)	20 ppm	4 h	Rat	NE
Sulfur dioxide (SO$_2$)	10 ppm	16 h/day, 20 wk	Rabbit	↑
	0.1–20 ppm	7 h/day, 5 days/wk, 2–5 wk	Rat	↑ at low conc. × time values, ↓ at high conc. × time values
Sulfuric acid (H$_2$SO$_4$)	1 mg/m^3 (0.3 μm)	1 h	Rabbit	↑
	3.6 mg/m^3 (1 μm)	4 h	Rat	↓
	0.25 mg/m^3 (0.3 μm)	1 h/day, 5 days/wk up to 240 days	Rabbit	↑
Ammonium sulfate [(NH$_4$)$_3$SO$_4$]	3.6 mg/m^2	4 h	Rat	NE
Lead	76, 161 mg/m^3	7 mo	Rabbit	NE
Silica	21.1 mg/m^3	5 h/day, 4 days/wk, 1 yr	Rat	↓
Chromium [Cr(VI)]	0.2 mg/m^3	Continuous, 42 days	Rat	↓
Diesel exhaust particles	0.2–4.1 mg/m^3	7 h/day, 5 days/wk, 18 wk	Rat	↓ at 4.1 mg/m^3
	0.35, 3.5, 7 mg/m^3	7 h/day, 5 days/wk, 30 mo	Rat	↓ at ≥3.5 mg/m^3
	4 mg/m^3	95 h/wk, 19 mo	Rat, Hamster	↓
Carbon black	7 mg/m^3	20 h/day, 7 wk, 1–6 days/wk	Rat	↓

a NE = no effect; ↑ = acceleration of clearance rate or time; ↓ = retardation of clearance rate or time; conc. = concentration.

From Schlesinger, R.B., *Crit. Rev. Toxicol.*, 20, 297, 1990.[37] With permission.

TABLE 5.55
Effects of Inhaled Toxicants on the Phagocytic Activity of Alveolar Macrophages

Toxicant	Exposure Concentration[a]	Exposure Duration	Aninal Species	Response[b]
Ozone (O_3)	1.2 ppm	2 h	Rabbit	↓
	0.1 ppm	2 h/day, 13 days	Rabbit	↓
	0.8 ppm	20 days	Rat	↑
	2.5 ppm	5 h	Rat	↓
	0.3–0.5 ppm	3 h	Rabbit	↓
	0.8 ppm	4 h	Rat	↓
Nitrogen dioxide (NO_2)	10.25 ppm	24 h	Rat	↓ at 25 ppm
	0.3, 1 ppm	2 h/day, 13 days	Rabbit	↓ at 0.3, ↑ at 1 ppm
	0.5 ppm	3–5 h/day, 5 days/wk, 1–3 mo	Mouse	↓ at 2 mo
Sulfur dioxide (SO_2)	1, 5, 10, 20 ppm	24 h	Rat	↑ at ≥5 ppm
Ethylene (CH_2O)	10, 20 ppm	24 h	Rat	↓ at 20 ppm
Chromium [Cr(VI)]	0.050 mg/m^3	28 days	Rat	↑
	0.025, 0.050, 0.200 mg/m^3	90 days, 6 h/day, 5 days/wk, 4–6 wk	Rat	↑ at 0.025–0.050 mg/m^3, ↓ at 0.200 mg/m^3
Calcium chloride (CaCl$_2$), Copper chloride (CuCl$_2$), Cobalt chloride (CoCl$_2$)	0.4–0.6 mg/m^3	6 h/day, 5 days/wk, 4–6 wk	Rabbit	NE
Cadmium (Cd)	1.5, 5.0 mg/m^3	0.5 h	Rat	↑ at 1.5 mg/m^2, ↓ at 5 mg/m^3
Nickel dust (Ni)	0.13 mg/m^3	5 h/day, 5 days/wk, 4–8 mo	Rabbit	NE
Diesel exhaust particles	0.25, 1.5, 6 mg/m^3	Up to 12 mo	Guinea pig, rat	↓

[a] *In vivo* exposures.

[b] ↓ = depression of phagocytic activity; ↑ = enhancement of phagocytic activity; NE = no effect.

From Schlesinger, R.B., *Crit. Rev. Toxicol.*, 20, 297, 1990.[37] With permission.

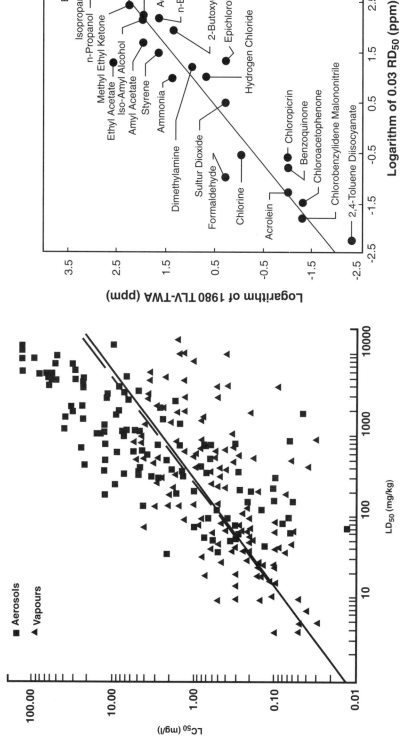

FIGURE 5.14 Correlation between time-weighted average threshold limit values (ACGIH) and RD_{50} values determined in mice for 26 irritants. Compiled from the data from Kane et al., *Am. Ind. Hyg. Assoc. J.*, 40, 207, 1979.[33] Figure reprinted from Parent, Richard A., *Comparative Biology of the Normal Lung*, 1992, CRC Press, Boca Raton, FL, with permission.

FIGURE 5.13 Double-logarithmic correlation of inhalation LC_{50} and oral LD_{50}. Solid line, least-squares regression; broken line, nonparametric regression. From Klimisch et al., *Regul. Toxicol. Pharmacol.*, 7, 21, 1987.[32] With permission.

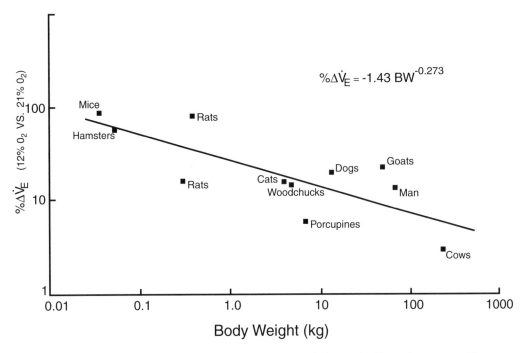

FIGURE 5.15 Ventilatory response to 12% inspired O_2 (or PI_{O_2} of 90 torr) in 10 species over a wide range of body size. From Boggs, D.F. and Tenny, S.M., *Respir. Physiol.,* 58, 245, 1984.[34] With permission.

SECTION 8. INHALATION EXPOSURE GENERATION

TABLE 5.56
Uniformity Test of Different Exposure Chambers

Chamber Type	Aerosol Size MMAD (µm)	Spatial Variation CV (%)
96-port nose-only	1	7
40-port nose-only	1	6
27″ Hinners	1	3–10
Hazleton 2000	1.2	5
Hazleton 1000	1.2	12
Horizontal flow	1.0	8–10
Horizontal flow	2–3	34–42
Diagonal flow	3	10–12

From *Concepts in Inhalation Toxicology,* Cheng, Y-S and Moss, O.R., Hemisphere Publishing, Taylor & Francis, Washington, D.C., 1989.[38] Reproduced with permission. All rights reserved.

TABLE 5.57
Ammonia Concentrations in an Inhalation Chamber

Animal Loading (%)	Chamber Air Flow (L/min)	No. of Air Changes per Hour	Hour of Sample (ppm NH₃ ± SE)		
			2	4	6
1	13	8	0.38 ± 0.08	0.48 ± 0.07	0.46 ± 0.13
1	26	16	0.20 ± 0.01	0.24 ± 0.02	0.45 ± 0.06
1	40	24	0.19 ± 0.04	0.24 ± 0.05	0.22 ± 0.03
3.1	13	8	0.84 ± 0.14	1.13 ± 0.14	1.11 ± 0.27
3.1	26	16	0.60 ± 0.09	1.04 ± 0.23	1.60 ± 0.22
3.1	40	24	0.19 ± 0.02	0.33 ± 0.05	0.39 ± 0.05
5.1	13	8	1.23 ± 0.18	1.51 ± 0.16	2.42 ± 0.38
5.2	26	16	0.66 ± 0.06	1.23 ± 0.20	2.05 ± 0.41
5.2	40	24	0.46 ± 0.08	1.02 ± 0.11	1.30 ± 0.27

From Phalen, R.F., *Inhalation Studies: Foundations and Techniques,* CRC Press, Boca Raton, FL, 1984.[11] With permission.

TABLE 5.58
Conversion Table for Gases and Vapors[a] (Milligrams per Liter to Parts per Million, and Vice Versa; 25°C and 760 mm Hg)

Molecular Weight	1 mg/l ppm	1 ppm mg/l	Molecular Weight	1 mg/l ppm	1 ppm mg/l	Molecular Weight	1 mg/l ppm	1 ppm mg/l
1	24,450	0.0000409	29	843	0.001186	57	429	0.002331
2	12,230	0.0000818	30	815	0.001227	58	422	0.002372
3	8,150	0.0001227	31	789	0.001268	59	414	0.002413
4	6,113	0.0001636	32	764	0.001309	60	408	0.002554
5	4,890	0.0002045	33	741	0.001350	61	401	0.002495
6	4,075	0.0002454	34	719	0.001391	62	394	0.00254
7	3,493	0.0002863	35	699	0.001432	63	388	0.00258
8	3,056	0.000327	36	679	0.001472	64	382	0.00262
9	2,717	0.000368	37	661	0.001513	65	376	0.00266
10	2,445	0.000409	38	643	0.001554	66	370	0.00270
11	2,223	0.000450	39	627	0.001595	67	365	0.00274
12	2,038	0.000491	40	611	0.001636	68	360	0.00278
13	1,881	0.000532	41	596	0.001677	69	354	0.00282
14	1,746	0.000573	42	582	0.001718	70	349	0.00286
15	1,630	0.000614	43	569	0.001759	71	344	0.00290
16	1,528	0.000654	44	556	0.001800	72	340	0.00294
17	1,438	0.000695	45	543	0.001840	73	335	0.00299
18	1,358	0.000736	46	532	0.001881	74	330	0.00303
19	1,287	0.000777	47	520	0.001922	75	326	0.00307
20	1,223	0.000818	48	509	0.001963	76	322	0.00311
21	1,164	0.000859	49	499	0.002004	77	318	0.00315
22	1,111	0.000900	50	489	0.002045	78	313	0.00319
23	1,063	0.000941	51	479	0.002086	79	309	0.00323
24	1,019	0.000982	52	470	0.002127	80	306	0.00327
25	987	0.001022	53	461	0.002168	81	302	0.00331
26	940	0.001063	54	453	0.002209	82	298	0.00335
27	906	0.001104	55	445	0.002250	83	295	0.00339
28	873	0.001145	56	437	0.002290	84	291	0.00344

TABLE 5.58 *(Continued)*
Conversion Table for Gases and Vapors[a] (Milligrams per Liter to Parts per Million, and Vice Versa; 25°C and 760 mm Hg)

Molecular Weight	1 mg/l ppm	1 ppm mg/l	Molecular Weight	1 mg/l ppm	1 ppm mg/l	Molecular Weight	1 mg/l ppm	1 ppm mg/l
85	288	0.00348	137	178.5	0.00560	189	129.4	0.00773
86	284	0.00352	138	177.2	0.00564	190	128.7	0.00777
87	281	0.00356	139	175.9	0.00569	191	128.0	0.00781
88	278	0.00360	140	174.6	0.00573	192	127.3	0.00785
89	275	0.00364	141	173.4	0.00577	193	126.7	0.00789
90	272	0.00368	142	172.2	0.00581	194	126.0	0.00793
91	269	0.00372	143	171.0	0.00585	195	125.4	0.00798
92	266	0.00376	144	169.8	0.00589	196	124.7	0.00802
93	263	0.00380	145	168.6	0.00593	197	124.1	0.00806
94	260	0.00384	146	167.5	0.00597	198	123.5	0.00810
95	257	0.00389	147	166.3	0.00601	199	122.9	0.00814
96	255	0.00393	148	165.2	0.00605	200	122.3	0.00818
97	252	0.00397	149	164.1	0.00609	201	121.6	0.00822
98	249.5	0.00401	150	163.0	0.00613	202	121.0	0.00826
99	247.0	0.00405	151	161.9	0.00618	203	120.4	0.00830
100	244.5	0.00409	152	160.9	0.00622	204	119.9	0.00834
101	242.1	0.00413	153	159.8	0.00626	205	119.3	0.00838
102	239.7	0.00417	154	158.8	0.00630	206	118.7	0.00843
103	237.4	0.00421	155	157.7	0.00634	207	118.1	0.00847
104	235.1	0.00425	156	156.7	0.00638	208	117.5	0.00851
105	232.9	0.00429	157	153.7	0.00642	209	117.0	0.00855
106	230.7	0.00434	158	154.7	0.00646	210	116.4	0.00859
107	228.5	0.00438	159	153.7	0.00650	211	115.9	0.00863
108	226.4	0.00442	160	152.8	0.00654	212	115.3	0.00867
109	224.3	0.00446	161	151.9	0.00658	213	114.8	0.00871
110	222.3	0.00450	162	150.9	0.00663	214	114.3	0.00875
111	220.3	0.00454	163	150.0	0.00667	215	113.7	0.00879
112	218.3	0.00458	164	149.1	0.00671	216	113.2	0.00883
113	216.4	0.00462	165	148.2	0.00675	217	112.7	0.00888
114	214.5	0.00466	166	147.3	0.00679	218	112.2	0.00892
115	212.6	0.00470	167	146.4	0.00683	219	111.6	0.00896
116	210.8	0.00474	168	145.5	0.00687	220	111.1	0.00900
117	209.0	0.00479	169	144.7	0.00691	221	110.6	0.00904
118	207.2	0.00483	170	143.8	0.00695	222	110.1	0.00908
119	205.5	0.00487	171	143.0	0.00699	223	109.6	0.00912
120	203.8	0.00491	172	142.2	0.00703	224	109.2	0.00916
121	202.1	0.00495	173	141.3	0.00708	225	108.7	0.00920
122	200.4	0.00499	174	140.5	0.00712	226	108.2	0.00924
123	198.8	0.00503	175	139.7	0.00716	227	107.7	0.00928
124	197.2	0.00507	176	138.9	0.00720	228	107.2	0.00933
125	195.6	0.00511	177	138.1	0.00724	229	106.8	0.00937
126	194.0	0.00515	178	137.4	0.00728	230	106.3	0.00941
127	192.5	0.00519	179	136.6	0.00732	231	105.8	0.00945
128	191.0	0.00524	180	135.8	0.00736	232	105.4	0.00949
129	189.5	0.00528	181	135.1	0.00740	233	104.9	0.00953
130	188.1	0.00532	182	134.3	0.00744	234	104.5	0.00957
131	186.6	0.00536	183	133.6	0.00748	235	104.0	0.00961
132	185.2	0.00540	184	132.9	0.00753	236	103.6	0.00965
133	183.8	0.00544	185	132.2	0.00757	237	103.2	0.00969
134	182.5	0.00548	186	131.5	0.00761	238	102.7	0.00973
135	181.1	0.00552	187	130.7	0.00765	239	102.3	0.00978
136	179.8	0.00556	188	130.1	0.00769	240	101.9	0.00982

TABLE 5.58 *(Continued)*
Conversion Table for Gases and Vapors[a] (Milligrams per Liter to Parts per Million, and Vice Versa; 25°C and 760 mm Hg)

Molecular Weight	1 mg/l ppm	1 ppm mg/l	Molecular Weight	1 mg/l ppm	1 ppm mg/l	Molecular Weight	1 mg/l ppm	1 ppm mg/l
241	101.5	0.00986	261	93.7	0.01067	281	87.0	0.01149
242	101.0	0.00990	262	93.3	0.01072	282	86.7	0.01153
243	100.6	0.00994	263	93.0	0.01076	283	86.4	0.01157
244	100.2	0.00998	264	92.6	0.01080	284	86.1	0.01162
245	99.8	0.01002	265	92.3	0.01084	285	85.8	0.01166
246	99.4	0.01006	266	91.9	0.01088	286	85.5	0.01170
247	99.0	0.01010	267	91.6	0.01092	287	85.2	0.01174
248	98.6	0.01014	268	91.2	0.01096	288	84.9	0.01178
249	98.2	0.01018	269	90.9	0.01100	289	84.6	0.01182
250	97.8	0.01022	270	90.6	0.01104	290	84.3	0.01186
251	97.4	0.01027	271	90.2	0.01108	291	84.0	0.01190
252	97.0	0.01031	272	89.9	0.01112	292	83.7	0.01194
253	96.6	0.01035	273	89.6	0.01117	293	83.4	0.01198
254	96.3	0.01039	274	89.2	0.01121	294	83.2	0.01202
255	95.9	0.01043	275	88.9	0.01125	295	82.9	0.01207
256	95.5	0.01047	276	88.6	0.01129	296	82.6	0.01211
257	95.1	0.01051	277	88.3	0.01133	297	82.3	0.01215
258	94.8	0.01055	278	87.9	0.01137	298	82.0	0.01219
259	94.4	0.01059	279	87.6	0.01141	299	81.8	0.01223
260	94.0	0.01063	280	87.3	0.01145	300	81.5	0.01227

[a] *Source:* Fieloner et al. (1921).[39]

From *Patty's Industrial Hygiene and Toxicology,* John Wiley & Sons, New York, 1991.[40] With permission.

TABLE 5.59
Characteristics of Nebulizers

Nebulizer	Operating Pressure (psi)	Flow Rate (L/min)	Output Concentrations (µg/L)	MMAD (µm)	GSD[a]
Laskin	20	84.0	4.8	0.7	2.1
In Tox	30	25.0	32.0	6.1	1.9
Solosphere	20		1.5	4.5	
Ohio	20		0.5	4.5	
DeVilbiss	20	16.0	14.0	3.2	1.8
Hospitak	20	11.0	23.0	1.0	2.1
Collision	20	7.1	7.7	2.0	2.0
Retec X-70 N	20	5.4	53.0	5.7	1.8
Lovelace	20	1.5	40.0	5.8	1.8

[a] GSD = geometric standard deviation.

From *Concepts in Inhalation Toxicology,* Moss, O.R. and Cheng, Y-S, Hemisphere Publishing, Taylor & Francis, Washington, D.C., 1989, p. 103.[41] Reproduced with permission. All rights reserved.

TABLE 5.60
Operating Characteristics of Compressed Air Nebulizers

Nebulizer	Applied Pressure (lb/in²)	Air Flow (L/min)	Aerosol Out (µl/L air)	Water Vapor Out (µ l/L air)	Volume Median Drop Diameter (µ)	G.S.D.[a]
Dautrebande with open vent	5	11.2	1.0	9.7	—	
	10	14.9	1.4	9.6	1.7	
	20	21.2	2.3	8.6	1.4	1.6–1.7
	30	27.3	2.4	8.2	1.3	
3-Jet Collison	15	6.1	8.7	12.6		
	20	7.1	9.0	14.8		
	30	9.4	9.0	19.4	About 2	About 2
	40	11.4	9.3	23.5		
	50	13.6	10.4	27.9		
De Vilbis® No. 40 with	15	12.4	15.5	8.6	4.2	
closed vent	20	16.0	14.0	7.0	3.2	1.8–1.9
	30	20.9	12.1	7.2	2.8	
Lovelace	20	1.34	(34)[b]	12	6.9	1.7
	30	1.81	(22)[b]	11	4.7	1.9
	40	2.28	(15)[b]	9	3.1	2.2
	50	2.64	(19)[b]	11	2.6	2.3
(Nebulizer chilled to 0°C)	20	1.34	55	1	—	—

[a] G.S.D = geometric standard deviation.

[b] Calculated.

From Phalen, R.F., *Inhalation Studies: Foundations and Techniques,* CRC Press, Boca Raton, FL, 1984.[11] With permission.

TABLE 5.61
Water Droplet Lifetimes

Size (µm)	Lifetime (sec) at 20% RH[a]
0.01	2×10^{-6}
0.1	3×10^{-5}
1.0	0.001
10.0	0.03
40.0	1.3

[a] At 50% RH, lifetime increases ~1.5 times; at 100% RH, lifetime increases 110–1000 times.

From *Concepts in Inhalation Toxicology,* Moss, O.R. and Cheng, Y-S, Hemisphere Publishing, Taylor & Francis, Washington, D.C., 1989, p. 105.[41] Reproduced with permission. All rights reserved.

TABLE 5.62
Characteristics of Dry Powder Generators

Generator	Delivery Mechanism	Dispersion Mechanism	Flow Rate (L/min)	Mass Concentration (mg/m³)	Test Material
NBS	Gravity	Venturi	50–85	1,500 and larger	Nonsticky powder
Wright Dust Feed	Rotating blade	Airstream	10–40	2–1100	Compactable powder
TSI model 3410	Rotating brush	Airstream	10–50	1–100	Nonsticky powder

TABLE 5.62 *(Continued)*
Characteristics of Dry Powder Generators

Generator	Delivery Mechanism	Dispersion Mechanism	Flow Rate (L/min)	Mass Concentration (mg/m³)	Test Material
MDA Micro Feed	Rotating disk	Venturi	30–50	10–300	Nonsticky powder
TSI model 3433	Rotating disk	Venturi	12–21	0.3–40	Nonsticky powder
Lovelace 4-in. FBG	Gravity	Fluidized bed	200	1–100	Nonsticky powder, fiber
TSI model 3400	Chain conveyor	Fluidized bed	5–15	10–100	Nonsticky powder
Jet-O-Mizer	Screw feed	Air mill	300–400	2–1000	Sticky powder
Battle Micronizer	Dual brush	Air mill	30–50	5–5000	Sticky powder
Microjet	Screw feed	Air mill	300–1000	2–1000	Fiber

From *Concepts in Inhalation Toxicology*, Moss, O.R. and Cheng, Y-S, Hemisphere Publishing, Taylor & Francis, Washington, D.C., 1989, p. 101.[41] Reproduced with permission. All rights reserved.

TABLE 5.63
Efficiencies in Terms of Residual Water Content of Selected Solid Desiccants Used for Drying 25°C Nitrogen Gas at 225 cc/min through a Bed 14 mm i.d. and 450 mm Deep

Desiccant	Avg. Efficiency (mg/l air)	Regeneration Time (h) and Temp. (°C)
Calcium sulfate (Drierito®)	0.067	1–2, 200–225
Silica gel	0.070	12, 118–127
Activated alumina	0.0029	6–8, 175–400
Anhydrous magnesium perchlorate	0.0002	48, 245
Molecular sieve SA (Union Carbide®)	0.0039	—

From Phalen, R.F., *Inhalation Studies: Foundations and Techniques,* CRC Press, Boca Raton, FL, 1984.[11] With permission.

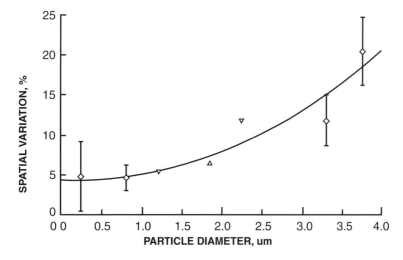

FIGURE 5.16 Spatial variations of aerosol concentrations in Hazelton 2000 exposure chambers as a function of aerosol particle size. Data are mean and standard deviation. From *Inhalation Toxicology,* Cheng, Y-S. and Moss, O.R., Hemisphere Publishing, Taylor & Francis, Washington, D.C., 1989, p. 50.[38] Reproduced with permission. All rights reserved.

REFERENCES

1. Tyler, W.S. and Julian, M.D., Gross and subgross anatomy of lungs, pleura, connective tissue septa, distal airways and structural units, in *Treatise On Pulmonary Toxicology,* vol. 1, *Comparative Biology of the Normal Lung,* Parent, R.A., Ed., CRC Press, Boca Raton, FL, 1992, chap. 4.

2. Schreider, J.P., Nasal airway anatomy and inhalation deposition in experimental animals and people, in: *Nasal Tumors in Animals and Man,* vol. III, *Experimental Nasal Carcinogenesis,* Reznik, G. and Stinson, Eds., CRC Press, Boca Raton, FL, 1983, pp. 1–26.

3. Pinkerton, K.E., Gehr, P., and Crapo, J.D., Architecture and cellular composition of the air-blood barrier, in *Treatise on Pulmonary Toxicology,* vol. 1, *Comparative Biology of the Normal Lung,* Parent, R.A., Ed., CRC Press, Boca Raton, FL, 1992, chap. 11.

4. Tenney, S.M. and Bartlett, D., Comparative quantitative morphology of the mammalian lung: trachea, *Respir. Physiol.,* 3, 130, 1967.

5. Gehr, P., Mwangi, D.K., Ammann, A., Maloiy, G.M.O., Taylor, C.R., and Weibel, E.R., Design of the mammalian respiratory system, V, scaling, morphometric pulmonary diffusing capacity to body mass: wild and domestic mammals, *J. Respir. Physiol.,* 44, 61, 1981.

6. Jones, J.H. and Longworth, K.E., Gas exchange at rest and during exercise in mammals, in *Treatise on Pulmonary Toxicology,* vol. 1, *Comparative Biology of the Normal Lung,* Parent, R.A., Ed., CRC Press, Boca Raton, FL, 1992, chap. 19.

7. Li-Fock, S.J. and Kaplowitz, M.R., Pleural liquid thickness *in situ* by light microscopy in five mammalian species, *J. Appl. Physiol.,* 59, 603, 1985.

8. Pinkerton, K.E., Mercer, R.R., Plopper, C.G., and Crapo, J.D., Distribution of injury and microdosimetry of ozone in the ventilatory unit of the rat, *J. Appl. Physiol.,* 1993.

9. Miller, F.J., Overton, J.H., Kimbell, J.S., and Russell, M.L., Regional respiratory tract absorption of inhaled reactive gasses, in *Toxicology of the Lung,* 2nd ed., Gardner, D.E., Crapo, J.D., and McClellan, R.O., Eds., Raven Press, New York, 1993, chap. 18.

10. Crapo, J.D., Young, S.L., Fram, E.K., Pinkerton, K.E., Barry, B.E., and Crapo, R.O., Morphometric characteristics of cells in the alveolar region of mammalian lungs, *Am. Rev. Respir. Dis.,* 128, 542, 1983.

11. Phalen, R.E., *Inhalation Studies: Foundations and Techniques,* CRC Press, Boca Raton, FL, 1984.

12. Schreider, J.P., Comparative anatomy and function of the nasal passages, in *Toxicology of the Nasal Passages,* Barrow, C.S., Ed., Hemisphere Publishing, New York, 1986, chap. 1.

13. Plopper, C.G., Mariassy, A.T., Wilson, D.W., Alley, J.L., Nishio, S.J., and Nettesheim, P., Comparison of nonciliated tracheal epithelial cells in six mammalian species: ultrastructure and population densities, *Exp. Lung. Res.,* 5, 281, 1983.

14. St. George, J.A., Harkema, J.R., Hyde, D.M., and Plopper, D.G., Cell populations and structural function relationships of cells in the airways, in *Toxicology of the Lung,* 2nd ed., Gardner, D.E., Crapo, J.D., and McClellan, R.O., Eds., Raven Press, New York, 1993, chap. 4.

15. Mariassy, A.T., Epithelial cells of the trachea and bronchi, in *Treatise on Pulmonary Toxicology,* vol. 1, *Comparative Biology of the Normal Lung,* Parent, R.A., Ed., CRC Press, Boca Raton, FL, 1992, chap. 6.

16. Plopper, C.G. and Hyde, D.M., Epithelial cells of bronchioles, in *Treatise on Pulmonary Toxicology,* vol. 1, *Comparative Biology of the Normal Lung,* Parent, R.A., Ed., CRC Press, Boca Raton, FL, 1992, chap. 8.

17. Stone, K.C., Mercer, R.R., Gehr, P., Stockstill, B., and Crapo, J.D., Allometric relationships of cell numbers and size in the mammalian lung, *Am. J. Respir. Cell. Mol. Biol.,* 6, 235, 1992.

18. Snipes, M.B., Long term retention and clearance of particles inhaled by mammalian species, *Crit. Rev. Toxicol.* 20, 174, 1989.

19. Boggs, D.F., Comparative control of respiration, in *Treatise on Pulmonary Toxicology,* vol. 1, *Comparative Biology of the Normal Lung,* Parent, R.A., Ed., CRC Press, Boca Raton, FL, 1992, chap. 20.

20. Mauderly, J.L., The effect of age on respiratory function of Fischer-344 rats, *Exp. Aging Res.,* 8, 31, 1982.

21. Sahebjami, H., Aging of the normal lung, in *Treatise on Pulmonary Toxicology,* vol. 1, *Comparative Biology of the Normal Lung,* Parent, R.A., Ed., CRC Press, Boca Raton, FL, 1992, chap. 21.

22. Mauderly, J.L., Ventilation, lung volumes and lung mechanics of young adult and old Syrian hamsters, *Exp. Aging Res.,* 5, 497, 1979.

23. Lai, Y.-L., Comparative ventilation of the normal lung, in *Treatise on Pulmonary Toxicology,* vol. 1, *Comparative Biology of the Normal Lung,* Parent, R.A., Ed., CRC Press, Boca Raton, FL, 1992, chap. 17.

24. Johanson, W.G., Jr. and Pierce, A.K., Lung structure and function with age in normal rats and rats with papain emphysema, *J. Clin. Invest.,* 52, 2921, 1973.

25. Henderson, R.F., Bronchoalveolar lavage: a tool for assessing the health status of the lung, in *Concepts in Inhalation Toxicology,* McClellan, R.O. and Henderson, R.F., Eds., Hemisphere Publishing, New York, 1989, chap. 15.

26. McDermott, M.R., Befus, A.D., and Bienenstock, J., The structural basis for immunity in the respiratory tract, *Int. Rev. Exp. Pathol.,* 23, 47, 1982.

27. Murray, M.J. and Driscoll, K.E., Immunology of the respiratory system, in *Treatise on Pulmonary Toxicology,* vol. 1, *Comparative Biology of the Normal Lung,* Parent, R.A., Ed., CRC Press, Boca Raton, FL, 1992, chap. 37.

28. Schlesinger, R.B., Deposition and clearance of inhaled particles, in *Concepts in Inhalation Toxicology,* McClellan, R.O. and Henderson, R.F., Eds., Hemisphere Publishing, New York, 1989, chap. 6.

29. Valberg, P.A. and Blanchard, J.D., Pulmonary macrophage physiology: origin, motility, endocytosis, in *Treatise on Pulmonary Toxicology,* vol. 1, *Comparative Biology of the Normal Lung,* Parent, R.A., Ed., CRC Press, Boca Raton, FL, 1992, chap. 36.

30. Stöber, W., McClellan, R.O., and Morrow, P.E., Approaches to modeling disposition of inhaled particles and fibers in the lung, in *Toxicology of the Lung,* 2nd ed., Gardner, D.E., Crapo, J.D., and McClellan, R.O., Eds., Raven Press, New York, 1993, chap. 19.

31. Wolff, R.K., Mucocilliary function, in *Treatise on Pulmonary Toxicology,* vol. 1, *Comparative Biology of the Normal Lung,* Parent, R.A., Ed., CRC Press, Boca Raton, FL, 1992, chap. 35.

32. Klimisch, H.-J., Bretz, R., Doe, J.E., and Purser, D.A., Classification of dangerous substances and pesticides in the European economic community directives: a proposed revision of criteria for inhalation toxicity, *Reg. Toxicol. Pharmacol.,* 7, 21, 1987.

33. Kane, L.E., Barrrow, C.S., and Alaire, Y., A short-term test to predict acceptable levels of exposure to airborne sensory irritants, *Am. Ind. Hyg. Assoc. J.,* 40, 207, 1979.

34. Boggs, D.F. and Tenney, S.M., Scaling respiratory pattern and respiratory drive, *Respir. Physiol.,* 58, 245, 1984.

35. Costa, D.L., Tepper, J.S., and Raub, J.A., Interpretations and limitations of pulmonary function testing in small laboratory animals, in *Treatise on Pulmonary Toxicology,* vol. 1, *Comparative Biology of the Normal Lung,* Parent, R.A., Ed., CRC Press, Boca Raton, FL, 1992, chap. 22.

36. Hahn, F.F., Chronic inhalation bioassays for respiratory tract carcinogenesis, in *Toxicology of the Lung,* 2nd ed., Gardner, D.E., Crapo, J.D., and McClellan, R.O., Eds., Raven Press, New York, 1993, chap. 16.

37. Schlessinger, R.B., The interaction of inhaled toxicants with respiratory tract clearance mechanisms, *Crit. Rev. Toxicol.,* 20, 297, 1990.

38. Cheng., Y-S. and Moss, O.R., Inhalation exposure systems, in *Concepts in Inhalation Toxicology,* McClellan, R.O. and Henderson, R.F., Eds., Hemisphere Publishing, New York, 1989, chap. 1.

39. Fieldner, A.C., Katz, S.H., and Kinney, S.P., Gas masks for gasses met in fighting fires, U.S. Bureau of Mines, Technical Paper No. 248, 1921.

40. Clayton, G.D. and Clayton, F.E., Eds., *Patty's Industrial Hygiene and Toxicology,* 4th ed., John Wiley & Sons, New York, 1991.

41. Moss, O.R. and Cheng, Y-S., Generation and characterization of test atmospheres: particles, in *Concepts in Inhalation Toxicology,* McClellan, R.O. and Henderson, R.F., Eds., Hemisphere Publishing, New York, 1989, chap. 3

ADDITIONAL RELATED INFORMATION

TABLE 5.64
Some Xenobiotic Metabolizing Enzymes in the Nasal Cavity

Enzyme	Test Reaction or Other Method for Detection	Test System	Notes
15-Lipoxygenase	Arachidonic acid metabolism	Human nasal cells	Nasal epithelial cells more active than bronchial cells
P-450	Diethylnitrosamine deethylase	Human nasal respiratory tissue microsomes	Nasal activity per nmol P-450 10–25 times that of liver
P-450	Five dealkylases	Human nasal respiratory tissue microsomes	HMPA and aminopyrine best substrates; ethoxycoumarin and ethoxyresorufin next best substrates; pentoxyresorufin poor substrate
Epoxide hydrolase	Safrole oxide hydrolase	Human nasal respiratory tissue homogenate	Activity higher than that in rats
Glutathione S-transferase	1-Chloro-2, 4-dinitro-benzene conjugation	Human nasal respiratory tissue homogenate	Activity higher than that in rats
DT-diaphorase	Dichlorophenol-indophenol metabolism	Human nasal respiratory tissue homogenate	Activity much less than that in rats
UDP-glucuronyl transferase	1-naphthol conjugation	Human nasal respiratory tissue homogenate	Absent in humans; present in rats
NADPH-cytochrome C-reductase	C Cytochrome C reduction	Human nasal respiratory tissue homogenate	Activity about 25% that of rat nasal mucosa
Rhodanese	Metabolism of cyanide to thiocyanate	Human nasal respiratory tissue homogenate	Activity in nonsmokers twofold higher than that in smokers
P-450PB-B; NADPH-cytochrome P-450 reductase	Immunohistochemistry	Male Holtzman rat olfactory and respiratory tissues, Bowman's glands, and seromucous glands	P-450PB-B is homologous with IIB1; Bowman's glands and apex of olfactory epithelial cells contained high concentrations of reductase
P450c	Immunocytochemistry	Male Alp/Apk rat olfactory epithelium; Bowman's glands	Homologous with P-450IA1; not induced by phenobarbital, clofibrate, or β-naphthoflavone
P-450βNF-B P-450PB-B P-450PCN-E	Immunohistochemistry	Male Holtzman rat olfactory epithelium; Bowman's glands, and seromucous glands	P-450βNF-B (homologuous with IA1) present in olfactory tissue at a higher level than in respiratory tissue; consistent with this, aryl hydrocarbon hydroxylase activity; PB-B (IIB1) intensely stained both tissues; PCN-E (IIIA) stained less intensely, but about equally in both tissues; apical portions of epithelial cells and subepithelial glands stained relatively intensely
P450d	Induction of encoding mRNA	S-D rat olfactory tissue microsomes	P-450d (IA2) but not P-450c (IA1) was induced to detectable levels
P-450olf1	cDNA library probe and sequence anaysis	S-D rat olfactory tissue microsomes	Termed IIG1; rabbit form may be P-450NMb; olfactory tissue specific
P-450olf2	Immunoblots	Wistar rat olfactory tissue	Homologous with IIA family
P-450IIE1	Immunohistochemistry	Male F344 rat	Glands in lamina propia heavily labeled; olfactory sustentacular cells apically labeled; ciliated cells of respiratory epithelium and nonsecretory cells of transitional epithelium labeled; luminal surface of olfactory epithelium in vomeral nasal organ labeled

TABLE 5.64 *(Continued)*
Some Xenobiotic Metabolizing Enzymes in the Nasal Cavity

Enzyme	Test Reaction or Other Method for Detection	Test System	Notes
Aromatase and 5a-reductase	Testosterone metabolism to estradiol and dihydrotestosterone	Measled S-D rat olfactory epithelium	Castration decreased estradiol production; activity restored by testosterone replacement
FAD-containing mono-oxygenase	Dimethylamine and N,N-dimethylaniline metabolism	Male F344 rat olfactory mucosa microsomes	Dimethylaniline apparently metabolized only by FAD-MO; dimethylamine metabolized by P-450, as well
Aldehyde dehydrogenase; formaldehyde dehydrogenase	Formaldehyde and acetaldehyde dehydrogenation; histochemistry	Male F344 rat respiratory and olfactory mucosa	Multiple forms; formaldehyde dehydrogenase most abundant in olfactory mucosa; epithelial cell cytoplasm and olfactory sensory cell nuclei; Bowman's and seromucous glands weakly positive; acetaldehyde dehydrogenase most abundant in respiratory mucosa; present in Bowman's glands and olfactory basal cells; absent from sensory cells and sustentacular cells
Carboxylesterase	Ester hydrolysis; histochemistry	F344 rat nasal tissue	k_m values ranged from 1–35 mM; V_{max} from 0.03 to 0.06; present in all nasal cells except olfactory neurons
Carbonic anhydrase	Histochemistry	Rat olfactory tissue	Present in receptor cells; absent in sustentacular cells
Epoxide hydrolase; UDP-glucuronyl transferase; glutathione S-transferase forms B, C, and E	Styrene oxide; 7-hydroxycoumarin; styrene oxide; immunohistochemistry	Male F344 or Holtzman rat nasal tissue homogenates	Epoxide hydrolase probably form A; GSH-T B, C, and E probably forms 5,5, 1,1, 3,3, respectively; GSH-T form C — which metabolizes ΔE^5-androstene-3, 17-dione — was at highest levels
Rhodanese	Cyanide metabolism to thiocyanate; immunohistochemistry	F344 rat nasal mucosa	Highest in apical portion of olfactory epithelium; absent from receptor cells; negligible in Bowman's glands; present in respiratory epithelium also
P-4503a, P-450 form 2, P-450 form 4, P-450 form 5	Immunochemistry; immunoblot; enzyme assays	Male New Zealand white rabbit nasal mucosa	Homologues IIE; Forms 2, 4, 5, by homology, are also termed IIB1, 1A2, and IVB1, respectively; forms 2 and 5 occur in both respiratory and olfactory tissue; form 4 found in olfactory tissue only; form 6 (homologous with IA1) absent in all tissues
FAD-containing mono-oxygenase	Immunoblot	Male New Zealand white rabbit olfactory and respiratory mucos	Approximately equal amounts in respiratory and olfactory tissues
P-450 form NMa, P-450 form NMb, P-450 form 2, P-450 form 3a, P-450 form 3b, P-450 form 4, P-450 form 6	Immunochemistry; testosterone metabolism; HMPA and phenacetin metabolism	Male New Zealand white rabbit nasal respiratory and olfactory epithelium	Only form 2 (IIBI) found in respiratory tissue; NMa very active for HMPA and phenacetin dealkylation; only 3% of liver P-450 is NMa; NMb (IIG1) occurs only in olfactory tissue; forms 3a and 4 are homologous with IIE1 and IA2, respectively; forms 3b and 6 (homologous to IIC3 and IA1, respectively) absent in nasal tissue

TABLE 5.64 *(Continued)*
Some Xenobiotic Metabolizing Enzymes in the Nasal Cavity

Enzyme	Test Reaction or Other Method for Detection	Test System	Notes
Carboxylesterase	Ester hydrolysis	Male and female New Zealand white rabbit nasal mucosa	Less activity than for mice, rats, or dogs. Activities in both mucosae similar to that in liver
P-450	p-Nitroanisole demethylase; aniline hydroxylase; carbon monoxide difference spectra	CD1 mouse nasal tissue microsomes	Compared to dog, rabbit, guinea pig, rat, and Syrian hamster, aniline better substrate in mouse than in any other species except Syrian hamsters
P-450; NADPH-cytochrome C-reductase	7-Ethoxycoumarin deethylase; carbon monoxide difference spectrum; cytochrome C-reductase	MFI mouse olfactory epithelium	Very high nasal activities relative to those in liver; activities higher in males than in females
Carboxylesterases	Ethylene glycol monomethylether acetate	Male and female B6C3F1₁Crl Br mouse nasal mucosa homogenates	Mouse activity greater than that of rats
Carboxylesterases	p-Nitrophenyl butyrate hydrolysis; histochemistry	B6C3F₁ mouse; both sexes; respiratory and olfactory tissue	Also examined rats; mouse and rat activity (V/k_m) similar; olfactory activity fivefold that of respiratory; V_{max} olfactory 0.5 µmol/min/mg protein, k_m 20–25 mM
P-450	p-Nitroanisole, O-demethylase, and aniline hydroxylase; carbon monoxide difference spectra	Syrian hamster nasal tissue microsomes	Very high activities relative to dog, rabbit, guinea pig, rat, and mouse; values (in nmol P-450 per mg protein): olfactory — 0.36, respiratory — 0.13, trachea — 0.26, liver — 1.10
Arylhydrocarbon oxidases/hydroxylase	Benzo(a)pyrene metabolism *in vivo*; olfactory and respiratory tissue microsomal activity	Syrian hamster nasal cavity	Also examined *in vitro* metabolism in 5 non-nasal tissues; olfactory tissue highest (4000 pmol/g tissue per hr); metabolites *in vivo* included tetrols, diols, quinones, oxides, and phenols
P-450; NADPH cytochrome C-reductase; cytochrome b5	7-Ethoxycoumarin and ethoxyresorufin dealkylase; hexabarbitone oxidase; aniline hydroxylase; cytochrome C-reductase; difference spectra	Syrian hamster olfactory tissue	Very high activities compared to those in rats and female mice; olfactory activities (but not P-450 content) higher than in liver
Carboxylesterases	Ester hydrolysis of acetate esters and lactones; ethyl acetate uptake *in vivo*	Syrian hamster olfactory nasal cavity	Hamster nasal activity much higher than rat or rabbit nasal activity with amyl acetate, but not with β-butyrolactone; ester uptake in hamster nose sensitive to enzyme inhibition (63–90%)
Alcohol dehydrogenase	Propanol metabolism *in vivo*	Syrian hamster tissue homogenates	k_m is 0.1 mM; V_{max} is 4 nmol/mg protein per min, 36 nmol/nose per min

From Schlesinger, R.B., Ben-Jebria, A., Dahl, A.R., Snipes, M.B., and Ultman, J., Disposition of inhaled toxicants, in *Handbook of Human Toxicology*, Massaro, E.J., Ed., CRC Press, Boca Raton, FL, chap. 12, pp. 493–550, 1997. With permission. Originally adapted from Dahl, A.R. and Hadley, W.M., Nasal cavity enzymes involved in xenobiotic metabolism: effects on the toxicity of inhalants, *Toxicology*, 21, 345, 1991.

TABLE 5.65
Summary of P-450 Isozymes Reported in the Rat and Rabbit Nasal Cavities

	Alternate Name		Nasal Tissue	
Isozyme	Rat	Rabbit	Rat	Rabbit
IAl	βNF-B	Form 6	Respiratory and olfactory	Absent
IA2	ISF-G,d	Form 4	Olfactory	Olfactory
IIA	olf2	—	Olfactory	Not reported
IIB1	PB-B,b	Form 2	Respiratory and olfactory	Respiratory and olfactory
IIC3	—	3b	Not reported	Absent
IIE1	j	3a,P-450ALC	Respiratory and olfactory	Olfactory
IIG1	olf1	P-450LM3c	Respiratory and olfactory	Not reported
IIIA	PCN-E			
IVB1	Form 5	Form 5	Not reported	Respiratory and olfactory

From Schlesinger, R.B., Ben-Jebria, A., Dahl, A.R., Snipes, M.B., and Ultman, J., Disposition of inhaled toxicants, in *Handbook of Human Toxicology,* Massaro, E.J., Ed., CRC Press, Boca Raton, FL, chap. 12, pp. 493–550, 1997. With permission. Originally adapted from Dahl, A.R. and Hadley, W.M., Nasal cavity enzymes involved in xenobiotic metabolism: effects on the toxicity of inhalants, *Toxicology,* 21, 345, 1991.

TABLE 5.66
Some P-450 Isozymes Reported in Lungs of Various Species

	Isozyme	Comments
Mouse	1A1	Induced in type II cells
	1A2	Induced in type II cells and endothelial cells
	2B1	Constitutive in type II cells and Clara cells
	2B2	Constitutive in type II cells and Clara cells
	4B1	Rabbit form activates ipomeanol and 2-aminofluorene
	"mN"	In Clara cells, metabolizes naphthalene
	"m50b"	In Clara cells, major naphthalene-metabolizing enzyme
Rat	1A1	Induced in bronchial epithelium, Clara cells, and type II cells
	2A3	Absent in rat liver
	2B1	Constitutive at highest levels in Clara cells
	2E1	Induced by hyperoxygen
	3A1/2	Induced in bronchial epithelium, Clara cells, and type II cells
	4B1	Absent in rat liver
	"FI"	Constitutive; induced by O_3
	"FII"	Cross reacts with rat anti 2B1 ; constitutive; induced by O_3
Rabbit	1A1	Highly inducible; occurs in endothelial cells without reductase
	2B1	With 4B1, accounts for 80% of uninduced P-450 in lung
	2E1, 2E2	2E1, 5% that of liver; 2E2, 2.5% that of liver
	4A4	P-450 prostaglandin ω-hydroxylase; occurs only in pregnant rabbits or after induction by progesterone
	4B1	Activates 2-aminofluorene and ipomeanol
Hamster	"MC"	Possibly IA1; highly inducible
	2B	Along with reductase, absent from mesothelium in adults
	4B	Present in mesothelium in adult
Human	1A1	Inducibility related to smoking and lung cancer
	2E1	Racial differences in 2E1 polymorphisms
	2F1	Ethoxycoumarin and pentoxyresorufin and 3-methylindole are substrates
	4B1	Unlike rabbit form, does not activate 2-aminofluorene

From Schlesinger, R.B., Ben-Jebria, A., Dahl, A.R., Snipes, M.B., and Ultman, J., Disposition of inhaled toxicants, in *Handbook of Human Toxicology,* Massaro, E.J., Ed., CRC Press, Boca Raton, FL, chap. 12, pp. 493–550, 1997. With permission. Originally adapted from Dahl, A.R. and Lewis, J.L., Respiratory tract uptake of inhalants and metabolism of xenobiotics, *Ann. Rev. Pharmacol. Toxicol.,* 32, 383, 1993.

6 Applied Inhalation Toxicology

Gary M. Hoffman, B.A., D.A.B.T.

CONTENTS

SECTION 1. EXPOSURES

All inhalation exposures involve the respiratory system as the major portal of entry for the test material. The test material normally is administered in the gaseous/vapor state or as an aerosol. In either case, the test material must be administered in a manner that provides stable, reproducible exposure concentrations. These exposure concentrations must be measured routinely to demonstrate that the actual exposure concentrations are within the desired ranges, or to provide information needed to bring the actual exposure concentrations within the desired ranges.

Administration of test materials in the gaseous/vapor state occur with chemicals that are normally a gas at room temperature or are solids or liquids with a vapor pressure high enough to generate the desired exposure concentration. The former are referred to as gases, while the latter are called vapors. Administration of test materials as gases is typically accomplished using flow dilution techniques. Administration of vapors is typically accomplished using gas scrubbing or evaporation-volatilization techniques. Because of the complexity and diversity of these systems and their unique application to specific studies, they cannot all be described here.

Administration of test materials as aerosols occur with chemicals that are normally liquids or solids at room temperature. These test materials do not possess a vapor pressure high enough to allow generation of the desired exposure concentration in the gaseous/vapor state. Aerosols originating from liquids can further be classified as liquid aerosols, while aerosols originating from solids can be classified as dusts. Administration of liquid aerosols is typically accomplished using spray atomization or evaporation-condensation techniques. Administration of dusts is typically accomplished using either a nonsegregating technique such as a dust feed or a segregating technique such as a sonic generator. Because of the complexity and diversity of these systems and their unique application to specific studies, they cannot all be described here.

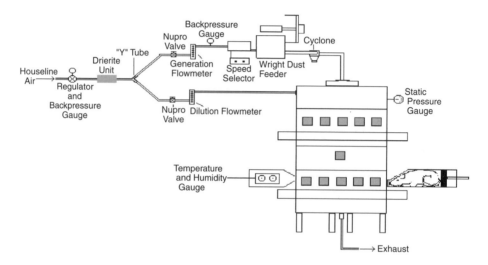

FIGURE 6.1 System for generation of a dust atmosphere into a 40-l nose-only exposure chamber. A Wright Dust Feeder is used to disperse the aerosolized powder through a cyclone, for removal of large particles, into the nose-only exposure chamber from which the test animals breathe.

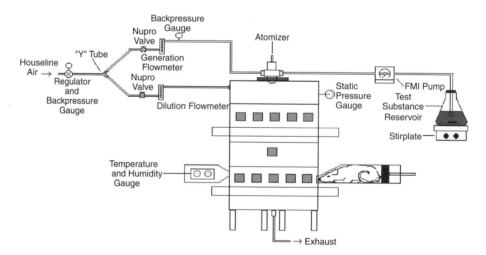

FIGURE 6.2 System for generation of a liquid aerosol atmosphere into a 40-l nose-only exposure chamber. A spray atomizer is used to disperse the aerosolized liquid, fed from a reservoir with a fluid metering pump, into the nose-only exposure chamber from which the test animals breathe.

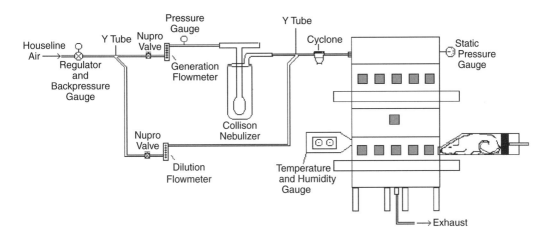

FIGURE 6.3 System for generation of a liquid aerosol atmosphere into a 40-l nose-only exposure chamber. A Collison Nebulizer is used to disperse the aerosolized liquid, through a cyclone for removal of large particles, into the nose-only exposure chamber from which the test animals breathe.

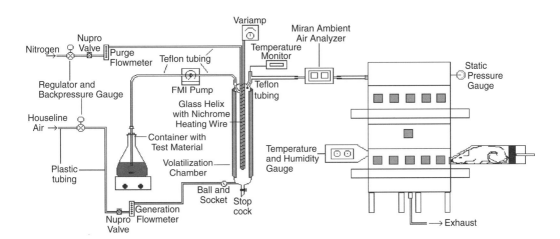

FIGURE 6.4 System for generation of a vapor atmosphere into a 40-l nose-only exposure chamber. A countercurrent volatilization chamber (heated with a nichrome wire, if needed) is used to disperse the vaporized liquid, fed from a reservoir with a fluid metering pump, into the nose-only exposure chamber from which the test animals breathe.

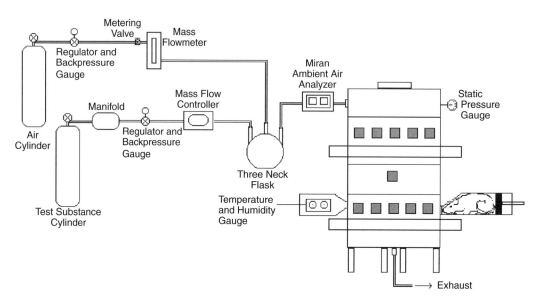

FIGURE 6.5 System for generation of a gas atmosphere into a 40-l nose-only exposure chamber. A mass flow controller is used to disperse the gas, fed from a pressurized cylinder, into the nose-only exposure chamber from which the test animals breathe.

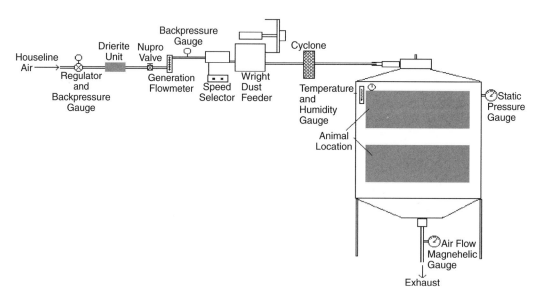

FIGURE 6.6 System for generation of a dust atmosphere into a 1000-l whole-body exposure chamber. A Wright Dust Feeder is used to disperse the aerosolized powder through a cyclone, for removal of large particles, into the whole-body exposure chamber within which the test animals breathe.

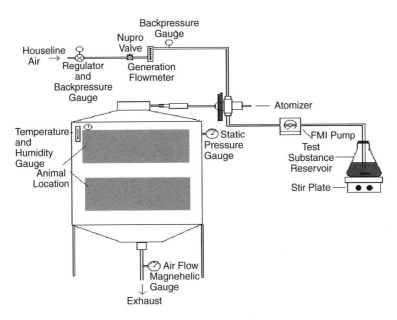

FIGURE 6.7 System for generation of a liquid aerosol atmosphere into a 1000-l whole-body exposure chamber. A spray atomizer is used to disperse the aerosolized liquid, fed from a reservoir with a fluid metering pump, into the whole-body exposure chamber within which the test animals breathe.

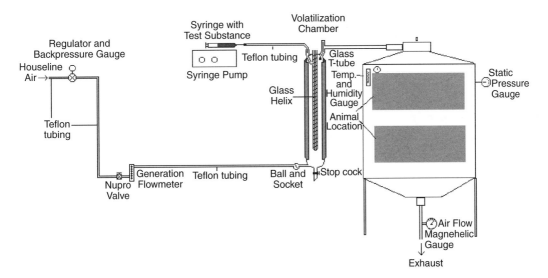

FIGURE 6.8 System for generation of a vapor atmosphere into a 1000-l whole-body exposure chamber. A countercurrent volatilization chamber (heated with a nichrome wire, if needed) is used to disperse the vaporized liquid, fed from a syringe pump, into the whole-body exposure chamber within which the test animals breathe.

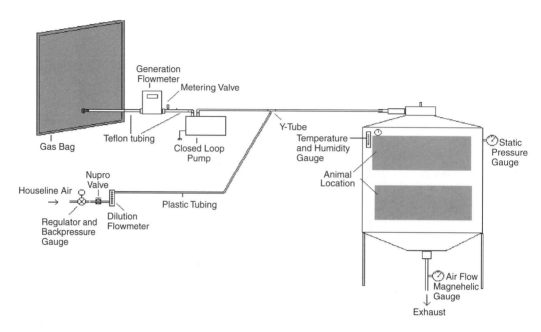

FIGURE 6.9 System for generation of a gas atmosphere into a 1000-l whole-body exposure chamber. A flowmeter is used to disperse the gas, fed from a gas bag with a vacuum pump, into the whole-body exposure chamber within which the test animals breathe.

SECTION 2. SAMPLING

All inhalation exposure concentrations must be measured routinely to demonstrate that the actual exposure concentrations are close to the targeted exposure concentrations, or to provide information needed to adjust the actual exposure concentrations close to the targeted exposure concentrations. Samples are routinely collected every hour, or sooner, during a single exposure inhalation study and every 1.5 h, or sooner, during a repeat exposure inhalation study. Gas and vapor exposures are typically measured using an infrared (IR) spectrophotometer or a gas chromatograph (GC). The IR is simpler to calibrate, only provides a total hydrocarbon concentration but does not quantify individual components in a complex mixture. The GC is more complex to calibrate but does quantify individual components in a complex mixture. In either case, the instrument would be directly

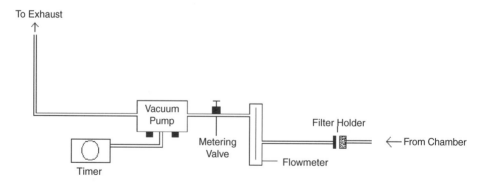

FIGURE 6.10 System for collection of filter paper samples of test atmospheres for gravimetric or analytical evaluation. A vacuum pump is used to draw the air sample through a glass fiber filter paper from the exposure chamber.

Chamber Monitoring Record

Study No.: _____
Date: _____
Group No.: _____
Test Material: _____

Prepared By: _____
Initial Review: _____
Final Review: _____

Time	Sample #	Generation Flowmeter (set)[1] (Lpm)	Dilution Flowmeter (set)[2] (Lpm)	Dust Feeder Speed ( )	Total Flow (Lpm)	Back-Pressure (psi)	Sample Flow (Lpm)	Sample Time (min.)	Sample Volume (liters)	Tare Wt. (mg)	Final Wt. (mg)	Net Wt. (mg)	Chamber Conc. (mg/L)	Adjust-ment	Initial/Date
T$_0$															

Balance Model: _____ Inh. # _____ Filter Paper: Brand: _____ Type: _____ Size: _____ cm Lot #: _____ Init/Date: _____

Comments:
1. Actual Generation Flow = _____ Lpm.
2. Actual Dilution Flow = _____ Lpm.

FIGURE 6.11 Example of a data sheet for recording data for a dust exposure with gravimetric air sampling.

calibrated using standards of the test material. Aerosol exposures are typically measured using gravimetric (weight difference) determination of test material collected onto a glass fiber filter. These filters may also be extracted for the test material using an appropriate solvent and then quantified with a gas chromatograph or liquid chromatograph. Aerosol exposures also require the evaluation of the particle size to assess the respirability for the test animals being exposed. Particle sizing is typically accomplished using cascade impactor techniques (with either gravimetric or analytical determination of the collected sample) or using photometric techniques such as laser-light interception. Particle sizing results are usually reported in terms of the mass median aerodynamic diameter (MMAD) and the geometric standard deviation (GSD).

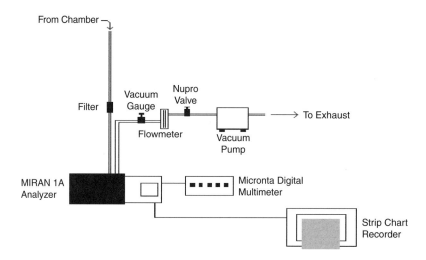

FIGURE 6.12 System for collection of air samples of test atmospheres for IR spectrophotometric evaluation. A vacuum pump is used to draw the air sample through a calibrated IR spectrophotometer from the exposure chamber.

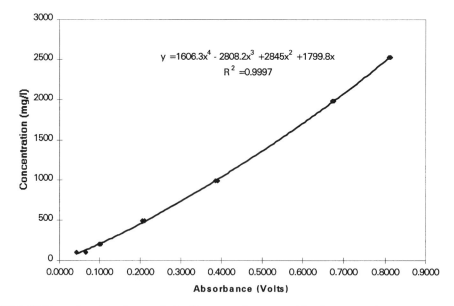

FIGURE 6.13 Example calibration graph for IR spectrophotometer. The IR spectrophotometer is calibrated by injecting known volumes of test material into a "closed-loop system" of known volume (5.64 l).

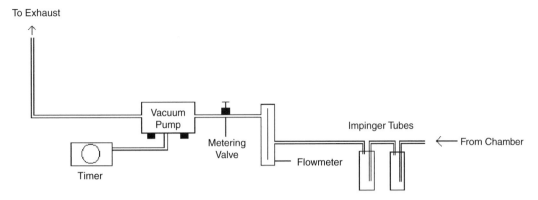

FIGURE 6.14 System for collection of impinger samples of test atmospheres for analytical evaluation. A vacuum pump is used to draw the air sample through tandem impingers (containing an appropriate solvent, e.g., water) from the exposure chamber.

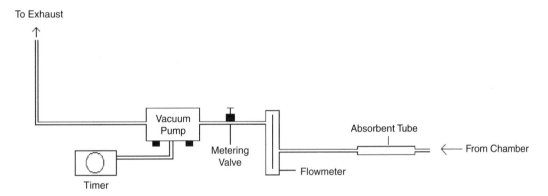

FIGURE 6.15 System for collection of absorbent tube samples of test atmospheres for analytical evaluation. A vacuum pump is used to draw the air sample through an absorbent tube (containing an appropriate medium, e.g., charcoal) from the exposure chamber.

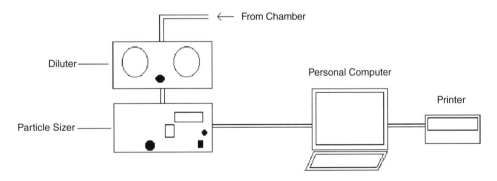

FIGURE 6.16 System for collection of aerosol samples of test atmospheres for particle size evaluation with the TSI Aerodynamic Particle Sizer. An internal vacuum pump is used to draw the air sample through a dilutor (100:1) and the particle sizer from the exposure chamber. The particle sizer uses a time-of-flight calibration based on the acceleration of particles through an orifice past a pair of laser beams.

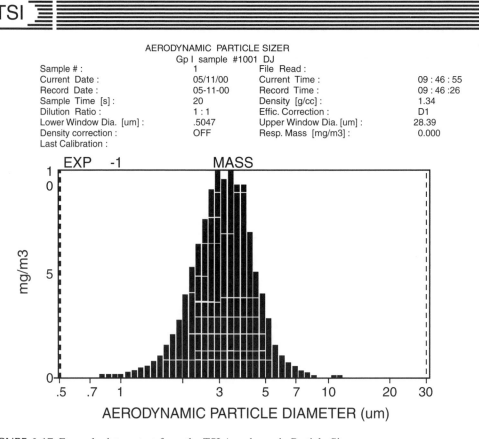

FIGURE 6.17 Example data output from the TSI Aerodynamic Particle Sizer.

```
TSI
```

AERODYNAMIC PARTICLE SIZER
Gp I sample #1001 DJ

Sample #:	1	File Read:	
Current Date:	05/11/00	Current Time:	09:47:37
Record Date:	05-11-00	Record Time:	09:46:26
Sample Time [s]:	20	Density [g/cc]:	1.34
Dilution Ratio:	1:1	Effic. Correction:	D1
Lower Window Dia. [um]:	.5047	Upper Window Dia.[um]:	28.39
Density correction:	OFF	Resp. Mass [mg/m3]:	0.000
Last Calibration:			

CONCENTRATION   CUMULATIVE PERCENT

DIA.	part/cm^3 NUMBER	um^2/cm^3 SURFACE	mg/m^3 MASS	NUMBER	SURFACE	MASS
<0.47	.327	.155	1.35E-5			
0.505	.270	.161	1.57E-5	1.60E-2	7.66E-4	1.36E-4
0.542	.387	.267	2.79E-5	3.89E-2	2.03E-3	3.78E-4
0.582	.555	.440	4.94E-5	7.19E-2	4.13E-3	8.07E-4
0.625	.810	.742	8.95E-5	.120	7.65E-3	1.58E-3
0.673	3.18	3.37	4.38E-4	.308	2.37E-2	5.38E-3
0.724	16.2	19.9	2.78E-3	1.27	.118	2.95E-2
0.778	25.1	35.6	5.34E-3	2.76	.287	7.58E-2
0.835	26.7	43.7	7.04E-3	4.34	.495	.137
0.898	29.7	56.1	9.72E-3	6.10	.762	.221
0.965	34.3	74.8	1.39E-2	8.13	1.12	.342
1.04	38.4	96.8	1.94E-2	10.4	1.58	.510
1.11	42.4	1.24E2	2.66E-2	12.9	2.16	.740
1.2	49.3	1.66E2	3.83E-2	15.8	2.95	1.07
1.29	53.5	2.08E2	5.16E-2	19.0	3.94	1.52
1.38	63.8	2.86E2	7.63E-2	22.8	5.30	2.18
1.49	67.6	3.50E2	.100	26.8	6.96	3.05
1.6	84.8	5.07E2	.156	31.8	9.37	4.40
1.72	91.5	6.31E2	.209	37.3	12.4	6.22
1.84	99.3	7.91E2	.281	43.1	16.1	8.65
1.98	1.15E2	1.06E3	.405	50.0	21.2	12.2
2.13	1.24E2	1.31E3	.539	57.3	27.4	16.8
2.29	1.20E2	1.47E3	.650	64.4	34.4	22.5
2.46	1.15E2	1.63E3	.774	71.2	42.1	29.2
2.64	1.10E2	1.79E3	.914	77.7	50.7	37.1
2.84	96.3	1.82E3	.996	83.4	59.3	45.8
3.05	75.5	1.65E3	.969	87.9	67.1	54.2
3.28	62.5	1.57E3	.995	91.6	74.6	62.8
3.52	47.6	1.39E3	.942	94.4	81.2	71.0
3.79	38.2	1.28E3	.938	96.7	87.3	79.1
4.07	23.5	9.11E2	.715	98.1	91.6	85.3
4.37	13.7	6.14E2	.518	98.9	94.6	89.8
4.7	8.69	4.50E2	.408	99.4	96.7	93.3
5.05	4.98	2.98E2	.290	99.7	98.1	95.8
5.42	2.19	1.51E2	.158	99.9	98.8	97.2
5.83	1.10	87.5	9.84E-2	99.9	99.2	98.1
6.26	.621	57.1	6.90E-2	1.000E2	99.5	98.7
6.73	.375	39.8	5.17E-2	1.000E2	99.7	99.1
7.23	.201	24.7	3.44E-2	1.000E2	99.8	99.4
7.77	.117	16.6	2.49E-2	1.000E2	99.9	99.6
8.35	2.49E-2	4.08	6.58E-3	1.000E2	99.9	99.7
8.98	1.35E-2	2.55	4.42E-3	1.000E2	99.9	99.7
9.65	1.18E-2	2.58	4.80E-3	1.000E2	99.9	99.8
10.4	1.57E-2	3.97	7.94E-3	1.000E2	1.000E2	99.8
11.1	8.44E-3	2.45	5.28E-3	1.000E2	1.000E2	99.9
12.	5.25E-3	1.76	4.07E-3	1.000E2	1.000E2	99.9
12.9	3.37E-3	1.31	3.25E-3	1.000E2	1.000E2	99.9
13.8	4.12E-3	1.85	4.93E-3	1.000E2	1.000E2	1.000E2
14.9	1.12E-3	.582	1.67E-3	1.00E2	1.000E2	1.00E2
16.	0.00	0.00	0.00	1.00E2	1.000E2	1.00E2
17.2	0.00	0.00	0.00	1.00E2	1.000E2	1.00E2
18.4	0.00	0.00	0.00	1.00E2	1.000E2	1.00E2
19.8	0.00	0.00	0.00	1.00E2	1.000E2	1.00E2
21.3	0.00	0.00	0.00	1.00E2	1.000E2	1.00E2
22.9	0.00	0.00	0.00	1.00E2	1.000E2	1.00E2
24.6	0.00	0.00	0.00	1.00E2	1.000E2	1.00E2
26.4	0.00	0.00	0.00	1.00E2	1.000E2	1.00E2
28.4	0.00	0.00	0.00	1.00E2	1.000E2	1.00E2
>30.5	0.00	0.00	0.00			
TOTALS	1.69E3	2.10E4	11.5			

FIGURE 6.18 Example data output from the TSI Aerodynamic Particle Sizer.

```
TSI ≡

                    AERODYNAMIC PARTICLE SIZER
                       Gp I sample #1001  DJ
       Sample #:               1          File Read:
       Current Date:        05/11/00      Current Time:          09:49:08
       Record Date:         05-11-00      Record Time:           09:46:26
       Sample Time [s]:        20         Density [g/cc]:        1.34
       Dilution Ratio:        1:1         Effic. Correction:     D1
       Lower Window Dia. [um]: .5047      Upper Window Dia.[um]: 28.39
       Density correction:    OFF         Resp. Mass [mg/m3]:    0.000
       Last Calibration:


       Particle Size Statistics (with no size distribution assumption)
       ---------------------------------------------------------------

       Number Count:
              median (CMAD)           2.056
              mean                    2.136
              count mean              1.961
              mode                    2.129
              standard deviation       .8695
              geo. standard deviation 1.528
              skewness                8.457E-3
              coeff. of variation [%] 40.70
       Surface Area:
              median (SMAD)           2.725
              mean                    2.840
              count mean              2.667
              mode                    2.839
              standard deviation      1.014
              geo. standard deviation 1.435
       Mass:
              median (MMAD)           3.055
              mean                    3.202
              count mean              3.018
              mode                    2.839
              standard deviation      1.155
              geo. standard deviation 1.411

       Particle Size Statistics (assuming log-normal distribution)
       ------------------------------------------------------------

       Number Count:
              median (CMAD)           2.056
              geo. standard deviation 1.528
              geo. mean               2.249
              mode                    1.718
       Surface Area:
              median (SMAD)           2.945
              geo. mean               3.222
              dia. of average surface 2.461
       Mass:
              median (MMAD)           3.525
              geo. mean               3.856
              dia. of average mass    2.692
```

FIGURE 6.19 Example data output from the TSI Aerodynamic Particle Sizer.

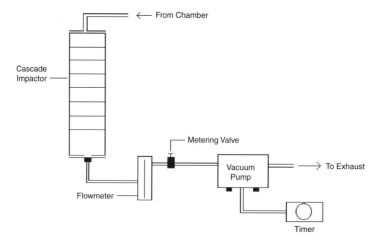

FIGURE 6.20 System for collection of aerosol samples of test atmospheres for particle size evaluation with a cascade impactor. A vacuum pump is used to draw the air sample through the multistage cascade impactor from the exposure chamber. The stages are individually assayed by gravimetric or analytical methodology.

Chamber Monitoring Record
ITP Cascade Impactor

Study No.: _____
Test Material: _____
Group: _____

Serial No.: _____
Sample No.: _____
Time of Sample: _____
Time Sampled (min.): _____

Prepared By: _____
Date: _____
Initial Review: _____
Final Review: _____

Impactor Stage	Stage Constant (μm)	Slide Weight Before (mg)	Slide Weight After (mg)	Δ Weight (μg)	Cumulative Mass (μg)
Filter		_____	_____	_____	_____
7	0.328	_____	_____	_____	_____
6	0.719	_____	_____	_____	_____
5	1.061	_____	_____	_____	_____
4	1.624	_____	_____	_____	_____
3	2.090	_____	_____	_____	_____
2	3.000	_____	_____	_____	_____
1	4.595	_____	_____	_____	_____
	10.000	_____	_____		
Initials					

Scale # _____ /Model # _____

Initial/Date _____

Chamber Concentration Calculation:

$$\frac{g}{(\underline{\quad} min) \, (\underline{\quad} Lpm)} \times \frac{1 \, mg}{1000 \, \mu g} = \underline{\quad} mg/L$$

FIGURE 6.21 Example data sheet for recording of data for particle size evaluation with a cascade impactor.

Maximum Likelihood Estimation of the MPD.
The following results are based on 5 cycles.

Prediction Equation:
    PROBIT(fraction of mass) = 3.887 + 2.662 * log(Stage Constant)

For the Input Data :

OBS	Stage Constant	Observed Mass (mic)	Cumulative Fraction of Mass	Predicted Cumulative Fraction
1	0.33	130.00	0.02	0.01
2	0.72	360.00	0.09	0.07
3	1.06	400.00	0.16	0.15
4	1.62	240.00	0.21	0.29
5	2.09	1060.00	0.40	0.40
6	3.00	950.00	0.57	0.56
7	4.50	530.00	0.67	0.74
8	10.00	1810.00	1.00	0.94

The chi-square value for testing the goodness of fit is 0.17, with p < 1.000.
    Since the significance was at least 0.05, the
    fit of the data and the model was good.

The GSD and associated 95% confidence interval :   2.375. (2.341, 2.411)

The MMAD50 and associated 95% confidence interval :   2.610. (2.585, 2.652)

The MMAD16 and MMAD84 are: 1.102 and 6.218

Based on the prediction equation :

Cutoff (microns)	% Mass Less Than the Cutoff
1	13.30
2	37.78
3	56.25
4	68.79
5	77.27
6	83.11
7	87.22
8	90.17
9	92.33
10	93.93

Sample # 1001

Plot of the observed and predicted cumulative mass.

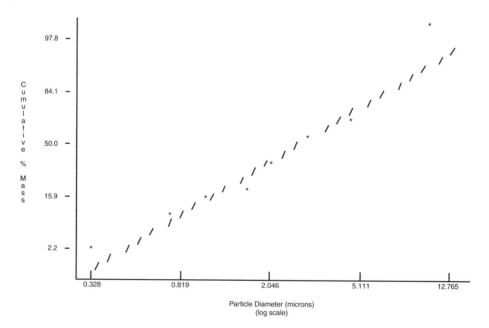

FIGURE 6.22 Example data evaluation for cascade impactor data using a computer program.

SECTION 3. TYPICAL EQUATIONS RELATED TO INHALATION TOXICOLOGY TESTING

1. The theoretical time that it takes a chamber to have an air change to a set of conditions is calculated:

$$\text{Air Change (min)} = V/F$$

where V = volume of the chamber (l)
   F = flow rate through the chamber (l/min)

2. The theoretical time that it takes a chamber to equilibrate to a set of conditions is known as the T_x and is calculated:

$$T_x \text{ (min)} = K \times V/F$$

where V = volume of the chamber (l)
   F = flow rate through the chamber (l/min)
   K = exponential constant = 4.6 (99% equilibration) = 2.3 (90% equilibration)

3. The minimum flow rate for a nose-only exposure chamber is known as the Q and is calculated:

$$Q \text{ (l/min)} = \text{animal number} \times \text{minute volume}$$

4. The volume-to-volume concentration of gas or vapor in air is calculated:

$$\text{Concentration (ppm)} = \text{volume of vapor or gas (µl)/volume of air (l)}$$

5. The conversion of concentration in ppm to weight-to-volume is calculated:

$$\text{Concentration (mg/m}^3) = \text{Concentration (ppm)} \times \text{MW}/24.5$$

where MW = molecular weight (g/mol)
   24.5 = gas constant (µl/µmol) at 25°C and 760 mmHg

6. The conversion of concentration in weight-to-volume to ppm is calculated:

$$\text{Concentration (ppm)} = \text{Concentration (mg/m}^3) \times 24.5/\text{MW}$$

where MW = molecular weight (g/mol)
   24.5 = gas constant (µl/µmol) at 25°C and 760 mmHg

7. The concentration of a pure gas metered into an exposure chamber is calculated:

$$\text{Concentration (ppm)} =$$
$$\text{Flow rate of gas (lpm)/Flow rate of chamber (lpm)} \times 10^6 \text{ µl/l}$$

8. The maximum attainable concentration in air for a volatile liquid is calculated:

$$\text{Concentration (ppm)} =$$
$$\text{Vapor pressure (mmHg)/Atmospheric pressure (mmHg)} \times 10^6 \ \mu l/l$$

where atmospheric pressure = 760 mmHg at sea level

9. Haber's rule for concentration and response relationship is calculated:

$$\text{Response} = C \times T$$

where C = exposure concentration
    T = time of exposure

10. The nominal concentration for an exposure is calculated:

$$\text{Nominal concentration (mg/m}^3\text{)} = W/V \times 1000 \ l/m^3$$

where W = quantity of test material consumed during the exposure (mg)
    V = volume of air through the chamber during the exposure (l)

$$\text{Nominal concentration (ppm)} = \text{concentration (mg/m}^3\text{)} \times 24.5/MW$$

where MW = molecular weight (g/mol)
    24.5 = gas constant ($\mu l/\mu mol$) at 25°C and 760 mmHg

11. The theoretical ventilation per minute of a resting mammal is known as the V_m and is calculated:

$$V_m\text{(ml/min)} = 2.18 \ M^{3/4}$$

where M = the mass of the animal (grams)

12. The theoretical dose level resulting from an inhalation exposure is calculated:

$$\text{Dose (mg/kg)} = C \times MV \times T \times D/BW$$

where C = concentration of test material in air (mg/m³)
    MV = minute volume of the test animal (ml/min)
    T = time of the exposure duration (min)
    D = deposition fraction into the respiratory tract
    BW = body weight of the test animal (g)

SECTION 4. GLOSSARY OF COMMON TERMS IN INHALATION TOXICOLOGY

Gas The airborne state of a chemical that boils at or below room temperature and pressure.

Vapor The airborne state of a chemical that is liquid at room temperature and pressure but is volatile.

Liquid aerosol The airborne state of a chemical that is liquid at room temperature and pressure but is nebulized into a particulate atmosphere.

Dust The airborne state of a chemical that is solid at room temperature and pressure but is dispersed into a particulate atmosphere.

Smoke The airborne state of a chemical that is combusted and allowed to condense into a particulate atmosphere.

Fume The airborne state of a chemical that is liquid or solid at room temperature and pressure but is heated and allowed to condense into a particulate atmosphere.

Mass median aerodynamic diameter (MMAD) The median-size particle based on mass measurement relative to a unit density sphere.

Geometric standard deviation (GSD) The relative dispersion of the MMAD such that a value approaching 1 indicates a monodisperse atmosphere.

Nose-only exposure A system for exposing test animals in which only their noses or snouts are exposed directly to the test material. The animals are restrained (e.g., in a tube) during the exposure. Two system designs are available:

> **Flow-past** Each restrained animal receives individually and continuously a flow of the contaminated air.

> **Non-flow-past** All restrained animals receive simultaneously and continuously a flow of the contaminated air.

Head-only exposure A system for exposing test animals in which only their heads are exposed directly to the test material. The animals are restrained (e.g., in a tube) during the exposure.

Whole-body exposure A system for exposing test animals in which their entire bodies are exposed directly to the test material. The animals are restrained (e.g., in a cage) during the exposure.

Intratracheal dosing A method of delivering, via a syringe and blunt needle, test material directly into the trachea of a test animal.

Bronchoalveolar lavage A method of washing the lungs, via the trachea, with an isotonic buffer to recover free cells and lung lining enzymes for evaluation of pulmonary toxicity.

7 Fundamental Neurotoxicology

Gene E. Schulze, Ph.D., D.A.B.T.

CONTENTS

0-8493-0370-2/02/$0.00+$1.50

SECTION 1. INTRODUCTION

Neurotoxicology is the subdiscipline of toxicology that focuses on the adverse effects of chemicals on the nervous system. Broadly defined, neurotoxicity is any adverse effect on the structure or function of the central and/or peripheral nervous system related to exposure to a chemical substance.[1-3] The foundation for understanding the toxic effects of chemicals on the nervous system, and therefore the science of neurotoxicology, is strongly influenced by contributions from the neurosciences. A thorough study of neurotoxicity includes several levels of analysis of chemical interactions within the nervous system: from the chemical or molecular level, progressing to the cellular and organ level, and ultimately to the whole animal or organismic level. Therefore, the science of neurotoxicology is truly multidisciplinary, founded on basic scientific principals drawn from toxicology, neurochemistry, neuropathology, electrophysiology, and psychology.

Neurotoxicity has become an important endpoint in hazard identification and in assessing the risks of chemicals.[2-4] This has occurred because of the realization that many chemicals may alter neural structure and/or function and the general lack of information regarding the effects of chemicals on the nervous system. The nervous system is of particular interest because mature neurons are generally incapable of regeneration, making most types of brain injury irreversible. In addition, the normal cascade of brain development during fetal and newborn life, in which clusters of neurons are actively dividing and migrating to anatomical areas where they differentiate and form anatomical and functional connections, may be exquisitely sensitive to disruption by chemicals, resulting in lasting and profound nervous system dysfunction.[5]

Regulatory activities have resulted in the publication of testing guidelines for assessing neurotoxicity. Under the authority of the Toxic Substances Control Act (TSCA), the Office of Toxic Substances of the U.S. EPA published testing guidelines for assessing the neurotoxic potential of industrial chemicals.[3] More recently, the Office of Pesticide Programs of the USEPA has proposed guidelines for assessing the neurotoxic potential of pesticides regulated under the Federal Insecticide Fungicide and Rodenticide Act (FIPRA).[2] Both sets of guidelines describe the use of a functional observational battery, assessment of motor activity, neuropathology, schedule-controlled operant behavior, and electrophysiology to characterize neurotoxicity in animals. The latter includes guidelines for assessment of delayed neurotoxicity and the use of neurotoxic esterase assays to evaluate the potential of acetylcholine esterase inhibitors to produce delayed neurotoxicity.

The scope of this chapter is to provide a brief overview on the history of neurotoxic exposures; indicators of neurotoxicity; regulatory testing strategies and requirements; anatomical, biochemical, and physiological manifestations of neurotoxicity; determinants of delayed neurotoxic effects; comparisons between neurotoxic endpoints; targets of neurotoxicant action; and review of the interspecies correlations important in assessing human risk for neurotoxicity. Readers are directed to the referenced material for more detailed information regarding topics covered in this chapter.

SECTION 2. HISTORICAL OVERVIEW

From a historical perspective, human neurotoxic exposure dates back to antiquity. Many plant and animal toxins produce their deleterious effects by interacting with the nervous system. Cobra venom, for instance, produces rapid death via action on the central nervous system, as does the venom from a black widow spider.[6] Of the inorganic species, lead has a long history of producing neurotoxic symptoms that to this day continue to be of public and governmental concern.[4] A brief historical overview of human exposure to neurotoxic agents is presented in Table 7.1.

Human exposure to potential neurotoxic substances continues to be of public concern. Table 7.2 illustrates the wide array of neuroactive chemicals to which modern workers may be exposed occupationally.

TABLE 7.1
Brief Historical Overview of Human Neurotoxic Exposures

Chemical	Year(s)	Exposure
Lead	370 BC	Lead toxicity first recognized in Greek mining industry
Manganese	1837	Chronic manganese poisoning first described in Scotland
Tetraethyl lead	1924	U.S. workers suffer neurological symptoms
Tri-*o*-Cresyl phosphate (TOCP)	1930	Chemical added to Ginger Jake produces paralysis
Apiol	1930s	European drug containing TOCP causes neuropathy
Thallium	1932	Contaminated barley poisons U.S. family
TOCP	1937	Contaminated cooking oil causes paralysis in South Africa
Tetraethyl lead	1946	Gas tank cleaners suffer neurological effects in England
Methyl mercury	1950s	Contaminated seafood causes neurotoxicity in Japan
Organotin	1950s	French drug containing diethyltin causes neurotoxicity
Clioquinol	1956	Drug causes neuropathy in Japan
Methyl mercury	1960s	Seed grain ingestion causes neurotoxicity in Iraq, Japan, and U.S.
n-Hexane	1969	Exposure causes neuropathy in Japan
Hexachlorophene	1971–72	Disinfectant produced toxicity in children in U.S. and France
Methyl-*n*-butyl ketone	1973	Industrial exposure produces polyneuropathy in U.S.
Chlordecone (Kepone)	1974–75	Industrial exposure produces severe neurological symptoms
Methylphenyltetrahydropyridine (MPTP)	1980s	Impurity in illicit drug synthesis produces Parkinson disease-like effects in the U.S.
Aldicarb	1985	Ingestion of contaminated melons produces neuromuscular deficits in the U.S. and Canada
Domoic acid	1987	Ingestion of contaminated mussels produces neurological illness in Canada
L-Tryptophane	1989	Ingestion of chemical contaminate associated with the production of L-tryptophan produces eosinophilia-myalgia syndrome in the U.S.

From U.S. EPA (1993).[4]

TABLE 7.2
Chemicals/Classes Cited by NIOSH Criteria Documents as Producing Nervous System Effects at Low Concentrations

Chemicals/Agents	Chemicals/Agents
Acrylamide	Mercury, inorganic
Alkanes	Methyl alcohol
Anesthetic gases, waste	Methyl parathion

TABLE 7.2 *(Continued)*
Chemicals/Classes Cited by NIOSH Criteria Documents as Producing Nervous System Effects at Low Concentrations

Chemicals/Agents	Chemicals/Agents
Carbaryl	Methylene chloride
Carbon disulfide	Nitriles
Carbon monoxide	Noise
Carbon tetrachloride	Parathion
Chloroform	Petroleum Solvents, refined
Cresol	Styrene
Dinitro-*o*-cresol	Tetrachloroethane (perchloroethane)
Ethylene dibromide	1,1,2,2-Tetrachloroethane
Fluorocarbon polymers, decomposition products	Thiols (*n*-Alkane, mono thiols, cyclohexanethiol, benzenethiol)
Formaldehyde	Toluene
Hydrogen cyanide and salts	1,1,1-Trichloroethane (methylchloroform)
Hydrogen sulfide	Tungsten and cemented tungsten products
Ketones	Xylene
Lead, inorganic/organic	Zinc oxide
Malathion	

From Anger (1989).[7] With permission.

TABLE 7.3
Expert Panels or Committees Making Recommendations for Neurotoxicity Testing

Study Group	Year	Recommendation
NRC	1975	Proposed a tiered evaluation of chemicals for potential neurotoxicity; tests include motor activity, functional observational battery, complex learned functions, behavioral teratology
NRC	1977	Recommended conditioned (i.e., schedule-controlled behavior) and unconditioned behavior (i.e., motor activity)
OECD	1982	Adopted acute and subchronic assays for delayed neurotoxicity of organophosphorus esters
NRC	1984	Neurobehavioral toxicity testing should include studies on behavior (conditioned and unconditioned) and morphology (neuropathology)
NRC	1986	Identified research needs to measure exposure using biological markers and better laboratory techniques
WHO/IPCS	1986	Recommended two levels of neurobehavioral testing (primary level, including functional observational battery and motor activity; secondary level, including schedule-controlled behavior, sensory function, and cognition)
EPA/FIFRA	1987	SAP subpanel recommends motor activity, functional observational battery, and neuropathology for pesticide testing
WHO/IPCS	1988	Steering committee develops protocol for international collaborative study on primary testing
OTA	1989	Workshop on Neurotoxicology in the Federal Government; Interagency Committee on Neurotoxicology (ICON) formed
OECD	1990	Proposed testing guidelines for neurotoxicity testing including functional observational battery and neuropathology; considered testing protocol for 14-day or 90-day studies which includes neruobehavioral observations and neuropathology where appropriate
EPA/FIFRA	1991	Adopted neurotoxicity guidelines for pesticide testing which included functional observational battery, motor activity, neuropathology, glial fibrillary acidic protein assay, revised delayed neurotoxicity testing, developmental neurotoxicity testing, schedule controlled operant behavior and peripheral nerve function testing.

Adapted from Tilson (1990).[8] With permission.

SECTION 3. REGULATORY REQUIREMENTS AND TESTING STRATEGIES

Concern regarding human exposure to environmental neurotoxic substances and a general lack of information regarding the neurotoxic properties of chemicals has lead governmental agencies to issue regulatory testing guidelines for assessing the neurotoxic potential of industrial chemical and pesticides.[2,3]

Regulatory assessment for neurotoxicity is currently required for industrial chemicals and pesticides. Pharmaceutical agents are tested on a case-by-case basis depending on the pharmacology and toxicity of the compound. In screening for neurotoxicity, a wide array of endpoints can be used and measured. Examples of various endpoints used for detecting neurotoxic action are given in Table 7.4.

Examples of endpoints that are routinely measured to assess neurotoxicity in animal safety studies are given in Table 7.5.

Regulatory guidelines issued by the U.S. EPA rely on utilization of a functional observational battery,[10] assessment of motor activity,[11,12] and neuropathological examinations[13] in rodents to screen industrial chemicals and pesticides for neurotoxic potential. A summary of measures contained in the functional observation battery are listed in Table 7.6. Similarly, a scheme for the neuropathological evaluation of selected nervous tissue from animals treated with a potential neurotoxic substance is illustrated in Table 7.7.

TABLE 7.4
Examples of Potential Endpoints of Neurotoxicity

Behavioral Endpoints
   Absence or altered occurrence, magnitude, or latency of sensorimotor reflex
   Altered magnitude of neurological measurements, such as grip strength or hindlimb splay
   Increases or decreases in motor activity
   Changes in rate or temporal patterning of schedule-controlled behavior
   Changes in motor coordination, weakness, paralysis, abnormal movement or posture, tremor, ongoing performance
   Changes in touch, sight, sound, taste, or smell sensations
   Changes in learning or memory
   Occurrence of seizures
   Altered temporal development of behaviors or reflex responses
   Autonomic signs

Neurophysiological Endpoints
   Change in velocity, amplitude, or refractory period of nerve conduction
   Change in latency or amplitude of sensory-evoked potential
   Change in EEG pattern or power spectrum

Neurochemical Endpoints
   Alteration in synthesis, release, uptake, degradation of neurotransmitters
   Alteration in second messenger-associated signal transduction
   Alteration in membrane-bound enzymes regulating neuronal activity
   Decreases in brain acetylcholine esterase
   Inhibition of neurotoxic esterase
   Altered developmental patterns of neurochemical systems
   Altered proteins (c-*fos*, substance P)

Structural Endpoints
Accumulation, proliferation, or rearrangement of structural elements
Breakdown of cells

TABLE 7.4 *(Continued)*
Examples of Potential Endpoints of Neurotoxicity

GFAP increases (adults)
Gross changes in morphology, including brain weight
Discoloration of nerve tissue
Hemorrhage in nerve tissue

From U.S. EPA (1993).[4]

TABLE 7.5
Examples of Parameters Recorded in Neurotoxicity Safety Studies

Clinical signs of neurotoxicity (onset and duration)
Body weight changes
Changes in behavior
Observations of skin, eyes, mucous membranes, etc.
Signs of autonomic nervous system effect (e.g., tearing, salivation, diarrhea)
Changes in respiratory rate and depth
Cardiovascular changes such as flushing
Central nervous system changes such as tremors, convulsion, or coma
Time of death
Necropsy results
Histopathological findings of the brain, spinal cord, and peripheral nerves

From Abou-Donia (1992).[9] With permission.

TABLE 7.6
**Summary of Measures in the Functional Observational Battery
and the Type of Data Produced by Each**

Home Cage and Open Field	Manipulative	Physiological
Posture (D)	Ease of removal (R)	Body temperature (I)
Convulsions, tremors (D)	Handling reactivity (R)	Body weight (I)
Palpebral closure (R)	Palpebral closure (R)	
Lacrimation (R)	Approach response (R)	
Piloerection (Q)	Click response (R)	
Salivation (R)	Touch response (R)	
Vocalizations (Q)	Tail pinch response (R)	
Rearing (C)	Righting reflex (R)	
Urination (C)	Landing foot play (I)	
Defecation (C)	Forelimb grip-strength (I)	
Gait (D,R)	Hindlimb grip-strength (I)	
Arousal (R)	Pupil response (Q)	
Mobility (R)		
Stereotypy (D)		
Bizarre behavior (D)		

Note: D, descriptive data; R, rank order data; Q, quantal data; I, interval data; C, count data. From U.S. EPA (1993).[4]

TABLE 7.7
General Neuropathology Test Scheme for "Potential" Neurotoxicants

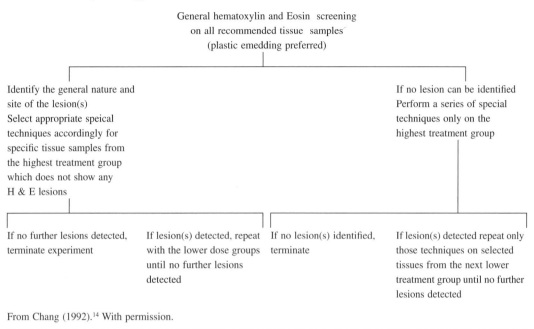

General hematoxylin and Eosin screening
on all recommended tissue samples
(plastic emedding preferred)

Identify the general nature and site of the lesion(s) Select appropriate speical techniques accordingly for specific tissue samples from the highest treatment group which does not show any H & E lesions

If no lesion can be identified Perform a series of special techniques only on the highest treatment group

If no further lesions detected, terminate experiment

If lesion(s) detected, repeat with the lower dose groups until no further lesions detected

If no lesion(s) identified, terminate

If lesion(s) detected repeat only those techniques on selected tissues from the next lower treatment group until no further lesions detected

From Chang (1992).[14] With permission.

SECTION 4. ANATOMICAL, BIOCHEMICAL, AND PHYSIOLOGICAL MANIFESTATIONS OF NEUROTOXICITY

A review of typical neuropathological effects in the central and peripheral nervous system of rats is given in Table 7.8.

There are various types of proteins that are specific for the nervous system. Therefore, chemically induced alterations in these proteins can serve as a biochemical marker for neurotoxicity.[16,17] In fact, the U.S. EPA has recommended the use of the glial fibrillary acidic protein assay as a biochemical marker for neurotoxicity. This protein assay can also be used to quantitate central nervous system damage. Other biochemical markers specific for various brain areas or cell types also exist, specific examples of which are given in Table 7.9.

One distinguishing property of nervous tissue is its ability to generate and propagate electrical signals. This property is probably its most important physiological function. In this regard, there are several ways to measure the electrical properties of the nervous system. These techniques may be used in various species and generally are noninvasive.[9] The use of these tests is also prescribed in the regulatory guidelines for assessing neurotoxicity.[2,3] Table 7.10 illustrates various noninvasive electrophysiological tests that can be used to detect and characterize neurotoxicity.

An insidious property of certain organophosphorus pesticides is their ability to produced delayed neurotoxicity in humans.[20] Experimental techniques have been developed to screen for this property by using the domestic hen as the test species. The hen has been found to be one of the most sensitive species for detecting delayed neurotoxicity.[21] The ability to produce delayed neurotoxicity resides in the pesticide's ability to inhibit the brain enzyme neurotoxic esterase.[20] A comparison of various organophosphorus pesticides in their potency to produce delayed neurotoxicity is presented in Table 7.11. Some physiochemical factors that influence the ability/potency of organophosphorus pesticides to produce this syndrome are illustrated in Table 7.12.

In screening chemicals for neurotoxicity, the general approach has been to utilize both behavioral and neuropathological endpoints.[22,23] The use of behavior and morphology in assessing neurotoxicity has been adopted because both endpoints are relevant indicators of nervous system damage.[24] However, behavior and neuropathology often show differing sensitivities for detecting neurotoxicity,[22–26] so this combination approach increases the probability of detecting neurotoxicity and provides a more comprehensive assessment of nervous system damage. Table 7.13 illustrates the differing sensitivities of behavior and morphology to damage by various chemical and physical agents.

TABLE 7.8
Prototypic Neurotoxic Pathology in the Central Nervous System and Peripheral Neuromuscular System of the Rat[a]

Anatomical Site	Axomopathy	Myelinopathy	Neuronopathy
CNS			
Cortical neurons[b]	0	0	±
*Ventral hypothalamus	0	0	++e
Subfornical organ	0	0	+e
Area postrema	0	0	+e
Lateral geniculate body	++d	±	±
Optic tract	+d	±	±
Optic nerve	0	±	±
Retina	0	±	±
Cerebellar vermis	++d	±	±
*Gracile nucleus[d]	++d	0	++s
*Cuneate nucleus	0	0	++s
Gracile tract (T6)	0	0	++s
Gracile tract (L5)	0	0	++s
*Ventromedial tract (medulla oblongata)	0	+	0
Ventromedial tract (T6)	+d	+	0
Ventromedial tract (L5)	++d	+	0
Dorsal spinocerebellar tract (medulla oblongata)	+d	+	0
Hypoglossal nucleus[b]	0	0	±
Descending tract of V	0	0	++s
Lumbar cord, anterior horn[b]	+p	0	+m
Mammillary bodies[d]	+d	0	0
PNS			
Gasserian ganglion[b]	0		++s
Lumbar dorsal root ganglia[b]	0	±	++s
Lumbar dorsal root	0	±	++s
Lumbar ventral root[e]	0	0	+m
Proximal sciatic nerve	±d	+	+
Tibial nerve at knee[e]	+d	+	+
Tibial calf muscle branches[f]	++d	++	+ +
Plantar nerves at ankle[e]	+d	+	+
Sural nerve at knee[g]	±d	+	++s
Gastrocnemius muscle[h]	+d	±	±
Lumbrical muscle spindles[i]	+d	0	+s
Lumbar neuromuscular junctions[h]	+d	0	0

TABLE 7.8 *(Continued)*
Prototypic Neurotoxic Pathology in the Central Nervous System and Peripheral Neuromuscular System of the Rat[a]

Anatomical Site	Axomopathy	Myelinopathy	Neuronopathy

[a] ++, Great vulnerability; +, less or late (for distal axonopathy) vulnerability; ±, variable or very late (for distal axonopathy) vulnerability; 0, no or little vulnerability; e, excitotoxin; s, sensory neuronopathy only; m, motor neuronopathy only; p, proximal axonopathy only; d, distal axonopathy only; *site that can be used to distinguish the three types of neurotoxic disease.

[b] Amount of neuronal lipofuscin increases with age.

[c] Aged animals display axonal changes in gracile nucleus (6 months plus), along with scattered myelin bubbles and remyelination in ventral root (1–2 years plus).

[d] Neuronal degeneration may be seen in normal animals.

[e] Plantar nerves are vulnerable to nerve entrapment; changes increase with age (6 months plus) and may spread to involve tibial nerve trunk.

[f] Best locus to prepare teased nerve fibers.

[g] Composed predominantly of sensory nerve fibers.

[h] Located on extrafusal muscle fibers only.

[i] Sensory innervation in midequatorial zone.

From Spencer and Schaumberg (1980).[15] With permission.

TABLE 7.9
Examples of Neurotypic and Gliotypic Proteins Suitable for Use as Biochemical Indicators of Neurotoxicity

See Table 8.18 for information.

TABLEL 7.10
Noninvasive Electrophysiological Tests for Neurotoxicity Testing

Peripheral	Needle electromyography
	Single/repetitive evoked muscle potentials
	Sensory/mixed nerve evoked potentials
	F-Wave
	H-Wave
Central	Spontaneous electroencephalogram
	Visual evoked potential
	Pattern reversal evoked potential
	Brainstem auditory evoked response
	Somatosensory evoked response
Cardiac	Electrocardiogram

From Ross (1989).[19] With permission.

TABLE 7.11
Examples of Organophosphorus Pesticides Producing Delayed Neuropathy

Compound	Hen (mg/kg)	Human Cases
Mipafox	25 IM	2
Haloxon	1000 PO	—
EPN	40–80 SC	3
Trichlornat	310 PO	2
Leptophos	400–500 PO	8
Desbromoleptophos	60 PO	—
DEF	1110 SC	—
Cyanofenphos	>100 PO	—
Isofenphos	100 PO	—
Dichlorvos	100 SC	—
Amiprophos	600 PO	—
Coumaphos	50 PO	—
Chlorpyrifos	150 PO	1
Salithion	120 PO	—
Methaminophos	—	9
Trichlorphon	—	Many

Adapted from Environmental Health Criteria 63 (1986).[20]

TABLE 7.12
Factors Influencing Organophosphorus-Induced Delayed Neuropathy

$$R^2\text{--}P{=}{=}X$$

with R^1 above and R^3 below P.

Group nomenclature for structural formula

   a. R_1 = Oxygen or sulfur

   b. R_2, R_3 = Variable groups such as alkoxy, aryl, or amide

   c. X = Acidic entity, such as halide, cyanide, thiocyanate, phenoxy, phosphate, or carboxylate

Factors which increase delayed neurotoxicity

   a. Phosphonates are more potent than phosphates

   b. Increase in chain length or hydrophobicity or R_2 and R_3

   c. Leaving groups which do not sterically hinder approach to the active site

Factors which decrease delayed neurotoxicity

   a. The converse of factors a to c above

   b. Bulky or nonplanar R or X groups

   c. A nitrophenyl X group

   d. More hydrophilic X groups

   e. Thioether linkages at X

From Cherniack (1988).[21] With permission.

TABLE 7.13
Comparison of Morphological and Behavioral Damage

Chemical	Morphology	Behavior
Methylmercury		
10 μg	Focal Purkinje cell loss	No change detected
50 μg	General Purkinje cell loss	Ataxia
Lead acetate		
400 mg/kg	Parietal pyramidal cell loss of spines	Learning deficit
Gestational X-irradiation (125R)		
6 wk		No hyperactivity
5 mo	Cortical pyramidal cell decreased spines	Hyperactivity
Perinatal carbon monoxide		
6 wk	No change detected	Hyperactivity
5 mo	Caudate interneuron increased spines	No hyperactivity
Gestational propylthiouracil	Synaptic count in cerebellum	Learning deficit

From Norton (1982).[26] With permission.

SECTION 5. TARGETS FOR NEUROTOXICANT ACTION

At the molecular level, neurotoxicants may act on nervous tissues by interacting with a variety of biochemical processes.[27–30] The most important property of nervous tissue is its ability to transmit information. This is accomplished by the propagation of electrical or chemical signals. These processes are vulnerable to disruption by chemicals. Electrical signals in the neuron are propagated by the movement of ions across the membrane through various ion-selective channels. These channels can often act as the focus of neurotoxicant action.[29] Chemical signals are propagated by the presynaptic release of neurotransmitters that diffuse across intercellular spaces and interact with receptors on adjacent cell membranes. These neurotransmitters, receptors, and associated second messenger, anabolic, and catabolic processes may also be the target for neurotoxicant action.[27,29,30] In addition, nervous tissue has a high metabolic demand and, because of its energy requirement, nervous tissue is extremely sensitive to compounds that interfere with energy metabolism.[32] Tables 7.14–16 provide examples of neurotoxins which interact with ion channels, cellular biochemistry, and neurotransmitter systems. Table 7.17 provides information regarding methods for characterizing neurotransmitter receptor binding sites that are used in neurotoxicity evaluations.

TABLE 7.14
Examples of Chemicals that Produce their Effect by Acting on Neuronal Ion Channels

Ion Channel	Blockers	Modulators
	Voltage-Activated Channels	
Sodium	Tetrodotoxin	Batrachotoxin
	Saxitoxin	Grayanotoxin
	Local anesthetics	Veratridine
	Pancuronium	Pyrethroids
	N-Alkylguanidines	DDT
		Goniopora toxin
		Sea anemone toxins
		Scorpion toxins
		Pronase
		N-Bromoacetamide

TABLE 7.14 *(Continued)*
Examples of Chemicals that Produce their Effect by Acting on Neuronal Ion Channels

Ion Channel	Blockers	Modulators
Potassium	Tetraethylammonium	
	Aminopyridines	
	Cesium	
	Local anesthetics	
Calcium	Dihydropyridines	Bay K8644
	Diltiazem	
	Verapamile	
	Enkephalins	
	Phenytoin	
	Polyvalent cations	
	Chemically Activated Channels	
Acetylcholine receptor	Local anesthetics	
	Histrionicotoxin	
	Amantadine	
	N-Alkyguanidines	
L-Glutamate receptor	Magnesium	
	2-amino-5-phosphonovaleric acid (2-APV)	
	γ-*d*-glutamylglycine	
	Barbiturates	
GABA receptor	Bicuculline	Baclofen
	Picrotoxin	Barbiturates
	Saclofen	Benzodiazepines
		Muscimol

From Narahasi (1992).[29] With permission.

TABLE 7.15
Examples of Subcellular Targets for Neurotoxin Action

Subcellular Target	Toxin	Biochemical Target
Nucleus	Actinomycin D	DNA replication
Ribosome	Cycloheximide Emetine	Protein Synthesis
Rough endoplasmic reticulum	Tunicamycin	Glycosylation
Mitochondria	Cyanide	Electron transport
Axon	*n*-Hexane	Axoplasmic transport
	Colchicine	Microtubules
	Cytochalasin	Neurofilaments
	Tetrodotoxin	Sodium channels
	TEA	Potassium channels
Presynaptic end plate	Hernicholinium	Choline uptake
	Botulinum toxin	Acetylcholine release
Synaptic cleft	Physostigmine	Acetylcholine esterase
Postsynaptic end plate	Bungarotoxin	Acetylcholine receptor

TABLE 7.16
Examples of Neurotransmitters and Neuropeptides which may be Disrupted by Neurotoxic Compounds

Neurotransmitter	Neuropeptide	Location of Neurons
GABA	Somatostatin	Cortex, hippocampus
	Cholecystokinin	Cortex
Acetylcholine	Vasoactive intestinal peptide	Parasympathetic system
	Substance P	Pontine
Norepinephrine	Somatostatin	Sympathetic system
	Enkephalin	Sympathetic system
	Neuropeptide Y	Medullary, pontine
	Neurotensin	Locus ceruleus
Dopamine	Cholecystokinin	Ventrotegmental
	Neurotensin	Ventrotegmental
Epinephrine	Neuropeptide Y	Reticular
	Neurotensin	Reticular
Scrotonin	Substance P	Medullary raphe
	TRH	Medullary raphe
	Enkephalin	Medullary raphe
Vasopressin	Cholecystokinin	Magnocellular
	Dynorphin	Hypothalamic
Oxytocin	Enkephalin	Magnocellular
Glutarnihe		Hypothalamic
Glycine		

From Cooper et al. (1986).[30] With permission.

TABLE 7.17
Agents Used to Characterize Neurotransmitter Receptor Binding

Labeled Ligand	Unlabeled Competitor	Neurotransmitter Receptor
DL-[Benzilic-4,4'-^{3}H]^{4}Quinuclidinyl benzilate	Atropine	Muscarinic cholinergic
[1-Phenyl-4-^{3}H]Spiroperidol	(+)Butaclamol	Dopamine
[Methylene-^{3}H(N)]Muscimol	GABA	GABA
[Methyl-^{3}H]Diazepam	Diazepam	Bcnzodiazepine
[1,2-^{3}H(N)]Serotonin	Serotonin	Serotonin
[G-^{3}H]Strychnine sulfate	Strychnine	Glycine
9-10-[9, 10-^{3}H(N)]Dihydro-α-ergocryptine	Ergocryptine	α-Adrenergic
Levo-[propyl-1,2,3-^{3}H]Dihydroalpernolol	Alprenolol	β-Adrenergic
[N-allyl-2,3-^{3}H]Naloxone	Levallorphan	Opiate
Opiate Subtypes		
[tyrosyl-3, 4-^{3}H(N)]DAGO	Etorphine	μ
[9-^{3}H(N)]Bremazocine	Etorphine	κ
[tyrosyl-3,5-^{3}H(N)]Enkephalin	Etorphine	δ
[piperidyl-3,4-^{3}H(N)]TCP	Phencyclidine	σ (PCP)

From Bondy and Ali (1992).[31] With permission.

SECTION 6. INTERSPECIES COMPARISONS

Animals are used in assessing neurotoxicity because it is believed that the effects observed in animals have human correlates.[33–36] These correlations are evident for the qualitative effects of various neurotoxicants including acrylamide (Table 7.18). However quantitative differences between species can be considerable. Table 7.19 compares the quantitative species differences of several psychoactive agents on the same endpoints in operant behavioral tests. Similarly, Table 7.20 compares various endpoints for use in developmental neurotoxicity testing across three species including human, whereas Table 7.21 compares qualitative and quantitative differences in the anatomic and behavioral effects of developmental methyl mercury exposure across species.

TABLE 7.18
General Signs of Acrylamide Toxicity in Humans and Comparable Changes Detected in Rats Using the Functional Observational Battery after Either 5-Day (20–45 mg/kg/day) or 90-day (1–23 mg/kg/day) Exposures

Human Signs	5-Day Exposure Rats	90-Day Exposure Rats
Numbness of lower limbs, ataxia, foot drop	Gait changes	Gait changes
Paresthsias, tenderness to touch	Increased tail pinch response	Decreased tail pinch response
Coldness	Hypothermia	
Excessive perspiration		
Desquarnation of hands and feet		
Muscle weakness of extremities	Increased landing foot splay	Increased landing foot splay
		Decreased grip strength
Weight loss	Weight loss	
Lassitude	Decreased arousal	
Hypersomnolence	Increased sleeping incidence	Increased sleeping incidence
Emotional changes		Increased handling reactivity
Positive Romberg's sign, loss of position senses	Decreased rearing, impaired righting	Decreased rearing, impaired righting
Muscle atrophy		
Urinary retention	Decreased urination, defecation	Decreased urination
(No direct correlate)	Pupil response inhibited	Pupil response inhibited

From Moser (1990).[37] With permission.

TABLE 7.19
Comparisons of Species Sensitivity to Drug-Induced Changes in Schedule-Controlled Operant Behavior

Drug	Measured	Sensitivity Order
d-Amphetamine	FI ↑[a]	Squirrel monkey = chimpanzee > pigeon = mouse > rat
	FR↓	Squirrel monkey = rat > chimpanzee = pigeon > mouse
Morphine	FR↓	Squirrel monkey = rhesus monkey > pigeon = rat > baboon > chimpanzee
	FR↓	Squirrel monkey > rhesus monkey = pigeon = rat = baboon > chimpanzee
Chlorpromazine	FR↓	Squirrel monkey > chimpanzee = rat > pigeon
δ-9-THC	FR↓	Pigeon > chimpanzee > rat
Phencyclidine	FR↓	Rhesus monkey > squirrel monkey > pigeon > mouse

[a] ↑ = Rate increase; ↓ = rate decrease; FI = fixed interval schedule of reinforcement; FR = fixed ratio schedule of reinforcement.

From McMillan (1990).[38] With permission.

TABLE 7.20
Comparisons of Endpoints in Developmental Neurotoxicology[a]

Functional Category	Rodents	Nonhuman Primates	Humans
Sensory	—	—	Sensory psychophysics
	PI-ASR	PI-ASR	PI-ASR
	Sensory-evoked potential	Sensory-evoked potential	Sensory-evoked potential
Motivational/arousal	Activity	Activity	Activity
	Sleep-wake	Sleep-wake	Sleep-wake
	—	—	Impulsivity
	Seizures	Seizures	Seizures
Cognition	—	—	Bayley MDI
	—	—	IQ
	—	Visual recognition memory	Visual recognition memory
	—	—	Language development
	Habituation	Habituation	Habituation
	Short-term memory	Short-term memory	Short-term memory
	Long-term memory	Long-term memory	Long-term memory
	Pavlovian conditioning	Pavlovian conditioning	Pavlovian conditioning
	SCOB	SCOB	SCOB
Motor	—	—	Bayley PDI
	Reflex dev.	Reflex dev.	Reflex dev.
	Locomotor dev.	Locomotor dev.	Locomotor dev.
	Motor control	Motor control	Motor control
	EMG	EMG	EMG
Social	Suckling	Suckling	Suckling
	Mother/infant contact	Mother/infant contact	Mother/infant contact
	Communication	Communication	Language
	Aggression	Aggression	Aggression
	Play	Play	Play
	Reproductive behavior	Reproductive behavior	Reproductive behavior

[a] Abbreviations: Dev., development; EMG, electromyograph-; MDI, mental development index; PDI, physical developmental index; PI-ASR, prepulse inhibition of acoustic startle response; SCOB schedule-controlled operant behavior.

From Stanton and Spear (1990).[39] With permission.

TABLE 7.21
Comparison of Neuropathological and Neurobehavioral Effects of Developmental Methyl Mercury Exposure Across Species

Human	Nonhuman Primate	Small Mammals
	High Brain Doses (12–20 ppm)	
Neuropathology		
Decrease in size of brain; damage to cortex, basal ganglia, and cerebellum; sparing of diencephalon; ventricular dilation; myelinated fibers; ectopic cells; gliosis; disorganized layers; misoriented cells; loss of cells.	Decrease in size of brain; damage to cortex and basal ganglia; sparing of diencephalon; gliosis; loss of cells (sparing of cerebellum); ventricular dilation; ectopic cells; disorganized layers.	Decrease in size of brain; damage to cortex, basal ganglia, hippocampus; and cerebellum; sparing of diencephalon; ventricular dilation; loss of myelin; misoriented cells; loss of cells.

TABLE 7.21 *(Continued)*

Comparison of Neuropathological and Neurobehavioral Effects of Developmental Methyl Mercury Exposure Across Species

Neurobehavior

Blindness, deafness, cerebral palsy, spacisticity, mental deficiency, seizures	Blindness, cerebral palsy, spacisticity, seizures.	Blindness, cerebral palsy, spasticity, seizures.

Moderate Brain Doses (3–11 ppm)

Neuropathology

No data	No data	Decrease in size of brain, damage to cortex and cerebellum, loss of myelin

Neurobehavior

Mental deficiency, abnormal reflexes and muscle tone, retarded motor development	Retarded development of object performance, visual recognition memory, and social behavior, visual disturbances, reduced weight at puberty (males)	Abnormal on water maze, auditory startle, visual evoked potentials, escape and avoidance, operant tasks, activity, response to drug challenge

Low Brain Doses (<3 ppm)

Neuropathology

No data	No data	Decrease in size of brain, and loss of cells.

Neurobehavior

Delayed psychomotor development	No data	Response to drug challenge, active-avoidance, operant tasks

From Burbacher et al. (1990).[40] With permission.

REFERENCES

1. Zbinden, G., Definition of adverse behavioral effects, in *Application of Behavioral Pharmacology in Toxicology,* Zbinden, G., Cuomo, V., Racagni, G., and Weiss, B., Eds., Raven Press, New York, 1983, 1–14.
2. U.S. Environmental Protection Agency, Federal Insecticide, Fungicide, and Rodenticide Act Testing Guidelines, National Technical Information Service, Springfield, VA, 1991.
3. U.S. Environmental Protection Agency, Toxic Substances Control Act Testing Guidelines. 40 CFR, Part 798, Subpart G., *Federal Register,* Vol. 50, No. 188, September 27, 1985.
4. U.S. Environmental Protection Agency, Draft report: Principles of neurotoxicity risk assessment, *Chemical Regulation Reporter,* Bureau of National Affairs, Inc., Washington, 1993, 900–943.
5. Claudio, L., An analysis of the U.S. Environmental Protection Agency neurotoxicity testing guidelines, *Reg. Toxicol. Pharmacol.,* 16, 202–212, 1992.
6. Russell, F.E. and Dart, R.C., Toxic effects of animal toxins, in *Casarett and Doull's Toxicology: The Basic Science of Poisons,* Amdur, M.O., Doull, J., and Klaassen, C.D., Eds., Pergamon Press, Elmsford, NY, 1991, 753–803.
7. Anger, W.K., Human neurobehavioral toxicology testing: current perspectives, *Toxicol, Ind. Health,* 5, 165–178,1989.
8. Tilson, H.A., Neurotoxicology in the 1990s, *Neurotoxicol. Teratol.,* 12, 293–300, 1990.
9. Abou-Donia, M.B., Principles and methods of evaluating neurotoxicity, in *Neurotoxicology,* Abou-Donia, M.B., Ed., CRC Press, Boca Raton, FL, 1992, 515.
10. Moser, V.C., Screening approaches to neurotoxicity: a functional observational battery, *J. Am. Coll. Toxicol.,* 8, 85–94, 1989.

11. Schulze, G.E., Large scale assessment of motor activity in rodents: validation of procedures for routine use in toxicity studies, *J. Am. Coll. Toxicol.,* 9, 455–463, 1990.

12. Crofton, K.M., Howard, J.L., Moser, V.C., Gill, M.W., Reiter, L.W., Tilson, H.A., and MacPhail, R.C., Interlaboratory comparison of motor activity experiments: implications for neurotoxicological assessments, *Neurotoxicol. Teratol.,* 13, 599–610, 1991.

13. Spencer, P.S. and Bischoff, M.C., Contemporary neuropathological methods in toxicology, in *Nervous System Toxicology,* Dixon, A.L., Ed., Raven Press, New York, 1982, 259–276.

14. Chang, L.W., Basic histopathological alterations in the central and peripheral nervous systems: classification, identification, approaches and techniques, in *Neurotoxicology,* Abou-Donia, M.B., Ed., CRC Press, Boca Raton, FL, 1992, 223–251.

15. Spencer, P.S. and Schaumburg, H.H., *Experimental and Clinical Neurotoxicology,* Williams & Wilkins, Baltimore, MD, 1980, chap. 50.

16. O'Callaghan, J.P., Neurotypic and gliotypic proteins as biochemical indicators of neurotoxicity, in *Neurotoxicology,* Abou-Donia, M.B., Ed., CRC Press, Boca Raton, FL, 1992, 61–90.

17. Lapadula, D.M. and Abou-Donia, M.B., Cytoskeletal Proteins, in *Neurotoxicology,* Abnou-Donia, M.B., Ed., CRC Press, Boca Raton, FL, 1992, 46–47.

18. O'Callaghan, J.P., Neurotypic and gliotypic proteins as biochemical markers of neurotoxicity, *Neurotoxicol. Teratol.,* 10, 452–455, 1988.

19. Ross, J.F., Application of electrophysiology in a neurotoxicity battery, *Toxicol. Ind. Health,* 5, 221–230, 1989.

20. Environment Health Criteria, *Organophosphorus Insecticides: A General Introduction,* World Health Organization, Geneva, 1986, 6.

21. Cherniack, M.A., Toxicology screening for organophosphorus-induced delayed neurotoxicity: complications in toxicity testing, *Neurotoxicology,* 9, 249–272, 1988.

22. Moser, V.C., Anthony, D.C., Sette, W.F., and MacPhail, R.C., Comparison of subchronic neurotoxicity of 2-hydroxyethyl acrylate and acrylamide in rats, *Fundam. Appl. Toxicol.,* 18, 343–352, 1992.

23. Tilson, H.A., Spencer, P.S., and Cabe, P.A., Acrylamide neurotoxicity in rats: a correlated neurobehavioral and pathological study, *Neurotoxicology,* 1, 89–104, 1979.

24. Broxup, B., Robinson, K., Losos, G., and Beyrouty, P., Correlation between behavioral and pathological changes in the evaluation of neurotoxicity, *Toxicol. Appl. Pharmacol.,* 101, 510–520, 1989.

25. Loeb, A.L. and Anderson, R.J., Detection of acrylamide neurotoxicity by behavioral but not electrophysiological methods, *Fed. Proc.,* 40, 678, 1981.

26. Norton, S., Behavior versus morphology as an indicator of central nervous system toxicity, in *Nervous System Toxicology,* Mitchell, C.L., Ed., Raven Press, New York, 1982, 255.

27. Ho, I.K. and Hoskins, B., Biochemical methods in neurotoxicological analysis of neuroregulators and cyclic nucleotides, in *Principles and Methods of Toxicology,* Hayes, A.W., Ed., Academic Press, New York, 1982, 375–402.

28. Miller, M.S. and Spencer, P.S., Single doses of acrylamide reduce anterograde transport velocity, *J. Neurochem.,* 43, 1401–1408, 1984.

29. Narahashi, T., Cellular electrophysiology, in *Neurotoxicology,* Abnou-Donia, M.B., Ed., CRC Press, Boca Raton, FL, 1992, 169.

30. Cooper, J.R., Bloom, F.E., and Roth, R.H., *The Biochemical Basis of Neuropharmacology,* 5th ed., Oxford University Press, New York, 1986, 359.

31. Bondy, S.C. and Ali, S.F., Neurotransmitter receptors, in *Neurotoxicology,* Abou-Donia, M.B., Ed., CRC Press, Boca Raton, FL, 1992, 129.

32. Norton, S., Toxic response to the central nervous system, in *Casarett and Doull's Toxicology: The Basic Science of Poisons,* Amdur, M.O., Doull, J., and Klaassen, C.D., Eds., Pergamon Press, Elmsford, NY, 1975, 179–205.

33. Paule, M.G., Schulze, G.E., and Slikker, W., Jr., Complex brain function in monkeys as a baseline for studying the effects of exogenous compounds, *Neurotoxicology,* 9, 463–472, 1988.

34. Buelke-Sam, J. and Mactutus, C.F., Workshop on the qualitative and quantitative comparability of human and animal developmental neurotoxicity, Work Group II Report: Testing methods in developmental neurotoxicity for use in human risk assessment, *Neurotoxicol. Teratol.,* 12, 269–274, 1990.

35. Driscoll, C.A., Streissguth, A.P., and Riley, E.P., Prenatal alcohol exposure: comparability of effects in humans and animal models, *Neurotoxicol. Teratol.,* 12, 231–237, 1990.

36. Reese, C., Francis, E.Z., and Kimmel, C.A., Qualitative and quantitative comparability of human and animal developmental neurotoxicants: a workshop study, *Neurotoxicology,* 11, 257–270, 1990.

37. Moser, V.C., Approaches for assessing the validity of a functional observational battery, *Neurotoxicol. Teratol.,* 12, 483–488, 1989.

38. McMillan, D.E., The pigeon as a model for comparative behavioral pharmacology and toxicology, *Neurotoxicol. Teratol.,* 12, 523–529, 1990.

39. Stanton, M.E. and Spear, L.P., Workshop on the qualitative and quantitative comparability of human and animal developmental neurotoxicity, Work Group 1 Report: Comparability of measures of developmental neurotoxicity in humans and laboratory animals, *Neurotoxicol. Teratol.,* 12, 261–267, 1990.

40. Burbacher, T.M., Rodier, P.M., and Weis, B., Methylmercury developmental neurotoxicity: a comparison of effects in humans and animals, *Neurotoxicol Teratol.,* 12, 191–202, 1990.

8 Applied Neurotoxicology

Rosemary C. Mandella, Ph.D., D.A.B.T.

CONTENTS

0-8493-0370-2/02/$0.00+$1.50
© 2002 by CRC Press LLC

SECTION 1. INTRODUCTION

Neurotoxicity is generally defined as an adverse change in the structure or function of the nervous system following exposure to a chemical, biological, or physical agent. An important concept in assessing neurotoxicity is that of the selective vulnerability of the nervous system to injuries. That concept is based on the structural complexity and cellular and molecular heterogeneity of the nervous system and means that neurotoxicants preferentially affect specific neuroanatomical regions and, within those regions, the target can be a specific type of neuronal or glial cell. Based on the selective vulnerability of the nervous system, neurotoxic injuries have been classified based on the neuronal structure or function affected. Examples of neurotoxicants responsible for each type of injury are presented in Tables 8.1 through 8.4.

1. *Neuronopathy*: The neurotoxic agent directly affects the cell body of the neuron (perikaryon). This often leads to the death of the neuron, including its cytoplasmic extensions (axons and dendrites) as well as the protective myelin sheath, and is irreversible.

2. *Axonopathy*: In this type of injury, the primary site of toxicity is the axon and it produces an effect that is the chemical equivalent of an axonal transection. This generally leads to the degeneration of the axon distal to the transection point, followed by the secondary degeneration of the myelin sheath. The cell body itself may be spared. Axonopathies have been further classified as "central-peripheral distal axonopathy" to indicate those injuries primarily involving the distal ends of long axons; "dying back" neuropathy which indicates that the distal axon progressively degenerates from the end of the axon back to the cell body; and "central-peripheral proximal axonopathy" in which the primary degeneration of the axon takes place proximal to the spinal cord. Since peripheral axons can regenerate, partial or complete recovery can occur after they are injured. This is generally not true for injuries to axons in the central nervous system.

3. *Myelinopathy*: Myelin is formed by oligodendrocytes in the central nervous system and Schwann cells in the peripheral nervous system and provides the electrical insulation for axonal neurotransmission. Injuries to the myelin sheath lead to slow or aberrant transmissions along the affected axon. Neurotoxicants may produce myelinopthay by separating the myelin lamellae, resulting in intramyelinic edema, or by causing the loss of myelin (demyelination).

4. *Neurotransmitter Effects*: Some substances may produce functional neurological changes by impairing the process of neurotransmission without producing structural changes in the neuron. These neurotoxicants may interrupt transmission of impulses, block or accentuate synaptic transmissions, or interfere with the second-messenger system.

TABLE 8.1
Examples of Chemicals Producing Neuronopathy

Neurotoxicant	Functional Effects	Morphological Effects	Ref.
Aluminum	Learning and memory deficits, tremor, incoordination, weakness, ataxia, seizures	Neurofibrillary aggregates, degeneration of cortical cells	1, 2
Domoic acid	Rigidity, stereotypy, loss of balance, memory loss, confusion, seizures	Neuronal loss, hippocampus and amygdala, layers 5 and 6 of neocortex	3–6
Doxorubicin	Ataxia	Degeneration of dorsal root ganglion cells, degeneration of peripheral nerves	7
Manganese	Parkinson-like disorder (loss of facial expression, tremors, rigidity, gait disturbances, ataxia)	Degeneration of basal ganglia, especially globus pallidus and striatum	8, 9
Methylmercury	Constriction of visual fields, cerebellar ataxia, paresthesias	Neuronal degeneration of the visual cortex, cerebellum, and dorsal root ganglia	10
1-Methyl-4-phenyl-1,2,3,6-tetrahydropyridine (MPTP)	Parkinsonism (loss of facial expression, tremors, rigidity, gait disturbances, ataxia)	Neuronal degeneration in the substantia nigra	11, 12
Trimethyltin	Aggression, hyperirritability, hyperreactivity, muscle weakness, tremors; convulsions	Necrosis of hippocampal neurons, also brain stem and spinal cord (mice) and areas of the limbic system (rats)	9, 13

TABLE 8.2
Examples of Chemicals Producing Axonopathy

Neurotoxicant	Functional Effects	Morphological Effects	Ref.
Acrylamide	Ataxia, tremor, possible paralysis, weakness, lethargy, paraesthesia, decreased pin-prick sensation	Central-peripheral distal axonopathy ("dying-back" type)	14, 15
Carbon disulfide	Sensory deficits and motor weakness	Neurofilament-filled axonal swellings in the distal axon, leading to axonal degeneration	16
Hexane	Sensory deficits and motor weakness	Neurofilament-filled axonal swellings in the distal axon, leading to axonal degeneration	16
3,3'-Iminodipropionitrile (IPDN)	Sensory deficits and motor weakness	Neurofilament-filled axonal swellings in the proximal axon, atrophy of distal axon	16, 17
Pyridinethione	Sensory deficits and motor weakness	Axonal swellings containing tubular and vesicular structures in the distal axon, leading to axonal degeneration	17
Tri-ortho-cresyl phosphate (TOCP)	Delayed peripheral neuropathy, spasticity	Central-peripheral distal axonopathy (peripheral nerves and spinal cord)	17

TABLE 8.3
Examples of Chemicals Producing Myelinopathy

Neurotoxicant	Functional Effects	Morphological Effects	Ref.
Acetyl-ethyl-tetramethyl-tetralin (AETT)	Hyperexcitability, limb weakness, ataxia, learning impairment	Intramyelinic edema in CNS and PNS; neuronal accumulation of ceroid-like pigments	18, 19
Cuprizone	Encephalopathy	Intramyelinic edema in CNS; degeneration of myelinated nerves in PNS	20
Hexachlorophene	Irritability, confusion, seizures, impaired vision, coma and death possible, especially in infants	Intramyelinic edema in CNS and PNS, vaculation of white matter in CNS, degeneration of optic nerve	21, 22
Tellurium	Hind-limb weakness	Demyelination in PNS	23
Triehyltin	Headache, visual disturbances, vertigo, paralysis	Intramyelinic edema in CNS, brain swelling	24

CNS = central nervous system; PNS = peripheral nervous system.

TABLE 8.4
Examples of Chemicals Producing Effects on Neurotransmission

Neurotoxicant	Functional Effect	Neurotransmission Effect
Amphetamine	Hyperactivity, restlessness, dizziness, tremor, irritability, stereotyped behavior	Interacts with catecholamine neurons to increase levels of norepinephrine and dopamine
Benzodiazepines	Motor incoordination, ataxia, mental confusion, lethargy	Potentiation of inhibitory effects of γ-aminobutyric acid (GABA)
Physostigmine	Cholinergic effects, e.g., miosis, tremors, confusion, excessive salivation and lacrimation, lethargy	Increases acetylcholine levels at nerve terminals by inhibition of acetylcholinesterase

SECTION 2. REGULATORY GUIDELINES

It is clear that neurotoxicants can elicit a broad spectrum of biochemical, structural, and functional abnormalities. This diversity must be taken into consideration in screening unknown chemicals for the potential to produce neurotoxicity. The approach taken by governmental regulatory agencies to address this diversity of effects combines neurobehavioral testing and neuropathology evaluations.

Behavior is the adaptive response of an organism to internal or external stimuli and, as such, represents the integrated end product of multiple neuronal subsystems. Thus, evaluation of behavior can serve as an indicator of the status of the functional components of the nervous system. In addition, since behavioral testing is noninvasive, it can provide a longitudinal assessment of the neurotoxic effcts of an agent, including persistence, delayed onset, or recovery. Typically, a functional observational battery (FOB) is employed to assess a wide range of neurobiological functions, including sensory, motor, and autonomic components and the measurement of motor activity using an automated device. Some regulations specify enhanced clinical observations (ECO) or detailed clinical observations (DCO), which include the observational components of the FOB without including the manipulative aspects.

Neuropathology evaluations generally call for *in situ* perfusion of tissue using an aldehyde fixative. Tissue samples collected should include all major regions of the nervous system. Paraffin embedding is considered acceptable for the central nervous system, but plastic embedding is required for the peripheral nervous system. If neuropathological lesions are detected, special stains may be used to characterize the abnormality further and determine the no-observable-effect level.

Tables 8.5 and 8.6 list the current guidelines for studies to screen for neurotoxicity. These represent tier 1 testing; additional morphological, chemical, or physiological evaluations may be necessary to provide a complete evaluation of neurotoxicity. Some of the guidelines apply to stand-alone neurotoxicity studies whose specific purpose is to evaluate neurotoxicity. These studies can be combined with any other toxicity study, as long as the basic requirements of both types of studies are met. In addition, elements of behavioral testing are increasingly being included in general toxicity tests with the growing emphasis on detecting subtle changes in the nervous system.

The test procedures for all of the guidelines generally include the following elements:

Animal Species: The preferred species is the laboratory rat. Other species, such as the mouse or dog, may be used under some circumstances, but neurobehavioral tests may have to be adapted to the species used.

Age: Young adult rats, approximately 6 weeks old, at the start of the study.

Number of Animals: At least 20 rats (10 males and 10 females) per dose or control group are generally used for neurobehavioral testing. Of those 20 animals, 10 (5 males and 5 females) are used for terminal neuropathology.

Treatment and Control Groups: At least three doses and a vehicle control are recommended.

Dose Selection: The high dose should produce significant neurotoxic effects or other clearly toxic systemic effects. The high dose need not be greater than 2 g/kg body weight for acute studies and 1 g/kg body weight for subchronic studies. The incidence of mortality in the high dose should not be such that it precludes a meaningful evaluation of the data. The mid and low doses should be fractions of the high dose to demonstrate any dose-related responses. There should be minimal or no effects at the low dose.

Route of Exposure: Selection of the route of exposure may be based on several criteria, including most likely route of human exposure, bioavailability, the likelihood of observing effects, practical difficulties, and the likelihood of observing nonspecific effects.

The types of evaluations, the numbers of animals for each evaluation, and the intervals for the evaluations for adult neurotoxicity testing are listed in Tables 8.5 and 8.6 for the U.S. Environmental Protection Agency (EPA) and the Organisation for Economic Cooperation and Development (OECD), respectively. These tables include stand-alone neurotoxicity studies as well as more general rodent studies that incorporate some elements of the neurotoxicity screens.

Divisions of the U.S. Food and Drug Administration (FDA) regulate pharmaceuticals and food additives. No specific protocol requirements have been issued for neurotoxicity testing of pharmaceuticals; testing requirements of drug candidates are generally determined on a case-by-case basis.

For food additives, the FDA Bureau of Foods has issued a draft revision of "Toxicological Principles for the Safety Assessment of Direct Food Additives and Color Additives Used in Food," also known as the "Redbook." The draft revision, which was issued for comment in 1993 and has not yet been issued in final form, addresses issues of neurotoxicity to a much greater extent than in the original 1982 version of the regulations. Neurotoxicity testing is discussed in Chapter III,C. Recommended Toxicity Tests, Section 2.i. In addition to stand-alone neurotoxicity studies, functional observational battery evaluations have been included in the 2–4 Week Toxicity Study in Rodents and the 90-Day Toxicity Study in Rodents. Although specifics regarding the number of animals and the recommended intervals are not stated, in practice, laboratories are generally conducting studies modeled on the requirements issued by the EPA.

TABLE 8.5
U.S. EPA Regulatory Guidelines for Neurotoxicity Testing

Duration/Study Type	Guideline No.	Date Issued	No. of Animals/Intervals			
			FOB	Motor Activity	ECO	Neuropathology
Acute Neurotoxicity Screen	OPPTS 870.6200	August 1998	10/sex/group, Preexposure, estimated time of peak effect (within 8 h of exposure), 7 and 14 days after exposure	10/sex/group, Preexposure, estimated time of peak effect (within 8 h of exposure), 7 and 14 days after exposure	None	5/sex/group, In situ perfusion of tissues 14 days after exposure
Subchronic Neurotoxicity Screen	OPPTS 870.6200	August 1998	10/sex/group, Preexposure, during the 4th, 8th, and 13th weeks of exposure (prior to exposure or, for feeding studies, at the same time of day)	10/sex/group, Preexposure, during the 4th, 8th, and 13th weeks of exposure (prior to exposure or, for feeding studies, at the same time of day)	None	5/sex/group, In situ perfusion of tissues after 13 weeks of exposure
90-Day Oral Toxicity in Rodents	OPPTS 870.3100	August 1998	10/sex/group, Near end of exposure period	10/sex/group, Near end of exposure period	10/sex/group, Preexposure, weekly during treatment	No specific neuropathology requirements
Chronic Toxicity in Rodents (12 months)	OPPTS 870.4100	August 1998	20/sex/group, Near end of exposure period	20/sex/group, Near end of exposure period	20/sex/group, Preexposure, weekly during treatment	No specific neuropathology requirements
21/28-Day Dermal Toxicity in Rodents	OPPTS 870.3200	August 1998	5–10/sex/group, Near end of exposure period	5–10/sex/group, Near end of exposure period	5–10/sex/group, Preexposure, weekly during treatment	No specific neuropathology requirements
90-Day Dermal Toxicity in Rodents	OPPTS 870.3250	August 1998	10/sex/group, Near end of exposure period	10/sex/group, Near end of exposure period	10/sex/group, Preexposure, weekly during treatment	No specific neuropathology requirements
90-Day Inhalation Toxicity in Rodents	OPPTS 870.3465	August 1998	10/sex/group, Near end of exposure period	10/sex/group, Near end of exposure period	10/sex/group, Preexposure, weekly during treatment	No specific neuropathology requirements

TABLE 8.6
OECD Regulatory Guidelines for Neurotoxicity Testing

Duration/Study Type	Guideline No.	Date Issued	No. of Animals/Intervals			
			FOB	Motor Activity	DCO	Neuropathology
Acute Neurotoxicity Study in Rodents	424	July 1997	10/sex/group; Preexposure, estimated time of peak effect (within 8 h of exposure), 7 and 14 days after exposure	10/sex/group; Preexposure, estimated time of peak effect (within 8 h of exposure), 7 and 14 days after exposure	Not required	5/sex/group; *In situ* perfusion of tissues
28-Day Neurotoxicity Study in Rodents	424	July 1997	10/sex/group; Preexposure, during the 4th week of exposure (as close as possible to the end of the exposure period)	10/sex/group; Preexposure, during the 4th week of exposure (as close as possible to the end of the exposure period)	Weekly	5/sex/group; *In situ* perfusion of tissues
90-Day Neurotoxicity Study in Rodents	424	July 1997	10/sex/group; Preexposure, once during the 1st or 2nd week of exposure, monthly thereafter	10/sex/group; Preexposure, once during the 1st or 2nd week of exposure, monthly thereafter	Not required	5/sex/group; *In situ* perfusion of tissues
Chronic Neurotoxicity Study in Rodents	424	July 1997	10/sex/group; Prior to exposure, at the end of the 1st month of exposure, every 3 months thereafter	10/sex/group; Prior to exposure, at the end of the 1st month of exposure, every 3 months thereafter	Not required	5/sex/group; *In situ* perfusion of tissues
28-Day Oral Toxicity Study in Rodents	407	July 1995	5/sex/group; 4th week of exposure	5/sex/group; 4th week of exposure	Preexposure and weekly during the study	No specific requirements
90-Day Oral Toxicity Study in Rodents	408	September 1998	10/sex/group; Toward end of exposure	10/sex/group; Toward end of exposure	Preexposure and weekly during the study	No specific requirements

SECTION 3. FUNCTIONAL OBSERVATIONAL BATTERY EVALUATIONS IN RATS

The FOB comprises a series of assessments designed to measure motor, sensory, and autonomic function, typically in the rat (Table 8.7). These assessments are conducted progressively at the following times: (1) when the rat is in its home cage; (2) while the rat is being handled and held during removal from the cage; (3) while the rat is moving freely in an open field; and (4) during manipulative tests. Since many of the assessments in the FOB are subjective, it is important to be aware of potential sources of bias. Factors to consider in controlling bias include the following:

1. Since many of the end points used in the FOB involve subjective ranking, it is necessary to have a scoring system with explicitly defined scales. An example of such a scoring system is presented in Table 8.8; similar scoring systems have been published.[25-28] In general, testing proceeds from evaluations that require no interaction with the subject (home cage observations) to those that require active manipulation of the subject (e.g., grip strength, landing foot splay).

2. Observers who conduct the FOB should be carefully trained to recognize different types of abnormal behavior in the rat as well as the importance of handling the animals in a gentle and consistent manner. The training is done most effectively using rats that have been treated with known neurotoxicants to illustrate the differences between control and treated animals. Training can often be combined with the collection of positive control data, used to provide evidence that the observational methods can detect major neurotoxic end points. Some of the chemicals used for this purpose are included in Table 8.9. Chemicals that produce transient neurological effects are preferred for training and collection of positive control data, as compared with chemicals that produce irreversible structural damage, since animals can then be used more than once and the number of animals used in training can be reduced.

3. A training video and reference manual for conducting an FOB has been produced under the sponsorship of the U.S. EPA and the American Industrial Health Council.*[29] These training materials are very useful in describing an array of abnormal behaviors and are an invaluable adjunct to in-life training.

4. The same observer should be used as much as possible to evaluate all the animals in a study. Since that is not always feasible, some demonstration of interobserver reliability is needed.

5. Observers who are conducting the FOB should be "blinded," i.e., unaware of the animal's assignment to a particular treatment group. In addition, the order of testing the animals should be randomized so there is no discernible pattern to the order in which treatment levels are tested.

6. Efforts should be made to ensure that variations in environmental test conditions are minimal and are not systematically related to treatment. These factors include lighting, temperature, humidity, noise level, odors, and environmental distractions. Others factors that should be controlled arise from the need to stagger dosing and evaluations over several days because of the length of time required to assess each animal in a study. In a typical study with four groups and 10 rats/sex/group, testing of the 80 rats occurs over a 4-day period such that 10 males and 10 females are tested each day. Time of day in which the FOB is conducted must therefore be controlled. Furthermore, the time of testing must be balanced against sex and treatment group. Thus 5 animals from each dose group (2 to 3 rats/sex/dose) must be tested in the same time frame on each day of testing.

---

* The training manual and video are available upon request from Dr. Virginia Moser at USEPA, Neutotoxicology, HERL, MD-74B, Research Triangle Park, NC 27711, Fax: (919) 541-5075; E-mail: moser.ginger@epamail.epa.gov.

Interpretation of the results of the FOB is complicated by the large amount of data that is generated and also by the different types of data that are collected. An examination of the scoring criteria shows that the data falls into the following types: continuous data (e.g., grip strength and landing foot splay), ranked or ordinal data (e.g., salivation, air-righting reflex), and descriptive or nominal data (e.g., home cage posture). One approach that has been presented to summarize FOB data and make it more accessible for statistical analysis uses the concept of functional domains of neurobehavior.[30] In this approach, certain measures of the FOB are grouped together under domains that represent broad neurobiological categories (Table 8.10). These data can then provide profiles of effects for different chemicals. For statistical analysis,[31] a severity score scheme can be set up that converts individual data for all measures to a 1 to 4 scale, based on data for control rats at each time point. For continuous data, the conversion process is based on the mean of the control samples with ranges defined by multiples of the standard deviation of the sample. For descriptive and some ranked data, score assignments are based on the frequency of occurrence of each score in the control group. After assigning severity scores to measures for each individual animal, the scores can be combined to produce a domain–related severity score that is amenable to statistical analysis. This approach has the advantage of not placing a disproportionate emphasis in interpreting the data on any one test measure. Examples of this type of analysis are presented in Table 8.11 for acrylamide, DDT, and parathion.

TABLE 8.7
Measures Included in the Functional Observational Battery

1. Assessment of the signs of autonomic function, including, but not limited to:
   a. Ranking of the degree of lacrimation and salivation
   b. Presence or absence of piloerection and exophthalmus
   c. Ranking or count of urination and defecation
   d. Pupillary size, such as constriction of the pupil in response to light
   e. Degree of palpebral closure
2. Description, incidence, and severity of any convulsions, tremors, or abnormal motor movements, both in the home cage and the open field
3. Ranking of reactivity to general stimuli, such as removal from the cage or handling, with a range of severity scores from no reaction to hyperreactivity
4. Ranking of the general level of activity during observation in the open field, with a range of severity scores from unresponsive to hyperactive
5. Description and incidence of posture and gait abnormalities observed in the home cage and open field
6. Ranking of any gait abnormalities, with a range of severity scores from none to severe
7. Forelimb and hind limb grip strength using an objective procedure
8. Quantitative measure of landing foot splay
9. Sensorimotor responses to stimuli of different modalities to detect gross sensory deficits; pain perception may be assessed by a ranking or measure to a tail pinch, tail flick, or hot plate; audition may be assessed by the response to a sudden sound, e.g., click or finger-snap
10. Body weight
11. Description and incidence of any unusual or abnormal behaviors, excessive or repetitive actions (sterotypes), emaciation, dehydration, hypotonia or hypertonia, altered fur appearance, red or crusty deposits around the eyes, nose, or mouth, and any other observations that may facilitate interpretation of the data
12. Additional measures that may also be included:
    a. Count of rearing activity on the open field
    b. Ranking of righting ability
    c. Body temperature
    d. Excessive or spontaneous vocalization
    e. Alterations in rate and ease of respiration, e.g., rales or dyspnea
    f. Sensorimotor responses to visual or proprioceptive stimuli

Source: U.S. Environmental Protection Agency, Health Effects Test Guidelines, OPPTS 870.6200, Neurotoxicity Screening Battery.

TABLE 8.8
Sample FOB Evaluation Scheme with Descriptions of Evaluations

- **Equipment Needed**
  Stopwatch
  Laboratory cart
  Absorbent paper
  Penlight
  Forceps
  Pencil or other blunt object
  Nalgene® or other container, approximately 18 in. × 15 in. × 5 in. (for air righting)
  Clean bedding
  A plastic container of slightly dampened sand, placed on a laboratory cart or other flat work surface (or ink pad or nontoxic paint and paintbrush) (for landing foot splay)
  Ruler
  Mouse trap, clipboard, or other "clicker"

- **Room Preparation**
  Turn on the white noise generator, set at 55 to 65 dB
  Monitor and record: room temperature, humidity, light intensity (lumens)
  Fill Nalgene or other container with bedding; using a ruler, measure 12 in. above the top of the bedding and mark this spot on the wall
  Measure 12 in. above the sand surface in the plastic container (or above flat surface covered with paper if using ink or paint)
  Calibrate the grip strength meters
  Place animals in cages in random order and identify only by a sequential number; this is done by a technician other than the one performing the FOB to prevent a potential source of bias

- **Examination Procedure**
  Record the initiation time of the FOB for each animal
  Record all of the observations in the appropriate columns of the FOB form
  Explain any abnormal behavior in the comments section as needed

- **In-Cage Observations**
  Posture — Score as follows:
      1 = Sitting or standing normally
      2 = Alert; sitting or standing oriented toward the observer
      3 = Asleep; may be curled up
      4 = Lying on side
      5 = Flattened; limbs may be spread
      6 = Crouched; sitting hunched with head hung down
  Vocalization — Score as follows:
      1 = No vocalizations present
      2 = Vocalizations present
  Palpebral Closure — Score as follows:
      1 = Eyelids open
      2 = Eyelids completely closed
      3 = Eyelids slightly drooping
      4 = Eyelids half closed

- **Handling Evaluations** — Remove the animal from its cage and evaluate for:
  Ease of Removal — Score as follows:
      1 = Very easy; sits quietly, accepts observer's touch
      2 = Easy; vocalization without resistance
      3 = Moderately difficult; rears, often follows observer's hand
      4 = Freezes; with or without vocalization
      5 = Difficult; runs around cage, is hard to pick up, attempts to bite or attack, with or without vocalization

TABLE 8.8 *(Continued)*
Sample FOB Evaluation Scheme with Descriptions of Evaluations

Ease of Handling — Score as follows:
>   1 = Very easy, totally limp
>   2 = Normal (easy; alert, the limbs may be pulled up against the body)
>   3 = Moderately difficult; vocalization without resistance to handling
>   4 = Freezes; rigid with or without vocalization
>   5 = Difficult; squirms or twists, attempts to bite, with or without vocalization

Chromodacryorrhea — Score as follows:
>   1 = Not present
>   2 = Present

Lacrimation — Score as follows:
>   1 = No lacrimation
>   2 = Moderate lacrimation
>   3 = Extreme lacrimation

Salivation — Score as follows:
>   1 = Not present
>   2 = Slight salivation (around mouth)
>   3 = Moderate salivation (facial and/or cervical area)
>   4 = Extreme salivation (on ventral surface)

Coat — Score as follows:
>   1 = Normal, well groomed
>   2 = Slightly soiled
>   3 = Moderately soiled
>   4 = Extremely soiled, crusty, unkempt

- **Weigh the animal and record the body weight**

- **Open Field Observations**
Place the animal on a clean laboratory cart for at least 2 min
Replace absorbent paper on the cart between each animal

Gait (manner of walking or moving on foot) — Score as follows:
>   1 = Normal
>   2 = Ataxia, uncoordinated movement, excessive sway, rock, or lurch
>   3 = Body drags or is flattened (animal's ventral surface makes contact with the cart surface)
>   4 = Limbs splayed or dragging; unable to support weight (specify hind or forelimbs)

Locomotion (ability to move from place to place) — Score as follows:
>   1 = Normal (animal moves easily around open field)
>   2 = Increased movement (animal moves mostly continuously, rarely stopping to sniff or groom)
>   3 = Decreased movement (reduced movement around field; movements may be sluggish)
>   4 = None (animal does not move around field even after gently prodding)

Arousal (evaluated after observing indicators of exploration, including locomotion, rearing, grooming, whisking, and
>   sniffing)
>   1 = Normal; alert with exploratory movements
>   2 = Low; slight stupor, some head or body movements
>   3 = Very low; stupor, little or no responsiveness to the environment
>   4 = High; slight excitement, tense, sudden darting or freezing
>   5 = Very high; hyperalert, sudden boost of running or movement

Exophthalmia
>   1 = Not present
>   2 = Present

Piloerection
>   1 = Not present
>   2 = Present

TABLE 8.8 *(Continued)*
Sample FOB Evaluation Scheme with Descriptions of Evaluations

Record number of fecal pellets on the paper (if unformed stool is noted, record a "U")

Record the number of pools of urine (if polyuria (apparently uncontrolled urination) is noted, record an "X")

Motor Movements (fasciculations, tremors, convulsions)

    1 = None

    2 = Slight

    3 = Extreme

Relevant information (e.g., limbs affected) will be recorded. Convulsions will be classified as tonic or clonic in the comment section. Any other unusual or abnormal movement or behavior will be described. This includes, but is not limited to, head weaving (movement from side to side), head bobbing (up and down movement), head tilt, backward movement, excessive or repetitive actions (stereotyped, e.g., sniffing, grooming, licking, circling), straub tail (tail is stiff and held in vertical position for extended periods).

- **Reflex Assessments**

Response to Visual Stimuli (evaluate by approaching the animal's head with a blunt object and holding the object 1 to 2 in. from the animal's head for a few seconds) — Score as follows:

    1 = Normal, slowly approaches, sniffs, and/ or turns away

    2 = No reaction

    3 = Freezes or pulls away slightly

    4 = Jumps or turns away abruptly to avoid

    5 = Attacks and/or bites

Response to a Sudden Sound (e.g., a click or finger snap above and behind the animal's head will be used to assess audition) — Score as follows:

    1 = Normal; flinches and/or flicks ears

    2 = No reaction

    3 = Exaggerated; jumps, flips, bites

Pupil Response (beam of a penlight is brought in from the side of the head and the pupil is observed; lights are turned off as necessary) — Score as follows:

    1 = Pupil constricts normally

    2 = Pupil size does not change

    3 = Miosis (specify right, left, or bilateral)

    4 = Mydriasis (specify right, left, or bilateral)

Pinna Reflex (to assess the sensitivity to a light touch, inside the ear, with a fine object) — Score as follows:

    1 = Ear flattens against head

    2 = Animal shakes head

    3 = No response

Proprioception (gently restrain the animal on a horizontal surface by grasping the thorax; gently pull back on the hind limb of the rat so that the dorsal surface of the paw is on the testing surface; release the hind limb) — Score as follows:

    1 = Returns leg to original position

    2 = Returns leg only partially to original position

    3 = No response, rat allows leg to remain in pulled back position

Pain Perception (tail pinch; using forceps, lightly pinch the animal's tail approximately 2 in. from the tip) — Score as follows:

    1 = Normal; turns and bites at the site or walks forward, away from the stimulus

    2 = No reaction

    3 = Apparent increased pain; jumps forward, with or without vocalization, or exhibits highly exaggerated, bizarre reaction, attacks, bites

- **Forelimb and Hind Limb Grip Strength** — Hold the animal with its forepaws resting within, but not touching the triangular pull bar of the grip strength meter. Grasp the animal by the base of its tail and slowly pull it across the bar. As the animal's forepaws grip the triangular pull bar, its grip strength will register on the display. Continue pulling the animal after it has released the triangular pull bar. The animal's hind limbs will then contact, and grip, the T-shaped push bar. The hind limb grip strength will register on the display. Repeat the measurements.

TABLE 8.8 *(Continued)*
Sample FOB Evaluation Scheme with Descriptions of Evaluations

• **Air Righting Reflex** — Hold the animal loosely by grasping the upper portions of the hind and forelimbs so that the animal is upside down and its body is horizontal to the Nalgene container on the counter. Using the mark on the wall, position the animal 12 in. above the bedding. Release the animal and observe its landing position. Score as follows:

    1 = Normal; lands on all four feet

    2 = Slightly uncoordinated (i.e., two legged or unsteady landing)

    3 = Lands on side

    4 = Lands on back

  Note: An obviously impaired animal or one of questionable viability should be excluded from the air righting reflex evaluation.

• **Landing Foot Splay Measurements** — Grasp the animal by the scruff of the neck and the base of the tail. Hold the animal above the sand at a height of 1 ft. Release the animal; measure the distance between the marks left by the animal's hind paws, measuring from the approximate middle of the animal's heel marks (or record the distance between ink or paint spots). Record the foot splay distance and repeat the test. [**Note:** An obviously impaired animal or one of questionable viability should be excluded from this evaluation.] Return the animal to its cage.

TABLE 8.9
Chemicals Commonly Used as Positive Control Materials for the FOB

Chemical	Effect
Acrylamide	Increased landing foot splay, decreased grip strength (especially hind limb), ataxia, decreased motor activity, tremors
Amphetamine	Increased arousal, increased locomotion, increased rearing, stereotypical behavior
Carbaryl	Autonomic signs (salivation, lacrimation, miosis), tremor, muscle fasciculations, altered
Physostigmine	gait, decreased activity, hypothermia, chewing motions
Parathion	
Chlorpromazine	Decreased activity, low arousal, flattened posture, altered gait, decreased grip strength
Dichlorodiphenyltrichloroethane (DDT)	Tremors, myoclonus, convulsions, increased response to auditory stimuli, gait abnormalities, hyperthermia
Triethyltin	Altered gait, decreased grip strength, decreased righting ability, decreased activity and arousal

Source: Adapted from Moser and Ross.[29]

TABLE 8.10
Measures of the FOB, Divided by Functional Domain

Functional Domain	FOB Measures
Activity	Home cage posture, palpebral closure, locomotion and rearing in open field, automated measure of motor activity
Autonomic	Lacrimation, salivation, pupil response, palpebral closure, defecation, urination
Convulsive	Tonic and clonic movements, tremors, myoclonus?
Excitability	Arousal, removal and handling reactivity, vocalizations
Neuromuscular	Gait, locomotion, forelimb and hind limb grip strength, landing foot splay, air righting
Sensorimotor	Tail-pinch response, auditory or click response, touch response, approach response
Physiological measures	Body weight, body temperature, piloerection

Source: Adapted from Moser.[30]

TABLE 8.11
Profile of FOB Effects across Functional Domains for Known Neurotoxicants

Functional Domain	FOB Measure Affected		
	Acrylamide[a]	p,p'-DDT[b]	Parathion[c]
Activity	Decreased motor activity, some decreased rearing, flattened posture in home cage	No consistent effects	Decreased motor activity, decreased rearing, flattened posture in home cage
Autonomic	No consistent effects	No consistent effects	Salivation, miosis
Convulsive	Some tremors, myoclonus	Tremors (mild to severe), some clonic convulsions, myclonus	Tremors, chewing
Excitability	No consistent effects	Some increased reactivity to removal from home cage, increased handling reactivity	Decreased arousal level
Neuromuscular	Altered gait (ataxia, uncoordinated placement of hind limbs, splaying of hind feet, knuckling of paws, dragging the hind limbs), increased landing foot splay, decreased hind limb and forelimb grip strength	Altered gait (ataxia, uncoordinated placement of limbs)	Altered gait (ataxia) and righting reflex, some decreases in forelimb and hind limb grip strength
Sensorimotor	No consistent effects	Increased click response, increased touch response	Decreased response to tail pinch, some decreases in click and touch response
Physiological measures	Decreased weight gain, hypothermia	Hyperthermia	Marked hypothermia

Note: Results were compiled from a collaborative study involving several laboratories. The findings presented are the significant observations generally found for the chemicals by the participating laboratories.

[a] Major effects observed after 4 weeks of dosing at 28.8 mg/kg via intraperitoneal injection.
[b] Acute effects observed 1 to 6 h after oral dose ranging from 58.0 to 195.8 mg/kg.
[c] Acute effects observed 1.5 to 3 h after oral dose ranging from 3.0 to 10.13 mg/kg.

Source: Based on data from Moser et al.[31]

SECTION 4. DETAILED CLINICAL OBSERVATIONS

In the last few years, many guidelines for acute, subchronic, and chronic studies have been revised to include DCO or ECO (see Tables 8.5 and 8.6). In practice, the DCO is generally conducted much the same as the observational components of the FOB, without the manipulative components (e.g., reactivity to stimuli, grip strength, landing foot splay, automated monitoring of motor activity). Evaluations are conducted outside the home cage, in a standard arena, and at similar times of day at each testing interval. An explicitly defined scoring system should be used and, like the FOB, environmental variables (e.g., temperature, humidity, odors, noise) should be minimized. An example of the measures generally included in the DCO is presented in Table 8.12.

TABLE 8.12
Measures Included in the Detailed Clinical Observational Battery

1. Response to handling
2. Changes in skin, fur, eyes, mucous membranes
3. Evaluation of respiration
4. Occurrence of secretions and excretions
5. Signs of autonomic activity (e.g., lacrimation, piloerectin, pupil size)
6. Changes in gait and posture
7. Ranking of general activity level
8. Description, incidence, and severity of any convulsions, tremors, or other abnormal motor movements
9. Description and incidence of any stereotyped behavior (e.g., excessive grooming, repetitive circling) or abnormal or bizarre behavior (e.g., self-mutilation, walking backward)

SECTION 5. MOTOR ACTIVITY

Monitoring motor activity via an automated activity recording device is an integral part of neurobehavioral assessment. The type of device is not specified by the regulatory agencies, although basic criteria for its capabilities and use must be met.

1. The device must be capable of detecting increases and decreases in activity; i.e., baseline activity as measured by the device must not be so low as to preclude detection of decreases or so high as to preclude detection of increases in activity. Positive control data demonstrating that this criterion has been met can be generated by treating animals with chemicals such as amphetamine or triadimefon to produce an increase in activity or chlorpromazine to produce a decrease in activity.
2. Each animal should be tested individually. When an animal is initially placed into a unit of the motor activity device it generally displays high activity as it explores the new environment. As the animal becomes acclimated during the test session, activity drops off asymptotically. To evaluate whether an animal displays this normal pattern of activity, the test session should be long enough for motor activity to approach asymptotic levels by the last 20% of the session for nontreated control animals.
3. Variations in environmental conditions (e.g., lighting, sound, activity) across treatment groups must be minimized.
4. Treatment groups must be counterbalanced across motor activity devices if multiple devices are used during a test session. Treatment groups must also be counterbalanced across time of day.

The most common devices for measuring motor activity include those that use photodetectors and video imaging. Video imaging devices generally measure the total distance traveled or the number of squares crossed in a set time interval. Photodetectors generally measure the number of beam breaks during the test session. The number of photobeams varies, as does the shape of the individual motor activity units (square, rectangular, and figure-8 are the most common).

Typical motor activity data for male Sprague–Dawley rats are presented in Figures 8.1 and 8.2. Motor activity was monitored using an automated Photobeam Activity System (San Diego Instruments, Inc., San Diego, CA) comprising 20 rectangular plastic shoe-box cages. Each individual cage was surrounded by a frame embedded with five photobeams. Each test session was 60 min in length; each session was divided into 12 5-min intervals. The number of beam breaks was plotted as a function of the time interval. Figure 8.1 shows the effects of chlorporomazine on motor activity. The control rats showed the expected asymptotic decrease in activity over the session, and there is a dose-dependent decrease in motor activity with increasing doses of chlorporomazine. Figure 8.2 shows the effect of amphetamine. The control rats again show the expected pattern of motor activity, but there is an inverse relationship between dose of amphetamine and increases in activity. The highest activity is seen at the low dose (2 mg/kg) and the activity remains high throughout the session. At the mid-dose (4 mg/kg), activity also remains high, without the normal asymptotic pattern, throughout the session, but total counts are less than those seen at the low dose. At the high-dose (8 mg/kg), activity is very similar to that of the control group. This illustrates an important point, namely, that the results of motor activity evaluations must not be considered in isolation from observational evaluations. In the case of amphetamine, the drug produces two effects, namely, an increase in activity and stereotypic behavior (e.g., compulsive sniffing or grooming). At the lower doses the effect of amphetamine on the motor pathways predominate and an increase in activity is seen. As the dose is increased a greater effect is observed on the pathways producing stereotypic behavior and the increase in motor activity is no longer apparent. Thus, the findings from the FOB may often be necessary to clarify seemingly discrepant motor activity data.

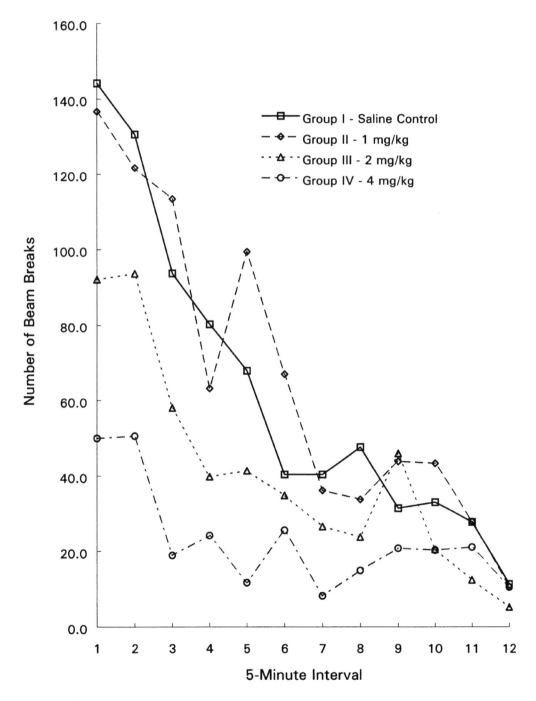

FIGURE 8.1 Mean motor activity values for male Sprague–Dawley rats treated with chlorpromazine.

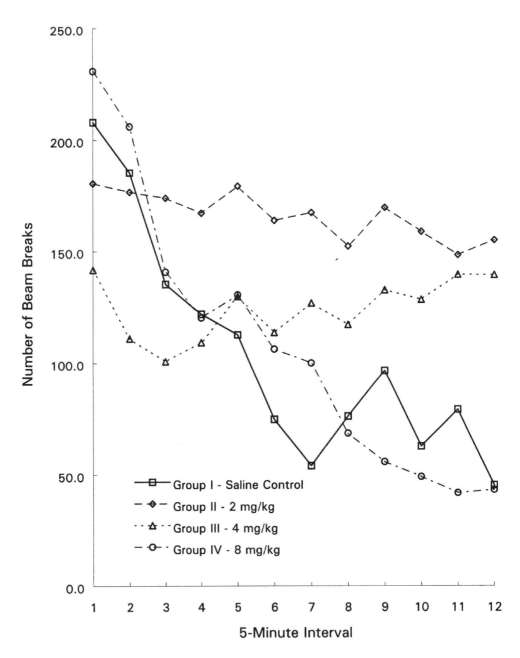

FIGURE 8.2 Mean motor activity values for male Sprague–Dawley rats treated with amphetamine.

SECTION 6. NEUROLOGICAL EVALUATIONS IN DOGS AND NONHUMAN PRIMATES

Dogs and monkeys are generally not used for neurotoxicity screening studies. The reasons for this center on questions of the appropriate use of animals in toxicity studies, as well as practical considerations. The cost and availability of these animals limit the number of animals that can be placed on study, thereby affecting the potential for detecting a neurotoxic effect. Cost and availability, as well as animal welfare issues, would also generally preclude the use of dogs and monkeys in validation studies with known neurotoxicant. In addition, some of the manipulative tests that are done with rodents are not easily done with the larger animals. This is especially true for nonhuman primates since handling monkeys can easily affect their behavior and may also pose a safety problem for the observer. The genetic background and breeding of rodents is also much more standardized that that of dogs and monkeys. Differences in the sources of the larger animals, housing conditions, socialization, interaction with humans, and ages can all have an effect on their neurological status.

However, under certain conditions it may be useful or necessary to evaluate systematically the neurological condition of a dog or monkey. This may occur, for example, during studies with pharmaceuticals that are targeted at the nervous system or when possible neurological effects are observed during general physical examinations and a more detailed evaluation is needed to describe the effect fully. Evaluation schemes for dogs and monkeys are presented in Tables 8.13 and 8.14, respectively. As with the rodent studies, the possibility for bias is of concern and factors such as environmental conditions should be controlled. Because of the smaller number of dogs and monkeys in a study and the individual variability in appearance that is inherent in the larger animals, performing "blinded" observations is much more difficult.

TABLE 8.13
Neurological Evaluation in the Dog

Behavior in Home Cage

Mental Status:

1. Normal, active (aware of surroundings, responds to presence of observer by moving or jumping around cage)
2. Normal, quiet (aware of surroundings, approaches observer)
3. Agitated (appears hypersensitive to stimuli, may respond aggressively to observer)
4. Low arousal (unresponsive to presence of observer, responds to physical stimuli)
5. Very low arousal (unresponsive to presence of observer or to physical stimuli)
6. Coma, unconsciousness

Posture:

1. Normal sitting or standing position
2. Sitting in a hunched position
3. Lying down, normal position
4. Lying on side
5. Lying down with limbs splayed

Out of Cage Evaluations

Observe the dog and note any abnormalities, e.g., position of the head, symmetry of facial muscles, position of the eyes, or excessive salivation or lacrimation. Check muscle tone (e.g., normal, rigid, flaccid) while handling the dog.

Reflex Activity

For evaluation of reflex activity, record any responses that are not exactly as expected (e.g., decreased but not absent).

Pupillary Reflex — Shine a penlight beam into the animal's eyes, one at a time. Hold the light beam for approximately 5 s and remove the light beam from the animal's eyes. The expected reaction is pupil constriction with the light and pupil dilation when the light is removed. Score as follows:

    1 = Present

    2 = Not present

TABLE 8.13 *(Continued)*
Neurological Evaluation in the Dog

Patellar Reflex — Lift one of the animal's hind legs, preventing the animal from placing any weight on the leg. Hold the leg loosely and tap the knee with a percussion hammer. The expected reaction is for the animal to kick its leg slightly in repsonse to the tap. Score as follows:

    1 = Present

    2 = Not present

Flexor Reflex — Firmly grasp one of the animal's forepaws and slowly pull forward. The expected reaction is for the animal to pull its leg back. Score as follows:

    1 = Present

    2 = Not present

Extensor Reflex — One of the animal's forepaws is placed in the palm of the examiners hands and the forepaw is pushed toward the dog. The expected response is for the animal to push against the hand. Score as follows:

    1 = Present

    2 = Not present

Corneal Reflex — The examiner holds a hand directly in front of and approximately 1 ft from the animal's face. The examiner moves his hand quickly toward the animal's face. The expected response is for the animal to blink its eyes.

Gait — Place the animal on the floor and observe. Score as follows:

    1 = Normal

    2 = Uncoordinated movement (ataxia)

    3 = Limbs splayed or dragging

Locomotor Activity — Place animal on the floor and observe. Score as follows:

    1 = Normal (moves easily around area, displays usual activity level)

    2 = Decreased movement (decreased exploratory movement, movements may appear sluggish)

    3 = No movement

Postural Reactions

Righting ability — Place the animal on its right side and observe its reactions. Repeat with the left side. The expected reaction is for the animal to right itself. Score as follows:

    1 = Able to achieve sternal recumbency or stand easily

    2 = Able to achieve sternal recumbency or stand only with unusual effort

    3 = Unable to achieve sternal recumbency or standing position

Visual Placing Response — Hold the animal around its midsection with its forelimbs free and facing away from the holder. Walk slowly toward a flat surface (table, laboratory cart) and observe the animal's ability to reach with its forelimbs to the surface (the expected response). Score as follows:

    1 = Reaches for surface with forelimbs

    2 = Does not reach for surface

Tactile Placing Response — Same procedure as visual placing response, except that the animal's eyes are covered. The animal is moved toward the surface until its legs bump gently against the edge. Observe ability to extend its legs toward the table in response to the tactile stimulus (expected response). Score as follows:

    1 = Reaches for the surface with forelimbs

    2 = Does not reach for the surface

Proprioceptive Positioning — While the animal is standing on all four feet, each foot is picked up in turn and replaced on the floor in a "knuckled over" position. The ability to correctly reposition the foot is noted. Score as follows:

    1 = Quickly and easily repositions feet

    2 = Difficulty in repositioning feet is noted (record which feet affected)

    3 = Cannot reposition feet correctly

Extensor Postural Thrust — Pick up the animal and hold it such that the hind feet dangle below it. Slowly lower the dog to the floor and note how readily and capably it bears weight on its hind legs. Move the animal from side to side and notice how well it keeps up with its hind feet. Score as follows:

    1 = Easily bears weight and movements coordinated with examiner

    2 = Easily bears weight but movements are not coordinated with examiner

    3 = Difficulty in bearing weight

TABLE 8.13 *(Continued)*
Neurological Evaluation in the Dog

Wheelbarrowing — Pick up the dog's hind legs and move the animal about the room. Note its ability to bear weight on its front legs and its coordination in moving right and left legs. Score as follows:

    1 = Easily bears weight and has coordinated movement

    2 = Easily bears weight but movements are uncoordinated

    3 = Difficulty in bearing weight

Hemistands/Hemiwalks — Pick up the front and hind legs on the left side and observe ability to bear weight on the right side. Prompt the animal to move on the front and hind right side and observe functional ability. Repeat for the left side. Score for each side as follows:

    1 = Easily bears weight and movements are coordinated

    2 = Easily bears weight but moves with difficulty

    3 = Difficulty in bearing weight

TABLE 8.14
Neurological Evaluation of Nonhuman Primates

Behavior in Home Cage

Observe each animal in its home cage. Eye contact with the animal should be avoided when possible, since this is stressful for the monkey.

Mental Status:

1. Normal, active (directs attention to the presence of the observer, moves energetically around cage, shows aggressive behavior, e.g., showing teeth)
2. Normal, quiet (directs attention to the presence of the observer, moves calmly around cage, but lacks normal aggressive behavior)
3. Low arousal state (no activity, does not respond to presence of the observer, responds to physical stimuli)
4. Very low arousal state (unconscious, no response to the observer or physical stimuli)

Posture:

1. Normal
2. Sitting in a hunched position
3. Lying down

Lacrimation:

1. Not present
2. Present
3. Excessive

Salivation:

1. Not present
2. Present
3. Excessive

Observe the animal for any of the following abnormal movements. Describe fully with regard to type, location, and severity:

    Tremors

    Convulsions

    Fasciculations

    Stereotypic behavior (e.g., circling, continuous rhythmic movements, compulsive grooming)

Cranial Nerve Function

Note any abnormal head positions (e.g., head tilt)

Movement of the facial muscles:

1. Symmetrical
2. Asymmetrical

Position of the eye lids:

1. Eyelids open
2. Eyelids slightly drooping
3. Eyelids half closed
4. Eyelids completely closed

TABLE 8.14 *(Continued)*
Neurological Evaluation of Nonhuman Primates

Pupillary light response — Shine a penlight beam into the animal's eyes, one at a time:
1. Pupils constrict
2. No response

Visual field — Hold an object in front of the monkey and move it laterally and up and down. Observe the ability of the monkey to follow the movements:
1. Follows all movements symmetrically
2. Asymmetry noted in following movements
3. Cannot move eyes laterally
4. Cannot move eyes up and down

Auditory response — Note the animal's response to a sudden sound produced by a "clicker" or other noisemaker:
1. Responds to noise
2. No response

Response to food — Present a small food treat to the animal (e.g., raisin, grape) and observe the ability of the animal to chew and swallow the treat.
1. Movements smooth and symmetrical
2. Difficulty with movements/not symmetrical
3. Unable to chew or swallow

Motor Function

Observe the motor ability of the primate while it is involved in various activities, e.g., ability to pick up a treat and place it in its mouth and ability to use limbs in climbing about the cage. Strength can be evaluated by presenting an examination probe to the animal and noting how firmly it grasps the probe. Any abnormalities should be noted with an indication of affected extremity.
1. Normal function and strength (normal use of extremities, no apparent differences between right and left sides, firmly grasps examination probe)
2. Normal strength, but appears to favor one side (note any physical reasons for this, e.g., sore on one foot)
3. Paresis (partial or incomplete paralysis, affected extremity may be used for some functions, but is unable to grasp examination probe firmly)
4. Paralysis (affected extremity not used for functions and unable to grasp examination probe)

SECTION 7. NEUROPATHOLOGY

Alterations in any of the structures comprising the nervous system are considered evidence of a neurotoxic effect. It is important to realize in evaluating structural effects of a compound that, in many cases, there is a lag time between exposure to a neurotoxicant and the ability to observe the lesion microscopically. Another factor to consider in microscopic evaluations is the potential for producing histological artifacts during the handling and processing of neuronal tissues. Neuronal tissue is somewhat delicate because of the lack of connective tissue and the high lipid content, and requires a great deal of care to visualize details at the microscopic level. Thus, regulated neurotoxicity studies generally include *in situ* tissue fixation by whole-body perfusion and the use of an aldehyde fixative (generally a combination of paraformaldehyde and glutaraldehyde).

In consideration of the diversity of the nervous system and the local specificity of action of neurotoxicants, it is essential that samples of the nervous system should be representative of all the major regions of the nervous system. A list of the areas generally sampled is found in Table 8.15. It is considered acceptable to embed the brain and spinal cord in paraffin, but it is essential that peripheral nerves be embedded in plastic for better observation of the details in those structures. General stains such as hematoxylin and eosin for paraffin-embedded tissues and toluidine blue for plastic-embedded tissues are acceptable, but additional stains are recommended to investigate further any observed changes in the nervous system. A list of some specialized stains is included in Table 8.16.

TABLE 8.15
Representative Areas of the Nervous System for Histopathological Evaluations

Brain

Section 1 (coronal incision rostral to olfactory tubercules): cerebral cortex, rhinal fissure, olfactory tracts

Section 2 (coronal incision through optic chiasm): cerebral cortex, corpus callosum, basal ganglia (globus pallidus, putamen, caudate nucleus), thalamus, hypothalamus, internal capsule, external capsule, lateral ventricles, third ventricle

Section 3 (coronal incision through infundibulum): cerebral cortex, corpus callosum, hippocampus, amygdala, thalamus, hypothalamus, lateral ventricles, third ventricle, internal capsule, external capsule

Section 4 (coronal incision at caudal margin of the mammillary body): cerebral cortex, hippocampus, medial geniculate nuclei, substantia nigra, cerebral aqueduct

Section 5 (coronal incision at caudal border of the trapezoid body): cerebellum, cerebellar peduncles, pyramidal tract, medulla, fourth ventricle

Section 6 (coronal incision through medulla immediately beneath the caudal edge of the cerebellum): medulla, pyramidal tract, olivary nuclei, central canal

Trigeminal ganglia

Eye, with Optic Nerve and Retina

Spinal Cord

Cervical (longitudinal and cross sections) — at cervical enlargement

Thoracic (longitudinal and cross sections)

Lumbar (longitudinal and cross sections) — at lumbar enlargement

Dorsal Root Ganglia and Associated Dorsal and Ventral Root Fibers

Cervical region

Lumbar region

Peripheral Nerves

Sciatic nerve (proximal region)

Tibial nerve (proximal, at the knee)

Tibial nerve and calf muscle (distal, at calf muscle)

Sural nerve

TABLE 8.16
Specialized Stains Used in Neurotoxicity Evaluations

Structure	Stain	Appearance
Nissl substance	Thionin stain	Nerve cells — bright blue
		Background — colorless
	Cresyl echt Violett for Nissl substance	Nissl substance — blue
Nerve fibers (axons and dendrites) and intracellular neurofibrils	Bielschowski's method for neurofibrils (silver stain)	Intracellular neurofibrils — black
	Bodian's method (silver stain)	Myelinated fibers, the finest nonmyelinated fibers of central and peripheral nervous system — black
	Sevier–Munger modification of Bielschowski's method (silver stain)	Nerve endings and neurofibrils — black Other elements — light brown
Neuroglia	Toluidine blue	Nerve cells
		Nucleus — pale blue
		Nissl bodies — dark blue
		Glia
		Astrocytes — pale blue
		Oligodendroglia — very dark blue

TABLE 8.16 *(Continued)*
Specialized Stains Used in Neurotoxicity Evaluations

	Cresyl echt Violett stain for nerve cells and glia	Nerve cells
		Nucleus — pale blue
		Nissl bodies — dark blue
		Glia
		Astrocytes — pale blue
		Oligodendroglia — very dark blue
	Holzer's stain for glia fibers	Glia fibers — blue
Myelin	Luxol fast blue method	Myelin fibers — blue to greenish blue
		Cells — pink to violet
	Luxol fast blue-periodic acid schiff-hematoxylin	Myelin sheath — blue green
		Capillary basement membranes — rose
		Nuclei — purple
	Luxol fast blue — Holmes' silver nitrate	Myelin sheath — blue to green
		Nerve fibers — black
	Luxol fast blue — Phosphotungstic acid hematolylin	Myelin — blue
		Glial fibers — purple
	Luxol fast blue — oil red O	Fat — red
		Myelin sheath — blue
Degenerated myelin	Marchi's method	Degenerating myelin — black
		Background — brown/yellow

Source: Carson, F., Nerve tissue, in *Theory and Practice of Histotechnology,* Sheehan, D.C. and Hrapchak, B.B., Eds., Battelle Press, Columbus, OH, 1980, chap. 14. With permission.

SECTION 8. NEUROCHEMICAL END POINTS
OF NEUROTOXICITY

Many different neurochemicals have been identified and measured in tissues of the nervous system. These include neurotransmitters, receptors, second messengers, and metabolic and catabolic enzymes. The presence of a change in a particular neurochemical parameter is not per se an indication of a toxic effect, since many neuroactive compounds can cause pharmacological changes. If, however, the neurochemical changes are correlated with neurophysiological, neuropathological, or neurobehavioral effects, then the neurochemical changes may be classified as neurotoxic effects. In most toxicity studies, neurochemical changes have been investigated to enhance the understanding of the mechanism of neurotoxic action, rather than to predict the neurotoxic potential of a particular agent. There are only a few cases in which neurochemical end points are used to screen for neurotoxicants and are included in neurotoxicity study guidelines. These end points are listed in Table 8.17. In addition to those parameters, a number of chemicals specific for neurons and glia are under investigation for possible use in predicting neurotoxic effects. Table 8.18 lists some of the neurotypic and gliotypic proteins for which alterations in levels have been associated with the actions of known neurotoxicants.

TABLE 8.17
Neurochemical End Points Used in Neurotoxicity Screening

Marker of Neurotoxicity	Localization	Neurotoxic Effects	Examples of Neurotoxicants	Ref.
Glial fibrillary acidic protein (GFAB)	Astrocytes	Astrocytes proliferate and hypertrophy in response to damage to the nervous system (reactive gliosis), resulting in an accumulation of GFAP; GFAP can be localized by immunocytochemistry and quantitated by immunoassays	MPTP Trimethyltiin Triethyltiin Tributyltin Methylmercury Domoic acid Bilirubin Kainate IDPN Methamphetamine	33, 34
Acetylcholinesterase activity	Synapses of cholinergic neurons in CNS and PNS	Acetylcholinesterase hydrolyzes the neurotransmitter acetylcholine; inhibition of enzyme activity prolongs the action of acetylcholine at the neurons synaptic receptors, resulting in exaggerated cholinergic effects; measurement of plasma and erythrocyte activity serves as a biomarker for peripheral effects	Organophosphate (OP) insecticides (e.g., parathion, malathion, and chlorpyrifos) Carbamate insecticides (e.g., aldicarb, carbaryl, carbofuran)	35
Neuropathy target esterase (NTE) or neurotoxic esterase	Neuronal membrane-bound enzyme	The enzyme hydolyzes phenyl valerate, although its cellular function is not known; the inhibition and "aging" of the phosphorylated NTE, i.e., the covalent binding of an organophosphate to the enzyme, is highly correlated with the initiation of organophosphate-induced delayed neurotoxicity (OPIDN); the hen is more sensitive than rodents and used in regulatory testing	OP compounds (e.g., mipafox, leptophos, methamidophos, trichlorphon, and chlorpyrifos), not all OPs that inhibit NTE cause OPIDN, but all OPs that cause OPIDN inhibit NTE	36

TABLE 8.18

Examples of Neurotypic and Gliotypic Proteins Altered by Neurotoxicants

Protein	Localization	Neurotoxicant	Area Affected	Ref.
Synapsin I	Synaptic vesicles, all CNS and PNS neurons	Bilirubin Trimethyltin	Cerebellum Hippocampus	34, 37
Protein III	Synaptic vesicles, all CNS and PNS neurons	Trimethyltin	Hippocampus	38
p38	Synaptic vesicles, all CNS and PNS neurons	Trimethyltin	Hippocampus	37
Purkinje cell-specific phosphoprotein (PCPP-260)	Cerebellar Purkinje cells	Bilirubin	Cerebellum	34
p68	Axonal intermediate filaments, all CNS and PNS neurons	Trimethyltin	Hippocampus	37
Protein-O-carboxymethyltransferase (PCM)	Cytosol, CNS neurons	Trimethyltin	Hippocampus	39
Neuron-specific enolase (NSE)	Cytosol, CNS and PNS neurons	Trimethyltin n-Hexane Toluene	Hippocampus Distal sciatic nerve Cerebellum	37, 40
Creatine kinase-B	Cytosol, CNS neurons	n-Hexane Toluene	Distal sciatic nerve Cerebellum	40
Myelin basic protein	Myelin, oligodendrocytes	Bilirubin Trimethyltin	Cerebellum Hippocampus	34, 41

SECTION 9. INTERNET WEB SITES RELATED TO NEUROTOXICITY

mbl.org Mouse brain library, includes brain sections for over a hundred mouse stains. Useful for structural correlates of genetically modified mice.

neuro.wustl.edu Web site created by Washington University Medical School in St. Louis. The neuromuscular disease center presents an exhaustive survey of neuromuscular disorder, including those caused by known toxicants.

neuroguide.com A searchable index of neuroscience resources available on the Internet.

rodentia.com Includes useful rat brain atlases.

SECTION 10. GLOSSARY

Akinesia Absence or the loss of the power of voluntary motion; immobility.

Ataxia Incoordination; the inability to coordinate the muscles in the execution of voluntary movement.

Axonopathy Neurological lesion in which the primary site of the lesion is the axon.

Catalepsy Condition in which there is waxy rigidity of the limbs that may be placed in various positions that will be maintained for a time.

Chromatolysis Response of the neuronal cell body to damage or transection of the axon, characterized by loss of stainable Nissl substance, particularly centrally, and the displacement of the nucleus from its central position to the periphery.

Clonic convulsion A convulsion in which the muscles alternately relax and contract.

Clonus A form of movement characterized by contractions and relaxations of a muscle, occurring in rapid succession.

Convulsion A violent spasm of the face, trunk, or extremities.

Demyelination   Destruction or loss of myelin from peripheral or central nerve axons.

Dysarthria   Disturbance of articulation due to emotional stress or to paralysis, incoordination, or spasticity of muscles used in vocalizing.

Dyskinesia   Difficulty in performing voluntary movements; a movement disorder characterized by insuppressible, stereotyped, automatic movements.

Dystonia   Abnormal tonicity (hyper- or hypo-) in any tissues.

Encephalopathy   Any disease of the brain.

Fasciculation   Involuntary contractions, or twitching, of groups of muscle fibers.

Gliosis   Response of the astrocytes in the central nervous system to damage, characterized by proliferation of fibrillary astrocytes and the formation of a network of cellular processes.

Hydrocephalus   A condition marked by an excessive accumulation of fluid, dilating the cerebral ventricles and thinning the brain.

Hyperkinesia   Excessive muscular activity.

Intramyelinic edema   Damage to myelin characterized by separation of the myelin lamellae.

Myclonus   Clonic spasms or twitching of a muscle or group of muscles.

Myelin   The lipoprotein material enveloping the axons of myelinated nerve fibers, composed of regularly alternating layers of lipids and protein; formed by Schwann cells in the peripheral nervous system and oligodendrocytes in the central nervous system.

Myelinopathy   Neurological lesion in which the protective myelin sheath is damaged either by separation of the myelin lamellae (intramyelinic edema) or by loss of myelin (demyelination).

Myotonia   Delayed relaxation of a muscle after an initial contraction.

Neuronopathy   Lesion affecting the cell body of the neuron.

Nissl substance   Material consisting of granular endoplasmic reticulum and ribosomes which occurs in nerve cell bodies.

Paraesthesia   An abnormal sensation, such as of burning, pricking, tickling, or tingling.

Perikaryon   Cell body of nerve cells, as distinguished from axons and dendrites.

Status spongiosus   Multiple fluid-filled spaces of microscopic size in the cerebral white matter.

Stereotypy   The constant repetition of gestures or movements that appears to be excessive or purposeless.

Tonic convulsion   A convulsion in which muscle contraction is sustained.

Tonic spasm   A continuous involuntary muscle contraction.

Wallerian degeneration   Degenerative process that occurs after transection of the axon. Proximal to the transection, the axon degenerates to the next node of Ranvier. If the transection is close to the neuronal cell body, there will be chromatolysis. Distal to the transection, both the axon and its myelin sheath disintegrate and are digested by the Schwann cells.

REFERENCES

1. Goyer, R.A., Toxic effects of metals, in *Casarett & Doull's Toxicology: The Basic Science of Poisons*, 5th ed., Klaassen, C.D., Ed., McGraw-Hill, New York, 1996, 722.
2. Lukiw, W.J. and McLachlan, D.R., Aluminum neurotoxicity, in *Handbook of Neurotoxicity*, Chang, L.W. and Dyer, R.S., Eds., Marcel Dekker, New York, 1995, chap. 4.
3. Norton, S., Toxic effect of plants, in *Casarett & Doull's Toxicology: The Basic Science of Poisons*, 5th ed., Klaassen, C.D., Ed., McGraw-Hill, New York, 1996, 846.
4. Tryphonas, L., Trulove, J., Nera, E., and Iverson, F., Acute neurotoxicity of domoic acid in the rat, *Toxicol. Pathol.*, 18, 1, 1990.
5. Tryphonas, L., Truelove, J., and Iverson, F., Acute parenteral neurotoxicity of domoic acid in cynomolgus monkeys, *Toxicol. Pathol.*, 18, 297, 1990.
6. Strain, S.M. and Tasker, R.A., Hippocampal damage produced by systemic injection of domoic acid in mice, *Neuroscience*, 44, 343, 1991.

7. Anthony, D.C., Montine, T.J., and Graham, D.G., Toxic responses of the nervous system, in *Casarett & Doull's Toxicology: The Basic Science of Poisons*, 5th ed., Klaassen, C. D., Ed., McGraw-Hill, New York, 1996, 466.

8. Chu, N.-S., Hochberg, F.H., Calne, D.B., and Olanow, C.W., Neurotoxicity of manganese, in *Handbook of Neurotoxicity*, Chang, L.W. and Dyer, R.S., Marcel Dekker, New York, 1995, chap. 3.

9. Abou-Donia, M.B., Metals, in *Neurotoxicology*, Abou-Donia, M.B., Ed., CRC Press, Boca Raton, FL, 1992, 387.

10. Chang, L.W. and Verity, M.A., Mercury neurotoxicity: effects and mechanisms, in *Handbook of Neurotoxicity*, Chang, L.W. and Dyer, R.S., Eds., Marcel Dekker, New York, 1995, chap. 1.

11. Langston, J.W., Ballard, P., Tetrud, J.W., and Irwin, I., Chronic parkinsonism in humans due to a product of meperidine-analog synthesis, *Science*, 219, 979, 1983.

12. Burns, R.S., Chiueh, C.C., Markey, S.P., Ebert, M.H., Jacobowitz, D.M., and Kopin, I.J., A primate model of parkinsonism: Selective destruction of dopaminergic neurons in the pars compacta of the subtantia nigra by *N*-methyl-4-phenyl-1,2,3,6-tetrahydropyridine, *Proc. Natl. Acad. Sci. U.S.A.*, 80, 4546, 1983.

13. Chang, L.W., Neurotoxicology of organotins and organoleads, in *Handbook of Neurotoxicity*, Chang, L.W. and Dyer, R.S., Eds., Marcel Dekker, New York, 1995, chap. 5.

14. Fullerton, P.M. and Barnes, J.M., Peripheral neuropathy in rats produced by acrylamide, *Br.. J. Ind. Med.*, 23, 210, 1966.

15. Spencer, P.S. and Schaumburg, H.H., Ultrastructural studies of the dying-back process, *J. Neuropathol. Exp. Neurol.*, 36, 300, 1997.

16. Graham, D.G., Amarnath, V., Eng, M.A., Kazaks, E.L., Valentine, W.M., and Anthony, D.C., Biomolecular basis for organic solvent neurotoxicity, in *Handbook of Neurotoxicity*, Chang, L.W. and Dyer, R.S., Eds., Marcel Dekker, New York, 1995, chap. 12.

17. Anthony, D.C., Montine, T.J., and Graham, D.G., Toxic responses of the nervous system, in *Casarett & Doull's Toxicology: The Basic Science of Poisons*, 5th ed., Klaassen, C.D., Ed., McGraw-Hill, New York, 1996, 476.

18. Akasaki, Y., Takauchi, S., and Miyoshi, K., Cerebellar degeneration induced by acetyl-ethyl-tetra-methyl-tetralin (AETT), *Acta Neuropathol.* (Berlin), 80, 129, 1990.

19. Spencer, P.S., Sterman, A.B., Horoupian, D.S., and Foulds, M.M., Neurotoxic fragrance produces ceroid and myelin disease, *Science*, 204, 633, 1979.

20. Love, S., Cuprizone neurotoxicity in the rat: morphologic observations, *J. Neurol. Sci.*, 84, 223, 1988.

21. Rose, A.L, Wisniewski, H.M., and Cammer, W., Neurotoxicity of hexachlorophene: new pathological and biochemical observations, *J. Neurol. Sci.*, 24, 425, 1975.

22. Tripier, M.F., Berard, M., Toga, M., Martin-Bouyer, G., Le Breton, R., and Garat, J., Hexachlorophene and the central nervous system; toxic effects in mice and baboons, *Acta Neuropathol.* (Berl.), 53, 65, 1981.

23. Anthony, D.C., Montine, T.J., and Graham, D.G., Toxic responses of the nervous system, in *Casarett & Doull's Toxicology: The Basic Science of Poisons*, 5th ed., Klaassen, C.D., Ed., McGraw-Hill, New York, 1996, 479.

24. Chang, L.W., Neurotoxicology of organotins and organoleads, in *Handbook of Neurotoxicity*, Chang, L.W. and Dyer, R.S., Eds., Marcel Dekker, New York, 1995, chap. 5.

25. McDaniel, K.L. and Moser, V.C., Utility of a neurobehavioral screening battery for differentiating the effects of two pyrethroids, permethrin and cypermethrin, *Neurotoxicol. Teratol.*, 15, 71, 1993.

26. Moser, V.C., McCormick, J.P., Creason, J.P., and MacPhail, R.C., Comparison of chlordimeform and carbaryl using a functional observtional battery, *Fundam. Appl. Toxicol.*, 11, 189, 1988.

27. O'Donoghue, J.L., Screening for neurotoxicity using a neurologically based examination and neuropathology, *J. Am. Coll. Toxicol.*, 8, 97, 1989.

28. Haggerty, G.C., Development of tier I neurobehavioral testing capabilities for incorporation into pivotal rodent safety assessment studies, *J. Am. Coll. Toxicol.*, 8, 53, 1989.

29. Moser, V.C. and Ross, J.F., Training video and reference manual for a functional observational battery, U.S. Environmental Protection Agency and American Industrial Health Council, 1996.

30. Moser, V.C., Applications of a neurobehavioral screening battery, *J. Am. Coll. Toxicol.*, 10, 661, 1991.

31. Moser, V.C., Becking, G.C., Cuomo, V., Frantik, E., Kulig, B.M., MacPhail, R.C., Tilson, H.A., Winneke, G., Brightwell, W.S., DeSalvia, M.A., Gill, M.W., Haggerty, G.C., Hornychova, M., Lammers, J., Larsen, J.-J., McDaniel, K.L., Nelson, B.K., and Ostergaard, G., The IPCS collaborative study on neurobehavioral screening methods: V. Results of chemical testing, *Neurotoxicology*, 18, 969, 1997.

32. Carson, F., Nerve tissue, in *Theory and Practice of Histotechnology*, Sheehan, D.C. and Hrapchak, B.B., Eds., Battelle Press, Columbus, OH, 1980, chap. 14.

33. O'Callaghan, J.P., Quantitative features of reactive gliosis following toxicant-induced damage of the CNS, *Ann. N. Y. Acad. Sci.*, 679, 195, 1993.

34. O'Callaghan, J.P., Neurotypic and gliotypic proteins as biochemical indicators of neurotoxicity, in *Neurotoxicology*, Abou-Donia, M.B., Ed., CRC Press, Boca Raton, FL, 1992, 61.

35. Costa, L.G., Interactions of neurotoxicants with neurotransmitter systems, *Toxicology*, 49, 359, 1988.

36. Abou-Donia, M.B., Organophosphorus ester-induced delayed neurotoxicity, *Annu. Rev. Pharmacol. Toxicol.*, 21, 511, 1981.

37. Brock, T.O. and O'Callaghan, J.P., Quantitative changes in the synaptic vesicle proteins synapsin I and p38 and the astrocyte-specific protein glial fibrillary acidic protein are associated with chemical-induced injury to the rat central nervous system, *J. Neurosci.*, 7, 931, 1987.

38. O'Callaghan, J.P. and Miller, D.B., Neuron-specific phosphoproteins as biochemical indicators of neurotoxicity: effects of acute administration of trimethyltin to adult rat, *J. Pharmacol. Exp. Ther.*, 231, 736, 1984.

39. Balaban, C.D., O'Callaghan, J.P., and Billingsley, M.L., Trimethyltin-induced neuronal damage in the rat brain: comparative studies using silver degeneration stains, immunocytochemistry, and immunoassay for neuronotypic and gliotypic proteins, *Neuroscience*, 26, 337, 1988.

40. Huang, J., Kato, K., Shibata, E., Asaeda, N., and Takeuchi, Y., Nerve-specific marker proteins as indicators of organic solvent neurotoxicity, *Environ. Res.*, 63, 82, 1993.

41. Veronesi, B., Pringle, J., and Mezei, C., Myelin basic protein-mRNA used to monitor trimethyltin neurotoxicity in rats, *Toxicol. Appl. Pharmacol.*, 108, 428, 1991.

9 Immunotoxicology: Fundamentals of Preclinical Assessment

Robert V. House, Ph.D. and Peter T. Thomas, Ph.D.

CONTENTS

0-8493-0370-2/02/$0.00+$1.50
© 2002 by CRC Press LLC

SECTION 1. INTRODUCTION

Immunotoxicology is the discipline concerned with detecting and understanding the effect of xenobiotics on the immune system. More specifically, it can be defined as the study of the consequences of exposure to drugs, chemicals, or environmental agents on the structure and function of the immune system. These consequences may be either temporary or permanent. This chapter summarizes information and procedures relevant to the practicing toxicologist conducting preclinical safety studies in which the immune system is a potential target. Although every effort has been made to present this information in a readily accessible format, the review is by no means inclusive, and presumes in the reader a basic understanding of the immune system and the fundamentals of toxicology assessment.

SECTION 2. THE IMMUNE SYSTEM AS A TARGET FOR TOXICITY

The immune system comprises a complex collection of interrelated cellular and molecular components that serve to recognize and protect the organism from foreign materials (primarily infectious agents). In the most simplistic terms, the essential functions of the immune system are to recognize, eliminate, and remember that which is foreign or "nonself." Recognition of nonself is generally useful, as when the challenge is obviously dangerous (e.g., infections or neoplasia), or potentially harmful (e.g., chemical autoimmunity). This capability is less obviously beneficial when the danger is less apparent (e.g., pollen, animal dander).

It is apparent that the essential function of the immune system is for survival. However, there are at least two features of this system that present a challenge when assessing the effect of potential toxicants. The first is that the vertebrate immune system is composed of dynamic cellular components that are constantly undergoing adaptation, differentiation, and proliferation. The second key feature is the immune system is regulated by exquisite regulatory and feedback mechanisms that can be upset in a positive or negative fashion.

SECTION 3. GUIDELINES, GUIDANCE, AND GUESSES: NAVIGATING THE REGULATORY ASPECTS OF PRECLINICAL IMMUNOTOXICOLOGY

A. OVERVIEW

The panel of validated assays and experimental approaches used in almost all modern immunotoxicology assessment has resulted from the seminal work of Luster et al.,[1] conducted under the aegis of the National Toxicology Program (NTP). The tier approach consists of a structured panel of assays designed to evaluate both the structural and functional integrity of the immune response of

TABLE 9.1
Original National Toxicology Program Tier Testing Approach

Parameter	Procedures
Screen (Tier I)	
Immunopathology	Hematology
	Weights — body, spleen, thymus, kidney, liver
	Cellularity — spleen
	Histology — spleen, thymus, lymph node
Humoral-mediated immunity	Enumeration of IgM antibody plaque-forming cells (PFC)
	Lymphocyte blastogenesis to lipopolysaccharide (LPS)
Cell-mediated immunity	Lymphocyte blastogenesis to mitogens and mixed lymphocyte reaction (MLR)
Nonspecific immunity	Natural killer (NK) cell activity
Comprehensive (Tier II)	
Immunopathology	Quantitation of splenic B- and T-cell numbers
Humoral-mediated immunity	Enumeration of IgG antibody PFC
Cell-mediated immunity	Cytotoxic T-lymphocyte (CTL) assay
	Delayed-type hypersensitivity (DTH) response
Nonspecific immunity	Macrophage function: quantitation of resident peritoneal cells and phagocytic activity
Host resistance challenge models	Syngeneic tumor cell models (B16F10; PYB6) bacterial models, viral models, parasite models

Source: Modified from Luster et al.[1]

an experimental animal (in the original work, rodents) following xenobiotic exposure. Initial assessment (screening) consists of a limited panel of assays designed to provide a "snapshot" of potential immune system alteration; if significant alteration in any of the parameters is observed, a second, more comprehensive panel of assays is available to evaluate the mechanism of action of immune dysfunction. The overall panel of assays is illustrated in Table 9.1.

The utility of the tier approach was further confirmed in a series of papers by Luster and colleagues[2-4] in which the results of tier testing with known immunosuppressant agents, as well as a number of industrial and environmental chemicals, were compared with the ability of these chemicals to alter host resistance. These papers thus provided information on the sensitivity and predictability of the various functional assays, using isolated cells and artificially constrained *in vitro* experimental systems, with actual observable deficits in immune function, specifically, the ability of the immune system to defend the host. These pivotal exercises resulted in experimental approaches in which selected assays could be combined to produce an expected level of predictability approaching 100%.

Although the tier approach was useful for its original intended purpose, the comparative studies by Luster et al. cited above suggested that it was not necessary to employ the entire tier panel to determine whether or not a test material has an effect (regardless of degree or mechanism of action). Although for the purposes of the present discussion, namely, evaluating the immune system in the context of preclinical drug development and safety testing, the tier approach will hereafter be referred to primarily from a historical perspective, it is important to remember that the overwhelming majority of regulatory mandates for testing new molecular entity (NME) drug candidates use components of the tier approach as a foundation.

At present, with the exception of agents regulated by the U.S. Environmental Protection Agency (EPA) and the Organisation for Economic Cooperation and Development (OECD) (which have issued formal testing guidelines), assessment of agents for potential immunotoxicity is not strictly mandated by law. However, all regulatory agencies appreciate the importance of immunotoxicology, and so have instituted so-called "guidance documents" to assist companies in determining when and how immunotoxicity assessment is to be performed. The following sections consider the various regulatory perspectives. Although some of the information below relates to regulation of environmental and industrial agents, it is important to consider in the present context for two reasons. First, there is enough overlap in regulation to make this inclusion necessary; for example, certain consumer products are regulated by the EPA. Second, it is instructive to observe how various regulatory agencies interpret the need for immunotoxicology testing.

B. Specific Documents

1. U.S. Environmental Protection Agency

The EPA has published two Health Effects Guidelines for immunotoxicity assessment. The first (OPPTS 880.3550, Biochemicals Test Guidelines), published in February of 1996, covers the immunotoxicology testing of biochemical pesticides.[5] A supporting document (OPPTS 880.3800, Immune Response) provides additional explanatory information.[6] These guidelines specify that immunotoxicology testing is to be included if subchronic (90-day) toxicology studies are required. A 30-day exposure by the relevant route (oral, dermal, or inhalation) is specified, and either mice or rats may be used. At least three dose levels, a negative control, and a positive control (as indicated) are specified, and the test should include a satellite group for assessing potential recovery from any observed effects. Testing mandated by these guidelines is fairly extensive and includes the following toxicological end points: hematology and clinical biochemistry; body and lymphoid organ weights; preservation of selected tissues for possible histopathological examination. In addition, specific immunotoxicity end points include assessment of humoral immunity (antibody-forming cell, or AFC, or ELISA may be used); assessment of cell-mediated immunity (cytotoxic T-lymphocyte, or CTL, mixed lymphocyte response, or MLR, delayed-type hypersensitivity, or DTH may be used); nonspecific cell-mediated immunity (natural killer, or NK cells or macrophages may be evaluated).

The second Health Effects Guideline, published in August of 1998 (OPPTS 870.7800, Immunotoxicity) is applicable to a wider range of materials, and is more commonly employed for testing EPA-regulated substances. The procedures in this document are more oriented toward the classical "Tier-type" screening assessment.[7] Studies mandated by this guideline employ a 28-day exposure by the most relevant route. At least three dose levels plus a negative control are included, and either mice or rats may be used. It is suggested to evaluate both species if the ADME is not known to be similar between the two species. Immunotoxicology parameters examined are to include spleen and thymus weight, spleen cell viability, and an antibody-forming cell assay (either the plaque or ELISA format may be used). If the AFC assay is suggestive of potential immunotoxicity, leukocyte phenotyping by flow cytometry may be required; if no evidence of immunotoxicity is seen in the AFC assay, assessment of NK cell function may be required. In general, the exact study design should be based on a case-by-case assessment and in consultation with the Agency whenever practical.

2. Organisation for Economic Cooperation and Development

The relevant OECD guideline for immunotoxicology is "Repeated Dose 28-day Oral Toxicity Study in Rodents (407)," the latest version of which was adopted in July of 1995. This guideline incorporates a number of standard toxicological end points that may also be used to assess potential immunotoxicity; these include total and differential leukocyte counts, histopathology of lymphoid organs/tissues (spleen, thymus, lymph nodes, and Peyer's patches), and spleen and thymus weights. In 1998, the Immunology Working Group (IWG) met to discuss potential future enhancements of the 407 guideline to provide more-detailed information. Some of the IWG recommendations for inclusion into the 407 guideline were enhanced histopathology for lymphoid cells and components of the lymphoid organs (e.g., morphometry, special stains), as well as the inclusion of a functional test (AFC or ELISA) if histopathology evaluation revealed evidence of potential immune system compromise. As of the preparation of this review, these suggestions have not been formally incorporated into the 407 guideline.

3. U.S. Food and Drug Administration

a. *Center for Drug Evaluation and Research*

The Center for Drug Evaluation and Research (CDER) is responsible for ensuring the safety of human pharmaceuticals produced primarily by synthetic or semisynthetic means (i.e., not biologicals). As of the preparation of this chapter, the immunotoxicology guidance document for CDER was in draft form and unavailable for public review. However, published information may provide insight into the possible nature of the CDER recommendations.[8-10] Signs observed in routine toxicology studies that may indicate possible immunotoxicity include hematological alterations such as anemia or leukopenia, histological changes such as atrophy or changes in resident cell types, evidence of more frequent infections in treated animals than in controls, evidence of neoplasia associated with immunosuppression, changes in clinical chemistry parameters (e.g., serum immunoglobulin levels), and pharmacokinetic signs including drug or metabolite accumulation in immune cells. Aspects of drug-related immunotoxicology of concern to CDER would include unintended immunosuppression, antigenicity, hypersensitivity, unintended immunostimulation, and autoimmunity; all of these sequelae have been associated with nonbiological pharmaceuticals.

Unintended immunosuppression is delineated because an increasingly sophisticated understanding of the immune response is resulting in a variety of NME designed specifically to suppress immunity. Unintended, drug-induced immunosuppression is relatively uncommon, but of sufficient concern to warrant consideration. Routine toxicology tests that may indicate immunosuppression include hematology (total counts and differentials), serum immunoglobulin levels, and descriptive histopathological examination of thymus, spleen, and draining lymph nodes (again echoing the general pattern of tier testing). In the event that results from these tests suggest immunosuppression, follow-up (Level I) tests should include assessment of leukocyte subsets by flow cytometric analysis, as well as the antibody-forming cell assay (plaque assay or ELISA platforms). If these follow-up tests are indicative of potential immune dysfunction, additional follow-up (Level II) tests should include an assessment of host resistance (infectious organisms or transplantable tumors), as well as mechanistic evaluation. The exact type of assays to be used, as well as the testing paradigm, should be carefully chosen on a case-by-case basis after consultation with the FDA.

A second area of concern to CDER is antigenicity; in the context of many biotechnology-derived pharmaceuticals, this refers to the propensity of the drug to induce a specific immune response directed against the drug itself. However, in the context of nonbiological drugs, antigenicity refers primarily to the induction of hypersensitivity reactions, or drug allergy. These reactions may be of any of the Type I to IV hypersensitivity reactions, and together they represent an important area of concern. Related to this concern is the adverse drug reaction known as pseudoallergy, whose mechanisms of action are not well understood. Although pseudoallergy does not appear to be immune mediated, it may be difficult to differentiate from true IgE-mediated hypersensitivity reactions.

Autoimmunity is the condition in which exposure to a drug is associated with the induction of an immune response against the patient's own (self) antigens; one classical example is drug-induced lupus. The mechanisms for drug-related autoimmunity are very poorly understood, and there are unfortunately no standard methods for prediction of this adverse effect. Closely related (if not, in fact, identical) with drug-induced autoimmunity is unintended immunostimulation. As with immunosuppression, NME are under development for the restoration or augmentation of a suboptimal immune response (e.g., repopulation of bone marrow following a transplant, treatment of AIDS). Unintended immunostimulation may be subtle and difficult to identify; moreover, its identification may be confounded by its overlap with the intended mechanism of action of a drug.

b. Center for Biologics Evaluation and Research

This center within the U.S. Food and Drug Administration (FDA) regulates the safety of human pharmaceuticals that are produced as biological agents, rather than synthesized. This includes blood and blood products, vaccines, and biotechnology products such as cytokines, therapeutic proteins, and monoclonal antibodies. As of the writing of this chapter, the Center for Biologics Evaluation and Research (CBER) does not have a guidance document for immunotoxicology testing; rather, all testing for potential immunotoxicity is to be evaluated on a case-by-case basis. In many cases, testing of drugs regulated by CBER would be covered by the CPMP/ICH "S6" document (see below).

c. Center for Devices and Radiological Health

Traditionally, immunotoxicology has been utilized to evaluate the effect of repeated exposure to test materials (drugs, chemicals, etc.) on the immune system; the precise regimen of exposure has been varied, but the repeated-dose nature of the exposure has not. However, it is being increasingly recognized that medical devices designed to remain in contact with the body (essentially a permanent exposure regimen) may present an even greater opportunity for either inducing a *de novo* immune response (to the device itself or to a different antigen), or of suppressing an unrelated immune response.[11-13]

In 1999, the Center for Devices and Radiological Health (CDRH), the branch of the FDA responsible for ensuring the safety of medical devices and for preventing unnecessary exposure to radiation from electronic products, published a guidance document entitled "Immunotoxicity Testing Guidance."[14] This document is intended to be used in conjunction with the CDRH Memorandum G95-1, which is an FDA-modified version of the International Standard ISO-10993 document "Biological Evaluation of Medical Devices — Part 1: Evaluation and Testing." The immunotoxicology guidance document describes a flowchart for determining whether immunotoxicology testing may be needed to support the safety of a medical device. There are also several tables summarizing potential immunotoxic effects based on body contact and contact duration. This includes type of body contact such as surface (skin, mucosal, or compromised surface); external communicating (blood path, tissue/bone/dentin); or implanted (tissue/bone, blood, body fluids). Testing approach/methods based on immunotoxic effect are also described (hypersensitivity, inflammation, immunosuppression, immunostimulation, and autoimmunity). Finally, a list of models that can be employed in evaluating immune responses (cross-referenced by immune parameter assessed and end point evaluated) is included.

d. Center for Food Safety and Applied Nutrition

The Center for Food Safety and Applied Nutrition (CFSAN) is responsible for the safety of food additives. In 1982, this center published a document entitled "Toxicological Principles for the Safety Assessment of Direct Food and Color Additives Used in Food," commonly known as "Redbook I." As of the preparation of this chapter, an updated document, generally known as "Redbook II," is currently in draft form.[15,16] This document features perhaps one of the most comprehensive sections on immunotoxicology testing of any guidance document, with various levels of recommended testing; these are classified as Retrospective Level I (expanded), Enhanced (expanded) Level I, Level II, and Enhanced (expanded) Level II.

In this scheme, Level I tests are those that do not require any exogenous manipulation of the immune system, such as immunization; this has the great advantage of utilizing the same animals used in a standard toxicity study. Level I tests include end points such as hematology, clinical chemistry, body and lymphoid organ weights, and standard histopathology. Expanded Level I tests are not as routine, but still do not require satellite groups of animals. These tests include such end points as evaluation of antibody classes, quantitation of autoantibodies, flow cytometry, lymphoproliferation, NK and macrophage function, cytokine assessment, and immunohistochemical staining. With careful planning, any of these tests could easily be incorporated into standard study designs, yet could provide a considerable amount of information on the structural integrity of the immune system, as well as a limited degree of knowledge regarding its functional competence.

Level II testing incorporates functional assessment of the immune system and usually requires the inclusion of satellite groups. Such assays include the AFC assay to measure B-cell function, and a delayed-type hypersensitivity to assess T-cell function. These assays provide additional information on the immune system not obtainable from the Level I tests, namely, the response to an immune "challenge" provided by an exogenous antigen. Enhanced Level II testing evaluates the overall immunocompetence of the test animal by means of host resistance to either an infectious organism or a transplantable tumor cell.

4. International Conference on Harmonisation of Technical Requirement for Registration of Pharmaceuticals for Human Use

The International Conference of Hormonisation (ICH) comprises representatives from Europe, the United States, and Japan, and was instituted as a forum for the pharmaceutical industry and regulatory agencies to discuss requirements for product registration in the three member regions. The ICH has published a document with direct relevance to immunotoxicology assessment, "Preclinical Safety Evaluation of Biotechnology-Derived Pharmaceuticals," commonly referred to as the "S6" Document.[17] Pertinent sections of the document include 3.6 (Immunogenicity) and 4.5 (Immunotoxicity Studies).

In Section 3.6, the S6 document recognizes the following: many biotech drugs are potentially immunogenic; detection of antibodies should not be the sole criterion for termination or modification of safety testing; and antibody formation in animals is not necessarily predictive for humans. In Section 4.5, it is noted that certain drug candidates may be intended to alter the immune response; that testing strategies may require screening studies followed by mechanistic studies; and that the standard, so-called tier approach is not recommended for biotechnology-derived pharmaceuticals. This latter point is perhaps one of the most important in that it places emphasis on science-based, case-by-case assessment of each compound based on its intended use and mechanism of action (particularly for immunotherapeutics). Unfortunately for investigators who lack expertise in immunotoxicology, the document does not provide specific instructions on how such assessment is to be performed.

5. Committee for Proprietary Medicinal Products

The Committee for Proprietory Medicinal Products (CPMP) was created by the European Commission to provide technical and scientific support for ICH activities. In July 2000, the CPMP published a document (CPMP/SWP/1042/99) entitled "Note for Guidance on Repeated Dose Toxicity," which includes guidance on immunotoxicology testing on agents intended for regulatory submission in Europe.[18] The document indicates that all new medicinal products should be screened for immunotoxic potential in at least one repeated dose toxicity study, preferably in a study of 28 days duration, although 14-day or 3-month studies may also be acceptable, based on circumstances. The interpretation of the results of such screening is "to be based on integrative analysis of changes in lymphoid cell populations as well as other types of toxicity," as well as the health status of the animals. In general, the testing approach outlined by the CPMP follows a tier approach (delineated as Initial Screening Phase and Extended Studies), although (somewhat paradoxically) the document advocates consideration of testing requirements on a case-by-case basis.

The initial screening phase consists of both nonfunctional and functional assessment of immune system integrity in rats or mice; all these end points, including the functional assays, are readily incorporated into standard toxicology assessment paradigms. Tests to be performed include hematology, lymphoid organ weights (thymus, spleen, draining and distant lymph nodes), lymphoid organ microscopy (thymus, spleen, draining and distant lymph nodes, Peyer's patches), bone marrow cellularity, NK cell activity, and distribution of lymphocyte subsets. (If these latter two functional assays are not available, the screening phase should include a primary antibody response to a T-cell-dependent antigen.) Alterations in these parameters may trigger additional testing. Whether this indicates changes in any parameter, all parameters, or a selective combination of certain parameters is not specified.

Extended studies to define mechanisms of any potential immunotoxicity are all functional in nature and are designed based on results of initial screening studies, and, again, should be determined on a case-by-case basis depending on the nature of the observations from the screening phases. Suggested tests for immune mechanistic functional assessment include delayed-type hypersensitivity response, mitogen- or antigen-stimulated lymphocyte proliferation, macrophage function, primary response to T-dependent antigen (e.g., AFC assay), and *in vivo* models of host resistance to infectious agents (bacteria, viruses, parasites) or tumor cells.

6. Japanese Immunotoxicology Regulatory Considerations

At present, the standard tier concept of immunotoxicity assessment is not utilized in Japan.[19] Current requirements for New Drug Applications in Japan include antigenicity studies, skin sensitization studies, and skin photosensitization studies. Several "indirect" immunotoxicity tests are used by some investigators, and include histopathological changes in lymphoid tissues, weight changes in lymphoid organs, bone marrow effects, and changes in hematology or blood chemistry. In general, "direct" immunotoxicity tests are not routinely performed in Japan because of a belief that the criteria for defining immunotoxicity are not clearly defined and the testing methods are not unified/standardized. However, this situation is expected to change in the near future.

C. Regulatory Considerations Meet the Real World

As will be easily recognized from the above sections, with the possible exception of the EPA and OECD, the concept of case-by-case assessment of immunotoxicity is integral to regulatory guidance. Naturally, the practice of this analysis will vary depending on the experience and needs of each immunotoxicologist. However, it may be instructive to provide an example of how such assessment has been done in the past. In 1998, Dean et al.[20] published the results of an informal poll of 15 pharmaceutical and biotechnology companies on how these companies actually incorporate immmunotoxicology assessment into the drug development process. The findings of this poll (taken and analyzed prior to publication of several of the more recent guidance documents) revealed:

- The decision to evaluate immunotoxicity of drugs is almost always performed on a case-by-case basis.
- The decision to evaluate immunotoxicity is driven by changes observed during standard toxicity testing, including hematology parameters (WBC and differential counts) or change in lymphoid organ weight, cellularity, or histopathology.
- Encountering immunotoxicity during preclinical development rarely results in project termination, but does assist in clinical development.
- Encountering immune effects during clinical development or postmarketing often results in termination of the project.
- The most frequent clinical immunotoxicity observed is systemic hypersensitivity following oral exposure. This is also the most difficult effect to predict.

SECTION 4. METHODS AND APPROACHES GENERALLY USED FOR PRECLINICAL IMMUNOTOXICOLOGY ASSESSMENT IN RODENTS

A. Overview

As amply demonstrated to this point, proper assessment of immunotoxic/immunomodulatory potential is dependent on a combination of standard toxicological end points and a carefully chosen panel of specific immune function assays. Whereas some investigators have demonstrated the potential for assessing immunotoxic potential using *in vitro* exposure to drugs,[21] for the immediate future the need will remain for whole-animal studies. The following sections examine specific approaches and techniques for evaluating the effect of test materials on the immune system. Although the title of this present chapter utilizes the traditional term *immunotoxicology* to describe this effect, any of the following methodologies can easily be used in the drug discovery development process to assess intentional immunomodulation as well.

B. CHOICE OF SPECIES

During the initial development of the discipline of immunotoxicology, the mouse was almost exclusively the model of choice, since much of the initial work in immunology was performed in this animal. Unfortunately, the mouse is not a common model for standard toxicology studies; in many cases this has necessitated extra studies with both rats and mice, which is wasteful of both animals and resources. More recently, the rat has gained prominence as a model for immunotoxicology testing, with several interlaboratory validation studies demonstrating the acceptability of this animal in detecting drug-induced immune modulation.[22-25] It is expected that this trend will continue, since it allows a more direct comparison between the assessment of the immune and other organ systems.

C. DESCRIPTIVE ASSESSMENT

1. Clinical and Anatomical Pathology

As previously mentioned, a considerable amount of information on the structural status of the immune system can be obtained from standard toxicology parameters, or from end points that can easily be incorporated into standard testing paradigms. A number of excellent reviews on the use of routine pathology for immunotoxicity assessment have recently been published.[23,26-28]

With an increasing number of biopharmaceutical agents under development and subsequent testing for safety, there is a need for more sophisticated methods of detecting subtle alterations in the structure of the immune system. In addition, immunotherapeutics require techniques that discriminate the precise location of deposition and action of these agents. Some of these techniques include immunohistochemistry (IHC), *in situ* hybridization, and *in situ* polymerase chain reaction techniques. An excellent overview of the benefits and challenges of these techniques has been published by Pilling.[29]

2. Flow Cytometry

Flow cytometry is a powerful tool that has revolutionized many areas of biological research. By using the high specificity available from monoclonal antibodies and the high accuracy of flow cytometers, both the structure and function of the immune system can be evaluated in great detail.[30] The early tier testing validation work of Luster el al.[2,3] found that surface marker analysis by flow cytometry was one of the most sensitive indicators of immunotoxicity. Perhaps for this reason, a number of regulatory agencies (FDA/CDER; CPMP; EPA) include flow cytometric analysis as a required or recommended end point for immunotoxicity assessment. However, a recent interlaboratory validation study conducted by Ladics et al.[31] found a considerable degree of variability within laboratories, even using a standardized protocol. This was also the conclusion of a workshop sponsored by the International Life Sciences Institute held in 1997,[32] whose recommendations indicated a lack of sufficient information on the use of flow cytometry in any type of immunotoxicity assessment. This lack of concrete information on the utility of flow cytometery in immunotoxicology suggests that, at present, great caution should be exercised in interpreting any such data; moreover, it argues that flow cytometry data are of little use in isolation from any supporting functional or observational pathology data.

Because of the complexity of the technology, as well as skill required for adequate interpretation of the resulting data, a truly useful description of methodologies for employing flow cytometry in immunotoxicology studies is beyond the scope of this chapter. Readers desiring a more thorough grounding in this subject are directed to any number of excellent reference books currently available.

D. FUNCTIONAL ASSESSMENT

1. Overview

Whether actively involved in immunotoxicology evaluation or using data gained from this type of study for understanding the total toxicological profile of a drug, it is important that one possess an understanding of the principles and techniques of immunology. This section describes the basic performance of several of the most useful assays for initial assessment of immunotoxicity: the AFC assay, generally considered to be a measure primarily of B-cell function (although in reality more of a measure of general immunocompetence); the NK cell assay for assessment of nonspecific host resistance; delayed-type hypersensitivity as a measure of T-cell function.

Since the majority of these assays employ at least basic mammalian cell culture, the section immediately following is intended to familiarize the beginner with the fundamentals of this technology.

2. Cell Culture Media and Supplements

a. Saline Solutions

Saline solutions serve two principal roles. First, they form the base for all cell culture media, providing water and inorganic salts. Mammalian cells can survive for limited periods of time in these solutions, although generally not for periods of longer than a few hours. For most studies, saline solutions are used primarily for washing cells, providing an isotonic/isosmotic environment. Three commonly encountered saline solutions in immunotoxicology are as follows:

- **Phosphate-buffered saline (PBS),** which is most commonly used for washing tissues and cells to remove blood, dead cells/debris, or other unwanted materials. When prepared without cations such as magnesium and calcium, PBS helps prevent clumping of cells and maintains a homogeneous single-cell suspension necessary for proper cell enumeration. The phosphate-based buffering system is used to maintain a physiological pH; PBS does not routinely contain a pH indicator, such as phenol red, although this reagent is available.
- **Hank's balanced salt solution (HBSS),** often used as physiological saline in place of PBS. It was originally formulated for pH equilibration in air (rather than the CO_2 atmosphere used in cell culture incubators), making it a good choice for short-term handling of cells on the benchtop. HBSS generally incorporates phenol red as a pH indicator.
- **Earles' balanced salt solution (EBSS),** originally formulated for pH equilibration in a CO_2 atmosphere, making it useful for short-term, nonsterile procedures that involve brief incubation periods. For many immunotoxicology studies, it is poorly suited to benchtop work, making it less commonly used than the aforementioned saline solutions.

b. Culture Media

There are numerous culture media available for cell isolation, growth, and maintenance. In many cases, the choice of which cell culture medium to use is determined by previous experiences as well as specific metabolic requirements of cell lines. One of the most commonly used culture media for immunotoxicology studies is RPMI-1640 (often referred to generically as RPMI), originally developed at Roswell Park Memorial Institute for the maintenance of human leukemic cell lines.

RPMI, when properly supplemented, is a versatile medium that can support a variety of cell types. Other culture media that may be encountered in the literature are all essentially modifications of basal media such as Eagle's Minimal Essential Medium (EMEM), Dulbecco's Minimal Essential Medium (DMEM), and Iscove's Minimal Essential Medium (IMEM). Certain target or indicator cells have been isolated in particular culture media; it is usually prudent to continue culturing these cells in the specified medium.

Cell culture media must be buffered to maintain optimal pH conditions. For immunotoxicology culture media, this function is usually performed by HEPES, a zwitterionic buffer incorporated into the original medium formulation at a concentration of 10 to 20 mM. Less often, sodium bicarbonate may be used as a buffer.

c. Serum

Serum is a highly complex fluid that provides a wide range of nutrients to cells *in vitro*. Because of the undefined nature of serum (and potential concomitant difficulties in reproducibility from a quality assurance/quality control standpoint), any ideal cell culture system would be totally serum free. Indeed, a number of serum-free culture supplements are commercially available, although few have been found to be universally acceptable. Among the sera used in immunotoxicology, the two most widely used are fetal bovine serum (FBS, occasionally but erroneously referred to as fetal calf serum, or FCS), useful for most species, and human serum, almost exclusively used in human and nonhuman primate studies.

- **FBS** is the most widely used serum supplement for immunotoxicology studies. FBS varies widely in quality, particularly in its ability to support cell growth, but sometimes also demonstrating an inhibitory effect on some immune functions *in vitro*. For this reason, it is imperative to lot-test FBS, even from known "good" suppliers, and to purchase large quantities of proven lots whenever practical. For immunotoxicology studies FBS is routinely heat-treated at 56°C for 30 min, ostensibly to inactivate endogenous complement, although there is some uncertainty regarding the utility of this procedure for most applications. For most studies, FBS is added to basal cell culture medium at a final concentration of 10%.
- **Human serum,** for some investigators, yields stronger and more reproducible results in primate studies than does FBS. Human AB negative serum is generally preferred, and is routinely heat-treated similarly to FBS. For most assays, human serum is added to basal culture medium at a final concentration of 5 to 10%.

d. Antimicrobials

Ideally, antimicrobial agents should not be included in cell culture medium. However, this is not an ideal world and, consequently, minor errors in sterile technique or errant breezes may compromise sterility. For *in vitro* immune function assays, this breach in aseptic culture can easily result in the compromise of critical studies. The most commonly encountered antimicrobial agents for cell culture are antibiotics (for control of bacterial and mycoplasma contamination) and antimycotics (for control of fungal infection).

Antibiotics generally used in immunotoxicology studies include gentamicin sulfate or a combination of penicillin and streptomycin. Both gentamicin and penicillin/streptomycin are effective in controlling both Gram-positive and Gram-negative bacteria; gentamicin is also effective in controlling mycoplasma. Gentamicin is used in culture at a final concentration of 5 to 50 µg/ml, and is stable in culture for approximately 5 days. Penicillin/streptomycin is used at a final concentration of 50 to 100 units/ml/50 to 100 µg/ml, and is stable in culture for approximately 3 days. One other agent that should be mentioned is Ciprofloxacin, which is sometimes used to "rescue" cell cultures contaminated with mycoplasma. Although such rescue may be vital for irreplaceable cell lines, it should be discouraged for routine culture practices.

Antimycotics are mentioned here only in reference to the observation that they should never be used in immunotoxicology studies. As a rule, gross contamination of culture with fungi represents a serious problem in culture technique or environment and steps must be taken to control the problem rather than to mask it. Moreover, many antifungal agents are toxic to mammalian cells.

e. Other Supplements

Mercaptoethanol is often added to culture medium at a final concentration of 0.05 mM. The precise role of this reagent is uncertain, although it appears to enhance viability during longer culture. It also apparently supplements macrophage function, making it especially useful in immune function assays.

Glutamine serves as a carbon source for cells in culture. It is relatively unstable at cell culture temperatures and should be added to culture medium immediately prior to use. Glutamine is generally added to culture medium at a final concentration of 5 mM.

Amino acids, except for certain specialty media, form an integral component of most prepared media. Particularly fastidious cells, however, may require additional supplementation with either essential or nonessential amino acids. When needed, they are generally added to medium at a final concentration of 1% of the stock solution.

3.   Preparation of Cells

With the exception of standard histopathological assessment and (occasionally) immunohistochemistry, *ex vivo* assessment of immune function in rodents requires that the lymphoid tissues (primarily the spleen, but occasionally the thymus or lymph nodes, and infrequently the bone marrow) be dissociated into single-cell suspensions. Dissociation destroys the functional architecture of the tissues and the effect of this disruption is unknown. However, there is currently no practical alternative, since it is necessary for standardizing the assays.

The technique described below has been used with excellent results (>90% viability in recovered cells) in the authors' laboratory. The procedure describes the preparation of single-cell suspensions from spleens, but is readily adaptable to thymus or lymph node cells.

Materials
- RPMI-1640 culture medium supplemented with 25 mM HEPES buffer, 10% FBS, 2 mM L-glutamine, and 50 µg/ml gentamicin
- Sterile petri dishes
- Sterile plungers from 1-ml syringes (for mice) or 3-ml syringes (for rats)
- 3-cc syringes fitted with 23-gauge needles
- Nylon macromesh (Spectrum Medical or equivalent), autoclaved
- 70% ethanol in wash bottle
- Sterile surgical instruments
- Sterile polypropylene centrifuge tubes

Procedure
1. Euthanize the animals by accepted technique. Place the animal on absorbent paper towels in a laminar flow hood, wet the animal's fur with 70% ethanol, and resect the skin of the torso (nonsterile tools may be used). Then, using sterile technique, open the body cavity and visualize the lymphoid tissue(s) of interest. Carefully isolate the tissue, removing as much fat and connective tissue as possible. Transfer the tissue to a sterile tube containing cell culture medium for transport to the cell culture laboratory.
2. Using sterile technique, transfer the tissue to a petri dish containing a piece of sterile nylon mesh (the mesh should be larger than the tissue sample, e.g., 1 in. square for a

mouse spleen). Transfer the medium in which the tissue was collected to the dish, wetting the mesh with a portion of it.

3. Using sterile scissors, make several incisions in the tissue. Then, using the syringe plunger as a pestle, gently rub the tissue across the mesh; keep the mesh constantly wet with culture medium to limit damage to the cells by friction. Continue rubbing the tissue until only connective tissue remains on the mesh.

4. Aspirate the cell suspension using the syringe/needle several times, breaking up any obvious clumps. Transfer the cell suspension back to the original collection tube and allow it to sit undisturbed for approximately 5 min. This will allow any remaining cell clumps, tissue fragments, and other debris to settle out.

5. Using a pipette, remove the suspension to a clean centrifuge tube (the debris remains behind). Centrifuge the cell suspension to pelletize the cells, and then remove the liquid. Tap the tube lightly to break up the cell pellet, then suspend the cells in a known volume of fresh culture medium. Mouse spleen suspensions of 5 ml and rat spleen suspensions of 10 ml are convenient volumes for subsequent procedures.

6. Determine cell number and viability by standard procedures, and then calculate the viable cell density of each preparation. Cells are now ready for use in assays.

4. IgM Antibody-Forming Cell Assay

Within a few days following *in vivo* injection of a foreign antigen, antibody molecules of the IgM class are produced and released into the systemic circulation. The AFC assay (alternatively referred to as the plaque-forming cell, or PFC assay) quantitates the production of specific antibody through enumeration of antibody-producing cells in the spleen following a primary antigenic stimulus such as sheep red blood cells (SRBC). Although the AFC response to SRBC is often classified as a measure of B-cell function, it is also useful for evaluating the proper overall function of the immune system, since the induction of this response requires cognate cell interaction and regulation by antigen-presenting cells such as macrophages, T cells, and various molecules including complement and cytokines. The primary antibody response is currently measured using either a PFC assay[33] or an ELISA.[34]

Materials
- RPMI-1640 culture medium, supplemented with 2 mM L-glutamine and 25 mM HEPES buffer
- SRBC in Alsever's solution
- Guinea pig complement (C')
- Dulbecco's phosphate-buffered saline (DPBS)
- DEAE dextran, 30 mg/ml in saline, pH 6.9
- Bacto-agar (agarose)
- Petri dishes, coverslips

Procedure
1. Immunize animals with an intravenous injection of washed SRBC in sterile saline 4 days prior to assay. Recommended inocula are approximately 1×10^8 SRBC for mice and approximately 2×10^8 SRBC for rats.

2. Euthanize the animals, remove the spleens, and prepare a single-cell splenocyte suspension in culture medium. Prepare two dilutions of the cell suspension in culture medium.

3. Wash SRBC by centrifugation (two to three times). After the final wash, retain approximately 100 μl of SRBC, then adjust the remaining cells to a final density of 10% in culture medium. Add C' to the reserved SRBC, mix well, and hold on ice until needed.

4. Prepare a solution containing 0.5% agar in DPBS, add DEAE-dextran (1.6 ml stock solution/100 ml agarose) and mix. Dispense the agar in 0.35-ml aliquots into polypropylene culture tubes, and maintain these tubes at 45°C.

5. For the assay, each tube contains 0.35 ml agarose solution, 100 µl cell suspension, and 25 µl C'. Add SRBC first and then the cell suspension, and immediately remove the tube from the water bath. Add the C' and mix the contents of the tube. Dispense the contents into a petri dish; then drop a coverslip so that an even matrix forms underneath. (Every effort should be made to avoid incorporating bubbles into the matrix, since bubbles can be mistaken for plaques by inexperienced personnel.)

6. Incubate the plates at 37°C for at least 3 h, and enumerate the plaques; a low-power magnifier such as a dissecting microscope is essential for this task. While the plates are incubating, determine cell number and viability of the original splenocyte suspensions.

7. The results are calculated as follows:
   a. Total number of plaques under each coverslip × 10 × dilution factor = PFC/ml of the original cell suspension (since 0.1 ml of the cell dilution is counted);
   b. PFC/ml × volume of original cell suspension = PFC/spleen;
   c. PFC/ml/number of viable cells/ml = PFC/10^6 viable splenocytes.

5. Anti-SRBC IgM ELISA

Materials
- SRBC in Alsever's solution
- Horseradish peroxidase (HRP)-conjugated, affinity-purified goat antimouse/antirat IgM antibody
- Peroxidase substrate (2-azino-bis-3-ethylbenzthiazoline-6-sulfonic acid, ABTS)
- ABTS buffer (phosphate-urea-hydrogen peroxide)
- PBS
- 96-well microplates
- General reagents and supplies for ELISA

Procedure
1. Immunize mice or rats with SRBC as for the plaque assay. After 5 days (mice) or 6 days (rats) later, obtain serum from both immunized and naive animals. Pool each as appropriate to use as standards or controls and freeze at –20°C.

2. Treat mice or rats with test material and vehicle (and a positive control, if necessary). On day 5 or 6 post-treatment (respectively), obtain serum from animals.

3. Prepare SRBC membrane antigen by lysis and solubilization. This antigen serves as the capture reagent in the ELISA.

4. Obtain anti-SRBC IgM antibodies to use as standards. Anti-SRBC must be of the appropriate species depending on the test animal.

5. Dilute membrane antigen to 1.0 g/ml in PBS and coat the wells of the microplates at approximately 4°C using 125 µl/well of the antigen preparation.

6. On the day of assay, wash the plates three times with 0.01% Tween-20 in water. Block unbound sites on the plates by incubating the plates with 200 µl/well of PBS/0.05% Tween-20, 3% bovine serum albumin, or 3% powdered milk.

7. Prepare serial twofold dilutions of test sera and antibody standards. Add to the plates and incubate for at least 1 h at room temperature.

8. Wash the plates three times, then add HRP-conjugated secondary antibody. Incubate for 1 h at room temperature, then wash the plates three times.

9. Add peroxidase substrate (ABTS) and incubate the plates at room temperature for 45 min. Stop the reaction by adding 3% oxalic acid to all wells.

10. Read the plates in a spectrophotometer at 405 nm and calculate the results based on curves prepared using the antibody standards.

Positive Control

Cyclophosphamide is routinely used as a positive immunosuppression control for the AFC assay (either plaque or ELISA format). For mice, cyclophosphamide is administered intraperitoneally at 80 mg/kg once approximately 24 h prior to euthanasia. For rats, it is administered intraperitoneally (ip) at 20 to 25 mg/kg daily for 4 to 5 days prior to euthanasia.

Notes

1. The AFC response varies depending on the day of analysis following immunization. Each species and strain should also be evaluated for the optimum response, although for intravenous injection the optimum assay period is usually 4 days following immunization.
2. The dose and route of antigen exposure alters the peak AFC response. Intravenous injections shift the optimum response to an earlier time, whereas an ip injection delays the peak response.
3. For quality control purposes each new test lot of complement should be tested and titrated prior to use. This step is also a requirement under certain immunotoxicology guidelines. Complement may be prepared fresh, but is commercially available in a lyophilized form that is more convenient.
4. The day of antigen administration relative to the last dose of chemical exposure should be considered when designing a study.
5. At the time of writing, SRBC membranes are not commercially available. Monoclonal and polyclonal antibodies specific for SRBC are commercially available from a variety of sources.
6. The direct comparability of results between the plaque assay and the ELISA is the source of some disagreement. The AFC assay measures antibody producing plasma cells in one organ (spleen) only, whereas the ELISA is a measure of systemic antibody production, which may have a different time course.
7. Other variations of the AFC assay may be performed to answer more-detailed, mechanistic questions. In particular, the method of Rittenberg and Pratt[35] directs the response to recognize haptens, and therefore is useful for evaluating T-independent antigens. A technique also exists in which immunization of the spleen cells is performed *in vitro*.[36] Although this technique has some advantages in mechanistic studies, it is labor-intensive and tricky to perform; its general utility in preclinical immunotoxicity assessment is thus limited.

6. Delayed-Type Hypersensitivity Assay

The delayed type hypersensitivity (DTH) assay is a measure almost exclusively of T-lymphocyte function. In this response, animals are sensitized via dermal contact to a strong contact sensitizer, and then challenged at a distant site with a lower concentration of the sensitizer. The secondary exposure to the antigen (or hapten) elicits an inflammatory response that includes lymphocyte proliferation and infiltration of the skin with fluid and various leukocytes. This response is measured indirectly by measuring changes in skin thickness; the pinna thus serves as the perfect site for challenge.

According to the early work of Luster et al.,[1] the DTH assay is not as accurate or as sensitive as either the mixed lymphocyte response (MRL) or the cytotoxic T-lymphocyte (CTL) assay. However, the assay is must easier technically than either of these other assays; moreover, it does not require specialized cell culture and thus is more accessible to most investigators. The assay described below is adapted from the method of Asherton and Ptak.[37]

Materials
- Hair clippers
- Oxazolone (4-ethoxymethylene-2-phenyl oxazolone; Sigma or equivalent)
- Acetone:olive oil (AOO) prepared in a 4:1 ratio (Sigma or equivalent)
- Positive displacement pipettor
- Micrometer (Oditest D1000 or equivalent)

Procedure
1. Randomize mice into groups of 8 to 10 animals/group. Shave the abdomen of all animals of as much fur as practical, taking care not to break the skin.
2. At least 24 h after fur removal, prepare a 2% (w/v) solution of oxazolone in the AOO carrier. Using a positive displacement pipettor, carefully apply 25 µl of this solution to the shaved abdomen of all animals. This represents the sensitization phase of the assay.
3. At 5 days following sensitization, measure the thickness of both the left and right pinnae of each animal. Ear thickness should be measured in the central portion of the pinna, taking care to avoid the very edge of the ear. Insofar as possible, the same approximate location should be measured each time.
4. Following this measurement, challenge the animals by applying 10 µl of oxazolone in AOO at a concentration of between 0.25 and 1% to the ventral and dorsal surfaces of the left pinna. The actual challenge concentration to be used may vary between laboratories, and should be determined empirically prior to actual use. The right pinna is challenged with 10 µl of AOO carrier on the dorsal and ventral surfaces. This represents the challenge phase of the assay.
5. At 24 and 48 h after challenge, measure the thickness of the left and right pinnae. Results of the assay are expressed as percent change in ear thickness according to the formula:
   Percent change = (thickness of challenged ear/thickness of contralateral control ear × 100).

Positive Control
If a positive control is required, a separate group of mice should be sensitized with oxazolone at a single concentration. Immediately following the challenge dosing, apply 30 µg of dexamethasone (Sigma or equivalent) in AOO to the pinna in a volume of 10 µl/ear.

Notes
1. It should be noted that the specific form of DTH that is measured in the assay described above (a contact hypersensitivity response) is different from that utilized in the original NTP validation studies, which was a tuberculin-type response;[38] however, the original procedure utilized intradermal injection of the pinnae with KLH (a protein antigen) and radiolabeling of the animal with [^{125}I]UdR, techniques that may not be standard in all laboratories.
2. The sensitization and challenge phases of this assay are usually timed to coincide with the test material dosing regimen, with either the day of challenge or the last day of ear measurement corresponding to the final day of test material exposure.
3. Perhaps more than most, this assay is subject to variability in results that are directly attributable to operator error. Care must be exercised to ensure that (a) the micrometer is not allowed to snap shut or to remain in place any longer than absolutely necessary to obtain a thickness determination and (b) that the reading be taken at the same location in each animal. Although the technique is not difficult to acquire, it does take practice to obtain reproducible results.
4. If more-detailed mechanistic immunotoxicology evaluation is desired, DTH techniques have been described that allow finer distinction of cellular alterations.[39]

7. Lymphocyte Blastogenesis (Mitogenesis)

A number of agents are capable of inducing lymphocyte activation, resulting in cellular proliferation. These agents may activate cells via a nonimmune capacity (concanavalin A, phytohemagglutinin, pokeweed mitogen), via receptors for bacterial cell components (lipopolysaccharide), via "simulated" immune reactions (monoclonal antibodies specific for the CD3 component of the T-cell antigen receptor, or anti-Ig molecules that trigger cell surface–bound Ig), or by using recall antigens (i.e., antigens that the host animal has had previous contact with or immunization to). This last option is particularly useful when assessing blastogenic response in human cells, since common recall antigens, such as candida antigen, or common vaccine components may be used. It also forms the basis for the lymphocyte transformation test, which can be used to detect drug allergy.[40]

Lymphocyte proliferation, by itself, does not assess specific effector function. However, the ability of lymphocytes to respond to activation signals in a physiological manner are widely used to assess overall immunocompetence. The advantages of this assay include (1) the assay is robust, and the basic technique is similar for all mammalian species routinely used in toxicology studies; (2) peripheral blood leukocytes may be used as the target cells, facilitating use of the assay in time-course studies or in other situations in which collection of cells at necropsy is not possible (e.g., human studies); (3) the ease of performance in a microplate format; and (4) the adaptability to mechanistic studies. Cells may be exposed to test material *in vitro*, which is of practical benefit when the test material may be too rare, expensive, or toxic to be used for *in vivo* exposure. The following procedure is adapted from Strong et al.[41]

Materials
- RPMI-1640 culture medium supplemented with 25 mM HEPES buffer, 10% FBS, 2 mM L-glutamine, and 50 µg/ml gentamicin
- Wash solution (DPBS/1% FBS)
- Cellular activators specific for the species under test; suggested agents and concentrations are provided in Table 9.2
- 96-well, flat-bottom microculture plates
- CellTiter Aqueous colorimetric indicator reagent (Promega), or equivalent
- Microplate spectrophotometer

Procedure
1. Prepare a single-cell suspension of the effector spleen cells, and adjust to a density of 2 × 10^6 viable cells/ml in culture medium.
2. Prepare stock solutions of mitogens to be used. The stock solution should be prepared at twice the final desired concentration to allow for dilution in culture. Prepare at least three dilutions to cover the expected optimal concentration; the concentrations listed in Table 9.2 should be taken only as suggestions, since the assay will perform slightly differently between laboratories and operators.
3. Add 100 µl of each mitogen dilution to replicate wells of 96-well microplates. Add an equivalent volume of culture medium only to replicate wells to serve as the nonstimulated control. In general practice, each microplate row will thus contain the cells from one animal, stimulated with one mitogen (i.e., three wells each of culture medium and three different mitogen dilutions).
4. Add 100 µl of the cell preparation to each well (cells from individual animals on different rows). If using a colorimetric reagent for the readout, the last row of each microplate must be left empty except for the last three to four wells, which will receive 200 µl each of culture medium.
5. Incubate the wells at 37°C in a 5% CO_2 atmosphere for approximately 72 h (total incubation time).

TABLE 9.2
Cell Activators Routinely Used in Lymphocyte Blastogenesis Assessment

		B Cells		T Cells
	Agents	**Suggested *In Vitro* Concentrations**	**Agents**	**Suggested *In Vitro* Concentrations**
Mouse	LPS	1–100 µg/ml	ConA	0.5, 1.0, 5.0 µg/ml
	anti-IgM + IL-4	Variable	PHA	0.5, 1.0, 5.0 µg/ml
	PWM[a]	Must be titrated	anti-CD3	Lot-specific (titrate)
Rat	STM	Must be titrated	PHA	0.5, 1.0, 5.0 µg/ml
	PWM	Must be titrated	anti-CD3	Lot-specific (titrate)
Primate	SAC	1:500 to 1:10,000	PHA	0.5, 1.0, 5.0 µg/ml
	PWM	Must be titrated	anti-CD3	Lot-specific (titrate)

[a] Pokeweed mitogen stimulates both B and T cells.
Abbreviations: anti-CD3 = anti-CD3 monoclonal antibody; ConA = concanavalin A; IL-4 = interleukin-4; LPS = bacterial lipopolysaccharide; PHA = phytohemagglutinin; PWM = pokeweed mitogen; SAC = *Staphylococcus aureus* Cowans I; STM = *Salmonella typhimurium* mitogen.

6. At 4 h prior to assay termination (i.e., at approximately 68 h of incubation), prepare the colorimetric indicator reagent as directed in the product insert. Add the colorimetric reagent to all wells, and then return the plates to the incubator for an additional 4 h.
7. Read the microplates on a spectrophotometer at the appropriate wavelength for the colorimetric agent used.

Positive Control
Cyclophosphamide, administered as described above for the AFC assay, has proved to be a reliable positive immunosuppression control for this assay.

Notes
1. The "traditional" end point for the lymphocyte proliferation assay has been the quantitation of radioactive thymidine incorporation into the proliferating cells. However, because of increasing concerns over the use (and, more importantly, the disposal) of low-level radioisotopes, a variety of other methods have been described. The colorimetric system recommended here has been found to work reliably and reproducibly in the authors' laboratory. Other colorimetric systems based on tetrazolium salts (MTT, XTT) will work, but have significant disadvantages.
2. Although proliferative assays can give relatively consistent results between rodents and humans, published reports[42] have revealed discrepancies for certain chemicals. Whenever possible, data from lymphocyte proliferation assays should be evaluated in conjunction with other tests to avoid this possibility.
3. Another type of lymphoproliferative assay is the mixed lymphocyte response (MLR), alternatively known as the mixed lymphocyte culture (MLC).[43] In this assay, leukocytes from animals on test are cocultured with leukocytes from a genetically dissimilar animal which have been metabolically inactivated with either gamma irradiation or a DNA intercalator such as mitomycin C. This assay is technically challenging, but has some limited advantages over assays using nonspecific cellular activators.

4. The actual method for reporting the results of these assays is known to have potentially significant effects on the data interpretation. This should be taken into careful consideration when incorporating these data into immunotoxicological profiles.

8. Natural Killer Cell Function

NK cell activity is measured *in vitro* by culturing single-cell suspensions of lymphoid cells with a tumor cell line known to be sensitive to NK-mediated cytotoxicity. The target cells are radiolabeled prior to the assay; thus, any cells which have been lysed will release their radioactivity into the culture medium, when it can subsequently be quantitated. The procedure described below is modified from the microculture method described by Reynolds and Herberman,[44] and is the standard approach for immunotoxicity assessment.

Materials
- RPMI-1640 culture medium supplemented with 25 mM HEPES buffer, 10% FBS, 2 mM L-glutamine, and 50 μg/ml gentamicin
- FBS
- DPBS
- Wash solution (DPBS/1% FBS).
- YAC-1 cell line (for rodent NK evaluation; ATCC #TIB 160) or K562 cell line (for primate NK evaluation; ATCC #243) maintained in log-phase growth
- 96-well, round-bottom microculture plates
- 0.1% solution of Triton X-100 in distilled H_2O
- ^{51}Cr as sodium chromate in sterile saline; specific activity of 200 to 500 mCi/mg
- Supernatant collection system

Procedure
1. Prepare a single-cell suspension of the effector spleen cells, and adjust to a density of 5 × 10^6 viable cells/ml in culture medium.
2. Prepare two serial 1:3 dilutions of the cell suspension in culture medium. Dispense 100 μl of each dilution in quadruplicate wells of 96-well, round-bottom microculture plates.
3. Centrifuge a log-phase culture of target cells and suspend the cell pellet in 0.5 ml FBS. Add 200 μl ^{51}Cr to the cells, mix well, and incubate at 37°C for 1 h. Wash the cells three times.
4. Suspend the target cells in culture medium, determine cell number and viability, and adjust the cells to a final density of 5 × 10^4 viable cells/ml in culture medium. Add the target cells to all wells in a volume of 100 μl/well. Include a row containing 100 μl target cell suspension and 100 μl culture medium/well (spontaneous release) and one row consisting of 100 μl target cell suspension and 100 μl 0.1% Triton X-100/well (total release).
5. Incubate the plates at 37°C, 5% CO_2 for 4 h. Harvest all wells with a supernatant collection system, and determine radiolabel release in a gamma counter.
6. Harvest supernatant fractions either manually or by using a semiautomatic harvesting system. Quantitate radiolabel released into the supernatant fractions in a gamma counter, and determine percent cytolysis using the formula: Percent cytolysis = (experimental release – spontaneous release)/(total release – spontaneous release) × 100.

Positive Controls
Immunosuppression control. A positive suppression control of the NK response should be included. Approximately 24 to 78 h prior to euthanasia, a separate group of animals are

injected intravenously with an optimum concentration of anti-asialo GM1 antibody. The exact amount to be given will vary from lot to lot. Treatment with an optimum dose of anti-asialo GM1 will result in an essentially complete abrogation of the NK response in rodents.[45]

Immunostimulation control. In some cases, it may be useful to include a positive control for NK cell augmentation. Although cytokines (IL-2 and IFN-γ) can enhance this response both *in vivo* and *in vitro*, an equally efficient, and more economical/reproducible, option is the use of interferon inducers such as polyinosinic:polycytidilic acid (poly I:C).[46] Poly I:C is administered intraperitoneally at a concentration of 100 µg/mouse or 500 to 1000 µg/rat approximately 24 h prior to assay.

Notes
1. NK activity is highest in young mice, declining after 12 weeks of age. Basal NK activity may be highly variable or undetectable in mice over 20 weeks old.
2. The target cells must be in log-phase growth to achieve adequate labeling with radioisotope.
3. The assessment of NK cell activity has been utilized most extensively in rodents and primates.
4. For laboratories unable to use radioisotopes, alternative methods have been developed using colorimetric, fluorometric, and flow cytometry end points. However, literature citations using these end points in immunotoxicology assessment are limited, and there has been no systemic comparison of these end points with the chromium release assay in this context.

9. Assessment of Macrophage Function

Macrophages, as previously described, are integral to the proper function of both specific and nonspecific host defense. Paradoxically, macrophage functional assessment is rarely included in initial screens of immunotoxicity. A notable exception is for drugs or devices that are expected to be trophic for macrophages, such as radioimaging agents. In situations in which such agents could potentially overwhelm the macrophages functional capacity (for example, by fully occupying the phagocytic mechanisms of the cell), it would be reasonable to suspect that the cell would be unable to perform its regulatory functions as well.

In the event that specific measurement of macrophage functional capability is warranted, a variety of assays are available to use (Table 9.3). Unfortunately, there are a number of technical challenges to working with this cells, including:

- *Limited supply.* Macrophages (and their circulating form, monocytes) comprise only a few percent of the total leukocyte population. This limits their use not only in rodent studies, but also in human and nonhuman primate experiments. Techniques are available for boosting recovery (e.g., injection of inflammatory substances into the peritoneal cavity), but these techniques artificially modify the cellular population that is collected.
- *Difficulty in isolation.* Monocytes/macrophages require special techniques to isolate, including density gradient centrifugation, elutriation, plastic adherence, magnetic bead phagocytosis, and a variety of other techniques. None of these enrichment techniques is ideal, since the enrichment processes invariably activate the cells to a degree.
- *Population heterogeneity.* Macrophage/monocytes are found in diverse compartments, and subtle differences in these populations may confound comparing the effect of the drug.
- *Inherent difficulty of the assays.* With the exception of measuring soluble macrophage products, such as cytokines or nitric oxide, macrophage functional assays are technically involved and do not always translate well between laboratories. Reproducibility may be a problem in assays utilizing target cells (e.g., cytotoxicity assays such as ADCC).

TABLE 9.3
Assays for Measuring Macrophage Function

Functional End Points	Elucidation of Effector/Regulatory Molecules
• Chemotaxis	• Cytokines (e.g., TNF/IL-1/IL-6)
• Cytolysis of tumor cells	• Nitric oxide
• Microbial killing	• Respiratory burst activity (NBT assay)
• Phagocytosis	• Prostaglandins and leukotrienes
• Antibody-dependent cellular cytotoxicity	

E. OTHER ANIMAL MODELS

1. OVERVIEW

Whereas rodent models have predominated in the evaluation of chemical-mediated immunomodulation and, at present, are the most common model for small-molecule drug-induced immunomodulation, rodents are far less desirable for evaluating biotechnology-derived therapeutics, particularly immunotherapeutics and vaccines.[47] This is true for two principal reasons. First, immunotherapeutics designed to modulate the primate immune system may not function properly in nonprimate models because of species differences. Second, and perhaps more relevant, human (or nonhuman primate) molecules may be recognized as foreign in nonprimates, leading to an immune response specific for the test material. Antibody produced may be neutralizing, partially or completely abrogating the physiological function of the molecules. At best, this situation profoundly complicates efficacy and toxicokinetic assessment; at worst, repeated dose with the test material could potentially lead to fatal anaphylaxis. In certain cases, it may be impractical, if not impossible, to conduct early safety assessment in primates, for example, when the relevant test material does not exist in sufficient quantities, or when appropriate test systems are not available in primates. In such cases, rodent homologues of the test material may be evaluated in rodents. However, this is an expensive and time-intensive approach and is not a viable alternative.

Although not as extensively developed as the corresponding rodent immunotoxicology assays, an increasing number of primate assays are now available (Table 9.4). In some cases the assays

TABLE 9.4
Representative Immunotoxicology Tests Available for Nonhuman Primates

Function Measured	Assay Used	Source
Structural integrity	Hematology/clinical chemistry	*Ex vivo*
	Histopathology	Necropsy
	Immunohistochemistry	Necropsy
	Flow cytometry	*Ex vivo*
B-cell function	Antibody production	*In vivo/ex vivo*
	Mitogenesis	*Ex vivo*
T-cell function	Delayed-type hypersensitivity	*In vivo*
	Cytokine analysis	*Ex vivo/in vitro*
	Mitogenesis and MLR	*Ex vivo*
Natural immunity	Natural killer (NK) cell function	*Ex vivo*
	Macrophage/neutrophil function	*Ex vivo*

are performed almost identically (except for certain reagents or target cells) to those used for rodents, such as the NK cell assay, macrophage function tests, immunoglobulin levels, cytokine production, and flow cytometric analysis of lymphocyte subsets.[48-50] All these tests can be performed on main study animals, and thus could be easily incorporated into a standard toxicology testing design.

Although the assays described above will provide much useful information, there will still be many instances in which it is necessary to assess directly the effect of a test material on the induction of a specific immune response; this assessment requires the immunization or sensitization of the animal with exogenous materials during the test material exposure period. For assessment of effects on humoral immunity, Tryphonas et al.[51] has described a system for measuring antibody production against different antigens. For assessment of effects on cellular immunity, a DTH assay has been described by Bleavins and de la Iglesia.[52]

2. Assessment of Cell-Mediated Immune Function in Primates by the DTH Assay

Cell-mediated immunity in primates may be assessed by a variety of assays including mitogenesis[53] and the mixed lymphocyte response.[54] However, these *ex vivo* assays may allow a certain degree of recovery from test material-related effects. The DTH is a completely *in vivo* model, allowing for the assessment of immune function in the presence of test material. The procedure described below is adapted from the method of Bleavins and de la Iglesia.[52]

Materials
- Freund's incomplete adjuvant (FIA) (available from Sigma Chemical, St. Louis, MO)
- *Trichophyton mentagrophytes* antigen and *Candida albicans* antigen (available from Hollister-Stier, Spokane, WA)
- Tetanus-diphtheria toxoid (available from Harry Schein, Inc., Melville, NY)
- Multitest CMI DTH kit (available from Connaught Labs, Swiftwater, PA)
- Calipers for measuring reaction site

Procedure
1. Prepare antigens for administration by preparing a 1:1 emulsion of FIA and antigens. Suggested antigen concentrations are 1000 protein nitrogen units (PNU) of *Trichophyton*, 1000 PNU of *Candida*, 1.2 Limes flocculation units (Lf) of diphtheria toxoid, and 6 Lf of tetanus toxoid. Immunize intradermally with this mixture a total of three times over a period of 7 days, using a separate site for each injection.
2. At 14 days following the final immunization, challenge the animals at a shaved epigastic site with the Multitest according to the provided instructions. Alternatively, a reference material may be prepared using the sensitizing antigens without FIA, injected intradermally in a volume of 0.1 ml.
3. At 24 and 48 h following challenge, measure the induration of the injection sites using calipers.

Positive Control
A separate group of animals sensitized with the antigen mixture is included. On the day of antigen challenge and on each subsequent day postchallenge the injection sites are treated with a topical corticosteroid cream such as 0.05% diflorasone diacetate.

Notes
1. Measurement of the induration of challenge sites at times later than 48 h has not been found to provide any additional information.

2. An alternative method for assessing DTH in primates has been described by Bugelski et al.[55] This method utilizes dermal sensitization to dinitrochlorobenzene (DNCB) and is performed similarly to the DTH in rodents described in a preceding section of this review. Although this method is much simpler than the intradermal sensitization described above, it is associated with some undesirable effects such as irritation and elevated liver and kidney enzymes.

3. As with other functional assays described in this chapter, careful consideration should be made of the timing of DTH assessment relative to test material dosing regimen. For extended duration studies, it may be necessary to provide a booster sensitization of the antigen.

3. Human Immunotoxicology

From the standpoint of preclinical safety assessment, the term *human immunotoxicology* is itself somewhat arcane since the purpose of safety assessment is to prevent this possibility. Nevertheless, unpredictable adverse drug reactions are recognized as unavoidable in this process.[56,57] Relatively common clinical findings that are suggestive of immunotoxicity include decreased white cell counts (one of the most common signs), "flu-like" symptoms, and hypersensitivity/allergy/pseudoallergy reactions. Of the latter finding, rashes are the most frequent, whereas anaphylaxis is rare. Clinical findings that are relatively rare include an increased incidence of lymphomas, infectious complications, and autoimmunity/systemic hypersensitivity.

Naturally, it is desirable to detect potential human immunotoxicity early in the development process; indeed, this is the sole purpose of preclinical immunotoxicology testing. However, a number of *in vitro* assays may be employed to evaluate potential human immune function. These assays may be useful for mechanistic evaluation of unanticipated reactions (e.g., potentially deleterious reactions such as idiosyncratic drug reactions, or conversely potentially beneficial actions that might suggest investigative options). Human *in vitro* assays may be necessary when species-related differences preclude the design of appropriate animal studies (examples would include humanized molecules, species-specific cytokines). Finally, these assays may be necessary when biochemical measurements alone are insufficient (as, for example, the induction of secondary immunosuppressive activity).

In vitro/ex vivo human immune function assays include most of those previously described for nonhuman primate studies such as basal or stimulated NK cell function, *in vitro* induction of cytotoxic T-lymphocyte (CTL) function (particularly the so-called redirected CTL response), cytokine production, macrophage and neutrophil functions, blastogenic response, and phenotypic analysis of leukocyte populations.

4. Assessment of Immunotoxicology in the Canine Model

The dog is frequently used as the nonrodent species for safety assessment studies. However, our knowledge of the canine immune system is arguably not as well developed as in the other experimental species; thus, there are considerably fewer reagents and techniques available. Related to this is the consequent dearth of baseline information on which to base comparisons of control and drug-treated animals. As a result immunotoxicology assessment in dogs has lagged behind rodents and nonhuman primates. From a practical standpoint, very little immune function information can be gained from the use of the dog that cannot be obtained from rodents. From an immunotoxicology perspective, the canine model may be most useful as a mechanistic tool in the relatively rare instances in which a species-related difference is observed. In the event that such assessment is desirable, a limited number of assays are listed in Table 9.5. It must be borne in mind, however, that these assays have not been extensively evaluated for sensitivity or predictivity in the context of immunotoxicology, and great caution must be exercised in the use of any resulting data in formulating safety or efficacy decisions.

TABLE 9.5
Available Models for Canine Immune System Assessment

Parameter Assessed	End Point Measured	Ref.
Structural integrity	Flow cytometry of leukocytes	58
Natural immunity	Natural killer cell activity	59
Humoral immunity	Quantitation of Ig subsets	60
	B-cell blastogenesis	61
	In vivo antibody response (KLH)	61
Cellular immunity	T-cell blastogenesis	61
	Quantitation of cytokines	(Limited number of reagents available)

5. Host Resistance: The Ultimate Determinant of Immunotoxicity?

As previously described, the early testing scheme developed by NTP included several models of host resistance in the Tier II tests; in fact, a comparison of the results obtained in host resistance assays formed an integral part of the validation process for most of the functional assays currently used in immunotoxicology assessment. Indeed, the ultimate purpose of the immune system (both specific and nonspecific aspects) is the defense of an organism from invaders, arguably rendering any other assessment secondary at best. Given the obvious advantages of host resistance assays, one would be justified in asking why these assays are not used more routinely (or, in fact, exclusively). Unfortunately, most host resistance assays are difficult to perform well, are labor, animal, and time intensive, and the results may be difficult to interpret for nonspecialists. Technical difficulties associated with these assays include:

- Species and strain differences in response to model organisms or cells. These differences may be subtle and difficult to differentiate.
- A requirement for basic facilities and experience in working with microbiological agents.
- A requirement for containment facilities for infectious organisms to prevent facility contamination.
- Difficulties associated with maintaining vigorous and reproducible microbial stock cultures, as well as titration of adequate infectious titers (challenge dose concentrations).

In spite of these difficulties, host resistance models are extremely useful in determining the true immunotoxic potential of test materials, and are recommended by several regulatory agencies for this purpose (see above). Some investigators choose to perform these assays exclusively, rather than in addition to less easily interpretable functional assays. Perhaps the greatest danger in this approach is that there is currently no "one size fits all" host resistance assay; that is, most of the assays that have been developed for this purpose evaluate only a few selected aspects of the overall immune response (Table 9.6). Therefore, if an investigator chooses to run only host resistance assays, it is vitally important that at least two (and preferably more) assays be run to evaluate CMI, HI, and natural host defense mechanisms.

A more frequently utilized approach is to perform the *in vivo/ex vivo* initial evaluation assays described above to determine whether or not a test material is associated with any evidence of immunomodulatory activity; if not, then host resistance assays would probably not provide any additional information. If, however, these functional assays suggest immune dysfunction, and the potential nature of this modulation is determined [e.g., cell-mediated immunity (CMI) is more affected than humoral immunity (HI), etc.], a specific host resistance assay may be employed to

TABLE 9.6
Host Resistance Models Employed in Rodent Immunotoxicology Studies

Model	Organism/Cell Used	Parameter(s) Evaluated	Ref.
Bacterial	*Listeria monocytogenes*	T-cell activation of lytic macrophages	62
	Streptococcus spp.	T-independent antibody production and subsequent phagocytosis by macrophages	63
Viral	Influenza virus	Lung defense by NK, CTL, interferon, and macrophages	64
	Cytomegalovirus	NK cells	65
	Reovirus	Production of gut IgA and virus-specific CTL	66
Parasite	*Leishmania* spp.	T cells and macrophages	67
	Trichinella spiralis	Primarily CMI; some HI	68
	Plasmodium yoelii	Antibody response	69
Fungal	*Candida albicans*	Depends on model setup	70
Tumor	B16-F10 melanoma	Macrophages and NK cells	71
	PYB6 sarcoma	CMI and NK cells	72

confirm this immune deficit, or conversely such an assay may provide evidence that a modest defect observed from the functional assays does not translate into a suppression of *in vivo* host resistance.

SECTION 5. QUALITY ASSURANCE CONSIDERATIONS

A. Laboratory Requirements Required to Meet (and Exceed) Good Laboratory Practice (GLP) Guidelines

There are numerous routine record-keeping activities in the immunotoxicology laboratory that must be performed to assure compliance with good laboratory practice (GLP) guidelines. Some of these laboratory requirements are described below and are summarized in Table 9.7.

1. Preparation and Tracking of Standard Operating Procedures

The use of current and relevant standard operating procedures (SOPs) is crucial for proper conduct of GLP-compliant immunotoxicology studies. Therefore, the preparation of detailed SOPs relevant

TABLE 9.7
Examples of Laboratory Record-Keeping Activities Necessary for GLP Compliance

Animal room temperatures, relative humidity	Cell line maintenance records
Animal room lighting conditions	Balance standardization
Refrigerator, freezer, CO_2 incubator conditions	Standard weight calibration
Equipment maintenance and use logs	Computer usage
Water analysis	Software validation
Food analysis	Test material use
Laboratory reagent labels	Employee training records

Source: Modified from Thomas et al.[73]

for all technical procedures and practices is the responsibility of personnel who are expert in these procedures. Once prepared, modified, and validated, these SOPs must be maintained in each laboratory in which GLP studies are conducted. Because technical changes are inherent in science (and especially in frontier technologies), SOPs are subject to modifications to enhance sensitivity and reproducibility, or to accommodate new paradigms. For this reason, it is important to ensure that only current copies of SOPs are available to laboratory personnel. Furthermore, when SOPs are revised or deleted, a system is necessary to guarantee that the outdated versions are recovered and replaced.

2. Animal Room Records

If *in vivo* studies are part of the immunotoxicology protocol (as they almost always will be), proper records include daily monitoring and recording of animal room temperature, relative humidity values, room air changes, and room illumination conditions (i.e., light/dark cycles).

3. Laboratory Equipment Use, Maintenance, and Monitoring

All equipment used to produce or collect raw data must be functioning properly, requiring constant vigilance. For example, the temperatures of laboratory refrigerators, freezers, water baths, refrigerated centrifuges, and incubators must be monitored and recorded. The speed of centrifuges must be verified; plate readers and cell counters must perform within specified limits. To ensure that all equipment is properly calibrated, it is a wise practice to set up routine schedules for the various types of calibrations. To confirm that these records are accurate, periodic calibration of thermometers and probes must be performed. Records associated with instrument calibration can be archived separately, whereas those pertinent to specific studies are maintained in the laboratory data books.

Besides the equipment monitoring and calibration described above, GLP regulations mandate complete written maintenance records be maintained for equipment used on GLP-regulated studies. Equipment manuals and usage logbooks are to be maintained with each piece of equipment. In general, regulatory agencies view equipment manuals as supplements to specific SOPs; therefore, the manual, usage logbook, and SOP should be kept in close proximity to the equipment.

4. Water and Food Analyses for Animal Studies

GLPs require that diets and water used for animal studies be free of unwanted chemicals or other materials that could interfere with the conduct or results of a study. Routine chemical analyses of the feed is often included as part of the study protocol. Records of periodic chemical and microbiological analyses of water samples are also needed and can be updated biannually. These data may prove invaluable in determining whether food or water contaminants adversely affected study results.

5. Reagent Inventory and Labeling

GLPs require that all laboratory reagents be labeled with identification of the material, its titer or concentration, storage conditions, and expiration date. The use of outdated reagents is not permitted and may invalidate study results. This requirement can be a major problem in the immunotoxicology laboratory because there are typically scores or even hundreds of chemicals, solutions, antibodies, cells, or etiological agents in use on a routine basis. It may be necessary to update retroactively all existing reagents and ensure that all new items are properly labeled as they are received. This requirement is particularly challenging when dealing with cell culture media and saline solutions, which are used at a fairly rapid rate and in large quantities.

6. Cell Lines

Cell lines used in standardized assays present a special challenge for GLP documentation. Because of their biological nature, cell lines are inherently more difficult to characterize and document than chemical reagents. To address this potential variability, certain documentation becomes necessary. At minimum, the derivation (species and origin) and subsequent manipulation (passage, cryopreservation) of the cells should be known; unfortunately, this information is not always available in detail. Whereas some of the cell lines routinely used in immunotoxicology studies (e.g., YAC-1, P815) are available from central cell banks (e.g., American Type Culture Collection), many investigators tend to use "hand me downs" from colleagues. In such cases, the cell line is essentially an accident waiting to happen. For example, subclinical mycoplasma contamination of a cell line may lead to a progressive variability and eventual loss of activity or viability in a cell line. Even worse, the infection may spread to other cells in the laboratory, necessitating their destruction. This can be catastrophic.

Other documentation for cell lines includes in-house tracking procedures (cryopreservation, thawing, storage, inventory), records on cell expansion and creation of master and working cell banks, and results of periodic characterization of the cells (genetic identity, microbial status). If the laboratory is conducting experimental infectivity (i.e., host resistance) assays, the bacterial, viral, and parasite models used should be characterized in an analogous manner.

7. Balance and Standard Weight Calibration

Standardized reference weights must be used before and after each weighing operation to ensure that the balance is properly calibrated. Furthermore, standardized reference weights should be verified periodically with known international standards. Laboratory reference weights should be sent out for verification, and all balances should be recalibrated on at least an annual basis.

8. Computer Usage and Security

The GLPs entrust the study director with the responsibility to verify the quality and integrity of the immunotoxicology data. Insofar as possible, all data should be captured and manipulated electronically. Because of possible inadvertent (or even intentional) alteration of computer hardware or software, it is necessary to restrict access to computers used to capture raw data, and to maintain a log of those using the computer. This may be done manually or electronically with passwords or data encryption programs.

9. Software Validation

Software and hardware programs must be verified in regard to data capture and manipulation. Verification programs to test the software and hardware limitations are often complex, time-consuming, and specific to the data being analyzed. Any computer maintenance or changes in software or hardware configurations must also be documented. The study director must ensure that changes in software or hardware do not affect the integrity of the data.

10. Test Material Documentation

Proper documentation of the test material used is one of the most important considerations in any GLP-regulated study. To assure that the correct test material is used, proper tracking is required from the time the material is first received in the laboratory until any residual test material is discarded. Improper tracking of test material (e.g., handling, storage) may invalidate an otherwise properly run experiment. Another important consideration concerns information regarding the stability, purity, and concentration of the test material. If a test material is suspended in a carrier, then the stability, purity concentration, and homogeneity testing of the test material/carrier mixture is also required by GLP. In the case of drugs or biological products, general guidance is provided in the various "Points to Consider" documents available from the FDA.

11. Personnel Training Records

Personnel working in the immunotoxicology laboratory require training in such diverse practices as cell culture, aseptic technique, basic microbiology, biosafety, radiation safety, and animal handling techniques (among others). Therefore, detailed training records are an integral part of the experimental record. GLP requirements mandate that study personnel be trained in their respective laboratory duties and that this training be documented. The study director should periodically review training records to guarantee that they are current and complete. As part of this process, detailed *curricula vitae* and job descriptions are required for all past and present employees involved in GLP-regulated studies.

B. QUALITY ASSURANCE AND QUALITY CONTROL

It is axiomatic that a laboratory conducting preclinical immunotoxicology studies to support drug development does so under GLP guidelines. It is perhaps less obvious that the need for strict quality control is at least as important, if not more so. The GLP guidelines outline the documentation processes by which data are collected, processed, and reported; they are less specific on the technical aspects of the assays themselves. Quality control (QC), properly executed, refers to internal procedures, independent of the quality assurance (QA) unit, that are established within the laboratory to guarantee a measure of interassay/interexperiment consistency. Much of the documentation required to comply with GLP regulations is also necessary for proper QC of laboratory operations. Examples of suggested documentation for the AFC assay are illustrated in Table 9.8. In addition to performing specific tasks, regular maintenance and updating of laboratory reagent inventories is essential for good QC. In an immunotoxicology laboratory, the number and variety of reagents can be daunting: chemical reagents, blood products (e.g., cell growth support characteristics of serum, donor information for SRBC), biologicals (e.g., bioactivity of cytokines, activity titers for complement and antibodies), and live organisms (e.g., identity and passage number for cell lines, infectivity data for bacterial and viral stocks).

It is understood that biological assays, in general, are susceptible to a certain degree of variability. However, time and money constraints, as well as the undesirability of wasting animal

---

TABLE 9.8
Documentation for the Antibody-Forming Cell (AFC) Assay Necessary for Meeting GLP Guidelines

Procedures	Reagents/Materials/Equipment
Test animal immunization[a]	Coulter Counter[e]
Spleen cell harvest[b]	Plasticware[f]
Spleen cell number/viability determination[c]	Cell culture media[g]
Reaction mixture incubation[d]	Immunological reagents (e.g., complement)[g]
Plaque enumeration[c]	

[a] Immunization date/time/route, animal number, SRBC concentration, technician identity.

[b] Animal number, date/time of organ collection, method of euthanasia, necropsy observations.

[c] Cell counts, technician identity, method of determination, verification of calculations.

[d] Incubation start/stop time, incubator identity, incubation conditions, identity of technician.

[e] Model, manufacturer, use/maintenance logs.

[f] Type, source, lot number, expiration (if applicable).

[g] Type, source, lot number, expiration, titer/activity used.

Source: Modified from Thomas et al.[73]

lives, preclude careless and sloppy work. Careful attention to the attendant myriad details, as well as an attempt to expect the unexpected, will pay dividends in the quality of data generated.

SECTION 6. SUMMARY AND PARTING THOUGHTS

A. Data Interpretation: The Holy Grail of Immunotoxicology

This chapter has attempted to provide the reader with a primer on the types of assays that are available to assess the effect of NME on the immune system, as well as the current status of regulatory expectations on such assessment for safety assessment of these compounds. However, there has been little instruction on how the resulting data are to be interpreted. Although a number of excellent reviews have recently been published on how immunotoxicology can be used for risk assessment and safety evaluation in humans, particularly from the standpoint of industrial or environmental exposure,[74-76] it is nearly impossible to codify rules for determining the ultimate effect of new drug candidates upon their entry into humans. A careful consideration of the guidelines described in this chapter, and an appreciation for the interactions between the specific and innate immune responses, and the immune system with other organs systems, will provide the most benefit in case-by-case evaluations.

B. Unanswered Questions in Immunotoxicology Assessment

Since its early development in the 1970s, the discipline of immunotoxicology has increased in scope and number of practitioners. Consequently, the foundation of baseline information and ideas has increased manyfold. The complexities of the immune system are now understood at a far finer detail, and this translates to a greater understanding of how xenobiotics can alter that response. Nevertheless, a number of important questions remain to be answered — questions that are vital if the promise of this discipline is ever to be fulfilled:

1. When does suppression of a normal immune response become pathological?
2. What is the relationship between statistical significance and biological relevance?
3. How does one recognize a superphysiological response?
4. What degree of immunostimulation is beneficial, and what degree is pathological? Does immunostimulation predispose to autoimmunity?
5. For immunomodulatory drugs, what differentiates toxicity from exaggerated pharmacology or efficacy?
6. Is the concept of immune reserve still valid? How does it relate to immunotoxicology and immunomodulation?

SECTION 7. GLOSSARY

ADCC (antibody-dependent cell-mediated cytotoxicity) Cell-mediated immunity in which a specific antibody binds to a target cell, targeting it for cytolytic activity by an effector cell (generally a macrophage).

Adjuvant A material that enhances an immune response. It generally refers to a mixture of oil and mycobacterial cell fragments (complete adjuvant).

Allogeneic From a different genetic background. In the context of immunotoxicology, this usually refers to the use of genetically dissimilar cells in *in vitro* assays to elicit a cell-mediated immune reaction.

Antibody Complex macromolecules produced by plasma cells that recognize specific antigens. Antibodies are also referred to as immunoglobulins (Ig). They consist of two basic units: the antigen-binding fragment (Fab) contains variable regions coding for antigen recognition; and the constant fragment (Fc), which determines the function of the antibody. Fc are designated IgA, IgD, IgE, IgG, and IgM. Cross-linking of antibody molecules on the surface of a cell leads to activation of complement, resulting in destruction of the target by lytic cells, or in phagocytosis by macrophages.

Antibody-forming cell (AFC) assay Also termed plaque-forming cell (PFC) assay. This assay measures the ability of animals to produce either IgM or IgG antibodies against a T-dependent or T-independent antigen following *in vivo* (or less frequently *in vitro*) immunization. Because of the involvement of multiple cellular and humoral elements in mounting an antibody response, the assay evaluates several immune parameters simultaneously. It is considered to be one of the most sensitive indicator systems for rodent immunotoxicology studies.

Antigen A molecule that is the subject of a specific immune reaction. Antigens are recognized in a cognate fashion by either immunoglobulins or the antigen receptor on the surface of T-cells. Antigens are usually proteinaceous in nature.

Antigen-presenting cell (APC) Cells that are responsible for making antigens accessible to immune effector and regulatory cells. Following internalization and degradation of the antigen (e.g., by phagocytes), a fragment of the antigen molecule is presented on the APC cell surface in association with histocompatibility molecules. The resulting complex is subsequently recognized by either B cells via surface-bound Ig molecules, or by T-cells via the T-cell antigen receptor. Induction of a specific immune response then proceeds. Representative APC include macrophages, dendritic cells, and certain B-cells.

Autoimmunity Reaction of the immune system against the host organism. In the context of drug development, autoimmunity may take the form of escape from tolerance, as when a drug modifies a host antigen, which is subsequently seen as foreign. Drug-induced autoimmunity may also result from bystander damage to host tissues from a drug-specific immune reaction.

B-cell/B lymphocytes Lymphocytes that recognize antigen via surface-bound Ig. B cells that have been exposed to cognate antigen subsequently proliferate and differentiate into plasma cells, which are responsible for producing specific antibody. B-cells differentiate in the bone marrow in mammals and in an organ known as the bursa in birds.

Bioassay A functional assay that depends on living cells as an indicator system. It may be performed either *in vivo* or *in vitro/ex vivo*.

Cell-mediated immunity (CMI) Antigen-specific reactivity mediated primarily by T–lymphocytes. CMI may take the form of immunoregulatory activity (mediate by CD4 helper T-cells) or immune effector activity (mediated by CD8 killer T-cells). Other forms of direct cellular activity in host defense (e.g., NK cells, macrophages) are not antigen specific and are more accurately referred to as natural immunity.

Cluster of differentiation (CD) A series of cell surface molecules used to denote cell types. These markers, used experimentally to identify cell types, serve various physiological roles *in vivo*.

Complement A group of approximately 20 protein precursor molecules that interact in a cascading fashion. Following activation, the various complement precursor molecules assemble into a complex that intercalates into the membrane of a cell, resulting is osmotic lysis of the target cell.

Cytokine Small peptides produced primarily by cells of the immune system, particularly helper T-cells. Cytokines are roughly grouped into nonexclusive categories including interleukins, tumor necrosis factors, interferons, colony-stimulating factors, and various miscellaneous cytokines. Related molecules include peptide growth factors, transforming growth factors, and chemokines. Cytokines form an interactive network with both hormones and neuropeptides. Cytokines may be referred to in the older literature as lymphokines.

Cytotoxic T-lymphocyte (CTL) A subset of CD8 T-cells that are able to kill target cells following the induction of a specific immune response. The mechanism of lysis appears to be a combination of direct lysis by extravasation of lytic molecules, as well as the induction of apoptosis in the target cell. Measurement of CTL activity is a sensitive indicator of CMI.

Delayed-type hypersensitivity (DTH) A form of CMI in which recall exposure to an antigen results in an inflammatory reaction mediated by T-cells.

Enzyme-linked immunosorbent Assay (ELISA) A type of immunoassay in which specific antibodies are used to capture and detect molecules of interest from a fluid matrix. The most common form is a "sandwich" ELISA in which the antibodies are bound to a substrate such as a plastic culture plate, and a second labeled antibody is used to detect the bound molecules.

Gut-associated lymphoid tissue (GALT) Lymphoid cells and tissues lining the mucosa that serve as the first point of contact with antigen encountered via this route. GALT comprises Peyer's patches, the appendix, tonsils, and mesenteric lymph nodes.

Hapten Low-molecular-weight molecules that are not antigenic by themselves, but which are recognized as antigens when bound to larger molecules, usually proteins.

Host defense The ability of an organism to protect itself against disease associated with exposure to infectious organisms, foreign tissue, or neoplasia. Host defense may be either specific or nonspecific (innate).

Humoral-mediated immunity (HMI) Specific immune responses that are mediated primarily by humoral factors including antibodies and complement. The induction of HMI generally, although not exclusively, requires the cooperation of cellular immune mechanisms.

Hypersensitivity A vigorous and often inappropriate immune response to seemingly innocuous antigens. Hypersensitivity is classed into subtypes depending on the mechanisms of action and the target cells or tissues.

Immune reserve The concept that the immune response exhibits multiple redundancies that are capable of accommodating acute reductions in isolated immune functions. This reserve would theoretically prevent a severe reduction in host resistance following a temporary immunosuppression of selected immune functions. This concept is important in interpretation of immunotoxicology data.

Immunoassay Refers to any assay that employs specific antibodies as reagents.

Immunostimulation Enhancement of immune function above an accepted baseline (control) level. Immunostimulation may be beneficial, e.g., therapeutics designed to restore a suboptimal immune response. It may conversely be detrimental, as would be the case with autoimmunity or hypersensitivity.

Immunosuppression Depression of immune function below an accepted baseline (control) level. Immunosuppression may result from inadvertent exposure to drugs or other chemical or physical agents, intentional modification for therapeutic reasons (e.g., organ transplantation), or following exposure to certain infectious agents (e.g., HIV). An important consideration in immunotoxicology is the ability to determine the amount of immunosuppression necessary to alter host defense. Immunosuppression may result in a state of immunodeficiency.

Immunotoxicology The discipline of synergistically applying cardinal principles of both immunology and toxicology to study the ability of certain treatments to alter the immune response.

Inflammation A nonspecific host defense mechanism characterized by the infiltration of leukocytes into the peripheral tissue, followed by the release of various mediators eliciting nonspecific physiological defense mechanisms. A normal prelude to a specific immune response, unchecked inflammation can result in extensive tissue damage.

Lymphoproliferation Proliferation of lymphocytes in response to stimulation with cellular activators such as antigens, mitogens, or allogeneic cells. Because proliferation is one of the initial consequences of activation, lymphoproliferation is used as a nonspecific indicator of immune responsiveness. This reaction is also referred to as "blastogenesis" or "mitogenesis."

Macrophage A bone marrow-derived cell present in the peripheral tissue that serves a wide variety of host defense functions, acting as both nonspecific phagocytes and killer cells, as well as regulators of specific immune reactions. Macrophages have different designations depending on the tissue in which they are located, such as Kuppfer cells in the liver, veiled cells in the lymphatic system, etc. When found in the circulation, macrophages take a slightly different form and are termed *monocytes*.

Major histocompatibility complex (MHC) Murine cell surface molecules that determine tissue compatibility and regulate self recognition and tolerance. Two major classes are recognized Class I (present on all nucleated cells) and Class II (present on B-cells, T-cells, and macrophages). MHC molecules direct the course of immune reactivity and are presented in association with antigens by APC. The human homologue is termed *human leukocyte antigen* (HLA).

Mitogen Molecules capable of inducing cellular activation; these may be protein or polysaccharide in nature.

Mixed lymphocyte response/reaction (MLR) An *in vitro* assay that measures the ability of lymphocytes to respond to the presence of allogeneic cells. This proliferation represents the initial stage of the acquisition of CTL function by CD8 T-cells, and thus serves as a measure of CMI. The MLR is a form of lymphoproliferation. Also referred to as mixed lymphocyte culture (MLC).

Mononuclear phagocyte system Previously known as the reticuloendothelial system (RES), this system is composed of all phagocytic cells of the body, including monocytes/macrophages and polymorphonuclear cells (i.e., neutrophils).

Natural (nonspecific) immunity Host defense mechanisms that do not require prior exposure to antigen; often are antigen-nonspecific in nature. Nonspecific immunity is mediated by NK cells, macrophages, neutrophils, γδT-cells, and complement.

Natural killer (NK) cells A population of lymphocytes distinct from T- and B-cells, also referred to as large granular lymphocytes (LGL) because of their microscopic appearance. NK cells exhibit cytotoxicity against virally infected cells and certain tumor cells. Assessment of NK cell function provides a good measure of nonspecific host defense.

New molecular entity (NME) A novel molecule under development for pharmaceutical purposes. The term encompasses both new chemical entities (NCE), such as small molecule drugs, and new biological entities (NBE).

Peripheral blood leukocytes (PBL) Leukocytes derived from the peripheral circulation. Because of their accessibility, these cells are often used in *ex vivo* immune function assessment in cases where terminal necropsy is impractical or undesirable (e.g., humans).

Skin immune system (SIS) Cells associated with the skin that participate in immunity. Includes Langerhans cells, dendritic cells, and keratinocytes. Alternatively known as skin-associated lymphoid tissue (SALT).

T-cell/T-lymphocyte Lymphocytes that recognize specific antigens via a complex of molecules known collectively as the T-cell antigen receptor (TCR). T cells are primarily responsible for the induction and maintenance of CMI, although they also regulate HMI and some nonimmune effector mechanisms. A variety of T-cell subpopulations exist, including T-helper cells, T-cytotoxic cells, T-inducer cells, and T-regulator cells. T-cells mature in the thymus.

Xenobiotic Any substance that is foreign to an organism. In the context of immunotoxicology, the term generally refers to nonbiological chemicals or drugs.

REFERENCES

1. Luster, M.I. et al., Development of a testing battery to assess chemical-induced immunotoxicity: National Toxicology Program's guidelines for immunotoxicity evaluation in mice, *Fundam. Appl. Toxicol.*, 10, 2, 1988.
2. Luster, M.I. et al., Risk assessment in immunotoxicology. I. Sensitivity and predictability of immune tests, *Fundam. Appl. Toxicol.*, 18, 200, 1992.
3. Luster, M.I. et al., Risk assessment in immunotoxicology. II. Relationship between immune and host resistance tests, *Fundam. Appl. Toxicol.*, 21, 71, 1993.
4. Luster, M.I. et al., Use of animal studies in risk assessment for immunotoxicology, *Toxicology*, 92, 229, 1994.
5. Document available at www.epa.gov/docs/OPPTS_Harmonized/880_Biochemicals_Test_Guidelines/Series/ 880-3550.pdf.
6. Document is available at www.epa.gov/docs/OPPTS_Harmonized/880_Biochemicals_Test_Guidelines/Series/880-3800.pdf
7. Document available at www.epa.gov/docs/OPPTS_Harmonized/870_Health_Effects_Test_Guidelines/Series/870-7800.pdf.
8. De Waal, E.J., Van De Laan, J.W., and Van Loveren, H., Immunotoxicity of pharmaceuticals: a regulatory perspective, *TEN*, 3, 165, 1996.
9. Van Der Laan, J.W. et al., Immunotoxicity of pharmaceuticals: current knowledge, testing strategies, risk evaluation and consequences for human health, *Drug Inf. J.*, 31, 1301, 1997.
10. Hastings, K.L., What are the prospects for regulation in immunotoxicology? *Toxicol. Lett.*, 102–103, 267, 1998.
11. Rodgers, K. et al., Immunotoxicity of medical devices, *Fundam. Appl. Toxicol.*, 36, 1, 1997.
12. Anderson, J.M. and Langone, J.J., Issues and perspective on the biocompatibility and immunotoxicity evaluation of implanted controlled release systems, *J. Control Release*, 57, 107, 1999.
13. Adachi, T. et al., Rat extracorporeal circulation model for evaluation of systemic immunotoxicity, *Toxicol. Lett.*, 115, 63, 2000.
14. Document available at www.fda.gov/cdrh/ost/ostggp/immunotox.pdf.
15. Hinton, D.M., Immunotoxicity testing applied to direct food and colour additive: US FDA "Redbook II" guidelines, *Hum. Exp. Toxicol.*, 14, 143, 1995.
16. Hinton, D.M., U.S. FDA "Redbook II" immunotoxicity testing guidelines and research in immunotoxicity evaluations of food chemicals and new food proteins, *Toxicol. Pathol.*, 28, 467, 2000.
17. Document available at www.ifpma.org/pdfifpma/s6.pdf.
18. Document available at www.eudra.org/humandocs/PDFs/SWP/104299en.pdf.
19. Maki, E., The practice of preclinical immunotoxicity testing in Japan, *Drug. Inf. J.*, 31, 1325, 1997.
20. Dean, J.H., Hincks, J.R., and Remandet, B., Immunotoxicology assessment in the pharmaceutical industry, *Toxicol. Lett.*, 102–103, 247, 1998.
21. Lebrec, H. et al., Immunotoxicological investigation using pharmaceutical drugs. *In vitro* evaluation of immune effects using rodent or human immune cells, *Toxicology*, 96, 147, 1995.
22. White, K.L. et al., Summary of an international methods validation study, carried out in nine laboratories, on the immunological assessment of cyclosporin A in the Fischer 344 rat, *Toxicol. In Vitro*, 8, 957, 1994.
23. ICCIS Group Investigators, Report of validation study of assessment of direct immunotoxicity in the rat, *Toxicology*, 125, 183, 1998.
24. Ladics, G.S. et al., Possible incorporation of an immunotoxicology functional assay for assessing humoral immunity for hazard identification purposes in rats on standard toxicology study, *Toxicology*, 96, 225, 1995.
25. Ladics, G.S. et al., Further evaluation of the incorporation of an immunotoxicological functional assay for assessing humoral immunity for hazard identification purposes in rats in a standard toxicology study, *Toxicology*, 126, 137, 1998.
26. Harleman, J.H., Approaches to the identification and recording of findings in the lymphoreticular organs indicative for immunotoxicity in regulatory type toxicity studies, *Toxicology*, 142, 213, 2000.
27. Kuper, C.F. et al., Histopathologic approaches to detect changes indicative of immunotoxicity, *Toxicol. Pathol.*, 28, 454, 2000.

28. Kuper, C.F. et al., Predictive testing for pathogenic autoimmunity: the morphological approach, *Toxicol. Lett.*, 112–113, 433, 2000.

29. Pilling, A.M., The role of the toxicologic pathologist in the preclinical safety evaluation of biotechnology-derived pharmaceuticals, *Toxicol. Pathol.*, 27, 678, 1999.

30. Burchiel, S.W. et al., Uses and future applications of flow cytometry in immunotoxicity testing, *Methods*, 19, 28, 1999.

31. Ladics, G.S. et al., Interlaboratory evaluation of the quantification of rat splenic lymphocyte subtypes using immunofluorescent staining and flow cytometry, *Toxicol. Methods*, 7, 241, 1997.

32. International Life Sciences Institute, Application of flow cytometry to immunotoxicity testing: summary of a workshop, ILSI Press, Washington, D.C., 1999.

33. Wilson, S.D., Munson, A.E., and Meade, B.J., Assessment of the functional integrity of the humoral immune response: the plaque-forming cell assay and the enzyme-linked immunosorbent assay, *Methods*, 19, 3, 1999.

34. Temple, L. et al., Comparison of ELISA and plaque-forming cell assays for measuring the humoral immune response to SRBC in rats and mice treated with benzo[a]pyrene or cyclophosphamide, *Fundam. Appl. Toxicol.*, 21, 412, 1993.

35. Rittenberg, M.B. and Pratt, K.L., Antitrinitorphenyl (TNP) plaque assay. Primary response of Balb/c mice to soluble and a particulate immunogen, *Proc. Soc. Exp. Med. Biol.*, 132, 575, 1969.

36. Mishell, R.I. and Dutton, R.W., Immunization of dissociated spleen cell cultures from normal mice, *J. Exp. Med.*, 126, 423, 1967.

37. Asherton, G. and Ptak, W., Contact and delayed hypersensitivity in the mouse. I. Active sensitization and passive transfer, *Immunology*, 14, 405, 1968.

38. Holsapple, M.P. et al., Characterization of the delayed hypersensitivity response to a protein antigen in the mouse, *Int. J. Immunopharmacol.*, 6, 399, 1984.

39. Yoshii, H. et al., A new assay system detecting antibody production and delayed-type hypersensitivity responses to trinitrophenyl hapten in an individual mouse, *Int. J. Immunopharmacol.*, 18, 31, 1996.

40. Nyfeler, B. and Pichler, W.J., The lymphocyte transformation test for the diagnosis of drug allergy: sensitivity and specificity, *Clin. Exp. Allergy*, 27, 175, 1997.

41. Strong, D.M. et al., *In vitro* stimulation of murine spleen cells using a microculture system and a multiple automated sample harvester, *J. Immunol. Methods*, 2, 279, 1973.

42. Herbert, T.B., Coriell, M., and Cohen, S., Analysis of lymphocyte proliferation data: do different approaches yield the same results? *Brain Behav. Immunol.*, 8, 153, 1994.

43. Bach, F.H. and Voynow, N.K., One-way stimulation in mixed lymphocyte cultures, *Science*, 153, 545, 1966.

44. Reynolds, C.W. and Herberman, R.B., *In vitro* augmentation of rat natural killer (NK) cell activity, *J. Immunol.*, 126, 1581, 1981.

45. Habu, S. et al., *In vivo* effects of anti-asialo GM1. I. Reduction of NK activity and enhancement of transplanted tumor growth in nude mice, *J. Immunol.*, 127, 34, 1981.

46. Djeu, J.Y. et al., Augmentation of mouse natural killer cell activity by interferon and interferon inducers, *J. Immunol.*, 122, 175, 1979.

47. Kennedy, R.C., Shearer, M.H., and Hildebrand, W., Nonhuman primate models to evaluate vaccine safety and immunogenicity, *Vaccine*, 8, 903, 1997.

48. Tryphonas, H. et al., Quantitation of serum immunoglobulins G, M and A in the rhesus monkey (*M. mulatta*) using human monospecific antisera in the enzyme-linked immunosorbent assay: developmental aspects, *J. Med. Primatol.*, 20, 58, 1991.

49. Chuang, L.F., Liu, Y., Killam, K., and Chuang, R.Y., Modulation by the insecticides heptachlor and chlordane of the cell-mediated immune proliferative responses of rhesus monkeys, *In Vivo*, 6, 29, 1992.

50. Verdier, F. et al., Determination of lymphocyte subsets and cytokine levels in cynomolgus monkeys, *Toxicology*, 105, 81, 1995.

51. Tryphonas, H. et al., Effects of toxaphene on the immune system of cynomolgus (*Macaca fascicularis*) monkeys. A pilot study, *Fundam. Chem. Toxicol.*, 38, 25, 2000.

52. Bleavins, M.R. and de la Iglesia, F.A., Cynomolgus monkeys (*Macaca fascicularis*) in preclinical immune function safety testing: development of a delayed-type hypersensitivity procedure, *Toxicology*, 95, 103, 1995.

53. Rappoocciolo, G. et al., A comparative study of natural killer cell activity, lymphoproliferation, and cell phenotypes in nonhuman primates, *Vet. Pathol.*, 29, 53, 1992.

54. Heise, E.R. et al., Mixed lymphocyte reactions in *Macaca fascicularis*, *J. Med. Primatol.*, 20, 67, 1991.

55. Bugelski, P.J. et al., Effects of sensitization to dinitrochlorobenzene (DNCB) on clinical pathology parameters and mitogen-mediated blastogenesis in cynomolgus monkeys (*Macaca fascicularis*), *Toxicol. Pathol.*, 18, 643, 1990.

56. Rieder, M.J., Mechanisms of unpredictable adverse drug reactions, *Drug Saf.*, 11, 196, 1994.

57. Uetrecht, J.P., New concepts in immunology relevant to idiosyncratic drug reactions: the "Danger Hypothesis" and innate immune system, *Chem. Res. Toxicol.*, 12, 387, 1999.

58. Williams, D.L., Studies of canine leucocyte antigens: a significant advance in canine immunology, *Vet. J.*, 153, 31, 1997.

59. Guenther, W. et al., NK activity of canine blood and marrow cells, *Tissue Antigens*, 43, 198, 1994.

60. Jones, R.D., Offutt, D.M., and Lonogmoor, B.A., Capture ELISA and flow cytometry methods for toxicologic assessment following immunization and cyclophosphamide challenge in beagles, *Toxicol. Lett.*, 115, 33, 2000.

61. Greeley, E.H. et al., The influence of age on the canine immune system, *Vet. Immunol. Immunopathol.*, 55, 1, 1996.

62. North, R., Importance of thymus-derived lymphocytes in cell-mediated immunity to infection, *Cell. Immunol.*, 7, 166, 1973.

63. Bradley, S.G. and Morahan, P.S., Approaches to assessing host resistance, *Environ. Health Perspect.*, 43, 66, 1982.

64. Lebrec, H. and Burleson, G.R., Influenza virus host resistance models in mice and rats: utilization for immune function assessment and immunotoxicology, *Toxicology*, 91, 179, 1994.

65. Selgrade, M.K., Daniels, M.J., and Dean, J.H., Correlation between chemical suppression of natural killer cell activity in mice and susceptibility to cytomegalovirus: rationale for applying murine cytomegalovirus as a host resistance model and for interpreting immunotoxicity testing in terms of risk of disease, *J. Toxicol. Environ. Health*, 37, 123, 1992.

66. Cuff, C.F. et al., Enteric reovirus infection as a probe to study immunotoxicity of the gastrointestinal tract, *Toxicol. Sci.*, 42, 99, 1998.

67. Birkland, T.P., Sypek, J.P., and Wyler, D.J., Soluble TNF and membrane TNF expressed on CD4+ T lymphocytes differ in their ability to activate macrophage antileishmanial defense, *J. Leukocyte Biol.*, 51, 296, 1992.

68. Luebke, R. et al., Host resistance to *Trichinella spiralis* in rats and mice: species-dependent effects of cyclophosphamide exposure, *Toxicology*, 73, 305, 1992.

69. White, W., Evans, C., and Taylor, D., Antimalarial antibodies of the immunoglobulin G2a isotype modulate parasitemias in mice infected with *Plasmodium yoelii*, *Infect. Immunol.*, 59, 3547, 1991.

70. Herzyk, D.J. et al., Single-organism model of host defense against infection: a novel immunotoxicologic approach to evaluate immunomodulatory drugs, *Toxicol. Pathol.*, 25, 351, 1997.

71. Fidler, I.J., Inhibition of pulmonary metastasis by intravenous injection of specifically activated macrophages, *Cancer Res.*, 34, 1074, 1974.

72. Urban, J.L. et al., Mechanisms of synteneic tumor rejection, susceptibility of host-selected progressor variants to various immunological effector cells, *J. Exp. Med.*, 155, 557, 1982.

73. Thomas, P.T., Boyne, R., and Sherwood, R.L., Nonclinical immunotoxicology studies: GLP considerations, in *Methods in Immunotoxicology*, Vol. 1, Burleson, G., Dean, J.H., and Munson, A.E., Eds., John Wiley & Sons, New York, 1995.

74. Selgrade, M.J.K., Use of immunotoxicity data in health risk assessments: uncertainties and research to improve the process, *Toxicology*, 133, 58, 1999.

75. Van Loveren, H. et al., Risk assessment and immunotoxicology, *Toxicol. Lett.*, 102–103, 261, 2000.

76. Vos, J.G. and Van Loveren, H., Experimental studies on immunosuppression: how do they predict for man? *Toxicology*, 129, 13, 1998.

ADDITIONAL RELATED INFORMATION

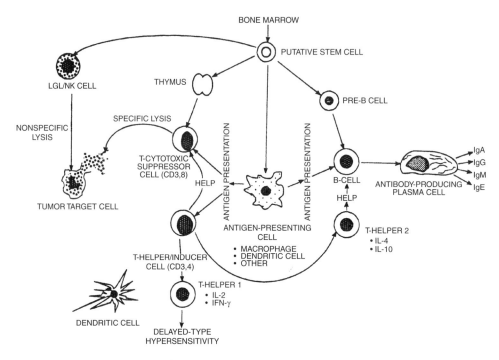

FIGURE 9.1 Cellular elements of the immune system.

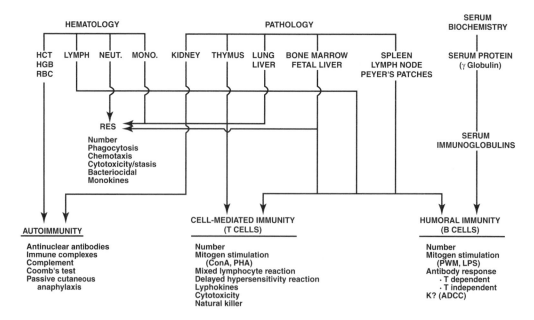

FIGURE 9.2 Relationship of immune function tests to routine toxicological parameters. From Norbury, K. and Thomas, P., in *In Vivo Toxicity Testing: Principles, Procedures and Practices,* Academic Press, New York, 1990, 410–448. With permission.

TABLE 9.9
Examples of Antemortem and Postmortem Findings that May Include Potential Immunotoxicity if Treatment Related

Parameter	Possible Observation (Cause)	Possible State of Immune Competence
	Antemortem	
Mortality	Increased (infection)	Depressed
Body weight	Decreased (infection)	Depressed
Clinical signs	Rales, nasal discharge (respiratory infection)	Depressed
	Swollen cervical area (sislodacryoadenitis virus)	Depressed
Physical examinations	Enlarged tonsils (infection)	Depressed
Hematology	Leukopenia/lymphopenia	Depressed
	Leukocytosis (infection/cancer)	Enhanced/Depressed
	Thrombocytopenia	Hypersensitivity
	Neutropenia	Hypersensitivity
Protein electrophoresis	Hypogammaglobulinemia	Depressed
	Hypergammaglobulinemia (ongoing immune response or infection)	Enhanced/Activated
	Postmortem	
Organ weights		
Thymus	Decreased	Depressed
Histopathology		
Adrenal glands	Cortical hypertrophy (stress)	Depressed (secondary)
Bone marrow	Hypoplasia	Depressed
Kidney	Amyloidosis	Autoimmunity
	Glomerulonephritis (immune complex)	Hypersensitivity
Lung	Pneumonitis (infection)	Depressed
Lymph node (see also spleen)	Atrophy	Depressed
Spleen	Hypertrophy/hyperplasia	Enhanced/activated
	Depletion of follicles	Depressed B cells
	Hypocellularity of periateriolar sheath	Depressed T cells
	Active germinal centers	Enhanced/activated
Thymus	Atrophy	Depressed
Thyroid	Inflammation	Autoimmunity

From Norbury, K. and Thomas, P., in *In Vivo Toxicity Testing: Principles, Procedures and Practices,* Academic Press, New York, 1990, 410–448. With permission.

TABLE 9.10
Examples of the Four Types of Hypersensitivity Responses[a]

Agents: Clinical Manifestations	Hypersensitive Reaction	Cells Involved	Antibody	Mechanism of Cell Injury
Food additives: GI allergy Penicillin: urticaria and dermatitis	Type I (anaphylactic)	Mast cell	IgE (and others)	Degranulation and release of inflammatory mediators such as histamine, proteolytic enzymes, chemotactic factors, prostaglandins, and leukotrienes
Cephalosporins: hemolytic anemia Aminopyrine: leukopenia Quinidine, gold: thrombocytopenia	Type II (cytotoxic)	Null (K) cells[b]	IgG, IgM	Antibody-dependent cellular cytotoxicity, or complement-mediated lysis
Hydralazine: systemic lupus erythomatosis Methicillin: chronic glomerulonephritis	Type III (immune complex)	PMNs[c]	IgG, IgM	Immune complex deposition in various tissues activates complement, which attracts PMNs causing local damage by release of inflammatory mediators
Nickel, penicillin, dinitrochlorobenzene, phenothiasines: contact dermatitis	Type IV (delayed hypersensitivity)	T cells (sensitized); macrophages	None	Release of lymphokines activates and attracts macrophages, which release mediators that induce inflammatory reactions

[a] Defined by Coombs and Gell (1968).[1]
[b] Also T cells, monocyte/macrophages, platelets, neutrophils, and eosinophils.
[c] Polymorphonuclear leukocytes.

From Norbury, K. and Thomas, P., in *In Vivo Toxicity Testing: Principles, Procedures and Practices*, Academic Press, New York, 1990. With permission.

10 Renal Toxicology: Renal Function Parameters for Adult Fischer-344, Sprague-Dawley, and Wistar Rats

William J. Powers, Jr., Ph.D., D.A.B.T.

CONTENTS

SECTION 1. INTRODUCTION

This chapter summarizes renal function parameters that were evaluated in both sexes of three rat strains (Fischer-344, Sprague-Dawley, and Wistar). These parameters can be used to characterize the nephrotoxicity potential of test compounds. The data in this chapter are from control (untreated) animals. Resting renal function parameters were evaluated using a battery of noninvasive procedures in unanesthetized animals. The renal response to specific stress was also evaluated using extracellular volume expansion and a urine concentrating ability test. In a separate group of animals, a battery of invasive procedures in anesthetized animals was used to evaluate specific renal functions, e.g., urine flow rate, glomerular filtration rate, fractional excretion of electrolytes, fractional reabsorption of water, and free water clearance, etc.

SECTION 2. METHODS

Fischer-344, Sprague-Dawley, and Wistar rats were received from Charles River Breeding Laboratory in Kingston, NY at approximately 6 weeks of age. Rats were housed singly in suspended stainless steel cages with a wire mesh front and bottom. The animals were maintained at a mean temperature of 72 ± 3°F, a humidity of 50 ± 5%, and a 12/12 hour light/dark cycle. Water was supplied *ad libitum* by an automatic watering system and Purina Certified Rodent Chow No. 5002 was also available *ad libitum*. Body weight and food consumption were recorded weekly.

A. RESTING RENAL FUNCTION

Each animal was placed in an individual metabolism cage for a 24-hour urine sample collection. The following parameters were analyzed and recorded: 24-hour urine volume, sodium, potassium, chloride, protein, glucose, alkaline phosphatase, lactate dehydrogenase, osmolality, pH, and creatinine. Individual animal blood and serum samples were analyzed for blood urea nitrogen (BUN), protein, creatinine, hematocrit (HCT), sodium, potassium, chloride, and osmolality.

B. EXTRACELLULAR VOLUME EXPANSION + 9-HOUR URINE COLLECTION

The extracellular volume space was expanded by intraperitoneal injection of isotonic saline (at 2.5% of body weight (v/w). Animals were then placed in individual metabolism units with food and water *ad libitum*. Urine was collected every 3 hours for a 9-hour period and analyzed for urine volume, sodium, potassium, chloride, osmolality, and creatinine.

C. URINE CONCENTRATING ABILITY

To measure the urinary concentrating ability, the animals were placed in the individual metabolism units with food *ad libitum*, but without drinking water. After the first 6-hour sample was discarded, two consecutive 24-hour urine samples were collected and analyzed for urine volume, sodium, potassium, chloride, osmolality, and creatinine.

D. INVASIVE PARAMETERS

A separate group of animals was used to evaluate specific renal parameters best measured using invasive techniques. The experimental procedure was as follows: Animals were anesthetized with

100 mg/kg intraperitoneal (IP) injection of inactin,[1]* then placed on a heated surgical table. The animal was then tracheotomized with Clay Adams polyethylene tubing (PE) 240 to maintain an open airway. A catheter was inserted into the jugular vein (PE 50) and an IV infusion started. The infusion solution was isotonic saline with 2.5 µCi [^{3}H]inulin/ml infused at approximately 0.02 ml/100 g body weight/min. A PE 50 catheter was placed in the carotid artery for blood sample collection. An inulin bolus consisting of 25 µCi [^{3}H]inulin in 0.3 ml of isotonic saline was injected IV. The bladder was catheterized with PE 60 tubing through a suprapubic incision. The animal was then allowed to equilibrate for 30 minutes. During the next hour the following measurements were made: urine flow rate and glomerular filtration rate [^{3}H]inulin clearance. Urine and plasma osmolality were determined along with urine/plasma inulin, sodium, potassium, and chloride ratios. Free water clearance and the fractional excretion of sodium, potassium, and chloride were also calculated. Kidneys were removed and weighed when each experiment was terminated (right and left kept separate). The following measurements were performed:

urine: volume, sodium, potassium, chloride, [^{3}H]inulin (liquid scintillation [^{3}H]inulin spectrophotometry), and osmolality
serum: hematocrit, sodium, potassium, chloride, and osmolality

SECTION 3. RENAL FUNCTION PARAMETERS

A. GLOSSARY AND ABBREVIATIONS

ALP alkaline phosphatase
Cr creatinine
Fischer-344 rat (F-344) inbred rat strain
GFR glomerular filtration rate (ml/min)
Hct hematocrit (%)
LDH lactate dehydrogenase
P_{Cl} plasma chloride (µEq/ml)
P_K plasma potassium (µEq/ml)
P_{Na} plasma sodium (µEq/ml)
P_{Osm} plasma osmolality (mOsm/kg)
Sprague-Dawley rat outbred rat strain
U_{Cl} urine chloride (µEq/ml)
U_K urine potassium (µEq/ml)
U_{Na} urine sodium (µEq/ml)
U_{Osm} urine osmolality (mOsm/kg)
U/P_{Cl} urine/plasma chloride ratio
U/P_{Inulin} urine/plasma inulin ratio
U/P_K urine/plasma potassium ratio
U/P_{Na} urine/plasma sodium ratio
$\dot{V}$ urine flow rate (ml/min)
Wistar rat outbred rat strain

---

* Inactin, supplied by Byk Gulden Konstanz, West Germany is the sodium salt of ethyl-(α-methyl-prophy)-malonyl-thiourea.

TABLE 10.1

Mean (±SD) Body Weights (g) for Fischer-344, Sprague-Dawley, and Wistar Rats (8–25 wk of age)[a]

Rat Strains	Age (wk)															
	8	9	10	11	12	13	14	15	16	17	18	19	20	21	24	25
F-344																
Males	224.8	239.3	252.7	268.6	280.0	289.0	294.4	303.9	312.3	321.5	323.6	328.9	328.3	328.1	340.6	343.1
SD	6.5	9.8	11.6	14.6	14.7	17.7	18.7	18.8	20.2	21.5	22.9	22.8	24.5	23.0	25.4	24.0
Sprague-Dawley																
Males	317.4	343.1	370.8	394.6	417.0	435.7	451.4	464.5	477.3	485.1	495.3	506.2	517.4	518.7	525.9	547.7
SD	16.6	16.9	21.2	23.4	27.4	26.8	28.7	32.4	33.1	35.7	38.1	40.6	42.7	45.3	49.8	46.9
Wistar																
Males	305.1	342.1	373.1	398.0	421.0	433.9	456.3	470.7	489.8	500.3	507.3	515.5	515.0	—	534.1	—
SD	10.6	8.5	10.0	9.0	9.1	11.6	12.3	12.6	16.9	13.6	14.1	17.2	20.3	—	21.4	—
F-344																
Females	143.8	146.6	151.9	159.9	163.1	166.6	166.0	169.3	173.4	177.7	176.3	179.5	180.5	179.4	184.6	183.4
SD	5.9	6.2	7.4	9.9	10.1	10.8	10.0	10.8	10.5	11.5	11.0	11.5	11.5	11.6	10.9	10.1
Sprague-Dawley																
Females	200.8	209.7	225.3	235.2	247.4	258.1	261.4	269.4	278.1	283.2	290.4	295.4	299.3	299.5	301.5	311.9
SD	14.0	19.5	17.8	21.0	24.5	25.2	26.9	30.4	31.6	30.4	31.5	32.0	32.6	31.6	33.9	35.6
Wistar																
Females	206.0	218.3	228.7	238.4	247.4	249.6	257.7	261.0	267.6	267.4	273.6	276.5	274.6	—	283.8	—
SD	16.2	17.5	17.9	17.9	20.5	22.0	23.3	24.3	23.7	25.7	24.7	23.8	24.0	—	24.9	—

[a] n = 6/group; — = data unavailable; F-344 = Fischer-344.

TABLE 10.2
Mean (±SD) Weekly Food Consumption (g) for Fischer-344, Sprague-Dawley, and Wistar Rats (for 13 wk)

Rat Strains	Week													
	0[a]	1	2	3	4	5	6	7	8	9	10	11	12	13
F-344														
Males	128.3	141.0	118.4	119.1	119.7	116.9	117.9	116.7	120.6	119.5	117.9	112.2	111.9	105.9
SD	7.9	10.2	9.7	9.6	9.7	7.6	7.8	8.6	10.3	10.3	8.9	8.7	7.9	12.7
Sprague-Dawley														
Males	174.5	206.3	182.8	181.3	183.6	185.3	185.6	176.4	180.4	180.4	183.6	178.5	173.4	168.2
SD	7.17	12.7	12.9	11.7	13.9	17.7	18.2	19.0	16.5	21.6	23.8	19.8	18.5	13.9
Wistar														
Males	223.3	189.9	190.6	189.5	191.7	188.9	189.4	195.3	185.8	188.6	189.3	180.8	184.1	—
SD	7.5	5.7	9.1	9.0	7.8	10.1	9.5	12.6	17.8	12.4	12.7	14.6	14.7	—
F-344														
Females	82.9	95.4	85.5	84.2	82.8	77.8	82.6	82.6	82.5	83.4	83.1	84.2	79.3	71.1
SD	6.8	8.8	9.6	7.3	6.2	5.6	5.4	5.0	6.6	6.5	5.2	5.9	4.4	5.4
Sprague-Dawley														
Females	129.1	155.8	142.5	139.8	136.6	134.8	138.0	137.1	137.9	136.4	136.1	126.8	119.5	124.5
SD	12.5	18.7	16.4	15.7	9.1	10.9	16.8	23.0	21.5	12.7	11.0	12.9	11.9	12.4
Wistar														
Females	167.5	133.9	141.1	131.4	136.5	147.3	130.3	130.0	128.7	129.7	127.2	126.3	133.8	—
SD	18.0	15.2	20.1	10.7	10.9	24.2	18.0	13.0	7.7	8.5	11.2	8.9	8.3	—

[a] = age at week 0 was approximately 8 wk; n = 6/group; F-344 = Fischer-344; — = data unavailable.

TABLE 10.3
24-Hour Mean Urinalysis Data with Standard Deviation (SD) and Standard Error of the Mean (SEM) in Adult Male Rats: Fischer-344, Sprague-Dawley, and Wistar Rats

Parameters	Strain								
	F-344			Sprague-Dawley			Wistar		
	Mean	SD	SEM	Mean	SD	SEM	Mean	SD	SEM
Volume, ml	5.92	2.15	0.88	14.83	7.63	3.12	12.68	4.06	1.66
Volume, ml/100 g body weight	1.78	0.556	0.227	2.824	1.339	0.547	2.453	0.761	0.311
Sodium (µEq/ml)	62.7	20.3	8.3	54.3	32.7	13.4	41.67	16.27	6.64
Potassium (µEq/ml)	197.67	32.87	13.42	168.0	75.2	30.7	146.0	37.5	15.3
Chloride (µEq/ml)	105.0	54.5	22.3	64.7	47.5	19.4	60.0	24.9	10.2
Protein (g/dl)	0.4833	0.0983	0.0401	0.5167	0.1941	0.0792	0.3667	0.0816	0.0333
Glucose (mg/dl)	7.33	17.96	7.33	0.00	0.00	0.00	0.00	0.00	0.00
ALP (IU)	154.2	54.4	22.2	87.1	53.7	21.9	141.4	43.4	17.8
LDH (IU)	3.83	9.39	3.83	34.17	83.69	34.17	0.00	0.00	0.00
Osmolality (mOsm/kg)	1312.3	210.5	86.0	1206	497	203	1197	325	133
pH	6.18	0.41	0.17	6.83	0.75	0.31	6.167	0.406	0.17
Creatinine (mg/dl)	144.2	22.8	9.3	142.0	61.9	25.3	165.7	60.7	24.8
Sodium/Cr µEq/mg Cr	43.2	124	5.07	35.78	7.88	3.22	25.37	7.55	3.08
Potassium/Cr µEq/mg Cr	137.2	11.6	4.72	117.29	15.55	6.35	91.10	16.1	6.59
Chloride/Cr µEq/mg Cr	70.3	35.3	14.40	39.5	25.0	10.20	36.9	14.7	5.99
Protein/Cr g/mg Cr	0.0039	0.00058	0.00024	0.0038	0.0012	0.00047	0.0023	0.0004	0.00016
Glucose/Cr mg/mg Cr	0.05	0.123	0.05	0	0	0	0	0	0

TABLE 10.4

24-Hour Mean Urinalysis Data with Standard Deviation (SD) and Standard Error of the Mean (SEM) in Adult Female Rats: Fischer-344, Sprague-Dawley, and Wistar Rats

Parameters	F-344			Sprague-Dawley			Wistar		
	Mean	SD	SEM	Mean	SD	SEM	Mean	SD	SEM
Volume, ml	8.82	4.32	1.76	8.43	3.43	1.40	18.22	8.07	3.29
Volume, ml/100 g body weight	4.93	2.41	0.98	2.839	1.119	0.457	6.48	2.46	1.00
Sodium (μEq/ml)	152.0	41.4	16.9	155.2	16.2	6.6	81.7	63.5	25.9
Potassium (μEq/ml)	304.0	91.2	36.8	324.2	50.8	20.7	179.7	97.9	40.0
Chloride (μEq/ml)	205.5	61.6	25.2	249.7	78.7	32.1	104.7	79.5	32.5
Protein (g/dl)	0.3333	0.0516	0.0211	0.4667	0.1211	0.0494	0.1833	0.0983	0.0401
Glucose (mg/dl)	9.3	14.5	5.9	8.33	.13.05	5.33	0.00	0.00	0.00
ALP (IU)	25.22	11.14	4.55	16.1	11.1	4.5	32.0	24.9	10.2
LDH (IU)	0.00	0.00	0.00	13.83	19.02	7.76	2.50	6.12	2.50
Osmolality (mOsm/kg)	1764	520	212	2286	650	266	1083	428	175
pH	7.00	0.632	0.26	7.83	1.17	0.48	7.50	1.23	0.50
Creatinine (mg/dl)	91.8	27.8	11.4	161.5	54.2	22.1	71.50	23.98	9.79
Sodium/Cr μEq/mg Cr	169.9	27.7	11.32	105.5	34.6	14.13	120.9	85.0	34.72
Potassium/Cr μEq/mg Cr	334.6	27.7	11.32	213.5	47.5	19.39	264.1	129.3	52.77
Chloride/Cr μEq/mg Cr	225.6	24.6	10.06	162.8	43.8	17.90	149.9	106.8	43.62
Protein/Cr g/mg Cr	0.0040	0.0015	0.00062	0.0031	0.00086	0.00035	0.0027	0.0015	0.0006
Glucose/Cr mg/mg Cr	0.0817	0.1266	0.0517	0.0417	0.0646	0.0264	0	0	0

TABLE 10.5

Mean Serum Chemistry/Hematology Parameters with Standard Deviation (SD) and Standard Error of Mean (SEM) in Adult Male Rats: Fischer-344, Sprague-Dawley, and Wistar Rats

	Strain								
	F-344			Sprague-Dawley			Wistar		
Parameters	Mean	SD	SEM	Mean	SD	SEM	Mean	SD	SEM
BUN (mg/dl)	17.333	0.848	0.346	16.15	2.08	0.85	20.63	2.14	0.87
Total protein (g/dl)	6.367	0.403	0.165	6.633	0.216	0.088	6.383	0.214	0.087
Creatinine (mg/dl)	0.830	0.172	0.070	0.860	0.145	0.059	1.015	0.154	0.0628
Osmolality, mOsm/kg H_2O	316.50	11.33	4.62	307.50	3.45	1.41	315.33	5.05	2.06
Potassium (mEq/l)	4.45	0.35	0.141	4.98	0.48	0.20	5.02	0.33	0.14
Chloride (mEq/l)	101.50	1.87	0.76	101.50	2.17	0.89	97.67	1.63	0.67
Sodium (mEq/l)	148.17	1.33	0.54	146.67	2.25	0.92	151.50	2.17	0.89
Hematocrit (%)	47.00	2.00	0.82	47.33	1.51	0.62	43.33	1.03	0.42

TABLE 10.6
Mean Serum Chemistry/Hematology Parameters with Standard Deviation (SD) and Standard Error of Mean (SEM) in Adult Female Rats: Fischer-344, Sprague-Dawley, and Wistar Rats

	Strain								
	F-344			Sprague-Dawley			Wistar		
Parameters	Mean	SD	SEM	Mean	SD	SEM	Mean	SD	SEM
BUN (mg/dl)	19.18	2.39	0.98	17.58	2.08	0.85	19.10	1.04	0.43
Total protein (g/dl)	6.550	0.321	0.131	7.333	0.665	0.272	6.867	0.225	0.092
Creatinine (mg/dl)	0.653	0.124	0.051	0.713	0.086	0.035	0.707	0.100	0.041
Osmolality, mOsm/kg H_2O	306.00	3.10	1.26	309.33	4.23	1.73	306.00	2.28	0.93
Potassium (mEq/1)	4.65	0.16	0.07	4.47	0.57	0.23	4.42	0.40	0.16
Chloride (mEq/1)	99.50	0.84	0.34	102.00	2.61	1.07	100.00	3.03	1.24
Sodium (mEq/l)	145.67	0.82	0.33	148.17	1.83	0.75	146.33	1.37	0.56
Hematocrit (%)	44.50	1.87	0.76	42.50	2.88	1.18	42.83	2.32	0.95

TABLE 10.7

Extracellular Volume Expansion Test: Urinalysis with Standard Deviations (SD) and Standard Error of the Mean (SEM) in Adult Male Rats: Fischer-344, Sprague-Dawley, and Wistar Rats

Parameters	Strain								
	F-344			Sprague-Dawley			Wistar		
	Mean	SD	SEM	Mean	SD	SEM	Mean	SD	SEM
Volume (ml)									
+3 h	2.67	1.71	0.70	3.65	2.20	0.90	4.13	2.69	1.10
+6 h	3.23	1.64	0.67	7.43	2.10	0.86	9.83	3.81	1.55
+9 h	2.72	0.68	0.28	3.95	1.39	0.57	3.42	1.46	0.60
Total 9-h volume	8.62	2.33	0.95	15.03	3.51	1.43	17.38	7.22	2.95
Volume, ml/100g body weight									
+3 h	0.772	0.474	0.193	0.675	0.411	0.168	0.778	0.501	0.205
+6 h	0.946	0.490	0.200	1.366	0.325	0.133	1.832	0.662	0.270
+9 h	0.804	0.228	0.093	0.726	0.240	0.098	0.636	0.257	0.105
Total 9-h volume	2.52	0.645	0.263	2.767	0.567	0.231	3.245	1.283	0.524
Sodium (μEq/ml)									
+3 h	150.3	36.2	14.8	145.0	50.4	20.6	89.0	37.2	15.2
+6 h	137.7	45.1	18.4	78.3	18.9	7.7	69.7	17.7	7.2
+9 h	130.7	12.5	5.1	100.7	38.1	15.5	106.3	14.1	5.8
Potassium (μEq/ml)									
+3 h	200.7	50.3	20.5	201.0	72.8	29.7	161.7	94.2	38.5
+6 h	123.3	66.5	27.1	102.0	21.9	8.9	81.3	22.4	9.1
+9 h	100.3	16.7	6.8	83.3	20.3	8.3	72.3	13.7	5.6

Chloride (µEq/ml)									
+3 h	266.7	66.9	27.3	238.2	98.0	40.0	177.0	74.1	30.2
+6 h	203.0	91.3	37.3	147.2	26.9	11.0	111.0	35.2	14.4
+9 h	158.8	20.3	8.3	105.7	45.3	18.5	113.3	18.3	7.5
Osmolality (mOsm/kg)									
+3 h	1235	306	125	1322	460	186	1055	613	250
+6 h	931	421	172	662	134	55	549	139	57
+9 h	876	127	52	692	83	34	662	195	80
Creatinine (mg/dl)									
+3 h	59.8	17.2	7.0	84.8	24.7	10.1	79.5	61.1	25.0
+6 h	58.0	26.6	10.9	41.3	12.2	5.0	38.3	14.6	5.9
+9 h	59.0	11.6	4.7	69.3	16.1	6.6	57.5	20.2	8.2
Sodium/Cr, µEq/mg Cr									
+3 h	260.2	62.2	25.38	173.5	35.9	14.65	148.0	69.7	28.5
+6 h	253.3	63.3	29.86	205.7	81.7	33.36	196.2	73.0	29.80
+9 h	229.6	54.5	22.24	156.0	70.4	28.74	198.2	54.9	22.39
Potassium/Cr, µEq/mg Cr									
+3 h	339.1	33.9	13.86	234.3	27.3	11.15	218.05	39.5	16.1
+6 h	213.8	46.5	18.96	255.0	54.3	22.15	222.	56.3	22.97
+9 h	172.4	25.7	10.51	123.9	34.8	14.22	131.5	24.2	9.88
Chloride/Cr, µEq/mg Cr									
+3 h	452.7	53.9	22.02	278.1	46.8	19.09	257.8	68.4	27.9
+6 h	359.6	62.3	25.42	374.5	100.8	41.14	305.7	110.6	45.14
+9 h	275.3	50.6	20.55	162.8	79.4	32.40	206.5	35.4	14.47

TABLE 10.8
Extracellular Volume Expansion Test: Urinalysis with Standard Deviations (SD) and Standard Error of the Mean (SEM) in Adult Female Rats: Fischer-344, Sprague-Dawley, and Wistar Rats

	Strain								
	F-344			Sprague-Dawley			Wistar		
Parameters	Mean	SD	SEM	Mean	SD	SEM	Mean	SD	SEM
Volume (ml)									
+3 h	2.82	1.40	0.57	1.72	1.04	0.43	5.00	4.16	1.70
+6 h	2.32	0.90	0.37	6.53	2.29	0.93	10.15	2.21	0.90
+9 h	1.88	0.40	0.16	2.32	0.63	0.26	3.22	1.37	0.56
Total 9-h volume	7.02	1.78	0.73	10.57	3.15	1.29	18.37	4.34	1.77
Volume ml/100 g body weight									
+3 h	1.549	0.852	0.348	0.592	0.401	0.164	1.847	1.556	0.635
+6 h	1.267	0.517	0.211	2.218	0.822	0.335	3.598	0.803	0.328
+9 h	1.021	0.205	0.064	0.785	0.256	0.104	1.140	0.492	0.201
Total 9-h volume	3.836	1.145	0.467	3.595	1.251	0.511	6.585	1.96	0.80
Sodium (µEq/ml)									
+3 h	126.3	17.7	7.2	136.3	48.2	19.7	60.8	28.2	12.6
+6 h	145.3	59.2	24.2	111.7	18.7	7.6	105.0	11.8	4.8
+9 h	126.3	54.9	22.4	158.0	49.8	20.4	114.0	27.4	11.2
Potassium (µEq/ml)									
+3 h	168.7	41.4	16.9	166.0	80.0	32.7	70.8	45.6	20.4
+6 h	119.3	47.1	19.2	102.7	57.4	23.4	54.7	15.2	6.2
+9 h	106.3	44.6	18.2	116.0	62.2	25.4	68.3	18.6	7.6

Chloride (µEq/ml)									
+3 h	204.2	33.9	13.9	225.7	111.7	45.6	98.2	72.5	32.4
+6 h	182.3	63.0	25.7	174.8	43.0	17.5	123.3	20.5	8.4
+9 h	149.7	53.1	21.7	142.8	50.1	20.5	95.5	46.5	19.0
Osmolality (mOsm/kg)									
+3 h	1055	281	115	1319	694	283	658	523	234
+6 h	894	353	144	723	370	151	445	96	39
+9 h	845	298	122	885	455	186	546	116	47
Creatinine (mg/dl)									
+3 h	40.0	15.5	6.3	78.5	48.6	19.8	43.4	45.2	20.2
+6 h	33.2	10.8	4.4	33.3	25.1	10.2	23.3	15.7	6.4
+9 h	33.8	5.6	2.3	55.3	29.3	12.0	40.7	7.7	3.2
Sodium/Cr, µEq/mg Cr									
+3 h	340.4	81.9	33.44	211.4	104.9	42.83	213.4	121.4	54.28
+6 h	432.1	72.0	29.38	423.3	158.9	64.86	553.3	195.7	79.91
+9 h	378.0	143.0	58.36	326.4	128.9	52.62	287.8	75.0	30.63
Potassium/Cr, µEq/mg Cr									
+3 h	436.5	60.5	24.68	227.8	82.7	33.76	198.3	69.1	30.91
+6 h	352.5	36.2	14.76	328.1	62.0	25.30	269.5	78.9	32.20
+9 h	310.7	92.8	37.87	213.6	46.7	19.06	174.8	59.7	24.37
Chloride/Cr, µEq/mg Cr									
+3 h	546.0	120.6	49.24	318.2	151.3	61.78	266.1	223.2	99.81
+6 h	550.2	47.8	19.52	625.8	167.1	68.22	628.8	196.0	80.03
+9 h	446.0	136.0	55.54	299.2	137.8	56.25	235.8	112.7	46.00

TABLE 10.9
48-Hour Urine Concentrating Test: Urinalysis with Standard Deviations (SD) and Standard Error of the Mean (SEM) in Adult Male Rats: Fischer-344, Sprague-Dawley, and Wistar Rats

Parameters	Strain								
	F-344			Sprague-Dawley			Wistar		
	Mean	SD	SEM	Mean	SD	SEM	Mean	SD	SEM
Volume (ml)									
+24 h	3.80	1.45	0.59	6.18	1.54	0.63	7.32	3.06	1.25
+49 h	1.62	0.48	0.19	2.13	0.27	0.11	2.95	1.51	0.62
Total	5.417	1.69	0.688	8.32	1.33	0.54	10.27	4.36	1.78
Volume ml/100 g body weight									
+24 h	1.09	0.362	0.148	1.125	0.253	0.103	1.318	0.562	0.230
+48 h	0.473	0.144	0.059	0.394	0.075	0.030	0.534	0.284	0.116
Total	1.563	0.427	0.174	1.519	0.217	0.088	1.852	0.811	0.331
Sodium (µEq/ml)									
+24 h	90.2	42.6	17.4	81.0	30.9	12.6	79.0	39.7	16.2
+48 h	196.2	55.1	22.5	144.3	41.8	17.1	132.7	38.0	15.5
Potassium (µEq/ml)									
+24 h	294.0	79.6	32.5	237.0	55.9	22.8	229.0	79.6	32.5
+48 h	453.8	97.2	39.7	292.7	44.5	18.2	281.0	83.5	34.1
Chloride (µEq/ml)									
+24 h	143.0	75.5	30.8	75.0	24.5	10.0	79.7	34.4	14.1
+48 h	234.2	80.1	32.7	106.7	65.1	26.6	91.2	51.0	20.8
Osmolality (mOsm/kg)									
+24 h	2171	472	193	1839	310	127	1937	591	241
+48 h	3618	502	205	3249	268	109	3251	550	225
Creatinine (mg/dl)									
+24 h	224.7	40.8	16.6	204.0	37.8	15.4	295.7	82.2	33.6
+48 h	399.7	37.6	15.3	599.5	48.8	19.9	536.2	149.1	60.9
Sodium/Cr, µEq/mg Cr									
+24 h	39.04	13.08	5.34	39.10	11.36	4.64	29.29	17.12	6.99
+48 h	48.43	9.93	4.05	24.26	7.57	3.09	24.97	5.59	2.28
Potassium/Cr, µEq/mg Cr									
+24 h	130.5	22.4	9.16	116.46	20.90	8.53	77.48	14.24	5.82
+48 h	113.8	21.5	8.79	49.10	8.51	3.47	52.72	10.52	4.29
Chloride/Cr, µEq/mg Cr									
+24 h	60.4	25.7	10.49	37.06	11.66	4.76	28.99	14.36	5.86
+48 h	58.0	16.0	6.51	18.39	11.50	4.69	16.61	8.55	3.49

TABLE 10.10

48-Hour Urine Concentrating Test: Urinalysis with Standard Deviations (SD) and Standard Error of the Mean (SEM) in Adult Female Rats: Fischer-344, Sprague-Dawley, and Wistar Rats

Parameters	F-344			Sprague-Dawley			Wistar		
	Mean	SD	SEM	Mean	SD	SEM	Mean	SD	SEM
Volume (ml)									
+24 h	4.48	0.35	0.15	6.70	1.80	0.73	6.63	1.18	0.48
+48 h	1.16	0.82	0.33	2.27	0.52	0.21	2.48	0.28	0.11
Total	5.65	0.89	0.363	8.97	2.05	0.84	9.12	1.40	0.57
Volume ml/100 g body weight									
+24 h	2.45	0.247	0.101	2.13	0.456	0.186	2.257	0.321	0.131
+48 h	0.632	0.44	0.179	0.732	0.170	0.069	0.849	0.088	0.036
Total	3.08	0.48	0.20	2.87	0.524	0.214	3.11	0.376	0.154
Sodium (µEq/ml)									
+24 h	248.0	14.3	5.8	250.0	38.7	15.8	214.5	90.0	36.8
+48 h	233.3	40.5	16.5	266.0	51.0	20.8	210.2	68.1	27.8
Potassium (µEq/ml)									
+24 h	510.7	18.4	7.5	445.0	97.3	39.7	447.0	132.1	53.9
+48 h	638.7	48.2	19.7	595.3	110.1	44.9	514.8	77.3	31.6
Chloride (µEq/ml)									
+24 h	343.5	28.5	11.6	280.0	67.5	27.6	268.3	122.1	49.9
+48 h	296.3	49.1	20.1	284.5	62.4	25.5	284.0	125.4	51.2
Osmolality (mOsm/kg)									
+24 h	2974	64	26	2750	412	168	2625	577	236
+48 h	4073	279	114	4126	688	281	3908	687	280
Creatinine (mg/dl)									
+24 h	223.8	12.1	4.9	160.0	20.6	8.4	192.3	29.1	11.9
+48 h	339.7	33.2	13.6	345.5	50.8	20.7	337.7	39.0	15.9
Sodium/Cr, µEq/mg Cr									
+24 h	111.18	10.36	4.23	156.5	16.8	6.84	109.6	45.6	18.64
+48 h	69.84	17.85	7.29	77.60	13.29	5.43	63.65	24.52	10.01
Potassium Cr, µEq/mg Cr									
+24 h	228.7	14.4	5.89	277.4	43.1	17.59	230.5	57.4	23.42
+48 h	189.4	22.0	8.97	173.2	26.2	10.68	153.9	27.3	11.13
Chloride/Cr, µEq/mg Cr									
+24 h	153.7	13.2	5.38	173.8	26.9	10.98	137.8	66.0	26.94
+48 h	88.3	20.0	8.15	83.3	17.4	7.11	85.3	38.9	15.90

TABLE 10.11
Kidney Weight Data with Standard Deviations (SD) and Standard Error of the Mean (SEM) in Adult Male Rats: Fischer-344, Sprague-Dawley, and Wistar Rats

	Strain										
	F-344			Sprague-Dawley			Wistar		
Parameters	Mean	SD	SEM	Mean	SD	SEM	Mean	SD	SEM
Left kidney weight (g)	1.230	0.067	0.027	1.808	0.247	0.101	1.860	0.172	0.070
Right kidney weight (g)	1.223	0.092	0.037	1.870	0.310	0.126	1.910	0.157	0.064
Total kidney weight (g)	2.453	0.153	0.062	3.68	0.551	0.225	3.77	0.327	0.133
Terminal body weight (g)	356.9	23.9	9.8	565.0	50.8	20.7	556.5	21.6	8.8
Kidney/body weight ratio × 1000	6.88	0.337	0.138	6.49	0.52	0.21	6.77	0.44	0.18

TABLE 10.12
Kidney Weight Data with Standard Deviations (SD) and Standard Error of the Mean (SEM) in Adult Female Rats: Fischer-344, Sprague-Dawley, and Wistar Rats

Parameters	Strain											
	F-344			Sprague-Dawley			Wistar		
	Mean	SD	SEM	Mean	SD	SEM	Mean	SD	SEM
Left kidney weight (g)	0.712	0.039	0.016	1.155	0.142	0.058	1.045	0.145	0.059
Right kidney weight (g)	0.712	0.028	0.011	1.188	0.166	0.068	1.065	0.129	0.052
Total kidney weight (g)	1.42	0.060	0.024	2.34	0.301	0.123	2.11	0.272	0.111
Terminal body weight (g)	189.8	9.6	3.9	322.5	38.1	15.6	293.7	28.1	11.5
Kidney/body weight ratio × 1000	7.51	0.28	0.11	7.32	0.97	0.40	7.18	0.57	0.23

TABLE 10.13

Renal Function Test Parameters with Standard Deviations (SD) and Standard Error of the Mean (SEM) in Adult Male Rats: Fischer-344, Sprague-Dawley, and Wistar Rats

Parameters	Strain								
	F-344			Sprague-Dawley			Wistar		
	Mean	SD	SEM	Mean	SD	SEM	Mean	SD	SEM
V̇ (ml/min)	0.00366	0.00181	0.00064	0.009012	0.00525	0.00186	0.003837	0.002206	0.000780
Hematocrit (%)	46.56	1.86	0.66	45.94	1.95	0.69	45.81	1.49	0.53
U_{Na} (μEq/ml)	113.3	57	20.2	144.5	64.4	22.8	89.4	65.6	24.8
U_K (μEq/ml)	255	120.6	42.6	322	206	73	273.1	94.6	35.7
U_{Cl} (μEq/ml)	231.7	150.8	53.3	236.4	143.7	50.8	174.7	153.8	58.1
P_{Na} (μEq/ml)	147.56	6.06	2.14	143.63	4.17	1.48	143.63	1.30	0.46
P_K (μEq/ml)	4.25	0.342	0.121	4.375	0.324	0.115	4.612	0.285	0.101
P_{Cl} (μEq/ml)	101.56	4.94	1.75	105.13	2.10	0.74	102.88	1.356	0.479
U_{Osm} (mOsm/kg)	1753	834	295	1747	598	226	1503	596	243
P_{Osm} (mOsm/kg)	303.8	39.6	14.0	308.6	31.1	11.0	306.8	18.1	6.4
GFR (ml/min)	1.844	0.912	0.323	3.62	1.94	0.69	3.322	0.880	0.311
U/P_{Inulin}	566	284	100	530	204	72	1129	569	210
U/P_{Na}	0.775	0.396	0.140	1.011	0.456	0.161	0.617	0.460	0.174
U/P_K	61.3	29.6	10.5	75.7	50.4	17.8	60.5	21.3	8.0
U/P_{Cl}	2.32	1.60	0.57	2.234	1.338	0.473	1.689	1.474	0.577
C_{H2O} (ml/min)	0.01842	0.01505	0.00532	−0.0430	0.0166	0.0063	−0.0209	0.0158	0.0065
FR_{H2O} (%)	99.77	0.107	0.038	99.75	0.1641	0.0580	99.90	0.0475	0.0168
FE_{Na} (%)	0.196	0.161	0.057	0.3084	0.3661	0.1294	0.0856	0.0874	0.0330
FE_K (%)	14.22	9.84	3.48	16.28	8.93	3.16	7.52	4.80	1.82

FE_{Cl} (%)	0.504	0.389	0.137	0.682	0.748	0.264	0.2324	0.2751	0.1040
$U_{Na} \times \dot{V}$ (μEq/min)	0.499	0.530	0.187	1.41	1.399	0.495	0.470	0.515	0.195
$U_{K} \times \dot{V}$ (μEq/min)	0.966	0.596	0.211	2.899	1.916	0.677	1.282	0.994	0.376
$U_{Cl} \times \dot{V}$ (μEq/min)	0.989	1.013	0.358	2.604	2.473	0.874	0.949	1.194	0.451
$\dot{V}$ (ml/min/g kidney weight)	1.805	1.014	0.359	2.649	1.758	0.622	1.101	0.575	0.203
U_{Osm} (mOsm/kg/g kidney weight)	856	406	144	496	150	57	435	171	70
GFR (ml/min/g kidney weight)	0.907	0.461	0.163	1.035	0.567	0.200	0.972	0.198	0.070
C_{H2O} (ml/min/g kidney weight)	−0.0092	0.0081	0.0029	−0.01235	0.00493	0.00187	−0.00593	0.00443	0.00181
FR_{H2O} (%/g kidney weight)	48.64	5.32	1.88	28.34	3.21	1.13	29.77	3.42	1.21
FE_{Na} (%/g kidney weight)	0.0963	0.0840	0.0297	0.0902	0.1074	0.03796	0.02470	0.02609	0.00986
FE_{K} (%/g kidney weight)	6.84	4.72	1.67	4.707	2.706	0.957	2.174	1.340	0.506
FE_{Cl} (%/g kidney weight)	0.284	0.210	0.074	0.2046	0.2278	0.0805	0.0660	0.0798	0.0302
$U_{Na} \times \dot{V}$ (μEq/min/g kidney weight)	0.2505	0.2875	0.1017	0.4152	0.4237	0.1498	0.1343	0.1519	0.0574
$U_{K} \times \dot{V}$ (μEq/min/g kidney weight)	0.472	0.313	0.111	0.837	0.566	0.20	0.363	0.258	0.098
$U_{Cl} \times \dot{V}$ (μEq/min/g kidney weight)	0.495	0.544	0.192	0.784	0.795	0.281	0.2673	0.3421	0.1293
Left kidney weight (g)	1.0329	0.1043	0.0369	1.717	0.155	0.055	1.630	0.231	0.082
Right kidney weight (g)	1.0386	0.1152	0.0407	1.839	0.225	0.080	1.766	0.232	0.082
Total kidney weight (g)	2.0715	0.2133	0.0754	3.556	0.370	0.131	3.396	0.406	0.144
Body weight (g)	326.0	30.5	10.8	544.2	26.9	9.5	551.9	48.8	17.2
Kidney/body weight ratio × 1000	6.349	0.137	0.048	6.524	0.464	0.164	6.156	0.523	0.185

TABLE 10.14
Renal Function Test Parameters with Standard Deviations (SD) and Standard Error of the Mean (SEM) in Adult Female Rats: Fischer-344, Sprague-Dawley, and Wistar Rats

Parameters	Strain								
	F-344			Sprague-Dawley			Wistar		
	Mean	SD	SEM	Mean	SD	SEM	Mean	SD	SEM
$\dot{V}$ (ml/min)	0.00325	0.00208	0.00078	0.00344	0.00248	0.00088	0.003414	0.003262	0.001233
Hematocrit (%)	43.56	6.30	2.23	44.13	4.49	1.59	44.71	3.05	1.15
U_{Na} (µEq/ml)	171.9	60.6	21.4	127	45.6	17.2	105.9	65.2	24.7
U_K (µEq/ml)	153	133	47	292.6	160.7	60.7	177.3	94.2	35.6
U_{Cl} (µEq/ml)	207.5	153.6	54.3	186.6	107.3	40.6	105.9	102.9	38.9
P_{Na} (µEq/ml)	144.50	5.71	2.02	148.75	6.32	2.23	147.43	4.04	1.53
P_K (µEq/ml)	3.537	0.334	0.118	4.075	0.282	0.100	4.329	0.160	0.061
P_{Cl} (µEq/ml)	101.875	1.356	0.479	103.13	1.25	0.44	107.29	2.812	1.063
U_{Osm} (mOsm/kg)	1025	546	223	1411	660	295	1150	536	219
P_{Osm} (mOsm/kg)	874.1	1485.9	525.4	403.5	65.5	23.1	316.3	18.2	6.9
GFR (ml/min)	0.587	0.245	0.087	1.219	0.739	0.261	1.483	0.463	0.175
U/P_{Inulin}	207	122	43	434	343	121	757	583	220
U/P_{Na}	1.19	0.414	0.146	0.843	0.280	0.106	0.716	0.437	0.165
U/P_{PK}	43.4	38.5	13.6	72.5	40.5	15.3	40.7	20.7	7.8
U/P_{Cl}	2.031	1.506	0.532	1.816	1.054	0.398	1.135	1.001	0.409
C_{H2O} (ml/min)	0.00565	0.00674	0.00275	−0.0131	0.01341	0.0060	−0.0084	0.00608	0.00248
FR_{H2O} (%)	96.93	1.6685	0.5899	97.045	7.114	2.5143	99.78	0.1571	0.0594
FE_{Na} (%)	1.53	2.368	0.835	0.478	0.7099	0.2683	0.2071	0.2844	0.1075

FE_K (%)	32.67	37.31	13.19	23.21	18.66	6.30	8.42	6.48	2.45
FE_{Cl} (%)	1.451	1.033	0.365	0.648	0.499	0.189	0.3783	0.5501	0.2283
$U_{Na} \times \dot{v}$ (μEq/min)	0.646	0.352	0.124	0.566	0.550	0.208	0.533	0.854	0.323
$U_K \times \dot{v}$ (μEq/min)	0.422	0.375	0.132	1.29	1.444	0.546	0.623	0.587	0.222
$U_{Cl} \times \dot{v}$ (μEq/min)	0.657	0.547	0.193	0.834	0.066	0.327	0.728	1.150	0.469
$\dot{V}$ (ml/min/g kidney weight)	2.39	1.37	0.48	1.792	1.335	0.472	1.843	1.718	0.649
U_{Osm} (mOsm/kg/g kidney weight)	801	492	201	744	339	152	617	260	106
GFR (ml/min/g kidney weight)	0.440	0.200	0.071	0.684	0.404	0.143	0.814	0.215	0.081
C_{H2O} (ml/min/g kidney weight)	−0.00467	0.00560	0.00228	−0.0070	0.00684	0.00906	−0.00448	0.00816	0.00129
FR_{H2O} (%/g kidney weight)	74.03	6.12	2.17	50.30	12.81	4.53	55.58	4.52	1.71
FE_{Na} (%/g kidney weight)	1.140	1.742	0.616	0.2149	0.2611	0.0987	0.1120	0.1514	0.0572
FE_K (%/g kidney weight)	24.96	27.87	9.85	11.69	7.65	2.89	4.54	3.37	1.27
FE_{Cl} (%/g kidney weight)	1.105	0.801	0.283	0.3259	0.2316	0.0875	0.2016	0.2983	0.1218
$U_{Na} \times \dot{v}$ (μEq/min/g kidney weight)	0.416	0.278	0.098	0.293	0.283	0.107	0.2858	0.4553	0.1721
$U_K \times \dot{v}$ (μEq/min/g kidney weight)	0.334	0.318	0.112	0.684	0.746	0.282	0.334	0.307	0.116
$U_{Cl} \times \dot{v}$ (μEq/min/g kidney weight)	0.511	0.465	0.164	0.447	0.457	0.173	0.3875	0.6141	0.2507
Left kidney weight (g)	0.6566	0.0542	0.0192	0.9685	0.1990	0.0704	0.8624	0.0605	0.0229
Right kidney weight (g)	0.6695	0.0520	0.0184	1.055	0.235	0.083	0.9426	0.0834	0.0315
Total kidney weight (g)	1.3261	0.1026	0.0363	2.023	0.432	0.153	1.805	0.138	0.052
Body weight	183.37	9.03	3.19	278.7	36.0	12.7	273.8	20.2	7.1
Kidney/body weight ratio × 1000	7.235	0.463	0.164	7.279	1.352	0.478	6.576	0.474	0.179

REFERENCE

1. AlliedSignal Inc., AlliedSignal Internal Report No. MA-179-81-1, October 3, 1983.

11 Reproductive Toxicology

Donald J. Ecobichon, Ph.D.

CONTENTS

0-8493-0370-2/02/$0.00+$1.50
© 2002 by CRC Press LLC

(See Chapter 12, Section 6, II, "Parental," for glossary of reproduction terms.)

SECTION 1. INTRODUCTION

Reproductive toxicology is "the study of the occurrence, causes, manifestations, and sequelae of adverse effects of exogenous agents on reproduction."[1] Reproductive "hazards" may encompass adverse health effects in the prospective mother, the father, and/or, of course, the developing embryo. The most striking features of reproduction are the myriad of rapidly multiplying cells, be they the gametes (ova, spermatozoa) or the tissues of the embryo, and the hypersusceptibility of such cells to a variety of agents at concentrations far lower than would be anticipated to elicit toxicity in other cell systems. This is a challenging field of toxicology, the spectrum of events caused by an *environment* (drugs, substances of abuse, industrial chemicals, pesticides, diet, lifestyles, etc.) resulting in effects as covert as alterations in normal levels of hormones with changes in performance (loss of libido, impotence, sterility, etc.) or more overt evidence of toxicity in the form of spontaneous abortion, embryonic or fetal death, reduced perinatal survival or teratogenicity (structural and/or functional anomalies) (Figure 11.1).

One must appreciate the concept of *toxic windows* during gamete production/function and in embryonic development, the narrow periods during which particular cell systems are susceptible to chemical-induced damage. In reproductive toxicology, it is insufficient to determine that the target site of the agent is the testis, the ovary, the conceptus, etc., but to examine the variety of direct and indirect events occurring during the reproductive/development cycle, each of these being characterized by multiple components (Table 11.1).

The challenge in reproductive toxicology is to design definitive tests capable of detecting any possible adverse biological effect caused by a potential toxicant in any segment of the reproductive cycles of male and/or female mammals. The achievement of this goal is complicated by such factors as species differences in response(s), gender differences in reproductive vulnerability, species variability in rates of embryonic development, as well as those interspecies variations in absorption, distribution, biotransformation, and elimination encountered in any mammalian toxicity study. Three questions must be answered concerning any proposed reproductive toxicity test. First, can it clearly identify chemicals causing reproductive/developmental toxicity? Second, can the test pinpoint the site of action of the potential toxicant, e.g., elicit the mechanism(s) of action by the endpoints of toxicity studied? Third, does the test ascertain the limit(s) of sensitivity, e.g., how toxic must the agent be to be detected?

A number of endpoints may be examined in the assessment of reproductive toxicology as is shown in Table 11.2. Because the teratogenic aspects of developmental toxicology are the topic of a separate section, this chapter restricts itself to the pre- and postconception aspects of reproductive toxicology.

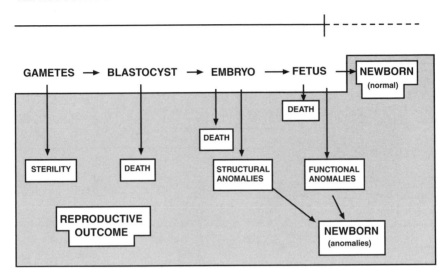

REPRODUCTIVE EXPOSURE

FIGURE 11.1 Physiological events during reproduction when exposure to physical or chemical agents or various forms of energy may induce adverse effects in reproductive outcomes.

TABLE 11.1
The Reproduction–Development Cycle

Fecundity	Embryo formation
Libido	Differentiation
Gametogenesis	Organogenesis
Gamete	Fetal maturation
Transport	Parturition
Function	Neonatal
Mating	Viability
Fertilization	Development
Zygote transport	Lactation
Implantation	Nutrition
Placental	Postnatal maturation
Formation	Sexual maturation
Function	Gametogenesis

From Ecobichon, D.J., *The Basis of Toxicity Testing*, CRC Press, Boca Raton, FL, 1992.[2] With permission.

TABLE 11.2
Endpoints in Assessing Reproductive Toxicity

Preconception evaluation
  Mating behavior
  Conception rates (preimplantation, fertilization)
  Animal weight
  Sperm and ovum production

TABLE 11.2 *(Continued)*
Endpoints in Assessing Reproductive Toxicity

Postconception evaluation
  Maternal weight gain
    Date of conception
    Date of delivery
  Implantation number
  Corpora luteal number
  Litter size
  Deaths (embryonic, fetal)
  Fetal viability (live fetuses)
  Malformation incidence (external, internal)
  Placental weight
  Pup weight
  Crown-rump length

Postnatal evaluation
  Problems at parturition
  Maternal-newborn relationship
  Ability of dam to rear young
  Postnatal growth and development
  Survival incidence (Day 0 to Day 21)
  Developmental landmarks — time of eye opening, hair growth, pinna opening, vaginal opening, etc.
  Functional testing—Day 21 or later

From Ecobichon, D.J., *The Basis of Toxicity Testing*, CRC Press, Boca Raton, FL, 1992,[2] Chap. 5, Table 7; and Haley, T.J. and Berndt, W.O., Eds., *Handbook of Toxicology*, Hemisphere Publishing Corp., Washington, D.C., 1987,[3] Chap. 7, p. 259. With permission.

SECTION 2. SPECIES DIFFERENCES

Reproductive toxicology requires detailed knowledge of species differences in reproductive biology and development. No surrogate animal species, used routinely in reproductive toxicity studies, mimics exactly the human in reproductive physiology. Consider the dramatic differences in uterine structure between multiparous animals and those bearing only one conceptus. Clearly, certain species lend themselves to the study of agent-induced actions on certain facets of reproduction. For decades, rodents (mice, rats) and rabbits have provided the bulk of reproductive toxicity data, because the species/strains are relatively well standardized: small size, high fertility (large litters), thereby providing adequate numbers of progeny for meaningful statistical analysis of the results. In addition, there is a massive database on chemical-induced reproductive toxicity in these species that cannot be ignored despite the fact that an investigator might want to use another species.[4] With other species, our knowledge of the reproductive cycle of the female may be far more extensive than that for the male. In such cases, only studies of selected endpoints in the female can be conducted with any assurity.

Characteristically, the first problem facing the investigator in reproductive studies is the vast interspecies variability in biological endpoints that must be considered when choosing a suitable animal model before any study. For the most commonly used test species, various parameters are listed in Table 11.3 for the breeding characteristics of the female of the species, with comparable data for the human.

TABLE 11.3
Breeding Characteristics of Female Laboratory Mammals Compared with the Human[a]

Parameters	Monkey[b]	Dog	Cat	Rabbit	Mouse	Guinea Pig	Hamster	Rat	Human
Age at puberty (days)	36 mo	6–8 mo	6–15 mo	5.5–8.5	35	55–70	35–56	37–67	12–15 yr
Breeding season	Oct.–Jan.	Spring–Fall	Feb.–July	All year	All year	All year	All year	All year	All year
Breeding life (years)	10–15	5–10	4	1–3	1	3	1	1	35
Breeding age (months)	54	9	10	6–7	2	3	2	2–3	180
Estrus cycle (days)	28	22	15–28	15–16	4–5	16–19	4	4–5	27–28
Duration of estrus (days)	1–6	7–13	4–19	30	1	1		1	2–8
Gestation period (days)	164	63	63	31	20	67	16	21	267
Litter size (number)	1	3–6	1–6	1–13	1–12	1–5	1–12	6–9	1
Birth weight (grams)	500–700	1100–2200	125	100	1.5	75–100	2.0	5.6	
Opening of eyes (days)	At birth	8–12	8–12	10	11	At birth	15	11	At birth
Weaning age (weeks)	16–24	6	6–9	18	3	2	3–4	3–4	
Weight at weaning (grams)	4400	5800	3000	1000–	11–12	250	35	10–12	

[a] Data obtained from various sources including: Ecobichon, D.J., *The Basis of Toxicity Testing*, CRC Press, Boca Raton, FL, 1992 [2] Chap. 2, Table 1; Spector, S., *Handbook of Biological Data*, W.B. Saunders Company, Philadelphia, PA, 1956,[5] various tables; Altman, P.L. and Dittmer, D.S., *Biology Data Book*, 2nd ed. Vol. I, Federation of American Societies for Experimental Biology, 1972,[6] various tables.

[b] Monkey = *Macaca mulatta*.

SECTION 3. GAMETOGENESIS

A. MALE GAMETOGENESIS

The testis is composed of a series of highly convoluted seminiferous tubules enclosed in a tunica and supported by connective tissue containing lymphatics, vasculature, phagocytic cells, and interstitial (Lehdig) cells.[7–10] A cross-sectional view of the seminiferous tubule has the appearance of a donut, with a basement membrane around the outer edge separated from the lumen by a parenchyma consisting of a myriad of morphologically distinct cells. Near the basement membrane are the stem or germ cells, immature sepermatogonia, and Sertoli cells. Further from the basement membrane are Sertoli and Leydig cells plus the migrating and developing spermatogonia, spermatocytes, spermatids, and spermatozoa.[10,11] Spermatogenesis begins during fetal life, stem cells being transformed to spermatogonia after birth, although these latter cells lie dormant until puberty when proliferative activity resumes (Table 11.4). These rapidly dividing, developing, and maturing cells are highly susceptible to chemical insult at many stages (Figure 11.2). Spermatogenesis can be divided into two separate stages: (1) *spermatocytogenesis*, during which the diploid Type A spermatogonia replicate by mitosis, each cell undergoing five mitotic divisions to form a host of Type B spermatogonia to be converted subsequently into primary spermatocytes and into haploid spermatids; (2) *spermiogenesis*, involving the differentiation of the spermatids into spermatozoa, the metamorphosis from a rounded cell into the characteristically shaped, mature spermatozoon having an elongated, condensed nucleus in the head, an acrosome, a reduction in cytoplasm, and a flagellum.[10,11,13] When spermiogenesis is completed, the spermatozoon is released into the lumen of the seminiferous tubule. Further maturation in the epididymis results in fertility and motility being conferred on the spermatozoon and the generation of suitable fluid vehicle.[9] This fluid is made up of secretions contributed by accessory glands (prostate), the seminiferous vesicles, and the epididymis. Agents may interfere with any of these functions or act on the epididymal tissue and/or the spermatozoon during this maturation period of 12 (rat) to 21 (human) days residence time.[9]

Considerable interspecies variability exists in the developmental/maturational stages of spermatogenesis in the testis in transit times through the various sections of the epididymis and in production rates of sperm (Table 11.5). All these factors must be considered in choosing an experimental model and the selection of time periods for treatment.

The evaluation of endpoints of toxicity in the male reproductive system includes the determination of testis and epididymal weights, morphological examination of both the testis and epididymis, assessment of sperm number in homogenized epididymis and testis, as well as sperm movement and morphology in minced sections of epididymis.[15] Additional parameters, including those of neurohormonal importance involving the hypothalamus and the anterior pituitary, are listed in Table 11.6.

Adult testicular function is largely influenced by the two gonadotrophic hormones, follicle-stimulating hormone (FSH) and luteinizing hormone (LH), both released from the anterior pituitary in response to the actions of the hypothalamic gonadotropin-releasing hormone (GnRH). Each of these glycoproteins has specific tissue targets as is shown in Table 11.7.[9,17] Sensitive radioimmune assays can be used for the measurement of circulating levels of these hormones, valuable additions to the evaluation of mechanisms of action of potential toxicants. Additional hormonal influence comes from testosterone and estradiol originating from the Leydig cells and inhibin from the Sertoli cells, each with their own specific target site, usually in a negative feedback capacity.

The evaluation of spermatoxoal function *in vivo* can be carried out by:

1. Serial matings of agent-exposed males with untreated virgin females over a period of several spermatogenic cycles (a cycle representing the period from spermatogonium to primary spermatocyte).[2]

2. Performing the classical, rodent, dominant lethal assay in which male mice or rats are treated with single, pulse-dose or short-term (5–7 days) doses of test agent at subtoxic levels and, subsequently, are serially mated with untreated virgin females throughout one complete spermatogenic cycle (Figure 11.3)[2] with assessment of fertility, fetal loss (pre- and postimplantational) in the near-term, pregnant females and offspring.

TABLE 11.4
Meiotic Stages During Oogenesis and Spermatogenesis

Division	Oogenesis	Spermatogenesis
First		
Prophase I		Primary spermatocytes are formed after several mitotic divisions at puberty. The first meiotic division takes 12–14 days and occurs in the testis. Spermatogenesis is an ongoing process with no "meiotic arrest."
Leptotene Zygotene Pachytene Diplotene	Occurs during fetal development	
	"Meiotic arrest" until after puberty	
Metaphase I Anaphase I Teleophase I Prophase II	Preovulatory changes	Second Secondary spermatocytes.
Metaphase II	Ovulation	Meiosis is completed in 24 days and results in four haploid spermatids.
Anaphase II Teleophase II	Fertilization	

From Dean, J., *Am. J. Ind. Med.,* 4, 31–49, 1983.[12] With permission.

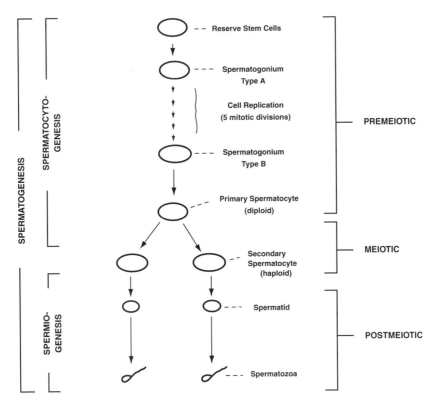

FIGURE 11.2 A general scheme of mammalian spermatogenesis, showing the premeiotic and meiotic stages of spermatocytogenesis (from reserve stem cells through the primary diploid spermatocyte to the haploid secondary sperm-atocyte) and the postmeiotic spermiogenesis with the development and maturation of the spermatozoa. Each cycle is completed in 35 to 64 days, depending on the species, with a new cycle being initiated at the Type A spermatogonium level every 12 to 13 days. (From Ecobichon, D.J., *The Basis of Toxicity Testing*, CRC Press, Boca Raton, FL, 1992,[2] Chap. 5, Fig. 2. With permission.)

TABLE 11.5
Species Variability in Parameters Involving Spermatogenesis[a]

Parameter	Mouse	Rat	Hamster	Rabbit	Dog	Monkey	Human
Spermatogenesis duration (days)	26–35	48–53	35	28–40			74
Duration of cycle of seminiferous epithelium (days)	8.6	12.9		10.7	13.6	9.5	16
Life span of:							
B-type spermatogonia (days)	1.5	2.0		1.3	4.0	2.9	6.3
L + Z spermatocytes (days)	4.7	7.8		7.3	5.2	6.0	9.2
P + D spermatocytes (days)	8.3	12.2		10.7	13.5	9.5	15.6
Golgi spermatids (days)	1.7	2.9		2.1	6.9	1.8	7.9
Cap spermatids (days)	3.5	5.0		5.2	3.0	3.7	1.6
Testis weight (grams)	0.2	3.7	1.8	6.4	12.0	4.9	34.0
Daily sperm production							
Per gram testis (×10^6)	54	14–22	22	25	20	23	4.4
Per individual (×10^6)	5–6	80–90	70	160	300	1100	125
Sperm reserve in cauda at sexual rest (×10^6)	49	440	575	1600		5700	420
Sperm storage in epididymal tissue (×10^6)							
Caput	20		200				
Corpus	7	300	175				420
Cauda	40–50	400	200				
Transit time through epididymis at sexual rest (days)							
Caput and corpus	3.1	3.0		3.0	?	4.9	1.8
Cauda	5.6	5.1		9.7	?	5.6	3.7
Ejaculate volume (ml)	0.04	0.2	0.1	1.0	?	?	3.0
Ejaculated sperm (10^6/ml)	5.0	?	?	150	?	?	80.0
Sperm transit time from vagina to tube	15–60 min	30–60 min		3–4 hr	20 min		15–30 min

[a] Data obtained from various sources including: Altman, P.L. and Dittmer, D.S., *Biology Data Book*, 2nd ed., Vol. I, Federation of American Societies for Experimental Biology, 1972,[6] various tables; Eddy, E.M. and O'Brien, D.A., *Toxicology of the Male and Female Reproductive Systems*, Working, P.K., Ed., Hemisphere Publishing Corp., New York, 1989,[14] Chap. 3, pp. 31–100; Blazak, W.F., *Toxicology of the Male and Female Reproductive Systems*, Working, P.K., Ed., Hemisphere Publishing Corp., New York, 1989,[15] Chap. 6, pp. 157–172; Zenick, H. and Clegg, E.D., *Principles and Methods of Toxicology*, 2nd ed., Hayes, A.W., Ed., Raven Press, New York, 1989,[16] Chap. 10, pp. 275–309; Spector, W.S., Ed., *Handbook of Biological Data*, W.B. Saunders Company, Philadelphia, PA: 1956,[5] various tables.

TABLE 11.6

Sites and Mechanisms of Action of Reproductive Toxicants in the Adult Male: Approaches for Detecting Altered Reproductive Function

Site of Action	Potentially Altered Mechanisms	Evaluative Tests
Hypothalamus	Neurotransmission	None at present
	Synthesis and secretion of GnRH	Hormone assay
	Receptors for LH, FSH, steroids	Receptor analysis
Anterior pituitary	Synthesis and secretion of LH, FSH, and PRL	Hormone assay and GnRH challenge
	Receptors for GnRH, LH, FSH, and steroids	Receptor analysis
Testis	Receptors for LH and PRL on Leydig cells	Receptor analysis
	Testosterone synthesis and secretion	*In vitro* production and hormone assay
	Vascular bed, blood flow	Morphology
	Blood-testis barrier	Morphology
	Receptors for FSH (Sertoli cells)	Receptor analysis
	Receptors for steroids	Receptor analysis
	Secretion of inhibin (ABP)	*In vitro* tests
	Sertoli cell function	*In vitro* tests
	Death of reserve spermatogonia	Germ cell count
	Spermatogonial mitosis	Germ cell count and % tubules without germ cells
	Spermatocyte meiosis	Spermatid counts and % of tubules with luminal sperm
	Spermatid differentiation	Sperm morphology
	Daily sperm production	Spermatid counts and seminal evaluation
Efferent ducts	Vascular bed	Morphology
	Resorption	?
Epididymis	Resorption	Sperm maturation
	Concentration of blood constituents	Biochemical analysis
	Secretion and interconversions	Biochemical analyses
	Enzyme activity	Biochemical analyses
	Agent transfer to luminal fluid	Assay for agent
	Smooth muscle contractility	Drug response both *in vitro* and *in vivo*
	Sperm transport	Sperm in ejaculate
Ductus deferens	Smooth muscle contractility	Response to drugs *in vitro* and *in vivo*
	Sperm transport	Sperm in ejaculate
Accessory sex gland	Secretion of agent(s)	Assays for agent(s)
	Secretion of spermicidal products	Evaluate sperm motility
Semen	Presence of agent(s)	Assay for agent(s)
	Spermicidal components	Evaluate sperm motility

Note: GnRH, gonadotrophin-releasing hormone; LH, luteinizing hormone; FSH, follicle-stimulating hormone; PRL, prolactin.

From Ecobichon, D.J., *The Basis of Toxicity Testing*, CRC Press, Boca Raton, FL, 1992,[2] Chap. 5, p. 89. With permission.

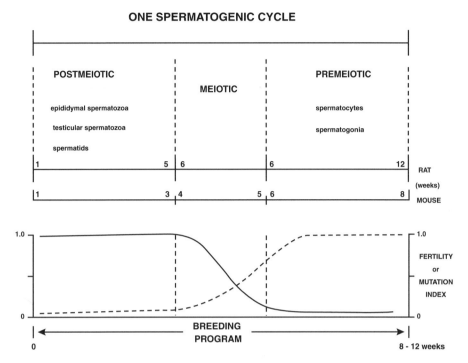

FIGURE 11.3 The dominant lethal assay. Treatment of male rodents (mouse, rat) with a reproductive toxicant may cause effects on cells at different stages of spermatogenesis. This schematic diagram illustrates the sequence of events in which male animals receive a brief (1–5 days) exposure to an agent capable of eliciting mutations. The extent of chromosomal damage is assessed subsequently by breeding the treated males serially with virgin females over an extended period (8 and 12 weeks for the mouse and rat, respectively). Indices (fertility, mutation, malformation, etc.) are developed to reflect the time point of damage to postmeiotic gametes (dotted line) or to premeiotic/meiotic gametes (solid line). Three exposure levels plus adequate controls should be used, with each male being mated serially with up to 50 virgin females over the time span of the study; three or four females are usually housed with the male at all times, being removed and replaced as they become pregnant. (From Ecobichon, D.J., *The Basis of Toxicity Testing*, CRC Press, Boca Raton, FL, 1992,[2] Chap. 5, Fig. 2. With permission.)

TABLE 11.7
Endocrine Control of Testicular Function in Adults

Hormone	Source	Major Target	Direct or Indirect Effect on Target(s)
Luteinizing hormone (LH)	Anterior pituitary	Leydig cells	Stimulate steroidogenesis (testosterone production)
Follicle-stimulating hormone (FSH)	Anterior pituitary	Sertoli cells	Stimulate protein synthesis (e.g., androgen-binding protein)
		Sertoli and/or germ cells	Maturation of spermatids into spermatozoa (spermiogenesis)
Testosterone	Leydig cells	Male accessory glands	Maintain structure and function
		Hypothalamus and pituitary	Negative feedback control on release of FSH and LH
Estradiol	Leydig cells	Anterior pituitary	Negative feedback control on release of FSH and LH
Inhibin	Sertoli cells	Anterior pituitary	Negative feedback control on release of FSH

From Overstreet, J.W. and Blazak, W.F., *Am. J. Ind. Med.*, 4, 5–15, 1983.[17] With permission.

B. Female Gametogenesis

The ovary consists of a collection of growing follicles (ova plus encasing granulosa and theca cells) lying in a dormant state in supporting tissue. The follicles arise from a population of primordial germ cells formed during embryonic/fetal development; these germ cells undergo numerous mitotic divisions resulting in several million oogonia, the bulk of which become atresic (Figure 11.4). A few oogonia undergo meiotic reduction to the haploid state and become surrounded by a single layer of granulosa cells, this structure being the primordial follicle which remains in an arrested, meiotic, prophase state until after puberty (Table 11.4). The other stages of meiosis will be completed after puberty and just before each ovulation. At puberty, primordial follicles are recruited into a pool of growing, primary follicles responsive to hormonal influence at the onset of each estrus cycle, one or more forming Graafian follicles and proceeding to the ovulatory follicle.[2] It is important to emphasize that the female mammal carries the entire complement of ova that will be used during her breeding life span. From this statement, it can be appreciated that ovarian tissue may be affected toxicologically while *in utero* (the developing female fetus of an exposed mother) or after exposure *ex utero* at any postpartum stage of development.

Interspecies variability is the rule of thumb for female mammals as in the male, the parameters listed in Table 11.8 requiring consideration before choosing any experimental model to assess the effects of potential toxicants on female gametogenesis and preimplantation/implantation. Postimplantation development, including teratogenesis, will be the topic of Chapter 12.

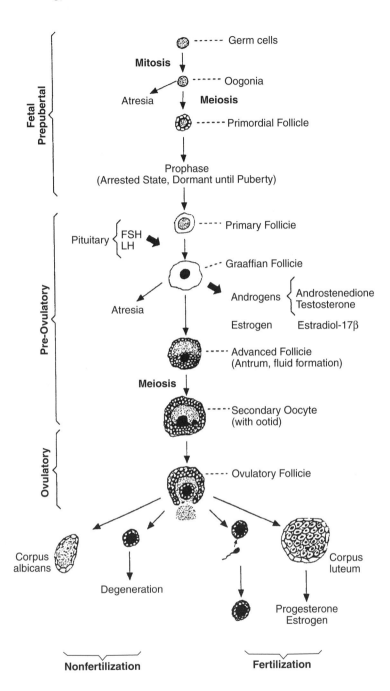

FIGURE 11.4 A general scheme of mammalian oogenesis, showing the fetal-prepubertal development of the primordial follicles that lie in an arrested state until puberty, at which time primary follicles begin to develop in response to preovulatory levels of pituitary follicle-stimulating hormone (FSH) and luteinizing hormone (LH), with the formation of the Graafian follicle and, subsequently, the advanced follicle which undergoes meiosis to produce a haploid oocyte. At the ovulatory stage, one mature ovum is released from each follicle. If the ovum is fertilized, the follicle becomes a steroid-secreting body, the corpus luteum, essential for the maintenance of the pregnancy. If fertilization does not occur, the follicle degenerates into a mass of cells, the corpus albicans. (From Ecobichon, D.J., *The Basis of Toxicity Testing*, CRC Press, Boca Raton, FL, 1992,[2] Chap. 5, Fig. 4. With permission.)

TABLE 11.8
Species Variability in Parameters Involving Oogenesis[a]

Parameter	Mouse	Rat	Guinea Pig	Hamster	Rabbit	Cat	Dog	Monkey	Human
Sexual maturity (days)	28	46–53	84	42–54	120–240	210–245	270–425	1642	
Duration of estrus (days)	9–20 h	9–20 h	6–11 h		30	4	9	4–6	2–8
Ovulation time (days)	2–3 h	9–20 h	10 h		10 h	24–56 h	1–3	9–20	15
Ovulation type[b]	S	S	S	S	I	I	S	S	S
No. ova released	8	10	?	7	10	4–6	8–10	1	1
Follicle size (mm)	0.5	0.9	0.8		1.8		10		
Ovum diameter (mm)	0.07–0.087	0.07–0.076	0.075–0.107		0.110–0.146	0.12–0.13	0.135–0.145	0.109–0.173	0.089–0.091
Zona pellucida (mm membrane thickness)			0.012		0.011–0.023	0.012–0.115	0.135	0.012–0.034	0.019–0.035
Transport time (to reach site of implantation) (days)	4.5	3.0	3.5	3.0	2.5–4	4–8	6–8	3.0	3.0
Implantation (days)	4.5–5.0	5.5–6.0	6.0	4.5–5.0	7–8	13–14	13–14	9–11	8–13
Rate of transport of sperm to oviduct (min)	15	15–30	15		5–10				5–60
Rate of transport of embryo to uterus (h)	72	95–100	80–85		60				80
Fertile life of spermatozoa in female tract (h)	6	14	21–22		30–32				24–48
Rate of transport of ova in female tract (h)	8–12	12–14	20	5–12	6–8				24
Segmentation (to form blastocele) (days)	2.5–4.0	4.5	5–6	3.25	3–4				5–8
Primitive streak (days)	7.0	8.5	10.0	6.0	6.5	13.0	13.0	18.0	
Duration of organogenesis (days)	7.5–16	9–17	11–25	7–14	7–20	14–26	14–30	20–45	
Gestational length (days)	20–21	21–22	65–68	16–17	31–32	58–71	57–66	164–168	

[a] Data obtained from various sources including: Ecobichon, D.J., *The Basis of Toxicity Testing*, CRC Press, Boca Raton, FL, 1992.[2] Chap. 5; Spector, S., *Handbook of Biological Data*, W.B. Saunders Company, Philadelphia, PA, 1956;[5] various tables; Altman, P.L. and Dittmer, D.S., *Biology Data Book*, 2nd ed., Vol. I. Federation of American Societies for Experimental Biology, 1972,[6] various tables; Eddy, E.M. and O'Brien. D.A., *Toxicology of the Male and Female Reproductive Systems*, Working, P.K., Ed., Hemisphere Publishing Corp., New York, 1989,[14] Chap. 3 pp. 31–100; Manson, J.M. and Kang, Y.J., *Principles and Methods of Toxicology*, 2nd ed., Hayes, A.W., Ed., Raven Press, New York, 1989.[18] Chap. 11, pp. 311–359.

[b] Ovulation type: I, induced; S, spontaneous.

SECTION 4. FERTILIZATION

Fertilization occurs when the ovum meets the upward migrating sperm in the region of the ampulla of the Fallopian tube. The spermatozoon must penetrate the vestments of the oocyte consisting of the thick acellular zona pellucida and several layers of granulosa cells. The success of the spermatozoon requires that it reach maturity at the appropriate time during incubation in the Fallopian tube, acquiring the capacity to fertilize the oocyte. The term capacitation is used to describe the poorly understood events leading to changes in the sperm surface and chemical changes within the cell (Table 11.9).[14] After capacitation, two distinct events occur: (1) the acrosome reaction, a series of fusions between specific sperm membranes which seems to release hydrolytic enzymes, including hyaluronidase and acrosin and may facilitate penetration of the granulosa cells (Table 11.10); and (2) activated motility, changes in the normal motility to provide the additional propulsive thrust needed to penetrate the zone pellucida through the digested pathway. In the perivitelline space, flagellar activity of the spermatozoon ceases on contact with the oolemma, and fusion with the vitellus begins in the midregion of the sperm head followed by phagocytosis of the sperm by the ooplasm.[17] Both capacitation and the acrosome reaction are required for sperm fusion with the oolemma; these reactions are necessary even when the zona pellucida has been removed from the oocyte.[19]

One can easily visualize that chemical-induced alterations in spermatozoon development at the time of capacitation, the acrosome reaction, and/or motility could influence reproductive success.

TABLE 11.9
Sperm Modification with Capacitation

Plasma membrane modifications
    Changes in surface components
        Loss of constituents adsorbed in excurrent ducts
        Changes in antibody and lectin binding
    Decrease in net negative surface charge
    Changes in lipid components
        Efflux of membrane cholesterol
        Decrease in cholesterol/phospholipid molar ratio
        Phospholipid methylation
        Cleavage of sterol sulfates
    Alterations in fluidity/mobility of membranes
        Changes in particle distribution
        Rearrangement of phospholipids
        Regionalized increases in fluidity
        Antigen redistribution
    Increased ion permeability
        Calcium
        Monovalent cations
Internal modifications
    Increase in intraacrosomal pH
    Altered cyclic nucleotide metabolism
    Increased endogenous protein carboxyl methylation

[a] From Eddy, E.M. and O'Brien, D.A., *Toxicology of the Male and Female Reproductive Systems*, Working, P.K., Ed., Hemisphere Publishing Corp., New York, 1989.[14] Chap. 3, Table 13. With permission.

TABLE 11.10
Factors Influencing Acrosome Reaction: Species Studied

Agents	Species
In vitro induction	
Triggers	
Influx of extracellular calcium	Mouse, hamster, guinea pig
Zona pellucida constituents	
ZP3 glycoprotein	Mouse
Heat-solubilized zonae	Hamster, rabbit
Additional ionic requirements	
Extracellular sodium	Guinea pig
Extracellular bicarbonate	Mouse, guinea pig
Alkaline pH	Guinea pig
Other agents stimulating reaction	
Albumin	Mouse, hamster
Glycosaminoglycans	Hamster, rabbit
Proteases	
Role in membrane vesiculation	Hamster
Matrix dispersion only	Mouse, guinea pig
Fatty acids or lysophospholipids	Hamster, guinea pig
Prostaglandins or hydroxyeicosatetraenoic acids	Hamster
Serotonin	Hamster
Molecular models	
Potential roles of calcium	
Modulation of enzyme activity	
Stimulation of adenylatecyclase	Mouse, guinea pig
Inactivation of Mg^{2+}-ATPase	Guinea pig
Direct effect on membrane fusion via charge neutralization	Guinea pig
Signal transduction mediated via second messengers	
Cyclic nucleotides	Hamster, guinea pig
Inhibitory guanine nucleotide-binding protein (G_1)	Mouse
Protein kinase C activity	Mouse
Transient accumulation of fusogenic lipids mediated by phospholipase A	Mouse, hamster, man

From Eddy, E.M. and O'Brien, D.A., *Toxicology of the Male and Female Reproductive Systems*, Working, P.K., Ed., Hemisphere Publishing Corp., New York, 1989,[14] Chap. 3, Table 14. With permission.

SECTION 5. MIGRATION *IN UTERO*

With successful fertilization of the ovum in the upper end of the Fallopian tube, the new embryo moves downward into the uterus where the myometrial smooth muscle and epithelial layers are being prepared to receive it as a consequence of the influence of progesterone secreted by the corpus luteum (Figure 11.5). By the time the fertilized ovum has reached the uterus, it has developed into the blastocyst (blastocoele), a sphere of single cells around a fluid-filled cavity in which the impregnated ovum is expanding (Table 11.11).

At this time point, the ovum adheres or implants on the uterine wall, initiating the development of a placental structure. The preimplantation interval (Table 11.8) is variable between species, but it represents a time when the rapidly duplicating cells may be hypersusceptible to chemical injury, the results of such damage being reflected in absence of implantation, early embryonic death, early fetal death/reabsorption, nonviability of newborn, and/or teratogenesis. Various quantifiable endpoints of reproductive toxicity are listed in Table 11.2 which can be converted into the various indices described below. In addition, because the female reproductive tract is highly dependent upon neuroendocrine centers (hypothalamus, anterior pituitary) for the secretion of appropriate growth hormones essential for specific action on the postpubertal ovary, studies of the accessory organs (oviduct, uterine muscle), cellular components of the Graffian follicle, etc., should not be ignored, leading to a long list of possible target sites and specific evaluative tests (Table 11.12).

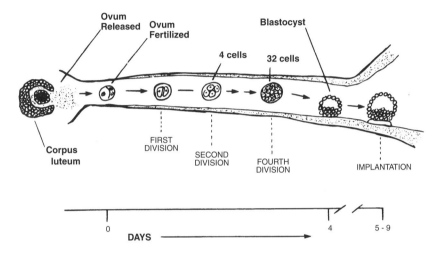

FIGURE 11.5 A schematic diagram illustrating the sequence of events after the successful fertilization of the mammalian ovum, denoting the cell divisions over the subsequent period of migration from the ampulla of the Fallopian tube to the uterus where the blastocyst begins to implant into the steroid-activated cells of the uterine muscle. The time course varies with species. (From Ecobichon, D.J., *The Basis of Toxicity Testing*, CRC Press, Boca Raton, FL, 1992,[2] Chap. 5, Fig. 5. With permission.)

TABLE 11.11
Zygote Cleavage Rates: Interspecies Comparisons[a]

Parameter	Mouse	Rat	Guinea Pig	Hamster	Rabbit	Monkey	Human[b]
First cleavage spindle (h)	21–48	24–35	27–38		24		
2–Cell (h)	21–43	24–48	23–48	24–36	21–25	26–49	42–55
4–Cell (h)	38–50	48–72	30–75	48–60	25–32	24–52	
8–Cell (h)	50–64	72–96	80–82	72	32–40		90–114
16–Cell (h)	60–70	96	107	66–72	40–47		
32–Cell (h)	68–80				48	96–144	114–136

[a] From Spector, W.S., Ed., *Handbook of Biological Data,* W.B. Saunders Company, Philadelphia PA, 1956,[5] various tables.

[b] Human data taken from *in vitro* culturing of inseminated (fertilized) ova, results reported in FitzGerald, L. and DiMattina, M., *Fertility Sterility*, 57, 641–647, 1992.[20] With permission.

TABLE 11.12

Sites and Mechanisms of Action of Reproductive Toxicants in the Adult Female: Approaches for Detecting Altered Reproductive Function

Site of Action	Possibly Altered Mechanisms	Evaluative Tests
Hypothalamus	Neurotransmission	None at present
	Synthesis/secretion of GnRH	Hormone analysis
	Receptors for FSH, LH, PRL	Receptor analysis
Anterior pituitary	Synthesis and secretion of LH, FSH, PRL	Hormone assay and GnRH challenge
	Receptors for GnRH, LH, FSH, and steriods	Receptor analysis
Ovary	Oocyte toxicity and increased atresia	Counts, morphology
	Abnormal meiosis	?
	Number of LH or FSH receptors in follicular of granulosa cells	Receptor analysis
	E_2 and P_4 synthesis/secretion	Hormone assay or *in vitro* tests
	Sensitivity to luteolysis	*In vitro* tests?
Ovum	Surface proteins interacting with sperm	Biochemical assays
	Altered zona pellucida	Sperm penetration tests
	Metabolic processes	?
	Syngamy	Morphology
	Implantation	Ratio implants/corporalutea
Uterine tube	Fimbria movement	?
	Ciliagenesis, cilia function	Morphology
	Number of E_2, P_4, receptors	Receptor analysis
	Sperm and ovum transport	Recovery and count
	Fluid environment	Biochemical analyses
Uterus	Number of E_2 and P_4 receptors	Receptor analysis
	PGE and PGF_2 secretion	PG assay
	Protein and glycoprotein secretion	Biochemical assays
	Sperm survival, transport	Recovery, count
	Luminal fluid	Biochemical analyses
	Exposure of sperm and embryo to agents in secretions	Specific assays for agent(s)
	Parturition	Incidence of dystocia
Cervix	Barrier to sperm	*In vitro* tests
Vagina	Exposure of sperm to agents in secretions	Assay for agent
Mammary Gland	Shedding of agent in milk	Assay for agent
	Altered milk composition	Biochemical analyses
	Decreased milk yield	Measure (weight of young, growth)

Note: GnRH, gonadotrophin-releasing hormone; LH, luteinizing hormone; FSH, follicle-stimulating hormone; PRL, prolactin; E_2, estradiol; P_4 progesterone; PG, prostaglandin.

From Ecobichon, D.J., *The Basis of Toxicity Testing*, CRC Press, Boca Raton, FL, 1992,[2] Ch. 5, p. 96. With permission.

SECTION 6. REPRODUCTION/DEVELOPMENTAL STUDIES

Because it is impossible to investigate the entire array of possible reproductive toxicity endpoints with one set of experiments, the task is usually broken up into manageable segments, using rodents as a suitable test species (Figure 11.6). Segment I testing provides the most comprehensive overview of reproductive toxicity, with the treatment of both sexes throughout gametogenesis (60 and 15 days for males and females, respectively) and usually mating the treated males or females with appropriate controls of the opposite sex. In some protocols, the treated males are mated with treated females, although determining the exact origin of the reproductive toxicity becomes difficult. Many different Segment I protocols have been developed, some in which only the female is treated whereas, in others, only the male is exposed to the potential toxicant.

Segment II testing pertains specifically to the screening of the capability of an agent to elicit toxicity during the period of organogenesis, the experiments beginning with normal conceptuses (untreated females bred with untreated males) and examines the influence exerted by given levels of the agent on cellular development during the organogenesis period only (days 6 to 15 for the mouse and rat and days 6 to 18 for the rabbit).

Segment III testing relates to the ongoing assessment of possible agent-induced effects during organogenesis in neonatal life, with particular endpoints assessing the effect(s) of the agent on delivery, lactation, neonatal survival, and vitality of the offspring up to and after the weaning age. Such studies permit testing for behavioral and cognitive deficits as well as other subtle target organ toxicity, including reproduction, that may become manifest as the animals develop.

Although the investigator may only be interested in gametogenesis and the fate of the fertilized ovum up to the point of implantation, protocols usually allow the pregnancy to progress to near term (gestational day 14–20). The data gathered at the necropsy of the euthanized dams and fetuses must be quantitated. To this end, a series of indices will be determined, and comparisons between control values and those determined for the agent-exposed animals carried out to assess the potential reproductive toxicity of the test chemical (Table 11.13). These same indices would be valid in both Segment II and III studies.

The most commonly conducted reproduction/development study follows a multigeneration protocol in which agent-exposed female rodents (mice, rats) are bred to untreated control males, the F_1 exposed females being retained as breeding animals for the next F_2 generation (Figure 11.7).[2] The sequence may be repeated again, F_2 exposed females being bred to untreated control males to provide an F_3 generation. Because a toxic effect may not occur in the original treated females, it may be "visited upon" the daughters and granddaughters, appearing in these offspring in the form of reproductive, behavioral, physiological, and/or biochemical anomalies. The question still remains as to how many generations should be studied. A two-generation study, if an appropriate dosage range has been chosen, should allow an investigator to confidently predict reproductive hazards associated with the chemical.

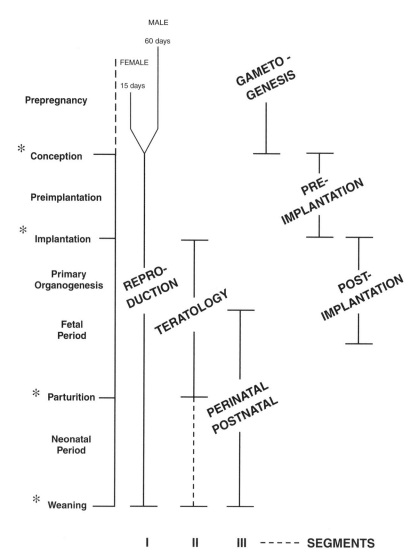

FIGURE 11.6 Various formats of testing reproductive toxicology in mammalian (rodent) species on distinct endpoints (*) in the reproductive cycle. In Segment I reproductive studies, either the male or female animals (or both) are exposed to the test agent for 60 to 15 days, respectively, before mating with either comparably treated or untreated control animals. The pregnant animals will be treated at the same dosage level(s) throughout gestation and parturition to the point of weaning the offspring. In Segment II teratology studies, healthy, untreated pregnant animals are exposed to the test agent from day 6 through day 15 (mouse or rat) or from day 6 through day 18 (rabbit) of gestation and are either: (1) euthanized on the day before parturiation and examined for anomalies; or (2) allowed to give birth, with examination both at birth and at weaning for anomalies. In Segment III perinatal/postnatal studies, the healthy, pregnant animals are treated with the test agent through at least 15 days of gestation and 21 days of lactation with effects on the newborn and postnatal offspring being quantified by a number of indices throughout development. Gametogenesis may be studied by treating either male or female animals throughout one gametogenic cycle followed by an extended breeding program with unexposed animals of the opposite sex. The *in vitro* culturing of pre- and /or postimplantation embryos in the presence of suitable concentrations of the test agent(s) in the incubation medium can be used as screening techniques to assess mechanisms of cytotoxicity on major organ systems up to approximately day 14 of *in utero* development. In all the studies above, at least three exposure groups plus controls, with adequate numbers of animals ($n = 10$ or 20) in each treatment group, should be used. (From Ecobichon, D.J., *The Basis of Toxicity Testing*, CRC Press, Boca Raton, FL, 1992,[2] Chap. 5, Fig. 1. With permission.)

TABLE 11.13
Fertility and Reproductive Indices Used in Single and Multigeneration Studies

Index	Derivation
Mating	$= \dfrac{\text{No. confirmed copulations}}{\text{No. of estrous cycles required}} \times 100$
Male fertility	$= \dfrac{\text{No. males impregnating females}}{\text{No. males exposed to fertile, nonpregnant females}} \times 100$
Female fertility	$= \dfrac{\text{No. of females confirmed pregnant}}{\text{No. of females housed with fertile male}} \times 100$
Female fecundity	$= \dfrac{\text{No. of females confirmed pregnant}}{\text{No. of confirmed copulations}} \times 100$
Implantation	$= \dfrac{\text{No. of implantations}}{\text{No. of pregnant females}} \times 100$
Preimplantation loss	$= \dfrac{\text{Corpora lutea} - \text{No. of implants}}{\text{No. of Corpora lutea}} \times 100$
Parturition incidence	$= \dfrac{\text{No of females giving birth}}{\text{No. of females confirmed pregnant}} \times 100$
Live litter size	$= \dfrac{\text{No of litters with live pups}}{\text{No. of females confirmed pregnant}} \times 100$
Live Birth	$= \dfrac{\text{No. viable pups born/litter}}{\text{No. pups born/litter}} \times 100$
Viability	$= \dfrac{\text{No. of viable pups born}}{\text{No. of dead pups born}} \times 100$
Survival	$= \dfrac{\text{No. of pups viable on day 1}}{\text{No. of viable pups born}} \times 100$
Pup death (day 1–4)	$= \dfrac{\text{No. of pups dying, postnatal days 1–4}}{\text{No. of viable pups born}} \times 100$
Pup death (days 5–21)	$= \dfrac{\text{No. of pups dying, postnatal days 5–21}}{\text{No. of viable pups born}} \times 100$
Sex ratio (at birth)	$= \dfrac{\text{No. of male offspring}}{\text{No. of female offspring}} \times 100$
Sex ratio (day 4) (day 21)	$= \dfrac{\text{No. of male offspring}}{\text{No. of female offspring}} \times 100$

From Ecobichon, D.J., *The Basis of Toxicity Testing,* CRC Press, Boca Raton, FL, 1992,[2] Chap. 5, p. 98. With permission.

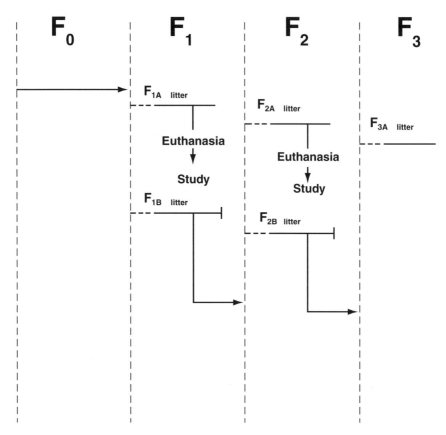

FIGURE 11.7 A typical, three-generation, reproductive study in which the agent-exposed, F_0 female animals are bred to untreated, control males with the production of F_{1A} litters that are euthanized at birth for morphological examination for anomalies. Having rested the F_0 females for 2 weeks while continuing the exposure, they are rebred with untreated males to produce F_{1b} litters which the treated females are allowed to rear. Females are selected from the F_{1B} litters, having been exposed to the test agent both transplacentally, via the milk and up to the time of puberty, and are bred with untreated control male animals to produce the next (F_2) generation. The F_{2A} litters are euthanized at birth and the F_{1B} females are rested and then rebred to produce the F_{2B} litters, providing a source of continuously agent-exposed females for the subsequent F_3 generation. (From Ecobichon, D.J., *The Basis of Toxicity Testing*, CRC Press, Boca Raton, FL, 1992,[2] Chap. 5, Fig. 7. With permission.)

SECTION 7. SCREENING ASSAYS

The challenge in reproductive toxicology is to construct a test that, in a short time (several weeks), would be able to separate the more potent reproductive and developmental toxicants from the less toxic agents.[21] A rapid screening test would be desirable and although several effects on organ culture, including growth inhibition of mammalian cell cultures, developmental anomalies in lower vertebrates and invertebrates, etc., have been assessed, the disadvantages of such assays have included the absence of maternal-fetal interaction, the difficulties of maintaining culture systems, and the problems of toxicant delivery.[22]

Several attempts have been made to develop an *in vivo* screening assay but most fall short of the ideal and, once again, become focused on one particular aspect of reproduction and development. One protocol, that of Chernoff and Kavlock,[22] was based on the hypothesis that most prenatal insults would manifest themselves postnatally as reduced viability and/or impaired growth. That particular test system, using gravid CD-1 mice, involved the administration of the maximum tolerated dose (MTD) of the test agents once or for up to 5 consecutive days during the period of major embryonic organogenesis (days 8–12). Of 28 test compounds known to be teratogenic, 15 showed some form of developmental toxicity, whereas, of 9 agents that showed no effect in standard tests, 3 demonstrated either reduced viability or weight. Four chemicals, known to elicit only fetal toxicity (reduced weight, supernumary ribs), caused weight reduction.

Traditional reproductive assessment by continuous breeding (RACB) protocols expose the F_0 animals to the test agent for 15 weeks during mating and produce up to 5 litters.[23] The usual developmental toxicity studies expose the pregnant females on gestation days 6–15.[2] In a recently published variation of the RACB protocol, described in Figure 11.8, the questions addressed were: (1) Would the design correctly identify reproductive and developmental toxicity? (2) What type(s) of effects would be found? (3) If adverse effects were produced, how much change would there be? (4) Would the test distinguish developmental from reproductive toxicity?[21] Comparisons with a standard developmental study and a 21-day screening assay revealed that this modified protocol could assess many of the endpoints found in the other designs. This modified protocol is closely related to the Chernoff-Kablock test protocol and unlike a Segment II study. The lack of pup/fetal dissection in this protocol means that the effect must be visible, skeletal and visceral malformations not being detected. However, the test protocol seemed to answer the questions posed above.

The OECD protocol, the "Combined Repeat Dose and Reproductive/Developmental Toxicity Screening Test (ReproTox)," a novel approach to generating data not only on systemic toxic effects with repeated dosing but also data on reproductive/developmental toxic effects in both males and females.[24] Characteristics of the ReproTox protocol include a longer dosing period than that used in 28-day repeated dose and teratogenicity studies; no hematological or serum chemical analyses in females; and extensive histopathology of the males, the females, and the offspring within a 54-day period. A schematic diagram of the time schedule of the test protocol is shown in Figure 11.9.[25] These authors examined the reliability of the protocol using cyclophosphamide as the test agent. The results showed that some 15 of 18 known toxicological properties of cyclophosphamide, except the adverse effects on spermatogenesis and fertility, could be identified.

Given that the fertilization-to-implantation period of development is highly susceptible to chemical insult, some unique protocols have been developed to assess reproductive/developmental toxicity in this early period (Figure 11.10).[26] In Protocol A, endpoints can be evaluated to assess the impact of the test agent on the cleavage-stage embryo, on implantation (day 4), and also on the postimplantation period of decidual development. In Protocol B, a refined variant of A, the treatment period is split into two phases: early administration (days 1–3) to assess preimplantation susceptibility; and treatment beginning on day 4 through day 8 to examine postimplantation effects. Protocol C involves a study of decidual cell response (DCR), manually stimulating the uterine cervix on proestrus/estrus (day 0) to initiate a pseudopregnancy after which the test agent is administered (days 1–8). On day 4, decidual induction is performed by surgically traumatizing the entire length of the uterine lining of one horn, leaving the other horn to serve as a control. On day 9, DCR will be evident by a marked increase in the weight of the traumatized horn. Protocol D is designed to study the effects of the test agent on the rate of embryo transport in the uterine horn before implantation.[26]

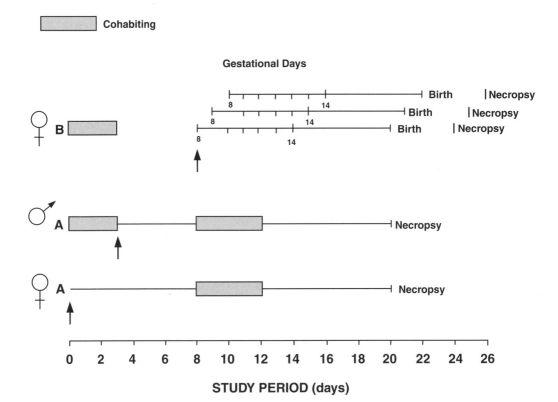

FIGURE 11.8 A schematic diagram illustrating the format of a short-term, reproductive and developmental toxicity screening assay. One group of male ($n = 10$) and two groups of female mice (designated A and B) are used at each dosage level. The untreated males and Group B females are caged together (cohabiting) for 3 days to provide time-mated females ($n = 10$ pregnant females/dosage) for treatment during organogenesis (gestational days 8 to 14), following which the dams are permitted to deliver, and the litters are evaluated on postnatal days 0, 1, and 4, necropsy taking place on day 4. The one group of male mice/dosage level begins treatment with the test agent after 3 days of mating with the Group B females. Group A female mice ($n = 10$/dosage level) are treated from day 0 to day 20 and, beginning at study day 8, are cohabited for five consecutive days with the males being treated. The Group A females are euthanized on study day 21 with necropsy being performed immediately. The treated males are euthanized on day 20 for study. The arrows indicate the time of initiating treatment; the hatched boxes indicate the time period of cohabitation. (Modified from Harris et al., *Fundam. Appl. Toxicol.*, 19, 186–192, 1992.[21])

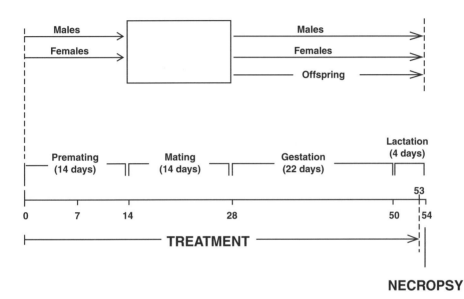

FIGURE 11.9 The protocol of the OECD Reproductive/Developmental Toxicity (Repro Tox) screening test. Male rats are dosed from 14 days before mating and throughout mating for a total of 42 days. Female rats are treated from 14 days before mating, during mating and the gestational period to postnatal (lactational) day 3. By random selection from the respective groups, one male to one female overnight mating was started on day 14 after the onset of treatment. The same pair are cohabited until sperm are found in the vaginal smear (day 0 of pregnancy), or for up to 14 days. Body weight and food consumption are measured once weekly. The live and dead pups are tallied, weighed, and sexed on lactational days 0 and 4 and are checked for any external anomalies. Necropsy occurs at lactational day 4 for the females and offspring. The male rats are necropsied on day 42 or 43, hematology and clinical chemistry being conducted in addition to a gross morphological examination. (Modified from Tanaka et al., *Fundam. Appl. Toxicol.,* 18, 89–95, 1992.[25])

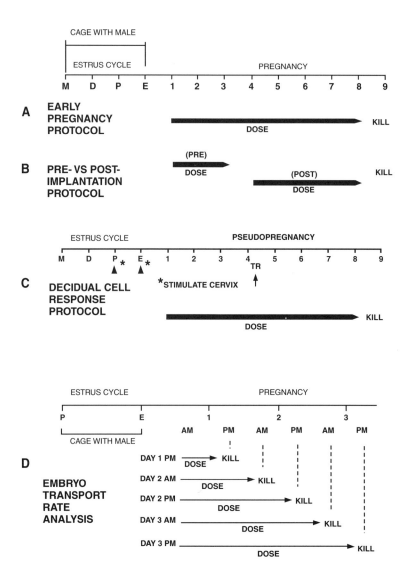

FIGURE 11.10 A schematic diagram illustrating experimental protocols to study toxicological mechanisms of implantation failure *in vivo* in rodents. Treatment throughout day 1 to day 8 *(Protocol A)* or treatment through day 1 to day 3 or day 3 to day 8 *(Protocol B)* will permit assessment of pre- and postimplantation effects of the test agent. *Protocol C* is designed to assess the possible biological effects of the test agent on the decidual cells in the uterus in an induced pseudopregnancy, treatment with the agent being initiated from day 1 through day 8. *Protocol D*, spanning only the first 3 days of pregnancy, is designated to monitor the effects of treatment on the rate of transport of the preimplantation embryo in the uterine horns by euthanizing treated pregnant animals every 12 h from day 1 through day 3, with microscopic examination of the opened uterus to establish the distance traveled by the embryo. (From Ecobichon, D.J., *The Basis of Toxicity Testing*, CRC Press, Boca Raton, FL, 1992,[2] Chap. 5, Fig. 8. With permission.)

SECTION 8. SPECIES SELECTION

Having considered the many facets of reproductive/developmental toxicology, one is still left with the question of which species is the best. There is no satisfactory answer; each species possesses unique features for the assessment of certain endpoints of toxicity. Table 11.14 provides a concensus of suitable species for specific reproductive endpoints.[2] Particular details for the conduction of specific reproductive tests may be found in appropriate chapters in Amdur et al.,[27] Haley and Berndt,[3] Hayes,[28] and Mattison.[29]

TABLE 11.14
Species Recommended for Evaluation of Reproductive Endpoints

Species	Male	Female
Mouse	Spermatogenesis	Embryogenesis (cleavage)
	Testicular pathogenesis	Ovarian pathogenesis
	Epididymal sperm	Estrus cycle
	Cellular biochemistry	Endometrium
	Fertility	
	In vitro fertilization	
Rat	Spermatogenesis	Embryogenesis (cleavage)
	Testicular pathogenesis	Ovarian pathogenesis
	Hormone profiles	Estrus cycle
	Hormone challenge	Endometrium
	Epididymal sperm	Fertility
	Cellular biochemistry	
Rabbit	Motility	Oviduct
	Ejaculation function	Hormone profiles
	Sperm function	*In vitro* fertilization
	Fertility	Embryogenesis (cleavage)
	Secondary sex organs	Hormone challenge
	Hormone profiles	
	Artificial insemination	
	In vitro fertilization	
Pig		Ovarian morphology
		Estrus cycle
		Fertility
		Hormone profiles
		In vitro fertilization
		Embryogenesis (cleavage)
Monkey		Menstrual cycle
		Oviduct
		Uterus
		Endometrium
		Fertility
		Hormone challenge
		Follicle development

From Ecobichon, D.J., *The Basis of Toxicity Testing*, CRC Press, Boca Raton, FL, 1992,[2] Chap. 5, p. 86. With permission.

REFERENCES

1. Johnson, E.M., Perspective on reproductive and developmental toxicology, *Toxicol. Ind. Health* 2, 453–482, 1986.

2. Ecobichon, D.J., Reproductive toxicology, in *The Basis of Toxicity Testing*, CRC Press, Boca Raton, FL, 1992, Chap. 5, pp. 83–112.

3. Haley, T.J. and Berndt, W.O., Eds., *Handbook of Toxicology*, Hemisphere Publishing, New York, 1987.

4. Schardein, J.L., *Chemically Induced Birth Defects*, Marcel Dekker, New York, 1985.

5. Spector, W.S., Ed., *Handbook of Biological Data*, W.B. Saunders, Philadelphia, 1956.

6. Altman, P.L. and Dittmer, D.S., *Biology Data Book*, 2nd ed., vol. 1, Federation of American Societies for Experimental Biology, Bethesda, MD, 1972.

7. Clermont, Y., Kinetics of spermatogenesis in mammals: seminiferous epithelium cycle and spermatogonial renewal. *Physiol. Rev.*, 52, 198–236, 1972.

8. Steinberger, E. and Steinberger, A., Spermatogenic function of the testis, in *Handbook of Physiology*, Hamilton, D.W. and Greep, R.O., Eds., Williams & Wilkins, Baltimore, 1975, Vol. 5, Section F, pp. 1–19.

9. Miller, R.K., Kellogg, C.K., and Saltzman, R.A., Reproductive and perinatal toxicology, in *Handbook of Toxicology*, Haley, T.J. and Berndt, W.O., Eds., Hemisphere Publishing, Washington, 1987, Chap. 7, pp. 195–309.

10. Robaire, B. and Hermo, L., Efferent ducts, epididymis and vas deferens: structure, functions and their regulation, in *The Physiology of Reproduction*, Knobil, E. and Neill, J., Eds., Raven Press, New York, 1988, Chap. 23, pp. 999–1080.

11. Russell, L.D., Normal testicular structure and methods of evaluation under experimental and disruptive conditions, in *Reproductive and Developmental Toxicity of Metals*, Clarkson, T.W., Nordberg, G.F., and Sagar, P.R., Eds., Plenum Press, New York, 1983, pp. 227–252.

12. Dean, J., Preimplantation development: biology genetics and mutagenesis, *Am. J. Ind. Med.,* 4, 31–49, 1983.

13. Oakberg, E.F., A description of spermiogenesis in the mouse and its use in analysis of the cycle of the seminiferous epithelium and germ cell renewal, *Am. J. Anat.*, 99, 391–413, 1956.

14. Eddy, E.M. and O'Brien, D.A., Biology of the gamete: maturation, transport, and fertilization, in *Toxicology of the Male and Female Reproductive System*, Working, P.K., Ed., Hemisphere Publishing, Washington, 1989, chap. 3, pp. 31–100.

15. Blazak, W.F., Significance of cellular endpoints in assessment of male reproductive toxicity, in *Toxicology of the Male and Female Reproductive Systems*, Working, P.K., Ed., Hemisphere Publishing, Washington, 1989, Chap. 6, pp. 157–172.

16. Zenick, H. and Clegg, E.D., Assessment of male reproductive toxicity: a risk assessment approach, in *Principles and Methods of Toxicology*, Hayes, A.W., Ed., Raven Press, New York, 1989, Chap. 10, pp. 275–309.

17. Overstreet, J.W. and Blazak, W.F., The biology of human male reproduction: an overview, *Am. J. Ind. Med.*, 4, 5–15, 1983.

18. Manson, J.M. and Kang, Y.S., Test methods for assessing female reproductive and developmental toxicology, in *Principles and Methods of Toxicology,* 2nd ed., Hayes, A.W., Ed., Raven Press, New York, 1989, Chap. 11, pp. 311–359.

19. Yanagimachi, R., Mechanisms of fertilization in mammals, in *Fertilization and Embryonic Development In Vitro*, Mastroianni, L., Jr. and Biggers, J.D., Eds., Plenum Press, New York, 1981, Chap. 5, pp. 81–182.

20. FitzGerald, L. and DiMattina, M., An improved medium for long-term culture of human embryos overcomes the *in vitro* developmental block and increases blastocyst formation, *Fertility Sterility*, 57, 641–647, 1992.

21. Harris, M., Chapin, R.E., Lockhart, A.C., and Jokinen, M.P., Assessment of a short-term reproductive and developmental toxicity screen, *Fundam. Appl. Toxicol.,* 1, 186–196, 1992.

22. Chernoff, N. and Kavlock, R.J., An *in vivo* teratology screen utilizing pregnant mice, *J. Toxicol. Environ. Health*, 10, 541–550, 1982.

23. Lamb, J.C., IV, Maronpot, R.R., Gulati, D.K., Russell, V.S., Hommel-Barnes, L., and Sabharwal, P.S., Reproductive and developmental toxicity of ethylene glycol in the mouse, *Toxicol. Appl. Pharmacol.*, 81, 100–112, 1985.

24. OECD, Guidelines for Testing Chemicals: Extended Steering Group Document No. 3, 1990.

25. Tanaka, S., Kawashima, K., Naito, K., Usami, M., Nakadate, M., Imaida, K., Takahashi, M., Hayashi, Y., Kurokawa, Y., and Tobe, M., Combined repeat dose and reproductive/developmental toxicity screening test (OECD): familiarization using cyclophosphamide, *Fundam. Appl. Toxicol.*, 18, 89–95, 1992.

26. Cummings, A.M., Toxicological mechanisms of implantation failure, *Fundam. Appl. Toxicol.*, 15, 571–579, 1990.

27. Amdur, M.O., Doull, J., and Klaassen, C.D., *Casarett and Doull's Toxicology, The Basic Science of Poisons*, 4th ed., Pergamon Press, Elmsford, NY, 1991.

28. Hayes, A.W., Ed., *Principles and Methods of Toxicology*, 2nd ed., Raven Press, New York, 1989.

29. Mattison, D.R., Ed., *Reproductive Toxicology*, Alan R. Liss, New York, 1983.

30. Amann, R.P., Use of animal models for detecting specific alterations in reproduction, *Fundam. Appl. Toxicol.*, 2, 13–16, 1982.

ADDITIONAL RELATED INFORMATION

TABLE 11.15
Comparison of Reproduction Guidelines

	U.S. FDA (1993)[a]	U.S. EPA (1996)[b]	OECD (1996)[c]	ICH (U.S. FDA, 1994)[d]
Number of Generations	Two generations, one litter per generation.	Two generations.	Two generations.	Two generations.
Animal Species	Rodent (rat or mouse)	Rat is preferred species. Justification and procedural adjustments needed for any other species.	Rat is preferred species. Justification and appropriate modifications are necessary if other species are used.	Rats is preferred species.
Age of Animals and Preparation	5–9 wk of age. Acclimate for 1 wk.	5–9 wk of age at start of dosing. Acclimate for 5 days.	6–9 wk old at start of dosing. Acclimate for 5 days.	
Number of Animals and Assignment	Parental (P) animals: Start with 30 males and 30 females (to obtain 20 pregnant females). F 1 generation: 25 males and 25 females.	Sufficient mating pairs to yield at least 20 pregnant females. Each test group should contain a similar number of mating pairs.	Sufficient mating pairs to yield at least 20 pregnant females.	Number of animals per sex per group sufficient to allow meaningful interpretation of the data.
Animal Care	Single housing of animals is recommended except during mating. Animal care should meet requirements of Institute of Laboratory Animal Resources (1996).	According DHHS/PHS NIH Publ. #86-23 (1985) "Guidelines for the Care and Use of Laboratory Animals" and other appropriate guidelines. Pregnant animals should be caged separately in delivery or maternity cages.	Animal room temperature should be 22°C(±3°C). Humidity should be 30– 70% (aim for 50–60%). Artificial light should provide 12 h dark and 12 h light. Use conventional diet. Provide unlimited water. Animals may be housed individually or in small groups of the same sex. Pregnant animals should be caged separately in delivery or maternity cages.	

Dose Levels	Minimum of 3 dose levels and concurrent control. *High dose:* provides some toxicity and <10% maternal mortality. Should comprise ≤5% of diet. *Low dose:* provides a minimum margin of safety. *Intermediate:* dose spaced between high and low.	At least 3 dose levels and concurrent control. Dose levels should be spaced to produce a gradation of toxic effects. It is desirable to have additional information on metabolism and pharmacokinetics. *Highest dose level:* should induce toxicity but not more than 10% mortality in parental animals. Dose should not exceed 1,000 mg/kg/day (or 20,000 ppm in the diet) unless potential human exposure data indicate the need for higher doses. *Intermediate dose level:* should produce minimal observable toxic effects. *Lowest dose level:* should not produce any evidence of toxicity.	At least 3 dose levels and concurrent control. Dose levels may be based on information from acute toxicity tests or results from repeated dose studies. *Highest dose level:* should induce toxicity but not death or severe suffering and no more than 10% mortality. *Lowest dose level:* should induce no toxic effects. *Intermediate dose levels:* Descending sequence of doses at two-to fourfold intervals. A fourth group is preferable to intervals greater than a factor of 10 between doses. *Desirable:* additional information on metabolism and pharmacokinetics. Characteristics of the vehicle should be considered: effects on absorption, distribution, metabolism, or retention of test substance, and effect on feed and water consumption, or the nutritional status of the animals.	At least 3 dose levels and concurrent control group. High dose level should be based on data from all available studies. Lower doses are selected in descending sequence. Dosage intervals should be close enough to reveal dosage-related trends that may be present.
Control Group	Concurrent control group required. In dietary study, control should be same diet. For carrier vehicle, volume given should equal the maximum amount of vehicle given.	Concurrent control, either untreated or sham treated. If administered in the diet, and diet causes decreased dietary intake, a pair-fed group may be needed.	Concurrent control, either untreated or sham treated. Handling of control group should be identical to treated groups. Vehicle should be given in the highest volume used. If administered in the diet, and diet causes decreased dietary intake, a pair-fed group may be needed.	

TABLE 11.15 *(Continued)*
Comparison of Reproduction Guidelines

	U.S. FDA (1993)[a]	U.S. EPA (1996)[b]	OECD (1996)[c]	ICH (U.S. FDA, 1994)[d]
Route of Administration	Oral route preferred: diet, drinking water, gavage.	Oral route preferred: diet, drinking water, gavage. If by gavage, doses should be based on individual body weight and adjusted weekly at a minimum.	Oral route preferred: diet, drinking water, gavage, single dose should be given to the animals.	Route of administration should be similar to those intended for human usage.
Dosing Schedule	Males and females are dosed 8–11 wk before mating, throughout mating and pregnancy to weaning of the F1a litter.	Animals should be treated 10 wk before mating. Dosing is continued during mating and pregnancy.	Animals should be treated 10 wk before mating. Dosing is continued during mating and pregnancy. Dosing of F1 begins at weaning.	Guidelines are split into two parts. 1. Treat males and females before mating, during mating, through implantation. Before mating, males are treated for 4 wk, females are treated for 2 wk. 2. Treat female from implantation through weaning. No provision of treatment of male.
Mating Procedures	Mate 1:1 for 2–3 wk. No further mating if mating has not occurred. 1:2 mating permitted if a male dies. Daily vaginal smears or plugs indicate copulation has occurred.	Mate 1:1 for up to 2 wk (or 3 estrus cycles). After 2 wk, animals are separated and not remated. Vaginal smears daily until evidence of copulation.	Mate 1:1 for up to 2 wk. Remating of females should be considered. Daily examination for presence of sperm or vaginal plugs. Pairs that fail to mate should be evaluated to determine the cause of apparent infertility.	Mate 1: 1 for up to 3 wk.
F1 Mating	Select 1 male and 1 female randomly from each litter and mate with pup of another litter (maximum 2 males and 2 females selected).	Select at least 1 male and 1 female randomly from each litter for mating with another pup of the same dose level but different litter to produce the F2 generation.	Select at least 1 male and 1 female randomly from each litter for mating with another pup of the same dose level but different litter to produce the F2 generation.	
2nd Mating	In cases of poor reproductive performance in controls or treatment-related alterations in the litter size, adults may be remated to produce F1b or F2b.	In cases of poor reproductive performance in controls or treatment-related alterations in the litter size, adults may be remated to produce F1b or F2b.	In cases of poor reproductive performance in controls or treatment-related alterations in the litter size, adults may be remated to produce F1b or F2b.	

Observation of Animals	Observe animals twice per day. Do thorough physical examination weekly.	Observe parental animals at least once per day. Do thorough physical examination weekly.	Do general clinical observations every day. Record all signs. At least twice per day, all animals should be observed for morbidity and mortality.	Observe parental animals at least once per day.
Weighing of Animals	Weigh animals on first day of administration, then weekly until necropsy, and at necropsy.	Parental and F1 animals are weighed on the first day of dosing and weekly thereafter. Parental animals should be weighed on gestation days 0, 7, 14, and 21.	Parental and F1 animals are weighed on the first day of dosing, weekly thereafter, and also during lactation on the same days as the weighing of the litters.	Weigh animals at least twice weekly.
Feed and Water Consumption	Measure feed consumption weekly (minimum). Water consumption should be measured as appropriate,	Measure feed consumption weekly (minimum) during mating and gestation. Water consumption should be measured weekly (minimum) if test substance is administered in the water,	Measure feed and water consumption weekly.	Measure feed intake at least weekly.
Estrus Cycle	Estrus cycle length and normality should be evaluated daily by vaginal smears for a minimum of 3 wk prior to mating.	Estrus cycle of P and F1 females should be evaluated by vaginal smears for a minimum of 3 wk prior to mating and throughout cohabitation.	Do vaginal smears on all P and F1 females prior to mating and optionally during mating.	Record vaginal smears daily, at least during mating.
Examination of Offspring	Examine litters as soon as possible after birth. Neonates should be observed, weighed, and sexed on postnatal days 0, 4, 7, 14, and 21. Measure anogenital distance in F2 if F1 sex ratio affected. Examine offspring for preputial separation (males) and vaginal opening (females).	Examine each litter as soon as possible after birth to determine the number and sex of pups, stillbirths, live births, and the presence of gross anomalies. Measure anogenital distance in F2 if F1 sex ratio affected. Examine offspring for preputial separation (males) and vaginal opening (females).	Examine each litter as soon as possible after birth to determine the number and sex of pups, still-births, live births, and the presence of gross anomalies. Weigh pups on days 0, 4, 7, 14, and 21. Measure anogenital distance in F2 if F1 sex ratio affected. Examine offspring for preputial separation (males) and vaginal opening(females).	Examine each litter to determine implantations, abnormalities, live births and dead offspring at birth. Weigh pups at birth. Determine pre- and post-weaning survival and growth/body weight.

TABLE 11.15 *(Continued)*
Comparison of Reproduction Guidelines

	U.S. FDA (1993)[a]	U.S. EPA (1996)[b]	OECD (1996)[c]	ICH (U.S. FDA, 1994)[d]
Standardization of Litter Size	Culling is optional. If culling is done, cull to 10 or 8 pups per litter based on historical litter size, on postnatal day 4 in a random manner.	Standardization of litter sizes is optional. If standardization occurs, litters may be culled to 4 males and 4 females or 5 males and 5 females randomly.	Standardization is optional. If standardization occurs, litters are culled to 4 males and 4 females randomly.	Value of culling is still under discussion.
Gross Necropsy	All parental and F1 animals and at least 2 male and 2 female pups per litter from unselected F1 and F2 weanlings should be examined macroscopically for structural abnormalities or pathological changes. Dead or moribund pups should be preserved and examined for possible defects and/or cause of death.	All parental and F1 animals and at least 3 male and 3 female pups per litter from unselected F1 and F2 weanlings should be examined macroscopically for structural abnormalities or pathological changes Dead or moribund pups should be preserved and examined for possible defects and/or cause of death.	All parental P and F1 animals and all F1 generation (unselected) pups should be examined macroscopically for structural abnormalities or pathological changes. Dead or moribund pups should be preserved and examined for possible defects and/or cause of death.	
Organ Weights of Parental Animals	Weigh organs from parental P and F1 animals: reproductive organs (uterus, ovaries, testes, epididymis, seminal vesicles, prostate), brain, liver, kidneys, adrenal glands, spleen, and known target organs.	Weigh organs from parental P and F1 animals: reproductive organs (uterus, ovaries, testes, epididymis, seminal vesicles, prostate) brain, liver, kidneys, adrenal glands, spleen, and known target organs.	Weigh organs from parental P and F1 animals: reproductive organs(uterus, ovaries, testes, epididymis, seminal vesicles, prostate), brain, liver, kidneys, adrenal glands, spleen, and known target organs.	
Organ Weights of Weanlings	Weigh brain, spleen, and thymus from F1 and F2 weanlings that are examined macroscopically.	Weigh brain, spleen, and thymus from F1 and F2 weanlings that are examined macroscopically.	Weigh brain, spleen, and thymus from F1 and F2 weanlings that are examined macroscopically.	

Tissue Preservation	For P and F1 parental animals, preserve vagina, uterus with cervix, ovaries with oviducts, 1 testis, 1 epididymis, seminal vesicles, prostate coagulating gland, target organs, grossly abnormal tissue. For F1 and F2 weanlings selected for macroscopic examination, preserve grossly abnormal tissue and target organs.	For P and F1 parental animals, preserve vagina, uterus with cervix, ovaries with oviducts 1 testis, 1 epididymis, seminal vesicles, prostate, coagulating gland, target organs, grossly abnormal tissue. For F1 and F2 weanlings selected for mating, preserve grossly abnormal tissue and target organs.	For P and F1 parental animals, preserve vagina, uterus with cervix, ovaries with oviducts, 1 testis, 1 epididymis, seminal vesicles, prostate, coagulating gland, target organs. For F1 and F2 weanlings not selected for mating, preserve grossly abnormal tissue and target organs.	
Histopathology	Do full histopathological examination of high-dose and control parental animals. If effects seen at high level, examine tissues from low and mid-dose levels. Do histology of developmental anomalies seen in weanlings with emphasis on organs of the reproductive system.	Do full histopathological examination of high-dose and control parental animals. If effects seen at high level, examine tissues from low-and mid-dose levels. Do histology of developmental anomalies seen in weanlings with emphasis on organs of the reproductive system.	Do full histopathological examination of high-dose and control P and F1 animals, organs demonstrating treatment-related changes in low- and mid-dose groups, and reproductive organs of low- and mid-dose animals suspected of reduced fertility.	
Report: Some End-Points for Females	Body and organ weights, female fertility index, gestation index, weaning index, sex ratio, viability indices, growth indices, maternal toxicity effects.	Body and organ weights, litter and pup weights, clinical observations, cycle length and stage of estrus, female fertility index, gestation index, viability index lactation index.	Body and organ weights, litter and pup weights, clinical observations, cycle length and stage of estrus, female fertility index, gestation index, viability index, lactation index.	Body weights, litter values, clinical signs, autopsy findings, abnormalities. Tabulation should be done in a clear, concise manner to account for every animal that was entered into the study.

[a] U.S. Food and Drug Administration, Center for Food Safety and Applied Nutrition, 1993, *Toxicological principles for the safety assessment of direct food additives and color additives used in food, "Redbook II" (draft)*, Washington, D.C., U.S. Food and Drug Administration, Center for Food Safety and Applied Nutrition.

[b] U.S. Environmental Protection Agency, 1996, *Health Effects Test Guidelines, OPPTS 870.3700, Prenatal Developmental Toxicity Study*, pp. 1–8, Washington, D.C., EPA 712-C-96-207.

[c] Organization for Economic Cooperation and Development, 1996, OECD, Guideline for Testing of Chemicals. Proposal for Updating Guideline 414. Prenatal Developmental Toxicity Study. Draft document, August 1996, pp. 1–11. Paris: Organization for Economic Cooperation and Development.

[d] U.S. Food and Drug Administration, 1994, International Conference on Harmonization; guideline on detection of toxicity to reproduction for medicinal products; availability, *Fed. Reg.*, Part IX, 59(183):48746–48752.

From Testing guidelines for evaluation of reproductive and developmental toxicity of food additives in females, Collins, T.F.X.. Sprando, R.L., Hansen, D.L., Shackelford, M.E., and Welsh, J.J., *International J. Toxicol*, 17, 299–336. Copyright 1998. Reproduced by permission of Taylor & Francis, Inc., http://www.routledge-ny.com.

12 Developmental Toxicology

Karen M. MacKenzie, Ph.D.
and Richard M. Hoar, Ph.D.

CONTENTS

0-8493-0370-2/02/$0.00+$1.50
© 2002 by CRC Press LLC

SECTION 1. STUDY DESIGNS

TABLE 12.1
Basic Developmental Toxicity Testing Protocol

Phase	Time	Developmental Toxicity Testing[a]
Acclimation period	Variable number of weeks	No exposure of the animals to the test agent
Cohabitation period	Day of mating determined (day 0)	No exposure of the animals to the test agent
Pre-embryonic period	Day of mating through day 5,[b] 6,[c] 7[d] of pregnancy	
Period of major embryonic organogenesis	Day 5, 6, or 7 through day 15[b,c] or 18[d] of pregnancy	Groups of pregnant animals exposed to the test agent
Fetal period	Day 15 or 18 through day 18,[b] 21,[c] or 30[d] of pregnancy	No exposure of the pregnant animals to the test agent
Term	Day 18,[b] 22,[c] or 31[d] of pregnancy	Females sacrificed (to preclude cannibalization of malformed fetuses), cesarean section performed, and young examined externally and internally

[a] Usually a sham-treated control group and three agent-treated groups are used with 20 to 25 mice or rats and 15 to 18 rabbits per group. The dose levels are chosen with the goal of no maternal or developmental effects in the low-dose group and at least maternal toxicity in the high-dose group (failure to gain or loss of weight during dosing, reduced feed and/or water consumption, increased clinical signs, or no more than 10% maternal death).

[b] Mice.

[c] Rats.

[d] Rabbits.

Modified from Johnson, 1990.[1]

SECTION 2. MATERNAL AND DEVELOPMENTAL TOXICITY

TABLE 12.2
Signs of Overt Maternal Toxicity

1. Daily (or isolated) body weight changes and/or effects on food and/or water consumption during the dosing period[a]
2. Changes in respiration, alertness, posture, spontaneous motor activity, color of mucous membranes, behavior (aggressive, depressed, lethargic, sedated), hair and coat appearance, color of urine, frequency of urination, and number and consistency of fecal pellets
3. Other signs such as nasal discharge, chromodacryarrhea, salivation, vaginal bleeding, tumor, convulsions, and coma
4. Death and necropsy findings

[a] Weight loss or failure to gain weight at any time during the dosing period may be followed by a rebound weight gain of sufficient magnitude to obfuscate an effect on maternal weight; therefore, maternal body weights should be determined daily.

Modified from Khera et al., 1989,[2] chap. 3.

TABLE 12.3
Endpoints of Developmental Toxicity in Female Rodents and Rabbits

Postconception evaluation
    Maternal weight gain (daily during treatment; not in rabbits)
    Clinical observations
Cesarean evaluations
    Implantation number
    Corpora lutea number (not in mice)
    Litter size
    Live fetuses
    Deaths (embryonic, fetal)
    Resorptions
    Pup weight, crown-rump length
    Incidence of malformations (external, visceral, skeletal)

Modified from Ecobichon, 1992,[3] chap. 5.

TABLE 12.4
Considerations for Establishing Cause and Effect Relationships[a]

1. Demonstration of consistency of association: the findings in studies using different methods and/or species and populations are similar.
2. Strength of the association between cause and effect: the effects appear more frequently in those exposed than in nonexposed individuals and the frequency and/or severity of the effects increases with increased exposure.
3. A temporal relationship exists between exposure and effect: effects appear after exposure at a time consistent with the mechanism of action.
4. There is a specificity of association: effects reported correlate with a single chemical exposure.
5. The observed effects are biologically plausible: the signs and symptoms are consistent with the mechanisms of toxicity, the life stage, and the target tissues/organs involved.

[a] Findings include death and/or resorption, reduced fetal body weight, malformation, and/or functional defect.

Modified from Johnson, 1986.[4]

TABLE 12.5
Arbitrary Classification of Chemicals Based on Teratogenic Potential

Criteria	Category A	Category B	Category C	Category D
1. Ratio: minimum maternotoxic dose to minimum teratogenic dose	Much greater than 1	Generally greater than 1, teratogenic range starts below the maternotoxic dose range[a] and overlaps it	≤ 1	No teratogenicity even at maternotoxic doses
2. Incidence of malformations	Dose related and high	Dose related and high	Dose relatedness of each malformation less obvious, incidence low	
3. Type of malformation at lower doses	Organ systems involved are specific	Characteristics, possibly specific, generally multiple	Nonspecific involving different organ systems	
4. Target cells	Specific cells	Specific cells	Nonspecific and generalized	Not known
5. Range of safety factor	1–400	1–300	1–250	1–100

[a] The maternotoxic dose range extends between the dose initiating signs of toxicity and the dose causing 50% mortality (LD_{50}).

Modified from Khera et al., 1989,[2] chap. 9.

TABLE 12.6
Category A: A Probable True or Selective Action in Animals

Chemical	Minimum Effective Dose,[a] (mg/kg), Route, and Days of Dosing during Pregnancy	Maternal Toxicity of the Minimum Effective Dose	Maternotoxic Dose, Acute, Species	LD_{50} (mg/kg)[b]	Salient Malformations
Mercaptopurine riboside	62.5 IP, 11	Not reported	Rat	2000–3000	Cleft palate; adactyly, ectrodactyly, syndactyly, or brachydactyly; short tail; kidneys absent, hypoplastic, or fused; adrenal extopic or absent[5]
Azaserine	2.5 IP; 11, 12, or 13	Not reported	Rat	75–100	Cleft palate; fused ribs and vertebrae; hemivertebrae; fused sternebrae; small or absent pelvis, femur, and fibula, syndactyly[6,7]
Ni(CO)$_4$	0.08 mg/L inhalation for 15 min	Not reported	Rat	0.58 mg/L for 15 min	Anophthalmia and microphthalmia[8]
Medroxyprogesterone acetate	3 or 10 SC, 10–12	None	Rabbit		Cleft palate[9]
Ethylenethiorea	30 PO, 13	None	Rat	60	Hydrocephalus and microphthalmia[10,11]
Mirex	5 or 6 PO, 6–15 or 8.5–15.5	None	Rat	Not reported	Subcutaneous edema[12] associated with tachycardia and first- and second-degree heartblocks[13]

[a] As published.
[b] By the same route and at about the same stage of gestation as used in teratologic assessments.

Modified from Khera et al., 1989,[2] chap. 9.

TABLE 12.7
Category A: Known Human Teratogens (Specific Malformations at Apparently Nonmaternotoxic Dosages in Humans)

Compound	Salient Malformations	Animal Species Manifesting Similar Malformations
1. Diethylstilbestrol	Adenocarcinoma	Mouse, rat, monkey epithelial lesions of vagina
2–5. Ethisterone, 17-methyltestosterone, testosterone, and norethindrone	Masculinization of newborn female	Mouse, rat, guinea pig, monkey
6. Iodine, thiouracil	Goitrous cretinism	Mouse, rat, rabbit, guinea pig
7. Organic mercury	Infantile cerebral palsy	Cat, monkey
8. Tetracycline	Discoloration of bone and teeth	Rat, dog
9. Thalidomide	Phocomelia, amelia, and others	Nonhuman primates

Modified from Khera et al., 1989,[2] chap. 9.

TABLE 12.8
Category B: High Incidence of Malformations Induced in Animals by a Wide Maternotoxic Dose Range

Chemical	Species	Salient malformations	Ref.
Copper citrate	Hamster	Cardiovascular	14
Hydrocortisone	Hamster	Cleft palate	15
Adriamycin	Rat	Esophageal and intestinal atresia and tracheoesophageal fistula, cardiovascular and other defects	16
Glycerol formal	Rat	Ventricular septal defect	17
Triamcinolone	Rat	Cleft palate	18
Vitamin A palmitate	Rat	Anophthalmia, cleft palate	19

Modified from Khera et al., 1989,[2] chap. 9.

TABLE 12.9
Criteria for Recognizing a New Developmental Toxin in Humans

1. An abrupt increase in the frequency of developmental toxicity usually heralded by, but not limited to, a particular defect or association with defects (syndrome)
2. Coincidence of this increase with a known environmental change, such as widespread use of a new drug or the accidental release of an environmental toxin
3. Known exposure to an environmental change at a particular stage of gestation yielding a characteristically consistent developmental toxicity
4. Absence of other factors common to all pregnancies yielding infants with the particular display of developmental toxicity

[a] Developmental toxicity includes death and/or abortion, reduced neonatal body weight, malformation, and/or functional deficit.

Modified from Wilson (1973).[20]

TABLE 12.10
Categories and Criteria Used in Classifying Drugs According to their Embryotoxic Potential in Humans[a]

1. Established as being embryotoxic
   a. Unquestionably produces a higher percentage of developmental defects or intrauterine death in infants of exposed than otherwise similar, nonexposed women
2. Suspected of being embryotoxic
   a. Apparent increase above background level of developmental defects or intrauterine death among infants of exposed women, based on large numbers of accumulated case reports
   b. Retrospective surveys indicate significant increase of defects or death among infants of exposed women, but "memory bias" of mothers introduces uncertainty
   c. Prospective surveys indicate significant increase among infants of exposed women, but total number of exposed cases relatively small in consecutive series
3. Possibly embryotoxic, under unusual conditions of dosage or in combination with other unidentified etiologic factors
   a. Questionable increase of defects or death among infants of exposed women based on large number of accumulated cases or on extensive epidemiologic surveys
   b. Strong indication from studies in more than one animal species that drug has definite embryotoxic potential, especially at high dosage
4. Not embryotoxic under any known conditions of human usage
   a. No increase in defects or death among infants born to exposed women in well-controlled epidemiologic surveys
   b. Extensively used by pregnant women over many years without substantiation of cause-effect relationship between use of the drug and adverse effects on the offspring

[a] Assuming exposure to therapeutic or higher dose during the first trimester.

From Wilson, 1977,[21] pp. 309–355. With permission.

TABLE 12.11
Chemicals Presenting a Risk to the Developing Fetus Based on Reliable Epidemiological and Teratological Evidence

Chemical	Adverse Reproductive Effects	Ref.
Anesthetic gases	Spontaneous abortion, congenital malformations (?)	22, 23
Ethylene oxide	Spontaneous abortion	24
Styrene	Spontaneous abortion, toxemia, congenital malformations	25–27
PCBs (yusho, oil disease)	Toxemia, low birth weight, stillbirth, missed abortion	28–30
Inorganic lead	Stillbirth, miscarriage, premature membrane rupture	31, 32
DDT	Premature birth	33
Carbon monoxide	Fetal and infant death, microcephaly, mental retardation	28
DES	Vaginal cancer in female offspring, urological anomalies in males	34, 35
Inorganic and organic mercury	Congenital cerebral palsy, prenatal mortality	28, 36

Modified from Khera et al. (1989),[2] chap. 7.

TABLE 12.12

Chemicals Presenting a Risk to the Developing Fetus Based on Suggestive Epidemiological and Teratological Evidence

Chemical	Adverse Reproductive Effects	Ref.
Benzene	Stillbirth, spontaneous abortion, aplastic anemia, perinatal death	28
Vinyl chloride	Congenital malformations of various kinds	28, 37
2,4-D	Spontaneous abortion, premature birth, toxicosis	38
Arsenic	Infant death, pulmonary hemorrhage, low birth weight	28, 39
Carbon disulfide	Spontaneous abortion	25

Modified from Khera et al., 1989,[2] chap. 7.

TABLE 12.13

Compounds with No Positive Report of Teratogenicity in Humans: A Comparison of Human Usage Levels and Dosages Found Teratogenic in Animals

Compounds	Human Exposure Level [mg (or as stated) per kg[a]]	Minimum Embryotoxic Dose, mg (or as Stated) per kg in Mouse (m), Hamster (h), Rat (r), Rabbit (rb) Dose in Animals	Approximate Ratio, Therapeutic Dose to Minimum Embryotoxic Dose
1. Acetazolamide	4	m 1000, h 600, r 400	1:100
2. Actinomycin D	0.015	r 0.025–0.1	1:2
3. Aldrin	0.002 µg	m 25, h 50	1:12,000
4. l-Asparaginase	50–200 IU	m and r 100 IU, rb 500 IU	1:1
5. Caffeine	20–25	m 250, r 75–100, rb 100	1:3
6. Carbamazepine	24	r 250	1:10
7. Carbaryl	0.01	guinea pig 300, dog 6–50	1:30,000
8. Chloramphenicol	50–80	r 2000–4000	1:25
9. Chlorpropamide	2–5	r 200	1:100
10. Codeine	2.4	m 100	1:40
11. Colchicine	0.06–0.07	m 0.5–1.0, rb 0.1–0.5	1:1.5
12. Cyclizine	1–2	r 75–100	1:40
13. Dexamethasone	0.024 in nasal spray	m 6, r 4	1:150
14. Dieldrin	0.0001	m 3.4, r 3.4, h 30	1: > 3000
15. Endrin	0.00001	m 2.5, r 0.58, h 5	1: > 3000
16. 5-Fluorouracil	12	r 12–37	1:1
17. Griseofulvin	10–20	r 500–1500	1:25
18. Haloperidol	0.04	m 14, h 80	1:350
19. Hydrocortisone	b	m 82.5, rb 10–50	
20. Hydroxyurea	20–30	r 137, cat 50, monkey 100	1:2.5
21. Meclizine	0.5–2	r 10–40	1:20
22. Medroxyprogesterone acetate	0.1–0.2	rb 75, m 30	1:375
23. Mescaline metaproterenol		guinea pig 0.45–3.25	1:33
24. Methadone	0.1–0.3	m 24, h 67	1:80
25. Methylprednisolone	b	m 4–8	
26. Mirex		r 1–6	
27. Mitomycin C		m 5–10	
28. Morphine	1.2–3.6	m 400	1: >100
29. Penicillin	up to 50,000 U	m 50,000–500,000 U	1:1

TABLE 12.13 *(Continued)*
Compounds with No Positive Report of Teratogenicity in Humans: A Comparison of Human Usage Levels and Dosages Found Teratogenic in Animals

Compounds	Human Exposure Level [mg (or as stated) per kg[a]]	Minimum Embryotoxic Dose, mg (or as Stated) per kg in Mouse (m), Hamster (h), Rat (r), Rabbit (rb) Dose in Animals	Approximate Ratio, Therapeutic Dose to Minimum Embryotoxic Dose
30. Perphenazine	0.3–0.6	r 20–150	1:200
31. Prednisolone	0.2–8	m 2.5, r 2.5, rb 0.1–0.25	80:1
32. Procarbazine	2–6	r 5–10, 10–40	1:1
33. Prochlorperazine	0.6–1.2	r 2.5–10	1:2
34. Pyrimethamine	0.5	h 160, r 12–40	1:24
35. Reserpine	0.001–0.025–	r 100, rb 0.16, guinea pig 10	1:160
36. Sodium chloride	0.18	m 1900	1: >3000
37. Sodium salicylate	72–108	m 500, r 250, cat 50, dog 400	2:1
38. Thioguanine	2	r 10	1:5
39. Trifluoperazine	0.1–1.0	r 20–25	1:20
40. Urethane	0.012	r 1000, m 15–1500	1:1000
41. Vinblastin	3.7 mg/m^2	m 2.5, r 0.25, h 0.25	
42. Vincristine	2 mg/m^2	h 0.1, m 0.15	

[a] Cited from Refs. 40 and 41 and other sources.

[b] Used for topical application.

SECTION 3. COMPARATIVE REPRODUCTIVE AND DEVELOPMENTAL PARAMETERS

TABLE 12.14
Reproductive Parameters for Various Species

Species	Age at Puberty	Sexual Cycle Type[a]	Sexual Cycle Duration (days)	Ovulation Time[b]	Ovulation Type[c]	Copulation Time[b]	Copulation Length	Implantation (days)	Gestation Period (days)
Mouse	5–6 wk	PE	4	2–3 h	S	Onset of estrus		4–5	19 (19–21)
Rat	6–11 wk	PE	4–6	8–11 h	S	1–4 h		5–6	21–22
Rabbit	6–7 mo	PE	Indefinite	10 h	I	Anytime[f]	Sec	7–8	31 (30–35)
Hamster	5–8 wk	PE	4	Early estrus	S	Estrus[g]	Sec	5+	16 (15–18)
Guinea Pig	8–10 wk	PE	16–19	10 h	S	Estrus	Sec	6	67–68
Ferret	8–12 mo	ME	Seasonal	30–36 h	I	Estrus	1–3 h	12–13	42
Cat	6–15 mo	PE	Seasonal[d]	24–56 h	I	3rd day[h]	1–2 h	13–14	63 (52–69)
Dog	6–8 mo	ME	9	1–3 days	S	Estrus	1–2 h	13–14	61 (53–71)
Monkey	3 y	PE	28	9–20 days	S	Anytime[i]		9	168 (146–180)
Man	12–16 yr	PE	27–28	14 day (13–15)	S	Anytime	15–30 min	7.5	267 (ovulation)

[a] PE = polyestrous; ME = monoestrus
[b] time from start of estrous cycle
[c] I = induced ovulation; S = spontaneous ovulation
[d] March to August
[e] after mating
[f] most receptive when in estrus
[g] 8–10 pm
[h] of estrus, most receptive
[i] most receptive 2 days before ovulation

Modified from Spector, 1956.[42]

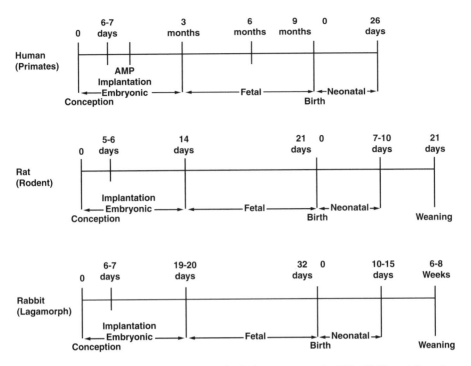

FIGURE 12.1 Developmental stages and timelines in the human, rat, and rabbit. AMP: anticipated menstural period. Average human menstural cycle is 28 days with ovulation occuring about 14 days. Rabbit ovulates following coitus. Modified from Miller et al., 1987,[79] chap. 7.

TABLE 12.15
Type of Placenta and Placentation for Various Species

Species	Functional Yolk Sac[a] (days/somites)	Circulation[b]	Gross Shape	Type of Placentation[c] Relation to Endometrium A	B	Implantation (days)
Mouse	5–9/20	I	Discoid	Deciduate	Hemochorial	4–5
Rat	8–12/20	I	Discoid	Deciduate	Hemochorial	5–6
Rabbit	7–11/20	I	Discoid	Deciduate	Hemochorial	7–8
Hamster	6–9/20	I	Discoid	Deciduate	Hemochorial	5+
Guinea pig	8–19/20	I	Discoid	Deciduate	Hemochorial	6
Ferret	Hemophagous organ	?	Discoid	Deciduate	Endotheliachorial	12–13
Cat	Hemophagous organ	?	Zonary to Discoid	Deciduate	Endotheliachorial	13–14
Dog	Hemophagous organ	?	Zonary to Discoid	Deciduate	Endotheliachorial	13–14
Monkey (Rhesus)	12–22/5	III	Discoid	Deciduate	Hemochorial	9
Man	12–21/5	III	Discoid	Deciduate	Hemochorial	7.5

[a] Histotrophic nutrition; yolk sac main source of nutrition until last day/somite indicated

[b] Placental vascular channels:

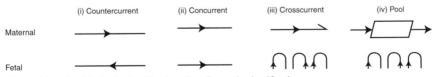

(i) Countercurrent   (ii) Concurrent   (iii) Crosscurrent   (iv) Pool

Maternal

Fetal

[c] Hemotrophic nutrition; A = Huxley's classification; B = Grosser's classification.

Modified from Spector, 1956;[42] Beck and Floyd, 1977;[43] Dawes, 1968,[44] chap. 2.

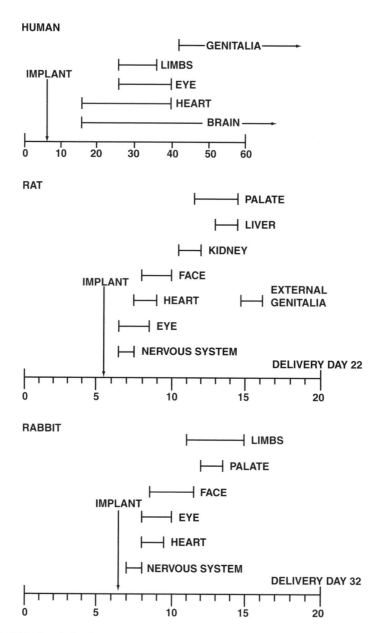

FIGURE 12.2 Critical periods of embryogenesis in the human, rat, and rabbit (days of gestation). When the emphasis is on appearance of birth defects rather than general developmental toxicity, be aware of the extremely short duration of the "target-window" in the animal surrogates. To produce birth defects rather than general developmental toxicity may require a concenteration of test agent which would kill the dam or destroy the pregnancy if delivered more than the one or two days included in the "target interval." Modified from Ecobichon, 1992,[3] chap. 5.

SECTION 4. EMBRYOLOGICAL DEVELOPMENT

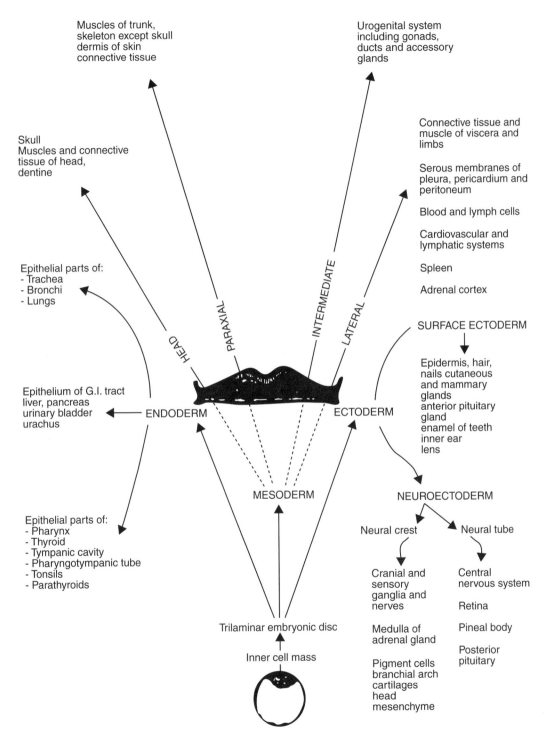

FIGURE 12.3 Derivation of various organs from primary germ layers of the embryonic cell mass. Modified from Moore, 1993,[80] p. 74.

TABLE 12.16
Derivation of Various Organs from Primary Germ Layers of the Embryonic Inner Cell Mass

Endoderm	Mesoderm	Ectoderm (Trophblast)
Liver	Vertebrae	Brain
Pancreas	Muscle	Spinal cord
Serous, mucous, and gastric glands	Dermis of skin, bone, and cartilage	Pituitary
Epithelium of digestive tube, respiratory system, and bladder	Connective tissue, blood, and blood vessels	Neural crest cells, retina, and lens
Thyroid	Urinary and reproductive apparatus	Adrenal medulla
Parathyroid	Epithelia of adrenal cortex, spleen, lymph nodes	Enamel of teeth
Pancreatic islets		Epithelium of oral, nasal, olfactory, genital, and anal cavities
Thymic corpuscles		Epithelium of skin and its derivatives — hair, nails, sweat, sebaceous, and mammary glands

Modified from Hafez, 1968.[45]

TABLE 12.17
Developmental Classification of Human Embryos

Developmental Stage	Witschi Standard Stages	Streeter Horizons	Carnegie Stages
Cleavage and blastula	1–7	I–III	1–3
Gastrula	8–11	IV–VII	4–6
Primitive streak	12	VIII	6–7
Neurula	13–17	IX–XII	7–12
Tailbud embryo	18–24	XII–XIII	12–13
Complete embryo	25	XIV	14
Metamorphosing embryo	26–33	XV–XXII	15–22
Fetus	34	XXIII	23
	34–36		Fetal Period

Modified from Hoar and Monie, 1981,[46] which includes refs. 47–51.

TABLE 12.18
Times of Some Key Developmental Events in Days

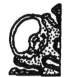

	Implantation	Primitive Streak	10-Somite Stage	Lower Limb Buds	Hand (Forepaw) Rays	Palatal Folds Uniting	Gestation Period
Man	7.5	17	25	32	37	57	267
Macaque	9	17	23	28	35	46	167
Guinea Pig	6.5	13	15	18.5	22	26	67
Rabbit	7.5	7.25	8.5	11	14.5	19.5	32
Rat	6	9	10.5	12	14	17	22
Mouse	5	8	1.5	10.3	12.3	15	19
Hamster	5	7	8	9.75	11	12	16

Modified from Hoar and Monie, 1981,[46] which includes refs. 48–50, 52–70.

TABLE 12.19
Development of Nervous System/Time in Days

   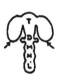

	Neural Plate	Neuropores Closed[a]	Three Brain Vesicles	Cerebral Hemispheres	Cerebellum	Olfactory Bulbs
Man	19	25–27	26	30	37	37
Macaque	20	25–27	25	29	36	38
Guinea Pig	13.5	15.25–15.5	15.3	17	19	23
Rabbit	8	9.5–10.5	9.5	11	15	14
Rat	9.5	10.5–11	10.5	12	14	13.5
Mouse	7	9.0–9.5	8	10	12	11
Hamster	7.5	8.5–9.0	8.5	9	11	11

Ref. as in Tables 12.17 and 12.18.

Abbreviations: AN, anterior neuropore; D, diencephalon; L, myelencephalon; M, mesencephalon; N, metencephalon; NT, notochord: P, prosencephalon; PN, posterior neuropore; R, rhombencephalon; T, telencephalon.

[a] Anterior neuropore first; posterior neuropore second.

Modified from Hoar and Monie, 1981.[46]

TABLE 12.20
Development of Eye and Ear/Time in Days

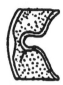 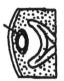

	Optic Vesicle Forming	Lens Separated	Optic Nerve Fibers Present	Otic Vesicle Forming	Cochlea Appearing	Otic Capsule Cartilaginous
Man	24	35	48	25	44	56
Macaque	23	32	39	25	37	42
Guinea Pig	15.5	18	21.5	15.5	20.5	22
Rabbit	9	11.5	15	9	13	20
Rat	10.5	12.5	14	11.5	13.5	15
Mouse	9.5	11.5	13	8.5	12	14.5
Hamster	8	10	11	8.5	10	11

Ref. 71 and as in Tables 12.17 and 12.18.

TABLE 12.21
Development of Respiratory System/Time in Days

  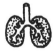

	Respiratory Diverticulum	Asymmetric Lung Buds	Major Bronchial Divisions	Surfactant Appears
Man	28	32	46	170
Macaque	27	29	36	140
Guinea Pig	16	18.5	21.5	—
Rabbit	10.5	12	15	27
Rat	12	13	15.5	19
Mouse	9.5	10.5	13	18
Hamster	9	9.5	10.5	—

Ref. 72 and 73 and as in Tables 12.17 and 12.18.

TABLE 12.22
Development of Heart and Great Arteries/Time in Days

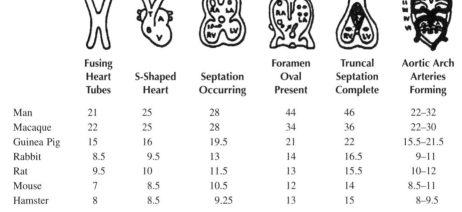

	Fusing Heart Tubes	S-Shaped Heart	Septation Occurring	Foramen Oval Present	Truncal Septation Complete	Aortic Arch Arteries Forming
Man	21	25	28	44	46	22–32
Macaque	22	25	28	34	36	22–30
Guinea Pig	15	16	19.5	21	22	15.5–21.5
Rabbit	8.5	9.5	13	14	16.5	9–11
Rat	9.5	10	11.5	13	15.5	10–12
Mouse	7	8.5	10.5	12	14	8.5–11
Hamster	8	8.5	9.25	13	15	8–9.5

Ref. 74 and as in Tables 12.17 and 12.18.

Abbreviations: A, primitive atrium; B, bulbus cordis: IF, interventricular foramen; LA, left atrium: LV, left ventricle; RA, right atrium; RV, right ventricle; T, truncus arteriousus; V, primitive ventricle.

Modified from Hoar and Monie, 1981.[46]

TABLE 12.23
Development of Gastrointestinal System/Time in Days

	Intestinal Pocket		Membranes Perforate		Liver			Stomach	Umbical Hernia	
	Forgut	Hindgut	Oral	Anal	Anlage	Epithelial Cords	Gall Bladder	Appears	Begins	Reduced
Man	20.5	21.5	28	49	24	26	26	31–32	45	65
Macaque	20.5		27–28		24–26		28–29	28–29	33–34	47–48
Guinea pig	14.5	15.5			16	16.5	19	16.5	23	
Rabbit	8.5	9	10	10	9.5	10.5	11.5	10.5	12.5	20
Rat	9.5	11	10	15	11	11.5		11.5	12.5	18
Mouse	7.8	8.5	8	14	8.8	9.5	9.7	11.5	11.0	16.3
Hamster	7.8	8	8.5	13	8.5	9	8.7	8.5	9.3	13
Standard Stages	13	15	15	31	16	16	17	18	27	34
Streeters Horizons	IX	XI	XI	XVIII	XI	XII	XII	XI–XII	XVII	XXIII

Ref. as in Tables 12.17 and 12.18.

Abbreviations: A, anal or cloacal membrane; DP, dorsal pancreas; FB, foregut or anterior intestinal portal; GB, gallbladder; H, heart; HG, hindgut or posterior intestinal portal; L, liver; O, oral or buccopharyngeal membrane; S, stomach; VP, ventral pancreas.

Modified from Hoar and Monie, 1981.[46]

TABLE 12.24
Development of Endocrine System/Time in Days

	Pharyngeal Pouches Appear	Para-Thyroid Thyroids	Thyroids	Thymus	Pancreas			Pituitary		Adrenal
					Ventral	Dorsal	Fused	Rathke's Pouch	Neuro-hypophysis	
Man	28	24–27	35–38	30–40	31–42	28	40–44		30–34	34
Macaque	24–29	28			29–30	28–29	35–36	28–29	30–31	23
Guinea pig	16–19	16.5				17.5		15.5	18.5	23
Rabbit	9–11.5	9.5	12.5	12.5	11.5	10	14	9.5	12	18
Rat	11–13	11–12	12.5	12.5	11.5	11	13	10.5	11.5	12.5
Mouse	8.3–9.8	8.5	11	12	9.7	9.5	11.5	8.5	11.5	11
Hamster	8	8.5	9	9	9.5	9.5	11.5	8.5	10	10
Standard Stages	16–19	15–16	25–36	19–27	17	17	27		23	23
Streeters Horizons	XI–XII	X–XI	XIV–XV	XII–XVI	XIII	XII	XVI	XII–XIII		XIII

Ref. as in Tables 12.17 and 12.18.

Abbreviations: AC, adult cortex; B, bone; DP, dorsal pancreas; EC, embryonic cortex; FC, foramen caecum; GB, gall bladder; M, medulla; PD, pars distals; PI, pars intermedia; PN, pars nervosa; VP, ventral pancreas.

Modified from Hoar and Monie, 1981c.[46]

TABLE 12.25
Development of Urogenital System/Time in Days

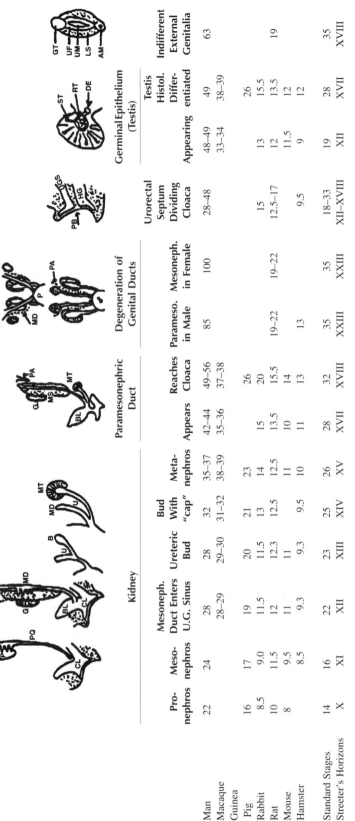

	Kidney						Paramesonephric Duct		Degeneration of Genital Ducts		Urorectal Septum Dividing Cloaca	Germinal Epithelium (Testis)		Indifferent External Genitalia
	Pro-nephros	Meso-nephros	Mesoneph. Duct Enters U.G. Sinus	Ureteric Bud	Bud With "cap"	Meta-nephros	Appears	Reaches Cloaca	Parameso. in Male	Mesoneph. in Female		Appearing	Testis Histol. Differentiated	
Man	22	24	28	28	32	35–37	42–44	49–56	85	100	28–48	48–49	49	63
Macaque			28–29	29–30	31–32	38–39	35–36	37–38				33–34	38–39	
Guinea Pig	16	17	19	20	21	23	26	26					26	
Rabbit	8.5	9.0	11.5	11.5	13	14	15	20			15	13	15.5	
Rat	10	11.5	12	12.3	12.5	12.5	13.5	15.5	19–22	19–22	12.5–17	12	13.5	19
Mouse	8	9.5	11	11	11	11	10	14				11.5	12	
Hamster		8.5	9.3	9.3	9.5	10	11	13	13		9.5	9	12	
Standard Stages	14	16	22	23	25	26	28	32	35	35	18–33	19	28	35
Streeter's Horizons	X	XI	XII	XIII	XIV	XV	XVII	XVIII	XXIII	XXIII	XII–XVIII	XII	XVII	XVIII

Ref. 75 and as in Tables 12.17 and 12.18.

Abbreviations: AM, anal membrane; B, ureteric bud; BL, urinary bladder; CL, cloaca; DE, ductus epididymidis; G, gonad; GT, genital tubercle; HG, hindgut; LS, labioscrotal swelling; MD, mesonephric duct; MS, mesonephros; MT, metanephros; P, pronephros; PA, paramesonephric duct; PB, perineal body; PQ, pronephric duct; RT, rete testis; ST, seminiferous tubule; U, ureter; UF, urogenital fold; UGS, urogenital sinus; UM, urogenital membrane.

Modified from Hoar and Monie, 1981.[46]

SECTION 5. HISTORICAL CONTROL DATA

TABLE 12.26
Historical Control Data — External Evaluations[76,77]

Rats			Rabbits	
External—88,270 Fetuses			External—20,071 Fetuses	
Incidence	Average (%)		Incidence	Average (%)
		General		
11	0.01	Anasarca		
19	0.02	Hematoma		
5	0.01	Local edema	5	0.02
		Skull		
7	0.01	Craniorachischisis		
		Domed head	12	0.06
26	0.03	Exencephaly	5	0.02
		Eyes		
7	0.01	Ablepharia		
16	0.02	Anophthalmia		
28	0.03	Microphthalmia		
9	0.01	Open eyelid		
		Mouth and Jaw		
9	0.01	Cleft palate	7	0.03
11	0.01	Agnathia		
6	0.01	Astomia		
18	0.02	Micrognathia		
15	0.02	Protruding tongue		
		Torso		
9	0.01	Anal atresia		
7	0.01	Gastroschisis	5	0.02
5	0.01	Omphalocele	14	0.07
		Spina bifida aperta	8	0.04
13	0.01	Umbilical hernia	9	0.04
		Extremities		
		Clubbed forefoot	8	0.04
		Ectrodactyly	5	0.02
		Forelimb flexion	10	0.05
		Hindlimb rotation	5	0.02
42	0.05	Tail malformation	11	0.05
		Miscellaneous		
27	0.03	Retarded growth		
		Twisted umbilicus	13	0.06

TABLE 12.27
Historical Control Data—Visceral Evaluations[76,77]

Rats			Rabbits	
Visceral — 37,868 Fetuses			Visceral — 19,310 Fetuses	
Incidence	Average (%)		Incidence	Average (%)
		Coronal Sections		
4	0.01	Cerebral ventricular enlargement	15	0.08
7	0.02	Hydrocephalus	10	0.05
7	0.02	Lens agenesis		
8	0.02	Folded retina		
10	0.03	Microphthalmia		
		Circumcorneal hemorrhage	6	0.03
		General		
		Fluid-filled abdominal cavity	6	0.03
		Blood Vessels		
		Enlarged aortic arch	8	0.04
		Interrupted aortic arch	6	0.03
14	0.04	Doubled azygous vein		
		Carotid-branching variation	73	0.38
9	0.03	Carotid-abnormal origin		
		Pulmonary trunk stenosis	6	0.03
16	0.04	Innominate agenesis		
		Subclavian artery-abnormal branch	56	0.39
		Subclavian artery-retroesophageal	10	0.05
		Truncus arteriosus persistent	15	0.08
		Heart		
		Atrium enlarged	8	0.04
5	0.01	Misshapen		
		Ventricular hypertrophy	10	0.05
6	0.02	Ventricular septal defect	19	0.10
		Lung and Trachea		
		Lung-agenesis	156	0.81
		Lung-altered lobation	67	0.35
19	0.05	Hypoplastic	6	0.03
		Liver		
		Altered lobation	12	0.06
		Gallbladder		
		Agenesis	27	0.14
		Hypoplastic	40	0.21
		Misshapen	19	0.10
		Enlarged	17	0.09
		Cystic	6	0.03
		Kidney		
435	1.15	Distended renal pelvis	48	0.25
37	0.10	Hydronephrosis	8	0.04
		Agenesis	12	0.06

TABLE 12.27 *(Continued)*
Historical Control Data—Visceral Evaluations[76,77]

Rats			Rabbits	
Visceral — 37,868 Fetuses			Visceral — 19,310 Fetuses	
Incidence	Average (%)		Incidence	Average (%)
5	0.01	Hemorrhagic displaced	8	0.04
394	1.04	Hypoplastic	6	0.03
		Ureters and Bladder		
76	0.20	Hydroureters		
		Ureter agenesis	6	0.03
348	0.92	Ureter convoluted		
1,087	2.87	Ureter distended	14	0.07
		Retrocaval	48	0.25
32	0.09	Bladder enlarged	5	0.03
		Male Reproductive Tract		
95	0.25	Displaced testis		

TABLE 12.28
Historical Control Data — Skeletal Evaluations[76,77]

Rats			Rabbits	
Skeletal — 41,917 Fetuses			Skeletal — 18,762 Fetuses	
Incidence	Average (%)		Incidence	Average (%)
		Skull		
		Bone island	47	0.25
		Enlarged fontanel	36	0.19
		Hyoid, ala(e) angulated	144	0.27
35	0.08	Hypoplastic interparietals		
10	0.03	Orbits misshapen		
		Intraparietals	6	0.03
31	0.08	Hypoplastic supraoccipitals		
		Sternebrae		
		Agenesis	19	0.10
		Asymmetric	10	0.06
		Duplicated	5	0.03
		Fused	172	0.92
13	0.03	Multiple fusions		
54	0.13	Split	56	0.30
197	0.47	Misaligned	99	0.53
27	0.06	Misshapen		
		Spinal Column		
5	0.01	Vertebral scrambling		
8	0.02	Fused cervical vert.		
9	0.02	Hypoplastic cervical vert.		
13	0.03	Agenesis thoracic vert.	17	0.09
9	0.02	Fused thoracic vert.	21	0.11

TABLE 12.28 *(Continued)*
Historical Control Data — Skeletal Evaluations[76,77]

Rats			Rabbits	
Skeletal — 41,917 Fetuses			Skeletal — 18,762 Fetuses	
Incidence	Average (%)		Incidence	Average (%)
		Hypoplastic thoracic vert.	8	0.04
		Misaligned thoracic vert.	24	0.13
		Hemivert. arch thoracic vert.	10	0.05
218	0.52	Dumbbell-shape thor. centra	38	0.20
268	0.64	Split thoracic centra	23	0.12
		Asymmetric thoracic centra	19	0.10
75	0.18	Misshapen thoracic centra		
		Lumbar Vertebra		
11	0.03	Agenesis	8	0.04
5	0.01	Misaligned	7	0.04
6	0.01	Lumbar centra-dumbbell		
14	0.03	Lumbar centra-split		
		Sacral Vertebra		
33	0.08	Fused		
6	0.02	Misaligned		
		Caudal Vertebra		
6	0.01	Agenesis		
27	0.07	Fused	9	0.05
		Misaligned	32	0.17
		Extra Vertebra		
7	0.02		92	0.49
		Lumbosacral Shift		
8	0.02			
		Missing Vertebra		
23	0.06		6	0.03
		Ribs		
23	0.06	Agenesis	19	0.10
		Branched/split	32	0.17
163	0.39	Cervical	83	0.44
		Clubbed	8	0.04
14	0.03	Fused	56	0.30
390	0.93	Hypoplastic	394	2.10
		Intercostal	10	0.06
113	0.27	Misshapen	9	0.05
1,341	3.21	Supernumerary	3,480	18.55
172	0.41	Wavy	56	0.30
		Thickened	98	0.52
		Short	482	2.57
21	0.05	Bent		
		13 present	615	3.28
		Ischium		
5	0.01	Hypoplastic		

TABLE 12.28 *(Continued)*
Historical Control Data — Skeletal Evaluations[76,77]

Rats			Rabbits	
Skeletal — 41,917 Fetuses			Skeletal — 18,762 Fetuses	
Incidence	Average (%)		Incidence	Average (%)
		Shoulder Girdle		
		Misshapen	16	0.09
		Ala, misshapen	5	0.29
		Appendicular Skeleton Forelimb		
5	0.01	Metacarpal agenesis	12	0.06
88	0.21	Metacarpal hypoplastic		
		Phalanx agenesis	24	0.13
		Hindlimb		
10	0.02	Phalanx agenesis		
18	0.04	Misaligned phalanx		

SECTION 6. GLOSSARY OF TERMS RELATING TO DEVELOPMENTAL TOXICOLOGY

Modified from Middle Atlantic Reproduction and Teratology Association (1989).[78]

GLOSSARY INDEX

I. FETAL AND NEWBORN

A. GENERAL

Aanasarca (edema) generalized accumulation of serum in the intercellular space

Hydramnios excessive amnionic fluid

Monozygotic twins two fetuses derived from one zygote (fertilized ovum); one placenta

Polysomatous monster (polysomus) doubling or tripling of the body of a fetus with each component having all or some of the body parts of a complete individual

    1. **Conjoined twins** double fetal monster ranging from two well-developed individuals (symmetrical conjoined twins) to those in which one incompletely developed fetus (unequal, parasitic twin) is attached to a more completely developed fetus (autosite)

2. **Parasitic twins**   thoracopagus

Rudiment   imperfectly or incompletely developed organ or body part having little or no function but which has functioned at an earlier stage of the same individual or in his ancestors

Subcutaneous hematoma   a circumscribed blood effusion in the subcutaneous tissue

B. HEAD

1. Cranium

Acephaly   congenital absence of the head

Acrania   partial or complete absence of the skull

Anencephaly   congenital absence of the cranial vault with missing or small brain mass

Cephalocele   a protrusion of a part of the cranial contents, not necessarily neural tissue

Craniorhachischisis   exencephaly and holorrachischisis (fissure of the spinal cord)

Cranioschisis   abnormal fissure of the cranium; may be associated with meningocele or encephalocele

Dilatation of lateral ventricle   enlargement of the lateral ventricle due to cerebrospinal fluid pressure; not so severe as to be called hydrocephaly

Domed head   dome-shaped head; may or may not be associated with hydrocephaly

Encephalocele   partial protrusion of brain through an abnormal cranial opening; not as severe as exencephaly

Exencephaly   brain outside of skull as a result of large cranial defect

Hydrocephaly   enlargement of the head caused by abnormal accumulation of cerebrospinal fluid in subarachnoid space (external hydrocephaly) or ventricular system (internal hydrocephaly)

Hydroencephalocele   brain substance expanded into a watery sac protruding through a cleft in the cranium; a hernia through a cranial defect of brain substance and meninges, in which fluid occupies the space between the two

Meningocele   hernial protrusion of the meninges through a defect in the skull

Meningoencephalocele   hernial protrusion of brain and meninges

Microcephaly   small head

2. Face

a. Eyes

Ablepharia   absence or reduction of the eyelid(s)

Aniridia   absence, complete or partial, of the iris

Anophthalmia   absence of eye(s)

Aphakia   failure of the lens to form

Cataract (opaque lens)   opacity of the crystalline lens

Coloboma   a cleft in the iris, ciliary body, choroid, or lids

Cyclopia   one central orbital fossa with none, one, or two globes

Exophthalmos   protrusion of the eyeball ("pop" eye)

Folded retina   detachment of the retina from the choroid

Macrophthalmia (buphthalmos)   enlarged eye(s)

Microphthalmia   small eye(s)

Open eye(s)   split or unfused eyelid(s); may be due to ablepharia

b. Ear (Pinna)

Anotia   absence of the external ear(s)

Ectopic pinna   displaced external ear

1. **Low set ear(s)**   low placement of the external ear

Microtia small external ear
Otocephaly absence of the lower jaw and ears united below the face
Synotia persistence of the external ears beneath the mandible

c. Nose

Absent or micro concha nasalis [enlarged nasal, turbinate(s)] See "Enlarged nasal turbinate(s)"
Arrhinia absence of nose
Enlarged nasal turbinate(s) Enlargement of the nasal passage(s) due to absent or micro concha
     nasalis
Naris (nostril) atresia absence or closure of nares
Nasal agenesis absence of the nasal cavity and external nose
Nasal atresia see "Naris (nostril) atresia"
Rhinocephaly a developmental anomaly characterized by the presence of a proboscis-like nose
     above the eyes, partially or completely fused into one
Septal agenesis absence of nasal septum
Single nostril single external naris

d. Mouth/Jaws

Aglossia absence of the tongue
Agnathia absence of lower jaw (mandible)
Astomia absence of oral orifice
Bifid tongue cleft tongue
Cheilognathopalatoschisis a cleft in the hard and soft palate, upper jaw and lip
Cleft face incomplete fusion of embryonic processes which normally unite in the formation of
     the face or one of its parts
Cleft lip incomplete fusion of the lip
Cleft palate incomplete fusion of the palatine shelves
High-arched palate a higher than normal palatal arch
Macroglossia enlarged tongue, usually protruding
Median facial cleft affects lips and maxilla or palate
Micrognathia shortened lower jaw (mandible); tongue may protrude
Microstomia small mouth opening
Protruding tongue tongue protruding from the mouth opening; could be the result of macro-
     glossia or micrognathia
Schistoglossia cleft tongue

C. TRUNK

1. General

Achondroplasia a hereditary defect in the formation of epiphysial cartilage, resulting in a form
     of dwarfism with short limbs, normal trunk, small face, normal vault, etc.
Exomphalos congenital herniation of abdominal viscera into umbilical cord
Gastroschisis fissure of abdominal wall (median line) not involving the umbilicus, usually
     accompanied by protrusion of the small and part of the large intestine, not covered by
     membranous sac
Omphalocele midline defect in the abdominal wall at the umbilicus, through which the intes-
     tines and often other viscera (stomach, spleen, and portions of the liver) protrude. These
     are always covered by a membranous sac. As a rule, the umbilical cord emerges from
     the top of the sac
    1. **Umbilical eventration** see "Umbilical hernia"

Situs inversus viscernum (totalis or partialis) total or partial transposition of viscera (due to incomplete rotation) to the other side of the body; heart most commonly affected (dextrocardia)

Thoracogastroschisis midline fissure in the thorax and abdomen

Thoracoschisis fissure of the chest wall

Umbilical hernia protrusion of viscera at the navel, covered by skin

2. Esophagus/Trachea

Ectopic esophagus displacement of the esophagus (description of position should be included)

Esophageal atresia discontinuity of the esophageal lumen usually associated with tracheoesophageal fistula

Esophageal stenosis constriction or narrowing of the esophageal lumen

Tracheal stenosis constriction or narrowing of the tracheal lumen

Tracheoesophageal fistula communication between esophageal and tracheal lumen

3. Heart/Major Vessels

Abnormal origin of right common carotid and right subclavian artery both arteries directly off the arch, associated with absence of innominate artery

Acardia absence of the heart

Atrioventricular (A-V) septal defect a defect that results in communication between an atrium and ventricle

Atrioventricular ostium (orifice) enlarged enlargement of an atrioventricular orifice

Atrioventricular valve enlarged see above

Cardiomegaly hypertrophy (enlargement) of the heart

Cor biloculare two-chambered heart

Cor triloculare three-chambered heart

Dextrocardia location of the heart in the right side of the thorax; a developmental disorder that is associated with total or partial situs inversus (transposition of the great vessels and other thoracoabdominal organs) or occurs as an isolated anomaly

    1. **Secondary dextrocardia** displacement of the heart to the right side of the thorax as a result of disease of the pleura, diaphragm, or lungs

Ectocardia displacement of the heart inside or outside the thorax

    1. **Ectopic cordis** displacement of heart outside of thorax caused by a failure of the midline to close (sternal cleft)

Enlarged pericardial sac enlargement of the sac (cavity) which envelops the heart

Exocardia abnormal position of the heart

Inferior vena cava defect

    1. **Dilated** lumen of the inferior vena cava enlarged or expanded

    2. **Displaced** inferior vena cava out of normal position

Levocardia displacement of the heart in the extreme left hemithorax

Innominate artery agenesis absence of the innominate artery (which normally arises from the arch of the aorta), associated with separate origin of the right common carotid artery and the right subclavial artery from the aortic arch

Interatrial septal defect (Foramen ovale apertum) A defect that results in communication between the atria. This defect is produced by abnormal development of the septum primum and septum secundum

Interventricular septal defect a defect of the septum between the ventricles of the heart; usually located at its membranous (superior) portion

Monocardium possessing a heart with only one atrium and one ventricle

Patent ductus arteriosus (ductus botalli) an open channel of communication between the main pulmonary artery and the aorta, may occur as an isolated abnormality or in combination with other heart defects

Right-sided descending aorta an aorta descending on the right side instead of the left side

Situs inversus see below

      1. **Cardiovascular situs inversus**   mirror-image transposition of the heart and vessels to the other side of the body

Teratology of Fallot an abnormality of the heart which includes pulmonary stenosis, ventricular septal defect, dextraposition of the aorta overriding the ventricular septum and receiving blood from both ventricles, right ventricular hypertrophy

Transposition of great vessels the aorta originates from the right ventricle whereas the pulmonary artery arises from the left ventricle; often associated with interventricular septal defect or a patent ductus ateriosus

Truncus communis a common aortic and pulmonary truncus; usually associated with other heart/vessels defects

4.   Lung

Agenesis of the lung (lobe) complete absence of a lobe of the lung

Aplasia of the lung the trachea shows rudimentary bronchi but pulmonary and vascular structures are absent

Atelectasis incomplete expansion of the lungs (or portion of the lung) at birth; collapse of pulmonary alveoli during postnatal life

Hypoplasia of the lung bronchial tree poorly developed and pulmonary tissue shows an abnormal histologic picture (total or partial); incomplete development, smaller

Unilobular lung in the rat fetus, a condition in which the right lung consists of one lobe instead of four separate lobes

5.   Abdomen/Abdominal Viscera

a.   Diaphragm

Diaphragmatic eventration elevation of the dome of the diaphragm

Diaphragmatic hernia diaphragmatocele protrusion of viscera, usually liver or intestine, through a defect in the diaphragm

b.   Stomach

Agastria absence of the stomach

Dextragastria having the stomach on the right side of the body

Gastromegaly abnormal enlargement of the stomach

c.   Liver

Hepatic lobe agenesis absence of a lobe of the liver

Hepatomegaly abnormal enlargement of the liver

Multilobular liver greater than normal number of liver lobes

d.   Gallbladder

Agenesis of gallbladder absence of the gallbladder. Note: Rats do not have a gallbladder

Multiple gallbladder more than one gallbladder (can be bilobed)

e.   Intestines

Agenesis of intestine absence of the intestine or section thereof

f. Kidneys

Absent or reduced renal papilla absent or smaller than usual apex of a Malpighian pyramid in the kidney

Agenesis of the kidney absence of the kidney(s)

Dilatation of renal pelvis abnormal distention of the pelvis due to urine retention or delayed development of renal papilla

Double kidney duplication of the renal pelvis and ureter in one kidney [in some cases the separation of the duplicated organ is incomplete (fused supernumerary kidney)]

Ectopic kidneys a congenital anomaly in which the kidney(s) is located in an abnormal position

    1. **Pelvic kidney**   location of the kidney in the pelvic region

Enlarged kidney(s) larger than normal size

Fused kidneys fusion of both kidneys

    1. **Cake (lump) kidney**   extreme fusion in which both kidneys unite to form one kidney

    2. **Disk (donut) kidney**   fusion of both the upper and lower poles

    3. **Horseshoe kidney**   fusion of the lower poles (common) or the upper poles (rare)

    4. **Sigmoid kidney**   fusion of the lower pole with the upper pole of the contralateral kidney

Hydronephrosis dilatation of the renal pelvis usually combined with destruction of renal parenchyma and often with dilatation of the ureters (bilateral, unilateral) (note: this is a pathology term and should have histological confirmation)

Renal hypoplasia incomplete development of the kidney

Supernumerary kidney a "kidney" in addition to the two usually present

g. Ureters

Aplasia of the ureter failure of the ureter(s) to develop

Convoluted ureters twisting (coiling) of the ureter(s)

h. Adrenals

Adrenal agenesis absence of the adrenal(s)

Adrenal hypoplasia underdeveloped adrenal(s)

Enlarged adrenals (adrenal hyperplasia, hypertrophy) larger than normal-sized adrenal(s)

i. Spleen

Accessory spleen an additional spleen

Asplenia absence of the spleen

Enlarged spleen larger than normal size

6. Urinary Bladder/Gonads/Anus

a. Urinary Bladder

Acystia absence of the urinary bladder

b. Gonads

Anorchism congenital absence of one or both testes

Cryptorchidism (undescended testes, ectopic testes) failure of the testes to descend into the scrotum (can be unilateral)

Hermaphroditism presence of both male and female sex organs in one individual

Hypospadias urethra opening on the underside of the penis or on the perineum (males), or into the vagina (females)

Pseudohermaphroditism possession of the sex organs of one sex (ovary or testis) but accompanied by some secondary sexual characteristics and external genitalia more or less similar to those of the opposite sex

c. Anus

Anal atresia congenital absence of the anus

Aproctia imperforation or absence of anus

Imperforate anus persistence of the anal membrane, so that the anus is closed (often associated with atresia of the lower portion of the rectum)

D. Skeletal System

1. General

Agenesis absence

Asymmetrical lack of correspondence in size, shape, or position of a pair of bones or bone parts on both sides of the median plane

Bent slightly curved

Bipartite ossification two ossification sites visible

Displaced (malpositioned) out of normal position

Duplicated a doubling

Fused bones joining of bones which should not be joined

Incomplete ossification (delayed, retarded) extent of ossification is less than what would be expected for that developmental age; not necessarily associated with reduced fetal or pup weight

Irregular ossification uneven calcification of cartilage matrix; abnormal sequence in appearance of ossification sites

Misshapen bones bone which differs in shape from normal

Missing absent

Rotated turning or tipping of a structure with the center of the point maintained

Shortened reduced in length

Thickened increased in extent from one surface to the opposite one

Unossified absence of ossification; existing structure present as a cartilagious or membraneous element

2. Skull

See "General" (Section 1)

Angulated hyoid abnormally shaped hyoid, in which greater cornua forms sharper than normal angles with hyoid body

3. Vertebrae

See "General" (Section 1)

Extra vertebrae in excess of the normal number of vertebrae

Hemivertebra presence of only one-half of a vertebral body

Lordosis anterior concavity in the curvature of the cervical and lumbar spine as viewed from the side

Lumbosacral shift condition when the lowest lumbar arch is aligned with the first sacral arch

Rachischisis absence of vertebral arches in limited area (partial rachischisis) or entirely (rachischisis totalis)

Scoliosis appreciable lateral curvature of the vertebral column

Spina bifida defect in closure of bony spinal canal

> 1. **Spinal bifida cystica** spina bifida associated with spinal cord and (Aperta) meninges' protrusion

2. **Spina bifida occulta** opening covered by skin; no protrusion of the spinal cord or meninges

4. Centra

See "General" (Section 1)
Dumbbell two ossification centers connected by a narrow isthmus
Hemicentra ossification of only one site within a centrum

5. Sternebrae

See "General" (Section 1)
Asymmetrical ossification sites are uneven, but not in a set pattern
Checkerboard ossification centers are bipartite and staggered giving checkerboard pattern
Hemisternebrae incomplete or accessory development of one side of a sternebral body

6. Ribs

See "General" (Section 1)
Bulbous having a bulge or balloon-like enlargement somewhere along its length
Displaced out of normal position
Rudimentary imperfectly developed rib-like structure
Short less than one-half the size of a normal rib
Thickened having a wide appearance
Wavy having curves; an undulating pattern

7. Extremities

See "General" (Section 1)
Abasophalangia absence of the proximal phalanx
Abrachius without arms, forelimbs
Adactyly absence of digits
Amelia see ectromelia
Amesophalangy absence of medial phalanx
Ankylosis inflexible, stiff joint
Aphalangia absence of a finger or a toe; corresponding metacarpals not affected
Apodia absence of one or both feet
Arthrogryposis persistent flexure or contracture of a joint; flexed paw (bent at wrist) is most common form of arthrogryposis
    1. **Dorsiflexed (hyperextension)** flexed dorsally
    2. **Plantar-flexed (hyperflexion)** flexed ventrally
Atelephalangy absence of a distal phalanx
Bowing of hindlimbs a bending outward of the limb(s)
Brachydactyly shortened digits
Club foot foot twisted out of shape or position, pes contortus, talipes
Dysmelia absence of a portion of one or several limbs
Ectrodactyly absence of all or of only a part of digit (partial ectrodactyly)
Ectromelia aplasia or hypoplasia of one or more bones of one or more limbs (this term includes amelia, hemimelia, and phocomelia)
Hemimelia absence of all or part of the distal half of a limb; could be: radial h., ulnar h., fibular h., or tibial hemimelia

Hyperflexed limbs excessive flexion of a limb
Macrobrachia abnormal size or length of the arm
Macrodactylia excessive size of one or more digits
Oligodactyly fewer than normal number of digits
Peromelia congenital absence or deformity of the terminal part of a limb or limbs
Phocomelia absence of proximal portion of limb(s) with the paws being attached to the trunk
    of the body by a single small irregularly shaped bone
Polydactyly extra digits
Sympodia (syrenomelus, sympus) fusion of the lower extremities
Synarthrosis a form of articulation, almost immobile, in which the bony elements are united
    by fibrous tissue
Syndactyly partially or entirely fused digits
Synmetacarpals/synmetatarsals fused metacarpals or metatarsals

8. Tail

Acaudia (anury) agenesis of the tail
Brachyury (short tail) tail that is reduced in length
Coiled tail tail with a spiral curvature
Curled tail tail with a "curved" type of bend
Filamentous threadlike
Fleshy tab filamentous extension from the tip of an otherwise normal tail
Kinked tail tail with a distinct bend
Rudimentary tail tail that exists only as a fleshy element

II. PARENTAL

A. MATERNAL

1. General

Abortifacient an agent which causes abortion
Abortion the premature expulsion from the uterus of the products of conception; of the embryo
    or of a nonviable fetus
Estrus phase of the sexual cycle of female mammals characterized by willingness to mate
Fecundity ability to produce offspring rapidly and in large numbers
Fertility capacity to conceive or induce conception
Infertility absence of the ability to conceive or to induce conception
Parity condition of a female with respect to the number of pregnancy(ies) which resulted in
    viable born offspring

2. Mammary Glands

Lactation (a) the secretion of milk; (b) the period of the secretion of milk
Supernumerary mammae accessory breast tissue and/or nipples (teats); mammae accessoriae

3. Vagina

Vaginal plug a mass of coagulated semen which forms in the vagina of animals after coitus;
    also called copulation plug or bouchon vaginal

4. Uterus

Ametria congenital absence of the uterus

Feticide the destruction of the fetus in the uterus
Hydrometra (uterine dropsy) excess fluid (clear, colorless) in the uterus
Pyometra pus within the uterus
Uterus the hollow muscular organ in female animals in which the developing embryo and fetus
     is nourished

5. Ovaries

Corpus luteum (corpora lutea, pl.) the yellow endocrine body formed in the ovary at the site
     of the ruptured graafian follicle
Follicle small excretory or secretory sac or gland
    1. **Atretic** a graafian follicle which has involuted
    2. **Graafian** a small spherical vesicular sac embedded in the cortex of the ovary, which
       contains an egg cell or ovum. Each follicle contains a liquid, liquor ovarii, and
       produces hormone folliculin or estrin
    3. **Ovarian** the egg and its encasing cells at any stage of its development
    4. **Primordial** an ovarian follicle consisting of an undeveloped egg enclosed by a
       single layer of cells
Luteal pertaining to or having the properties of the corpus luteum, its cells, or its hormone
Luteinic (a) pertaining to or having the properties of the corpus luteum; (b) pertaining to
     luteinization
Luteinization the process taking place in the follicular cells of graafian follicles which have
     matured and discharged their egg; the cells become hypertrophied and assume a yellow
     color, the follicles becoming corpora lutea

6. Pregnancy

Ectopic pregnancy implantation (and possible development) of a blastocyst outside of the
     uterine cavity
Multigravida a female pregnant for the second (or more) time
Multipara a female that has had two or more pregnancies which resulted in birth of viable
     offspring
Nulliparous a female that never has born viable offspring
Pseudopregnancy (a) false pregnancy: condition occurring in animals in which anatomical and
     physiological changes occur similar to those of pregnancy; (b) the premenstrual stage
     of the endometrium so called because it resembles the endometrium just before implan-
     tation of the blastocyst
Unigravida (primigravida) a female pregnant for the first time
Unipara (primipara) a female who has borne only one offspring
Uniparental pertaining to one of the parents only
Uniparous (primiparous) producing only one ovum or offspring at one time

7. Parturition

Delivery expulsion or extraction of the fetus and placenta at birth
Parturition the act or process of giving birth
Dystocia abnormal labor
Labor function of female organism by which the product of conception is expelled from the
     uterus through the vagina to the outside world
    1. **Complicated** labor in which convulsions, hemorrhage, or some other untoward
       event occurs
    2. **Delayed** labor which occurs later than the expected date

3. **Premature (early)**   labor which occurs before the normal end of gestation

Perinatal occurring shortly before, during, or shortly after birth

Postparturition (postpartum) after birth, or after delivery

8. Products of Conception

Blastocyst the mammalian conceptus in the postmorula stage

Conceptus the sum of derivatives of a fertilized ovum at any stage of development from fertilization until birth

Implantation (nidation) attachment of the blastocyst to the epithelial lining of the uterus, including its penetration through the uterine epithelium, and its embedding in the endometrium

Morula the solid mass of blastomeres (embryonic cells) formed by cleavage of a fertilized ovum

9. Placental Membranes

Amniochorial pertaining to the amnion and chorion

Amnion the inner of the fetal membranes; a thin, transparent sac which holds the fetus suspended in the amniotic fluid

Chorion the outermost of the fetal membranes, consisting of an outer trophoblastic epithelium lined internally by extraembryonic mesoderm; its villous portion, vascularized by allantoic blood vessels, forms the placenta

Oligohydramnios (oligoamnios) reduction in the amount of amniotic fluid

Polyhydramnios excessive amount of amniotic fluid

Yolk sac an extraembryonic membrane composed of endoderm and splanchnic mesoderm; it is the organ in which the first red blood cells are formed. In rodents, it is the primary absorptive surface (gut) prior to formation of the placenta.

10. Ova

Gamete a male (spermatozoon) or female (ovum) reproductive cell

Implantation (nidation) attachment of the blastocyst to the epithelial lining of the uterus, including its penetration through the uterine epithelium, and its embedding in the endometrium

11. Embryo

Conceptus the whole product of fertilization until birth; the embryo or fetus and the extraembryonic membranes

Embryogenesis the growth and development of the embryo

Embryogenic (a) pertaining to the development of the embryo; (b) producing an embryo

Embryo the early or developing stage of any organism, especially the developing product of fertilization of an egg after the long axis appears and until all major structures are presented

Embryonal pertaining to embryo

Embryonic pertaining to the embryo as defined above

Embryopathology the science of abnormal embryos or of defective development

Extraembryonic not occurring as a part of the embryo proper; applied specifically to the fetal membranes

Presomite embryos before the appearance of somites

Somite one of the paired masses of mesoderm arranged segmentally alongside the neural tube of the embryo, forming the vertebral column and segmental musculature

Teratoma a tumor containing a disorderly arrangement of tissues and organs, as a result of faulty embryonic differentiation and organization produced through abnormal inductive influences

12. Fetus

Conjoined twins a double fetal monster, ranging from two well-developed individuals joined by a superficial connection of varying extent, to those in which only a small part of the body is duplicated

Fetal pertaining to a fetus

Fetoplacental pertaining to the fetus and placenta

Fetus the unborn offspring in the postembryonic period

Neonatal pertaining to a newborn offspring (in the human, the first 4 weeks of life)

Neonate newly born; a newborn offspring

Polysomia a doubling or tripling of the body of a fetus

Teras a fetal monster (plural: terata)

B. Paternal

1. General

Androgen a class of steroid hormones produced in the gonads and adrenal cortex that regulate masculine sexual characteristics

Cycle of the seminiferous epithelium the complete series of successive cellular associations occurring in the seminiferous epithelium

Daily spermatozoal production the total number of sperm produced per day by the two testes

Duration of spermatogenesis the interval between the time a stem spermatogonium becomes committed to produce spermatozoa and its subsequent release from the germinal epithelium into the lumen (about 72 days in the human and fewer in most animals)

Efficiency of spermatozoal production the number of sperm produced per day per gram of testicular parenchyma

Ejaculate the total seminal sample obtained during ejaculation

Ejaculation the expulsion of semen through the urethra

Fecundate (fertilize) to impregnate

Meiosis cell division occurring in maturation of the sex cells (gametes) by means of which each daughter nucleus receives half the number of chromosomes characteristic of the somatic cells of the species

Nonmotile spermatozoon a sperm that does not move a discernible distance during visual observation

Percentage of motile sperm the percentage of sperm that are motile, regardless of pattern (progressive, circular, or backward)

Percentage of progressively motile sperm the percentage of sperm that move forward (excluding circularly motile and backward motile sperm)

Semen a mixture of sperm and fluids from the excurrent ducts and accessory sex glands

Seminiferous epithelium the normal cellular components within the seminiferous tubule consisting of Sertoli cells, spermatogonia, primary spermatocytes, secondary spermtocytes, and spermatids

Sertoli cells cells in the testicular tubules providing support, protection, and nutrition for the spermatids

Sperm morphology the characteristic features (shape, form) comprising sperm

Spermatogenetic cellular stage one of a series of characteristic cellular groupings of different types of germ cells found in a specific area of a seminiferous tubule

Spermatocytogenesis the first stage of spermatogenesis in which spermatogonia develop into
    spermatocytes and then into spermatids

Spermatogenesis the process of formation of spermatozoa, including spermatocytogenesis and
    spermiogenesis

Spermiation the second stage of spermatogenesis in which the spermatids transform into
    spermatozoa

Spermiogenesis the second stage of spermatogenesis in which the spermatids transform into
    spermatozoa

Testosterone the hormone produced by the interstitial cells of the testes, which functions in
    the induction and maintenance of male secondary sex characteristics

Total spermatozoa the total number of spermatozoa in an ejaculate

III. MODIFYING TERMINOLOGY

A. Development

Agenesis absence of an organ or part of an organ

Anomaly (anomalous) any deviation (malformation or variation) from the norm

Aplasia lack of development of an organ, frequently used to designate complete suppression
    or failure of development of a structure from the embryonic primordium

Bifurcate forked

Bifurcation (a) division into two branches; (b) site where a single structure divides into two

Bilobate having two lobes

Defect an imperfection

    1. **Acquired** an imperfection gained secondarily after birth, not hereditary or innate

    2. **Congenital** an imperfection present at birth, due to abnormal embryonic development

Deflection a turning, or state of being turned, aside

Deformity distortion of any part or general disfigurement of the body

Development gradual growth or expansion, especially from a lower to a higher stage of
    complexity

    1. **Arrested** cessation of the developmental process at some stage before its normal
       completion

    2. **Postnatal** that which occurs after birth

    3. **Prenatal** that which occurs before birth

    4. **Regulative** the development of an embryo; the determination of the various organs
       and parts being gradually attained through the action of inductors

Deviation variation from the regular standard or course

Dislocation the displacement of any part from the original position

Displacement removal from the normal position or place; ectopia

Diverticulum a pouch or pocket leading off a main cavity or tube

Dysgenesis defective development; malformation

Dysplasia (a) abnormal development of tissue; (b) alteration in size, shape, or organization of
    adult cells

Ectopic out of the normal place

Evagination an outpouching of a layer or part

Fissure any cleft or grove, normal or abnormal

Imperforate not open; abnormally closed

Macro (prefix) meaning large

Malformation defective or abnormal formation; deformity. A permanent structural deviation
    which generally is incompatible with, or severely detrimental to, normal survival or
    development

Malposition abnormal or anomalous position

Micro (prefix) meaning small

Morphogenesis the various processes occurring during development by which the shape and the structure of a particular organ or part of the body is established

Morphology the science of the form and structure of an organism, or any of its parts, without regard to function

Pendulous hanging loosely; swinging freely

Variation a minor divergence beyond the usual range of structural constitution

B. CONSISTENCY

Maceration the softening of a solid by soaking. In obstetrics, the degenerative changes with discoloration and softening of tissues, and eventual disintegration of a conceptus retained in the uterus after its death.

Mummification conversion into a state resembling that of a mummy, such as occurs in dry gangrene, or the shriveling and drying up of a dead fetus

Pachynsis abnormal thickening

C. COLOR

Albinic unpigmented, having no color

Albinism congenital absence of pigment in the skin, hair, and eye; may be total or partial

Cyanosis bluish discoloration, applied especially to skin and mucous membranes

Icteroid (ictericious) having a yellow hue; seemingly jaundiced

IV. COMMON LABORATORY TERMS

A. GENERAL

Aberration a minor structural change. It may be a retardation (a provisional delay in morphogenesis), a variation (external appearance controlled by genetic and extragenetic factors), or a deviation (resulting from altered differentiation).

Abortion the termination of pregnancy before the conceptus is capable of *ex utero* survival

Anomaly or abnormality a morphologic or functional deviation from normal limits. It can be a malformation or a variation.

Average pup (fetus) weight Total weight of living pups (fetuses) in litter/number of living pups (fetuses) in litter

Birth delivery at term

Cannibalism the eating of one's own kind, frequently observed in the postpartum period of rabbits or rats

Conceptus term used when the stage of prenatal development at the time of initial insult is not known; also referred to as *embryo-fetus*

Day "0" of lactation usually referred to as "postpartum day 0" day of birth

Day "0" of pregnancy day on which positive evidence of mating has been ascertained

Dead fetus a nonliving fetus *in utero*

Developmental toxicity any adverse effect on development (morphologic, physiologic, or functional) initiated prenatally and appearing during the lifetime of the progency

Embryo-fetus used when the stage of prenatal development at the time of conception is not known; also referred to as conceptus

Embryotoxicity signifies embryonic loss during the early preimplantation or postimplantation stages of pregnancy

Fetotoxicity any prenatally initiated toxic manifestation observed in a fetus (death, body weight reduction, delayed ossification, or functional defect), which may or may not be related to toxic effects in the mother and which, although initiated *in utero,* appears during prenatal or postnatal development. Any of these effects resulting from the direct action of a test agent on the embryo or fetus (as defined in Dorland's *Medical Dictionary*) and occurring at doses far below those toxic for the mother should be regarded as suggestive of true, or selective, embryo- or fetotoxicity.

Maternal toxicity transitory or permanent pathologic state of health or alteration in maternal physiology and/or behavior with the potential to cause adverse effects in the offspring during embryofetal or postnatal development

Positive evidence of mating sperm or semen plug in vagina

Postpartum after delivery

Pregnant an animal with uterine evidence of implantation or an animal which delivers a conceptus

Premature birth birth before expected time but capable of surviving *ex utero*

Reproductive toxicity deals with toxic effects on any aspect of reproduction of offspring proceeding from the development of gametes and their fusion

Resorption a conceptus which, having implanted in the uterus, subsequently died and is being or has been resorbed
   1. **Early** evidence of implantation without recognizable embryo/fetus
   2. **Late** dead embryo or fetus with external degenerative changes

Retarded development an organ, fetus, or newborn which has not developed concomitantly with its chronological age

Retarded growth growth of fetus or neonate which is not concomitant with chronological age; small for age

Runt normally developed fetus or newborn that is significantly smaller than the rest of the litter

Stillbirth birth of dead fetus

Teratogen an intrinsic or extrinsic factor or an alteration in maternal homeostasis that induces, during prenatal development, a permanent structural or functional abnormality in the fetus, which is detected in a prenatal or postnatal examination. If malformations are induced at apparently nonmaternotoxic doses, the agent is a true, or selective, teratogen.

Term the expected date of birth

Threshold level the highest level of a chemical or test substance, obtained by the best possible estimates from experimental data, that is judged insufficient to produce an adverse effect on prenatal and postnatal development in humans or animals

Weaning date day on which animal is separated from its mother

REFERENCES

1. Johnson, E.M., The effects of riboviron on development and reproduction: A critical review of published and unpublished studies in experimental animals, *J. Am. Coll. Toxicol.,* 9, 551, 1990.
2. Khera, K.S., Grice, H.C., and Clegg, D.J., *Current Issues in Toxicology: Interpretation and Extrapolation of Reproductive Data to Establish Human Safety Standards,* Springer-Verlag, New York, 1989.
3. Ecobichon, D.J., *The Basis of Toxicity Testing,* CRC Press, Boca Raton, FL, 1992.
4. Johnson, E.M., Perspectives in reproductive and developmental toxicity, *Toxicol. Ind. Health,* 2, 453–482, 1986.
5. Kury, G., Chaube, S., and Murphy, M.L., Teratogenic effects of some purine analogues on fetal rats, *Arch. Pathol.,* 86, 395, 1968.
6. Murphy, M.L. and Karnofsky, D.A., Effect of azaserine and other growth inhibiting agents on fetal development of the rat, *Cancer,* 9, 955, 1956.

7. Murphy, M.L., Dagg, C.P., and Karnofsky, D.A., Comparison of teratogenic chemicals in the rat and chick embryos, *Pediatrics,* 19, 701, 1957.

8. Sunderman, F.W., Jr., Allpass, P.R., Mitchell, J.M., Baslet, R.C., and Albert, D.M., Eye malformations in rats: Induction by prenatal exposure to nickel carbonyl, *Sci.,* 203, 550, 1979.

9. Andrew, F.D. and Staples, R.E., Prenatal toxicity of medroxyprogesterone acetate in rabbits, rats and mice, *Teratol.,* 15, 25, 1977.

10. Khera, K.S., *N,N*-Ethylenethiourea: Teratogenic study in rats and rabbits, *Teratol.,* 7, 243, 1973.

11. Khera, K.S. and Tryphonas, L., Ethylenethiourea-induced hydrocephalus: Pre- and postnatal pathogenesis in rats given a single oral dose during pregnancy, *Toxicol. Appl. Pharmacol.,* 42, 85, 1977.

12. Khera, K.S., Villeneuve, D.C., Terry, G., Panopio, L., Nash, L., and Trivett, G., Mirex: A teratogenicity, dominant lethal and tissue distribution study in rats, *Food Cosmet. Toxicol.,* 14, 25, 1976.

13. Grabowski, C. and Payne, D.B., An electrocardiographic study of cardiovascular problems in Mirex-fed rat fetuses, *Teratol.,* 22, 167, 1980.

14. DiCarlo, F.J., Jr., Syndromes of cardiovascular malformations induced by copper citrate in hamsters, *Teratol.,* 21, 89, 1980.

15. Shah, R.M. and Chaudhry, A.P., Hydrocortisone-induced cleft palate in hamsters, *Teratol.,* 7, 191, 1973.

16. Thompson, D.J., Molello, J.A., and Strebing, R.J., Teratogenicity of adriamycin and daunomycin in the rat and rabbit, *Teratol.,* 17, 151, 1978.

17. Aliverti, V., Bonanomi, L., Giavini, E., Leone, V.G., and Mariam, L., Effects of glycerol formal on embryonic development in the rat, *Toxicol. Appl. Pharmacol.,* 56, 93, 1980.

18. Walker, B.E., Induction of cleft palate in rats with antiinflammatory drugs, *Teratology,* 4, 39, 1971.

19. Hayes, W.C., Cobel-Geard, S.R., Hanley, T.R., Jr., Murray, J.S., Freshour, N.L., Rao, K.S., and John, J.A., Teratogenic effects of vitamin A palmitate in Fischer 344 Rats, *Drug Chem. Toxicol.,* 4, 283, 1981.

20. Wilson, J.G., *Environment and Birth Defects,* Academic Press, New York, 1973.

21. Wilson, J.B., Embryotoxicity of drugs in man, in *Handbook of Teratology,* Wilson, J.G. and Fraser, F.C., Eds., chap. 8, pp. 309–355, Plenum Press, New York, 1977.

22. Spence, A.A. and Knill-Jones, R.P., Is there a health hazard in anaesthetic practice?, *Br. J. Anaesth.,* 50, 713, 1978.

23. Vessey, M.P. and Nunn, J.F., Occupational hazards of anaesthesia, *Br. Med. J.,* 281, 696, 1980.

24. Hemminki, K., Mutanen, P., Saloniemi, I., Niema, M.L., and Vainio, H., Spontaneous abortions in hospital staff engaged in sterilizing instruments with chemical agents, *Br. Med. J.,* 285, 1461, 1982.

25. Hemminki, K., Franssila, E., and Vainio, H., Spontaneous abortions among female chemical workers in Finland, *Int. Arch. Occup. Environ. Health,* 45, 123, 1980.

26. Holmberg, P.C., Central-nervous-system defects in children born to mothers exposed to organic solvents during pregnancy, *Lancet,* ii, 177, 1979.

27. Murray, F.J., John, J.A., Balmer, M.F., and Schwetz, B.A., Teratologic evaluation of styrene given to rats and rabbits by inhalation or by gavage, *Toxicol.,* 11, 335, 1978.

28. Barlow, S.M. and Sullivan, F.M., *Reproductive Hazards of Industrial Chemicals: An Evaluation of Animal and Human Data,* Academic Press, London, 1982.

29. Bercovici, B., Wassermann, M., Cucos, S., Ron, M., Wassermann, D., and Pines, A., Serum levels of polycholorinated biphenyls and some organochlorinated insecticides in women with recent and former missed abortions, *Environ. Res.,* 28, 169, 1983.

30. Wassermann, M., Ron, M., Bercovici, B., Wassermann, D., Cucos, S., and Pines, A., Premature delivery and organochlorine compounds: polychlorinated biphenyls and some organochlorine insecticides, *Environ. Res.,* 28, 106, 1982.

31. World Health Organization (WHO), *Lead,* Environmental Health Criteria, 2, U.N. Environment Program and World Health Organization, Geneva, 1977.

32. Fahim, M.S., Fahim, Z., and Hall, D.G., Effects of subtoxic lead levels on pregnant women in the state of Missouri, *Res. Commun. Chem. Pathol. Pharmacol.,* 13, 309, 1976.

33. O'Leary, J.A., Davies, J.E., Edmundson, W.F., and Feldman, M., Correlation of prematurity and DDE levels in fetal whole blood, in *Epidemiology of DDT,* Davies, J.F. and Edmundsen, W.F., Eds., Futura Publishing, Mount Kisco, New York, 1972, 55.

34. Herbst, A.L., Ulfelder, H., and Poskanzer, D.C., Adenocarcinoma of the vagina: Association of maternal stilbestrol therapy with tumor appearance in young women, *N. Engl. J. Med.,* 284, 878, 1971.

35. Gill, W.B., Schumacher, G.F.B., and Bibo, M., Pathological semen and anatomical abnormalities of the genital tract in human male subjects exposed to diethylstilbestrol in utero, *J. Urol.*, 117, 447, 1977.

36. Tsubaki, T. and Irukayama, K., *Methylmercury Poisoning in Minamata and Niigata, Japan,* Elsevier Press, Amsterdam, 1977.

37. Infante, P.F., Oncogenic and mutagenic risks in communities with polyvinyl chloride production facilities, *Ann. N.Y. Acad. Sci.,* 271, 49, 1979.

38. Carmelli, D., Hofherr, J., Tomsic, J., and Morgan, R.W., A case-control study of the relations between exposure to 2, 4-D and spontaneous abortions in humans, *SRI International, 1981.*

39. Nordstrom, S., Beckman, L., and Nordenson, I., Occupational and environmental risks in and around a smelter in northern Sweden. V. Spontaneous abortion among female employees and decreased birth weight in their offspring, *Hereditas,* 90, 291, 1979.

40. Goodman, L.S. and Gilman, R., *The Pharmacological Basis of Therapeutics. A Textbook of Pharmacology, Toxicology and Therapeutics for Physicians and Medical Students,* 4th ed., MacMillan, New York, 1970.

41. McEvoy, G.K. and McQuarrie, G.W., *American Hospital Formulatory Service,* American Society of Hospital Pharmacists, Bethesda, MD, 1984.

42. Spector, W.S., *Handbook of Biological Data,* WADC Technical Report 56–273, 1956.

43. Beck, F. and Lloyd, J.B., Comparative placental transfer, in *Handbook of Teratology,* Wilson, J.G. and Fraser, F.D., Eds., chap. 5, pp. 155–183, Plenum Press, New York, 1977.

44. Dawes, G.S., *Foetal and Neonatal Physiology: A Comparative Study of the Changes at Birth,* Year Book Medical Publishers, Chicago, 1968.

45. Hafez, E.S.E., *Reproduction in Farm Animals,* Lea & Febiger, Philadelphia, 1968.

46. Hoar, R.M. and Monie, I.W., Comparative development of specific organ systems, in *Developmental Toxicology,* Kimmel, C.A. and Buelke-Sam, J., Eds., Raven Press, New York, 1981, 13.

47. O'Rahilly, R., *Development Stages in Human Embryos. Part A: Embryos of First Three Weeks (Stages 1–9) Publication 631,* Carnegie Institute, Washington, 1973.

48. Streeter, G.L., Developmental horizons in human embryos (XI–XII), *Contrib. Embryol.,* 30, 211–245, 1942.

49. Streeter, G.L., Developmental horizons in human embryos (XIII–XIV), *Contrib. Embryol.,* 31, 27–63, 1945.

50. Streeter, G.L., Developmental horizons in human embryos (XV–XVIII), *Contrib. Embryol.,* 32, 133–203, 1948.

51. Witschi, E., *Development of Vertebrates,* W.B. Saunders, Philadelphia, 1956.

52. Altmann, P.L. and Dittmer, D.S., *Growth,* Federation of American Societies of Experimental Biology, Washington, 1962.

53. Hamilton, W.J. and Mossman, H.W., *Human Embryology,* 4th ed., Heffer, Cambridge, 1972.

54. Monie, I.W., Comparative development of the nervous, respiratory, and cardiovascular systems, *Environ. Health Perspect.,* 18, 55–60, 1976.

55. O'Rahilly, R. and Meucke, E.C., The timing and sequence of events in the development of the human urinary system during the embryonic period proper, *Z. Anat. Entwickl. Gesch.,* 139, 99, 1972.

56. Shepard, T.H., *Catalog of Teratogenic Agents,* 2nd ed., Johns Hopkins University Press, Baltimore, 1976.

57. Hendrickx, A.G. and Sawyer, R.H., Embryology of the rhesus monkey, in *The Rhesus Monkey,* Vol. 2, Bourne, G.H., Ed., Academic Press, New York, 1975, 141–169.

58. Heuser, C.H. and Streeter, G.L., Development of the macaque embryo, *Contrib. Embryol.,* 29, 15–55, 1941.

59. Halman, M.T. and Prickett, M., The development of the external form of the guinea-pig (*Cavia cobaya*) between the ages of eleven days and twenty days of gestation, *Am. J. Anat.,* 49, 351–373, 1931/31.

60. Scott, J.P., The embryology of the guinea pig. 1. Table of normal development, *Am. J. Anat.,* 60, 397–432, 1937.

61. Edwards, J.A., The external development of the rabbit and rat embryo, in *Advances in Teratology,* Woollam, D.H., Ed., Academic Press, New York, 1968, 239–263.

62. Minot, C.S. and Taylor, E., Normal plates of the development of the rabbit, in *Normentafeln Zur Entwicklungsgeschichte der Wirbelthieri,* Keibel, F. and Gischer, G., Eds., Jena, 1905, 5.

63 Monie, I.W., Comparative development of rat, chick and human embryos, in *Teratologic Workshop Manual (Supplement),* Pharmaceutical Manufacturers Association, Berkeley, 1965, 146–162.

64. Waterman, A.J., Studies of the normal development of the New Zealand White strain of rabbit, *Am. J. Anal.,* 72, 473–515, 1943.

65. Farris, E.J. and Griffith, J.R., *The Rat in Laboratory Investigation,* 2nd ed., Haffner, New York, 1962.
66. Nelson, O.E., *Comparative Embryology of the Vertebrates,* McGraw-Hill, New York, 1953.
67. Otis, E.M. and Brent, R., Equivalent ages in mouse and human embryos, *Anat. Rec.,* 120, 33–63, 1954.
68. Snell, G.D. and Stevens, L.C., The early embryology of the mouse, in *Biology of the Laboratory Mouse,* Green, E.L., Ed., Blakiston, Philadelphia, 1966, 205–245.
69. Boyer, C.C., Chronology of development for the golden hamster, *J. Morphol.,* 92, 1–37, 1953.
70. Boyer, C., Embryology, in *The Golden Hamster,* Hoffman, R.A., Robinson, P.F., and Magalhaes, H., Eds., Iowa State University Press, Ames, Iowa, 1968, 73–89.
71. Pei, Y.F. and Rhodin, J.A.G., The prenatal development of the mouse eye, *Anat. Rec.,* 168, 105–126, 1970.
72. Boyden, E.A., Development of the lung in the pig-tail monkey (*Macaca nemestrina*), *Anat. Rec.,* 186, 15–37, 1976.
73. Meyrick, B. and Reid, L.M., Ultrastruture of alveolar lining and its development, in *Development of the Lung,* Hodson, W.A., Ed., Marcel Dekker, New York, 1977, 135–214.
74. Sissman, N.J., Developmental landmarks in cardiac morphogenesis: comparative chronology, *Am. J. Cardiol.,* 25, 141–148, 1970.
75. Fraser, B.A. and Sato, A.G., Differentiation of the male and female gonad and external genitalia in the human embryo, *Congenital Anomalies,* 27, 324, 1987.
76. Middle Atlantic Reproduction and Teratology Association, *Historical Control Data for Development and Reproductive Toxicity Studies Using the Crl:CD Rat,* Lang, P.L., Ed., Charles River Laboratories, Wilmington, MA, 1993.
77. Middle Atlantic Reproduction and Teratology Association, *Historical Control Data for Development and Reproductive Toxicity Studies using the New Zealand White Rabbit,* Lang, P.L., Ed., Hazleton Research Products, Denver, PA, 1993.
78. Middle Atlantic Reproduction and Teratology Association, *A Compilation of Terms Used in Developmental Toxicity Evaluations,* 1989.
79. Miller, R.K., Kellogg, C.K., and Saltzman, R.A., Reproductive and perinatal toxicology, in *Handbook of Toxicology,* Haley, T.J. and Bendt, W.O., Eds., Hemisphere Publishing, Washington, 1987.
80. Moore, K.L., *The Developing Human,* W.B. Saunders Co., Philadelphia, 1993.

BIBLIOGRAPHY

Christian, M.S., Galbraith, W.M., Voytek, P., and Mehlman, M.A., *Assessment of Reproductive and Teratogenic Hazards,* Princeton Scientific Publishers, Inc., Princeton, 1983.

Kalter, H., *Issues and Reviews in Teratology,* Vol. 2, Plenum Press, New York, 1984.

Kimmel, C.A. and Buelke-Sam, J., *Developmental Toxicology,* Raven Press, New York, 1981.

Manson, J.M. and Wise, L.D., Teratogens, in *Cassarett and Doull's Toxicology,* Amdur, M.O., Doull, J., and Klaassen, C.D., Eds., Pergamon Press, New York, 1991, chap. 7.

National Institute of Child Health and Human Development, *An Evaluation and Assessment of the State of the Science: Genetics and Teratology,* U.S. Department of Health and Human Services, Public Health Service, National Institutes of Health, 1991.

Thomas, J.A., Toxic responses of the reproductive system, in *Cassarett and Doull's Toxicology,* Amdur, M.O., Doull, J., and Klaassen, C.D., Eds., Pergamon Press, New York, 1991, chap. 16.

Tyl, R.W., Developmental toxicology, in *General & Applied Toxicology,* Vol. II, Ballantyne, B., Marrs, T., and Turner, P., Eds., Stockton Press, New York, 1993, chap. 44.

Wilson, J.G. and Fraser, F.D., Eds., *Handbook of Teratology,* Plenum Press, New York, 1977.

ADDITIONAL RELATED INFORMATION

TABLE 12.29
Comparison of Developmental Toxicity Guidelines

	U.S. FDA (1993)[a]	U.S. EPA (1996)[b]	OECD (1996)[c]	ICH (U.S. FDA, 1994)[d]
Species and Strain	Rat, mouse, hamster, rabbit. Preferred: rat and rabbit. Choice should be based on pharmacokinetic differences.	Use most relevant species. Use laboratory species and strains commonly used in prenatal developmental toxicity testing.	Use most relevant species. Use laboratory species and strains commonly used in prenatal developmental toxicity testing. Preferred rodent: rat. Preferred nonrodent: rabbit.	Use most relevant species. Usually 2 species; justify use of only 1 species. Preferred rodent: rat. Preferred nonrodent: rabbit.
Age and Sex	Young, mature, nonpregnant females of uniform size and age.	Use young adults. Use nulliparous females.	Use young adults. Animals should be of uniform weight and age. Use animals that have not been subjected to previous experimental procedures.	Use young, mature adults, virgin females.
Animal Care	Single housing, except during mating. Feed and water ad libitum. Diet should meet nutritional requirements. Animal care should meet requirements of Institute of Laboratory Animal Resources (1996).	Animal care should meet requirements of DHHS/PHS NIH Pub. #86-23 (1985).	Detailed information on temperature, humidity, lighting, diets, water. Cages: Mating should be carried out in cages suitable for purpose; after copulation, cage animals separately.	

Number of Animals	At least 20 pregnant females at or near term in each group.	Each test and control group should contain at least 20 animals with implantation sites at necropsy.	Each test and control group should contain at least 20 animals with implantation sites at necropsy.	Each group should contain 16–20 litters.
Dose Levels	Use 3 dose levels and concurrent control group. *High dose level:* some developmental toxicity or <10% maternal toxicity. ≤5% of diet for non-nutritive additives. *Low dose level:* no effects; level expected to provide a minimum margin of safety. *Intermediate dose level:* spaced to allow arithmetic or geometric progression between high and low doses. Minimal effects expected.	Use 3 dose levels and concurrent control group. Dose levels should be spaced to produce gradation of toxic effects. *High dose level:* <1000 mg/kg/day oral or dermal, or 2 mg/L by inhalation unless potential human exposure indicates need for higher exposure.	Use 3 dose levels and concurrent control group. Dose levels should be spaced to produce gradation of toxic effects. *High dose level:* <10% maternal mortality. *Intermediate dose level:* minimal observable toxic effects. Optimal for intermediate dose: two- to fourfold interval. 4th group preferable to using very large intervals. *Low dose level:* no maternal or developmental toxicity.	Use at least 3 dose levels and concurrent control group. High dose level should be based on data from all available studies. Lower doses are selected in descending sequence. Dosage intervals should be close enough to reveal dosage-related trends that may be present.
Control group	When a test substance is administered in a vehicle, the vehicle alone should be administered to control animals. Use sham control group if data are insufficient on the toxic properties of the vehicle.	Concurrent control should be sham-treated or vehicle control.	Concurrent control should be sham-treated or vehicle control.	Concurrent control should be sham-treated or vehicle control.
Route of Administration	Resembles route of human exposure (diet or drinking water), or gavage.	Usually orally by intubation. If other route is used, provide justification and reason for selection.	Usually orally by intubation. If other route is used, provide justification and reason for selection.	Route of administration should be similar to those intended for human usage.
Dosing Schedule	Minimum: From implantation to 1 day before cesarean day. Or entire time of gestation (if part of reproduction study).	Minimum: From implantation to cesarean. Or from fertilization to cesarean.	From implantation to 1 day prior to expected day of delivery.	From implantation to the closure of the hard palate (day 15–18).
Observation of Maternal Animals	At least twice each day. Record signs of overt toxicity.	At least each day. Record signs of overt toxicity.	At least each day. Record signs of overt toxicity.	At least each day. Record signs of overt toxicity.

TABLE 12.29 (Continued)
Comparison of Developmental Toxicity Guidelines

	U.S. FDA (1993)[a]	U.S. EPA (1996)[b]	OECD (1996)[c]	ICH (U.S. FDA, 1994)[d]
Weight of Maternal Animals	Weigh before first dose, weekly until necropsy, and at time of necropsy, except if dosed by gavage (daily or every 3 days).	Weigh at day 0, at termination, and at least at 3-day intervals during dosing.	Weight at day 0, at termination, and at least at 3-day intervals during dosing.	Record body weight and body weight changes at least twice weekly.
Feed and Fluid Consumption	Minimum: Weekly feed consumption measurement. Fluid consumption measurement as appropriate.	Feed consumption recorded on same days as body weights.	Feed consumption recorded on same days as body weights.	Feed consumption at least once weekly.
Necropsy	Necropsy all adults. Any dam showing signs of imminent abortion or premature delivery should be necropsied	Necropsy all adults. Females showing signs of abortion or premature delivery should be killed and subjected to a thorough macroscopic examination.	Necropsy all adults. Females showing signs of abortion or premature delivery should be killed and subjected to a thorough macroscopic examination.	Necropsy all adults.
Cesarean Section	Intact uterus is removed and weighed. Dams are evaluated blindly.	Evaluate dams blindly.	Examine dams macroscopically for structural abnormalities or pathological changes that may have influenced the pregnancy.	Preserve organs with macroscopic findings for possible histological evaluation.
Examination of Uterus and Placenta	Examine for fetal deaths and number of live fetuses. Determine number of corpora lutea. Examine uterus for resorption sites by ammonium sulfide stain. Weigh intact uterus.	Remove uteri and ascertain pregnancy status. Examine nongravid uteri by ammonium sulfide stain. Weigh gravid uterus. Determine number of corpora lutea. Examine uterus for embryo or fetal deaths and viable fetuses.	Remove uteri and ascertain pregnancy status. Examine nongravid uteri by ammonium sulfide stain. Weigh gravid uterus. Determine number of corpora lutea. Examine uterus for embryo or fetal deaths and viable fetuses.	Count corpora lutea, numbers of live and dead implantations, and gross evaluation of placenta.

Examination of Fetuses	Weigh and sex each fetus. Examine each fetus for external anomalies. Fix half fetuses for skeletal examination and half for visceral examination. For rabbits, each fetus should be examined for both skeletal and visceral anomalies.	Weigh and sex each fetus. Examine each pup for external anomalies. For rodents, examine half for skeletal and half for visceral anomalies. For rabbits, each fetus should be examined for both skeletal and visceral anomalies.	Weigh and sex each fetus. Examine each pup for external anomalies. For rodents, examine half fetus for skeletal and half for visceral anomalies or examine each fetus for visceral and skeletal anomalies. For rabbits, each fetus should be examined for both skeletal and visceral anomalies	Weigh and sex each fetus. Examine each pup for external anomalies. For rodents, examine half fetus for skeletal and half for visceral anomalies or examine each fetus for visceral and skeletal anomalies. For rabbits, each fetus should be examined for both skeletal and visceral anomalies. If no effects are noted in the high dose animals there is no need to test lower doses.
Test Report	Species and strain, body weight and weight change, feed and fluid consumption, clinical observations, necropsy findings, corpora lutea counts, implantation data, live fetuses, dead fetuses, incidence per litter of all divergences from normal fetal development (external, soft-tissue, skeletal), adequate statistical treatment.	Species and strain, maternal toxic response data, body weight and weight change, feed and water consumption, necropsy findings, corpora lutea counts, implantation data, developmental endpoints (number of live offspring, sex ratio, fetal body weight, external, soft-tissue, or skeletal alteration), adequate statistical treatment.	Species and strain, maternal toxic response data, body weight and weight change, feed and water consumption, necropsy findings, corpora lutea counts, implantation data, developmental endpoints (number of live offspring, sex ratio, fetal body weight, external, soft-tissue, or skeletal alteration), adequate statistical treatment.	Tabulation of individual values in a clear, concise manner to account for every animal. Tabulations of body weight, food consumption, litter values, clinical signs, autopsy values, abnormalities.

[a] U.S. Food and Drug Administration, Center for Food Safety and Applied Nutrition, 1993, *Toxicological principles for the safety assessment of direct food additives and color additives used in food, "Redbook H" (draft)*, Washington, D.C., U.S. Food and Drug Administration, Center for Food Safety and Applied Nutrition.

[b] U.S. Environmental Protection Agency, 1996, *Health effects test guidelines, OPPTS 870.3700, Prenatal developmental toxicity study*, pp. 1–8, Washington, D.C.: EPA 712-C-96-207.

[c] Organization for Economic Cooperation and Development, 1996, OECD Guideline for Testing of Chemicals, Proposal for Updating Guideline 414, Prenatal Developmental Toxicity Study, Draft document, August 1996, pp. 1–11, Paris, Organization for Economic Cooperation and Development.

[d] U.S. Food and Drug Administration, 1994, International Conference on Harmonisation; Guideline on detection of toxicity to reproduction for medicinal products; availability, *Fed. Reg.*, Part IX, 59(183):48746–48752.

From Testing guidelines for evaluation of reproductive and developmental toxicity of food additives in females, *International J. Toxicol.*, Collins, T.F.X., Sprando, R.L., Hansen, D.L., Shackelford, M.E., and Welsh, J.J., Eds., 17: 299–336. Copyright 1998. Reproduced by permission of Taylor & Francis, Inc., http://www.routledge-ny.com.

13 Endocrine Toxicology: Male Reproduction

Suresh C. Sikka, Ph.D., H.C.L.D.
and Rajesh K. Naz, Ph.D.

CONTENTS

0-8493-0370-2/02/$0.00+$1.50
© 2002 by CRC Press LLC

SECTION 1. INTRODUCTION

Endocrine disrupters are natural products or synthetic chemicals that interfere with the biosynthesis, secretion, transport, binding, action, or elimination of hormones in the body. They affect cellular homeostasis, reproduction, development, and/or its physiology. Effects may be reversible or irreversible, immediate (acute) or latent. Dose, timing, and duration of exposure at critical periods of life are important considerations for assessing the adverse effects of an endocrine disrupter. In males, these cause reproductive system abnormalities, including reduced sperm production, impaired fertility, testicular and prostate cancers, abnormal sexual development, alteration in pituitary and thyroid gland functions, immune suppression, and neurobehavioral effects. Endocrine disrupters are also popularly known as *gender benders,* mainly because evidence has shown disturbing trends in reproductive health. Contrary to the belief of some environmentalists that the human species is approaching a fertility crisis, there is available data that refute such conclusions.[1-3] The fact remains that one in six couples has trouble conceiving, with males equally responsible for their infertility.

The evidence that such environmental chemicals cause infertility is still largely circumstantial. There are many missing links in the causal chain that would connect these endocrine disrupters to receptor binding, which results in altered reproductive health that may lead to infertility. Lists of such potential estrogenic chemicals continue to grow, although it is not known what exact levels and combinations of these chemicals may be hazardous to male reproductive functions. There is still not enough evidence to determine whether this decline in semen quality is geographically localized or is a global phenomenon. Certain synthetic chemicals termed *endocrine impostors* exert a variety of toxic effects on the gonads, fertility, sexual, and reproductive function, in addition to behavioral and other effects. Recent discoveries of deformed frogs in Minnesota lakes and fertility problems in alligators found in Lake Apopka in Florida have been attributed to embryonic exposure to environmental pollutants.[4] Many agents in the environment have now been classified as male reproductive toxicants and have been the subject of a number of reviews.[5-11] Thus, etiology, diagnosis, and treatment of male factor infertility remains a real challenge.

The recent development of intracytoplasmic sperm injection (ICSI), a technique introduced in the early 1990s, is the most important breakthrough in the treatment of male factor infertility. This is due to many well-controlled clinical studies and basic scientific knowledge of the physiology, biochemistry, and molecular and cellular biology of the male reproductive system and identification of greater numbers of men with male factor problems. In addition, the latest genetic tools of investigations, e.g., Y-chromosome deletions and gene microarray analyses, have further strengthened the hypothesis that the decline in male reproductive health and fertility may be related to the presence of certain toxic chemicals in the environment. These chemicals mimic or otherwise disrupt the hormonal balance in the body by interfering in their production, or binding to specific hormone receptors during fetal and neonatal development.

SECTION 2. BACKGROUND

Over the past several years, many investigators have expressed serious concerns about the estrogenic effects of environmental toxicants, such as polychlorinated biphenyls (PCBs), dichlorodiphenyltrichloroethane (DDT), dioxin, and pesticides.[7,12-15] The potential reproductive health hazards of these chemicals include testicular, penile, or prostate cancer, undescended testis, Sertoli-cell-only pattern, and hypospadias, which cause poor gonadal function, low fecundity rates, and abnormality in sexual development.[12,16,17] It was in the mid-1970s that dibromochloropropane (DBCP) exposure was found to cause impaired testicular function, male infertility, embryo/fetal loss, birth defects, childhood cancer, and other postnatal structural or functional abnormalities. Even after three decades, the database for establishing safe exposure levels or risk assessment for such outcomes remains very limited.

There is ample evidence that *in utero* exposure to certain potent synthetic estrogens such as DES has an adverse reproductive effect on the progeny of women exposed to DES during their pregnancies. The pesticide DDT (1,1,1-trichloro-2,2-bis[4-chlorophenyl]ethane) and its metabolites have affected Western gull populations in Southern California as a result of testicular feminization of male embryos leading to abnormal sex ratios. More recently, the decline in the birthrate and increasing male reproductive tract abnormalities of alligators in Lake Apopka in Florida have been reported.[4]

Poor semen quality (low sperm number, motility, and morphology) over the past 50 years has been attributed to environmental toxicants, many of which act as "estrogens."[18] This "estrogen hypothesis" has recently inspired a number of debates and scientific investigations.[2,8,17] In spite of the fact that it takes only one sperm to fertilize an egg, problems in the production, maturation, and fertilization ability of sperm due to these endocrine disrupters are the most common cause of male infertility. The human male produces relatively fewer sperm on a daily basis compared with many of the animal species used for toxicity testing. In fact, in many men over age 30, the lower daily sperm production rate already places them close to the subfertile or infertile range.[19] Thus, a less dramatic decrease in sperm numbers or semen quality in humans can have serious consequences for reproductive potential.

Current advances in the knowledge of gonadal function and dysfunction and sperm motion and function have resulted in increased understanding of reproductive toxicity and infertility. Although any discussion of gonadal function and toxicity is of special relevance to humans, this understanding is the result of extensive research in many animal species employing various experimental models.

SECTION 3. GENERAL STRUCTURE, FUNCTION, AND REGULATION OF THE MALE REPRODUCTIVE TRACT

A. COMPOSITION OF THE TESTIS

The testes are the male gonads, which usually exist in pairs and are the sites of spermatogenesis and androgen production. These are the potential target sites for an environmental toxicant that disrupts endocrine function. The testes develop abdominally at the renal level and descend into the scrotum. Each testis arises from a primitive gonad on the medial surface of the embryonic mesonephros. Primitive germ cells migrate to the medial surface from the yolk sac, cause the coelomic

TABLE 13.1
Testicular Size and Associated Clinical Conditions

	Testicular Size	
Clinical Condition	Volume (ml)	Dimensions (cm)
Severe hypogonadism (e.g., Klinefelter's syndrome)	2	2.0×1.2
	4	2.5×1.5
Moderate hypogonadism (e.g., gonadotrophin deficiency or maturation arrest)	6	2.9×1.8
	10	3.4×2.1
	15	4.1×2.5
Normal size (may include obstructive or idiopathic oligozoospermia)	20	4.3×2.8
	25	4.7×3.1
	30	5.2×3.3

Source: Sikka, S.C., Testicular toxicology, in *Endocrine and Hormonal Toxicology,* Harvey, et al., Eds., Chapter 5, 1999 © John Wiley & Sons Limited, 1999, 96. Reproduced with permission.

epithelial cells to proliferate, and form the sex cords that lead to the formation of major components of the testis. Spermatozoa are the haploid germ cells responsible for fertilization and species propagation. Various compartments of the testis are under endocrine influences from the pituitary and hypothalamus via paracrine and autocrine regulations. Measurement of testicular size is an important index of their normal development and can be associated with many clinical conditions (Table 13.1).

1. Seminiferous Tubules

About 80% of the testicular mass consists of highly coiled "seminiferous tubules" within which spermatogenesis takes place. The remaining 20% consists of Leydig cells and Sertoli cells, important for establishing normal spermatogenesis. These tubules are formed by a very complex stratified epithelium containing spermatogenic cells and supporting cells called Sertoli cells. The epithelium is surrounded by a lamina propria composed of a double-layered basal lamina, three to five inner layers of myofibroblast and one or more outer layers of fibroblasts. The proliferation of the mesenchyme separates the sex cords from the underlying coelomic epithelium by the seventh week of fetal development. These sex cords become the seminiferous tubules that develop a lumen after birth. During the fourth month, sex cords become U-shaped, and their ends anastomose to form the rete testis, which provides communication with the epididymis. The primordial sex cells are referred to as prespermatogonia, and the epithelial cells of the sex cords as Sertoli cells.

2. Sertoli Cells

Sertoli cells, also called "nurse cells," provide nourishment to the developing sperm during spermatogenesis. These cells form a continuous and complete lining within the tubular wall and establish the blood–testis barrier by virtue of tight junctions. The luminal environment is under the influence of follicle-stimulating hormone (FSH) and inhibin. Besides providing nourishment to the developing sperm cells, Sertoli cells have several other functions including:

1. Destruction of defective sperm cells
2. Secretion of fluid that helps in the transport of sperm into the epididymis
3. Release of hormone inhibin that helps regulate FSH and sperm production

The formation of a competent blood–testis barrier by differentiating Sertoli cells is essential to the establishment of normal spermatogenesis during puberty. Thus, interference by endocrine disrupters leading to spermatogenic impairment and infertility may indeed reflect changes in the function of the Sertoli cell population and not necessarily pathology in the germ cells themselves, thus creating a Sertoli-cell-only testes (Figure 13.3).

3. Leydig Cells

The origin of these cells is from interstitial mesenchymal tissue during the eighth week of human embryonic development. These cells are located in the connective tissue area marked by angular interstices between the seminiferous tubules. Their main function is to produce testosterone and steroidal intermediates from cholesterol via a series of enzymatic pathways.[20] This steroidogenesis is under the control of luteinizing hormone (LH) from the pituitary.

B. SPERMATOGENESIS AND SPERMIATION

Spermatogenesis is a chronological process that takes about 42 days in the rodent and 72 days in men. During this period, relatively undifferentiated primitive stem cells called spermatogonia undergo several mitotic divisions to generate a large population of diploid cells called primary spermatocytes. These produce secondary spermatocytes and spermatids (the haploid germ cells) by two meiotic cell divisions. Spermiogenesis is the morphological transformation of undifferentiated round spermatids into elongated flagellar germ cells capable of motility (Figure 13.1). The germ cells comprise an acrosome covered head, which contains the condensed DNA; a midpiece containing densely packed mitochondria; and a long flagellum called the tail region. The release of mature germ cells from the seminiferous tubules is known as spermiation. The timing of the whole process of spermatogenesis, from spermatogonial division through spermiation, is species and strain dependent (Table 13.2). Extensive studies on spermatogenesis in the rodent testis have been carried out, but still very little is known about the details of these phenomena in primate and human testes.[21]

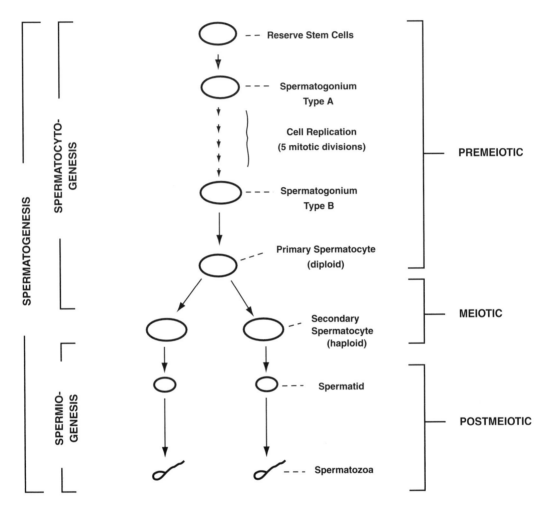

FIGURE 13.1 A general scheme of mammalian spermatogenesis, showing the premeiotic and meiotic stages of spermatocytogenesis (from reserve stem cells through the primary diploid spermatocyte to the haploid secondary spermatocyte) and the postmeiotic spermiogenesis with the development and maturation of the spermatozoa. Each cycle is completed in 35 to 75 days, depending on the species, with a new cycle being initiated at the Type A spermatogonium level every 12 to 13 days. (From Ecobichon, D., in *CRC Handbook of Toxicology,* Derelanko, M.J. and Hollinger, M.A., Eds., CRC Press, Boca Raton, FL, 384, 1995. With permission.)

TABLE 13.2
Species Variability in Parameters Involving Spermatogenesis

Parameter	Mouse	Rat	Hamster	Rabbit	Dog (Beagle)	Monkey (Rhesus)	Human
Spermatogenesis duration	34–35	48–53	35	50	62	70	74
Duration of cycle of seminiferous epithelium (days)	8.6	12.9	8.7	10.7	13.6	9.5	16
Life span of:							
B-type spermatogonia (days)	1.5	2.0		1.3	4.0	2.9	6.3
L + Z spermatocytes (days)	4.7	7.8		7.3	5.2	6.0	9.2
P + D spermatocytes (days)	8.3	12.2		10.7	13.5	9.5	15.6
Golgi spermatids (days)	1.7	2.9		2.1	6.9	1.8	7.9
Cap spermatids (days)	3.5	5.0		5.2	3.0	3.7	1.6
Testis weight (g)	0.2	3.7	1.8	6.4	12.0	4.9	34.0
Daily sperm production							
Per gram testis ($\times 10^6$)	54	14–22	22	25	20	23	4.4
Per individual ($\times 10^6$)	5–6	80–90	70	160	300	1100	125
Sperm reserve in cauda at sexual rest ($\times 10^6$)	49	440	575	1600		5700	420
Sperm storage in epididymal tissue ($\times 10^6$)							
Caput	20		200				420
Corpus	7	300	175				
Cauda	40–50	400	200				
Transit time through epididymis at sexual rest (days)							
Caput and corpus	3.1	3.0		3.0	?	4.9	1.8
Cauda	5.6	5.1		9.7	?	5.6	3.7
Ejaculate volume (ml)	0.04	0.2	0.1	1.0	?	?	>2.0
Ejaculated sperm (10^6/ml)	5.0	?	?	150	?	?	80.0
Sperm transit time from vagina to tube	15–60	30–60	?	3–4 h	20 min	?	15–30 min

Source: Adapted from Ecobichon.[60]

C. Epididymis and Sperm Maturation

The epididymis is the single convoluted tubule through which the testicular sperm must pass. The mesonephric ducts in the region of the epigenital tubules become convoluted and develop to form the epididymis. Functionally, the epididymis is divided into three major regions: (a) caput, or the head, (b) corpus, or the body, and (c) cauda, or the tail. Sperm mature and acquire significant motility as they traverse the caput and corpus, and they become stored in the cauda regions. The regional expression of many different genes, proteins, and other biochemicals in the epididymis suggests a linear maturational mechanism for sperm as they transverse this organ.

D. Vas Deferens and Sperm Transport

The vas deferens, also derived from mesonephric tubules, is a thick, muscular tube that carries sperm from the epididymis to the ejaculatory ducts in the prostate and penis. The first part of the vas deferens, originating at the cauda epididymis, is convoluted. As it approaches the prostate, adjacent to the seminal vesicles, it becomes dilated and is called the ampulla. The normal growth and development of the vas during puberty is also an androgen-dependent event.

E. Sex Gland Secretions and Ejaculation

The primary function of the seminal vesicles and prostate, also called the sexual accessory glands, is to provide a fluid environment and nutrients for sperm motility and survival. Approximately 95% of semen is made up of these secretions, while 5% is made up of sperm cells. Seminal vesicles arise as an extensive out-pocketing of the mesonephric ducts at the level of the prostate, thus sharing common embryological origins with the vas deferens and the epididymis. The prostate arises as buds from the primitive posterior urethra, penetrates the surrounding mesenchyme, and consists of various zones. The central zone surrounds the ejaculatory ducts before they enter into the urethra. The peripheral zone is the primary site of prostatic neoplasms, while the transition zone is the primary site for the formation of benign prostatic hyperplasia (BPH). The seminal vesicles contribute the greatest proportion of fluid to ejaculate. The exact roles of many of the substances in seminal fluid are not well understood. Prostatic fluid contains many important enzymes and polyamines, which help in lysis of the seminal coagulum and liquefaction of the ejaculate. The growth of the prostate is under control of androgens, mainly dihydrotestosterone (DHT), and the androgen-responsive elements (AREs). The AREs regulate the expression of androgen-responsive genes.

F. Penis/Ejaculatory Tract

This is the end organ of the male reproductive tract, meant for copulation and transfer of seminal fluid for fertilization. Corpus cavernosum, spongiosum, and endothelial-lined smooth muscle sinusoids are the main components of the body of the penis. Arterial and venous blood supply, as well as innervation to the penis play a significant role in erection and ejaculation. Nitric oxide (NO) has recently been shown to be the most important noncholinergic, nonadrenergic neurotransmitter responsible for penile erection. The normal growth of the penis during puberty is considered to be, in part, an androgen-dependent event and thus may be affected by endocrine disrupters.

G. Hormonal Regulation of Male Reproductive Function

1. Hypothalamic–Pituitary–Gonadal Axis

The growth, development, and functioning of the mammalian male reproductive system depend upon a normal hypothalamic–pituitary–gonadal (HPG) axis (Figure 13.2). The hypothalamus synthesizes and releases, in a pulsatile fashion, the decapeptide gonadotropin-releasing hormone (GnRH) that regulates the production and release of the pituitary hormones LH and FSH. These glycoprotein pituitary hormones regulate the gonadal function, including androgen biosynthesis and spermatogenesis. The HPG axis is under negative feedback control (long loop and short loop) mechanisms regulated by circulating steroidal hormones and inhibin (Table 13.3). The growth and function of male reproductive organs is regulated by the action of the androgens testosterone (T) and DHT, mediated via the androgen receptors (AR). The following classes of chemicals have androgen antagonistic properties by interfering with the AR and affecting reproductive development and function.

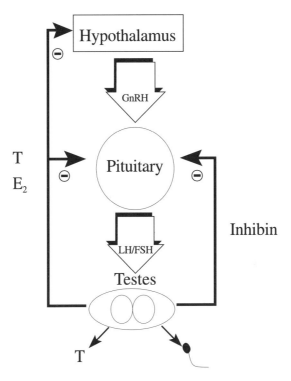

FIGURE 13.2 The hypothalamus–pituitary–gonadal axis. GnRH, which is secreted from the hypothalamus, stimulates LH and FSH secretion from the pituitary. LH stimulates testosterone secretion and sperm production by the testes, and FSH stimulates inhibin B secretion and potentiates the effects of LH on sperm production. Testosterone inhibits GnRH, LH, and FSH secretion, while inhibin B inhibits FSH secretion via feedback inhibition mechanisms. (T = testosterone, E_2 = estradiol.)

TABLE 13.3
Endocrine Control of Testicular Function in Adults

Hormone	Source	Major Target	Direct or Indirect Effect or Target(s)
Luteinizing hormone (LH)	Anterior pituitary	Leydig cells	Stimulate steroidogenesis (testosterone production)
Follicle-stimulating hormone (FSH)	Anterior pituitary	Sertoli cells	Stimulate protein synthesis (e.g., androgen-binding protein)
		Sertoli and/or germ cells	Maturation of spermatids into spermatozoa (spermiogenesis)

TABLE 13.3 *(Continued)*
Endocrine Control of Testicular Function in Adults

Hormone	Source	Major Target	Direct or Indirect Effect or Target(s)
Testosterone	Leydig cells	Male accessory grands	Maintain structure and function
		Hypothalamus and pituitary	Negative feedback control on release of FSH and LH
Estradiol	Leydig cells	Anterior pituitary	Negative feedback control on release of FSH and LH
Inhibin	Sertoli cells	Anterior pituitary	Negative feedback control on release of FSH

Source: Overstreet, J.W. and Blazak, W.F., *Am. J. Ind. Med.*, 4, 5–15, copyright 1983. © John Wiley & Sons Limited. Reproduced with permission.

2. Antiandrogens

These are the chemicals that prevent binding of androgens to the AR without activation. Examples of antiandrogens are the pharmaceutical hydroxyflutamide and the pesticides procymidone, vinclozolin, and DDT metabolite *p,p'*-DDE. Estradiol and DES, in addition to their high affinity for the estrogen receptor, also have significant affinity for the AR. It is possible that the mechanism by which estrogenic chemicals impair development of the male reproductive system may be via antiandrogenic properties rather than estrogen receptor activation. Administration of vinclozolin to pregnant rats from gestation day 14 to postnatal day 3 produced male offspring with a variety of reproductive defects characteristic of interference with AR action (e.g., reduction of anogenital distance, impaired penis development, existence of vaginal pouches, prostate gland agenesis, and reduced or absent sperm production).

3. Estrogens

Recent reports of reduced sperm production, improper development of the penis, cryptorchidism, and testicular tumors by the Danish Environmental Protection Agency indicate that the human male reproductive system, as well as that of certain wildlife species, has been compromised by environmental toxicants in specific geographic locations. It has been hypothesized that these effects are due to exposure *in utero* to exogenous chemicals with estrogenic activity. Estrogenic environmental chemicals octylphenol, octylphenol phenoxylate, and butyl benzyl phthalate, as well as DES resulted in reduced rat testicular weight and sperm production.[13] The male offspring exposed to DES *in utero* had increased incidence of genital malformations, including epididymal cysts and testicular abnormalities such as small testes and microphallus. With exposure *in utero* to relatively high levels of a potent exogenous estrogen, about one-third of the men who were recontacted have clinically detectable reproductive system effects. The types of effects that were observed are consistent with those that would be predicted from studies with rodents.

4. Receptor Agonists

A group of halogenated aromatic hydrocarbons (Ah) that affect the male reproductive tract can activate the Ah receptor. Dioxin (2,3,7,8-TCDD) affects the developing male reproductive system in rodents even at lower doses because of impaired testosterone biosynthesis and impairment of central nervous system sexual differentiation. The low androgen level is not accompanied by increased LH levels, indicating impairment of the feedback mechanism for control of LH synthesis and release and action as a direct Ah receptor agonist. Observed effects include decreased anogenital distance, delayed testis descent, impaired spermatogenic function, decreased accessory sex gland weights, and feminization of male sexual behavior.

SECTION 4. ENDOCRINE DISRUPTERS AND MALE REPRODUCTION

A. ENVIRONMENTAL/OCCUPATIONAL AGENTS

Any chemical, physical, or biological agent that alters physiological control processes and affects the normal functioning of the gonads can cause reproductive toxicity. The effect may be mild or severe, and the duration may vary from transient dysfunction to permanent gonadal damage. This can occur either by a direct chemical action of the agent or indirectly via the metabolic products formed during the reaction process. A potential gonadotoxic agent can interrupt the normal function of the male reproductive system at (1) any level of the HPG axis, (2) directly at the gonadal level, or (3) by altering post-testicular events, such as sperm motility or function or both. Any disruption of these events by toxicants may lead to hypogonadism, infertility, and/or decreased libido/sexual function (Table 13.4). Endocrine disrupters are widespread in the environment, have an ability to bioaccumulate, and resist biodegradation. Many agricultural products (phytoestrogens), industrial chemicals, and heavy metals have significant environmental consequences as a result of their multiple routes of exposure.[6,22]

TABLE 13.4
Summary of the Most Common Gonadotoxic Agents

Class	Agents	Adverse effects/comments
(A) Environmental/Occupational Agents		
Organochemicals and pesticides	DBCP DDT PCBs Dioxins Methyl chloride	↓ Fertility, ↓ Libido, embryo fetal loss, birth defects, cancer; estrogenic effects, poor semen quality
Heavy metals	Lead Mercury Cadmium Cobalt Chromium	↓ HPG axis, ↓ spermatogenesis, CNS effects, testicular damage
Recreational drugs	Nicotine Alcohol Marijuana Steroids	↓ Spermatogenesis, poor sperm function, ↓ HPG axis
(B) Pharmacological Agents		
Antimicrobials	Tetracyclines Sulfas Gentamycin Neomycin Nitrofurantoin	↓ Sperm function, ↓ spermatogenesis, testicular damage
Antineoplastic	Nitrogen mustard Cyclophosphamide Cisplatin Procarbazine	↓ Sperm motility
Radiation	X-rays, γ-rays	Germ cell and Leydig cell damage
Other drugs	Cimetidine GnRH analogues KTZ, Leuprolide Cyclosporine Lithium Flutamide Gossypol	↓ HPG-axis, ↓ sperm; ↓ libido, ↓ steroidogenesis

TABLE 13.4 *(Continued)*
Summary of the Most Common Gonadotoxic Agents

Class	Agents	Adverse effects/comments
(C) Biological Agents		
	Hyperthermia	↑ ROS, spermatogenesis, ↓ testicular damage, poor sperm morphology
	Infection/inflammation	↑ ROS, ↑ WBC, ↓ SOD, ↑ IL-8, ↓ sperm function
	Oxidative stress	↑ ROS, ↑ LPO, ↑ cytokines, ↓ T, ↓ sperm function
	Age-related	↑ ROS, ↓ HPG, ↑ LPO, ↓ spermiation

Abbreviations: DBCP = dibromochloropropane; DDT = dichlorodiphenyltrichloroethane; KTZ = keto-conazole; ROS = reactive oxygen species; LPO = lipid peroxidation; SOD = superoxide dismutase

Source: Sikka, S.C., in *Endocrine and Hormonal Toxicology,* Harvey, et al., Eds., © John Wiley & Sons Limited, New York, copyright 1999, 100. Reproduced with permission.

1. Agricultural and Industrial Chemicals

Many agricultural and industrial chemicals that affect the male reproductive system include DDT (*o,p*-dichlorodiphenyl-trichloroethane), epichlorhydrin, ethylene dibromide, and dioxins. Methyl chloride is used in the production of organosilicates and gasoline antiknock additives.[23] Dibromo-chloropropane (DBCP) is a nematocide widely used in agriculture. DDT, a commonly used pesticide, and its metabolites (*p,p′*-DDT, and *p,p′*-DDE) have estrogenic effects in males by blocking the androgen receptors.[16] The plasma/tissue concentration of an estrogenic toxicant depends upon the detoxification and elimination mechanisms in the organism.[24] These agents can disrupt the hypothalamic–pituitary–gonadal axis, affecting the endocrine and reproductive functions. Such organic solvents have been reported to induce changes in semen quality, testicular size, and serum gonadotropins.[15,25] In addition to impaired spermatogenesis, endocrine disrupters may affect sperm motility and morphology secondary to various hormonal alterations. Morphological sperm abnormalities due to secretory dysfunction of the Leydig and Sertoli cells may impair the sperm-fertilizing capacity.

2. Heavy Metals

Heavy metals, mainly lead, cadmium, cobalt, mercury, boron, aluminum, chromium, arsenic, and lithium, exert adverse reproductive effects in human and experimental animals.[26] *Lead* exposure in paint and battery-plant workers suppressed testosterone and sperm production. Testicular biopsies revealed peritubular fibrosis, and vacuolation, suggesting a direct testicular effect. Lead can also disrupt the hormonal feedback mechanisms at the hypothalamic–pituitary level; however, these effects can be reversed when lead is removed from the system.[27] *Mercury* exposure is common during the manufacture of thermometers, thermostats, mercury vapor lamps, paint, electrical appliances, and mining. It alters spermatogenesis and decreases fertility in experimental animals. *Boron* is extensively used in the manufacture of glass, cements, soaps, carpets, crockery, and leather products and has a major adverse reproductive effect on the testes and the hypothalamic–pituitary axis in a manner similar to lead.[28] *Cadmium,* another heavy metal widely used in the electroplating, battery electrode, galvanizing, plastics, alloys, and paint pigment industries and also present in soil, coal, water, and cigarette smoke, is a testicular toxicant. In animal studies, cadmium has been shown to cause strain-dependent severe testicular necrosis in mice.[29] Cadmium alters DNA binding and blocks transcription of sulfhydryl-containing proteins. It can also induce the expression of heat shock proteins, oxidative stress response genes, and heme oxygenase induction mechanisms. Further studies are needed to delineate the specific toxic mechanisms involved in oligozoospermia, decreased libido, and fertility impairment due to heavy metal toxicity.

B. Pharmacological Agents

Radiation therapy, as well as numerous pharmacological drugs and chemotherapeutic agents, is known to adversely affect testicular function (Table 13.4).

1. Chemotherapeutic Agents

Specific antimicrobials, (e.g., tetracycline derivatives, sulfa drugs, nitrofurantoin, erythromycin) and cancer chemotherapeutic agents (e.g., mechlorethamine) can be toxic to germinal epithelium, or impair spermatogenesis and spermatozoal function resulting in infertility.[30,31] Postmeiotic germ cells are specifically sensitive to cyclophosphamide treatment, with abnormalities observed in progeny.[32] Chronic low-dose cyclophosphamide treatment in men affects sperm decondensation due to the alkylation of nuclear proteins or DNA. This is likely to affect pre- and postimplantation loss or contribute to congenital abnormalities in offspring. Although combination therapy with alkylating agents improves survival in patients with Hodgkin's disease, lymphoma, and leukemia, such therapy induces germinal aplasia resulting in sterility in many adults.[33] The severity of testicular damage and recovery is usually related to the dose, duration, and category of chemotherapeutic agent used.[34] The prepubertal and young adolescent testes are less sensitive to chemo- and radiation therapy than is the postpubertal testis, which may depend upon the androgenicity of dividing cells.

2. Anabolic Steroids

Abuse of anabolic steroids to build stamina and muscle mass is very common among athletes and has resulted in severe oligozoospermia and decreased libido. These steroids cause feedback inhibition of the hypothalamus–pituitary axis resulting in hypogonadotropic hypogonadism and severe impairment of normal sperm production and infertility in this population.[35] These defects can be reversed within 4 months to 1 year after cessation of chronic anabolic steroid use.

3. Radiation Therapy

Radiotherapy (X-rays, neutrons, and radioactive materials) is routinely used for the treatment of seminomatous germ cell tumors and lymphomas. Testicular damage due to radiation exposure is generally more severe and difficult to repair than that induced by chemotherapy.[36] A direct dose of irradiation to the testes greater than 0.35 Gy causes reversible aspermia, but doses in excess of 2 Gy will likely lead to permanent azoospermia. The time taken for damage and recovery not only depends upon dose but also on duration and developmental stage of the germ cells in the testes. Germ cells are the most radiosensitive. At higher radiation doses (>15 Gy), Leydig cells will also be affected. In addition to direct damage to the testes, whole-body irradiation can also damage the hypothalamic–pituitary axis and affect reproductive functions leading to sterility.[37]

4. Other Pharmacological Drugs

Numerous pharmacological agents and many clinically approved drugs have gonadotoxic effects, especially at higher doses. Administration of GnRH agonists and related analogues leads to suppression of gonadotropins and spermatogenesis. This approach has been utilized for the development of potential male contraceptive agents. Ketoconazole, an antifungal agent, inhibits testosterone biosynthesis primarily by inhibiting the activities of steroidogenic enzymes in Leydig cells without any direct effect at the pituitary level.[38] Cyclosporine has been the drug of choice for immunosuppression in patients who undergo organ transplantation, but it has hypoandrogenic effects mediated through the hypothalamic–pituitary axis.

C. Biological Conditions

Certain pathophysiological conditions have significant gonadotoxic effects.

1. Hyperthermia

Progressive germ cell damage occurs in the cryptorchid testis secondary to the increased temperature of the extrascrotal location. Elevated testicular temperature is also considered to be responsible for testicular dysfunction in men with varicocele. Hyperthermia results in impaired Leydig cell function, a gradual loss in size of seminiferous tubules, and peritubular hyalinization with fibrosis of the testis, which is accompanied by characteristic structural changes, notably the retention of cytoplasmic droplets in the ejaculated sample. This finding signifies elevated levels of reactive oxygen species (ROS) and sperm dysfunction.[39] Germinal cells respond to heat by producing unique patterns of heat shock proteins, and these may prove to be useful markers of susceptibility to thermal and oxidative stress.

2. Chronic Infection/Inflammation

An infection/inflammation of the genitourinary tract in an infertile man is suspected when the semen analysis shows an increased number of leukocytes (>1 to 2 million white blood cells/ml semen). Acute and subacute infection and inflammation of the male gonads and accessory sex glands can be associated with disturbances in both sex gland function and sperm quality. Some of these conditions (e.g., chlamydia infection, mumps orchitis, tuberculosis, syphilis, leprosy) can cause irreversible sterility, are invariably symptomatic, and are associated with leukocytospermia/bacteriospermia. Chronic infection and inflammation of the reproductive tract can also contribute to the infertile state; the impact of such asymptomatic or "silent infections" is sometimes more severe. The pathophysiology involves damage to the seminiferous tubules or obstruction to the passage of sperm at the level of the epididymis or ejaculatory duct.

The precise role of genital tract infection, the site of origin of leukocytes, their migratory pattern and mode of action, and the contribution that bacteria or viruses and the subsequent genitourinary inflammation have on sperm function are not well described. Elevated leukocytes/granulocytes are believed to release various proinflammatory/bioactive cytokines, in addition to hydrogen peroxide, and other reactive oxygen species. These cause oxidative stress and peroxidative damage to spermatozoa.

3. Aging and Gonadotoxicity

Age-related degenerative disorders of the testis, especially in some industrialized societies, may be increasing as suggested by the reports of declining sperm count over the last two generations. Spermatogenic failure, reduced sperm output, and low seminal volume occur with senescence in a variety of animal species and in humans. Germ cell degeneration with age starts with the spermatids leading to sclerosis of tubules and consists of thickened and highly collagenized tunica propria with an increased number of myoid cells. These are phagocytosed by Sertoli cells accompanied by decreased vascularity and Sertoli cell abnormalities that would lead to faulty spermiation and spermatogenic failure. A significant decrease in Leydig cell numbers and androgen biosynthesis with a concurrent rise in serum FSH and LH has also been observed in the older population. This is sometimes referred to as "andropause." Most of these changes are strikingly similar to those seen in men with idiopathic testicular failure, probably due to induced gonadotoxicity.

4. Oxidative Stress

The presence of retained cytoplasmic droplets on spermatozoa due to (a) imperfect spermiation in the aging testis and (b) chronic infection and inflammation of the genito-urinary tract is associated with oxidative stress and reduced fertility potential. Midpiece anomalies are linked to ROS-induced membrane lipid peroxidation (LPO) and high creatine kinase (CK) activity in immature sperm. This has recently been attributed to genetic defects in the mitochondrial genome that controls oxidative phosphorylation. Increased intracellular levels of lipofuscin pigment, lipids, and multiple nuclei seen in the gonads of older men can be associated with mitochondrial dysfunction compounded by ROS-induced oxidative stress.[40,41] It is difficult to differentiate such gonadal anomalies and post-testicular effects due to aging and/or occupational exposures. Development of new methods and approaches for studying this problem is warranted.

D. RECREATIONAL AGENTS

Many agents used for recreational purposes when consumed in excess impair reproductive functions.

1. Alcohol Consumption

Chronic high-level consumption of alcohol in men with alcohol dependence syndrome has been shown to decrease sperm concentration, affect normal morphology, and impair sexual function. Tobacco, nicotine, caffeine, and other recreational drugs can further influence the effect of alcohol on gonadal function and sperm quality. Caffeine consumption has been shown to increase the risk of dyspermia. Alterations in the HPG axis are the key mechanisms of alcohol-induced gonadotoxicity. Avoidance of chronic, heavy alcohol use can reverse these effects.

2. Cigarette Smoking

The number of cigarettes, the nicotine dose, duration, age of the smoker, and the levels of serum cotinine (the active metabolite of nicotine) are some of the parameters that may explain the variability of effects on reproductive functions in smokers.[42] A detrimental effect of smoking on sperm concentration, motility, and morphology may be caused by impaired spermatogenesis secondary to various hormonal alterations.[43] Smoking and the presence of varicocele have also been proposed as having an additive, detrimental effect on sperm motility and density.

3. Marijuana, Cocaine, Heroin, and Methadone

Like nicotine, many other recreational drugs affect the HPG axis. These drugs decrease sperm number and motility, and negatively impact normal sperm form. Decreased testosterone and altered gonadotropin levels due to feedback inhibition of the HPG axis resulting in hypogonadotropic hypogonadism are the likely mechanisms of their gonadotoxic effects. These defects can be reversed within 4 months of nonuse.

SECTION 5. MECHANISM(S) OF ACTION OF ENDOCRINE DISRUPTERS

There are several potential target sites and cellular processes at which a given gonadotoxic agent could exert endocrine-related effects and disrupt organ function. This is due to the fact that the complexity of these processes involves several hormonal communications. Such impaired hormonal control could occur as a consequence of altered hormone synthesis, storage/release, transport/clearance, receptor recognition/binding, or postreceptor responses.[44]

A. Altered Hormone Biosynthesis

Many agents (e.g., aminoglutethimide, cyanoketone, ketoconazole) possess the ability to inhibit steroid hormone biosynthesis in the testes by directly inhibiting specific enzymatic steps in the steroidogenic pathway or by regulating at the transcriptional and/or translational levels.[38] Some fungicides also block estrogen biosynthesis by directly inhibiting aromatase activity. In addition, some endocrine disrupters alter protein hormone biosynthesis induced by gonadal steroids. Both estrogen and testosterone have been shown to affect pituitary hormone synthesis through changes in the glycosylation of LH and FSH.[45] Many endocrine disrupters affect the biological activity of these glycoprotein hormones directly or indirectly via altering biogenic amines (e.g., dopamine) or via altering GnRH at the hypothalamic–pituitary level. Any environmental compound that mimics or antagonizes the action of these steroid hormones could presumably alter glycosylation and biosynthesis of LH and FSH.

B. Altered Hormone Storage and/or Release

Unlike protein hormones, steroid hormones are not stored intracellularly within membranous secretory granules. Testosterone is produced and released by the Leydig cells of the testis on activation of the LH receptors by circulating LH. Any compounds that block the LH receptor or the activation of the $3',5'$-cyclic AMP–dependent cascade involved in testosterone biosynthesis can rapidly alter the secretion of this hormone. The release of many protein hormones is dependent on the activation of second messenger pathways, such as cAMP, phosphatidylinositol 4,5-bisphosphate (PIP2), inositol 1,4,5-trisphosphate (IP3), tyrosine kinase, and ionic calcium. Interference with these processes consequently will alter their serum levels and thus availability of such hormones.

C. Altered Hormone Transport and Clearance

Both protein and steroid hormones are transported in blood in the free and/or bound state. Steroid hormones are transported in the blood by specialized transport (carrier) proteins known as steroid hormone-binding globulin (SHBG). These binding proteins are produced in the liver. Any alteration in the concentration of these binding globulins in the blood may either increase or decrease the bioavailability of these steroid hormones at the target sites. For example, DDT analogues are potent inducers of hepatic microsomal monooxygenase activities *in vivo*. Induction of this monooxygenase activity can cause a decrease in androgen as a result of enhanced clearance. Similarly, treatment with lindane (gamma-hexachlorocyclohexane) increases the clearance of estrogen.

D. Altered Hormone Receptor Recognition and Binding

Hormones directly interact with their receptors (intracellular or membrane bound) to elicit responses at their respective target sites. Specific binding of the natural ligand to its receptor is the first critical step in hormone action. Sex steroids, adrenal steroids, thyroid hormones, vitamin D, and retinoic acid first bind to intracellular (nuclear) receptors in a ligand-dependent manner to regulate gene transcription through their interaction with specific DNA sequences (response elements). A number of environmental agents (e.g., methoxychlor, chlordecone, DDT, some PCBs, and alkylphenols) either alter receptor recognition by mimicking the natural ligand and acting as an agonist or by inhibiting binding and acting as antagonist to disrupt estrogen receptor interaction. The dicarboximide fungicide vinclozolin exerts its antiandrogenic effect via its metabolite that alters affinity for the androgen receptor. DDT metabolite *p,p'*-DDE also binds to the androgen receptor and blocks testosterone-induced cellular responses.[46] Certain environmental estrogens (e.g., *o,p*-DDT, alkylphenols, and chlordecone) can inhibit binding to both estrogen and progesterone receptors, with equal affinity for the two receptors.[47]

Receptors for protein hormones are located on and in the cell membrane. Binding of these hormones to their receptors elicits signal transduction across the membrane that is mediated by the activation of second-messenger systems. Some examples include alterations in G protein–mediated cAMP-dependent protein kinase A (e.g., after LH stimulation of the Leydig cell); phosphatidylinositol regulation of protein kinase C and inositol triphosphate (e.g., GnRH stimulation of gonadotrophs; thyrotropin-releasing hormone stimulation of thyrotrophs); tyrosine kinase (e.g., insulin binding to the membrane receptor); and calcium ion flux mechanisms. Many xenobiotics thus disrupt signal transduction of peptide hormones by interfering with one or more of these processes.

E. ALTERED HORMONE POSTRECEPTOR ACTIVATION

Binding of an agonist or an endogenous ligand to its receptor initiates a cascade of events leading to appropriate signal transduction across the membrane and cellular response. In the case of nuclear receptors, the initiation leads to message transcription and appropriate protein biosynthesis. A variety of environmental agents interfere with such postreceptor second-messenger systems. For example, calcium/calmodulin-mediated cellular responses are dependent on the flux of calcium ions through the membrane which is altered by a variety of environmental toxicants. Antiestrogen tamoxifen inhibits protein kinase C activity, while phorbol esters enhance protein kinase C activity by mimicking the diacylglycerol pathway. Steroid hormone postreceptor activation can also be modified by indirect mechanisms, e.g., TCDD exposure downregulates steroid and glucocorticoid receptors.[48] Consequently, because of the diverse pathways of endocrine disruption, any assessment must consider the net result of all influences on hormone receptor function and feedback regulation.

G. INDUCTION OF OXIDATIVE STRESS

Exposure to many types of environmental contaminants, chronic disease state, aging, or gonadal injury can induce a state of oxidative stress associated with an increased rate of cellular damage that results in gonadotoxicity. Oxidative stress is a condition induced by oxygen and oxygen-derived free radicals commonly known as reactive oxygen species (ROS).[19] Normally, adequate levels of cellular antioxidants, mainly superoxide dismutase (SOD), catalase, glutathione (GSH) peroxidase and reductase will maintain the free radical scavenging potential in the testes. Oxidative stress is the result of an imbalance between ROS generation and intrinsic ROS scavenging activities. A situation in which there is a shift in this balance toward pro-oxidants, because of either generation of excessive ROS or diminished antioxidant capacity, is referred to as oxidative stress status (OSS). Its assessment may play a critical role in monitoring testicular toxicity and infertility.[10,41] The major ROS species with toxic manifestations to the male reproductive system include superoxide (O_2^-), hydroxyl (OH^-), hydrogen peroxide, and nitric oxide ($NO^.$) radicals. These can contribute to hormonal imbalance, gonadal dysfunction, and poor sperm motility/function leading to infertility.[39] Nitric oxide and superoxide radicals combine to form highly reactive peroxynitrite radicals that induce endothelial cell injury.[50,51] This may result in altered blood flow to the testis and impair testicular function. Free radicals damage DNA through oxidation of primarily guanine bases via peroxyl or alkoxyl radicals that result in DNA strand breaks affecting cross-linking. ROS also induce oxidation of critical sulfhydryl (–SH) groups in proteins and DNA, as well as alter cellular integrity and function with an increased susceptibility to attack by toxicants.

SECTION 6. LABORATORY ASSESSMENT OF MALE REPRODUCTIVE TOXICITY

Essentially, a complete evaluation of toxicity has four components: (1) hazard identification, (2) dose–response assessment, (3) human-exposure assessment, and (4) risk characterization. The hazard identification and dose–response data are derived from experimental animal studies that may be supplemented with data from *in vitro* studies. This information is then extrapolated to assess the effect on human populations and the data integrated for risk characterization. In the clinical setting, a detailed history and physical examination is followed by semen analysis, testicular biopsy, and endocrine assessment of the HPG axis. Many specialized *in vitro* and *in vivo* models can evaluate the effects of potential gonadotoxic agents and are excellent research tools. Although *in vitro* testing systems have significantly advanced the knowledge of testicular toxicology, *in vivo* systems are still an essential part of the risk assessment process.

A. SEMEN ANALYSIS

Semen analysis represents a critical component of the initial evaluation of the infertile male and is indicative of normal or abnormal spermatogenesis, sperm morphology, and sperm motility (Table 13.5). In combination with specialized sperm function tests, it can be a good measure of infertility. The World Health Organization manual is considered to be the guideline describing complete semen analysis.[52,53]

TABLE 13.5
Human Semen Analysis: Normal Ranges

Semen Characteristic	Units	Normal	Borderline	Pathological
Volume	ml	2.0–6.0	1.5–2.0	< 1.5
pH	pH units	> 7.2	7.0–7.2	< 7.0
Sperm Concentration	10^6/ml	> 2.0	10–20	< 10
Total Sperm Count	10^6/ejaculate	> 80	20–80	< 20
Sperm Motility (0.5–2.0 h after ejaculation)	% Motile	> 50	35–50	< 35
Progression (at 37°C)	Scale 0–4	3 or 4	2	< 2
Straightline velocity	μm/s	> 25	20–25	< 20
Sperm morphology	% Normal	≥ 50	35–50	< 35
Head defects	Per 100 sperm	< 35	35–50	> 50
Midpiece defects	Per 100 sperm	≤ 20	21–25	> 25
Tail defects	Per 100 sperm	≤ 20	21–25	> 25
Sperm vitality	% live	> 75	50–75	< 50
WBC	10^6/ml	0	< 1	> 1
Fructose (total)	mg %	> 100.0	50–100	< 50
Antisperm antibody	% Immunobead (IgG, IgA, or IgM) binding to motile spermatozoa	0–20	20–50	> 50

Source: Adapted from Mortimer.[52]

B. TESTICULAR BIOPSY

The primary indication for testis biopsy is to aid in the diagnosis of obstruction of the male reproductive system in azoospermic men.[21] Testis biopsy is also performed to identify the quality of spermatogenesis or to identify the presence of sperm cells that may be aspirated and used for assisted reproduction (Figure 13.3). Aspirated spermatozoa are then used for intracytoplasmic sperm injection (ICSI) in male factor infertility due to azoospermia or severe oligozoospermia. Standard evaluation of testicular biopsy is carried out by light microscopy and can be combined with DNA flow cytometry for a more objective evaluation of spermatogenic arrest.[40,54] Electron and laser microscopy of the germinal epithelium have also been employed to evaluate testicular and sperm damage.

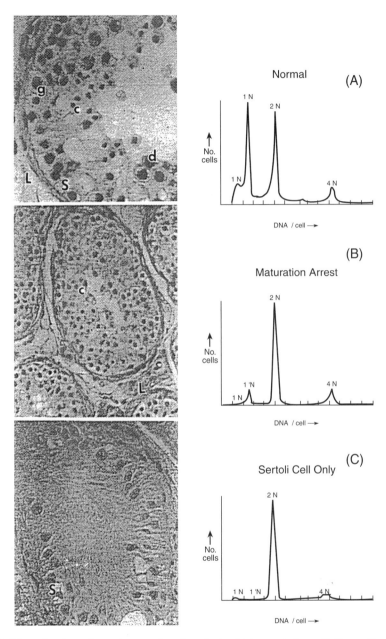

FIGURE 13.3 Plate showing photomicrographs of testicular histomorphology (left panel) and DNA-flow cytometric histogram (right panel). Labels on the figures show the location of spermatogonia (g), spermatocytes (c), spermatids (d), Sertoli cells (S), and Leydig cells (L). Panel (A) shows normal spermatogenesis; panel (B) shows maturation arrest at the primary spermatocyte stage (about 70% are diploid cells); and panel (C) shows severe germinal aplasia (Sertoli cell only syndrome) where about 90% cells are diploid. (Modified from Sharlip, I.D. and Chan, S.L., Testicular biopsy and vasography, in *Male Infertility and Sexual Dysfunction*, Wayne, J.G., Ed., Hellstrom, Springer Verlag, New York, 1997.)

C. ENDOCRINE ASSESSMENT

Patients with primary testicular failure may have significantly elevated gonadotropins, especially FSH, due to the absence of negative feedback (see Figure 13.2). Abnormally low gonadotropin levels are secondary to hypothalamic or pituitary dysfunction. Blood tests for evaluation of the HPG axis are routinely employed and recommended not only for men presenting with infertility, but also to evaluate the mechanisms of action of potential gonadotoxic agents (Table 13.6).[20]

TABLE 13.6
Evaluation of Effect of Hormonal Disrupters in the Adult Male

Potential Sites	Effects	Evaluative Tests
Testis Leydig cells	Necrosis	Weight, histopathology, receptor analysis, RIA LH/PRL
	T biosynthesis/secretion	*In vitro* production and hormone assay
Sertoli cells	FSH/Inhibin/Steroids	Receptor analysis, RIA
	Sertoli/Leydig cell function	*In vitro* tests (co-culture)
	Blood-testis barrier	Morphology
Seminiferous tubules	Spermatogonial mitosis	Germ cell count and % tubules without germ cells
	Spermatocyte meiosis	Spermatid counts and % tubules with luminal sperm
	Spermatid differentiation	Germ-cell culture, morphology
Epididymis	Sperm maturation	Histopathology, biochemical tests
Brain	Hypothalamic–pituitary axis	Pituitary cell-culture, hypothalamus perfusion, histopathology, hormone challenge, accessory sex-organ weights
Seminal Fluid	Daily sperm production	Spermatid counts, semen evaluation
Blood	HPG axis	Hormones/ABP assays

Abbreviations: LH = luteinizing hormone; PRL = prolactin; FSH = follicle stimulating hormone; ABP = androgen binding protein; HPG = hypothalamic–pituitary–gonadal.

Source: Adapted from Sikka and Naz.[9]

D. IN VITRO MODELS

Many *in vitro* models (e.g., Sertoli–germ cell co-cultures; Sertoli cell–enriched cultures; germ cell–enriched cultures; Leydig cell cultures; Leydig–Sertoli cell co-cultures; and peritubular and tubular cell cultures) can be used alone or in combination to investigate specific cellular and molecular mechanisms in the testis.[42,55] A toxic agent or its metabolites, as well as the precursors or selective inhibitors, can be individually administered to isolated cell types to evaluate specific toxicity mechanisms.[56-59] These tools also help to evaluate the interactions of adjacent cell types and to screen a class of compounds for new product development. However, certain dynamic processes, e.g., spermiation associated with spermatogenesis, are difficult to evaluate by such *in vitro* approaches.

E. IN VIVO MODELS

In vivo assessment of testicular toxicity involves multigenerational studies in an animal model.[60] It has a complex design because testicular function, mainly spermatogenesis, is a very complicated process. The spermatogenic cycle is highly organized throughout the testis and the duration varies with different species (see Table 13.2). In the rat, it requires 52 days. To test the sensitivity of all stages of spermatogenesis, the exposure should last the full duration of the cycle. If a toxicant affects the immature spermatogonia, a change in mature sperm may not be detectable before 7 to 8 weeks. Effects on more mature germ cells would be detected sooner. Because germ cells are continuously dividing and differentiating, the staging of spermatogenesis has proved to be an extremely sensitive tool to identify and characterize even subtle toxicological changes (Figure 13.4). For accurate identification of stage-specific lesions of the seminiferous epithelium, critical evaluation of morphological structures is very important. Various stereomicroscopic preparations have been developed to achieve this stage-specific identification and characterization.[61]

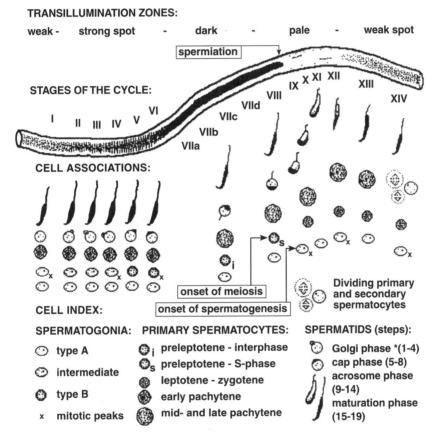

FIGURE 13.4 Schematic tracing of a living unstained rat seminiferous tubule under a transilluminating stereomicroscope. The transillumination zones are a reflection of increasing chromatin condensation of the late (steps 12 to 19) spermatids and their arrangement in the seminiferous epithelium. This is related to the stages of the cycle. The most obvious alteration in transillumination is seen at spermiation at stage VIII. Another distinct point is at stage VI, when the late spermatids lose their bundle arrangement and the dark spot absorption pattern changes into the dark zone. It is of interest that the onset of spermatogenesis and meiosis occurs at the same stage (VIII) of the cycle when the most mature spermatids spermiate. (From Parvinen, M., Toppari, J., and Lahdetie, J., in *Male Reproductive Toxicology,* Academic Press, San Diego, 1993, 143. With permission.)

F. SPERM NUCLEAR INTEGRITY ASSESSMENT

Recent attention has been focused on assessment of sperm structural morphology and physiology as important end points in reproductive toxicology testing. The structural stability of sperm nuclei depends upon their unique packaging, either during spermatogenesis or sperm maturation. It appears to be enhanced by the oxidation of protamine sulfhydryl groups to inter- and intramolecular disulfide bonds.

1. Sperm Activation Assay

This assay is based upon decondensation of sperm nuclei *in vitro* that can be induced by exposure to disulfide reducing agents. The time taken to induce extensive decondensation (assay end) is evaluated and is considered to be inversely proportional to the stability of the sperm nucleus.[62] Many tests are being developed based upon evaluation of sperm structural integrity and decondensation characteristics.[56] The time taken for sperm decondensation varies by species and follows the order human > primate> hamster> mouse > rat.

2. DNA Stability Assay or Sperm Chromatin Structure Assay (SCSA)

This assay is based upon direct evaluation of sperm chromatin integrity and provides information about genetic damage to sperm.[56] A shift in DNA pattern (from double-stranded intact DNA to denatured single stranded) can be induced by a variety of mutagenic and chemical agents and evaluated either by DNA flow cytometric analysis (see Figure 13.3) or by sperm chromatin structure assay.

3. A Single-Cell Gel Electrophoresis (Comet) Assay

This assay uses fluorescence intensity measurements by microscopy and image analysis. A shift in the DNA pattern can also be evaluated by acridine orange staining, where double-stranded DNA is stained green and single-stranded DNA is stained red. Animals exposed to known mutagens demonstrate increased amounts of single-stranded DNA, indicating an increase in genetic damage.

4. DNA Flow Cytometry

This is a very useful tool that permits rapid, objective assessment of a large number of cells.[40,54,62] Comet assay, when combined with centrifugal elutriation, can provide a useful *in vitro* model to study differences in metabolism and the susceptibility of different testicular cell types to DNA damaging compounds. Thus, new findings through these systems should lead to greater knowledge about why a chemical or class of chemicals can cause testicular toxicity.

G. Y Chromosome Deletion

The Y chromosome is necessary for both gonadal development and spermatogenesis. This chromosome is acrocentric with 60 million base pairs (bp). Most infertile men with Y deletions have severe defects of spermatogenesis. Definable genetic abnormalities using screens for Y chromosome microdeletions and standard karyotype have been observed in 20 to 30% of men with severe oligozoospermia and azoospermia. Karyotype analysis and microdeletion evaluation of the Y chromosome are indicated in such cases. The testicular histologies in a small number of such cases have revealed either Sertoli cell only or germ cell arrest phenotype. Common defects associated with azoospermia factor (AZF) include deletions of the AZFb or AZFc (DAZ) region of the Y chromosome. The Y chromosome deletion detection system (e.g., Promega Corp., Madison, WI) provides a standardized screening panel amplifying only specific informative nonpolymorphic sequence tag sites (STS) on the q arm of the Y chromosome. The amplification products (80 to 400 bp) of the four multiplex polymerase chain reactions can be separated by agarose gel electrophoresis and visualized by ethidium bromide staining. Failure to amplify specific regions of the Y chromosome is indicative of specific deletions in the test samples and is probably associated with infertility (Figure 13.5).

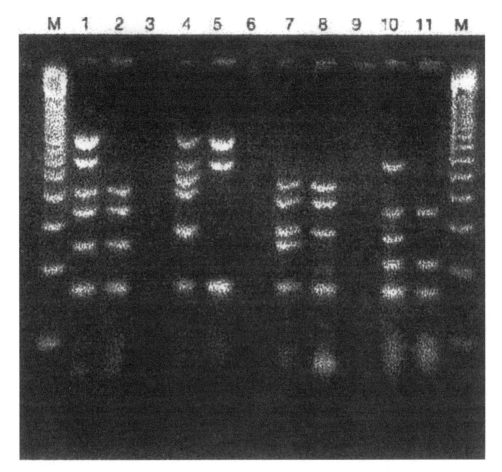

FIGURE 13.5 Y chromosome deletion analysis. The amplification products from Multiplex A (lanes 1 and 2), Multiplex B (lanes 4 and 5), Multiplex C (lanes 7 and 8) and Multiplex D (lanes 10 and 11) reactions are shown. Control human male genomic DNA from Promega (lanes 1, 4, 7, 10) is compared to a test male genomic DNA (lanes 2, 5, 8, 11). Markers (M) are the 50 bp DNA Step Ladder. Nothing was loaded in lanes 3, 6, 9. The gel is 4% Nu Sieve® 3:1 agarose. (From Y-Chromosome Deletion Detection System, Promega Corporation. With permission.)

H. Gene Microarray Technology

With the advent of sequence information for the entire mammalian genome, it is now possible to analyze gene expression and gene polymorphisms on a genomic scale employing gene array technology.[63,64] Gene array analysis is a relatively new, quick, and easy way to compare the expression levels of many nucleic acid species simultaneously in normal and abnormal or affected tissues. The genomic library provides a comprehensive tool for assessing the expression pattern of known genes in tissue samples. DNA microarray or DNA chips are fabricated on glass or membrane substrates by high-speed robotics. There are many commercial organizations that provide complete, ready-to-use array systems for such evaluations. The information obtained from these commercial arrays has been used to interrogate gene expression associated with male infertility. The whole-genome arrays will soon be a powerful tool identifying and characterizing toxicants in environmental and pharmaceutical science. In defined model systems, treatment with known agents, such as polycyclic aromatic hydrocarbons, dioxin-like compounds, peroxisome proliferators, oxidant stress, or estrogenic chemicals may provide a gene expression "signature" on a microarray, which represents the cellular response to these agents. These same systems can then be treated with unknown toxic agents to determine if one or more of these standard signatures are elicited. cDNA microarrays could also be used to determine cross talk between combinations of agents (i.e., dioxin and estrogen). Microarray technology could in the long run provide a relatively inexpensive, quick way to screen for potential bioactive agents and will help elucidate the mechanism of action of an agent. It is also likely that new molecular targets of toxicant action will be identified that may be used to detect changes in exposed human populations, information essential for the risk assessment process.

SECTION 7. CONCLUSIONS AND PERSPECTIVES

Much recent evidence in both human and wildlife support the theory that endocrine disruption causes increased incidences of cancers, reproductive anomalies, and infertility. Through controlled dose–response studies, it appears that many compounds (e.g., alkyl phenol ethylates and their degradation products, chlorinated dibenzodioxins and difurans, and polychlorinated biphenyls, or PCBs) can induce irreversible induction of male sex characteristics in females (imposex), which can lead to sterility and reduced reproductive performance. However, this hypothesis is called into question for several reasons based upon the fact that production, secretion, and elimination of hormones is highly regulated by the body via homeostatic and negative feedback control mechanisms. Therefore, minor increases of hormones following dietary absorption and in association with liver detoxification of these xenobiotics may be inconsequential in disrupting endocrine homeostasis. In addition, low ambient concentrations of chemicals along with low-affinity binding of purported xenobiotics to target receptors probably are insufficient to activate an adverse response in adults. Finally, the long-term data are not available for mixtures of chemicals that may be able to affect endocrine function. More research is needed to confirm or refute this hypothesis.

In conclusion, a variety of extraneous and internal factors can induce reproductive toxicity leading to poor sperm quality and male factor infertility. Several of these influences (e.g., glandular infection, environmental toxicants that are mainly estrogenic chemicals, nutritional deficiencies, aging, ischemia, and oxidative stress) disrupt the hormonal milieu. Partial androgen insensitivity, mainly due to altered androgen-to-estrogen balance, may contribute to significant oligozoospermia (Table 13.7). The role of chronic inflammation on the reproductive organs is not completely understood, as it is asymptomatic and difficult to demonstrate objectively. There is an urgent need to develop reliable animal models to characterize all the factors involved. In addition, the medical management of poor sperm quality is lacking. The application of sophisticated and expensive assisted reproductive techniques such as ICSI to male factor infertility, regardless of cause, does not necessarily treat the cause and may inadvertently pass on adverse genetic consequences. Thus, a clinician should always assess the potential environmental risks at the time of patient evaluation in an attempt

TABLE 13.7
Nomenclature for Some Semen Variables Commonly Used in Andrology

Normozoospermia	Normal semen sample
Oligozoospermia	Sperm concentration fewer than 20×10^6/ ml
Asthenozoospermia	More than 50% spermatozoa with poor (< 2 grade) forward progression
Teratozoospermia	Fewer than 30% spermatozoa with normal morphology
Oligoasthenoteratozoospermia	Signifies disturbance of above three variables (combinations of only two prefixes may also be used)
Azoospermia	No spermatozoa in the ejaculate
Aspermia	No ejaculate

Source: Adapted from *WHO Laboratory Manual for the Examination of Human Semen and Sperm-Cervical Mucus Interaction.*[53]

to identify the etiology of reproductive toxicity. If an association between occupation/exposure and infertility is established, plans to control and prevent exposure to others should be initiated.

REFERENCES

1. Brake, A. and Krause, W., Decreasing quality of semen, *Br. Med. J.,* 305, 1498–1503, 1992.
2. Fisch, H., Goluboff, E. T., Olson, J. H., Feldshuh, J., Broder, S. J., and Barad, D. H., Semen analyses in 1283 men from the United States over a 25-year period: no decline in quality, *Fertil. Steril.,* 65,1009–1014, 1996.
3. Olsen, G. W., Bodner, K. M., Ramlow, J. M., Ross, C. E., and Lipshultz, L. I., Have sperm counts been reduced 50 percent in 50 years? A statistical model revisited, *Fertil. Steril.,* 63, 887–893, 1995.
4. Guillette, L. J., Gross, T. S., Masson, G. R., Matter, J. M., Percival, H. F., and Woodward, A. R., Developmental abnormalities of the gonad and abnormal sex hormone concentrations in juvenile alligators from contaminated and control lakes in Florida, *Environ. Health Perspect.,* 102(8), 680–688, 1994.
5. Cheek, A. O. and McLachlan, J. A., Environmental hormones and the male reproductive system, *J. Androl.,* 19, 5–10, 1998.
6. Jorgensen, N., Toppari, J., Grandjean, P., and Skakkebaek, N. E., Environment and male reproductive function, in *Male Reproductive Function,* Wang, C., Ed., Kluwer Academic Publisher, Boston, chap. 17, pp. 321–337, 1999.
7. Kavlock, R. J. and Perreault, S. D., Multiple chemical exposure and risks of adverse reproductive function and outcome, in *Toxicological of Chemical Mixtures: From Real Life Examples to Mechanisms of Toxicology Interactions,* Yang, R. S. H., Ed., Academic Press, Orlando, FL, 1994, 245-297.
8. Lamb, D. J., Hormonal disruptors and male infertility: are men at serious risk?, *Reg. Toxicol. Pharmacol.,* 26, 001–007, 1997.
9. Sikka, S. C. and Naz, R. K., Endocrine disruptors and male infertility, in *Endocrine Disruptors — Effect on Male and Female Reproductive Systems,* CRC Press, Boca Raton, FL, 1999, chap. 8, pp. 225–246.
10. Sikka, S. C., Testicular toxicology, in *Endocrine and Hormonal Toxicology,* Harvey, P., Rush, K., and Cockburn, A., Eds., John Wiley & Sons, West Sussex, England, Chap. 5, 91–110, 1999.
11. Stone, R., Environmental estrogens stir debate. News and comment, *Science,* 256, 308–310, 1994.
12. Colborn, T., vomSaal, F. S., and Soto, A. M., Developmental effects of endocrine-disrupting chemicals in wildlife and humans, *Environ. Health Perspect.,* 1101(5), 378-384, 1993.
13. McLachlan, J. A. and Arnold, S. F., Environmental estrogens, *Am. Sci.,* 84, 452–461, 1996.
14. Parvinen, M., Lahdetie, J., and Parvinen, L. M., Toxic and mutagenic influences on spermatogenesis, *Arch. Toxicol.,* 7, 147–150, 1984.
15. White, T. E., Rucci, G., Liu, Z., and Gasiewicz, T. A., Environmentally persistent alkylphenolic compounds are estrogenic, *Endocrinology,* 135, 175–182, 1994.
16. Kelce, W. R., Monosson, E., Gamcsik, M. P., Laws, S. C., and Gray, L. E., Jr., Environmental hormone disrupters: evidence that vinclozolin developmental toxicity is mediated by antiandrogenic metabolites, *Toxicol. Appl. Pharmacol.,* 126, 276–285, 1994.
17. Sharpe, R. M. and Skakkebaek, N. E., Are estrogens involved in falling sperm counts and disorders of the male reproductive tract? *Lancet,* 351, 1392–1395, 1993.
18. Working, P. K., Male reproductive toxicity: comparison of the human to animal models, *Environ. Health Perspect.,* 77, 37–44, 1998.
19. Schrader, S. M. and Kanitz, M. H., Occupational hazards to male reproduction, in *State of the Art Reviews in Occupational Medicine: Reproductive Hazards,* Gold, E., Schenker, M., and Lesley, B., Eds., Hanley and Belfus, Philadelphia, PA, 405–414, 1994.
20. Ewing, L. L., Zirkin, B. R., and Chubb, C., Assessment of testicular testosterone production and Leydig cell structure, *Environ. Health Perspect.,* 38, 19-27, 1981.
21. Parvinen, M., Lahdetie, J., and Parvinen, L. M., Toxic and mutagenic influences on spermatogenesis, *Arch. Toxicol.,* 7, 147–150, 1984.
22. Safe, S. H., Environmental and dietary estrogens and human health: is there a problem? *Environ. Health Perspect.,* 103, 346–351, 1995.

23. Whorton, M. D., Krauss, R. M., and Marshall, S., Infertility in male pesticide workers, *Lancet*, 2, 1259–1261, 1977.

24. Bulger, W. H., Nuccitelli, R. M., and Kupfer, D., Studies on the *in vivo* and *in vitro* estrogenic activities of methoxychlor and its metabolites role of hepatic mono-oxygenase in methoxychlor activation, *Biochem. Pharmacol.*, 27, 2417–2423, 1978.

25. Schrader, S. M., Principles of male reproductive toxicology, in *Environmental Medicine*, Brooks, S. M. and Gochfeld, M., Eds., Mosby, St. Louis, MO, 1995, 95–100.

26. Snow, E. T., Metal carcinogenesis: mechanistic implications, *Pharmacol. Ther.*, 53, 31–65, 1992.

27. Winter, C., Reproductive and chromosomal effects of occupational exposure to lead in males, *Reprod. Toxicol.*, 3, 221–233, 1989.

28. Weir, R. J. and Fisher, R. S., Toxicological studies on borox and boric acid, *Toxicol. Appl. Pharmacol.*, 23, 251–264, 1972.

29. King, L. M., Andrew, M. G., Sikka, S. C., and George, W. J., Murine strain differences in cadmium-induced testicular toxicity, *Toxicologist*, 36(2), 186, 1997.

30. Schlegel, P. N., Chang, T. S. K., and Maeshall, F. F., Antibiotics: potential hazards to male fertility, *Fertil. Steril.*, 55, 235–242, 1991.

31. Shalet, S. M., Effects of cancer chemotherapy on testicular function of patients, *Cancer Treatment Rev.*, 7, 41–152, 1980.

32. Qiu, J., Hales, B. F., and Robaire, B., Adverse effects of cyclophosphamide on progeny outcome can be mediated through post-testicular mechanisms in the rat, *Biol. Reprod.*, 46, 926–931, 1992.

33. Sherins, R. J. and DeVita, V. T., Jr., Effect of drug treatment for lymphoma on male reproductive capacity, *Annu. Intern. Med.*, 79, 216–220, 1973.

34. Meistrich, M. L., Quantitative correlation between testicular stem cell survival, sperm production, and fertility in mouse after treatment with different cytotoxic agents, *J. Androl.*, 3, 58–68, 1982.

35. Jarow, J. P. and Lipshultz, L. I., Anabolic steroid-induced hypogonadotropic hypogonadism, *Am. J. Sports Med.*, 18, 429–431, 1990.

36. Oats, R. D. and Lipshultz, L. I., Fertility and testicular function in patients after chemotherapy and radiotherapy, in *Advances in Urology*, Vol. 2, Lytton, B., Ed., Mosby Year Book, Chicago, 1989, 55–83.

37. Ogilvy-Stuart, A. and Shalet, S. M., Effect of radiation on the human reproductive system, *Environ. Health Perspect.*, 101, 109–116, 1993.

38. Sikka, S. C., Gonadotoxicity, in *Male Infertility and Sexual Dysfunction*, Hellstrom, W. J. G., Ed., Springer-Verlag, New York, 1997, 292–306.

39. Aitken, R. J. and Clarkson, J. S., Cellular basis of defective sperm function and its association with the genesis of reactive oxygen species by human spermatozoa, *Reprod. Fertil.*, 81, 459–469, 1987.

40. Evenson, D. P., Flow cytometry evaluation of male germ cells, in *Flow Cytometry: Advanced Research and Clinical Applications*, Vol. 1, Yen, A., Ed., CRC Press, Boca Raton, FL, 1989, 218–246.

41. Sikka, S. C., Rajasekaran, M., and Hellstrom, W. J. G., Role of oxidative stress and antioxidants in male infertility, *J. Androl.*, 16, 464-468, 1995.

42. Sofikitis, N. V., Miyagawa, I., Zavos, P., Sikka, S. C., Hellstrom, W. J. G., Effect of smoking on testicular function, semen quality and sperm fertilizing capacity, *J. Urol.*, 154, 1030–1034, 1995.

43. Vine, M. F., Tse, C. J., Hu, P. C., and Truong, K. Y., Cigarette smoking and semen quality, *Fertil. Steril.*, 65, 835–842, 1996.

44. Creasy, D. M., Hormonal mechanisms in male reproductive tract toxicity, in *Endocrine and Hormonal Toxicology*, Harvey, P. W. Y., Rusk, K., and Cockburn, A., Eds., John Wiley & Sons, West Sussex, England, chap. 16, pp. 355–405, 1999.

45. Wilson, C. A., Leigh, A. J., and Chapman, A. J., Gonadotrophin glycosylation and function, *J. Endocrinol.*, 125, 3–14, 1990.

46. Kelce, W. R., Stone, C. R., Laws, S. C., Gray, L. E., Jr., Kemppainen, J. A., and Wilson, E. M., Persistent DDT metabolite *p,p′*-DDE is a potent androgen receptor antagonist, *Nature*, 375, 581–585, 1995.

47. Mueller, G. C. and Kim, U. H., Displacement of estradiol from estrogen receptors by simple alkylphenols, *Endocrinology*, 102, 1429–1435, 1978.

48. Safe, S., Astroff, B., Harris, B., Zacharewski, T., Dickerson, R., Romkes, M., and Biegel, L., 2,3,7,8-Tetrachlorodibenzo-*p*-dioxin (TCDD) and related compounds as antiestrogens; characterization and mechanism of action, *Pharmacol. Toxicol.*, 69, 400–409, 1991.

49. Gagnon, C., Iwasaki, A., deLamirande, E., and Kavolski, N., Reactive oxygen species and human spermatozoa (review), *Ann. N.Y. Acad. Sci.*, 637, 436–444, 1991.

50. Koppenol, W. H., Moreno, J. J., Pryor, W. A. et al., Peroxynitroite, a cloaked oxidant formed bt nitric oxide and superoxide, *Chem. Res. Toxicol.*, 5, 834–842, 1992.

51. Rosselli, M., Dubey, R. K., Imthurn, B., Macase, E., and Keller, P. J., Effects of nitric oxide on human spermatozoa: evidence that nitric oxide decreases sperm motility and induces sperm toxicity, *Hum. Reprod.*, 10, 1786–1790, 1995.

52. Mortimor, D., *Practical Laboratory Andrology*, Oxford University Press, Oxford, 1994.

53. *WHO Laboratory Manual for the Examination of Human Semen and Sperm–Cervical Mucus Interaction*, 3rd ed., Cambridge University Press, Cambridge, 1992.

54. Evenson, D. P., Jost, L. K., Baer, R. K., Turner, T. W., and Schrader, S. M., Individuality of DNA denaturation patterns in human sperm as measured by the sperm hormatin structure assay, *Reprod. Toxicol.*, 5:115-125, 1991.

55. Steinberger, A. and Clinton, J. P., Two-compartment cultures of Sertoli cells — applications in testicular toxicology, in *Methods in Toxicology*, Part A, *Male Reproductive Toxicology*, Chapin, R. E. and Heindel, J. J., Eds., Academic Press, New York, 1993, 230–245.

56. Darney, S. P., *In vitro* assessment of gamete integrity, in *In-Vitro Toxicology: Mechanisms and New Toxicology — Alternative Methods in Toxicology*, Vol. 8, Goldberg, A. M., Ed., Ann Liebert, New York, 199, 63–75.

57. Georgellis, A., Toppari, J., Veromaa, T., Rydstrom, J., and Parvinen, M., Inhibition of meiotic divisions of rat spermatocytes *in vitro* by polycyclic aromatic hydrocarbons, *Mutat. Res.*, 231, 125–135, 1990.

58. Gray, T. J. B., Application of *in vitro* systems in male reproductive toxicology, in *Physiology and Toxicology of Male Reproduction*, Lamb, J. C. IV and Foster, P. M. D., Eds., Academic Press, San Diego, CA, 1988, 250–253.

59. Lamb, J. C. IV and Chapin, R. E., Testicular and germ cell toxicity: *in vitro* approaches, *Reprod. Toxicol.*, 7, 17–22, 1993.

60. Ecobichon, D. J., Reproductive toxicology, in *CRC Handbook of Toxicology*, Derelanko, M. J. and Hollinger, M. A., Eds., CRC Press, Boca Raton, FL, 1995, 379–402.

61. Chapin, R. E., Phelps, J. L., Somkuti, S. G., and Heindel, J. J., The interaction of Sertoli and Leydig cells in the testicular toxicity of tri-*o*-cresyl phosphate, *Toxicol. Appl. Pharmacol.*, 104, 483–495, 1990.

62. Perrault, S. D., Barbee, R. R., Elstein, K. H., Zucker, R. M., and Keeler, C. L., Interspecies differences in the stability of mammalian sperm nuclei assessed *in vivo* by sperm microinjection and *in vitro* by flow cytometry, *Biol. Reprod.*, 39, 157-167, 1988.

63. Gentalen, E., Chee, M., A novel method for determining linkage between DNA sequences: hybridization to paired probe arrays, *Nucl. Acids Res.*, 27(6), 1485–1491, 1999.

64. Gerry, N. P., Witowski, N. E., Day, J., Hammer, R. P., Barany, G., and Barany, F., Universal DNA microarray method for multiplex detection of low abundance point mutations, *J. Mol. Biol.*, 292(2), 251–262, 1999.

14 Endocrine Toxicology: The Female Reproductive System

Patricia B. Hoyer, Ph.D.
and Patrick J. Devine, Ph.D.

CONTENTS

SECTION 1. INTRODUCTION — IMPACT OF ENVIRONMENTAL CHEMICALS

The female must perform two distinct reproductive functions: development and support of female germ cells, and maintenance of the fetus until it can survive in the outside world. Reproductive toxicology involves detecting and understanding potentially detrimental influences on reproductive success. This field has been developing in response to observations linking clustered effects in humans to specific types of exposure. There are several examples of how xenobiotics in the form of pharmaceuticals can impact reproductive function in humans. One example is the effect of the sedative thalidomide prescribed to women in the 1950s for morning sickness during early pregnancy.[1] A greatly increased incidence of children born with developmental organ and limb malformations was traced to *in utero* exposure to thalidomide. This drug was reported to have been responsible for 8000 malformed children over a 2-year period. Whereas thalidomide is an example involving developmental limb defects, reproductive effects in humans have been seen with the synthetic estrogen diethylstilbestrol (DES). From the 1940s to 1960s, DES was widely prescribed for high-risk pregnancies. In 1971, Herbst et al.[2] observed an increased incidence of rare vaginal clear cell adenocarcinoma in daughters of these women who had been exposed *in utero* to DES. Subsequent research has demonstrated that prenatal exposure to DES can also cause fertility defects, teratogenesis, and neoplasia throughout the male and female reproductive tract.[3] Thalidomide and DES represent therapeutic exposures; however, there is also evidence of reproductive effects that have been documented following occupational exposures. In the early 1990s in Korea, a disproportionate number of female workers in an electronics plant who had been exposed to 2-bromopropane (2BP) were discovered to suffer from amenorrhea and hot flashes. Subsequent animal studies have determined that 2BP causes ovarian follicle damage.[4] The more recent attention focused on endocrine disruptors has made it clear that there is an incomplete understanding of how xenobiotic chemicals can affect and damage the female reproductive system. With the trend toward women starting families later in life, the effect of longer-term environmental exposure on fertility must be considered. The world has experienced rapid technological and industrial advancement in the last part of the 20th century, making it increasingly important to design and improve approaches for identifying chemicals, drugs, and mixtures that are potentially detrimental to reproductive function in women.

SECTION 2. REPRODUCTIVE LIFE SPAN IN WOMEN — FETAL DEVELOPMENT, PUBERTY, AND MENOPAUSE

A. FETAL DEVELOPMENT

The indifferent gonadal anlage forms at about week 5 of gestation with the arrival of primordial germ cells that migrate from their site of origin near the yolk sac. In the genetic female, there is an absence of the Y chromosome, and the indifferent gonad develops into an ovary. Additionally, in the absence of Müllerian-inhibiting factor, the female reproductive tract develops from the Müllerian ducts into the oviducts, uterus, and vagina. Finally, in the absence of testosterone, the Wolffian ducts regress. Germ cells (oogonia) proliferate during fetal development, but develop into oocytes and enter the prophase of the first meiotic division where they become arrested until shortly before ovulation. As a result, oogenesis does not occur postnatally and a female is born with the entire cohort of germ cells she will ever have.

B. Puberty

Puberty, the time at which sexual reproduction becomes possible, generally occurs between the ages of 9 and 16 in humans. Puberty is identified in women as the first menstruation, which usually occurs prior to the first ovulation. From birth and throughout the prepubertal period, waves of follicular development in the ovary occur; however, all follicles become atretic. Thus, puberty marks the time at which oocytes can be recruited and developed to ovulation.

The onset of puberty is evident as a gradual increase in the secretion of the gonadotropins, luteinizing hormone (LH), and follicle-stimulating hormone (FSH) by the pituitary, acting on instructions from the hypothalamus. This increase may result from the removal of an inhibitory influence on hypothalamic gonadotropin-releasing hormone (GnRH) release. This change in the "setpoint" of the inhibitory influence must occur because increasing amounts of steroids (which provide negative feedback on the release of GnRH and the gonadotropins) are secreted by the ovary as puberty approaches. Thus, the initiation of puberty in females may involve the "resetting" or desensitization of the hypothalamus to negative feedback by ovarian steroid hormones.

C. Menopause

Ovarian failure (menopause) in women is associated with the cessation of ovarian cyclicity. The average age of menopause in the United States is 50, and this is a direct consequence of depletion of the follicular reserve. Menopause is preceded by a period of increasingly irregular cycles (the perimenopausal period). This progressive failure in ovarian function is accompanied by a gradual increase in circulating levels of FSH (and eventually LH), and a decline in circulating 17β-estradiol concentrations. It is thought that the absence of estrogen is the cause of most of the clinical symptoms associated with menopause, such as osteoporosis and increased risk of cardiovascular disease.[5] Recently, this loss of estrogen has also been implicated in other health risks such as depression,[6] colon cancer,[7] Alzheimer's disease,[8] and macular degeneration.[9]

SECTION 3. FEMALE REPRODUCTIVE SYSTEM — HYPOTHALAMIC/PITUITARY/OVARIAN AXIS

The major functions of the ovary are production of the female germ cell, the oocyte, and production of female sex steroid hormones. The ovary of the mature female contains highly dynamic structures that undergo major changes during the monthly cycle. Specifically, the ovary contains two endocrine glands: the follicle and the corpus luteum. The follicle is responsible for gametogenesis (oogenesis) and production of the hormone 17β-estradiol (steroidogenesis). The other endocrine system, the corpus luteum, is derived from follicular tissue following ovulation and is present on the ovary of the nonpregnant female only during the second half of the menstrual cycle, but is maintained if pregnancy occurs. The corpus luteum produces the steroid hormone progesterone, which is responsible for implantation and the maintenance of pregnancy.

A. Ovarian Steroids

The major ovarian steroids are the estrogens (primarily 17β-estradiol) and progesterone. 17β-Estradiol is responsible for follicular maturation, and hyperplasia of the endometrium and uterine vasculature during the follicular phase. In the endometrium, 17β-estradiol also stimulates synthesis of receptors for 17β-estradiol and progesterone (a priming for hormonal regulation in pregnancy). Additionally, 17β-estradiol provides both negative and positive feedback on the hypothalamus and pituitary for regulation of LH and FSH secretion. During puberty, 17β-estradiol promotes breast development, maturation of the external genitalia, and the female pattern of fat distribution. Progesterone facilitates implantation by preparing the uterus to accommodate a blastocyst and provides maintenance of pregnancy by inhibiting uterine contractions and endometrial sloughing. Additionally, progesterone provides negative feedback on the hypothalamus and pituitary for inhibition of release of the gonadotropins. In prepubertal females, progesterone promotes development of breast alveoli.

B. Regulation of Gonadotropin Release

Tonic secretion of LH and FSH from the anterior pituitary can be affected by the inhibitory actions of 17β-estradiol and progesterone in a classical long loop of negative feedback (Figure 14.1). Because both steroids participate in the inhibition of gonadotropin release, the absence of either 17β-estradiol or progesterone alone will cause basal LH and FSH levels to increase. Additionally, inhibin produced by granulosa cells in developing follicles also contributes to the selective inhibition of FSH release. In contrast to tonic LH secretion, which is controlled by a negative feedback mechanism, an LH surge that triggers ovulation is produced by a neuroendocrine reflex arc of positive feedback that is not clearly understood. This is known to be stimulated by increasing, marked elevations in circulating 17β-estradiol levels that are produced by the largest developing preovulatory (Graafian) follicle (see Figure 14.1). As a result, when levels become sufficiently elevated, 17β-estradiol shifts from its inhibitory role in regulating LH and FSH release, and initiates the LH surge (which triggers ovulation). In contrast to 17β-estradiol, progesterone inhibits the LH surge. This ensures that estrogen output in early pregnancy does not stimulate ovulation.

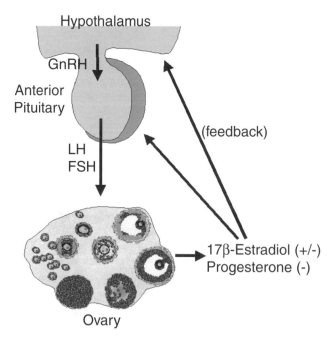

FIGURE 14.1 Hypothalamic–pituitary–ovarian axis. GnRH stimulates the anterior pituitary to synthesize and secrete LH and FSH. These in turn cause progression of development of ovarian follicles and corpora lutea, which produce 17β-estradiol and progesterone, and these feed back onto the anterior pituitary and hypothalamus.

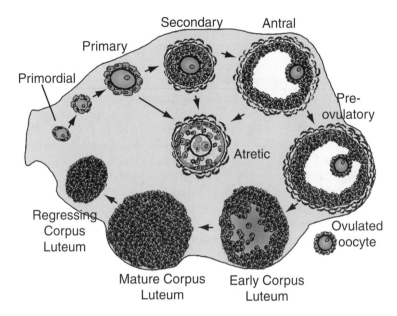

Primordial
Primary
Secondary
Antral
Pre-ovulatory
Atretic
Ovulated oocyte
Regressing Corpus Luteum
Mature Corpus Luteum
Early Corpus Luteum

FIGURE 14.2 Development of ovarian follicles. Primordial follicles are activated to grow and develop from primary through secondary and antral stages of follicular development until ovulation. Most follicles degenerate by the process of atresia before reaching the ovulatory stage. Those follicles that do ovulate luteinize to become corpora lutea, which support pregnancy if fertilization occurs.

SECTION 4. OVARIAN PHYSIOLOGY — FOLLICULAR DEVELOPMENT

At birth, the ovary contains its full complement of germ cells since oogonia are only formed during fetal development. Oogonia become oocytes when they begin the early stages of meiosis and many are incorporated into primordial follicles. Oocytes not incorporated into follicles degenerate. The oocyte, arrested in an early stage of meiosis, will remain in this state of suspended animation until it becomes activated for follicular development. Therefore, in some oocytes, this period of arrest can last for years. In the mature ovary, once a follicle begins to develop it is committed to one of two fates (Figure 14.2). If the hormonal milieu is appropriate, it will continue to develop to ovulation. However, most (greater than 99.9%) follicles never ovulate; instead, they degenerate by a process called atresia, which can occur at any stage of follicular development. In women, about 6 million oogonia are formed during fetal development; at birth the ovary contains approximately 2 million oocytes incorporated into primordial follicles; about 400,000 primordial follicles are present in the ovaries by the time of puberty; yet, only about 400 follicles are destined to ovulate.

The stages of follicular development toward ovulation involve a continuum of events, each providing further maturation of the follicular cells (see Figure 14.2). Upon receipt of an as yet unknown signal for development, the primordial follicle is activated and becomes a primary follicle. As the follicle develops, there is proliferation of the granulosa cells surrounding the oocyte, and acquisition of a layer of theca interna cells surrounding the granulosa layer. Follicles progress from the primary stage to the secondary stage when multiple layers of granulosa cells are present around the oocyte. When the follicle develops sufficiently, an antrum (fluid-filled space) develops within the granulosa cell layer. The antral follicle continues to grow, and at its most mature stage prior to ovulation is known as a Graafian (preovulatory) follicle. Following ovulation, the cells remaining, which had formed the structure of the follicle, infiltrate and differentiate (luteinize) to form a solid gland, the corpus luteum (see Figure 14.2). Resumption of meiosis in the oocyte occurs only at the time of impending ovulation. Meiosis progresses through the first division, producing a secondary oocyte and the first polar body, which degenerates. Meiosis then continues to the beginning of the second division, which is only completed if fertilization occurs.

Granulosa cells surround the developing gamete, and help support its development and maturation. In early development of an antral follicle, granulosa cells are regulated by FSH. One of the effects of FSH is to stimulate expression of aromatase (the enzyme that converts androgens to estrogens). In the late stages of follicular development (preovulatory), granulosa cells also acquire receptors for LH (under the combined influence of FSH and 17β-estradiol). This prepares these cells to receive the appropriate signal for ovulation in the form of the LH surge. Theca interna cells are vascularized and are responsible for the synthesis of androgens (testosterone and androstenedione), which is regulated by LH.[10] Androgens synthesized and secreted by theca cells diffuse across the basal lamina membrane to the adjacent granulosa cells to be converted by aromatase to estrogens (termed the two-cell theory of steroid synthesis).

Luteal cells formed by luteinization of the theca and granulosa cells following ovulation primarily produce progesterone. Synthesis and secretion of progesterone in these cells is stimulated by LH. Additionally, maintenance of the corpus luteum (tropic support) requires the presence of LH as well. In humans, the corpus luteum also synthesizes and secretes 17β-estradiol; however, progesterone output is much greater. In the nonpregnant female, at the end of the menstrual cycle, the corpus luteum undergoes luteolysis and progesterone production falls. Conversely, in pregnancy, the corpus luteum receives a signal from the developing conceptus in the form of human chorionic gonadotropin (hCG), which binds to the LH receptor. This rescues the corpus luteum so that it will continue to secrete progesterone for establishment and early maintenance of pregnancy.

SECTION 5. SITES OF DISRUPTION OF REPRODUCTIVE FUNCTION

An endocrine disrupter or reproductive toxicant can have detrimental effects to reproduction in women at a number of levels. Toxicants can have direct effects on the ovary or reproductive tract, or they can inhibit ovulation or development of the oocyte (ovotoxicity) or preparation of the reproductive tract to receive and support the embryo. The mechanism(s) by which chemicals are ovotoxic could be due to direct ovarian toxicity or to an indirect effect on the hypothalamus and/or pituitary. In the former case, ovarian failure would produce rather than result from changes in circulating FSH levels, and FSH levels should increase as a result of loss of negative feedback from the ovarian hormones usually produced by developing follicles. Conversely, if the effect is at the hypothalamic–pituitary level, alterations in gonadotropin secretion should precede ovarian changes. In one long-term study, female B6C3F$_1$ mice were treated with the occupational chemical 4-vinylcyclohexene (VCH) for 30 days (age 28 to 58 days).[11] At that time, compared with controls, more than 90% of primordial follicles had been lost. Circulating FSH levels were not increased before the 240 day time point. Therefore, the ovary was suggested as a direct target because ovarian changes significantly preceded the rise in circulating FSH levels.

The level and duration of exposure to an environmental chemical may determine the effects of reproductive toxicants. Individuals are only rarely exposed acutely to high levels of reproductive toxicants. These can usually be readily identified. However, the possible effects of chronic, low-dose exposures are of particular concern, because they are more likely to occur and are more difficult to identify. These types of exposures may cause reproductive or fertility problems that go unrecognized for years because of the potential for cumulative damage. Manifestations of such injury could include infertility, early menopause, or eventual development of ovarian cancer.

Another factor involving the overall effects of reproductive toxicants is the lifetime stage at which exposure occurs (Figure 14.3). Temporary infertility can occur in an adult cyclic woman following damage to the ovaries, whereas exposure during childhood might induce sterility by chemical-induced destruction of germ cells. Further, exposures *in utero* may cause improper

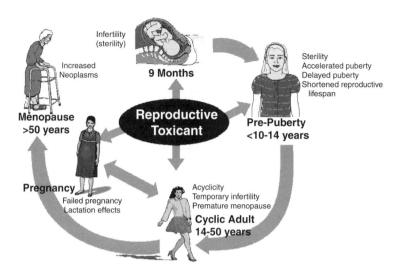

FIGURE 14.3 Reproductive life span of females. Exposure to reproductive toxicants can have a long-term impact on female reproductive capacity. The effect can vary depending upon whether the damage occurred during fetal development, childhood (prepuberty), regular adulthood (cyclic adult), or pregnancy. (Reprinted from Boekelheide, K. et al., *Comprehensive Toxicology,* Vol. 10, *Reproductive and Endocrine Toxicology,* Copyright 1997, p. 253, with permission from Elsevier Science.)

development of ovarian follicles or permanent alterations in the reproductive tract, as occurred in response to DES. The remainder of this chapter primarily focuses on potential reproductive effects that can be caused by direct impairment of the ovary.

SECTION 6. CONSEQUENCES OF OVARIAN TOXICITY

Chemicals that extensively destroy primordial and primary follicles can cause irreversible infertility (premature menopause in humans) since, once destroyed, they cannot be replaced. Furthermore, destruction of primordial follicles will have a delayed effect on cyclicity that is undetected until there are no follicles left to be recruited for development. Alternatively, damage to large growing or antral follicles can cause a reversible disruption of cyclicity by impacting on ovarian steroid production and ovulation. This effect is generally reversible because more follicles can ultimately be recruited for development from the pool of primordial follicles that remain.

SECTION 7. SPECIFIC OVARIAN TOXICANTS — HUMAN EFFECTS AND ANIMAL STUDIES

A. CHEMOTHERAPEUTIC AGENTS

Destruction of oocytes contained in ovarian follicles can be caused by a variety of environmental or pharmacological chemicals.[12] The toxic effects of chemotherapeutic drugs in women cancer patients surviving chemotherapy have become important issues. Since the beginning of antineoplastic therapy to treat a variety of diseases and malignancies, the ability of these agents to produce ovarian failure has been known. Nitrogen mustard, chlorambucil, and vinblastine have been reported to cause sterility in women.[13-15] Cyclophosphamide (CPA), an alkylating agent in cancer chemotherapy, is also known to cause premature ovarian failure in women.[16] These observations in humans have motivated a variety of studies with CPA in rodents to elucidate better its mechanism of ovotoxicity. Miller and Cole[17] studied the ovaries in mice treated with low doses of CPA for 1 year.

There were reduced numbers of oocytes, especially in primordial follicles, and corpora lutea. Effects on other tissues such as the kidney, spleen, thymus, or lymph nodes were found. Estrous cyclicity was destroyed and cysts/tumors were observed in the ovarian germinal epithelium. In a short-term study, susceptibility to CPA was greatest in primordial follicles in C57Bl/6N and D2 mice and SD rats.[18] Plowchalk and Mattison[19] observed a time- and dose-dependent relationship between CPA and ovarian toxicity by looking at changes in ovarian structure and function. In C57Bl/6N mice given a single intraperitoneal (ip) injection of increasing concentrations of CPA, primordial follicle numbers were reduced in a dose-dependent manner. The loss of primordial follicles was essentially complete at 3 days and the estimated ED_{50} (concentration that produced 50% follicle loss) was 122 mg/kg body weight. From these animal studies, it appears that premature ovarian failure in women treated with CPA is likely to be via destruction of primordial follicles.

B. CIGARETTE SMOKING

Epidemiological studies conducted over the last four decades have demonstrated a relationship between smoking and impaired fertility. Cigarette smoke is a well-known reproductive toxicant. One study reported that rates of pregnancy were reduced to 75% in light smokers and 57% in heavy smokers when compared with nonsmokers. Furthermore, smokers required 1 year longer to conceive than did nonsmokers.[20] Along with the impact on fertility, there are also effects of cigarette smoke on pregnancy and the fetus. Prenatal exposure to cigarette smoke has been associated with retarded intrauterine growth and premature deliveries.[5] Additionally, conception in women whose mothers smoked while pregnant was significantly reduced when compared with women whose mothers had not.[21] Decreased follicular levels of 17β-estradiol were seen in smoking women when compared with nonsmokers, and cultured human granulosa cells secrete decreased amounts of 17β-estradiol in the presence of an extract of cigarette smoke.[22] Thus, these effects may relate to the infertility associated with cigarette smoking.

Women smokers have also been reported to experience a 1- to 4-year-earlier age for the onset of menopause (Figure 14.4).[5] The earlier onset of menopause among smokers may be induced by several possible mechanisms. Cigarette smoke is a complex mixture of alkaloids (nicotine), polycyclic aromatic hydrocarbons (PAH), nitroso compounds, aromatic amines, and protein pyrolysates, many of which are carcinogenic.[23] Direct oocyte destruction caused by one or more of these chemicals is the most logical mechanism by which cigarette smoke induces early menopause. Of additional concern is the finding in animal studies that exposure of mice *in utero* to cigarette smoke resulted in a reduced number of ovarian primordial follicles in female offspring.[24]

C. POLYCYCLIC AROMATIC HYDROCARBONS

Many animal studies have demonstrated ovotoxic effects of PAHs. High levels of PAHs are present in cigarette smoke, including benzo[*a*]pyrene (BaP), 3-methylcholanthrene (3-MC), and 9,10-dimethyl-1,2-benzanthracene (DMBA).[25] In mouse studies, oocyte destruction was shown to occur in response to these three chemicals[26] and ovarian tumors resulted.[27,28] Mattison and Thorgeirsson[29] reported oocyte destruction after single, high doses of these chemicals in mice. Multiple doses of these compounds can also destroy small follicles, although effects are observed at much lower doses.[30]

An effect of DMBA and BaP on antral follicles has also been reported in mice. DMBA was reported to decrease small follicles initially, with a secondary effect on large follicles.[31] In a morphological assessment of ovaries collected from mice that were dosed with PAHs, Mattison et al.[32] reported that BaP, 3-MC, and DMBA all destroyed primordial follicles; however, only DMBA decreased antral follicles. Yet, in a subsequent study in mice, BaP decreased numbers of corpora lutea, and this effect was reversible. These observations are consistent with disrupted ovulation and targeting of BaP to antral follicles, which were reduced in number at the higher doses. The

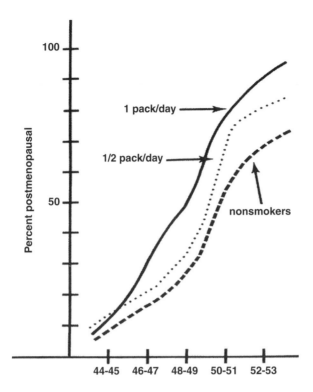

FIGURE 14.4 Effect of smoking on age of menopause. Toxicants in cigarette smoke appear to destroy small oocytes. No major effects on fertility are noted during the reproductive life span, but shortening of reproductive life span occurs. (From Mattison, D.R. and Schulman, J.D., *Contemp. Obste. Gynecol.*, 15, 157, 1980. With permission.)

discrepancy in findings between the two studies is not easily understood; however, it is apparent that under certain conditions, PAHs can also damage antral follicles.

D. OCCUPATIONAL CHEMICALS

1,3-Butadiene (BD) and the related olefins isoprene and styrene are released during the manufacture of synthetic rubber and thermoplastic resins, and the estimated annual occupational exposure of U.S. employees is 3700 to 1,000,000 people.[33] These chemicals have also been reported in cigarette smoke and automobile exhaust. Chronic animal inhalation studies have shown that carcinogenesis caused by BD is higher in mice than rats. At lower doses, female mice exposed daily by inhalation for as long as 2 years exhibited ovarian atrophy, granulosa cell hyperplasia, and benign and malignant granulosa cell tumors.[34] Thus, ovarian effects of BD appear to occur at lower concentrations than are required to produce effects in other tissues. In a short-term study, dosing of B6C3F1 mice (ip) daily for 30 days with the BD metabolite 1,3-butadiene diepoxide resulted in a depletion of primordial (98%) and growing (primary to preantral, 87%) follicles, compared with control animals.[35] The results of this study demonstrated direct ovarian targeting of the ovary by the diepoxide of BD, and provided evidence that this was the ovotoxic form of the chemical.

There are mixed opinions about the risk of human exposure to BD-induced toxicity. According to Bond et al.,[36] there is not enough evidence for an association between occupational exposure and human lymphatic and hematopoietic cancers. They have shown that the metabolic activation of BDE (the carcinogenic form) occurs to a greater extent in mice than in rats and humans.

Furthermore, they concluded that because concentrations encountered in the environment or work-place are usually below 2 ppm, a carcinogenic risk to humans is not likely. However, the potential cumulative toxic effects of long-term exposure to low concentrations over the course of years was not discussed. This is particularly important when the target cells are of a nonrenewing type (for example, ovarian follicles).

The dimerization of BD forms 4-vinylcyclohexene (VCH). The VCH family of compounds are occupational chemicals released at low concentrations during the manufacture of rubber tires, plasticizers, and pesticides.[33] VCH and its diepoxide metabolite VCD have been shown in mice and rats to (1) produce extensive destruction of primordial and primary follicles,[37] (2) cause premature ovarian failure,[11] (3) increase the risk for development of ovarian tumors,[19] and (4) affect normal ovarian development of female offspring exposed *in utero*.[12] Because no significant effects on other tissues have been reported in studies with this class of chemicals, the damage they produce appears to be highly selective, and does not involve widespread toxicity. Ovarian damage caused by VCH and its related epoxide metabolites has been demonstrated by a variety of exposure routes, including dermal,[38] oral,[39] inhalation,[40] and intraperitoneal injection.[37] It is therefore important to consider the potential risks for human exposure.

E. PHTHALATES

Di-(2-ethylhexyl)phthalate (DEHP) is widely used in the production of many polyvinyl chlo-ride–based plastics, including medical and food packages. DEHP can leach out of plastics and contaminate food or the surrounding environment. Decreased rates of pregnancy, increased rates of miscarriage, and anovulation have been associated with occupational exposure of Russian women to phthalates. Also, repeated oral exposure of female SD rats to DEHP caused disruptions of reproductive function, in the form of delayed ovulation, reduced granulosa cell size in antral follicles, decreased circulating 17β-estradiol, progesterone, and LH levels, and increased FSH.[41] From the responses to DEHP in rats, the authors concluded that these reproductive effects resulted from a specific targeting of large antral follicles, because of suppressed granulosa cell 17β-estra-diol production.

F. HALOGENATED ARYL HYDROCARBONS

Endocrine disrupters that display estrogenic/antiestrogenic effects have been actively studied in their ability to target developmental and uterine sites of action, although intracellular mechanisms involved in these actions remain poorly understood. The effects of 2,3,7,8-tetrachlorodibenzo-*p*-dioxin (TCDD) on sexual development and fertility have been studied in depth.[42] There is much evidence for a hypothalamic–pituitary site of action, although this compound also has been shown to cause direct ovotoxicity.[43] Reductions in ovulation and alterations in the estrous cycle were observed following a single oral dose of TCDD in female rats. The mechanism by which TCDD directly targets the ovary might be due to inhibition of 17β-estradiol production in granulosa cells, as suggested by *in vitro* studies.[44] It is possible this chemical has targeted effects at several sites.

The PCB compound 3,3,4,4-tetrachlorobiphenyl (TCB) has been shown to be teratogenic in the mouse and embryolethal in the rat, as well as to have transplacental ovarian toxicity in the mouse.[45] Follicles in all stages of development were reduced 40 to 50% in female offspring at 28 days of age when mice were exposed *in utero* on day 13 of gestation. Interestingly, during a 5-month period of testing, this extent of follicular damage did not adversely affect reproductive function in these offspring.

G. OTHER OVOTOXIC AGENTS

The alkylating agents 1,4-di(methanesulfonoxy)-butane (Myleran), trimethylenemelamin (TEM), and isopropyl methanesulfonate (IMS) have been shown to destroy oocytes in small follicles in

(SECXC57BL)F1 mice within several days of a single ip injection.[46] Daily oral administration of nitrofurazone over 2 years caused ovarian lesions, including development of benign mixed tumors and granulosa cell tumors in mice. Hexachlorobenzene, a persistent halogenated hydrocarbon identified as a contaminant in human follicular fluid, is of particular concern in view of its ability to destroy primordial follicles in rhesus and cynomolgus monkeys.[47] Dobson and Felton[48] reported a variety of other compounds that were capable of producing significant primordial follicle loss in mice, including methyl and ethyl methanesulfonate, busulfan, and urethane. Additionally, of a number of fungal toxins and antibiotics tested, procarbazine HCl and 4-nitroquinoline-1-oxide were ovotoxic. Finally, dibromochloropropane, urethane, N-ethyl-N-nitrosourea, and bleomycin demonstrated primordial follicle killing, with bleomycin being the most potent. In general, all these ovotoxic chemicals are also known to possess mutagenic–carcinogenic effects. The results of an *in vitro* mutagenicity study testing a number of industrial and laboratory chemicals using *Escherichia coli* demonstrated a high correlation between alkylating activity and increased mutagenicity.[49] Thus, these studies have further provided a correlation between ovotoxicity and subsequent development of tumorigenesis. To what extent these two events are linked is not clearly understood at this time.

SECTION 8. MECHANISMS OF OVOTOXICITY

In determining mechanisms involved in ovotoxicity, it is first important to determine whether selective or distinct follicular populations are targeted. In studies investigating the mechanism(s) by which 4-vinylcyclohexene diepoxide (VCD) is ovotoxic, rats were dosed daily for 30 days. Morphological evaluation of ovaries from control and treated rats revealed that significant loss of small follicles had occurred in follicles in the primordial, primary, and secondary stages (Figure 14.5). However, at a shorter time of dosing, reduced numbers of primordial and primary follicles were seen on day 15; yet the number of secondary follicles was unchanged. Thus, these findings supported that primordial and primary follicles are directly targeted by VCD and that the loss of secondary follicles seen on day 30 was the result of fewer primordial and primary follicles from which to recruit.

A. CELL DEATH

Only a select few follicles in the ovary will ever develop completely and be ovulated.[10] Instead, the vast majority begin development, but are lost by a process of cell death, called atresia. Atretic follicles at all stages of development can be morphologically distinguished from healthy follicles. Follicular atresia in rats has been shown to occur via a mechanism of physiological cell death, apoptosis.[50] Thus, morphological changes of a cell undergoing atresia are those characteristic of apoptosis.

It has been proposed that xenobiotic-induced premature ovarian failure can be due to increased rates of atresia. However, there appears to be a relationship among the dose of a given chemical, the duration of treatment, and the type of cell death that follows. Chemicals such as acetaminophen, carbon tetrachloride, or hydrogen peroxide used to treat hepatocytes at low doses can cause apoptosis, whereas, at higher doses, necrosis results.[51-53] This suggests that mechanisms of cellular damage in response to xenobiotics differ as a function of dose. In a previous study, a single dose of VCD in rats was protective against the normal rate of atresia (follicle loss by apoptosis).[54] This was in marked contrast to VCD-induced apoptosis (acceleration of atresia) that is seen after 15 days of daily dosing.

In other studies investigating ovotoxicity in rats and mice, morphological evidence consistent with both types of cell death has been reported. Ovaries collected from mice dosed with a relatively high dose of cyclophosphamide (CPA, 500 mg/kg) demonstrated necrotic damage in oocytes contained in primordial follicles.[14] This effect was specific for the oocyte because surrounding

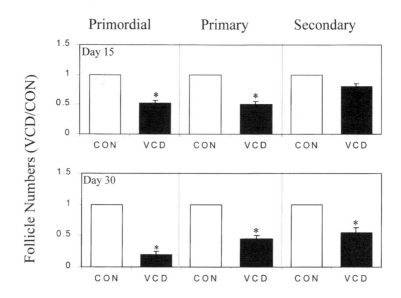

FIGURE 14.5 Reductions of small follicle numbers by repeated dosing with 4-vinylcyclohexene diepoxide. Female Fischer 344 rats (age day 28) were dosed daily with vehicle control (open bars) or VCD (80 mg/kg, ip, closed bars) for 15 or 30 days. Ovaries were collected and processed for histological counting of primordial, primary, and secondary follicles. *$p < 0.05$ different from control ($n = 5$/group) (unpublished results).

granulosa cells appeared unchanged. Conversely, atretic changes in primordial follicles were reported at lower doses (100 mg/kg). In rats treated with the phthalate DEHP, antral follicle damage was observed in association with retarded ovulation.[41] The morphological changes in these follicles were also consistent with atresia.

In studies in mice treated with PAHs (80 mg/kg BaP, 3-MC, or DMBA), oocyte morphology consistent with necrosis was observed in primordial follicles.[55] These changes caused by 3-MC and BaP were seen in the absence of visible effects in the associated granulosa cells. Of the three, DMBA produced more visible toxicity by more extensively destroying follicles and disrupting ovarian architecture.

Taken together, the reports related to mechanisms of cell death during ovotoxicity suggest that dose and duration of exposure impact the outcome. This provides further rationale for designing animal studies using low-dose repeated exposure to mimic the nature of human exposures more closely.

B. Intracellular Sites of Damage

In general, intracellular sites targeted by ovotoxic chemicals have not been identified. Many epoxidated compounds have been associated with increased mutagenicity in *in vitro* bacterial assays. The ability of epoxides to produce DNA adducts and induce sister chromatin exchanges has also been demonstrated at the molecular level.[56,57] However, whether or not DNA damage is the event that initiates ovotoxicity has not been determined for most of these chemicals. It has been proposed that plasma membrane damage is more highly correlated with ovotoxicity than DNA damage. This observation was supported by comparing alkylating properties with genetic activity in a variety of epoxide-containing chemicals.[58] Thus, the cellular event(s) initiated directly by ovotoxic chemicals may be at the level of proteins involved in signaling pathways or regulatory mechanisms associated with cell death/viability determination, rather than as a direct result of DNA damage. As with the type of cell death, this also may vary with dose and duration of exposure.

SECTION 9. EVALUATION OF POTENTIAL TOXICANTS — MODELING AN APPROACH

A novel reproductive toxicant is likely to be identified by observing reduced numbers of offspring in multigenerational studies being performed to measure transplacental effects in nonreproductive organs. Observation of this phenomenon would then lead to a more thorough characterization of the target for toxicity.[59] This reduction in live births could be due to direct fetotoxicity or to an effect on placental function, maternal ovarian function, or testicular function in males. To determine the general target, animal studies should be designed to examine each process that could be involved (Figure 14.6). A first approach might involve dosing of the female only, to determine which gender is affected. Treated females mated with untreated males can be sacrificed just before parturition, and the number of live and dead offspring, implantation sites, and resorption sites can be counted in the uterus. Corpora lutea can also be counted in the maternal ovaries as an indication of the number of ovulations. If the number of corpora lutea is similar to the number of offspring, but reduced compared with numbers in untreated females, a direct ovarian effect impacting on ovulation would be suggested. If the number of corpora lutea is greater than the number of implantation sites, this data would suggest an effect on fertilization, the placenta, or the uterus. If fewer offspring than implantations are observed, an effect on the uterus or fetus could be proposed. If the number of implantation sites is equal to the number of offspring, but less than the number of corpora lutea, an effect on fertilization is most likely. Increased numbers of resorption sites or dead fetuses would point to fetotoxicity but might reflect a placental effect. If it is determined that the impairment is on ovulation, the ovary can be examined as a target site. Histological examination of the numbers of follicles at different stages of follicular development and measurement of circulating 17β-estradiol and progesterone levels can help identify the effect of the chemical on the ovary. Overall, this points out the importance of being watchful of potential reproductive effects in multigenerational studies undertaken for other reasons.

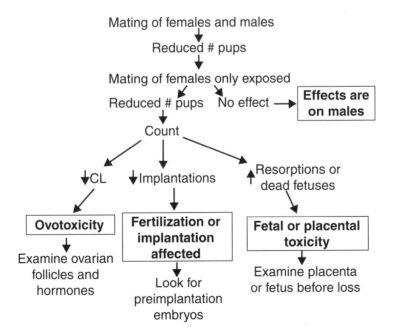

FIGURE 14.6 Approach for evaluating reproductive effects. The specific target of a reproductive toxicant can be determined in laboratory animals by determining which specific events are altered during reproduction. This can be accomplished by monitoring the number of corpora lutea, preimplantation embryos, implantation sites, pups, and/or live offspring during mating of treated females with untreated males.

SECTION 10. SUMMARY AND CONCLUSIONS

In summary, environmental chemicals that impact ovarian function can directly disrupt endocrine balance by decreasing the production of ovarian hormones and interfering with ovulation. These effects are rather immediate, target large antral follicles, and can be reversed once there is no longer exposure to the chemical. On the other hand, ovarian function can be irreversibly impaired by exposure to chemicals that destroy small preantral follicles. This produces an indirect disruption of endocrine balance, once hormonal feedback mechanisms have been affected. The manifestation of this type of ovarian toxicity is delayed until irreversible ovarian failure (early menopause) has occurred. This particular type of ovotoxicity is of particular concern in women because of health risks known to be associated with menopause. Future research should be aimed at understanding specific mechanisms of ovotoxicity, and improving the ability to predict human risk from the wide variety of exposures to these chemicals in the environment.

ACKNOWLEDGMENTS

This work has received support from the National Institutes of Environmental Health Services (Center Grant ES06694, R01ES08979, R01ES09246), Arizona Disease Control Research Commission (9809), Chemical Manufacturers' Association, and the March of Dimes.

REFERENCES

1. Seegmiller, R. E., Selected examples of developmental toxicants, in *Reproductive and Endocrine Toxicology*, Vol. 10, Boekelheide, K., Chapin, R. E., Hoyer, P. B., and Harris, C., Eds., Elsevier Science, New York, 1997, chap. 45.
2. Herbst, A. L., Ulfelder, H., and Poskanzer, D. C., Adenocarcinoma of the vagina. Association of maternal stilbestrol therapy with tumor appearance in young women, *N. Eng. J. Med.*, 284, 878, 1971.
3. Hendry, W. J., DeBrot, B. L., Zheng, X. L., Branham, W. S., and Sheehan, D. M., Differential activity of diethylstilbestrol versus estradiol as neonatal endocrine disrupters in the female hamster (*Mesocricetus auratus*) reproductive tract, *Biol. Reprod.*, 61, 91, 1999.
4. Yu, X., Kamijima, M., Ichihara, G., Li, W., Kitoh, J., Xie, Z., Shibata, E., Hisanaga, N., and Takeuchi, Y., 2-Bromopropane causes ovarian dysfunction by damaging primordial follicles and their oocytes in female rats, *Toxicol. Appl. Pharmacol.*, 159, 185, 1999.
5. Mattison, D. R., Plowchalk, B. S., Meadows, M. J., Miller, M. M., Malek, A., and London, S., The effect of smoking on oogenesis, fertilization, and implantation, *Semin. Reprod. Endocrinol.*, 7, 291, 1989.
6. Sowers, M. F. R. and LaPietra, M. T., Menopause: its epidemiology and potential association with chronic diseases, *Epidemiol. Rev.*, 17, 287, 1995.
7. Fernandez, E., La Vecchia, C., Braga, C., Talamini, R., Negri, E., Parazzini, F., and Franceschi, S., Hormone replacement therapy and risk of colon and rectal cancer, *Cancer Epidemiol. Biomarkers Prev.*, 7, 329, 1998.
8. Waring, S. C., Rocca, W. A., Petersen, R. C., O'Brien, P. C., Tangalos, E. G., and Kokmen, E., Postmenopausal estrogen replacement therapy and risk of AD: a population-based study, *Neurology*, 52, 965, 1999.
9. Smith, W., Mitchell, P., and Wang, J. J., Gender, oestrogen, hormone replacement and age-related macular degeneration, *Aust. N. Z. J. Ophthalmol.*, 25, S13–S15, 1997.
10. Hirshfield, A. N., Development of follicles in the mammalian ovary, *Int. Rev. Cytol.*, 124, 43, 1991.
11. Hooser, S. B., Douds, D. P., DeMerell, D. G., Hoyer, P. B., and Sipes, I. G., Long-term ovarian and gonadotropin changes in mice exposed to 4-vinylcyclohexene, *Reprod. Toxicol.*, 8, 315, 1994.
12. Hoyer, P. B. and Sipes, I. G., Assessment of follicle destruction in chemical-induced ovarian toxicity, *Annu. Rev. Pharmacol. Toxicol.*, 36, 307,1996.
13. Sobrinho, L. G., Levine, R. A., and DeConti, R. C., Amenorrhea in patients with Hodgkin's disease treated with antineoplastic agents, *Am. J. Obstet. Gynecol.*, 109, 135, 1971.

14. Damewood, M. D. and Grochow, L. B., Prospects for fertility after chemotherapy or radiation for neoplastic disease, *Fertil. Steril.,* 45, 443, 1986.

15. Chapman, R. M., Gonadal injury resulting from chemotherapy, *Am. J. Ind. Med.,* 4, 149, 1983.

16. Koyama, H., Wada, T., Nishizawa, Y., Iwanaga, T., Aoki, Y., Terasawa, T., Kosaki, G., Yamamoto, T., and Wada, A., Cyclophosphamide-induced ovarian failure and its therapeutic significance in patients with breast cancer, *Cancer,* 39, 1403, 1977.

17. Miller, J. J. and Cole, L. J., Changes in mouse ovaries after prolonged treatment with cyclophosphamide, *Proc. Soc. Exp. Biol. Med.,* 133, 190, 1970.

18. Shiromizu, K., Thorgeirsson, S. S., and Mattison, D. R., Effect of cyclophosphamide on oocyte and follicle number in Sprague Dawley rats, C57BL/6N and DBA/2N mice, *Pediatr. Pharmacol.,* 4, 213, 1984.

19. Plowchalk, D. R. and Mattison, D. R., Reproductive toxicity of cyclophosphamide in the C57GBL/6N mouse. 1. Effects on ovarian structure and function, *Reprod. Toxicol.,* 6, 411, 1992.

20. Baird, D. D. and Wilcox, A. J., Cigarette smoking associated with delayed conception, *J. Am. Med. Assoc.,* 253, 2979, 1985.

21. Weinberg, C. R. and Wilcox, A. J., Reduced fecundability in women with prenatal exposure to cigarette smoking, *Am. J. Epidemiol.,* 125, 1072,1989.

22. VanVoorhis, B. J., Syrop, C. H., Hammit, D. H., Dunn, M. S., and Snyder, G. D., Effects of smoking on ovulation induction for assisted reproductive techniques, *Fertil. Steril.,* 58, 981, 1992.

23. Stedman, R. L., The chemical composition of tobacco and tobacco smoke, *Chem. Rev.,* 68, 153, 1968.

24. Vahakangas, K., Rajaniemi, H., and Pelkonen, O., Ovarian toxicity of cigarette smoke exposure during pregnancy in mice, *Toxicol. Lett.,* 25, 75,1985.

25. Beverson, R. B., Sandler, D. P., Wilcox, A. J., Schreinemachhers, D., Shore, D. L., and Weinberg, C. R., Effect of passive exposure to smoking on age at natural menopause, *Br. Med. J.,* 293, 792, 1986.

26. Mattison, D. R., Difference in sensitivity of rat and mouse primordial oocytes to destruction by polycyclic aromatic hydrocarbons, *Chem. Biol. Interact.,* 28, 133, 1979.

27. Krarup, T., 9,10-Dimethyl-1,2-benzoanthracene induced ovarian tumors in mice, *Acta Pathol. Microbiol. Scand.,* 70, 241, 1967.

28. Krarup, T., Oocyte destruction and ovarian tumorigenesis after direct application of a chemical cacinogen (9,10-dimethyl-1,2-benzanthacene) to the mouse ovary, *Int. J. Cancer,* 4, 61, 1969.

29. Mattison, D. R. and Thorgeirsson, S. S., Ovarian aryl hydrocarbon hydroxylase activity and primordial oocyte toxicity of polycyclic aromatic hydrocarbons in mice, *Cancer Res.,* 39, 3471, 1979.

30. Borman, S. M., Christian, P. J., Sipes, I. G., and Hoyer, P. B., Ovotoxicity in female Fischer rats and B6 mice induced by low-dose exposure to three polycyclic aromatic hydrocarbons: comparison through calculation of an ovotoxic index, *Toxicol. Appl. Pharmacol.,* 167, 191, 2000.

31. Bengtsson, M., Hamberger, L., and Rydstrom, J., Metabolism of 7,12-dimethylbenz(a)anthracene by different types of cells in the human ovary, *Xenobiotica,* 18, 1255, 1988.

32. Mattison, D. R., Shiromizu, K., Pendergrass, J. A., and Thorgeirsson, S. S., Ontogeny of ovarian glutathione and sensitivity to primordial oocyte destruction by cyclophosphamide, *Pediatr. Pharmacol.,* 3, 49, 1983.

33. IARC (International Agency for Research on Cancer), 4-Vinylcyclohexene, in: *IARC Monographs on the Evaluation of Carcinogenic Risks to Humans: Some Industrial Chemicals,* Vol. 60, Lyon, France, 1994, 347.

34. Melnick, R. L., Huff, J., Chou, B. J., and Miller, R. A., Carcinogenicity of 1,3-butadiene in C57BL/6 X C3HF1 mice at low exposure concentrations, *Cancer Res.,* 50, 6592, 1990.

35. Doerr, J. K., Hooser, S. B., Smith, B. J., and Sipes, I. G., Ovarian toxicity of 4-vinylcyclohexene and related olefins in B6C3F1 mice: role of diepoxides, *Chem. Res. Toxicol.,* 8, 963, 1995.

36. Bond, J. A., Recio, L., and Andjelkovich, D., Epidemiological and mechanistic data suggest that 1,3-butadiene will not be carcinogenic to humans at exposures likely to be encountered in the environment or workplace, *Carcinogenesis,* 16, 165, 1995.

37. Smith, B. J., Mattison, D. R., and Sipes, I. G., The role of epoxidation in 4-vinylcyclohexene-induced ovarian toxicity, *Toxicol. Appl. Pharmacol.,* 105, 372, 1990.

38. National Toxicology Program (NTP), Toxicology and carcinogenesis studies of 4-vinyl-1-cyclohexene diepoixide in F344/N rats and B6C3F1 mice, NTP Technical Report, 1989, 362.

39. Grizzle, T. B., George, J. D., Fail, P. A., Seely, J. C., and Heindel, J. J., Reproductive effects of 4-vinylcyclohexene in Swiss mice assessed by a continuous breeding protocol, *Fundam. Appl. Toxicol.*, 22, 122, 1994.

40. Bevan, C., Stadler, J. C., Elliot, G. S., Frame, S. R., Baldwin, J. K., Leung, H-W., Moran, E., and Panepinto, A. S., Subchronic toxicity of 4-vinylcyclohexene in rats and mice by inhalation exposure, *Fundam. Appl. Toxicol.*, 32, 1, 1996.

41. Davis, B. J., Maronpot, R. R., and Heindel, J. J., Di-(2-ethylhexyl)phthalate suppresses estradiol and ovulation in cycling rats, *Toxicol. Appl. Pharmacol.*, 128, 216, 1994.

42. Safe, S. H. and Krishnan, V., Chlorinated hydrocarbons: estrogens and antiestrogens, *Toxicol. Lett.*, 82, 731, 1995.

43. Li, X., Johnson, D. C., and Rozman, K. K., Reproductive effects of 2,3,7,8-tetrachlorodibenzo-*p*-dioxin (TCDD) in female rats: ovulation, hormonal regulation, and possible mechanism(s), *Toxicol. Appl. Pharmacol.*, 133, 321, 1995.

44. Moran, F. M., Enan, E., Vandevoort, C. A., Stewart, D. R., Conley, A. J., Overstreet, J. W., and Lasley, B. L., 2,3,7,8-Tetrachlorodibenzo-*p*-dioxin (TCDD) effects on steroidogenesis of human luteinized granulosa cell in vitro, *Biol. Reprod. Suppl. 1*, 56, 65, 1997.

45. Ronnback, C., Effect of 3,3′,4,4′-tetrachlorobiphenyl (TCB) on ovaries of foetal mice, *Pharm. Toxicol.*, 69, 340, 1991.

46. Generoso, W., Stout, S. K., and Huff, S. W., Effects of alkylating chemicals on reproductive capacity of adult female mice, *Mutat. Res.*, 13, 171,1971.

47. Jarrell, J. F., McMahon, A., Villeneuve, D., Franklin, C., Singh, A., Valli, V. E., and Bartlett, S., Hexachlorobenzene toxicity in the monkey primordial germ cell without induced porphyria, *Reprod. Toxicol.*, 7, 41,1993.

48. Dobson, R. L. and Felton, J. S., Female germ cell loss from radiation and chemical exposures, *Am. J. Ind. Med.*, 4, 175, 1983.

49. Hemminki, K., Falck, K., and Vainio, H., Comparison of alkylation rates and mutagenicity of directly acting industrial and laboratory chemicals, *Arch. Toxicol.*, 46, 277, 1980.

50. Tilly, J. L., Kowalski, K. I., Johnson, A. L., and Hsueh, A. J. W., Involvement of apoptosis in ovarian follicular atresia and post-ovulatory regression, *Endocrinology*, 129, 2799, 1991.

51. Hirata, K., Ogata, I., Ohta, Y., and Fujiwara, K., Hepatic sinusoidal cell destruction in the development of intravascular coagulation in acute liver failure of rats, *J. Pathol.*, 158, 157, 1989.

52. Pritchard, D. J. and Butler, W. H., Apoptosis — The mechanism of cell death in dimethylnitrosamine-induced hepatotoxicity, *J. Pathol.*, 158, 253, 1989.

53. Shen, W., Kamendulis, L. M., Ray, S. D., and Corcoran, G. B., Acetaminophen-induced cytotoxicity in cultured mouse hepatocytes: correlation of nuclear Ca^{2+} accumulation and early DNA fragmentation with cell death, *Toxicol. Appl. Pharmacol.*, 111, 242,1991.

54. Borman, S. M., VanDePol, B. J., Kao, S. W., Thompson, K. E., Sipes, I. G., and Hoyer, P. B., A single dose of the ovotoxicant 4-vinylcyclohexene diepoxide is protective in rat primary ovarian follicles, *Toxicol. Appl. Pharmacol.*, 158, 244, 1999.

55. Mattison, D. R. and Schulman, J. D., How xenobiotic compounds can destroy oocytes, *Contemp. Obstet. Gynecol.*, 15, 157, 1980.

56. Citti, L., Gervasi, P. G., Turchi, G., Bellucci, G., and Bianchini, R., The reaction of 3,4-epoxy-1-butene with deoxyguanosine and DNA in vitro: synthesis and characterization of the main adducts, *Carcinogenesis*, 5, 47, 1984.

57. deRaat, W. K., Induction of sister chromatid exchanges by styrene and its presumed metabolite styrene oxide in the presence of rat liver homogenate, *Chem. Biol. Interact.*, 20, 163, 1978.

58. Turchi, G., Bonatti, S., Citti, L., and Gervasi, P. G., Alkylating properties and genetic activity of 4-vinylcyclohexene metabolites and structurally related epoxides, *Mutat. Res.*, 83, 419, 1981.

59. Diawara, M. M., Chavez, K. J., Hoyer, P. B., Williams, D. E., Dorsch, J., Kulkosky, P., and Franklin, M. R., A novel group of ovarian toxicants: the psoralens, *J. Biochem. Mol. Toxicol.*, 13, 195, 1999.

ADDITIONAL RELATED INFORMATION

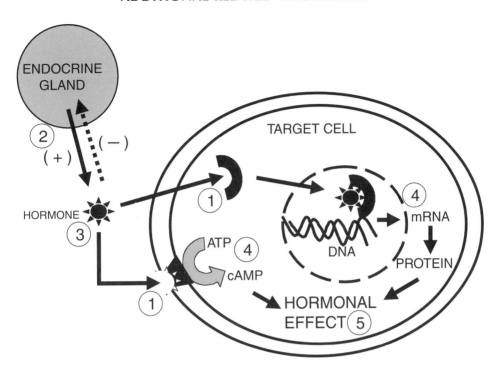

FIGURE 14.7 A generalized schematic of mammalian hormonal regulation showing major points for potential disruption/modulation. Endocrine disrupters/modulators are defined as exogenous substances that can alter or modulate endocrine function resulting in adverse effects at the level of the organism, its progeny, and/or populations of organisms. The site of action most focused on for these substances is at the target cell hormone receptor (1). A substance that has an affinity for binding to either a peptide-hormone membrane receptor or a steroid-hormone cytoplasmic receptor might act either as an agonist inducing the hormonal action or as an antagonist, preventing the natural hormone from inducing its effect. However, endocrine disrupters/modulators need not interact with a receptor to affect hormonal regulation. They may affect the synthesis and secretion of the hormone or its regulatory control at the endocrine gland (2) or the transport or elimination of the hormone (3) resulting in increased or decreased levels of hormone reaching the target cell. Endocrine disrupters/modulators might interfere with or alter the cellular mechanisms through which the hormone exerts its effect (4). For steroid hormones this involves gene activation and synthesis of specific proteins or for peptide hormones, activation of a second-messenger sequence producing cellular effects such as enzyme activation and alteration of cell membrane permeability. Endocrine disrupters/modulators may alter the temporal expression of the hormonal effect (5) such as causing the premature expression of the hormonal effect at a critically sensitive period during sexual development.

TABLE 14.1
Overview of Major Mammalian Hormones

Source	Hormone	Target	Major Effect
Anterior pituitary	Growth hormone (GH)	Multiple sites	Stimulates bone and muscle growth and metabolic functions
	Adrenocorticotropic hormone (ACTH)	Adrenal cortex	Stimulates secretion of adrenal cortex hormones
	Thyroid stimulating hormone (TSH)	Thyroid	Stimulates secretion of thyroid hormone
	Follicle-stimulating hormone (FSH)	Ovaries Testes	Stimulates production of ova and sperm
	Lutenizing hormone (LH)	Ovaries Testes	Stimulates ovulation and production of estrogen, progesterone, and testosterone
	Prolactin (LTH)	Mammary Ovary	Stimulates milk production and maintains estrogen and progesterone secretion
	Melanocyte-stimulating hormone (MSH)	Melanocyte	Stimulates dispersal of pigment
Hypothalamus/posterior pituitary	Oxytocin	Uterus Mammary	Stimulates contraction of uterus and secretion of milk
	Antidiuretic hormone (ADH)	Kidney	Promotes water retention
Thyroid	Triiodothyronine (T_3) and thyroxin (T_4)	Multiple	Stimulates and maintains metabolism
	Calcitonin	Bone	Lowers blood calcium
Parathyroid	Parathyroid hormone	Bone Kidney Digestive tract	Raises blood calcium
Ovary	Estrogens (estradiol)	Uterus Multiple sites	Stimulates growth of uterine lining, promotes development and maintenance of secondary sex characteristics
Ovary/placenta	Progesterone	Uterus Breast	Promotes growth of uterine lining
Placenta	Chrorionic gonadotropin	Anterior pituitary	Stimulates release of FSH and LH
Testis	Androgens (testosterone)	Multiple sites	Supports spermatogenesis, promotes development and maintenance of secondary sex characteristics
Adrenal cortex	Glucocorticoids (cortisol)	Multiple sites	Raises blood glucose
	Mineralocorticoids (aldosterone)	Kidney	Maintains sodium and phosphate balance
Adrenal medulla	Epinephrine (adrenalin)	Muscle	Raises blood glucose, increases metabolism and constricts certain blood vessels
	Norepinephrine	Liver Blood vessels	
Pineal gland	Melatonin	Multiple sites	Regulates biorhythms, influences reproduction in some species
Pancreas	Insulin	Multiple sites	Lowers blood glucose
	Glucagon	Liver Fatty tissue	Raises blood glucose
Thymus	Thymosin		Stimulates T lymphocytes
Gastrointestinal Tract			
Duodenum	Secretin	Pancreas	Stimulates secretion of pancreatic enzymes
	Cholescystokinin	Gallbladder	Stimulates release of bile
Stomach	Gastrin	Stomach Intestinal tract	Stimulates acid secretion and contraction of intestinal tract

TABLE 14.2
EDSTAC Recommended Endocrine Disrupter Tier 1 Screening Protocols[a]

Assay	Estrogen Agonism	Estrogen Antagonism	Androgen Agonism	Androgen Antagonism	Thyroid-Related Effects	Steroid Synthesis	Aromatase Inhibition	5-α-Reductase Inhibition	HPG4[b]
In vitro									
Estrogen receptor binding	x	x							
Androgen receptor binding			x	x					
Steroidogenesis						x			
Placental aromatase							x		
In vivo									
3-day uterotrophic	x		(x)[c]						
20-day pubertal female	x	x			x	x	x		x
Hershberger			x	x					LH[d]
Hershberger + T	(x)[e]			x				x	LH[d]
14-day intact male	x			x	x	x	(x)[f]	x	x
20-day pubertal male	x		x	x	x	x		x	x
Frog metamorphosis	?[g]	?[g]	?[g]	?[g]	x	x	?[g]	?[g]	x
Fish gonadal recrudescence	x	x	x	x	?[g]	x	x	?[g]	x

[a] From: Goldman, J.M., Laws, S.C., Balchak, S.K., Cooper, R.L., and Kavlock, R.J., 2000, Endocrine-disrupting chemicals: Prepubertal exposures and effects on sexual maturation and thyroid activity in the female rat. A focus on the EDSTAC Recommendations, *Critical Reviews in Toxicology*, 30, 135, CRC Press, Boca Raton. With permission. Originally adapted from United States EPA, 1998, EDSTAC Final Report, Chap 5. Screening and Testing, http://www.epa.gov/scipol/oscpendo/history/chap5v14.pdf. p. 5–3.

[b] HPG — indicates that the model has an intact hypothalamic–pituitary–gonadal axis (except for the Hershberger assay which does not), and that effects on hypothalamic–pituitary control of gonadal endocrine function would be evaluated.

[c] It is likely that aromatizable androgens would be detected in this assay; however, given that there are no examples of environmental androgens, this point cannot be empirically demonstrated.

[d] Agents that affect LH levels would be detected in the assay.

[e] Empirical demonstration that the assay detects estrogens is limited. The biology of the system suggests that they will be detected.

[f] Empirical demonstration that aromatase inhibitors are detected is limited. Its sensitivity to aromatase inhibitors is lacking, a placental aromatase assay would be added to this option.

[g] The biology of these organisms suggests that these effects may be detectable. However, there are no empirical data to support the sensitivity of the assay for these endpoints. The final EDSTAC report is available at www.epa.gov/opptintr/opptendo/finalrpt.htm.

TABLE 14.3
Reported Female Pubertal Parameters in Various Strains of Rats[a,b]

Strain	Control VO (day)	Age-1st E	Age-1st Di	BW at VO
Holtzman	36.8 ± 0.2	NR	NR	NR
Holtzman	35.6 ± 0.7	NR	36.6 ± 0.7	129.7 ± 2.6
Holtzman	35.6 ± 0.8	NR	36.7 ± 0.8	114.9 ± 4.1
Holtzman	34.4 ± 1.2[c]	NR	NR	NR
	35.0 ± 0.3			
	35.6 ± 1.2			
Sprague-Dawley	35.5 ± 1.0	35.9 ± 0.9	NR	115.9 ± 5.5
Sprague-Dawley	38.4 ± 0.4	NR	NR	180 ± 8[de]
Sprague-Dawley*	35.2 ± 0.3	NR	36.6 ± 0.2	90 ± 2[e]
Sprague-Dawley	34.0 ± 0.2	NR	35.0 ± 0.4	124.3 ± 4.4[d]
Sprague-Dawley*	31.7 ± 0.4	NR	33.0 ± 0.4	NR
Sprague-Dawley	33.6 ± 0.5	NR	NR	125.9 ± 1.2
Sprague-Dawley	31.9 ± 0.4[c]	NR	NR	126.1 ± 2.1[f]
	36.1 ± 0.4			
	37.9 ± 0.5			
	38.3 ± 0.5			
Sprague-Dawley	34.2 ± 0.7[g]	NR	NR	129.1 ± 3.0[h]
	through			
	37.2 ± 1.5			
Sprague-Dawley	33.4 ± 0.8[i]	NR	NR	NR
Wistar	41.7 ± 0.5	NR	NR	NR
Wistar	37.4 ± 3.1	NR	NR	104.8 ± 20.5
Wistar	37.0 ± 0.8	NR	NR	123 ± 2.4
Wistar	36.7 ± 0.3	NR	NR	NR
Wistar	34.3 ± 0.8	35.1 ± 0.8	NR	101 ± 3
Wistar	35.4 ± 1.0	NR	NR	NR
Wistar (R-Amsterdam substrain)	39.3 ± 0.5[c]	39.5 ± 0.4	NR	90.8 ± 2.0
	38.2 ± 0.8	38.5 ± 0.9		90.6 ± 2.0
Wistar (R-Amsterdam substrain)	38.6 ± 0.4[g]	NR	NR	93.9 ± 2.8[gj]
	through			through
	42.1 ± 0.3			105.9 ± 1.8
Fischer 344	36.5 ± 1.5	NR	NR	86.6 ± 3.2
Long-Evans	39.0 ± 3.0	NR	NR	NR
Long-Evans	32–34[c]	33–34[c]	NR	97–116[c]
Long-Evans	35.0 ± 0.3	NR	NR	130 ± 2
Long-Evans	36.2 ± 0.5	NR	NR	NR
Long-Evans	30.6 ± 0.2	NR	NR	114 ± 1.8

Note: Above data are taken from selected papers that are representative for each of the listed rat strains. VO, vaginal opening; E, vaginal estrus; Di, vaginal diestrus; NR, not reported.

[a] Values are group means ± standard errors of the mean.

[b] All cited studies employed light:dark photoperiods of 12 h:12 h or 14 h:10 h with the exception of two studies (*) which reported 10 h:14 h.

[c] Numbers represent the range of control group means for different experimental blocks.

[d] body weight (BW) at 1st Di.

[e] Estimate from graphed data.

[f] BW at d35.

From Goldman, J.M., Laws, S.C., Balchak, S.K., Cooper, R.L., and Kavlock, R.J., 2000, Endocrine-disrupting chemicals: Prepubertal exposures and effects on sexual maturation and thyroid activity in the female rat. A focus on the EDSTAC Recommendations, *Critical Reviews in Toxicology,* 30, 135, CRC Press, Boca Raton, FL. With permission.

TABLE 14.4
Ontogeny of Receptors and Hormones in the Male Rat

Steroid or Protein	GD-18 to Birth	PND 1–15	PND 16–25	PND 26–35	PND 36–45	PND 46–55	PND 56–65	PND 66–90
GnRH pulsatility	+		+++	+++	+++	+++	Pulsatile	Pulsatile
GnRH receptor	gd-16-birth +	+	+	+++	+++	+++	++	→
LH receptor	gd-15 +	+	++	++	+++	+++	+++	+++
FSH	+	+	+	+++	+++	++	++	++
FSH receptor semi-tubules	+	+++ pnd 10–15	+++	++	→			
Prolactin	+	+	+	+++	+++	→		
Inhibin B		+ pnd-3, ++ pnd10–15	+++	++	+			
TSH (plasma)	+++	+ to +++	++	+++	+++	++	++	++
T3		+ to ++	+++	+++	++	++	+	
T4		+ to ++	+++	+++	+++	++	++	
AR testes	+	++	+	++	++	+++	+++	+++

Note: ↓ = decreased to adult levels, + = low level, ++ = moderate level, and +++ = high level. Blank cells represent undetermined levels. AR, androgen receptor; GD, gestation day; GnRH, gonadotropin-releasing hormone; PND, postnatal day

From Stoker, T.E., Parks, L.G., Gray, L.E. and Cooper, R.L., 2000, Endocrine-disrupting chemicals: Prepubertal exposures and effects on sexual maturation and thyroid function in the male rat. A focus on EDSTAC recommendations, *Critical Reviews in Toxicology*; 30, 197, CRC Press, Boca Raton, FL. With permission.

TABLE 14.5
Estrogen Receptor IC$_{50}$ Values and Relative Binding Affinities for Various Substances

Substance	Mean IC$_{50}$ (M)	Relative Binding Affinity (%)	Log Relative Binding Affinity
17β-Estradiol	8.99×10^{-10}	100.0	2.00
17α-Estradiol[a]	2.93×10^{-8}	3.068	0.49
Estriol	9.25×10^{-9}	9.719	0.99
Estrone	1.23×10^{-8}	7.309	0.86
Alachlor	$>1 \times 10^{-4}$	—	—
Aldosterone	$>1 \times 10^{-4}$	—	—
Aldrin	$>6 \times 10^{-4}$	—	—
Benzyl alcohol	$>1 \times 10^{-2}$	—	—
Benzylbutyl phthalate	$>1 \times 10^{-3}$	—	—
Bis-(2-ethylhexyl) phthalate	$>1 \times 10^{-3}$	—	—
2,2-Bis-(4-hydroxyphenyl)-butane (bisphenol B)	1.05×10^{-6}	0.086	−1.07
Bisphenol A	1.17×10^{-5}	0.008	−2.11
Caffeine	$>1 \times 10^{-4}$	—	—
Corticosterone	$>1 \times 10^{-4}$	—	—
o,p'-DDD	$>3 \times 10^{-4}$	—	—
o,p'-DDT	6.43×10^{-5}	0.001	−2.85
p,p'-DDT	$>1 \times 10^{-3}$	—	—
Dibutyl phthalate	$>1 \times 10^{-3}$	—	—
2,4'-Dichlorobiphenyl	3.65×10^{-4}	0.0002	−3.61
2,4-Dichlorophenoxyacetic acid (2,4-D)	$>1 \times 10^{-4}$	—	—
Dieldrin	$>1 \times 10^{-4}$	—	—
Diethyl phthalate	$>1 \times 10^{-3}$	—	—
Diethylstilbestrol	2.25×10^{-10}	399.556	2.60
5-α-Dihydrotestosterone[a]	$>1 \times 10^{-3}$	—	—
Dihydroxymethoxychlor olefin	3.40×10^{-8}	2.644	0.42
2,2'-Dihydroxybenzophenone	$>1 \times 10^{-4}$	—	—
4,4'-Dihydroxybenzophenone	2.60×10^{-5}	0.003	−2.46
4,4'-Dihydroxystilbene[a]	3.20×10^{-7}	0.281	−0.55
Dopamine	$>1 \times 10^{-4}$	—	—
Ethinyl estradiol[b]	4.73×10^{-10}	190.063	2.28
2-Ethylhexyl 4-hydroxybenzoate[a]	4.95×10^{-6}	0.018	−1.74
4-Ethylphenol	1.34×10^{-3}	0.00007	−4.17
Eugenol	$>1 \times 10^{-3}$	—	—
Hepatochlor	$>1 \times 10^{-4}$	—	—
2-Hydroxy-4-methoxybenzophenone	$>1 \times 10^{-4}$	—	—
4-Hydroxytamoxifen	5.13×10^{-10}	175.244	2.24
Kepone	7.00×10^{-6}	0.013	−1.89
Lindane	$>1 \times 10^{-4}$	—	—
Melatonin	$>1 \times 10^{-4}$	—	—
Methoxychlor	1.44×10^{-4}	0.001	−3.20
Metolachlor	$>1 \times 10^{-4}$	—	—
Mirex	$>1 \times 10^{-4}$	—	—
Nafoxidine	1.25×10^{-7}	0.719	−0.14
4-Nonylphenol[a]	2.40×10^{-6}	0.037	−1.43
1,8-Octanediol	$>1 \times 10^{-4}$	—	—

TABLE 14.5 *(Continued)*
Estrogen Receptor IC$_{50}$ Values and Relative Binding Affinities for Various Substances

Substance	Mean IC$_{50}$ (M)	Relative Binding Affinity (%)	Log Relative Binding Affinity
4-Octylphenol	1.95×10^{-5}	0.005	−2.34
4-Phenethylphenol	4.40×10^{-5}	0.002	−2.69
Phenolphthalin	4.25×10^{-4}	0.0002	−3.67
2-Phenylphenol	$>1 \times 10^{-4}$	—	—
3-Phenylphenol	2.45×10^{-4}	0.0004	−3.44
4-Phenylphenol	9.80×10^{-5}	0.001	−3.04
Progesterone	$>1 \times 10^{-3}$	—	—
Propyl 4-hydroxybenzoate	1.50×10^{-4}	0.0006	−3.22
4-Stilbenol	$>1 \times 10^{-4}$	—	—
Tamoxifen citrate	5.55×10^{-8}	1.620	0.21
4-*tert*-Amylphenol	1.65×10^{-4}	0.0005	−3.26
4-*tert*-Butylphenol	3.68×10^{-4}	0.00024	−3.61
Testosterone	$>1 \times 10^{-3}$	—	—
2′,3′,4′,5′-tetra-chloro-4-biphenylol[a]	3.95×10^{-7}	0.228	−0.64
Thalidomide	$>1 \times 10^{-3}$	—	—
Triphenyl phosphate	$>1 \times 10^{-4}$	—	—

Note: Data in this table were derived from a standardized estrogen receptor competitive-binding assay. Uteri from ovariectomized Sprague–Dawley rats were the source of the estrogen receptor. The IC$_{50}$ = substance molar concentration giving 50% inhibition of [^{3}H]-estradiol binding. The relative binding affinity was calculated by dividing the IC$_{50}$ of estradiol by the IC$_{50}$ of the substance and is expressed as a percent (estradiol = 100). Refer to the reference paper by Blair et al. for details on the method used and receptor relative binding affinities for additional substances.

[a] substance exhibited a U-shaped binding curve.

[b] synthetic estrogen.

Adapted from Blair, R.M., Fang, H., Branham, W.S., Hass, B.S., Dial, S.L., Moland, C.L., Tong, W., Shi, L., Perkins, R., and Sheehan, D.M., The estrogen receptor relative binding affinities of 188 natural and xenochemicals: structural diversity of ligands, *Toxicol. Sci.,* 54, 138, 2000.

15 Genetic Toxicology

Richard H.C. San, Ph.D., Ramadevi Gudi, Ph.D., Valentine O. Wagner III, M.S., Robert R. Young, M.S., and David Jacobson-Kram, Ph.D., D.A.B.T.

CONTENTS

0-8493-0370-2/02/$0.00+$1.50
© 2002 by CRC Press LLC

SECTION 1. INTRODUCTION

This chapter on genetic toxicology is designed to serve as a reference guide to toxicologists and regulatory specialists developing mutagenicity data for product evaluation and regulatory submission. The individual sections are designed to provide a general understanding of the principles of each test and a consideration of factors that must be weighed in assay performance and data evaluation. In addition, historical data are provided that can aid in the determination of the validity of individual test results. Finally, a summary is provided of regulatory requirements for regulatory agencies in the United States, in the European Community, and in Japan.

Reviews are provided for the most commonly performed genetic toxicology tests, including bacterial mutation assays in *Salmonella* and *Escherichia coli*, mammalian mutagenesis in Chinese hamster ovary and mouse lymphoma cells, *in vitro* cytogenetics in continuous cell lines and in human peripheral blood lymphocytes, *in vivo* cytogenetics, the mouse micronucleus test, unscheduled DNA synthesis and mutation analysis in transgenic mice.

SECTION 2. BACTERIAL MUTAGENESIS ASSAY

Of the microbial test systems that have been developed over the past 20 years, the *S. typhimurium* and the *E. coli* tester strains are the most widely used for detecting gene mutations. The bacterial mutation assay has proved to be a reliable and economical assay for routine screening of chemicals for mutagenic activity.[1-5]

The *S. typhimurium* and *E. coli* strains each have a defect in one of the genes involved in histidine and tryptophan biosynthesis, respectively. The defect renders the cell dependent (auxotrophic) on exogenous histidine or tryptophan. Unless the cell experiences a mutation that reverts the dysfunctional gene back to the wild-type (prototrophic) genotype, the cell becomes disabled when the exogenous histidine or tryptophan is exhausted. For this reason, this assay is referred to as a reverse or back mutation assay. Since base substitution mutations are reverted only by base substitution mutagens and frame-shift mutations are reverted only by frame-shift mutagens, it is necessary to use more than one tester strain to detect both types of mutagens. The *S. typhimurium* strains detect reversion from his– to his+ at a single site in one of the 12 steps of histidine biosynthesis. The *E. coli* strains detect reversion from trp– to trp+ at the *trpE* gene in a site blocking tryptophan biosynthesis prior to the formation of anthranilic acid. To adequately assess the mutagenic potential of a chemical, it is important to select an appropriate battery of tester strains. The strain battery that was globally adopted in 1997 by the Organisation for Economic Cooperation and Development (OECD)[6] and the International Conference on Harmonisation (ICH)[7] requires selection of one strain from each of five categories, as follows:

1. TA98
2. TA100
3. TA1535
4. TA1537, TA97, or TA97a
5. TA102, WP2 *uvr*A, or WP2 *uvr*A (pKM101).

To detect cross-linking agents strain TA102 or WP2 (pKM101) must be used.

Strains TA98, TA1537, TA97, and TA97a are reverted by frame-shift mutagens. Strains TA100, TA1535, TA102, and the *E. coli* strains WP2 *uvr*A or WP2 *uvr*A (pKM101) are reverted by base substitution mutagens.[8,9] Strain TA102 and the *E. coli* strains possess A-T base pairs at the site of the mutation unlike the other strains that possess G-C base pairs at their mutation sites. In addition, TA102 has been shown to be useful for detecting oxidative mutagens such as bleomycin that are not detected by other *Salmonella* tester strains. The *uvr*B mutation has not been introduced into this strain; therefore, with an intact excision repair system, it can detect cross-linking agents such as mitomycin C.[10]

To increase their sensitivity to mutagens, additional mutations have been incorporated in each strain. Mutations in the *uvr*A gene of *E. coli* and in the *uvr*B gene of *S. typhimurium* are partial deletions of each respective gene.[11] The *uvr* genes code for a series of DNA excision repair proteins involved in removal of T-T dimers induced by ultraviolet (UV) light. Cells with this type of mutation are unable to repair damage induced by UV light and other types of mutagens. The presence of either of these mutations can be detected by demonstrating sensitivity to UV light. The pKM101 plasmid codes for an error-prone DNA repair system.[12,13] The proposed mechanism by which this plasmid increases sensitivity to mutagens is by modifying an existing bacterial DNA repair polymerase complex involved with the mismatch-repair process.[14-16] Cells containing this plasmid are resistant to ampicillin. The *rfa* wall mutation prevents the *S. typhimurium* cells from synthesizing an intact polysaccharide cell wall.[17] Therefore, large molecules such as benzo[*a*]pyrene that are normally excluded are able to penetrate the cell. Cells containing this mutation are sensitive to crystal violet.

Although the tester strains described above are capable of detecting a wide range of direct-acting mutagens, they are incapable of detecting promutagens until the promutagens are converted to their mutagenic forms by NADPH-dependent mammalian microsomal enzymes. Since bacteria do not possess the microsomal enzymes necessary for promutagen activation, the required metabolic activity must be supplied exogenously. Ames and co-workers[18] developed an exogenous metabolic activation system derived from the microsomal fraction of mammalian tissue homogenates. The supernatant (referred to as S9) from centrifugation of the liver homogenate at $9000 \times g$ is combined with necessary cofactors for use as an S9 mix in the bacterial mutagenesis assay.

Bacterial mutation assays can either be performed using the more common plate incorporation procedure or the preincubation modification of the assay. In the plate incorporation procedure, a 100-µl aliquot of tester strain, 50 to 500 µl of test article or vehicle or positive control and 500 µl of S9 mix or buffer are added to 2.0 ml of molten selective top agar. After mixing, the mixture is overlaid onto the surface of a Vogel–Bonner bottom agar plate. After the plates have solidified, the plates are inverted and incubated for approximately 48 h at $37 \pm 2°C$ prior to counting of revertant colonies.

The standard plate incorporation assay using Aroclor 1254 induced rat liver S9 is not effective for detecting all classes of promutagens. The preincubation modification described by Yahagi et al.[19] has greatly enhanced the utility of the bacterial mutation assay. A number of chemicals are more readily detected using the preincubation approach. These include various nitrosamines,[19] certain azo compounds,[20] and classical mutagens such as aflatoxin B_1, benzidine, and benzo(*a*)pyrene.[21] The preincubation methodology allows for maximum interaction between tester strain, S9, and test chemical, which could explain its increased sensitivity to certain chemicals, especially for volatile chemicals and for test materials that are labile in aqueous systems.

In the preincubation mutagenesis assay, the tester strains are incubated with the test article in a liquid environment prior to plating. A 50 to 500 µl aliquot of test article or vehicle or positive control, 500 µl of S9 mix or buffer and 100 µl of tester strain are added to glass culture tubes. The mixture is allowed to incubate for the appropriate period of time (e.g., 20 or 60 min at $37 \pm 2°C$). Selective top agar (2.0 ml) is then added to each tube and the mixture is overlaid onto the surface of a Vogel–Bonner minimal bottom agar plate. After the plates have solidified, the plates are inverted and incubated for approximately 48 h at $37 \pm 2°C$ prior to counting of revertant colonies.

The following criteria must be met for the mutagenicity assay to be considered valid:

1. *Tester strain integrity.* The presence of the *rfa* wall mutation must be confirmed in the *Salmonella* strains by demonstrating sensitivity to crystal violet. The presence of the *uvr*A or *uvr*B mutation must be confirmed by demonstrating sensitivity to UV light. The presence of the pKM101 plasmid must be confirmed by demonstrating resistance to

TABLE 15.1
Historical Solvent Controls[a]: Bacterial Mutagenicity Assay
(Plate Incorporation Method)

		Revertants per Plate								
		Salmonella typhimurium						Escherichia coli		
S9	Parameter	TA98	TA100	TA1535	TA1537	TA97	TA102	WP2 uvrA	WP2 uvrA (pKM101)	WP2 (pKM101)
−	Mean	17	123	13	6	—	253	13	170	42
	SD	6	32	5	3	—	51	3	50	9
	Minimum	5	69	3	2	—	183	6	82	31
	Maximum	41	208	31	19	—	362	23	255	57
+	Mean	21	123	11	7	—	302	13	182	52
	SD	7	29	4	3	—	86	3	22	10
	Minimum	9	74	3	1	—	173	5	138	37
	Maximum	49	224	27	15	—	460	24	207	75

[a] Solvent controls including but not limited to deionized water, dimethylsulfoxide, ethanol, and acetone.

ampicillin. The presence of the pAQ1 plasmid must be confirmed by demonstrating resistance to tetracycline.

2. *Spontaneous revertant background frequency.* Based on historical control data, all tester strain cultures must exhibit a characteristic number of spontaneous revertants per plate in the solvent controls. Each laboratory must define its own acceptable rate based on historical frequency. Historical solvent control values for the plate incorporation method and the preincubation method are shown in Tables 15.1 and 15.2, respectively. Table 15.3 shows the consistency of the solvent control values among the four most commonly used solvents.

3. *Tester strain titers.* To ensure that appropriate numbers of bacteria are plated, all tester strain culture titers must be equal to or greater than 3×10^9 cells/ml.

4. *Positive control values.* Each mean positive control value must exhibit at least a twofold increase over the respective mean vehicle control value for each tester strain. Two positive

TABLE 15.2
Historical Solvent Controls[a]: Bacterial Mutagenicity Assay (Preincubation Method)

		Revertants per Plate								
		Salmonella typhimurium						Escherichia coli		
S9	Parameter	TA98	TA100	TA1535	TA1537	TA97	TA102	WP2 uvrA	WP2 uvrA (pKM101)	WP2 (pKM101)
−	Mean	20	117	13	6	—	—	11	173	43
	SD	10	25	4	2	—	—	2	22	18
	Minimum	8	66	5	2	—	—	5	126	22
	Maximum	54	215	22	12	—	—	16	208	84
+	Mean	30	126	13	7	—	—	12	204	45
	SD	13	29	5	3	—	—	3	54	10
	Minimum	11	85	3	3	—	—	6	145	25
	Maximum	58	229	31	14	—	—	19	359	68

[a] Solvent controls including but not limited to deionized water, dimethylsulfoxide, ethanol, and acetone.

TABLE 15.3
Historical Negative Control Values without S9 Activation

													Revertants per Plate					
	Acetone				DMSO				Ethanol				Water			
Strain	Mean	SD	Min	Max	Mean	SD	Min	Max	Mean	SD	Min	Max	Mean	SD	Min	Max
TA98	16	7	6	52	17	7	3	59	18	7	4	57	16	6	5	46
TA100	125	26	69	231	118	21	71	288	117	22	70	196	120	21	65	262
TA1535	10	4	4	26	10	4	3	34	9	3	2	24	10	4	3	35
TA1537	6	3	1	17	5	2	0	15	5	2	1	13	5	3	0	22
TA97	—	—	—	—	119	16	95	154	—	—	—	—	121	24	55	165
TA102	—	—	—	—	302	56	208	428	252	22	226	295	314	43	273	413
WP2 *uvr*A	17	6	9	36	15	5	6	48	16	5	5	37	16	5	3	44
WP2 *uvr*A (pKM101)	221	40	143	308	214	50	134	371	224	63	134	387	220	59	97	384
WP2 (pKM101)	70	45	13	159	59	29	15	181	60	29	21	166	66	33	18	162

Note: SD = standard deviation; Min = minimum value; Max = maximum value.

control chemicals are routinely included for each tester strain in each assay: one that is directly acting and positive in the absence of an exogenous source of metabolic activation and one that is indirectly acting and requires metabolic activation to its active form. A commonly used positive control chemical in the presence of exogenous metabolic activation is 2-aminoanthracene for *Salmonella* tester strains TA98, TA100, TA1535, TA1537, TA97, and TA97a and for *E. coli* tester strains WP2 *uvr*A and WP2 *uvr*A (pKM101). Sterigmatocystin is a positive control used for tester strains TA102 and WP2 (pKM101) with metabolic activation. For positive control chemicals in the absence of exogenous metabolic activation, the following are commonly used: sodium azide for TA100; and TA1535, 2-nitrofluorene for TA98; 9-aminoacridine for TA1537, TA97, and TA97a; and methyl methanesulfonate for all *E. coli* tester strains. Mitomycin C is commonly used for tester strain TA102 without activation.

5. *Toxicity.* A minimum of three nontoxic dose levels is required to evaluate assay data. A dose level is considered toxic if it causes a >50% reduction in the mean number of revertants per plate relative to the mean solvent control value (this reduction must be accompanied by an abrupt dose-dependent drop in the revertant count) or a reduction in the background lawn. In the event that fewer than three nontoxic dose levels are achieved, the affected portion of the assay is repeated with an appropriate change in dose levels.

All conclusions are based on sound scientific judgment; however, as a guide to interpretation of the data, the following criteria may be considered. Although there is no evidence supporting a specific requirement for a two- or threefold increase over background, this arbitrary rule is the most common method used in the evaluation of data. For a test article to be evaluated positive, it must cause a dose-related increase in the mean revertants per plate of at least one tester strain over a minimum of two increasing concentrations of test article. Data sets for tester strains TA98, TA100, TA102, TA97, TA97a, and all *E. coli* tester strains are judged positive if the increase in mean revertants at the peak of the dose response is equal to or greater than two times the mean solvent control value. Data sets for tester strains TA1535 and TA1537 are judged positive if the increase in mean revertants at the peak of the dose response is equal to or greater than three times the mean solvent control value. Ideally, the most appropriate determinant of a positive (mutagenic) response is a reproducible, statistically significant dose-related increase in revertant colonies. Several statistical procedures have been published; however, a recommended choice has yet to be established.[22,23]

SECTION 3. *IN VITRO* ASSAY SYSTEMS FOR GENE MUTATION IN MAMMALIAN CELLS

The two standard *in vitro* assays for gene mutation in mammalian cells utilize either cultured mouse lymphoma L5178Y cells or Chinese hamster ovary (CHO) cells. Both assays are designed to detect forward mutations at specific loci and are designated the Thymidine Kinase[+/-] (TK[+/-]) Mouse Lymphoma Mutation Assay[24] and the CHO/Hypoxanthine-Guanine Phosphoribosyl Transferase (HGPRT) Mutation Assay,[25] according to their respective target genes, TK and HGPRT. The protocols for the two assays differ somewhat but follow the same basic principles.[24-26] The two assays have the following steps in common:

1. Preparation of cells for treatment;
2. A preliminary cytotoxicity test;
3. Treatment with the test article in the presence and absence of an exogenous metabolic activation system (Aroclor 1254-induced rat liver S9 plus enzyme cofactors);
4. An expression period during which mutations are fixed in DNA and endogenous levels of wild-type enzyme decrease;
5. A selection period during which cells are cloned in the presence of a selective agent;
6. Cytotoxicity and cloning efficiency determinations; and
7. Data collection, calculations to determine mutant frequency, cytotoxicity and cloning efficiency and assessment of the response to the test article.

The two assays differ procedurally in certain areas, such as the way cells are cultured and cloned and the time for the expression and selection periods. However, the major difference in the two assays is in the specific target gene for mutation.

The TK[+/-] Mouse Lymphoma Mutation Assay utilizes a strain (TK[+/-]-3.7.2C clonal line) of mouse lymphoma cells that has been made heterozygous at the TK locus. These cells contain the TK enzyme, which is involved in a salvage pathway for incorporation of exogenous thymidine into the cell through phosphorylation of thymidine. Trifluorothymidine (TFT), the selective agent used in this assay, can also be phosphorylated by the TK enzyme, and, as a consequence, cells containing the enzyme are sensitive to the cytostatic and cytotoxic effects of TFT. Forward mutations of the single functional TK gene can result in the loss of TK activity and, thus, the acquisition of TFT resistance. These mutant cells can be quantitated after an appropriate expression period by cloning in a soft agar medium supplemented with the selective agent TFT.

The CHO/HGPRT Mutation Assay was designed to select for mutations at the X-chromosome-linked and, therefore, hemizygous HGPRT gene. The HGPRT enzyme catalyzes phosphorylation of purines in one of the purine salvage pathways. The selective agent used in this assay, 6-thio-guanine (6-TG), is also a substrate for this enzyme and cells that retain the functional HGPRT enzyme are susceptible to the cytotoxic effects of 6-TG. Forward mutations that result in the loss of the functional HGPRT gene render cells resistant to 6-TG. These mutant cells can be quantitated following an expression period by cloning in culture medium supplemented with 6-TG, the selective agent.

The major difference in the protocols for the two assays involves the way the cells are cultured. For the TK[+/-] Mouse Lymphoma Mutation Assay, cells are initially cultured, treated, and allowed an expression period in suspension culture. Following this, mutant cells are quantitated with an electronic colony counter after cloning in a soft agar medium containing TFT. For the CHO/HGPRT Mutation Assay, cells are cultured, treated, allowed an expression period, and cloned in the presence of 6-TG as cells or colonies attached to plastic culture dishes. After selection, mutant colonies are fixed, stained, and counted by eye. In the authors' laboratory, a 2-day expression period followed by a 10- to 12- day selection period is used in the TK[+/-] Mouse Lymphoma Mutation Assay, and a 7- to 9-day expression period followed by a 7- to 9-day selection period is used in the CHO/HGPRT Mutation Assay.

Both assays detect point mutations involving base substitutions, deletions, frameshifts, and rearrangements within the locus and, thus, can be used interchangeably for detection of these types of lesions. However, the TK[+/−] Mouse Lymphoma Mutation Assay offers the additional advantage of being able to detect clastogenic lesions involving multiple genes and multilocus deletions. These different mutational end points, point mutations vs. chromosomal mutations, can be distinguished by TK-deficient mutant colony size. After treatment with many mutagenic substances, TK-deficient mutant colonies exhibit a characteristic frequency distribution of colony sizes, which can be determined through the use of an electronic colony counter with sizing capability. The precise distribution of large and small mutant colonies appears to be the characteristic mutagenic "fingerprint" of carcinogens in this system.[27,28] Clive et al.[27,29-33] have presented cytogenetic and molecular evidence to substantiate the hypothesis that the small colony variants carry chromosome aberrations associated with chromosome 11, the chromosome on which the TK locus is distally located in the mouse.[34,35] In general, large mutant colonies are karyotypically similar to the parental cells, whereas small mutant colonies have readily recognizable chromosome rearrangements or multilocus deletions involving chromosome 11. Thus, the TK[+/−] Mouse Lymphoma Mutation Assay makes it possible to detect a variety of genetic lesions, ranging from point mutations to multilocus mutations, and to construct a mutational spectrum for any agent giving a mutagenic response in this system.

For either assay, maintenance of an acceptable background mutant frequency is essential. Cells are routinely cleansed for removal of spontaneous mutant cells by supplementing medium with thymidine, hypoxanthine, methotrexate, and glycine (for cleansing TK[+/−] mouse lymphoma cells) or hypoxanthine, aminopterin, and thymidine (for cleansing CHO cells). An acceptable background mutant frequency range must be established in any laboratory conducting these assays. This can be accomplished by including untreated and solvent controls. Once a historical database has been established for a particular solvent, the untreated control can be dropped. However, the untreated control should be included when new solvents are used. In the authors' laboratory, the background mutant frequency for mouse lymphoma cells ranges from 18 to 93 mutants/10^6 surviving cells with a mean of 40.2 to 46.6 mutants/10^6 surviving cells depending on the treatment and activation system used (see Table 15.3). The background mutant frequency for CHO cells ranges from 0.5 to 24.3 mutant cells/10^6 surviving cells with a mean of 5.5 to 6.1 depending on the treatment and activation system used (Table 15.4).

Two positive controls, one directly acting and one requiring metabolic activation, are also included with each assay. For the CHO/HGPRT Mutation Assay, ethyl methanesulfonate (EMS), a directly acting mutagen, and benzo(*a*)pyrene, which requires metabolic activation, are routinely used. For the TK[+/−] Mouse Lymphoma Mutation Assay, methyl methanesulfonate (MMS), a direct-acting mutagen that induces both large and small colonies, and dimethylbenz(*a*)anthracene, which

TABLE 15.4

Historical Control Values for Mammalian Gene Mutation Assays (Mutant Frequency Per 10^6 Surviving Cells)

Cells/locus	S9	Untreated Cells		Solvent controls	
		Mean ± SD	Range	Mean ± SD	Range
CHO/(HGPRT)	−	6.1 ± 5.6	0.5–24.3	5.5 ± 4.9	0.5–18.1
	+	6.0 ± 4.8	0.5–20.3	5.5 ± 4.5	0.6–16.4
Mouse lymphoma (TK)	−	40.9 ± 13.6	18.0–84.0	40.2 ± 13.2	20.0–80.0
	+	44.1 ± 14.2	18.0–93.0	46.6 ± 14.8	23.0–93.0

requires metabolic activation, are used. In addition, MMS serves as a control for the ability to detect small mutant colonies.[36]

For both assays, the toxic effects of the treatment must be determined to decide on the range of doses for treatment in the definitive assay, as well as to identify meaningful results from the definitive assay. Doses that produce more than 90% reduction in surviving cells as compared with the negative controls are not used to determine mutagenic effects of the treatment material, since that degree of toxicity alone is known to induce mutations in these systems. Currently, achievement of 70 to 90% reduction in surviving cells is considered optimal for detecting mutagenic activity from a cytotoxic test agent. For test compounds that do not induce toxicity, demonstration by chemical analysis that appropriate doses were used becomes more critical.

Cytotoxicities are determined in different ways in the two assays. For the TK$^{+/-}$ Mouse Lymphoma Mutation Assay, cytotoxicity is expressed as % Total Growth which is determined by multiplying the % Suspension Growth from the expression period by the % Cloning Growth from the selection period. The % Suspension Growth is determined by comparing the growth of treated cells vs. negative control cells during the 2-day expression period when the cells are growing in suspension culture. The % Cloning Growth is determined by comparing the number of colonies generated by treated cells vs. the number of colonies generated by negative control cells during the selection phase of the assay when the cells are growing in soft agar medium supplemented with TFT. For the CHO/HGPRT Mutation Assay, cytotoxicity is expressed as % Relative Cloning Efficiency and is determined by comparing the number of colonies generated by treated cells with the number of colonies generated by negative control cells through the expression phase of the assay.

Certain other considerations are important to the validity of these assays. In general, test compounds are tested up to a concentration of 5 mg/ml or up to or in slight excess of the limits of solubility or up to doses that produce 90% reduction in surviving cells as compared with the negative controls. Doses that produce little or no toxicity should also be included. In addition, control of pH and osmolality is critical since excesses of either will induce false-positive results. New lots of S9, serum, and medium must be screened for their ability to support growth and background mutation frequencies within historically acceptable levels. For the TK$^{+/-}$ Mouse Lymphoma Mutation Assay, cloning conditions are best judged by the recovery of small colony mutants as determined by sizing of positive control colonies.

The validity of the assay is determined by the background mutant frequency of the negative controls, plating efficiency of solvent controls, and the mutant frequencies of the positive controls. For the TK$^{+/-}$ Mouse Lymphoma Mutation Assay, the following criteria are required:

1. The mutant frequency of the positive controls must be at least 100 mutants/10^6 clonable cells over that of the appropriate solvent control cultures;
2. The spontaneous mutant frequency of the solvent control cultures must be between 20 and 100/10^6 surviving cells; and
3. The plating efficiency of the solvent controls must be greater than 50%.

For the CHO/HGPRT Mutation Assay, the following criteria are required:

1. The positive control must induce a mutant frequency at least three times that of the solvent control and must exceed 40 mutants/10^6 clonable cells;
2. The spontaneous mutant frequency in the solvent and untreated controls must fall within the range of 0 to 25 mutants/10^6 clonable cells; and
3. The cloning efficiency of the untreated and solvent controls must be greater than 50%.

Statistical methods, such as analysis of variance or linear regression for the TK$^{+/-}$ Mouse Lymphoma Mutation Assay and a transformation test by Snee and Irr for the CHO/HGPRT Mutation

Assay (see Nestmann et al.[26]), may be used for interpretation of results of these assays. However, interpretation is generally based on the presence of a dose-related increase in mutant frequency.

For the TK$^{+/-}$ Mouse Lymphoma Mutation Assay, the following criteria are used in the authors' laboratory as guidelines in evaluation of the assay results. An assay is considered positive if the test compound produces a concentration-related increase in mutant frequency with more than one dose level in the 10% or greater Total Growth range exhibiting a mutant frequency which is at least 100 mutants/10^6 clonable cells over the background level. The assay is considered negative if the test compound does not produce a concentration-related increase in mutant frequency or an increase of less than 55 mutants/10^6 clonable cells above the background level in dose levels in the 10% or greater Total Growth range. The assay is considered equivocal if the test compound does not produce a concentration-related increase in mutant frequency, but any one dose level in the 10% or greater Total Growth range exhibits a mutant frequency that is between 55 and 99 mutants/10^6 clonable cells over the background level.

For the CHO/HGPRT Mutation Assay, the following criteria are used as guidelines for interpretation of assay results. An assay is considered positive if the test compound produces a dose-dependent increase in mutant frequencies with at least two consecutive doses showing mutant frequencies elevated above 40 mutants/10^6 clonable cells. If a single point above 40 mutants/10^6 clonable cells is observed at the highest dose, the assay will be considered equivocal. If no culture exhibits a mutant frequency of >40 mutants/10^6 clonable cells, the assay will be considered negative.

SECTION 4. ASSAY SYSTEMS FOR CHROMOSOME DAMAGE

Cytogenetic assays permit the direct visualization of test article-induced chromosome damage and can be performed both *in vitro* and *in vivo*. Following exposure of the cells to the test article, metaphases are evaluated microscopically for chromatid- and chromosome-type deletions or rearrangements. Cytogenetic assays can be used to assess mutagenic exposures of workers or general populations as well as for screening of chemicals for clastogenic activity.

A. *In Vitro Methods*

The *in vitro* assay systems most frequently used for screening chemicals for clastogenic potential include Chinese hamster cells (ovary, CHO or lung, CHL) or human peripheral blood lymphocytes (PBL), which are stimulated to divide using phytohemagglutin. To mimic the metabolism and detoxification that may occur *in vivo*, the *in vitro* assay is conducted both in the absence and presence of an exogenous source of metabolic activation. The most commonly used activation system is a mixture of Aroclor 1254-induced rat liver S9 and enzyme cofactors. Following exposure of cells to a test article, dividing cells are arrested in metaphase using a spindle inhibitor such as colcemid. Metaphase cells are collected at a time selected to assure that cells are in the first metaphase after chemical exposure. Additional sample times are normally selected to allow evaluation of cells whose cycle may be delayed and may require more time to reach metaphase. In the event that multiple sample times are not used, the effect of the test article on the normal cell cycle kinetics must be taken into account when selecting the single sampling time.

It is essential that any laboratory conducting such assays establish acceptable ranges for the negative control groups. For *in vitro* assay systems, controls often include a negative control consisting of untreated cells as well as a control consisting of solvent vehicle alone. For those laboratories with very large historical databases, it may be sufficient to perform only the solvent control for comparison purposes. For small databases or instances requiring the use of an unusual or infrequently used solvent, both the negative and solvent controls are necessary to demonstrate that the solvent did not alter the spontaneous background frequency encountered with the particular target cell line. In the authors' laboratory, the background rate of CHO cells ranges from 0 to 6%

TABLE 15.5
**Historical Control Values for *In Vitro* Cytogenetics Test Systems
(% aberrant cells)**

Cells	S9	Untreated Cells		Solvent Controls	
		Mean ± SD	Range	Mean ± SD	Range
CHO	−	1.2 ± 1.1	0–5	1.4 ± 1.3	0–6
	+	1.3 ± 1.2	0–5	1.5 ± 0.9	0–4.5
Human PBL	−	0.1 ± 0.2	0–2	0.2 ± 0.4	0–2
	+	0.1 ± 0.3	0–1	0.1 ± 0.3	0–1

aberrant cells with a mean of between 1.2 and 1.5%, depending upon treatment and activation system (Table 15.5). However, it should be noted that the presence or absence of S9 has little effect on the percentage of aberrant cells in untreated or solvent-treated cells. The percentage of damaged cells routinely seen with cultured human PBL is lower than that observed with established cell lines, ranging from 0 to 2%, with a mean of approximately 0.2%.

Positive controls are routinely included in each assay. Two positive control chemicals are required: one that is direct acting and positive in the absence an exogenous source of metabolic activation and one that is indirect acting and requires metabolic activation to its active form. The most commonly used positive controls for the *in vitro* cytogenetics assay systems are *N*-methyl-*N'*-nitro-nitrosoguanidine or mitomycin C for the nonactivation test system and cyclophosphamide or benzo(*a*)pyrene for the S9 activation test system. The purpose of these controls is to demonstrate the ability of the target cells to respond to chemical insult. A statistically significant increase in percent aberrant cells in the positive control relative to the solvent control is a criterion for a valid test. Dose levels for positive controls should be selected to yield a moderate level of activity, thereby allowing for evaluation of the sensitivity of the test system.

The toxic effects of treatment must be reported to justify dose selection. Methods most frequently used include mitotic inhibition, cell growth inhibition, or reduction in cloning efficiency. A minimum of 50% toxicity must be achieved in the high-dose group for toxic substances, unless limited by solubility, in which case the lowest precipitating dose level will be the highest dose selected for evaluating chromosome aberrations or other special considerations. The number and types of structural chromosome aberrations found should be presented for each replicate treatment condition. This information allows consideration of the reproducibility between the replicates as well as the consequence of the damage observed. The percentage of structurally damaged cells (percent aberrant cells) in the total population of cells examined is calculated for each group. The frequency of structural aberrations per cell (mean aberrations per cell) also is calculated and reported for each group as a measurement of the severity of damage. Chromatid and isochromatid gaps are presented in the data but are not included in the total percentage of cells with aberrations or in the frequency of structural aberrations per cell.[37,38]

Statistical analysis of the percent aberrant cells may be performed using a variety of methods; one of the most common is the Fisher's exact test. Fisher's test is used to compare pairwise the percent aberrant cells of each treatment group with that of the solvent control. The Cochran–Armitage test has been recommended as a trend test for dose responsiveness.[39]

All conclusions are based on sound scientific judgment; however, as a guide to interpretation of the data, the test article is considered to induce a positive response when the percentage of cells with aberrations is increased in a dose-responsive manner with one or more concentrations being statistically elevated relative to the solvent control group.

A number of special considerations, mandated by the chemical properties of the test article, are required with the *in vitro* cytogenetics assays. Materials are normally tested up to or in slight excess of their limit of solubility in the treatment medium. However, because of potentially artifactual results that can be obtained under nonphysiological testing conditions, chemicals are not tested in excess of 10 mM concentrations (or 5 mg/ml).[40] The pH of treatment medium must also be monitored during the exposure period because of potential artifacts that may be observed under treatment conditions of low or high pH, particularly in the S9-activated test system.[41] Similarly, ionic strength must be monitored and controlled because of the artifactual responses observed with nonclastogens when tested at concentrations that result in high osmolality.[42]

B. *In Vivo Methods*

The two most frequently used end points for *in vivo* evaluation of clastogenic potential are the bone marrow metaphase assay and the bone marrow micronucleus test. Both assays may be conducted using either mice or rats. To maximize delivery of the test article to the bone marrow, intraperitoneal administration is the preferred route of administration. Alternatively, the route may be selected to represent the expected route of human exposure. A high dose level is selected to represent the maximum tolerated dose (MTD), defined as that dose demonstrating signs of bone marrow toxicity or other clear signs of systemic effects. The MTD is defined as a dose producing signs of toxicity such that higher dose level would be expected to produce mortality.

1. Metaphase Analysis

In the bone marrow metaphase analysis assay, dividing bone marrow cells are arrested in metaphase by an intraperitoneal injection of colchicine. Metaphase cells are collected at two time points following dose administration. As in the *in vitro* assay, sample times are selected to assure analysis of first-division metaphase cells, both nondelayed and delayed. Cells are evaluated microscopically for chromosome aberrations as is done in the *in vitro* assay.

Animals exposed to vehicle alone are used as negative controls and the spontaneous background rate is very low. The percentage of damaged cells routinely seen in either rat or mouse bone marrow ranges from 0 to 2% (Table 15.6). No difference is observed between species or sexes.

TABLE 15.6
Historical Control Values for
Bone Marrow Metaphase Analyses
(% aberrant cells)

		Aberrant Cells	
Species	**Sex**	**Mean ± SD**	**Range**
Rat	Male	0.1 ± 0.4	0–2
	Female	0.2 ± 0.5	0–2
Mouse	Male	0.2 ± 0.6	0–2
	Female	0.1 ± 0.5	0–2

Positive controls are routinely included in each assay; the most frequently encountered is cyclophosphamide or mitomycin C. The purpose of this control group is to demonstrate an ability of the target cells to respond to chemical insult. Although not essential, the positive control is optimally given by the same route as the test article. Because of variation caused by uptake, distribution, and metabolism of the chemical and cell cycle kinetics of the target cells, the magnitude of the positive response is greatly affected by the metaphase collection time. As in the *in vitro* systems, dose levels for positive controls should be selected to yield a moderate level of activity, thereby allowing for evaluation of the sensitivity of the test system.

For data analysis, the mitotic index and the total number and types of aberrations should be presented for each animal. As with the *in vitro* assay systems, gaps are presented in the data but are not included in the total percentage of cells with one or more aberrations or in the average number of aberrations per cell.[37,38] The percentage of damaged cells in the total population of cells scored is calculated for each treatment group. The severity of damage within the cells is reported as the average number of aberrations per cell for each treatment dose. Male and female animals should be analyzed separately.

As always, conclusions are based on sound scientific judgment; however, as a guide to interpretation of the data, the test article is considered to induce a positive response when the number of aberrant cells is significantly increased in a dose-responsive manner relative to the vehicle control. A significant increase at the high dose only with no dose response is considered suspect. A significant increase at one dose other than the high dose with no dose response is considered equivocal. The test article is judged negative if no statistically significant increases in percent aberrant cells are observed relative to the vehicle control group at any sampling time.

2. Micronucleus Test

The micronucleus test is often used as a substitute for the technically more difficult and more laborious bone marrow metaphase assay. Since micronuclei are formed by intact chromosomes or chromatid fragments that are not incorporated into the nuclei of daughter cells during cell division, their presence is used to detect agents that are either clastogens or that alter integrity or function of the spindle apparatus. Because of the strong correlation between chromosomal breakage and micronuclei formation, the two assay systems are considered to be equivalent for screening purposes.[43,44] Although the micronucleus test may be performed in both rats and mice, mice are the preferred species.

In the micronucleus test, bone marrow smears are prepared at one to two time points following dose administration, usually 24 and 48 h after exposure. Should more than two treatments be employed, bone marrow may be sampled at a single time point, 24 h after the last doses.[45]

Smears are evaluated microscopically for micronucleated polychromatic erythrocytes (MPCE). The ratio of polychromatic erythrocytes (PCE) to normochromatic erythrocytes (NCE) is also measured as an indicator of bone marrow toxicity.

In general, the mean incidence of MPCE must not exceed 5/1000 PCE (0.5%) in the negative (vehicle) control. In the authors' laboratory, historical control values range between 0 to 8 MPCE/1000 PCE for individual animals with a mean of 0.5 MPCE/1000 PCE (or 0.05%). No significant difference exists between males and females (Table 15.7).

Positive controls are routinely included for every assay. As in the bone marrow metaphase assay, the positive control is usually given by the same route as the test article. The positive control response is greatly influenced by the route of administration, which can affect uptake and distribution as well as optimum sampling time.[46] The positive control must be statistically elevated relative to the concurrent negative control for the test to be valid.

TABLE 15.7
Historical Control Values for the Mouse Micronucleus Test

Parameter	Ratio of PCE/Total Erythrocytes		MPCE/1000 PCE Scored	
	Males	Females	Males	Females
Mean	0.57	0.60	0.45	0.48
SD	0.09	0.09	0.84	0.77
Range	0.12–0.85	0.13–0.86	0–8	0–5

For evaluation of the data, the incidence of MPCE/2000 PCE should be presented for each animal and treatment group. Statistical significance is determined using appropriate statistical methods. The Kastenbaum–Bowman tables, which are based on the binomial distribution, have been recommended.[47] All analyses should be performed separately for each sex. To quantify the test article effect on erythropoiesis, an indicator of bone marrow toxicity, the proportion of PCE to total erythrocytes also should be presented for each animal and treatment group.

As a guide to interpretation of the data, the test article is considered to induce a positive response if a dose-responsive increase in MPCE is observed and one or more dose levels are statistically elevated relative to the vehicle control at any sampling time. If a single treatment group is significantly elevated at one sacrifice time with no evidence of a dose response, the assay is considered a suspect or unconfirmed positive, and a repeat experiment will be recommended. The test article is judged negative if no statistically significant increases in MPCE above the concurrent vehicle control values are observed at any sampling time.

For both the bone marrow metaphase assay and the micronucleus test, it is important to collect and analyze bone marrow samples at multiple time points.[37,44,45,48] To allow for metabolic activation and because many clastogens cause substantial cell cycle delay, no single sampling time is optimal. In the event of negative findings, it may be necessary to demonstrate that the target cells (i.e., bone marrow) were exposed to the test article. This may be achieved by a measure of bone marrow toxicity (mitotic inhibition or depressed PCE/total erythrocyte ratio), or in its absence, tissue distribution data. In some cases, blood serum levels may be sufficient to document exposure.

SECTION 5. DNA DAMAGE AND REPAIR ASSAYS

Monitoring unscheduled DNA synthesis (UDS) in primary cultures of rat hepatocytes presents several advantages over other cell types used to monitor possible interactions between a test article and DNA. First, the target cells possess the ability to metabolize many promutagens/procarcinogens to their active form, thus eliminating the need for an exogenous source of metabolic activation. Second, rat hepatocytes in culture are nearly 100% nondividing, so no metabolic blocks are needed to inhibit replicative DNA synthesis. Third, the target cells are epithelial in origin. Since most human cancers are carcinomas, an assay using epithelial cells to monitor genetic damage may be more relevant to the *in vivo* situation than a similar assay using fibroblasts.

A. *In Vitro* UDS Assay

The use of primary hepatocytes obtained from young adult (6- to 12-week-old) Sprague–Dawley or Fischer rats has been demonstrated to be sensitive to the DNA-damaging activity of a variety of chemicals.[49-51] Primary rat hepatocytes are isolated from the liver by perfusion with ethylene glycol-bis(β-aminoethyl ether) N,N,N',N'-tetraacetic acid (EGTA) solution followed by collagenase solution. At 90 to 180 min after plating onto coverslips, the cells are washed with culture medium, re-fed with serum-free culture medium (for the UDS assay, the medium contains 10 μCi/ml tritiated-thymidine, ^{3}H-TdR) and exposed to the test article for approximately 18 to 20 h at 37°C. The cells on coverslips are then processed for autoradiography. The cells are evaluated on the basis of incorporation of ^{3}H-TdR into hepatocyte DNA, as evidenced by the presence of silver grains over the nucleus, presumably as a consequence of DNA repair. If possible, a total of 150 nuclei are scored per dose level, with 50 nuclei (if possible) scored from each of three replicate cultures. Nuclei undergoing replicative DNA synthesis at the time of ^{3}H-TdR labeling are completely blackened with grains, and are not counted. Cells exhibiting toxic effects of treatments, such as irregularly shaped or very darkly stained nuclei, are not counted. A net nuclear grain count is calculated for each nucleus scored by subtracting the mean of the cytoplasmic area counts from the nuclear area count. For each treatment group, a mean net nuclear grain count and standard

TABLE 15.8
**Historical Control Values for the *In Vitro*
UDS Assay (Net Nuclear Grain Counts[a])**

Untreated Cells		Solvent Controls	
Mean ± SD	Range	Mean ± SD	Range
−1.7 ± 1.1	−3.8–0.5	−1.5 ± 1.1	−4.0 to 0.8

[a] Solvent controls including but not limited to deionized water, dimethylsulfoxide, ethanol, and acetone.

deviation (SD), as well as the proportion of cells in repair (percentage of nuclei showing ±5 net nuclear grain counts) are determined.

Selection of dose levels for the UDS assay is based upon toxicity of the test article. Toxicity may be assessed in a number of ways; the most common is by measuring the amount of lactate dehydrogenase (LDH) that has leaked from the cells into the culture medium relative to the solvent control. Leakage of this enzyme increases with the loss of cell membrane integrity. The treated cultures are also observed microscopically for toxic effects.

To establish acceptable ranges for the negative control groups, a negative control consisting of untreated cells as well as a control consisting of solvent-treated cells is typically included in each assay. For laboratories with very large historical databases, it may be sufficient to perform only the solvent control for comparison purposes. For small databases or instances requiring the use of an unusual or infrequently used solvent, both the negative and solvent controls are necessary to demonstrate that the solvent did not alter the response of the cells. In the authors' laboratory, the historical untreated and solvent control values are shown in Table 15.8. A positive control is routinely included in each assay to demonstrate that the target cells are responsive to DNA damage; 7,12-dimethylbenz(*a*)anthracene (DMBA) and 2-acetylaminofluorene (2-AAF) are examples of positive controls that are commonly used.

For an assay to be considered valid, the proportion of cells in repair in the untreated and solvent-treated controls must be less than 15%, and the net nuclear grain count must be less than 1. In addition, the mean net nuclear grain count of the positive control must be at least 5 counts over that of the solvent control.

All conclusions are based on sound scientific judgment; however, the following is offered as a guide to interpretation of the data. Any mean net nuclear count that is increased by at least 5 counts over the solvent control is considered significant.[49,50] A test article is judged positive if it induces a dose-related increase with no less than one dose significantly elevated above the solvent control. A significant increase in the mean net nuclear grain count in at least two successive doses in the absence of a dose response is also considered positive. A significant increase in the net nuclear grain count at one dose level without a dose response is judged equivocal. A test article is considered negative if no significant increase in the net nuclear grain counts is observed. The percentage of cells in repair (cells with ±5 net nuclear grains) may also be used in making a final evaluation of the activity of the test article.

B. *IN VIVO/IN VITRO* UDS ASSAY

In light of the change in the profile of hepatocyte metabolism immediately following removal of the cells from the animal,[52] the *in vivo/in vitro* UDS assay is designed to account for complex patterns of metabolic activation, detoxification, uptake distribution, and excretion of chemicals. The experimental design is based on procedures as described by Mirsalis et al.[53] and Butterworth et al.[54] Hepatocytes are isolated at two time points (2 to 4 h and 12 to 16 h) following the administration (by gavage, intravenous injection, or intraperitoneal injection) of test article as well as positive and negative (solvent) controls. The collection of hepatocytes at two time points is an attempt to permit detection of maximum UDS response that occurs shortly after treatment (e.g., with dimethylnitrosamine, or DMN, or methyl methanesulfonate, or MMS) as well as those occurring at 12 to 16 h post-treatment (e.g., with DMN, 2-acetylaminofluorene, or 2-AAF, or 2,6-dinitrotoluene).

Hepatocytes are isolated according to the procedures described for the *in vitro* UDS assay. At 90 to 180 min after plating, the cells are washed once in serum-containing culture medium and re-fed with serum-free medium containing ^{3}H-TdR. After 4 h the radioactive medium is removed and the plates washed in serum-free medium plus 0.25 mM thymidine. The cells are then incubated for 17 to 20 h in culture medium plus 0.25 mM thymidine. After incubation, the cells are processed for autoradiography and silver grain counting according to procedures described for the *in vitro* UDS assay.

Commonly used positive controls include MMS and DMN for the 2 to 4 h time point, and DMN and 2-AAF for the 12 to 16 h time point. While 2-AAF can be used as the positive control via oral gavage, the level of UDS elicited is quite often very marginal. Because of its limited solubility in an aqueous vehicle, 2-AAF cannot be used as the positive control via the intravenous route. In light of these limitations, the authors' laboratory has conducted experiments and demonstrated that DMN can be used as the positive control (via oral gavage or intravenous injection) for both the early sampling time (2 to 4 h) and the late sampling time (12 to 16 h).[55] A substantial amount of the data in the published literature is based on chemicals (including chemicals commonly used as positive controls) administered by gavage (e.g., Mirsalis and Butterworth,[56] Ashby et al.[57]). While the use of intraperitoneal injection is acceptable and considered more relevant in some situations, the optimal dose (for positive controls as well) may vary with the route of administration used. It is therefore important to consider the appropriate dose level for the positive control while selecting the route of administration.

The historical solvent control data, criteria for a valid test, and criteria for data evaluation are essentially the same as those presented for the *in vitro* UDS assay.

SECTION 6. TRANSGENIC ASSAY SYSTEM FOR *IN VIVO* MUTAGENESIS

An *in vivo* mutation system has been developed using transgenic mice.[58] Transgenic C57BL/6 and B6C3F1 mice (Big Blue®, Stratagene Cloning Systems, La Jolla, CA) have been constructed such that each cell of every tissue contains multiple copies of a bacteriophage lambda shuttle vector at an identical chromosomal integration site. These lambda shuttle vectors contain a *lacI* gene as a target for mutagenesis testing. The shuttle vector carrying the target gene is recovered from genomic DNA using an *in vitro* packaging extract. The packaging extract contains enzymes that recognize and excise the shuttle vector from within the genomic DNA and that mediate the packaging into infectious phage particles. Each packaged phage represents a single rescued target gene. Packaged phage are plated with *E. coli* cells and form plaques on the bacterial lawn.

The *lacI* gene was selected as the target gene because its mutations are easily detected, it is highly sensitive to missense mutations, and because it has been widely studied as a target for *in vitro* mutagenesis. The *lacI* gene codes for the production of the Lac repressor protein. This repressor protein binds to the *lac* operator and blocks the transcription of the *lacZ* reporter gene. Mutation in the target gene will render the resulting Lac repressor protein inactive, the *LacZ* gene will be expressed, and its protein product, β-galactosidase, will be produced. For detection of mutants using a color screening system, a chromogenic substrate, X-gal, is included in the plating agar. The β-galactosidase produced in mutant plaques cleaves the X-gal and the resulting plaques appear blue in color. Plaques formed from phage-carrying nonmutant target genes produce an active Lac

TABLE 15.9
Background Mutant Frequencies
(Big Blue C57B1/6 Mouse)

Organ	Mutant Frequency[a]
Bone Marrow	14×10^{-6}
Heart	24×10^{-6}
Kidney	31×10^{-6}
Liver	33×10^{-6}
Lung	24×10^{-6}
Spleen	16×10^{-6}

[a] Color screening system for mutant detection.

repressor protein, which suppresses the production of β-galactosidase and are colorless. Additional selectable systems are under development for detection of mutants. While selectable systems will reduce the time and cost of the assay, complete characterization and comparison to the color screening system will be required to document the effect of selective pressure on sensitivity or recovery of mutants.

The transgenic mouse mutation system is highly adaptable to screening for mutagenic potential.[59] Mutation analysis can be performed on any organ or tissue. Mutational spectrum analysis also permits a detailed mechanistic analysis of mutagenesis at the molecular level. The mutant frequency is determined for each animal and tissue analyzed as the ratio of mutant to nonmutant plaques. Treatment groups are compared with the vehicle control group by organ using the Kastenbaum–Bowman tables for determination of statistical significance of mutant frequencies.[60]

Spontaneous mutant frequencies must be accumulated historically for each organ or tissue. In general, background mutant frequencies range from 10 to 40×10^{-6} (Table 15.9). To reduce animal to animal variability, a minimum of 300,000 plaques should be analyzed from each tissue.[61] The most commonly used positive controls are ethynitrosourea, methylnitrosourea, or benzo(*a*)pyrene. The positive control group must be statistically elevated relative to the concurrent negative control group to achieve a valid test.

The following criteria are used as guidelines in evaluation of this type of study. The test article is considered to induce a positive response when the mutant frequency is significantly increased in a dose responsive manner relative to the vehicle control. A significant increase at the high dose only with no dose response is considered suspect. A significant increase at one dose other than the high dose with no dose response is considered equivocal.

SECTION 7. REGULATORY GUIDELINES

A. FDA-REGULATED PRODUCTS

1. Pharmaceuticals

The International Conference on Harmonisation (ICH) of Technical Requirements for Registration of Pharmaceuticals for Human Use has developed guidelines for a number of disciplines to bring global harmony to safety testing of human drugs. In July 1997, the ICH adopted Harmonised Tripartite Guideline S2A, entitled "Guidance on Specific Aspects of Regulatory Genotoxicity Tests for Pharmaceuticals." This guideline provides direction on methodology for performing and evaluating specific genotoxicity tests. In 1998, the ICH adopted Harmonised Tripartite Guideline S2B, entitled "A Standard Battery for Genotoxicity Testing of Pharmaceuticals." This guideline provides direction on which mutagenicity tests should be performed. These efforts have been quite successful in that now the same set of tests can be used to register a new drug in the United States, Europe, and Japan.

*a. Guidance on Specific Aspects of Regulatory Genotoxicity Tests
    for Pharmaceuticals*

This guideline focuses on bacterial reverse mutation assays, *in vitro* assays for chromosomal aberrations, forward mutations in cultured mammalian cells, and *in vivo* assays for chromosomal aberrations in bone marrow cells of rodents. The specifics of the guidance have been reviewed in the previous sections on the individual assays.

*b. Harmonised Tripartite Guideline S2B: A Standard Battery for Genotoxicity
    Testing of Pharmaceuticals*

This guideline gives explicit guidance for selection of genotoxicity tests that will support the registration of a new pharmaceutical worldwide. The following standard test battery is recommended:

- A test for gene mutations in bacteria;
- An *in vitro* test with cytogenetic evaluation of chromosomal damage with mammalian cells or an *in vitro* mouse lymphoma tk assay;
- An *in vivo* test for chromosomal damage using rodent hematopoietic cells.

The guideline goes on to states, "for compounds giving negative results, the completion of this 3-test battery performed and evaluated in accordance with current recommendations, will usually provide a sufficient level of safety to demonstrate the absence of genotoxic activity. Compounds giving positive results in the standard test battery may, depending on their therapeutic use, need to be tested more extensively.

The guideline also gives examples of situations in the 3-test battery may need modification. These are summarized below:

- Limitations to the use of bacterial test organisms. Such limitations would include situations where the test material is highly toxic to bacteria, as might be expected with an antibiotic. Alternatively, if it is known that the test material is specifically designed to interact with elements of eukaryotic cells such as a topoisomerase inhibitor, then the bacterial test would not be appropriate. Under such circumstances the guideline directs the use of a four-test battery, i.e., the bacterial mutation assay, *in vitro* cytogenetics, the mouse lymphoma gene mutation assay, and the *in vivo* cytogenetics assay.
- Compounds bearing structural alerts for genotoxic activity. If a compound that is structurally similar to a known mutagen gives negative results in the standard three-test battery, it should be tested further. Additional testing would depend on the nature of the chemical and the known reactivity and metabolism of the structurally related mutagen.
- Limitations to the use of standard *in vivo* tests. For certain compounds, standard *in vivo* tests may be inappropriate. Such compounds include drugs that are not systemically absorbed and do not reach the target tissue, bone marrow. Examples listed in the guideline include radioimaging agents, aluminum-based antacids, and some dermally applied pharmaceuticals.
- Additional genotoxicity testing in relation to the carcinogenicity bioassay. The guideline calls for additional genotoxicity testing in cases where the standard three-test battery is negative and there are findings in a carcinogenicity study that cannot be explained by a specific nongenotoxic mechanism. Additional types of tests that are mentioned include unscheduled DNA synthesis in liver, mutation in transgenes of transgenic animals, and molecular characterization of genetic changes in tumor-related genes.
- Structurally unique chemical classes. If a test material represents a new class of compounds that may be new to regulatory agencies, it should be tested in all four assays.

The guideline also states that, in general, confirmatory studies that replicate the original study are not required.

2. Food Additives

The FDA Center for Food Safety and Applied Nutrition (CFSAN) recently published draft Toxicological Principles for the Safety Assessment of Direct Food Additives and Color Additives Used in Food, or "Redbook II."[62] In chapter IV C1, Short-Term Tests for Genetic Toxicity, the agency recommends a battery consisting of gene mutation in *Salmonella typhimurium*, gene mutation in mammalian cells *in vitro* and cytogenetic damage *in vivo*. For the *Salmonella* assay they recommend strains TA98, TA100, TA1535, and TA1537. Use of other strains requires justification. For the gene mutation assay, FDA recommends the mouse lymphoma TK$^{+/-}$ assay. Although other less validated assays may be acceptable, they require justification. For the *in vivo* chromosome aberration assay, the FDA recommends "concurrent detection of micronuclei of circulating erythrocytes and chromosomal aberrations in marrow cells of the mouse."

Although CFSAN has not finalized "Redbook II" and has not published intentions to follow other guidelines, it is likely that it also will follow the ICH guidance.

3. Medical Devices

In 1995, the Center for Devices and Radiological Health (CDRH) announced its intention to substitute ISO 10993 Part-1 "Biological Evaluation of Medical Devices" for the Tripartite Biocompatibility Guidance, which had been used to that time. The ISO guidelines call for a three-test battery with one test for gene mutations, one test for chromosomal breakage, and one for DNA damage/repair. Two of the three tests should be performed in mammalian cells. The *de facto* battery that developed was a bacterial reverse mutation assay (Ames test), an *in vitro* assay for chromosomal aberrations in either CHO cells or human peripheral blood lymphocytes, and an *in vitro* rat hepatocyte UDS assay. A number of laboratories chose to perform sister chromatid exchange (SCE) analysis in place of UDS. It is the authors' opinion that the SCE assay is highly susceptible to artifacts and can result in false-positive determinations.

Although CDRH has not officially changed guidance, it appears more recently to be following ICH guidelines. This has the effect of substituting an *in vivo* micronucleus test in place of the UDS assay. Typically, these tests are performed on extracts of the medical device material. The extracts are prepared based on USP guidelines and generally include a polar (saline) and nonpolar (DMSO or ethanol) solvent.

4. Products of Recombinant DNA Technology

The FDA Center for Biologics Evaluation and Research has not definitively stated whether genetic toxicology testing is required on recombinant DNA products. Mutagenicity testing is listed, along with other types of studies, as conditionally required for vaccines, monoclonal antibodies, blood-derived products, hormones, cytokines, and other regulatory factors. The authors' experience has been that a "pharmaceutical type" battery is often required for monoclonal antibodies that are linked to an imaging moiety by way of a chelating agent. In general, the farther removed a biologic product is from an endogenous material, the more likely it is that testing will be required.

B. EPA-REGULATED PRODUCTS

1. New Chemicals

EPA-regulated materials requiring mutagenicity testing are covered under either the Toxic Substances Control Act (TSCA) or under the Federal Insecticide, Fungicide and Rodenticide Act

TABLE 15.10
Criteria Triggering TSCA PMN Test Battery

1. More than 1000 workers exposed
2. More than 100 workers exposed by inhalation to more than 10 mg/kg/day
3. More than 100 workers exposed by inhalation to 1–10 mg/day for more than 100 days per year
4. More than 250 workers exposed by routine dermal contact for more than 100 days per year
5. Presence of the chemical in any consumer product where (a) the physical state of the chemical in the product and (b) the manner of use would make exposures likely
6. More than 70 mg/year exposure via surface water
7. More than 70 mg/year of exposure via air
8. More than 70 mg/year exposure via groundwater
9. More than 10,000 kg/year release to environmental media
10. More than 1000 kg/year release to surface water after calculated estimates of treatment

(FIFRA). TSCA regulates new chemicals (Section 5) and those that were already in commerce at the time the act was passed (Section 4). Although TSCA does not require toxicology testing for submission of a Pre-Manufacture Notice (PMN), the agency has indicated that, if the material in question meets certain criteria relating human exposure or release into the environment (Table 15.10) then a battery of safety tests should be performed. For the genetic toxicology component the battery includes an *Salmonella* gene mutation assay and a mouse micronucleus.

2. Existing Chemicals

Toxicology testing for existing chemicals is administered through test rules or consent orders. Because Section 4 chemicals often have wide distribution in the environment and/or widespread human exposure, the base set has, in addition to *Salmonella* and the micronucleus test, an *in vitro* gene mutation assay. Positive responses in the two gene mutation assays trigger a study for "interaction with gonadal DNA." The category includes end points such as SCE, alkaline elution, and UDS. Positive evidence of interaction with gonadal DNA triggers a specific locus test, either the visible or biochemical assay. A positive response in an *in vivo* bone marrow cytogenetics assay triggers a dominant lethal assay, and a positive response in a dominant lethal triggers a heritable translocation assay. Chronic studies for carcinogenicity are triggered by (1) positive responses in all three base set tests, (2) positive responses in the *Salmonella* and the *in vivo* chromosomal effects assay, or (3) positive responses in the *in vitro* gene mutation assay and the *in vivo* chromosomal effects assay. Single positive responses or positive responses in the two *in vitro* assays results in a "data review."[63]

3. Agricultural Chemicals

The Office of Pesticide Program (OPP) mutagenicity testing scheme is similar to the TSCA requirements. The test battery consists of a *Salmonella* mutagenicity assay, a mouse lymphoma gene mutation assay, and an *in vivo* bone marrow cytogenetics assay, either metaphase or micronucleus. If one chooses the CHO or V79 HGPRT gene mutation assay in place of mouse lymphoma, OPP then requires an additional assay for *in vitro* chromosomal aberrations.

C. JAPANESE REGULATORY AGENCIES

1. Pharmaceuticals

The Ministry of Health and Welfare is a signatory to the ICH guidelines and therefore follows the guidance described above.

2. Agricultural Chemicals

The Ministry of Agriculture, Forestry and Fisheries requires three major end points to be analyzed on agricultural chemicals. These include reverse mutation in bacteria, *in vitro* chromosomal aberrations, and primary DNA damage as measured by a bacterial repair test, the Rec-assay.[64]

3. New Chemicals

The Ministry of Health and Welfare, the Ministry of International Trade and Industry, and the Agency of Environment published guidelines for toxicity testing of new chemicals. Two mutagenicity studies are required and include a reverse mutation assay in bacteria and chromosomal aberrations in cultured mammalian cells. A mouse micronucleus is also specified as one of seven additional toxicity screening tests.[64]

4. Workplace Chemicals

The Ministry of Labor regulates registration of new chemical substances, marketing of chemicals, raw materials, intermediates, by-products, and waste generated in the workplace.[64] Only a single mutagenicity test is required for these materials, a *Salmonella* mutagenicity assay along with *E. coli* strain WP2 *uvr*A. If the bacterial assay shows "strong mutagenicity potential," an *in vitro* chromosomal aberration assay will be additionally required.

D. EUROPEAN ECONOMIC COMMUNITY

1. Pharmaceuticals

Negative results in a *Salmonella* mutagenicity assay alone, or in combination with an *in vitro* cytogenetics assay, is generally sufficient to begin clinical trials. To receive a product license, the EEC Committee on Proprietary Medicinal Products (CPMP) follows the ICH guidelines described above.

2. Pesticide Registration and Chemical Notification

A base set comprising *Salmonella* and/or *E. coli* and an *in vitro* cytogenetics assay is required for premanufacturing or preimport notification of new chemicals to be manufactured in quantities between 1 and 10 tons/year. For chemicals with more than 10 tons/year in commerce or where 50 tons in aggregate are in commerce, a mammalian gene mutation assay and *in vivo* cytogenetics assay are added. The 7th Amendment to directive 79/831/EEC will require a *Salmonella* assay only on chemicals manufactured in quantities between 100 kg and 1 ton/year.[66]

REFERENCES

1. McCann, J., Choi, E., Yamasaki, E., and Ames, B. N., Detection of carcinogens as mutagens in the *Salmonella*/microsome test: assay of 300 chemicals, *Proc. Natl. Acad. Sci. U. S. A.*, 72, 5135, 1975.
2. Sugimura, T., Yahagi, T., Nagao, M., Takeuchi, M., Kawachi, T., Hara, K., Yamasaki, E., Matsushima, T., Hashimoto, Y., and Okada, M., Validity of mutagenicity tests using microbes as a rapid screening method for environmental carcinogens, in *Screening Tests in Chemical Carcinogenesis*, Montesano, R., Bartsch, H., and Tomatis, L., Eds., IARC Scientific Publications No. 12, Lyon, France, 1976, 81.
3. Dunkel, V. C., Collaborative studies on the *Salmonella*/microsome mutagenicity assay, *J. Assoc. Off. Anal. Chem.*, 62, 874, 1979.
4. Dunkel, V. C., Zeiger, E., Brusick, D., McCoy, E., McGregor, D., Mortelmans, K., Rosenkranz, H. S., and Simmon, V. F., Reproducibility of microbial mutagenicity assays: I. Tests with *Salmonella typhimurium* and *Escherichia coli* using a standardized protocol, *Environ. Mutagen*, 6(Suppl. 2), 1, 1984.

5. Dunkel, V. C., Zeiger, E., Brusick, D., McCoy, E., McGregor, D., Mortelmans, K., Rosenkranz, H. S., and Simmon, V. F., Reproducibility of microbial mutagenicity assays: II. Testing of carcinogens and non-carcinogens in *Salmonella typhimurium* and *Escherichia coli, Environ. Mutagen,* 7(Suppl. 5), 1–248, 1985.

6. OECD Guideline 471, Genetic Toxicology: Bacterial Reverse Mutation Assay, Ninth Addendum to OECD Guidelines for the Testing of Chemicals, OECD, Paris, February 1998.

7. International Conference on Harmonisation (ICH) of Technical Requirements for Registration of Pharmaceuticals for Human Use, Guidance on Specific Aspects of Regulatory Genotoxicity Tests for Pharmaceuticals, S2A document recommended for adoption at step 4 of the ICH process on July 19, 1995, *Fed. Regis.,* 61, 18198–18202, April 24, 1996.

8. Maron, D. M. and Ames, B. N., Revised methods for the *Salmonella* mutagenicity test, *Mutat. Res.,* 113, 173, 1983.

9. Wilcox, P., Naidoo, A., Wedd, D. J., and Gatehouse, D. G., Comparison of *Salmonella typhimurium* TA102 with *Escherichia coli* WP2 tester strains, *Mutagenesis,* 5, 285, 1990.

10. Levin, D. E., Hollstein, M., Christman, M. F., Schwiers, E. A., and Ames, B. N., A new *Salmonella* tester strain (TA102) with A-T base pairs at the site of mutation detects oxidative mutagens, *Proc. Natl. Acad. Sci. U. S. A.,* 79, 7445–7449, 1982.

11. Ames, B. N., McCann, J., and Yamasaki, E., Methods for detecting carcinogens and mutagens with the *Salmonella*/mammalian-microsome mutagenicity test, *Mutat. Res.,* 31, 347, 1975.

12. Eisenstadt, E., Miller, J. K., Kahng, L. -S., and Barnes, W. M., Influence of *uvr*B and pKM101 on the spectrum of spontaneous UV- and γ-ray-induced base substitutions that revert *his*G46 and *Salmonella typhimurium, Mutat. Res.,* 220, 113, 1989.

13. McCann, J., Springarn, N. E., Kobori, J., and Ames, B. N., Detection of carcinogens as mutagens: bacterial tester strains with R factor plasmids, *Proc. Natl. Acad. Sci. U. S. A.,* 72, 979–983, 1975.

14. Walker, G. C., Plasmid (pkM101)-mediated enhancement of repair and mutagenesis: dependence on chromosomal genes in *Escherichia coli* K-12, *Mol. Gen. Genet.,* 152, 93, 1977.

15. Shanabruch, W. G. and Walker, G. C., Localization of the plasmid (pkM101) gene(s) involved in rec A+ lex A+ dependent mutagenesis, *Mol. Gen. Genet.,* 179, 289, 1980.

16. Langer, P. J., Shanabruch, W. G., and Walker, G. C., Functional organization of plasmid pkM101, *J. Bacteriol.,* 145, 1310, 1981.

17. Ames, B. N., Lee, F. D., and Durston, W. E., An improved bacterial test system for the detection and classification of mutagens and carcinogens, *Proc. Natl. Acad. Sci. U. S. A.,* 70, 782, 1973.

18. Ames, B. N., Durston, W. E., Yamasaki, E,. and Lee, F. D. Carcinogens are mutagens: a simple test system combining liver homogenates for activation and bacteria for detection, *Proc. Natl. Acad. Sci. U. S. A.,* 70, 2281, 1973.

19. Yahagi, T., Nagao, M., Seino, Y., Matsushima, T., Sugimura, T., and Okada, M., Mutagenicities of N-nitrosamines on *Salmonella, Mutat. Res.,* 48, 121, 1977.

20. Prival, M. J. and Mitchell, V. D., Analysis of a method for testing azo dyes for mutagenic activity in *Salmonella typhimurium* in the presence of flavin mononucleotide and hamster liver S-9, *Mutat. Res.,* 97, 103, 1982.

21. Matsushima, T., Genotoxicity of new Japanese chemicals, in *Mutation and the Environment,* Part E, Wiley-Liss, New York, 1990, 251.

22. Kier, L. E., Brusick, D., Auletta, A. E., Von Halle, E. S., Brown, M. M., Simmon, V. F., Dunkel, V., McCann, J., Mortelmans, K., Prival, M., Rao, T. K., and Ray, V., The *Salmonella typhimurium*/mammalian microsomal assay. A report of the U. S. Environmental Protection Agency Gene-Tox Program, *Mutat. Res.,* 168, 69, 1986.

23. Claxton, L. D., Allen, J., Auletta, A., Mortelmans, K., Nestmann, E., and Zeiger, E., Guide for the *Salmonella typhimurium*/mammalian microsome tests for bacterial mutagenicity, *Mutat. Res.,* 189, 83, 1987.

24. Clive, D., Caspary, W., Kirby, P. E., Krehl, R., Moore, M., Mayo, J., and Oberly, T. J., Guide for performing the mouse lymphoma assay for mammalian cell mutagenicity, *Mutat. Res.,* 189, 143, 1987.

25. Li, A. P., Carver, J. H., Choy, W. N., Hsie, A. W., Gupta, R. S., Loveday, K. S., O'Neill, J. P., Riddle, J. C., Stankowski, L. F., Jr., and Yang, L. L., A guide for the performance of the Chinese hamster ovary cell/hypoxanthine-guanine phosphoribosyl transferase gene mutation assay, *Mutat. Res.,* 189, 135, 1987.

26. Nestmann, E. R., Brillinger, R. L., Gilman, J. P. W., Rudd, C. J., and Swierenga, S. H. H., Recommended protocols based on a survey of current practice in genotoxicity testing laboratories: II. Mutation in Chinese hamster ovary, V79 Chinese hamster lung and L5178Y mouse lymphoma cells, *Mutat. Res.,* 246, 255, 1991.

27. Clive, D., Johnson, K. O., Spector, J. F. S., Batson, A. G., and Brown, M. M. M., Validation and characterization of the L5178Y TK$^{+/-}$ Mouse Lymphoma Mutagen Assay System, *Mutat. Res.,* 59, 61, 1979.

28. DeMarini, D. M., Brockman, H. E., deSerres, F. J., Evans, H. E., Stankowski, L. F., Jr., and Hsie, A. W., Specific-locus mutations induced in eukaryotes (especially mammalian cells) by radiation and chemicals: a prospective, *Mutat. Res.,* 220, 11, 1989.

29. Hozier J., Sawyer, J., Moore, M., Howard, B., and Clive, D., Cytogenetic analysis of the L5178Y TK$^{+/-}$, TK$^{-/-}$ Mouse Lymphoma Mutagenesis Assay System, *Mutat. Res.,* 84, 168, 1981.

30. Glover, P. and Clive, D., Molecular spectra of L5178Y TK$^{-/-}$ mutants induced by diverse mutagens, *Environ. Mutagen,* 14, 71, 1989.

31. Applegate, M. L., Moore, M. M., Broder, C. B., Burrell, A., Juhn, G., Kasweck, K. L., Lin, P. -F., Wadhams, A., and Hozier, J. C., Molecular dissection of mutations at the heterozygous thymidine kinase locus in mouse lymphoma cells, *Proc. Natl. Acad. Sci. U. S. A.,* 87, 51, 1990.

32. Clive, D., Glover, P., Applegate, M., and Hozier, J., Molecular aspects of chemical mutagenesis in L5178Y TK$^{+/-}$ mouse lymphoma cells, *Environ. Mutagen,* 5, 191, 1990.

33. Glover, P., Krehl, R., Poorman-Allen, P., and Clive, D., Distinctive aspects of mammalian cell mutagenesis. II. Most mutations induced by most mutagens involve several kilobases of DNA, *Environ. Mutagen,* 19, 20, 1992.

34. Kozak, C. A. and Ruddle, F. H., Assignment of the genes for thymidine kinase and galactokinase to *Mus musculus* chromosome 11 and the preferential segregation of this chromosome with Chinese hamster/mouse somatic cell hybrids, *Somatic Cell Genet.,* 3, 121, 1977.

35. Hozier, J., Scalzi, J., Sawyer, J., Carley, N., Applegate, M., Clive, D., and Moore, M. M., Localization of the mouse thymidine kinase gene to the distal portion of chromosome 11, *Genomics,* 10, 827, 1991.

36. Moore, M. M., Clive, D., Howard, B. E., Batson, A. G., and Turner, N. T., *In situ* analysis of trifluorothymidine-resistant (TFT^r) mutants of L5178Y/TK$^{+/-}$ mouse lymphoma cells, *Mutat. Res.,* 151, 147, 1985.

37. Preston, R. J., Dean, B. J., Galloway, S., Holden, H., McFee, A. F., and Shelby, M., Mammalian *in vivo* cytogenetic assays. Analysis of chromosome aberrations in bone marrow cells, *Mutat. Res.,* 189, 157, 1987.

38. Swierenga, S. H. H., Heddle, J. A., Sigal, E. A., Gilman, J. P. W., Brillinger, R. L., Douglas, G. R., and Nestmann, E. R., Recommended protocols based on a survey of current practice in genotoxicity testing laboratories, IV. Chromosome aberration and sister-chromatid exchange in Chinese hamster ovary, V79 Chinese hamster lung and human lymphocyte cultures, *Mutat. Res.,* 246, 301, 1991.

39. Margolin, B. H., Resnick, M. A., Rimpo, J. Y., Archer, P., Galloway, S. M., Bloom, A. D., and Zeiger, E., Statistical analyses for *in vitro* cytogenetic assays using Chinese hamster ovary cells, *Environ. Mutagen.,* 8, 183, 1986.

40. Scott, D., Galloway, S. M., Marshall, R. R., Ishidate, M., Jr., Brusick, D., Ashby, J., and Myhr, B. C., Genotoxicity under extreme culture conditions. A report from ICPEMC Task Group 9, *Mutat. Res.,* 257, 147, 1991.

41. Morita, T., Watanabe, Y., Takeda, K., and Okumura, K., Effects of pH in the *in vitro* chromosomal aberration test, *Mutat. Res.,* 225, 55, 1989.

42. Galloway, S. M., Deasy, D. A., Bean, C. L., Kraynak, A. R., Armstrong, N. J., and Bradley, M. O., Effects of high osmotic strength on chromosome aberrations, sister-chromatid exchanges and DNA strand breaks, and the relation to toxicity, *Mutat. Res.,* 189, 15, 1987.

43. Kliesch, V., Danford, N., and Adler, I. -D., Micronucleus test and bone marrow chromosome analysis. A comparison of two methods *in vivo* for evaluating chemically induced chromosomal alterations, *Mutat. Res.,* 80, 321, 1981.

44. Heddle, J. A., Hite, M., Kirkhart, B., Mavournin, K., MacGregor, J. T., Newell, G. W., and Salamone, M. F., The induction of micronuclei as a measure of genotoxicity. A Report of the U. S. Environmental Protection Agency Gene-Tox Program, *Mutat. Res.,* 123, 61, 1983.

45. MacGregor, J. T., Heddle, J. A., Hite, M., Morgolin, B. H., Ramel, C., Salamone, M. F., Tice, R. R., and Wild, D., Guidelines for the conduct of micronucleus assays in mammalian bone marrow erythrocytes, *Mutat. Res.,* 189, 103, 1987.

46. Hayashi, M., Sutou, S., Shimada, H., Sato, S., Sasaki, Y. F., and Wakata, A., Difference between intraperitoneal and oral gavage application in the micronucleus test. The 3rd collaborative study by CSGMT/JEMS-MMS, *Mutat. Res.,* 223, 329–344, 1989.

47. Hart, J. W. and Engberg-Pedersen, H., Statistics of the mouse bone-marrow micronucleus test: counting, distribution and evaluation of results, *Mutat. Res.,* 111, 195, 1983.

48. Preston, R. J., Au, W., Bender, M. A., Brewen, J. G., Carrano, A. V., Heddle, J. A., McFee, A. F., Wolff, S., and Wassom, J. S., Mammalian *in vivo* and *in vitro* cytogenetic assays: a report of the U. S. EPA's Gene-Tox Program, *Mutat. Res.,* 87, 143, 1981.

49. Williams, G. M., Carcinogen-induced DNA repair in primary rat liver cell cultures, a possible screen for chemical carcinogens, *Cancer Lett.,* 1, 231, 1977.

50. Williams, G. M., The detection of chemical mutagens/carcinogens by DNA repair and mutagenesis in liver cultures, in *Chemical Mutagens,* Vol. VI, De Serres, F. J. and Hollaender, A., Eds., Plenum Press, New York, 1979, 71.

51. Probst, G. S., McMahon, R. E., Hill, L. E., Thompson, C. Z., Epp, J. K., and Neal, S. B., Chemically-induced unscheduled DNA synthesis in primary rat hepatocyte cultures: a comparison with bacterial mutagenicity using 218 compounds, *Environ. Mutagen.,* 3, 33, 1981.

52. Michalopoulos, G., Sattler, C. A., Sattler, G. L., and Pitot, H. C., Cytochrome P-450 induction by phenobarbital and 3-methylcholanthrene in primary cultures of hepatocytes, *Science,* 193, 907, 1976.

53. Mirsalis, J. C., Tyson, K. C., and Butterworth, B. E., The detection of genotoxic carcinogens in the *in vivo–in vitro* hepatocyte DNA repair assay, *Environ. Mutagen.,* 4, 553, 1982.

54. Butterworth, B. E., Ashby, J., Bermudez, E., Casciano, D., Mirsalis, J., Probst, G., and Williams, G., A protocol and guide for the *in vivo* rat hepatocyte DNA-repair assay, *Mutat. Res.,* 189, 123, 1987.

55. San, R. H. C., Sly, J. E., and Raabe, H. A., Unscheduled DNA synthesis in rat hepatocytes following *in vivo* administration of dimethylnitrosamine via different routes, *Environ. Mol. Mutagen.,* 27(Suppl. 27), 58, 1996.

56. Mirsalis, J. C. and Butterworth, B. E., Detection of unscheduled DNA synthesis in hepatocytes isolated from rats treated with genotoxic agents: an *in vivo–in vitro* assay for potential carcinogens and mutagens, *Carcinogenesis,* 1, 621, 1980.

57. Ashby, J., Lefevre, P. A., Burlinson, B., and Penman, M. G., An assessment of the *in vivo* hepatocyte DNA-repair assay, *Mutat. Res.,* 156, 1, 1985.

58. Provost, G. S., Kretz, P. L., Hamner, R. T., Matthews, C. D., Rodgers, B. J., Lundberg, K. S., Dycaico, M. J., and Short, J. M., Transgenic systems for *in vivo* mutation analysis, *Mutat. Res.,* 288, 133, 1993.

59. Kohler, S. W., Provost, G. S., Fieck, A., Kreta, P. L., Bullock, W. O., Sorge, J. A., Putman, D. L., and Short, J. M., Spectra of spontaneous and mutagen-induced mutations in the lacI gene in transgenic mice, *Proc. Natl. Acad. Sci. U. S. A.,* 88, 7958, 1991.

60. Kastenbaum, M. A. and Bowman, K. O., Tables for determining the statistical significance of mutation frequencies, *Mutat. Res.,* 9, 527, 1970.

61. Young, R. R., Rodgers, B., Provost, G. S., Short, J. M., and Putman, D. L., Interlab comparison of liver spontaneous mutant frequency from lambda/*lac*I transgenic mice, *Environ. Mutagen,* 21(Suppl. 22), 79, 1993.

62. FDA, Toxicological Principles for Safety Assessment of Direct Food Additives and Color Additives Used in Food, "Redbook II," 1993.

63. Auletta, A., Dearfield, K. L., and Cimino, M. C., Mutagenicity test schemes and guidelines: U. S. EPA Office of Pollution Prevention and Toxics and Office of Pesticide Programs, *Environ. Mutagen,* 21, 38, 1993.

64. Sofuni, T., Japanese guidelines for mutagenicity testing, *Environ. Mutagen.,* 21, 2, 1993.

65. CPMP, Commission of the European Communities: The Rules Governing Medicinal Products in the European Community, Vol. III, *Guidelines on the Quality, Safety and Efficacy of Medicinal Products for Human Use,* 1989, 103.

66. Kirkland, D. J., Genetic toxicology requirements: official and unofficial views from Europe, *Environ. Mutagen,* 21, 8, 1993.

ADDITIONAL RELATED INFORMATION

TABLE 15.11
The Genetic Code

Codon	Amino Acid	Codon	Amino Acid
UUU or UUC	phenylalanine	UAA or UAG	nonsense (ochre) nonsense (amber)
UUA or UUG	leucine	CAU or CAC	histidine
CUU, CUC, CUA, or CUG	leucine	CAA or CAG	glutamine
AUU, AUC, or AUA	isoleucine	AAU or AAC	asparagine
AUG	methionine	AAA or AAG	lysine
GUU, GUC, GUA, or GUG	valine	GAU or GAC	aspartic acid
UCU or UCC	serine	GAA or GAG	glutamic acid
UCA or UCG	serine	UGU or UGC	cysteine
CCU, CCC, CCA, or CCG	proline	UGA	nonsense (umber)
ACU, ACC, ACA, or ACG	threonine	CGU, CGC, CGA, or CGG	arginine
GCU, GCC, GCA, or GCG	alanine	AGU or AGC	serine
UAU or UAC	tyrosine	AGA or AGG	arginine
		GGU, GGC, GGA, or GGG	glycine

16 Carcinogenesis

Michael J. Derelanko, Ph.D., D.A.B.T., F.A.T.S.

CONTENTS

SECTION 1. INTRODUCTION

Cancer ranks as the toxic effect of most concern to the public. Because of this, considerable effort and financial resources are spent annually to identify potential human carcinogens. The purpose of this chapter is to supply basic information pertaining to carcinogenesis in rodents which is essential for understanding and interpreting the results of chronic rodent carcinogenicity studies.

This chapter is divided into six sections. Section 2 provides an overview of mechanisms hypothesized to be involved in chemical carcinogenesis. Section 3 presents data on spontaneous carcinogenesis in several strains of mice and rats commonly used in chronic bioassays. Information pertaining to the design of the chronic rodent carcinogenicity study and the susceptibility of various rodent organs/tissues to chemically induced carcinogenesis can be found in Section 4. Basic tumor pathology is presented in Section 5. Section 6 provides a glossary of terms associated with carcinogenesis.

Information pertaining to cancer in humans can be found in the chapter on Risk Assessment elsewhere in this book.

SECTION 2. MECHANISMS OF CARCINOGENESIS

It is currently believed that the development of malignant tumors does not result from a single event but from a multistep process consisting of discrete but interrelated biological events. Evidence for a multistage process of carcinogenesis exists for a variety of animal organ systems including skin, liver, urinary bladder, lung, kidney, intestines, and pancreas.[1]

In the multistage model of carcinogenesis, development of a single cell into a malignant tumor occurs in three stages: initiation, promotion, and progression. Initiation involves an irreversible change in a normal cell (usually an alteration of the genome) allowing for unrestricted growth. The initiated cell may remain latent for months or years. During this period of latency, the initiated cell is phenotypically indistinguishable from surrounding cells. Further development of the initiated cell into a neoplastic cell requires a period of promotion. Under the influence of a promoter, tumor formation is accelerated through clonal expansion of initiated cells. Promoters, which do not directly interact with DNA, are a diverse group of agents believed to act via a variety of proposed mechanisms most often resulting in increased cell proliferation. The process of promotion is considered reversible and requires prolonged and repeated exposure to promoter agents.

Progression is the final step in which preneoplastic foci develop into malignant cells. In this stage, tumor development is characterized by karyotopic changes, increased growth rate and invasiveness. The reader is referred to the following review articles for a more detailed discussion of multistage carcinogenesis: Pitot and Dragon,[2] Maronpot,[1] Pitot,[3] and Butterworth and Goldsworthy.[4]

This section presents basic characteristics of initiator, promoter, and progressor agents, provides a brief overview of the multistage carcinogenesis model, and offers a classification of carcinogenic chemicals according to proposed mode of action.

TABLE 16.1
Characteristics of Initiation, Promotion, and Progression

Initiation	Promotion	Progression
• Irreversible	• Reversible	• Irreversible
• Additive	• Nonadditive	• Karyotypic abnormalities appear accompanied by increase growth rate and invasiveness
• Dose response can be demonstrated; Does not exhibit a readily measurable threshold	• Dose response having a measurable threshold can be demonstrated	• Benign and/or malignant tumor observed
• No measurable maximum response	• Measurable maximum effect	• Environmental factors influence early stage of progression
• Initiators are usually genotoxic	• Promoters are usually not mutagenic	• Progressors may not be initiators
• One exposure may be sufficient	• Prolonged and repeated exposure to promoters required	• Progressors act to advance promoted cells to a potentially malignant stage
• Must occur prior to promotion	• Promoter effective only after initiation has occurred	• Spontaneous progression can occur
• Requires fixation through cell division	• Promoted cell population dependent on continued presence of promoter	
• Initiated cells are not identifiable except as foci lesions following a period of promotion	• Causes expansion of the progeny of initiated cells producing foci lesions	
• "Pure" initiation does not result in neoplasia without promotion	• "Pure" promoters not capable of initiation	
• Spontaneous (fortuitous) initiation can occur	• Sensitive to hormonal and dietary factors	

Adapted from Pitot, 1991[3] and Maronpot, 1991.[1]

Multistage Carcinogenesis

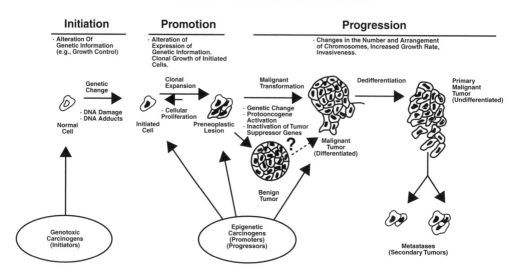

FIGURE 16.1 A model of the process of multistage carcinogenesis showing the three stages of initiation, promotion, and progression. In this model, an initiator irreversibly alters genetic information of a normal cell. With prolonged exposure to a promoter, clonal expansion of the initiated cell occurs, usually the result of enhanced cellular proliferation, "fixing" the genetic change caused by the initiator and resulting in the formation of a preneoplastic foci. This step can be reversible with insufficient exposure to the promoter. The critical step in carcinogenic process involves progression of the preneoplastic cells to malignancy. Under the influence of progressor agents, karyotypic changes occur accompanied by increased growth rate and invasiveness leading to metastasis. This process is considered irreversible. During progression, both benign and malignant tumors are usually observed. Controversy exists as to whether a "true" benign tumor can progress to malignancy or whether the "BENIGN" tumor that progresses to malignancy contains malignant cells localised *in situ* which have not yet invaded beyond the basement membrane of the developing tumor (adapted from Echobichon[5]).

TABLE 16.2
Defense Mechanisms and Self-Limiting Processes That Could Prevent Initiation or Progression

- Mutagens may be metabolized to nonmutagenic metabolites
- Genotoxic carcinogens may bind to materials other than DNA such as proteins or glutathione
- Error–free DNA repair processes may repair damage to DNA before the damage is fixed by DNA replication.
- Damage to DNA may occur at sites not involved in carcinogenesis
- Damage to DNA may result in cell death before cell replication
- Initiated cells may be destroyed by the immune system
- Other critical events in multistage carcinogenesis do not occur or do not occur at critical times

Adapted from Maynard et al.[29]

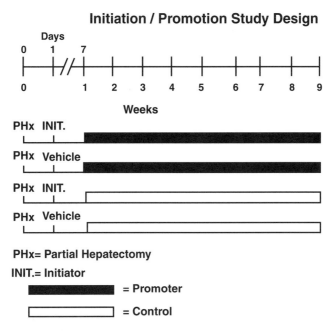

FIGURE 16.2 Schematic of a typical study designed to assess initiating and promoting potential of chemicals. To simulate cell proliferation, a partial hepatectomy (~70% of the liver) is performed on four groups of rats on the first day of the study (day 0).To investigate initiating activity, the suspect chemical in vehicle or vehicle alone is administered 24 h after hepatectomy (day 1).The single administration of the suspect chemical is generally by the oral route although other exposure routes are used. Beginning on day 7 of the study and continuing for 8 weeks, a known promoter is administered to the animals (usually sodium phenobarbital, 500 ppm) in drinking water or water alone. At the end of 8 weeks, the animals are sacrficed and livers examined microscopically for the presence of foci of altered hepatocytes which have been selectively strained for γ-glutamyl transpeptidase as a marker. The response is quantitiated as the number of foci per area of tissue. An increase in the number of foci only in the group treated with the promoter indicates that the suspect chemical is a "pure" initiator. An increase in foci in rats both with and without promoter treatment indicates that the suspect chemical possesses both initiating and promoting activity. Using the same study design, a chemical can be assessed for promoting potential by giving a known initiator on Day 1 of the study (usually diethylnitrosamine, 50 mg/kgPO) and administering the suspect chemical in drinking water during the 8-week promotional period (adapted from Yager et al.[6]).

TABLE 16.3
Classification of Carcinogenic Chemicals Based on Mode of Action

Classification[a]	Mode of Action	Examples
I. Genotoxic	Agents which interact with DNA.	
1. Direct acting (primary carcinogen; activation-independent)	Organic chemicals; direct alteration of DNA, chromosome structure or number; metabolic conversion not required; generation of reactive electrophiles and covalent binding to DNA.	bischloromethylether, β-propiolactone, ethylene imine
2. Procarcinogen (secondary carcinogen; activation-dependent)	Organic chemicals; requires biotransformation to a direct acting carcinogen (proximate carcinogen).	nitrosamines, ethylene dibromide, vinyl chloride
3. Inorganic carcinogen	Direct effects on DNA may occur through interference with DNA replication.	nickel, cadmium

TABLE 16.3 *(Continued)*
Classification of Carcinogenic Chemicals Based on Mode of Action

Classification[a]	Mode of Action	Examples
II. Epigenetic	Agents for which there is no direct evidence of interaction with DNA.	
4. Cytotoxin	Cytolethal; induction of regenerative cell proliferation; mutations may occur secondarily through several mechanisms including: release of nucleases, generation of reactive oxygen radicals, DNA replication before adduct repair; preferential growth of preneoplastic cells may be caused by selective killing of normal cells or expression of growth control genes (oncogenes).	nitrilo triacetic acid, chloroform
5. Mitogen	Stimulation of mitogeneic cell proliferation directly or via a cellular receptor; mutations may occur secondarily as a result of increased cell proliferation; preferential growth of preneoplastic cells may be caused through alteration of rates of cell birth or death.	phenobarbital, α-hexachloro-cyclohexane
6. Peroxisome Proliferator	Generation of reactive oxygen radicals through pertubation of lipid metabolism; growth control genes may be activated directly or via a cellular receptor.	fenofibrate, diethylhexyl phthalate, clofibrate
7. Immunosuppressor	Enhancement of the development of virally induced, transplanted and metastatic neoplasms possibly through impairment or loss of natural and acquired tumor resistance.	azathioprine, cyclosporin A, 6-mercaptopurine
8. Hormones and Hormonal-Altering Agents	Chronic stimulation of cell growth through activation of regulatory genes; other potential modes of action include: promotional effects resulting from alteration of hormonal homeostasis, inhibition of cell death (apoptosis), generation of reactive radicals.	estrogens, diethylstilbestrol, synthetic androgens
9. Solid-State Carcinogen	Generally only mesenchymal cells/tissues affected; physical size and shape of agent is critical; mechanism of action uncertain.	polymers (plastic), metal foils (gold), asbestos
10. Cocarcinogen	*Simultaneous* adminisitration enchances the carcinogenic process caused by a genotoxic carcinogen; possible mechanisms include: enhanced biotransformation of a procarcinogen, inhibition of detoxification of a primary carcinogen, enhanced absorption or decreased elimination of a genotoxic carcinogen.	phorbol esters, catechol, ethanol
11. Promoter	Administration *subsequent* to a genotoxic agent promotes tumor formation through enchancement of the clonal expansion of preneoplastic cells; multiple and diverse mechanisms proposed.	phorbol esters, saccharin, croton oil
12. Progressor	Development of initiated/promoted cells influenced; associated with alterations in biochemical and morphological characteristics, increased growth rate, invasiveness, and metastases; direct or indirect induction of structural (karyotypic) changes to chromosomes.	aasenic salts, benzene, hydoxyurea

[a] Classifications shown are not rigid. For example, a chemical may be both genotoxic and mitogenic or cytotoxic; phorbol ester can be both a promoter and a cocarcinogen.

Adapted from Weisburger and Williams, 1980.[7] Additional sources: Pitot and Dragon,[2] Pitot,[8] Pitot,[3] Maronpot,[1] and Butterworth and Goldsworthy.[4]

SECTION 3. SPONTANEOUS CARCINOGENESIS

Spontaneous carcinogenesis occurs in rodents as well as humans. A degree of background tumor formation is always observable in control animals from chronic rodent carcinogenicity studies. Certain organs/tissues seem to be more susceptible to spontaneous tumor formation than others. The incidence of spontaneous tumor formation in these organs varies by species and strain. It is of interest that organs most susceptible to spontaneous tumor formation are not always the ones most susceptible to chemically induced carcinogenesis as occurs in chronic rodent bioassays (see Section 4).

A chemical is considered to be carcinogenic in a chronic rodent study when it causes the formation of tumors in excess of background or produces a unique tumor not believed to occur spontaneously in the strain of rodent studied. Therefore, knowledge of the incidence of spontaneous tumor formation is essential for interpreting the results of chronic rodent bioassays. This section provides an overview of spontaneous tumor formation reported for several strains of mice and rats routinely used in carcinogenicity studies. This information is presented as a reference of spontaneous tumor formation likely to be encountered in chronic rodent studies. Because many factors such as diet, housing conditions, or duration of study influence spontaneous tumor formation,[9] the reader is cautioned that it would be inappropriate to use the data presented here to draw conclusions about the carcinogenic potential of any chemical. Information on spontaneous tumor formation from which such conclusions are drawn should most appropriately be obtained from concurrent controls and historical data for the specific species and strain used as developed in and maintained by the laboratory in which the study was conducted.

The tumor incidence data provided in this section are not specific for tumor type. The reader is referred to the cited sources for more detailed descriptions of spontaneous tumor formation in the species and strains presented.

TABLE 16.4
Reported Percent Incidence[a] of Spontaneous Tumor Formation by Organ/Tissue in Various Mouse Strains

	CD-1		B6C3F1	
Organ/Tissue	Male	Female	Male	Female
Adrenal	0–27.9(%)	0–3.8	<1.0–1.4	<1.0
Body cavities	—	—	<1.0	<1.0
Brain	—	0–2.0	<0.1–0.1	0–0.1
Circulatory system	—	—	<1.0–2.9	<1.0–2.4
Heart	—	—	0. 1–<1.0	0–0.1
Intestines	—	—	<1.0	<1.0
Kidney	0–2.8	0–1.4	<1.0	<0.1–<1.0
Leukemia/lymphoma	0–8.6	1.4–25.0	1.6–19.0	1.7–33.2
Liver	0–17.3	0–7.1	15.6–40.1	2.5–10.5
Lung/trachea	0–26.0	0–38.6	9.2–22.5	3.5–7.1
Mammary gland	—	0–7.3	—	<1.0–1.3
Ovary	NA	0–4.8	NA	<1.0
Pancreas	—	—	0.1–2.1	<0.1–<1.0
Pancreatic islets	0–2.1	0–1.4	<1.0	<1.0
Pituitary	0–0.8	0–10.0	<1.0	3.2–13.1
Skin/subcutaneous	0–2.8	0–2.0	<0.1–1.9	0.1–1.6
Stomach	0–4.9	0–3.8	0.3–1.1	<1.0
Testes[b]	0–2.0	NA	<1.0	NA

TABLE 16.4 *(Continued)*
Reported Percent Incidence[a] of Spontaneous Tumor Formation by Organ/Tissue in Various Mouse Strains

	CD-1		B6C3F1	
Organ/Tissue	Male	Female	Male	Female
Thyroid	0–2.0	—	1.0–1.1	<1.0–1.7
Urinary bladder	0–2.0	0–1.4	0–0.1	<0.1–1.0
Uterus/vagina	NA	0–13.3	NA	1.2–1.9

[a] Range.
[b] Includes prostate and seminal vesicles.

Adapted from Gad and Weil.[10] Additional sources: Chu,[11] Fears et al.,[12] Page,[13] Gart et al.,[14] Tarone, et al.,[15] Rao et al.,[16] and Lang.[17]

TABLE 16.5
Reported Percent Incidence[a] of Spontaneous Tumor Formation by Organ/Tissue in Various Rat Strains

	F-344		Sprague-Dawley		Wistar	
Organ/Tissue	Male	Female	Male	Female	Male	Female
Adrenal	2.4–38.1(%)	4.0–12.0	1.4–7.6	2.7–4.3	0–48.6	0–57.1
Body cavities	<1.0–9.0	0.3–1.9	1.1–1.4	1.8	–	–
Brain	0.8–8.1	<1.0	1.4–2.7	0.9–1.6	0–8.0	0–6.0
Circulatory system	0.4–3.8	<1.0	0.5	—	0–3.3	0–2.5
Heart	<1.0	<1.0	—	—	0	0
Intestines	<1.0	<1.0	—	0.5	0–3.1	0–3.8
Kidney	<1.0	<1.0	1.6	0.9	0–2.5	0–2.0
Leukemia/lymphoma	6.5–48.0	2.1–24.6	1.9–2.2	1.4–1.6	0–12.0	0–16.0
Liver	0.5–3.4	0.5–3.9	1.1	0.5–2.2	0–5.0	0–12.0
Lung/trachea	<1.0–3.0	<1.0–2.0	1.6	2.2	0–5.7	0–2.1
Mammary gland	0–1.5	8.5–41.0	0.5–2.3	36.4–45.1	0–6.7	1.3–45.0
Ovary	NA	<1.0	NA	1.1	NA	0–4.3
Pancreas	0.2–6.0	0	—	—	0–51.7	0–1.7
Pancreatic islets	0.8–4.9	0.8–1.3	0.9–2.7	0.5	0–25.0	0–4.0
Pituitary	4.7–34.7	0.3–58.6	11.2–33.2	37.3–57.6	2.3–58.3	6.7–68.0
Preputial gland	1.4–2.4	1.2–1.8	—	—	—	—
Skin/subcutaneous	5.7–7.8	2.5–3.2	2.8–6.5	3.2–3.8	0–21.9	0–5.0
Stomach	<1.0	<1.0	–	–	0	0–2.2
Testes[b]	2.3–90.0	NA	4.2–4.3	NA	0–22.0	NA
Thyroid	3.6–12.0	4.7–10.0	1.9–3.8	1.8	0–21.7	2.5–22.4
Urinary bladder	<1.0	<1.0	0.5	—	0–2.0	0–2.0
Uterus/vagina	NA	5.5–24.6	NA	3.3–4.5	NA	1.1–25.3

[a] Range.
[b] Includes prostate and seminal vesicles.

Adapted from Gad and Weil.[10] Additional sources: Chu,[11] Fears et al.,[12] Page,[13] Gart et al.,[14] Tarone et al.,[15] Goodman et al.,[18] Bombard et al.,[19] Walsh and Poteracki,[20] Haseman,[21] Rao et al.,[22] and Poteracki and Walsh.

TABLE 16.6
Tumor Classification and Background Rates in F344 Rats and B6C3F1 Mice

| | Background Rate (%) | | | | | Background Rate (%) | | | |
| | Mice | | Rats | | | Mice | | Rats | |
Site	F	M	F	M	Site	F	M	F	M
1. Skin, breast papilloma	0.1	0.3	0.5	1.8	52. Lung squamous carcinoma	0.0	0.0	0.1	0.2
2. Respiratory, oral papilloma	0.0	0.0	0.2	0.2	53. Oral, GI squamous carcinoma	0.1	0.2	0.1	0.2
3. GI papilloma	0.8	0.6	0.2	0.2	54. Urinary, reproductive squam carcinoma	0.0	0.0	0.2	0.1
4. Urinary, reproductive papilloma	0.1	0.1	0.2	0.2	55. Skin, GI basal cell carcinoma	0.1	0.0	0.2	0.4
5. Skin, breast adenoma	1.5	1.8	0.9	0.1	56. Urinary transitional cell carcinoma	0.0	0.0	0.1	0.1
6. Respiratory, oral adenoma	3.8	9.8	1.2	1.8	57. Skin, breast adenocarcinoma	1.3	0.1	1.9	0.2
7. Liver adenoma	3.6	9.7	0.1	0.1	58. Lung adenocarcinoma	0.0	0.0	0.0	0.0
8. GI adenoma	0.4	0.7	1.0	4.5	59. Oral, GI adenocarcinoma	0.1	0.5	0.1	0.5
9. Urinary, reproductive adenoma	0.3	0.1	1.9	2.4	60. Urinary, reproductive adenocarcinoma	0.3	0.0	1.1	0.3
10. Pituitary adenoma	8.3	0.4	26.5	15.8	61. Endocrine, brain adenocarcinoma	0.1	0.1	0.5	0.2
11. Endocrine adenoma	0.5	1.2	0.3	0.7	62. Islet cell carcinoma	0.1	0.0	0.2	1.2
12. Skin, urinary adenoma	0.0	0.1	0.0	0.2	63. Bile duct carcinoma	0.0	0.0	0.0	0.0
13. Reproductive, endocrine adenoma	0.1	0.0	0.1	0.2	64. Hepatocellular carcinoma	3.6	18.9	2.1	3.1
14. Tubular cell adenoma	0.0	0.1	0.1	0.2	65. Alveolar, broncheolar carcinoma	1.8	5.6	0.4	0.9
15. Follicular, clear cell adenoma	1.9	1.2	6.2	6.9	66. Chromophobe carcinoma	0.1	0.0	0.4	0.2
16. Cortical adenoma	0.4	1.2	2.3	1.0	67. Tubular cell adenocarcinoma	0.0	0.1	0.0	0.2
17. Skin, breast, liver cystadenoma	0.1	0.3	0.4	0.0	68. Thyroid follicular cell carcinoma	0.3	0.2	0.5	0.9
18. GI, urinary, reproductive cystadenoma	0.3	0.0	0.0	0.0	69. Cortical carcinoma	0.0	0.1	0.2	0.1
19. Endocrine cystadenoma	0.1	0.0	0.1	0.0	70. Clear cell carcinoma	0.0	0.0	2.4	2.8
20. Acinar cell adenoma	0.0	0.0	0.1	1.4	71. Adnexal, sebaceous carcinoma	0.0	0.0	0.2	0.3
21. Keratoacanthoma	0.1	0.1	0.3	1.6	72. Thymoma	0.0	0.0	0.0	0.0
22. Tubular adenoma	0.4	0.0	0.2	0.0	73. Granulousa cell carcinoma	0.3	NA	0.5	NA
23. Interstitial cell tumor	NA	0.4	NA	83.3	74. Interstitial cell carcinoma	NA	0.0	NA	1.0
24. Pheochromocytoma	0.9	1.4	4.4	18.6	75. Pheochromocytoma, malignant	0.1	0.1	0.4	1.6
25. Skin, breast fibroma	0.0	1.2	1.4	4.5	76. Skin sarcoma	1.2	4.6	0.8	1.7
26. Blood, bone fibroma	0.0	0.0	0.0	0.1	77. Other sites sarcoma	0.3	0.2	0.4	0.5
27. Fibroma, other sites	0.0	0.0	0.3	0.0	78. Blood, bone sarcoma	0.3	0.3	0.2	0.6
28. Lipoma	0.2	0.1	0.3	0.7	79. Liposarcoma	0.0	0.0	0.0	0.1
29. Leiomyoma	0.3	0.0	0.2	0.1	80. Leiomyosarcoma	0.6	0.3	0.4	0.2
30. Endometrial stromal polyp	1.3	0.0	17.9	0.0	81. Endometrial stromal sarcoma	0.3	0.0	1.0	0.1
31. Fibroadenoma	0.2	0.0	22.4	2.0	82. Carcinosarcoma	0.0	0.1	0.0	0.1
32. Hemangioma	1.1	1.2	0.1	0.2	83. Mesothelioma, osteosarcoma	0.4	0.3	0.4	3.2

(33.–51. continued on following page)   (84.–102. continued on following page)

TABLE 16.6 *(Continued)*
Tumor Classification and Background Rates in F344 Rats and B6C3F1 Mice

Site	Mice F	Mice M	Rats F	Rats M	Site	Mice F	Mice M	Rats F	Rats M
33. Osteoma	0.1	0.0	0.0	0.1	84. Teratoma	0.1	0.1	0.0	0.0
34. Hamartoma	0.0	0.0	0.0	0.0	85. Hemangiosarcoma	1.7	2.6	0.1	0.3
35. Ganglioneuroma	0.0	0.1	0.3	0.5	86. Granular cell tumor	0.0	0.0	0.1	0.1
36. Chromophobe adenoma	1.3	0.0	12.2	5.0	87. Glioma	0.0	0.0	0.2	0.3
37. Skin, breast carcinoma	0.1	0.1	0.3	0.4	88. Oligodendroglioma	0.0	0.0	0.2	0.2
38. Blood, bone carcinoma	0.1	0.0	0.1	0.1	89. Astrocytoma	0.0	0.0	0.5	0.5
39. Lung carcinoma	0.0	0.0	0.0	0.0	90. Olfactory neuroblastoma	0.0	0.0	0.0	0.0
40. Oral, GI carcinoma	0.0	0.1	0.0	0.0	91. Neurofibrosarcoma	0.2	0.4	0.3	0.5
41. Urinary carcinoma	0.0	0.0	0.0	0.0	92. Lymphoma	8.3	3.4	1.4	1.7
42. Reproductive carcinoma	0.1	0.0	1.5	1.7	93. Lymphocytic lymphoma	3.8	1.6	0.3	0.3
43. Pituitary carcinoma	0.4	0.0	2.2	1.1	94. Histiocytic lymphoma	4.8	2.6	0.2	0.3
44. Endocrine carcinoma	0.0	0.0	0.0	0.1	95. Mixed lymphoma	6.2	2.3	0.0	0.0
45. Brain carcinoma	0.1	0.0	0.4	0.1	96. Malignant reticulosis	0.1	0.1	0.0	0.0
46. Skin, breast papillary carcinoma	0.1	0.0	0.1	0.0	97. Leukemia	0.4	0.2	3.1	4.3
47. Lung papillary carcinoma	0.0	0.0	0.0	0.0	98. Myelomonocytic leukemia	0.0	0.0	1.7	2.1
48. GI, urinary papillary carcinoma	0.0	0.0	0.0	0.0	99. Lymphocytic leukemia	0.5	0.1	0.8	1.3
49. Uterus, ovary papillary carcinoma	0.0	NA	0.1	NA	100. Plasmacytic leukemia	0.1	0.1	7.5	10.9
50. Thyroid papillary carcinoma	0.0	0.0	0.0	0.1	101. Granulocytic leukemia	0.1	0.1	0.2	0.2
51. Skin squamous carcinoma	0.1	0.2	0.7	1.2	102. Monocytic leukemia	0.0	0.0	1.8	2.2

Note: The information in this table was developed from the NCI/NTP Carcinogenesis Bioassay Data Base (CBDS) system and includes only experiments completed by 1983. Rates are averages in all control groups in relevant experiments (for 312 chemicals) and are rounded to one decimal place. Some designations include multiple sites for the subject tumor.

From Linkov et al.,[30] with permission from Oxford University Press.

TABLE 16.7
Spontaneous Neoplasms Occurring in Three or More Control Wistar Rats

Neoplasm	Male No.	Male %[a]	Male % Range	Female No.	Female %[a]	Female % Range
Endocrine						
Pituitary adenoma	156	33.6	18.3–51.7	234	50.3	43.1–58.3
Carcinoma				10	2.2	0–5.4
Adrenal pheochromocytome — benign	45	9.7	4.0–21.7	6	1.3	0–3.3
Pheochromocytoma — malignant	8	1.7	0–3.3	2	0.4	0–1.0
Cortical adenoma	16	3.4	0–9.5	19	4.1	0–7.0
Cortical carcinoma	1	0.2	0–1.0	4	0.9	0–1.7
Thyroid C cell adenoma	27	5.8	3.3–11.4	39	8.4	5.8–10.0
C cell carcinoma	2	0.4	0–0.8	2	0.4	0–2.0
Follicular adenoma	18	3.9	1.7–6.9	13	2.9	2.0–3.3
Follicular carcinoma	4	0.9	0–1.7	7	1.5	0–3.3
Pancreatic islet cell adenoma	25	5.4	0–25.0	8	1.7	0.8–4.0
Islet cell carcinoma	7	1.5	0–6.7	3	0.7	0–1.5
Parathyroid adenoma	9	1.9	0–4.0			

TABLE 16.7 *(Continued)*
Spontaneous Neoplasms Occurring in Three or More Control Wistar Rats

Neoplasm	Male			Female		
	No.	%[a]	% Range	No.	%[a]	% Range
Integumentary						
Mammary fibroadenoma	12	2.6	0–6.7	168	36.1	18.0–45.0
Adenoma				18	3.9	2.0–6.7
Adenocarcinoma				31	6.7	1.7–12.4
Keratoacanthoma	52	11.2	2.0–21.9	3	0.7	0–1.9
Fibroma	21	4.5	1.0–9.2	14	3.0	1.9–5.0
Fibrosarcoma	15	3.2	0.8–6.2			
Papilloma	15	3.2	1.0–8.3	2	0.4	0–0.8
Squamous cell carcinoma	6	1.3	0–3.3	5	1.1	0–3.3
Lipoma	5	1.1	0–4.0			
Liposarcoma	2	0.4	0–1.5	1	0.2	0–0.8
Trichofolliculoma	7	1.5	0–4.2	1	0.2	0–0.8
Pilomatrixoma	2	0.4	0–1.0	1	0.2	0–1.0
Schwannoma	2	0.4	0–0.8	2	0.4	0–2.0
Basal cell tumor	3	0.7	0–2.0	3	0.7	0–2.0
Histiocytic sarcoma	3	0.7	0–1.9			
Zymbal's gland carcinoma	3	0.7	0–1.7	1	0.2	0–0.8
Reproductive						
Testicular interstitial cell tumor	49	10.5	8.3–15.2			
Prostatic adenoma	3	0.7	0–1.5			
Uterine/vaginal stromal polyp				72	15.5	7.7–20.8
Stromal sarcoma				5	1.1	0–4.0
Schwannoma				11	2.4	0–5.0
Granular cell tumor				13	2.8	0–6.2
Endometrial adenoma				4	0.9	0–3.1
Granulosa cell tumor				7	1.5	1.0–2.0
Gastrointestinal						
Pancreatic acinar cell adenoma	62	13.3	0–51.7	3	0.7	0–1.7
Acinar cell carcinoma	16	3.4	0–16.7			
Hepatocellular adenoma	13	2.8	0–5.0	10	2.2	0–4.2
Carcinoma	5	1.1	0–2.0	1	0.2	0–0.08
Cholangioma				3	0.7	0–2.0
Intestinal adenocarcinoma	6	1.3	0–3.1	4	0.9	0–2.3
Intestinal leiomyoma	2	0.4	0–1.7	4	0.9	0–2.3
Hematopoietic/lymphatic						
Thymoma — benign	14	3.0	0–5.0	35	7.5	0–14.6
Thymoma — malignant	2	0.4	0–2.0	5	1.1	0–3.3
Lymphoma	6	1.3	0–4.6	11	2.4	0–7.7
Granular cell leukemia	5	1.1	0–2.0	7	1.5	0–3.1
Histiocytic sarcoma	5	1.1	0–3.1	3	0.7	0–1.7
Nervous						
Granular cell meningioma	11	2.4	0–3.3	7	1.5	0–3.1
Astrocytoma	4	0.9	0–2.0	3	0.7	0–1.5
Oligodendroglioma	2	0.4	0–1.0	2	0.4	0–1.0
Urinary						
Renal cell adenoma	8	1.7	0–2.5	3	0.7	0–1.5
Renal cell carcinoma	2	0.4	0–0.8	1	0.2	0–0.8
Renal mesenchymal tumor	4	0.9	0–1.7	11	2.4	0–3.8

TABLE 16.7 *(Continued)*
Spontaneous Neoplasms Occurring in Three or More Control Wistar Rats

Neoplasm	Male No.	%[a]	% Range	Female No.	%[a]	% Range
Cardiovascular						
Cardiac schwannoma	2	0.4	0–1.5	5	1.1	0–2.0
Hemangioma	8	1.7	0–3.3	6	1.3	0–1.5
Hemangiosarcoma	16	3.4	0–3.3	3	0.7	0–2.5
Musculoskeletal						
Osteosarcoma	1	0.2	0–2.0	3	0.7	0–2.0

a = Percent of population.(male or female), Range is between studies

From Poteracki and Walsh[31] with permission from Oxford University Press. Note: table reports neoplasms from 930 control rats (465 male, 465 female) from five carcinogenicity bioassays conducted between 1990 and 1995.

TABLE 16.8
Ranking of Mouse Organs Based on Incidence of Spontaneous Tumor Formation (Benign and Malignant)

Males Organ	Incidence[a]	Females Organ	Incidence[a]
1. Liver	28.7 (%)	1. Blood/lymphoid tissue[b]	29.1
2. Lung/trachea	24.3	2. Lung/trachea	22.9
3. Adrenal	14.7	3. Pituitary	11.6
4. Blood/lymphoid tissue[b]	13.8	4. Liver	8.8
5. Stomach	3.0	5. Uterus/vagina	7.6
6. Circulatory system	2.9	6. Mammary gland	4.3
7. Skin/subcutaneous	2.4	7. Ovary	2.8
8. Pancreas	2.1	8. Circulatory system	2.4
9. Thyroid	1.6	9. Adrenal	2.2
10. Kidney	1.5	10. Stomach	2.1
11. Pancreas (islets)	1.2	11. Skin/subcutaneous	1.8
Testes	1.2	12. Thyroid	1.7
12. Urinary bladder	1.1	13. Kidney	1.4
13. Pituitary	0.5	14. Urinary bladder	1.2
14. Intestines	0.4	15. Brain	1.1
15. Brain	0.1	16. Pancreas	< 1.0
15. Heart	0.1	16. Pancreas (islets)	0.8
15. Body cavities	0.1	17. Body cavities	0.3
		18. Intestines	0.2
		19. Heart	0.1

[a] Mean of highest reported percent incidence of spontaneous tumor formation for various mouse strains.
[b] Leukemia/lymphoma.

TABLE 16.9
Ranking of Rat Organs Based on Incidence of Spontaneous Tumor Formation (Benign and Malignant)

Males		Females	
Organ	Incidence[a]	Organ	Incidence[a]
1. Pituitary	42.1(%)	1. Pituitary	61.4
2. Testes	38.8	2. Mammary gland	43.7
3. Adrenal	31.4	3. Adrenal	24.5
4. Pancreas	28.9	4. Uterus/vagina	18.1
5. Blood/lymphoid tissue[b]	20.7	5. Blood/lymphoid tissue[b]	14.1
6. Thyroid	12.5	6. Thyroid	11.4
7. Skin/subcutaneous	12.1	7. Liver	6.0
8. Pancreas (islets)	10.9	8. Skin/subcutaneous	4.0
9. Brain	6.3	9. Brain	2.7
10. Body cavities	3.5	10. Lung/trachea	2.1
10. Mammary gland	3.5	11. Pancreas (islets)	1.9
11. Lung/trachea	3.4	11. Ovary	1.9
12. Liver	3.2	11. Intestines	1.9
13. Circulatory system	2.5	12. Preputial gland	1.8
14. Preputial gland	2.4	12. Circulatory system	1.8
15. Intestines	2.1	13. Pancreas	1.7
16. Kidney	1.7	14. Body cavities	1.4
17. Stomach	1.2	15. Urinary bladder	1.1
18. Urinary bladder	0.9	15. Stomach	1.1
19. Heart	0.2	16. Kidney	1.0
		17. Heart	<0.1

[a] Mean of highest reported percent incidence of spontaneous tumor formation for various rat strains.
[b] Leukemia/lymphoma.

SECTION 4. CHEMICAL CARCINOGENESIS

The chronic rodent carcinogenicity study is one of the most elaborate, labor-intensive, and costly of all toxicology studies. To evaluate the carcinogenic potential of chemicals, animals are exposed to a substance of concern throughout their lifetime during which time the appearance of unique and/or excess tumors are noted. Although some tumors are observable grossly, the ultimate identification and morphological characterization is made through histopathological examination of generally 45 organs/tissues per animal. Considering the typical study consists of 400 rodents, as many as 9000 microscopic sections can be evaluated just in the control and high-dose groups. In addition, data collected on physical examinations, body weights, food consumption, hematology, clinical chemistry, and necropsy during as many as 24 months must be compiled and analyzed. The cost of a chronic carcinogenicity study in one species ranges from 0.7 to 1.5 million U.S. dollars depending on the route of exposure. The seriousness of the endpoint evaluated is usually justification for the time and money expended since in the eyes of the public, cancer is the most feared of all human diseases.

Widespread and routine evaluation of chemicals for carcinogenic potential has been performed for over three decades beginning in earnest in the mid-1960s.[1] Despite many problems associated with the chronic rodent carcinogenicity study, discussion of which is beyond the scope of this book, the rodent bioassay is considered the best available method for identifying potential carcinogens.[1]

Most of the substances known to be carcinogenic to humans have been found to cause cancer in animals.[24] The converse of this, that most of the substances shown to cause cancer in animals will cause cancer in humans under realistic conditions of exposure, is the subject of much debate.

As pointed out by Maronpot,[1] the original National Cancer Institute (NCI) chronic rodent carcinogenicity bioassay was intended to screen for potential carcinogens and was not intended to define carcinogen potency, mechanisms of tumor formation, or human relevance. However, results of these studies are often used in this way for human risk assessment. The reader should bear in mind that these studies only demonstrate that certain chemicals are capable of causing cancer in animals under specific conditions of exposure. The judgment as to whether a chemical poses a carcinogenic risk should only be made after factors such as route and duration of exposure, genotoxic potential, comparative species metabolism, as well as other information relevant to human exposure are considered.[1]

This section presents information on the basic design of the chronic rodent carcinogenicity study and the reported susceptibility of various organs/tissues of rodents to chemically induced tumor formation. The reader is referred to the cited sources for more detailed discussion of the chronic rodent carcinogenicity study, its conduct and interpretation. The 2-year rodent bioassay has been the "gold standard" for evaluation of chemical carcinogenicity for over 25 years. However, it has come under criticism because of its high cost, requirements for high doses and questionable relevance to humans. As this book went to press, several alternative bioassays were under investigation which use transgenic animals designed to address these concerns (e.g., Tg.AC and p53 6-month transgenic mouse assays).

TABLE 16.10
Typical Basic Design of a Chronic Carcinogenicity Study[a]

Animals

Species	Usually rats, mice and, occasionally hamsters
Strain	Common laboratory strains (e.g., rats: F-344, Sprague–Dawley; mice: CD-1, $B_6C_3F_1$)
Age	<6–8 wk
Housing	Individual or group

Study Design

No. animals/group	50/sex/group[b]
No. groups	3 dose levels/1 control[c]
Exposure route	Oral, dermal, or inhalation as appropriate to potential human exposure
Study duration	Average lifespan of strain used, at least 18 mo for mice, 24 mo for rats

Observations

Mortality/moribundity	2 times/day
Gross clinical observations	At least daily
Detailed physical examinations	1 time/wk
Body weights	Weekly (weeks 1–13), monthly thereafter
Food consumption	Weekly (weeks 1–13), monthly thereafter
Water consumption	Weekly (weeks 1–13), monthly thereafter (when test substance is administered in drinking water)
Hematology	CBC, blood smear, at 3, 12, and 18 mo (20/sex/group) and at termination (all survivors). Differential blood counts for control and high-dose and additional groups if effects observed at high-dose level
Clinical chemistry	3 times during test period, generally pretest (base line), 12 mo, and at termination (10/sex/group)
Urinalysis	May be performed along with hematology (10/sex/group)
Ophthalmoscopic exam	Pretest and at termination

TABLE 16.10 *(Continued)*
Typical Basic Design of a Chronic Carcinogenicity Study[a]

Gross necropsy	All animals (including spontaneous deaths)
Organ weights	10/sex/group to include liver, kidney, adrenals, brain, and gonads, and others if suspected target organs
Histopathology	Control and high-dose groups, other groups if positive findings in high-dose group (see Table 16.11 for organs/tissues frequently observed), suspected target organs/tissues—all groups, all gross lesions and tumors

[a] Based in part on U.S. Environmental Protection Agency Guidelines.[25]

[b] Additional animals per group if interim sacrifices are planned.

[c] Additional control groups may be needed depending on known or suspected toxicity of the vehicle used. Dose levels should be spaced to produce a gradation of effects. The highest dose should elicit signs of toxicity without substantially altering the normal life span due to effects other than tumors. The lowest dose level should produce no evidence of toxicity. Ideally, the intermediate dose level(s) should produce minimal observable toxic effects.

TABLE 16.11
Organs/Tissues Typically Selected for Histopathological Examination in Chronic Carcinogenicity Studies

Adrenals	Kidney(s)	Spleen
Aorta	Lacrimal gland[a]	Sternum
Bone marrow (sternal/femoral)	Liver	Stomach
Brain	Lung(s)	Testes
Medulla/pons	Lymph nodes (representative)	Thymus
Cerebellum		Thyroid
Cerebral cortex	Mammary gland	Trachea
Esophagus	Nasal turbinates[a]	Urinary bladder
Eye(s)	Nerve (peripheral)	Uterus
Femur	Ovaries	Vagina[a]
Gall bladder (if applicable)	Pancreas	Zymbal's Gland[a]
Harderian gland[a]	Parathyroids	Other
Heart	Pituitary	Accesory genital organs
Intestines	Salivary gland	All gross lesions/tumors
Duodenum	Skeletal muscle	
Jejunum	Skin	
Ileum	Spinal cord	
Cecum	Cervical	
Colon	Midthoracic	
Rectum	Lumbar	

[a] Occasionally selected.

TABLE 16.12

National Toxicology Program's Levels of Evidence of Carcinogenicity Used for Interpretative Conclusions Regarding Chronic Rodent Carcinogenicity Study Results

Clear Evidence of Carcinogenic Activity

Demonstrated by studies that are interpreted as showing a dose-related (i) increase of malignant neoplasms, (ii) increase of a combination of malignant and benign neoplasms, or (iii) marked increase of benign neoplasms if there is an indication from this or other studies of the ability of such tumors to progress to malignancy.

Some Evidence of Carcinogenic Activity

Demonstrated by studies that are interpreted as showing a chemically related increased incidence of neoplasms (malignant, benign, or combined) in which the strength of the response is less than that required for clear evidence.

Equivocal Evidence of Carcinogenic Activity

Demonstrated by studies that are interpreted as showing a marginal increase of neoplasms that may be chemically related.

No Evidence of Carcinogenic Activity

Demonstrated by studies that are interpreted as showing no chemically related increases in malignant or benign neoplasms.

Inadequate Study of Carcinogenic Activity

Demonstrated by studies that, because of major qualitative or quantitative limitations, cannot be interpreted as valid for showing either the presence or absence of carcinogenic activity.

From Maronpot, R.R., *Handbook of Toxicologic Pathology*, Academic Press, San Diego, 1991.[1] With permission.

TABLE 16.13

Top Ten Organs/Systems Developing Tumors in Carcinogenesis Studies — Mice[a]

Ranking	Males	Females
1	Liver	Liver
2	Lung	Lung
3	Forestomach	Forestomach
4	Circulatory system	Hematopoietic system
5	Hematopoietic system	Circulatory system
6	Thyroid gland	Mammary gland
7	Harderian gland	Ovary
8	Adrenal gland	Thyroid gland
9	Kidney	Uterus/cervix
10	Five sites[b]	Harderian gland

Note: See Table 24.14 for a ranking of human organs/systems based on frequency of occurrence of site-specific cancers.

[a] Based on 379 long-term chemical carcinogenesis studies from the National Toxicology Program (NTP) Data Base.

[b] Heart, nasal cavity, preputial gland, skin, urinary bladder.

Modified from Huff et al.[26]

TABLE 16.14
Top Ten Organs/Systems Developing Tumors in Carcinogenesis Studies — Rats[a]

Ranking	Males	Females
1	Liver	Liver
2	Kidney	Mammary gland
3	Zymbal gland	Zymbal gland
4	Forestomach	Thyroid gland
5	Thyroid gland	Forestomach
6	Skin	Urinary bladder
7	Hematopoietic system	Clitoral gland
8	Urinary bladder	Hematopoietic system
9	Intestines	Kidney
10	Nasal cavity	Uterus/cervix

Note: See Table 24.14 for a ranking of human organs/systems based on frequency of occurrence of site-specific cancers.

[a] Based on 379 long-term chemical carcinogenesis studies from the National Toxicology Program (NTP) Data Base.

Modified from Huff et al.[26]

TABLE 16.15
Frequency of Carcinogenic Response to Chemicals by Organ/System — Rats and Mice[a]

	Number Positive at Site (%)[b]	
	Chemicals Evaluated as Carcinogenic in Rats ($n = 354$)[c]	Chemicals Evaluated as Carcinogenic in Mice ($n = 299$)[c]
Liver	143 (40%)	171 (57%)
Lung	31 (9%)	83 (28%)
Mammary gland	73 (21%)	14 (5%)
Stomach	60 (17%)	42 (14%)
Vascular system	26 (7%)	47 (16%)
Kidney/ureter	45 (13%)	12 (4%)
Hematopoietic system	35 (10%)	39 (13%)
Urinary bladder/urethra	37 (10%)	12 (4%)
Nasal cavity/turbinates	33 (9%)	4 (1%)
Ear/Zymbal's gland	30 (9%)	2
Esophagus	29 (8%)	7 (2%)
Small intestine	21 (6%)	3 (1%)
Thyroid gland	20 (6%)	10 (3%)
Skin	20 (6%)	1
Peritoneal cavity	17 (5%)	7 (2%)
Oral cavity	16 (5%)	1
Large intestine	15 (4%)	
Central nervous system	15 (4%)	2
Uterus	11 (3%)	5 (2%)
Subcutaneous tissue	10 (3%)	1

TABLE 16.15 *(Continued)*
Frequency of Carcinogenic Response to Chemicals by Organ/System — Rats and Mice[a]

	Number Positive at Site (%)[b]	
	Chemicals Evaluated as Carcinogenic in Rats ($n = 354$)[c]	Chemicals Evaluated as Carcinogenic in Mice ($n = 299$)[c]
Pancreas	9 (3%)	
Adrenal gland	7 (2%)	4 (1%)
Pituitary gland	7 (2%)	4 (1%)
Clitoral gland	7 (2%)	2
Preputial gland	2	7 (2%)
Testes	6 (2%)	1
Harderian gland		6 (2%)
Spleen	6 (2%)	
Ovary		4 (1%)
Gall bladder		3 (1%)
Bone	3	
Mesovarium	2	
Myocardium		2
Prostate	2	
Vagina	1	

[a] Based on 354 and 299 chemicals considered carcinogenic to rats and mice, respectively, in long-term chemical carcinogenesis studies from the carcinogenic potency database (CPDB).

[b] Percentages not given when fewer than 1% of the carcinogens were active at a given site.

[c] Chemicals have been excluded for which the only positive results in the CPDB are for "all tumor bearing animals," i.e., there is no reported target site.

From Gold et al.[27] With permission.

TABLE 16.16
Animal Neoplastic Lesions of Questionable Significance to Humans

- Male rat renal tumors with α_2-globulin nephropathy
- Rodent urinary bladder neoplasia
- β_2-receptor stimulant-induced rat mesovarian leiomyomas
- Rodent stomach carcinoid tumors associated with prolonged acid secretion suppression
- Rodent thyroid follicular cell tumors
- Canine mammary neoplasia related to progestagen administration
- Rodent mammary neoplasia related to estrogen administration
- Rat uterine endometrial carcinomas related to dopamine agonists
- Leydig cell tumors in rat testes
- Mouse ovarian tubulostromal adenomas

Source: Alison et al.[32] With permission.

SECTION 5. TUMOR PATHOLOGY

The primary goal of the chronic rodent carcinogenicity study is to assess the development of tumors in animals exposed to a chemical of concern as compared with controls. Four types of neoplastic responses are considered to be evidence of chemically induced carcinogenesis:[28] 1) a greater incidence of tumors in exposed animals than occurs spontaneously in controls; 2) the earlier development of tumors in exposed animals than observed in controls; 3) the formation of unique tumors in exposed animals which do not occur spontaneously in controls; and 4) an increased multiplicity of tumors in exposed animals compared with controls. In the chronic rodent bioassay, the ultimate discovery and identification of any tumors must come from histopathological examination. Basic information on tumor pathology is presented in this section.

TABLE 16.17
Capacity of Tissues to Undergo Hyperplasia

High capacity
    Surface epithelium
    Hepatocytes
    Renal tubules
    Fibroblasts
    Endothelium
    Mesothelium
    Hematopoietic stem cells
    Lymphoid cells
Moderate capacity
    Glandular epithelium
    Bone
    Cartilage
    Smooth muscle of vessels
    Smooth muscle of uterus
Low capacity
    Neurons
    Skeletal muscle
    Smooth muscle of GI tract

From Maronpot, R. R., *Handbook of Toxicologic Pathology*, Academic Press, San Diego, 1991.[1] With permission.

TABLE 16.18
Selected Examples of Presumptive Preneoplastic Lesions

Tissue	Presumptive Preneoplastic Lesion[a]
Mammary gland	Hyperplastic alveolar nodules (HANs), atypical epithelial proliferation, lobular hyperplasia, intraductal hyperplasia, hyperplastic terminal duct
Liver	Foci of cellular alteration, hepatocellular hyperplasia, oval cell proliferation, cholangiofibrosis
Kidney	Karyocytomegaly, atypical tubular dilation, atypical tubular hyperplasia
Skin	Increase in dark basal keratinocytes, focal hyperplasia/hyperkeratosis
Pancreas (exocrine)	Foci of acinar cell alteration, hyperplastic nodules, atypical acinar cell nodules

[a] Many of these presumptive preneoplastic lesions are seen in carcinogenicity studies utilizing specific animal model systems. Generalizations about these presumptive preneoplastic lesions are inappropriate outside the context of the specific animal model system being used.

From Maronpot, R. R., *Handbook of Toxicologic Pathology*, Academic Press, San Diego, 1991.[1] With permission.

TABLE 16.19
Comparative Features of Benign and Malignant Neoplasms

	Benign	Malignant
General effect on the host	Little; usually do not cause death	Will almost always kill the host if untreated.
Rate of growth	Slow; may stop or regress	More rapid (but slower than "repair" tissue); autonomous; never stop or regress
Histologic features	Encapsulated; remain localized at primary site	Infiltrate or invade; metastasize
Mode of growth	Usually grow by expansion, displacing surrounding normal tissue	Invade, destroy, and replace surrounding normal tissue
Metastasis	Do not metastasize	Most can metastasize
Architecture	Encapsulated; have complex stroma and adequate blood supply	Not encapsulated; usually have poorly developed stroma; may become necrotic at center
Danger to host	Most without lethal significance	Always ultimately lethal unless removed or destroyed *in situ*
Injury to host	Usually negligible but may become very large and compress or obstruct vital tissue	Can kill host directly by destruction of vital tissue
Radiation sensitivity	Radiation sensitivity near that of normal parent cell; rarely treated with radiation	Radiation sensitivity increased in rough proportion to malignancy; often treated with radiation
Behavior in tissue	Cells cohesive and inhibited by mutual contact	Cells do not cohere; frequently not inhibited by mutual contact
Resemblance to tissue of origin	Cells and architecture resemble tissue of origin	Cells atypical and pleomorphic; disorganized bizarre architecture
Mitotic figures	Mitotic figures rare and normal	Mitotic figures may be numerous and abnormal in polarity and configuration
Shape of nucleus	Normal and regular; show usual stain affinity	Irregular; nucleus frequently hyperchromatic
Size of nucleus	Normal; ratio of nucleus to cytoplasm near normal	Frequently large; nucleus to cytoplasm ratio increased
Nucleolus	Not conspicuous	Hyperchromatic and larger than normal

From Maronpot, R. R., *Handbook of Toxicologic Pathology*, Academic Press, San Diego, 1991.[1] With permission.

TABLE 16.20
Selected Taxonomy of Neoplasia

Tissue	Benign Neoplasia[a]	Malignant Neoplasia[b]
Epithelium		
Squamous	Squamous cell papilloma	Squamous cell carcinoma
Transitional	Transitional cell papilloma	Transitional cell carcinoma
Glandular		
Liver cell	Hepatocellular adenoma	Hepatocellular carcinoma
Islet cell	Islet cell adenoma	Islet cell adenocarcinoma
Connective tissue		
Adult fibrous	Fibroma	Fibrosarcoma
Embryonic fibrous	Myxoma	Myxosarcoma
Cartilage	Chondroma	Chondrosarcoma
Bone	Osteoma	Osteosarcoma
Fat	Lipoma	Liposarcoma

TABLE 16.20 *(Continued)*
Selected Taxonomy of Neoplasia

Tissue	Benign Neoplasia[a]	Malignant Neoplasia[b]
Muscle		
Smooth muscle	Leiomyoma	Leiomyosarcoma
Skeletal muscle	Rhabdomyoma	Rhabdomyosarcoma
Cardiac muscle	Rhabdomyoma	Rhabdomyosarcoma
Endothelium		
Lymph vessels	Lymphangioma	Lymphangiosarcoma
Blood vessels	Hemangioma	Hemangiosarcoma
Lymphoreticular		
Thymus	(not recognized)	Thymoma
Lymph nodes	(not recognized)	Lymphosarcoma (malignant lymphoma)
Hematopoietic		
Bone marrow	(not recognized)	Leukemia
		Granulocytic
		Monocytic
		Erythroleukemia
Neural tissue		
Nerve sheath	Neurilemmoma	Neurogenic sarcoma
Glioma	Glioma	Malignant glioma
Astrocytes	Astrocytoma	Malignant astrocytoma
Embryonic cells	(not recognized)	Neuroblastoma

[a] "-oma," benign neoplasm.

[b] "Sarcoma," malignant neoplasm of mesenchymal origin; "carcinoma," malignant neoplasm of epithelial origin.

From Maronpot, R. R., *Handbook of Toxicologic Pathology,* Academic Press, San Diego, 1991.[1] With permission.

SECTION 6. GLOSSARY OF TERMS RELATED TO CARCINOGENS*

Activation (oncogene activation) The alteration of a protooncogene so it produces an abnormal protein or an overabundance of its normal protein product. In either case, the altered activity of the gene represents at least one critical step, in the process of oncogenesis.

Adduct The covalent linkage or addiction product between an alkylating agent and cellular macromolecules such as protein, RNA, and DNA.

Alkylating agent A chemical compound that has positively charged (electron-deficient) groups that can form covalent linkages with negatively charged portions of biological molecules such as DNA. The covalent linkage is referred to as an adduct and may have mutagenic or carcinogenic effects on the organism. The alkyl species is the radical that results when an aliphatic hydrocarbon loses one hydrogen atom to become electron-deficient. Alkylating agents react primarily with guanine, adding their alkyl group to N7 of the purine ring.

Altered focus A histologically identifiable clone of cells within an organ that differs phenotypically from the normal parenchyma. Foci of altered cells usually result from increased cellular proliferation, represent clonal expansions of initiated cells, and are frequently

* Reprinted from Maronpot, R.R., *Handbook of Toxicologic Pathology,* Academic Press, San Diego, 1991, pp. 127–129[1] With permission.

observed in multistage animal models of carcinogenesis. Foci of cellular alteration are most commonly observed in the liver of carcinogen-treated rodents and are believed by some to represent preneoplastic lesions.

Amplification (gene amplification) Increase in the number of specific genes or groups of genes frequently observed in different types of transformed cells. Because of the increase in gene copy number, there is increased production of the product encoded by the gene that has been amplified. Gene amplification is one form of oncogene activation.

Anaplasia Lack of normal organizational or structural differentiation of cells or tissues. Anaplastic cells are typically poorly differentiated.

Anticarcinogenesis The prevention or diminution of neoplasm formation by administration of an agent other than the carcinogen. Anticarcinogenic agents may be effective when given before, during, or after administration of the carcinogenic agent.

Antioncogene Synonym for tumor suppressor gene, an antioncogene has an effect opposite to that of an oncogene. *See* oncogene.

Benign A classification of anticipated biological behavior of neoplasms in which the prognosis for survival is good. Benign neoplasms grow slowly, remain localized, and usually cause little harm to the patient.

Bioassay An *in vivo* or *in vitro* test to quantitate the potency or activity of an agent in affecting a biological process relative to standards or positive controls of known activity. A bioassay presumes that the dose response of the organism is known. An example of a bioassay would be to measure the quantity of an active metabolite in the serum by testing the toxicity of the serum on cells of known sensitivity. It is not technically correct to refer to standard rodent carcinogenicity tests as bioassays, since they typically do not employ positive controls and practical considerations preclude accurate determination of low-dose responses to carcinogens.

Carcinogen An agent that causes neoplasia.

Carcinogenesis The process of generation of benign and malignant neoplasia in the broadest possible sense.

Carcinogenicity test The administration of an agent to a test species to determine if that agent directly or indirectly causes an increased incidence of neoplasms relative to untreated or vehicle-treated controls.

Chalone A postulated tissue-specific hormone-like substance produced by normal cells that inhibits cell replication.

Choristoma A mass of well-differentiated cells from one organ included within another organ, e.g., adrenal tissue present in the lung.

Chromosomal aberration A numerical or structural chromosomal abnormality.

Co-carcinogen An agent not carcinogenic alone but that potentiates the effect of a known carcinogen.

Cocarcinogenesis The augmentation of neoplasm formation by simultaneous administration of a genotoxic carcinogen and an additional agent (co-carcinogen) that has no inherent carcinogenic activity by itself.

Codon A group of three DNA bases that codes for a specific amino acid. Codons constitute the alphabet of the genetic code.

Direct carcinogen Carcinogens that have the necessary structure to directly interact with cellular constituents and cause neoplasia. Direct acting carcinogens do not require metabolic conversion by the host to be active. They are considered genotoxic because they typically undergo covalent binding to DNA.

Dysplasia Disordered tissue formation characterized by changes in size, shape, and orientational relationships of adult types of cells. Primarily seen in epithelial cells.

Electrophilic Related to an electron-attracting atom or chemical compound in an organic reaction.

EMTD Estimated maximum tolerated dose. Since the maximum tolerated dose is difficult to determine in advance, it is estimated from preliminary animal toxicity tests. *See* MTD.

Enhancer 1. *Tumor enhancer* — An agent that increases the neoplastic response to a carcinogen or to a cryptogenic form of initiation. The term is more generic than such terms as cocarcinogen or tumor promoter and makes no implications regarding the agent's actual or temporal mechanism of action. 2. *Molecular biology usage* — A DNA sequence located in the noncoding region of a gene that functions to increase the activity of promoter sequences responsible for initiation of DNA transcription.

Epigenetic Change in phenotype without a change in DNA structure. One of two main mechanisms of carcinogen action, epigenetic carcinogens are nongenotoxic, i.e., they do not form reactive intermediates that interact with genetic material in the process of producing or enhancing neoplasm formation.

Exon The regions of the genome containing structural genes that undergo transcription into messenger RNA. *See* intron.

Genome The total gene complement present in the normal set of chromosomes characteristic of an organism.

Genotoxic carcinogen An agent that interacts with cellular DNA either directly in its parent form (direct carcinogen) or after metabolic biotransformation.

Hamartoma A localized overgrowth of differentiated cells that have an altered growth pattern in relation to the organ in which they are found, e.g., a nodule of disorganized striated muscle fibers within a region of normal skeletal muscle.

Hyperplasia A numerical increase in the number of phenotypically normal cells within a tissue or organ.

Hypertrophy Increase in the size of an organelle, cell, tissue, or organ within a living organism. To be distinguished from hyperplasia, hypertrophy refers to an increase in size rather than an increase in number. Excessive hyperplasia in a tissue may produce hypertrophy of the organ in which that tissue occurs.

Initiation The first step in carcinogenesis whereby limited exposure to a carcinogenic agent produces a latent but heritable alteration in a cell, permitting its subsequent proliferation and development into a neoplasm after exposure to a promoter.

Initiator A chemical, physical, or biological agent that is capable of irreversibly altering the genetic component (DNA) of the cell. While initiators are generally considered to be carcinogens, they are typically used at low noncarcinogenic doses in two-stage initiation-promotion animal model systems. Frequently referred to as a "tumor initiator."

In situ **carcinoma** A localized intraepithelial form of epithelial cell malignancy. The cells possess morphological criteria of malignancy but have not yet gone beyond the limiting basement membrane.

Intron Noncoding region of a gene that contains regulatory sequences important for transcription. Introns are spliced out during transcription and are thus not translated into protein products.

Keloid Benign (presumably nonneoplastic) overgrowths of dermal scar tissue occasionally observed in humans and horses following trauma. These proliferative lesions can attain considerable size and tend to occur following surgical removal.

Malignant A classification of anticipated biological behavior of neoplasms in which the prognosis for survival is poor. Malignant neoplasms grow rapidly, invade, and destroy, and are usually fatal.

Metabolic cooperation A direct exchange of molecules between two cells in contact with one another. Such exchange is thought to occur through gap junctions in the cell membranes of the adjacent cooperating cells.

Metaplasis The substitution in a given area of one type of fully differentiated cell for the fully differentiated cell type normally present in that area, e.g., squamous epithelium replacing ciliated epithelium in the respiratory airways.

Metastasis The dissemination of cells from a primary neoplasm to a noncontiguous site and their growth therein. Metastases arise by dissemination of cells from the primary neoplasm via the vascular or lymphatic system and are an unequivocal hallmark of malignancy.

Mitogenesis The generation of cell division or cell proliferation.

MTD Maximum tolerated dose. Refers to the maximum amount of an agent that can be administered to an animal in a carcinogenicity test without adversely affecting the animal due to toxicity other than carcinogenicity. Examples of having exceeded the MTD include excessive early mortality, excessive loss of body weight, production of anemia, production of tissue necrosis, and overloading of the metabolic capacity of the organism.

Mutation A structural alteration of DNA that is hereditary and gives rise to an abnormal phenotype. A mutation is always a change in the DNA base sequence and includes substitutions, additions, rearrangements, or deletions of one or more nucleotide bases. Mutations in exons lead to altered protein products. Mutations in introns can lead to altered amounts of protein.

Oncogene The activated form of a protooncogene. Oncogenes are associated with development of neoplasia.

Preneoplastic lesion A lesion usually indicative that the organism has been exposed to a carcinogen. Presence of preneoplastic lesions indicates that there is enhanced probability for development of neoplasia in the affected organ. Preneoplastic lesions are believed to have a high propensity to progress to neoplasia.

Procarcinogen An agent that requires bioactivation in order to give rise to a direct acting carcinogen. Without metabolic activation these agents are not carcinogenic.

Progression Processes associated with the development of an initiated cell to a biologically malignant neoplasm. Sometimes used in a more limited sense to describe the process whereby a neoplasm develops from a benign to a malignant proliferation or from a low grade to a high grade of malignancy. Progression is that stage of neoplastic development characterized by demonstrable changes associated with increased growth rate, increased invasiveness, metastases, and alterations in biochemical and morphologic characteristics of a neoplasm.

Promoter 1. *Use in multistage carcinogenesis* — An agent which is not carcinogenic itself but when administered after an initiator of carcinogenesis stimulates the clonal expansion of the initiated cell to produce a neoplasm. 2. *Use in molecular biology* — A DNA sequence that initiates the process of transcription and is located near the beginning of the first exon of a structural gene.

Promotion The enhancement of neoplasm formation by the administration of a carcinogen followed by an additional agent (promoter) that has no intrinsic carcinogenic activity by itself.

Protein kinase An enzyme that catalyzes the phosphorylation of proteins. Protein kinases are critical parts of signal transduction in cells and, therefore, are important in control of cellular function.

Protooncogene A normal cellular structural gene that, when activated by mutations, amplifications, rearrangements, or viral transduction, functions as an oncogene and is associated with development of neoplasia. Protooncogenes regulate functions related to normal growth and differentiation of tissues.

Provirus The DNA copy of the RNA of a retrovirus which is ultimately integrated into the chromosomal DNA of the cell.

Proximate carcinogen Metabolite of a carcinogen intermediate in the conversion to an ultimate carcinogen.

Regulatory gene A gene that controls the activity of a structural gene or another regulatory gene. Regulatory genes usually do not undergo transcription into messenger RNA.

Restriction fragment length of polymorphism (RFLP) A method used to identify unique DNA sequences on two homologous chromosomes. RFLP is used to identify allelic differences between complementary DNA sequences.

Sister chromatid exchange The morphological reflection of an interchange between DNA molecules at homologous loci within a replicating chromosome.

Somatic cell A normal diploid cell of an organism as opposed to a germ cell, which is haploid. Most neoplasms are believed to begin when a somatic cell is mutated.

Stop study Generally refers to an animal carcinogenicity study wherein exposure to the potential carcinogen is limited to 3, 6, 9, or 12 months, after which the animals are held for several additional months without further treatment.

Structural gene A gene that encodes a specific protein product that is produced by a cell.

Suppressor gene A regulatory gene that normally functions to suppress growth by inhibiting the activity of structural genes responsible for growth.

Syncarcinogenesis The synergistic enhancement of neoplasm formation by simultaneous or sequential administration of two different agents.

Teratoma A benign neoplasm composed of tissues from all three germ layers. Teratomas are believed to arise as areas of tissue that, in early embryonic life, escape normal regulatory control mechanisms for organization and subsequently grow slowly in a disorganized manner.

Threshold The level of an agent below which no physiological, biochemical, or pathological effect can be measured.

Transcription Production of messenger RNA from a single stranded DNA template.

Transduction Excision of viral nucleic acid sequences from infected cells together with cellular DNA sequences and their subsequent packaging into mature viral particles. Transduction permits the transfer of DNA from one cell to another with the virus acting as the vector.

Transfection The direct transfer of DNA sequences into a cell.

Transformation Typically refers to tissue culture systems where there is conversion of normal cells into cells with altered phenotypes and growth properties. If such cells are shown to produce invasive neoplasms in animals, malignant transformation is considered to have occurred.

Translation Process whereby messenger RNA directs the synthesis of protein.

Translocation Displacement of one part of a chromosome to a different chromosome or to a different site on the same chromosome.

Ultimate carcinogen That form of the carcinogen that actually interacts with cellular constituents to cause the neoplastic transformation. The final product of metabolism of the procarcinogen.

Weight-of-evidence An approach for assessing the potential carcinogenic hazard of an agent by considering all available information relative to the biological action of the agent.

Xenobiotic A biologically active drug, hormone, or chemical substance not produced endogenously by the organism. A substance foreign to the organism.

REFERENCES

1. Maronpot, R. R., Chemical carcinogenesis, in *Handbook of Toxicologic Pathology,* Haschek, W. M. and Rousseaux, C. G., Eds., Academic Press, San Diego, 1991, chap. 7.
2. Pitot, H. C. and Dragon, Y. P., Stage of tumor progression, progressor agents, and human risk, *Proc. Soc. Exp. Biol. Med.,* 202, 37, 1993.
3. Pitot, H. C., Endogenous carcinogenesis: The role of tumor promotion, *Proc. Soc. Exp. Biol. Med.,* 198, 661, 1991.
4. Butterworth, B. E. and Goldsworthy, T. L., The role of cell proliferation in multistage carcinogenesis, *Proc. Soc. Exp. Biol. Med.,* 198, 683, 1991.

5. Ecobichon, D. J., *The Basis of Toxicity Testing,* CRC Press, Boca Raton, 1992, chap. 6.

6. Yager, J. P., Zurlo, J., and Ni, N., Sex hormones and tumor promotion in liver, *Proc. Soc. Exp. Biol. Med.,* 198, 667, 1991.

7. Weisburger, J. H. and Williams, G. M., Chemical carcinogens, in *Cassarett and Doull's Toxicology: The Basic Science of Poisons,* 2nd ed., Doull, J., Klaassen, C. D., and Amdur, M. O., Eds., Macmillan, New York, 1980, chap. 6.

8. Pitot, H. C., The dynamics of carcinogenesis: implications for human risk, *C.I.I.T. Activities,* Chemical Industry Institute of Toxicology, vol. 13, no. 6, 1993.

9. Haseman, J. K., Huff, J. E., Rao, G. N., and Eustis, S. L., Sources of variability in rodent carcinogenicity studies, *Fundam. Appl. Toxicol.,* 12, 793, 1989.

10. Gad, S. C. and Weil, C. S., *Statistics and Experimental Design for Toxicologists,* Telford Press, New Jersey, 1986.

11. Chu, K., *Percent Spontaneous Primary Tumors in Untreated Species Used at NCI for Carcinogen Bioassays,* NCI Clearing House, 1977, cited in Gad and Weil.[10]

12. Fears, T. R., Tarone, R. E., and Chu, K. C., False-positive and false-negative rates for carcinogenicity screens, *Cancer Res.,* 27, 1941, 1977, cited in Gad and Weil.[10]

13. Page, N. P., Concepts of a bioassay program in environmental carcinogenesis, in *Environmental Cancer,* Kraybill, H. F. and Mehlman, M. A., Eds., Hemisphere, New York, 1977, pp. 87–171, cited in Gad and Weil.[10]

14. Gart, J. J., Chu, K. C., and Tarone, R. E., Statistical issues in interpretation of chronic bioassay tests for carcinogenicity, *J. Natl. Cancer Inst.,* 62, 957, 1979, cited in Gad and Weil.[10]

15. Tarone, R. E., Chu, K. C., and Ward, J. M., Variability in the rates of some common naturally occurring tumors in Fischer 344 rats and (C57BL/6NXC3H/HEN) F' (B6C3F$_1$) mice, *J. Natl. Cancer Inst.,* 66, 1175, 1981, cited in Gad and Weil.[10]

16. Rao, G. N., Haseman, J. K., Grumbein, S., Crawford, D. D., and Eustis, S. L., Growth, body weight, survival and tumor trends in (C57BL/6 × C3H/HeN)F$_1$ (B6C3F1) mice during a nine-year period, *Toxicol. Pathol.,* 18, 71, 1990.

17. Lang, P. L., Spontaneous neoplastic lesions in the Crl:CD-1® (ICR) BR mouse, Charles River Laboratories, Wilmington, MA, 1987.

18. Goodman, D. G., Ward, J. M., Squire, R. A., Chu, K. C., and Linhart, M. S., Neoplastic and nonneoplastic lesions in aging F344 rats, *Toxicol. Appl. Pharmacol.,* 48, 237, 1979, cited in Gad and Weil.[10]

19. Bomhard, E., Karbe, E., and Loeser, E., Spontaneous tumors of 2000 Wistar TNO/W. 70 rats in two-year carcinogenicity studies, *J. Environ. Pathol. Toxicol. Oncol.,* 7, 35, 1986.

20. Walsh, K. M. and Poteracki, J., Spontaneous neoplasms in control Wistar rats, *Fundam. Appl. Toxicol.,* 22, 65, 1994.

21. Haseman, J. K., Patterns of tumor incidence in two-year cancer bioassay feeding studies in Fischer 344 rats, *Fundam. Appl. Toxicol.,* 3, 1, 1983.

22. Rao, G. N., Haseman, J. K., Grumbein, S., Crawford, D. D., and Eustis, S. L., Growth, body weight, survival, and tumor trends in F344/N rats during an eleven-year period, *Toxicol. Pathol.,* 18, 61, 1990.

23. Altman, N. H. and Goodman, D. G., Neoplastic diseases, in *The Laboratory Rat:* vol. I. *Biology and Diseases,* Baker, H. J., Lindsey, J. R., and Weisbroth, S. H., Eds., Academic Press, New York, 1979, chap. 13.

24. Wilbourn, J., Haroun, L., Haseltine, E., Kaldor, J., Partensky, C., and Vainio, H., Response of experimental animals to human carcinogens: an analysis based upon IARC monographs program, *Carcinogenesis,* 7, 1853, 1986, cited in Ecobichon.[5]

25. United States Environmental Protection Agency Health Effects Testing Guidelines, *Code of Federal Regulations,* 40, part 798, 1989.

26. Huff, J., Cirvello, J., Haseman, J., and Bucher, J., Chemicals associated with site-specific neoplasia in 1394 longterm carcinogenesis experiments in laboratory rodents, *Environ. Health Perspect.,* 93, 247, 1991.

27. Gold, L. S., Slone, T. H., Manley, N. B., and Bernstein, L., Target organs in chronic bioassays of 533 chemical carcinogens, *Environ. Health Perspect.,* 93, 233, 1991.

28. Pintadosi, S. and Sullivan, J. B., Chemical and environmental carcinogenesis, In: *Hazardous Materials Toxicology: Clinical Principles of Environmental Health,* Sullivan, J. B. and Krieger, G. R., Eds., Williams and Wilkins, Baltimore, 1992, chap. 8.

29. Maynard, R. L., Cameron, K. M., Fielder, R., McDonald, A., and Wadge, A., Setting air quality standards for carcinogens: an alternative to mathematical quantitative risk assessment-discussion paper, *Human & Experimental Toxicology,* 14, 175,1995.

30. Linkov, I., Wilson, R., and Gray, G. M., Anticarcinogenic responses in rodent bioassays are not explained by random effects, *Toxicol. Sci.,* 43, 1, 1998.

31. Poteracki, J. and Walsh, K. M., Spontaneous neoplasms in control Wistar rats: a comparison of reviews. *Toxicol. Sci.,* 45, 1,1998.

32. Alison, R. H., Capen, C. C., and Prentice, D. E., Neoplastic lesions of questionable significance to humans, *Toxicol. Path.,* 22, 179, 1994.

17 Animal Histopathology

John C. Peckham, D.V.M., M.S., Ph.D.

CONTENTS

SECTION 1. GENERAL INFORMATION

TABLE 17.1
Solutions Commonly Used for Tissue Fixation[1-3]

Fixative Solution	Primary Chemical(s)	Use	Tissue Recommended (Time)	Advantages/Disadvantages	Comments
Formalin-saline (10%)	Formaldehyde (37–40% gas in water), Sodium chloride	General fixative for light microscopy	All (1–3 days), CNS (1–4 wk)	Easily used, rapid penetration, formic acid formation	Specimen <5 mm thickness, volume of tissue to fixative 1:>10. Move to 70% alcohol
Neutral buffered formalin (10%)	Formaldehyde (37%), Sodium phosphate buffers	General fixative for light microscopy	All (1–7 days), CNS (1–4 wk)	Easily used, rapid penetration, longer storage without formic acid formation	Specimen <5 mm thickness, volume of tissue to fixative 1:>10. Move to 70% alcohol
Formalin ammonium bromide	15% Formalin, Ammonium bromide	Special fixative for nervous system	CNS (3–30 days)	Preferred for Cajal gold stain for astrocytes	
Bouin's	Picric acid, Formaldehyde (37%), Acetic acid (15:5:1)	Brilliant colors, sharp nuclear details	Ovaries, testis, thyroid, adrenal (4–18 h)	Rapid fixation, must be replaced with 70% alcohol	Specimens thin, collect within minutes of death
Zenker's	Mercuric chloride, Potassium dichromate, Sodium sulfate	Brilliant colors, sharp nuclear details	Eye (6–18 h)	Rapid fixation, less shrinkage, poor penetration	Collect within minutes of death
Zenker acetic formalin	Zenker base, Formaldehyde (37%), Acetic acid	Brilliant colors, sharp nuclear details	Bone with marrow (6–18 h)	Good for hematopoietic tissues	Specimens thin
Carnoy's	Absolute alcohol, Chloroform, Acetic acid	Sharp nuclear details	All (1–3 h)	Rapid penetration, quick fixation, lysis of erythrocytes	Small specimens, Transfer to alcohol
Helley's (Zenker's formalin)	Zenker base, Formaldehyde (37%)	Brilliant colors, sharp nuclear details	Bone marrow (6–18 h)	Good for hematopoietic tissues	Specimens thin
Glutaraldehyde (2–6%)	Glutaraldehyde (25%), Phosphate buffers	General fixative for electron microscopy	All (6–24 h)	Rapid fixation, used for perfusion fixation of deep tissues, e.g., CNS	Secondary fixation: Osmium tetroxide, specimens <1 mm^3, collect within minutes of death or perfuse
Karnovsky's	Paraformaldehyde, Glutaraldehyde (50%), Phosphate buffers	General fixative for electron microscopy	All (1–2 h)	Rapid fixation, used for perfusion fixation of deep tissues; e.g., CNS	Specimens <1 mm^3 collect within minutes of death or perfuse, keep fixative 4°C, store in sucrose buffer

TABLE 17.2
Stains Commonly Used in Histopathology[1-4]

Procedure	Dye(s)	Use or Structures Stained	Result
Hematoxylin and eosin (H & E)	Hematoxylin, eosin or phloxine-eosin	General light microscopy	Nucleus: blue / Cytoplasm: red / Red blood cell: red
Masson trichrome	Iron hematoxylin, acid fuchsin, Ponceau 2R, light green	General light microscopy	Nucleus: black / Cytoplasm: red / Collagen: green / Reticular fibers: green
Mallory's phosphotungstic acid hematoxylin (PTAH)	Hematoxylin, phosphotungstic acid	General light microscopy	Nucleus: blue / Muscle fibers: blue / Collagen: red / Fibrin: blue
Verhoeff's Van Gieson	Alcoholic hematoxylin, ferric chloride, Verhoeff iodine	Elastic fibers	Elastic fibers: black / Collagen: red / Nucleus: blue / Background: yellow
Weigert's elastic	Resorcin-basic fuchsin, iron hematoxylin, Van Gieson's solution, (acid fuchsin, picric acid)	Elastic fibers	Nucleus: blue / Cytoplasm: yellow / Collagen: red / Elastic fibers: black
Gomori's reticulum	Ammoniacal silver, ferric ammonia sulfate, gold chloride	Reticulum fibers	Reticulum fibers: black / Background: gray
Wilder's reticulum	Ammoniacal silver, gold chloride, Mayer's Hematoxylin	Reticulum fibers	Reticulum fibers: black / Collagen: red / Nucleus: blue
McManus periodic acid-Schiff (PAS) with and without diastase digestion	Periodic acid Schiff's reagent, light green or hematoxylin, either Harris's or Mayer's	Carbohydrates: glycogen, glycoproteins, glycolipids in cytoplasm, basement membrane, or capsule of fungi	Glycogen: rose to purple / Mucin: blue / Basement membrane: pink

TABLE 17.2 (*Continued*)
Stains Commonly Used in Histopathology[1-4]

Procedure	Dye(s)	Use or Structures Stained	Result
PAS-Alcian blue	Periodic acid Schiff's reagent alcian blue, pH 2.5 or pH 1.0	Acid mucopolysaccharides, glycosaminoglycans in mucus and cartilage	Polysaccharides: red Mucosubstances: red Acid mucopolysaccharides: blue
PAS-Hematoxylin	Periodic acid Schiff 's reagent, Harris hematoxylin, light green	Carbohydrates: glycogen, glycoproteins, glycolipids in cytoplasm, basement membrane, or capsule of fungi	Glycogen: rose to purple Mucin: blue Basement membrane: pink
PAS-MS	Periodic acid Schiff 's reagent; methenamine silver	Reticulum fibers	Reticular fibers: blue
Mowry's colloid iron	Ferric chloride, colloid iron, acetic acid, ferrocyanide	Acid mucopolysaccharides in cytoplasm and mucins	Hyaluronic acid: blue Sialomucin: blue
Armed Forces Institute of Pathology: Mucosubstances	Aldehyde fuchsin Mucicarmine, Mayer's hematoxylin	Mucosubstances in mast cells and mucins Mucosubstances in mucin	Mast cells, hyaluronic acid, sialomucin, sulfated mucosubstances
Mayer's mucicarmine			Mucin: red Nucleus: blue
May-Grunwald Giemsa	Giemsa	Polychromasia	Mast cells: blue Nucleus: blue
Nocht Azure Eosin	Azure A, eosin B	Polychromasia	Cytoplasm: red to blue Nucleus: blue Secretory granules: red Bacteria: blue Mast cells: blue
Tomlinson-Grocott	Toluidine blue	Polychromasia	Nucleus: blue Cytoplasm: red to blue Mast cells: dark blue
Lipid (requires frozen sections and fixation without lipid solvents)	Sudan black B	Neutral lipids and triglycerides in cytoplasmic fat	Compound lipids: blue black

Stain	Substance	Reagents	Results
Lipid (requires frozen sections and fixation without lipid solvents)	Neutral lipids and triglycerides in cytoplasmic fat	Sudan IV or Sudan red	Neutral lipids: red
Armed Forces Institute of Pathology: Fat (requires frozen sections and fixation without lipid solvents)	Neutral lipids and triglycerides in cytoplasmic fat	Oil red O	Simple neutral lipids: red
Bennhold	Amyloid	Congo red, Mayer's hematoxylin	Amyloid: pink to red Nucleus: blue
Lillie's amyloid	Amyloid	Crystal violet	Amyloid: red-purple Background: blue-purple
Feulgen's	Deoxyribonucleic acid (DNA) in nuclei	HCl, Schiff's reagent	Nuclear DNA: red
RNA (with and without ribonuclease)	Ribonucleic acid (RNA)	Methylene blue or toluidine blue	RNA: blue staining (which is lost after pretreatment with ribonuclease)
Kluver-Berrera	Nervous tissue: nerve fibers	Luxol fast blue, cresyl violet	Myelin: greenish blue Cells pink to violet
Einarson	Nervous tissue: neurons	Gallocyanin	Nissl substance: dark blue Cytoplasm: pale blue
Bodian silver	Nervous tissue: argyrophilic granules and nerve fibers	Protargol, hydroquinone	Argyrophilic granules: black Nerve fibers: black Nucleus: black Background: gray
Gridley's fungus	Fungi	Chromic acid, Feulgen reagent, aldehyde Fuchsin, metanil yellow	Fungi: deep purple Elastic tissue: purple Mucin: purple Background: yellow
Grocott's fungus	Fungi	Methenamie silver, nitrate, gold chloride, light green	Fungi: black Mucin: grey Background: pale green
Brown and Brenn Gram	Bacteria: bacterial wall	Crystal violet, Gram's iodine solution, basic fuchsin	Bacteria: Gram-positive: blue Gram-negative: red Nucleus: red Background: yellow
Ziehl-Neelsen acid fast	Acid fast bacteria, acid fast pigment	Carbol fuchsin, acid alcohol, methylene blue	Acid fast bacteria: red Acid fast pigment: red Nucleus: blue

TABLE 17.2 (*Continued*)
Stains Commonly Used in Histopathology[1-4]

Procedure	Dye(s)	Use or Structures Stained	Result
Von Kossa's calcium	Silver nitrate, sodium thiosulfate (Hypo), nuclear fast red	Calcium salts, bone	Calcium salts: black / Nucleus: red / Cytoplasm: light pink
Phosphate (acid fixatives cannot be used when identifying calcium phosphate)	Silver nitrate, hydroquinone	Bone, ossification: calcification	Calcium phosphate: black
Perl's iron	Potassium ferrocyanide, HCL, nuclear fast red	Iron (ferric ions)	Iron (ferric ions): dark blue precipitate / Nucleus: red
Lead citrate	Lead citrate	Electron microscopy	Organelle ultrastructure detailed by electron dense deposits
Uranium acetate	Uranium acetate	Electron microscopy	Organelle ultrastructure detailed by electron dense deposits
Janigan	Thioflavine-T	Fluorescence microscopy: juxtaglomerular cells	Juxtaglomerular cell granules: golden yellow
Vassar-Culling	Thioflavine-T	Fluorescence microscopy: amyloid	Amyloid: white or yellow
Acridine orange fluorescence	Acridine orange	Fluorescence microscopy: fungi, nucleic acids, virus particles	Fungi: bright orange / DNA: yellowish-green / RNA: reddish-orange
Immunofluorescence	Antibodies coupled to fluorescent dyes, such as fluorescein isothiocynate or rhodamin	Fluorescence microscopy: various antigenic structures	Positive antigen-antibody fluorescence
Histochemistry; acid phosphatase	Glycerophosphate, lead nitrate, ammonium sulfide	Light and electron microscopy	Lysosomes: black
Histochemistry; dehydrogenases	Monotetrazole	Light and electron microscopy	Mitochondria: dark dense precipitate
Histochemistry; peroxidases	3,3'-Diaminoazobenzidine	Light and electron microscopy	Peroxidase sites: dense precipitate
Immunohistochemistry; peroxidase	Peroxidase bound to antibody, 3,3'-Diaminoazobenzidine	Light and electron microscopy	Antigen sites: dense precipitate
Immunohistochemistry; ferritin	Ferritin bound to antibody	Light and electron microscopy	Antigen sites: dense precipitate
Avidin-Biotin-Enzyme complexes	Biotinylated antibody, avidin-enzyme complex chromagen	Light microscopy	Antigen sites: dense or colored precipitate

TABLE 17.3
Common Abbreviations and Codes Used in Histopathology

Code	Finding or Observation
+ (1)	= Minimal grade lesion
++(2)	= Mild or slight grade lesion
+++ (3)	= Moderate grade lesion
++++ (4)	= Marked or severe grade lesion
+++++ (5)	= Very severe or massive grade lesion
(No Entry)	= Lesion not present or organ/tissue not examined
+	= Tissue examined microscopically
-	= Organ/tissue present, no lesion in section
A	= Autolysis precludes examination
B	= Primary benign tumor
I	= Incomplete section of organ/tissue or insufficient tissue for evaluation
M	= Primary malignant tumor
M	= Organ/tissue missing, not present in section
N	= No section of organ/tissue
N	= Normal, organ/tissue within normal limits
NCL	= No corresponding lesion for gross finding
NE	= Organ/tissue not examined
NRL	= No remarkable lesion, organ/tissue within normal limits
NSL	= No significant lesion, organ/tissue within normal limits
P	= Lesion present, not graded (for example, cyst, anomaly)
R	= Recut of section with organ/tissue
U	= Unremarkable organ/tissue, within normal limits
WNL	= Organ/tissues within normal limits
X	= Not remarkable organ/tissue, normal
X	= Incidence of listed morphology, lesion present

TABLE 17.4
Frequently Used Grading Schemes for Histopathology[5,6]

Severity Degree	Proportion of Organ Affected	(A) Grade	Percentage of Organ Affected	(B) Grade	Percentage of Organ Affected	(C) Grade	Percentage of Organ Affected	(D) Grade	Percentage of Organ Affected	(E) Grade	Quantifiable Finding
Minimal	Very small amount	1	(A1) < 1–25% (A2) < 1–15%	1	<1%			1	<1%	1	1–4 foci
Slight	Very small to small amount			2	1–25%	1	1–25%				
Mild	Small amount	2	(A1) 26–50% (A2) 16–35%			2	26–50%	2	1–30%	2	5–8 foci
Moderate	Middle or median amount	3	(A1) 51–75% (A2) 36–60%	3	26–50%	3	51–76%	3	31–60%	3	9–12 foci
Marked	Large amount	4	(A1) 76–100% (A2) 61–100%							4	>12 foci
Moderately severe	Large amount			4	51–75%						
Severe	Very large amount			5	76–100%	4	76–100%	4	61–90%		
Very severe or massive	Very large amount							5	91–100%		

TABLE 17.5
Goals for Protocol Tissue Availability During Histopathology[d 7,8]

| Organ or lesion | Fischer 344 Rat[a,b] | | B6C3F₁ Mouse [c] | |
	Fair Range (%) >Fair = Good	Historical Availability	Fair Range (%) >Fair = Good	Historical Availability
Gross lesions	<100	Unknown	<100	Unknown
Adrenal cortex	96–97.9	98.7 (m)[a]	92–95.9	97.0 (m)
		98.7 (f)[a]		98.6 (f)
Adrenal medulla	96–97.9	97.0 (m)[a]	92–95.9	95.9 (m)
		96.1 (f)[a]		96.9 (f)
Bone with marrow	96–97.9	97.1 (m)[a]	92–95.9	99.2 (m)
		97.1 (f)[a]		99.4 (f)
Brain	96–97.9	99.7 (m)[a]	96–97.9	99.7 (m)
		99.8 (f)[a]		99.5 (f)
Clitoral gland	92–95.9	90.3 (f)[a]		100.0 (f)
Epididymis	92–95.9	98.3 (m)[a]	88–93.9	98.9 (m)
Esophagus	92–95.9	95.6 (m)[b]	88–93.9	
		96.3 (f)[b]		
Gallbladder			84–91.9	87.3 (m)
				90.2 (f)
Heart	96–97.9	99.9 (m)[a]	96–97.9	99.8 (m)
		99.9 (f)[a]		99.8 (f)
Intestine, large		95.6 (m)[b]		
		96.8 (f)[b]		
Cecum	88–93.9		88–93.9	
Colon	88–93.9		88–93.9	
Rectum	88–93.9		88–93.9	
Intestine, small		96.3 (m)[b]		
		97.8 (f)[b]		
Duodenum	88–93.9		88–93.9	
Ileum	88–93.9		88–93.9	
Jejunum	88–93.9		88–93.9	
Islets, Pancreas	92–95.9	98.5 (m)[a]	88–93.9	97.7 (m)
		99.0 (f)[a]		97.5 (f)
Kidney	96–97.9	99.7 (m)[a]	96–97.9	99.6 (m)
		99.7 (f)[a]		99.4 (f)
Larynx	92–95.9		88–93.9	
Liver	96–97.9	99.8 (m)[a]	96–97.9	99.7 (m)
		99.9 (f)[a]		99.7 (f)
Lung	96–97.9	99.8 (m)[a]	96–97.9	99.7 (m)
		99.9 (f)[a]		99.8 (f)
Lymph node	92–95.9		88–93.9	
Nasal cavity	96–97.9	97.6 (m)[a]	96–97.9	98.1 (m)
		96.8 (f)[a]		98.4 (f)
Ovary	96–97.9	99.6 (f)[a]	92–95.9	97.0 (f)
Pancreas	92–95.9	98.8 (m)[a]	88–93.9	98.3 (m)
		99.2 (f)[a]		98.3 (f)
Parathyroid	60–79.9	89.4 (m)[a]	50–69.9	76.9 (m)
		88.0 (f)[a]		77.9 (f)
Pituitary gland	92–95.9	98.3 (m)[a]	84–91.9	91.1 (m)
		99.0 (f)[a]		94.5 (f)

TABLE 17.5 *(Continued)*
Goals for Protocol Tissue Availability During Histopathology[d 7,8]

Organ or lesion	Fischer 344 Rat[a,b]		B6C3F₁ Mouse [c]	
	Fair Range (%) >Fair = Good	Historical Availability	Fair Range (%) >Fair = Good	Historical Availability
Preputial gland	92–95.9	95.4 (m)[a]		100.0 (m)
Prostate	92–95.9	98.6 (m)[a]	88–93.9	97.5 (m)
Salivary gland	96–97.9	97.9 (m)[a]	92–95.9	99.3 (m)
		97.4 (f)[a]		98.5 (f)
Seminal vesicle	92–95.9		88–93.9	
Skin	96–97.9		96–97.9	
Spleen	96–97.9	99.5 (m)[a]	92–95.9	98.9 (m)
		99.7 (f)[a]		98.9 (f)
Forestomach and stomach	92–95.9	98.8 (m)[b]	92–95.9	
		98.6 (f)[b]		
Testis	96–97.9	99.6 (m)[a]	92–95.9	99.4 (m)
Thymus		84.9 (m)[a]		77.1 (m)
Chronic	60–79.9	87.5 (f)[a]	50–69.9	86.6 (f)
Subchronic	96–97.9		92–95.9	
Thyroid	94–97.9	98.9 (m)[a]	92–95.9	98.5 (m)
		99.4 (f)[a]		98.5 (f)
Trachea	92–95.9	94.7 (m)[b]	88–93.9	
		95.6 (f)[b]		
Urinary bladder	92–95.9	98.0 (m)[a]	92–95.9	97.6 (m)
		98.4 (f)[a]		96.7 (f)
Uterus	92–95.9	99.1 (f)[b]	92–95.9	

[a] 7142 rats, 3572 males (m), 3570 females (f).

[b] 3919 rats, 1936 males (m), 1983 females (f).

[c] 7596 mice, 3807 males (m), 3789 females (f).

[d] The goal that 100% of all protocol organs and lesions will be available for histopathology is rarely possible because of sampling errors, lost tissues, and very small organs.

SECTION 2. COMMON MICROSCOPIC POSTMORTEM CHANGES IN LABORATORY RATS[9]

Adrenal gland, cortex
> Condensation of cells of zona glomerulosa (40 min*)
> Karyoklasis (clumping of chromatin) in epithelial cells of zona fasiculata and zona reticularis (8 h)

Adrenal gland, medulla
> Nuclear condensation and pyknosis (2 h)
> Increased cytoplasmic vacuolation (2 h)

Ampullary gland
> Sloughed and disruption of epithelium (< 20 min)

Blood
> Hemolysis and pigmentation of adjacent tissues (> 16 h)

---

* Time of onset after death.

Blood vessel (major)

    Aorta — formation of clear and pale staining areas between elastic laminae (< 20 min)

    Aorta — darkening and condensation of smooth muscle nuclei (16 h)

Bone (sternum)

    Bone and cartilage — no remarkable postmortem changes at 16 h.

Bone marrow

    Pyknosis of megakaryocytes (2 h)

Brain

    Increased clear space around oligodendroglia in white matter (2 h)

    Formation of clear space around cortical astrocytes (4 h)

    Increased numbers of shrunken hyperchromatic neurons (8 h)

    Pyknosis of oligodendroglia in corpus callosum (8 h)

    Pyknosis of cells in granular layer of the cerebellum (12 h)

    Increased foamy and vacuolated cytoplasm of cortical neurons (12 h)

Brown fat (perithymic)

    Granular cytoplasm (4 h)

    Blood-filled vessels (8 h)

    Condensed nuclei (8 h)

    Formation of intracellular soap, basophilic deposits (8 h)

Bulbourethral gland

    Increased granularity and lack of uniformity to the epithelial cell cytoplasm (12 h)

Clitoral gland

    No remarkable postmortem changes at 16 h

Coagulating gland

    Pyknosis of villous epithelium (20 min)

    Pyknosis of basal epithelium (20 min)

    Disruption of epithelium (4 h)

Ductus (vas) deferens

    Formation of intercellular clear clefts between adjacent epithelial cells (20 min)

Epididymis

    Formation of intercellular clear clefts between adjacent epithelial cells (16 h)

Esophagus

    Pale cytoplasm of polyhedral epithelial cells (40 min)

    Formation of interfiber clear spaces in muscle (40 min)

    Formation of vesicular spaces within collagen of the submucosa (8 h)

    Pyknosis of fibrocyte nuclei in submucosa (8 h)

    Absence of mitotic figures in basal epithelium layer (12 h)

Eye

    Shrinkage of nuclei and formation of clear spaces and clefts in the substantia propria of cornea (20 min)

    Absence of mitotic figures in anterior epithelium of the cornea (40 min)

    Condensation of nuclei in the retina (8 h)

Fat

    No remarkable postmortem changes at 16 h

Fat, brown (*see* Brown Fat)

Harderian gland

    Pyknosis of glandular epithelial cells (4 h)

    Karyorrhexis of glandular epithelial cells (12 h)

Heart

    Condensation and darkening of endothelial nuclei (20 min)

    Formation of interfiber clear spaces in muscle (40 min)

Intestine, large — cecum
>   Loss of superficial epithelial cells (< 20 min)
>   Saprophytic bacilli in the lamina propria (< 20 min)
>   Formation of interfiber clear spaces and pyknosis of myofiber nuclei (1 h)
>   Disruption and sloughing of crypt epithelium (1 h)
>   Basophilia of the lamina propria caused by the presence of large numbers of bacilli (1 h)
>   Loss of crypt epithelial cells (2 h)
>   Loss of cells in lamina propria (8 h)

Intestine, large — colon
>   Loss of superficial epithelial cells (< 20 min)
>   Saprophytic bacilli in the lamina propria (< 20 min)
>   Formation of interfiber clear spaces and pyknosis of myofiber nuclei (40 min)
>   Disruption and sloughing of crypt epithelium (2 h)
>   Loss of crypt epithelial cells (4 h)
>   Basophilia of the lamina propria caused by the presence of large numbers of bacilli (4 h)
>   Pyknosis of remaining epithelial cells (8 h)
>   Loss of cells in lamina propria (12 h)

Intestine, small — duodenum
>   Loss of villar epithelium (< 20 min)
>   Formation of interfiber clear spaces and pyknosis of myofiber nuclei (40 min)
>   Loss of cells in the villous lamina propria (4 h)
>   Lateral separations in crypt epithelium (4 h)
>   Loss of epithelium from crypts (12 h)
>   Loss of cells in basal lamina propria (12 h)

Intestine, small — ileum
>   Loss of villar epithelium (< 20 min)
>   Formation of interfiber clear spaces and pyknosis of myofiber nuclei (40 min)
>   Lateral separations in crypt epithelium (40 min)
>   Loss of cells in the villous lamina propria (1 h)
>   Loss of cells in basal lamina propria (2 h)
>   Pyknosis of Peyer's patch lymphocytes (4 h)
>   Loss of epithelium from crypts (12 h)
>   Total loss of mucosal epithelium (12 h)

Intestine, small — jejunum
>   Loss of villar epithelium (< 20 min)
>   Loss of cells in the villous lamina propria (< 20 min)
>   Formation of interfiber clear spaces and pyknosis of myofiber nuclei (40 min)
>   Lateral separations in crypt epithelium (1 h)
>   Loss of cells in basal lamina propria (12 h)
>   Loss of epithelium from crypts (> 16 h)

Islets, pancreatic
>   Pyknosis of peripheral islet cells (4 h)
>   Pyknosis of most of islet cells (16 h)

Kidney
>   Pyknosis and vacuolated cytoplasm of distal convoluted tubular epithelium (40 min)
>   Pyknosis of majority of nuclei of ascending and descending tubules of loops of Henle at corticomedullary junction (2 h)
>   Contraction of nuclei and increased granularity of cytoplasm of proximal convoluted tubular epithelium (4 h)
>   Separation and sloughing of pelvic urothelium (4 h)
>   Majority of glomerular cell nuclei pyknotic (8 h)

Formation of clear space around loops of Henle deep in medulla (8 h)
Pyknotic nuclei in collecting tubule epithelium of cortex (12 h)
Lacrimal gland (exorbital)
Nuclear condensation of acinar epithelium (12 h)
Liver
Sinusoidal accumulation of blood (resembles congestion) (< 20 min)
Presence of saprophytic bacilli (2 h)
Lung (immersion-fixed)
Parenchymal blood accumulation (resembles congestion) (< 20 min)
Separation of bronchiolar epithelium from lamina propria (< 20 min)
Presence of proteinaceous fluid in alveolar spaces (40 min)
Pyknosis of a majority of alveolar cells (4 h)
Pyknosis and sloughing of bronchiolar epithelium (16 h)
Lung (airway-perfused)
Parenchymal blood accumulation (resembles congestion) (40 min)
Pyknosis of a majority of alveolar cells (40 min)
Separation of bronchiolar epithelium from lamina propria (1 h)
Presence of proteinaceous fluid in alveolar spaces (2 h)
Lymph node, mandibular
Decreased density or rarefaction in cortical lymphocytes (20 min)
Cleavage lines resembling "dull-knife distortion" (1 h)
Pyknosis of cortical lymphocytes (4 h)
Lymph node, mesenteric
Decreased density or rarefaction in cortical lymphocytes (20 min)
Cleavage lines resembling "dull-knife distortion" (1 h)
Pyknosis of cortical lymphocytes (2 h)
Mammary gland (female)
Formation of clear spaces at base of acinar epithelial cells (1 h)
Pyknosis of acinar epithelium (2 h)
Sloughing of epithelial cells into ducts (4 h)
Mammary gland (male)
Increased foamy, vacuolated appearance of acinar cell cytoplasm (4 h)
Pyknosis of acinar epithelium (4 h)
Ovary
Formation of clear spaces around follicles (40 min)
Individualization of luteal cells (4 h)
Pancreas, exocrine
Vacuolar spaces in acinar epithelium (40 min)
Loss of central chromatin (hollow nuclei) in pancreatic duct epithelium (1 h)
Formation of clear interstitial spaces around acini (4 h)
Disappearance of eosinophilic, proteinaceous luminal duct contents (4 h)
Parathyroid gland
Formation of clear spaces at base of chief cells (1 h)
Peripheral nerve, sciatic nerve
Slight nuclear contraction of Schwann cells (2 h)
Pituitary gland, pars distalis
Increased pyknotic pituicytes (2 h)
Pallor or disappearance of pituicyte cytoplasm (4 h)
Pituitary gland, pars intermedia
Increased pyknotic pituicytes (4 h)
Pallor or disappearance of pituicyte cytoplasm (4 h)

Preputial gland

    No remarkable postmortem changes at 16 h

Prostate, dorsal

    Pale or clear luminal contents (< 20 min)

Prostate, ventral

    Pale or clear luminal contents (16 h)

Salivary gland, parotid

    Vacuole and clear space formation in the basal portion of the ductular epithelium (40 min)

    Pyknosis of ductular epithelium (1 h)

    Pyknosis and karyoklasis (clumping of chromatin) of acinar epithelium, which resembles very acute necrosis (12 h)

Salivary gland, sublingual

    Pyknosis and disruption of ductular epithelium (8 h)

Salivary gland, submaxillary

    Loss of tubuloalveolar (serous) cell nuclei (2 h)

    Tubuloalveolar (serous) cell dispersion that resembles very acute necrosis (2 h)

    Disintegration and disruption of interlobular duct epithelium which resembles very acute necrosis (4 h)

    Mucus-producing acini were unremarkable at 16 h

Seminal vesicles

    Pyknosis of epithelium (1 h)

    Detachment and change to cuboidal appearance of epithelial cells with disruption of epithelial surface (2 h)

    Appearance of fractures and lucent or paler areas in lumen contents (8 h)

Skeletal muscle

    Fiber disorganization and "fracturing" into small haphazard cleavage spaces (20 min)

    Formation of interfiber clear spaces (1 h)

    Condensed and hyperchromatic endomysial nuclei (1 h)

Skin

    Chromatin clumping and karyorrhexis of sebaceous cells (40 min)

    Pyknosis of dermal fibrocytes (2 h)

    Epidermis and dermis were unremarkable at 16 h

Spleen

    Pyknosis of megakaryocytes (< 20 min)

    Decreased density or rarefaction of lymphocytes in white pulp (40 min)

    Cleavage lines resembling "Dull-knife distortion" (40 min)

    Pyknosis of most white pulp lymphocytes (8 h)

    Generalized pyknosis of red pulp (12 h)

Stomach, forestomach

    Pyknosis of basal epithelial cells (4 h)

    Pyknosis of fibrocytes in superficial lamina propria (4 h)

    Formation of clear spaces around fibrocytes in superficial lamina propria (4 h)

    Formation of interfiber clear spaces and pyknosis of myofiber nuclei (8 h)

Stomach, glandular

    Loss of superficial epithelium from mucosal ridges (< 20 min)

    Separation of glandular epithelium from basement membrane (40 min)

    Formation of interfiber clear spaces and pyknosis of myofiber nuclei (1 h)

    Separation of crypt epithelium from basement membrane (2 h)

    Lateral separations in glandular epithelium (4 h)

    Pyknosis of crypt epithelium (4 h)

Testes
    Individualization of interstitial cells (1 h)
    Pyknosis of interstitial cells (2 h)
    Formation of clear spaces around seminiferous tubules (8 h)
Thymus
    Large medullary extravasations of erythrocytes, which resemble antemortem thymic
        hemorrhages and apparently result from the loss of blood from leaky thymic vessels (<
        20 min)
    Cleavage lines resembling "dull-knife distortion" (4 h)
    Nuclear contraction of cortical lymphocytes (4 h)
    Decreased density or rarefaction in cortical lymphocytes (16 h)
Thyroid gland
    Pale, foamy and/or bubbly colloid (< 20 min)
    Pyknosis of parafollicular "C" cells (40 min)
    Epithelial cells free in colloid (1 h)
    Pyknosis of follicular epithelium (2 h)
    Disruption of follicular epithelium (4 h)
    Pyknosis of epithelium in largest follicles occurred later than in small- to medium-sized
        follicles (8 h)
Tongue
    Formation of interfiber clear spaces in skeletal muscle (40 min)
    Perinuclear clear spaces (halo) in polyhedral cell layer of the mucosa (4 h)
    Contraction and darkening of muscle cell nuclei (4 h)
    Absence of mitotic figures in basal epithelial cell layer (12 h)
Trachea
    Disruption or sloughing of epithelium into glandular lumen (4 h)
    Pyknosis of superficial epithelium (8 h)
    Loss or sloughing of superficial epithelium (8 h)
    Loss of cilia (12 h)
    Pyknosis of glandular epithelium (12 h)
    Formation of intracellular soap, basophilic deposits in fat cells, deep in the mucosa (16 h)
Urinary bladder
    Formation of vacuoles in transitional epithelium (< 20 min)
    Formation of interfiber clear spaces and pyknosis of myofiber nuclei (1 h)
    Disruption and sloughing of the surface transitional epithelium (4 h)
Uterus
    Separation of glandular epithelium from basement membrane (20 min)
    Formation of interfiber clear spaces and pyknosis of myofiber nuclei (4 h)
    Sloughing of superficial endometrial epithelium (8 h)
    Cervix had no remarkable postmortem changes at 16 h
Vagina
    No remarkable postmortem changes at 16 h

SECTION 3. HISTOPATHOLOGIC FINDINGS IN CONTROL
LABORATORY MICE[10–31,80]

Adrenal gland, cortex
    Amyloidosis (amyloid deposition) — associated with systemic amyloidosis (see Kidney)
    Atrophy, diffuse — low incidence (CD-1: males 5%, females < 1%)

Accessory cortical nodules — common in adrenal capsule or adjacent connective tissues (CD-1 mice: 2–5%)

Extramedullary hematopoiesis — usually occurs in association with leukemoid reactions and myeloid hyperplasia (*see* Bone marrow)

Pigmentation, ceroid (lipofuscin) — accumulates in residual X-zone cells

Hyperplasia, eosinophilic cell, focal (CD-1: 2000 males 10.8%, 2000 females 8.8%)

Hyperplasia, subcapsular (Type A) spindle cells: common in mice of all ages; incidence up to 80% in aged CD-1 females (CD-1: 2000 males 16.6%, 2000 females 33.6%)

Hyperplasia, subcapsular vacuolated (Type B) cells: proliferation of large polyhedral vacuolated cells; usually associated with spindle cell hyperplasia

X-zone (inner cortex) — normal basophilic cells in young mice of both sexes; involution complete by about 10 days of age in males, may be seen up to 30 weeks of age in females; characterized in females by marked vacuolation, especially in nonbred females

Tumors

    Cortical adenoma, all types — low incidence

        (CD-1; 891 males 0.9%, 890 females 0.5%)

        (CD-1; 2000 males 1.3 %, 2000 females < 1%)

        (B6C3F$_1$; 2240 males 2.4%, 2306 females 0.3%)

    Type A cell adenoma

    Type B cell adenoma

    Cortical carcinoma (adenocarcinoma), all types: very low incidence

        (B6C3F$_1$; three reported in 2240 males 0.1%; and one reported in 2306 females < 0.1%,)

        (CD-1; none, 891 males; three in 890 females 0.3%)

        (CD-1 mice, 2000 males none, 2000 females < 1%)

Adrenal gland, medulla

    Hyperplasia — low incidence (CD-1 mice, 1–8%; males > females)

    Hypertrophy

    Tumors

        Ganglioneuroma — very rare; none reported in more than 10,000 CD-1 and B63F$_1$ mice

        Pheochromocytoma (benign) — low incidence

            (CD-1; five in 891 males 0.6%, and three in 890 females 0.3%)

            (CD-1 mice, 2000 males < 1%, 2000 females < 1%)

            (B6C3F$_1$; 2240 males 1.2%, 2306 females 0.7%)

        Pheochromocytoma, malignant — very low incidence

            (CD-1 none in 891 males, one in 890 females 0.1%)

            (B6C3F$_1$; two reported in 2240 males 0.1%; and none reported in 2306 females 0.0%)

Blood vessels

    Amyloidosis — frequent vascular finding especially in lungs and liver (*see* Kidney)

    Angiectasis — common finding especially in uterus, ovary, liver, spleen, and lymph nodes.

    Arteritis (polyarteritis nodosa, periarteritis, perivasculitis) — frequent finding, most often in kidney, heart, mesentery, uterus, testis, and urinary bladder (RF; 311 females 18.0%)

    Hyalinization, arterial — amyloid-negative eosinophilic deposits within the media of arterial walls (RF; 311 females 14.1%)

    Mineralization — foci of calcification in the wall of the aorta are common in some strains such as DBA (*see* Heart)

    Tumors

        Hemangioma and hemangiosarcoma — common especially in subcutaneous tissue, liver, spleen, and uterus

Hemangioma (angioma, hemangioendothelioma), all sites (B6C3F$_1$; 2343 males 1.5%, 2486 females 1.6%)

Hemangiosarcoma (angiosarcoma, hemangioendotheliosarcoma) all sites (B6C3F$_1$; 2343 males 2.7%, 2486 females 1.9%)

Bone

Exostosis (hyperostosis) (*see* Hyperplasia)

Fracture callus — common in ribs and extremities, especially feet and tail from restraining or fighting

Hyperplasia (exostosis, hyperostosis) — sporadically associated with chronic infections; observed also as a focal thickening of ventral thoracic vertebrae from gavage

Inflammation (osteomyelitis) — common in bones of feet and tail associated with wounds from fighting

Necrosis, sternal — reported in sternebrae of nearly all of 427 female RF mice older than 15 months of age

Osteodystrophy (fibro-osseous lesions) common in B6C3F$_1$ female mice; incidence up to 40% in females and < 1% in males (B6C3F$_1$; 2543 males none, 2522 females 1.0%)

Osteitis fibrosis — uncommon, associated with hyperparathyroidism and severe renal disease

Tumors

Ossifying fibroma — occasional, reported in jaw of CD-1 mice

Osteoma, all sites — uncommon in CD-1 mice (CD-1; one in 891 males 0.2%, and two in 890 females 0.2%)

Osteosarcoma, all sites (CD-1; two in 891 males 0.2%, and two in 890 females 0.2%) (B6C3F$_1$; 2343 males 0.1%, 2486 females 0.6%)

Bone marrow

Atrophy (hypoplasia, aplasia) — unusual finding

Fibrosis — occasional small foci in the marrow space

Hyperplasia, erythroid — associated with anemia

Hyperplasia, megakaryocytic — usually accompanies myeloid hyperplasia

Hyperplasia, myeloid (leukemoid reaction) — associated with neutrophilia, abscesses, acute pyelonephritis, pneumonia, extensive necrosis, neoplasms, anemia, and systemic infections; accompanied by extramedullary hematopoiesis

Tumors

Leukemia, myelogenous (myeloid, granulocytic)

(CD-1; 891 males 1.8%, 890 females 1.9%)

(B6C3F$_1$; 2343 males 0.7%, 2486 females 2.1%)

Brain and meninges (central nervous system)

Cyst, epithelial — squamous cell cysts are uncommon; most often observed in the spinal cord

Chromatolysis — occasional finding characterized by dispersion and dissolution of Nissl substance.

Dark cells — common finding; foci of neurons which appear shrunken and basophilic without changes in the surrounding parenchyma or glial cells are regarded as artifacts

Gitter Cells — microglial macrophages usually associated with myelin breakdown

Infarction — uncommon focal finding as a result of vascular blockage, usually observed as a healing area of chronic inflammation

Inflammation — frequent finding as small foci of chronic inflammatory cells, lymphocytes, and plasma cells in the brain and meninges

Malacia — necrosis of neural tissues with loss of architecture, breakdown of myelin or neuropil, and accumulation of foamy macrophages (gitter cells)

Mineralization, cerebral — common small basophilic deposits; usually in thalamus; in up to 5% of CD-1 mice

Necrosis — ischemic neuronal injury, occasional finding of shrunken, hyaline, densely eosinophilic cell bodies and small, basophilic nuclei which results from a variety of causes including ischemia, anoxia, seizures, epilepsy, and some metabolic disturbances

Pigmentation, melanin (melanosis) — common in meninges of olfactory bulb and optic nerves of pigmented strains

Vacuolation — vacuoles are a frequent finding associated with a variety of causes including artifacts, intramyelinic edema, spongy degeneration, spongiform encephalopathies, uremia, retrovirus (Murine Leukemia Virus) infection and probably ageing

Tumors

Central nervous system tumors are rare in most mice; usual incidence 0.05–0.1% (B6C3F$_1$; 2303 males none, 2378 females none)

Astrocytoma — rare but most reported in VM and BRVR strains, up to 1.5% (B6C3F$_1$; 2849 males none, 2826 females none)

Lipoma — uncommon lesion consisting of lipocyte foci in the choroid plexus reported in BALB/c and other strains may be a hamartoma (malformation) not neoplastic (B6C3F$_1$; one in 2849 males 0.04%, 2826 females none)

Meningioma — uncommon but reported in CD-1, in B6C3F$_1$, and most often in C3H strains

(CD-1; one in 891 males 0.1%, none in 890 females)

(B6C3F$_1$; 2849 males none, one in 2826 females 0.04%)

Oligodendroglia — rare finding, most reported in BALB/c (B6C3F$_1$; one, malignant, in 2849 males 0.04%, and one, benign in 2826 females 0.04%)

Clitoral gland

Small in mice; often examined only if grossly abnormal

Atrophy — minor degrees are common in aged mice

Cysts — minor degrees are common in aged mice

Dilatation — commonly cysts accompany atrophy

Enlargement — commonly result of cysts or inflammation

Inflammation, suppurative (abscess) — common finding

Tumors — none reported (B6C3F$_1$; 2486 females none)

Coagulating gland

Inflammation, suppurative — usually associated with prostatic, urinary bladder, or kidney inflammation

Tumors

Adenoma — uncommon finding

(CD-1; three in 891 males 0.3%)

(B6C3F$_1$; none in 2343 males)

Adenocarcinoma — rare, none in CD-1 mice (B6C3F$_1$; none in 2343 males)

Ductus (vas) deferens (*see* Epididymis)

Ear

External ear (pinna or auricle and auditory canal)

Inflammation, auricular cartilage (proliferative chondritis)

Inflammation, chronic — frequent finding as a result of wounds and fighting; *see* skin for additional lesions

Tumors — same as Skin

Middle ear

Inflammation (otitis media) occasional finding, often associated with sinusitis and upper respiratory infections; tympanic cavity usually contains purulent exudate

Inner ear

    Inflammation (otitis interna) often extending from middle ear; can result in encephalitis and lost of balance or circling behavior; may be associated with active necrotizing arteritis in adjacent tissues

    Zymbal's gland (auditory sebaceous glands)

        Tumors — none reported in CD-1 mice (B6C3F$_1$; one, adenoma, in 2855 males 0.04%, and one, carcinoma, in 2838 females 0.04%)

Epididymis

    Changes commonly observed are secondary to testicular atrophy and include: lack or diminished spermatozoal contents, intraepithelial cysts formation, tubular debris

    Inflammation, granulomatous (spermatic granuloma) — common

    Tumors — very rare

        Hemangioma (angioma, hemangioendothelioma) — (CD-1; one in 891 males 0.1%)

        Leiomyoma — one has been reported in a B6C3F$_1$ mouse

        Sarcoma — three (0.1%) reported in 2823 B6C3F$_1$ mice

Esophagus

    Inflammation — common in association with gavage injuries during dosing; severity and frequency range from small foci of macrophages to large areas of necrosis and abscess-formation; perforations can lead to extensive inflammation of subcutis or pleura.

    Tumors — unusual; squamous cell tumors have been reported in some strains (B6C3F$_1$; one papilloma, in 3789 females 0.03%; one carcinoma in 2855 males 0.04%; and one carcinoma in 2838 females 0.04%)

Eye

    Atrophy, retina — frequent finding from a variety of causes including genetics, light exposure and retroorbital blood sampling; low incidence: CD-1; high incidence: C3H (up to 100%), CBA, Swiss

    Cataract, lens — very common finding (over 25%) in CD-1 mice based on ophthalmologic examinations

    Degeneration, retina — associated with atrophy

    Dystrophy, corneal (*see* Mineralization)

    Inflammation, globe (panophthalmitis) — occasional finding; usual intraocular findings consist of small lymphocyte and plasma cell infiltrates in ciliary body and sclera; more severe after retroorbital blood sampling; most severe after fight wounds; may result in phthisis bulbi (severe atrophy)

    Inflammation, conjunctiva (conjunctivitis) — suppurative inflammation occurs sporadically, especially abscesses of the meibomian glands

    Inflammation, cornea (keratitis) — sporadic occurrence of acute or chronic inflammation results in opacities

    Opacity, cornea (*see* Inflammation and Mineralization)

    Mineralization, cornea (corneal dystrophy) — subepithelial mineralization of the cornea is a common finding in CD-1 mice with an incidence up to 10%; also, increased in some strains such as DBA, BALB/c, and C3H (*see* Heart)

    Iris, mineralization — sporadic finding in CD-1 mice

    Phthisis bulbi — shrinkage or severe atrophy of the globe; usually the result of chronic inflammation or trauma

    Tumors — intraocular tumors are very rare in mice

Forestomach

    Erosion (*see* Ulcer)

    Diverticulum — rare finding

    Ulcer — erosions and ulcers (focal necrosis) with accompanying inflammation of the squamous mucosa are very common lesions; vary in severity; severe ulceration is accompanied by acute and chronic inflammation, penetration of the inflammatory changes into the stomach wall, and in some animals, peritonitis.

Hyperkeratosis — associated with hyperplasia; occurs as a diffuse change in anorectic mice

Hyperplasia, squamous (acanthosis, hyperkeratosis, parakeratosis) — most proliferative or hyperplastic changes of the squamous mucosa are reactive, focal, and associated with gastric inflammation; occasionally the entire forestomach is affected; focal hyperplasia commonly involves the junction with the glandular stomach

Inflammation (gastritis) — common finding often associated with erosion or ulceration; vary from focal acute or chronic inflammation to perforation of the stomach wall; foci of lymphocytes and plasma cells in the submucosa are common

Necrosis — superficial necrosis (erosion) and deep necrosis (ulceration) are common findings (*see* Ulcer)

Tumors — squamous cell tumors are common

    Squamous papillomas — low incidence; up to 1% in CD-1 mice
        (B6C3F$_1$; 2252 males 0.3%, 2486 females 0.5%)
        (B6C3F$_1$; 3807 males 1.6%, 3789 females 3.6%)

    Squamous carcinomas — very low incidence
        (CD-1; three in 891 males 0.3%, and one in 890 females 0.1%)
        (B6C3F$_1$; none, 2252 males, two in 2486 females 0.1%)
        (B6C3F$_1$; 3807 males 0.2%, 3789 females 0.2%)

    Leiomyoma — very low incidence (B6C3F$_1$; none, 3807 males, two in 3789 females < 0.1%)

    Mast cell tumor (B6C3F$_1$; two, benign, < 0.1% and one, malignant, < 0.1% in 3807 males, and one, benign, in 3789 females < 0.1%)

Gallbladder

Degeneration, hyaline — eosinophilic droplets are commonly present in epithelial cells of aged B6C3F$_1$ mice

Inflammation (cholecystitis) — foci of inflammatory cells occasionally occur within the walls of bile ducts and the gallbladder

Tumors — unusual
    (B6C3F$_1$; two adenomas 0.08% and one sarcoma 0.04% in 2484 males; one papilloma in 2590 females, 0.04%); (CD-1; papillomas, one in 891 males 0.1%, one in 890 females 0.1%)

Harderian gland

Atrophy — common focal or diffuse finding associated with cystic dilatation of glandular lumens

Cysts — occasional finding

Ectasia, glandular (cystic dilatation) — focal or diffuse dilatation of glandular lumens with epithelial atrophy

Hyperplasia, focal — occasional finding of small, noncompressive lesions with both cellular hyperplasia and hypertrophy

Inflammation (adenitis) — focal inflammatory cells, especially small aggregates of lymphoid cells are common, 20% incidence was observed in 274 C57BL/6 female mice; incidence increases with age

Tumors

    Adenoma — low incidence
        (< 2% of CD-1 mice; up to 8% of B6C3F$_1$; < 3% of C3H)
        (CD-1; 891 males 10.2%, 890 females 6.95%)
        (B6C3F$_1$; 2343 males 2.1%, 2486 females 1.3%)

Adenocarcinoma — very low incidence (< 1% of CD-1 mice)
  (CD-1; 891 males 0.5%, 890 females 0.2%)
  (B6C3F$_1$; two reported in 2343 males 0.1%, and one reported in 2486 females < 0.1%)
Myoepithelioma — infrequent in most strains, but more common in BALB mice, especially females

Heart

Amyloidosis — common finding in CD-1 mice; often associated with cardiac atrial thrombosis (*see* Kidney)
Atrial thrombosis — common finding associated with pulmonary chronic venous congestion
  (RF; 427 females 6.8%)
  (CD-1; 2000 males 4.5%, 2000 females 1%)
Fibrosis — usually associated with necrosis (CD-1; 2000 males < 1%, 2000 females < 1%)
Inflammation (myocarditis) — minor aggregates of inflammatory cells and fibrosis are common; more severe changes are usually associated with necrosis and infectious diseases (CD-1; 2000 males 3.4%, 2000 females 2.5%)
Mineralization (dystrophic cardiac or myocardial calcification, cardiac calcinosis) — the heart as well as the tongue, cornea, and aorta are frequent sites of soft-tissue calcification in some strains: DBA, C3H, BALB/c, CBA, and C3N with incidence of 100% in DBA/2; uncommon in CD-1 and B6C3F$_1$ mice; incidence and severity is modified by age, sex, parity, and diet
Myocardial degeneration — occasional finding occurring as vacuolation of myocytes
Myocardial necrosis (focal necrosis; acute, necrotizing inflammation; acute focal inflammation; focal subacute or chronic inflammation; focal fibrosis) — a frequent localized lesion accompanied by inflammatory cells and fibrosis; incidence at 18 months of age, 30–40% in CD-1
Pigmentation, melanin (melanosis) — common in heart valves of pigmented strains, such as C57BL
Valvular inflammation — uncommon
Tumors
  Hemangioma (angioma, hemangioendothelioma) — very rare (B6C3F$_1$; none in 3807 males, none in 3789 females)
  Hemangiosarcoma, (angiosarcoma, hemangioendotheliosarcoma) — very rare (B6C3F$_1$; 3798 males < 0.1%, 3779 females < 0.1%)
  Mesothelioma (CD-1; one in 891 males 0.1%, none in 890 females)
  Rhabdomyosarcoma — very rare
  Secondary metastatic or multiple systemic tumors are common

Intestines (unspecified, NOS)

Amyloidosis — frequent finding in CD-1 mice, especially in jejunum (*see* Kidney)
Arteritis — occasional finding in mesenteric blood vessels of CD-1 mice; fibrinoid necrosis usually present
Ectopic pancreatic tissue — sporadic finding in duodenum
Dilatation — frequent finding in animals found dead, probably from bacterial gas production; dilatation of the colon, occasional finding of unknown cause
Hyperplasia, lymphoid — occasional finding from immunological stimulation such as systemic illness (CD-1; 2000 males 1%, 2000 females 1%)
Hyperplasia, mucosal — normal physiological thickening of the intestines occurs in pregnant and lactating mice

Metazoan parasites

Nematodiasis — pin worms are common findings in the colon and occasionally in the ileum with no inflammation

Tumors

Adenoma — very low incidence, < 0.3% in CD-1 mice; most often in duodenum

Adenoma, small intestine

(CD-1; two in 891 males 0.2%, one in 890 females 0.1%)

(B6C3F$_1$; 3807 males 0.8%, 3789 females 0.4%)

Adenomatous polyp, small intestine (B6C3F$_1$; 3807 males 0.2%, 3789 females 0.1%)

Adenoma, anus (CD-1; one in 891 males 0.1%, none in 890 females)

Adenocarcinoma — very low incidence < 0.1% in CD-1 mice

Adenocarcinoma, small intestine (CD-1; none in 891 males, two in 890 females 0.2%)

(B6C3F$_1$; 2148 males 0.7%, two in 2234 females 0.1%)

(B6C3F$_1$; 3807 males 1.0%, 3789 females 0.3%)

Adenocarcinoma, large intestine (B6C3F$_1$; one in 3807 males < 0.1%, none in 3789 females)

Leiomyoma — occasional finding

Leiomyoma, large intestine (B6C3F$_1$; none in 3807 males, two in 3789 females < 0.1%)

Leiomyosarcoma — occasional finding

Leiomyosarcoma, large intestine (B6C3F$_1$; none in 3807 males, two in 3789 females < 0.1%)

Sarcoma, unspecified — occasional finding

Sarcoma, large intestine (CD-1; one in 891 males 0.1%, none in 890 females)

Squamous cell carcinoma — occasional finding

Squamous cell carcinoma, large intestine (CD-1; none in 891 males, one in 890 females 0.1%)

Squamous cell carcinoma, anus (CD-1; one in 891 males 0.1%, none in 890 females)

Squamous cell carcinoma, rectum (B6C3F$_1$; one in 3807 males < 0.1%, none in 3789 females)

Islets, pancreatic

Atrophy, beta cell — diabetes mellitus is rare in CD-1 mice; genetically determined occurrence in some strains, for example db/db

Hyperplasia-uncommon in CD-1 mice, common in C3H; large islets are common in aged B6C3F$_1$ mice

Tumors

Islet cell adenoma — low incidence, 0.5% in CD-1 (CD-1; 891 males 0.3%, 890 females 0.6%) (B6C3F$_1$; 2237 males 0.4%, 2200 females 0.4%)

Islet cell carcinoma — uncommon in CD-1 mice (B6C3F$_1$; none, 2237 males, two in 2200 females 0.1%)

Joints

Arthrosis — common in CD-1 mice

Inflammation (arthritis) — occasional lesions, usually adjacent to wounds or septic foci

Osteoarthritis — degenerative lesions with inflammation; low incidence (0–5%, CD-1 mice)

Subluxation — occasional lesion of intervertebral joints resulting in distortion of the tail

Prolapsed intervertebral disc — rare, reported in CD-1 mice

Kidney

Amyloidosis — common site, usually associated with systemic amyloidosis; additional sites include intestines, myocardium, nasal submucosa, parotid salivary gland, thyroid gland, adrenal cortex, spleen, lungs, liver, tongue, testes, ovary, uterus, aorta, skin, pancreas, and lymph node (primarily mesenteric); considered cause of illness or death in 6.5% of 766 male and 8.1% of 766 female CD-1 mice over 12 months of age; various incidences: (CD-1 mice, 10–40%) (B6C3F$_1$; 2543 males 1.9%, 2522 females 0.2%)

Cysts (polycystic disease) — common finding associated with dilatation of tubules; cortical cysts are common in CD-1; congenital cysts of varying size have high frequencies in several strains such as BALB

Endstage — marked or severe glomerular, tubular, and interstitial changes with inflammation

Extramedullary hematopoiesis — usually occurs in the perirenal fat associated with leukemoid reactions and myeloid hyperplasia (*see* Bone marrow)

Glomerulonephritis (glomerulonephropathy, glomerulosclerosis) — common finding in certain strains of older mice such as AKR, BALB/c, and CBA; low incidence as significant lesion in most strains

(RF; 427 females 84%; 311 females 95.1%)

(CD-1; males 4%, females 12%)

(CD-1; 2000 males 24.9%, 2000 females 24.9%)

(B6C3F$_1$; 2543 males 1.2%, 2522 females 2.4%)

Hydronephrosis — common finding; can occur in high prevalence among certain strains or be secondary to urinary obstruction or pyelonephritis; various incidences: (CD-1 mice, up to 10%) (B6C3F$_1$; 2543 males 0.6%, 2522 females 0.2%)

Hyperplasia, tubular epithelium, focal — occasional finding

Infarction — common finding; low incidence (CD-1 mice, 2–4%)

Inflammation, nonsuppurative — common finding of lymphocyte aggregates which tend to accumulate around renal interlobular arteries, 3% incidence was observed in 274 C57BL/6 female mice

Interstitial (tubulointerstitial) nephritis — tubular degeneration and interstitial fibrosis with lymphocytic infiltrates and sometimes mineral deposits (CD-1; males 5.5%, females 3.8%)

Mineralization (nephrocalcinosis, calcification) — small foci of mineral deposits are common (CD-1; males 5.0%, females 2.4%)

Necrosis, tubular — kidneys of mature male mice of certain genotypes such as DBA and C3H are exquisitely sensitive to chloroform fumes which result in tubular necrosis and mineralization

Obstructive uropathy (urologic syndrome, obstructive genitourinary disease) (*see* Urethra)

Papillary necrosis — usually occurs in kidneys with severe damage associated with amyloidosis

Pyelonephritis — occasional finding in CD-1 mice, usually associated with inflammation of the lower urinary tract, including pyelonephritis in males which accompanies inflammation of the prostate, seminal vesicles, coagulation gland, and urinary bladder; also, occurs in some animals with urethral mucous plugs; embolic suppurative nephritis is infrequent (B6C3F$_1$; 2543 males 1.6%, 2522 females 1.5%)

Tumors

Adenoma — very low incidence (< 1%; CD-1 mice)

(CD-1; three in 891 males 0.3%, and one in 890 females 0.1%)

(B6C3F$_1$; 3791 males 0.3%, 3767 females 0.1%)

Adenocarcinoma — very low incidence (< 0.1%; CD-1 mice)
(CD-1; one in 891 males 0.1%, one in 890 females 0.1%)

Carcinoma — very rare
(CD-1; two in 891 males 0.2%, none in 890 females)
(B6C3F₁; one in 3791 males < 0.1%, and one in 3767 females < 0.1%)

Lipoma — very rare (CD-1; one in 891 males 0.1%, none in 890 females)

Nephroblastoma — very rare; none reported in CD-1 mice

Transitional cell carcinoma — very rare in mice
(CD-1; none in 891 males, none in 890 females)
(B6C3F₁; one in 244 males 0.4%, none in 246 females)

Lacrimal gland — ectopic Harderian gland tissue, occasional finding *(see* Harderian gland)

Larynx *(see* Trachea)

Liver

Amyloidosis — common site in systemic amyloidosis; occurs in 10–20% of CD-1 mice in blood vessels and along sinusoids *(see* Kidney)

Angiectasis (telangiectasis) — common finding, especially in females, up to 10% of CD-1 mice; widely dilated vascular spaces lined by normal-appearing endothelium which results in blood filled cystic spaces and distortion of the sinusoids (also *see* Sinusoidal dilatation); incidence reported as telangiectasis (CD-1; 2000 males < 1%, 2000 females < 1%)

Congestion — common-finding dependent on the mode of death and length of time before tissue fixation; frequently centrilobular and more pronounced after cardiac failure

Cytomegaly — common finding in hepatocytes of aged mice

Dilatation, sinusoidal, focal — common in aged mice; consists of widely dilated sinusoids, sometimes cystic, which retains the shape and position of the sinusoids

Enlargement (hepatocytic hypertrophy)

Extramedullary hematopoiesis — frequent finding as foci along sinusoids or around central veins and portal vessels; usually associated with leukemoid reactions and myeloid-hyperplasia *(see* Bone marrow)

Fatty change (fatty metamorphosis, lipidosis) — fat vacuoles in hepatocytes occur in 5% of CD-1 mice; usually midzonal in untreated mice, increases with age and obesity; may accompany hepatocytic cellular alteration; focal cytoplasmic vacuolative changes of hepatocytes adjacent to the cleft of the median lobe has been termed tension lipidosis; microvesicular fatty change has been associated with Reye's-like syndrome in BALB/c ByJ mice

Hepatocytic cellular alteration, focal — occasional finding of foci from one to several lobules in diameter consisting of hepatocytes; identified as clear cell, eosinophilic, basophilic, and mixed cell foci (CD-1; 2000 males < 1%, 2000 females < 1%)

Hepatocytic, degeneration, vacuolation (may be included in some reports as fatty change; See fatty change) (CD-1; 2000 males 2.5%, 2000 females 2%)

Hyperplasia, hepatocellular (nodular) — occasional finding of diffuse or focal areas larger than a lobule consisting of normal or hypertrophic hepatocytes (CD-1; 2000 males 1.3%, 2000 females < 1%)

Hypertrophy, hepatocytic — common finding in aged mice associated with cytomegaly, karyomegaly, and intranuclear inclusions

Inclusion bodies, intranuclear — common finding of eosinophilic inclusions in the nuclei of hepatocytes resulting from invaginations of the cytoplasm; increased with age

Inclusion bodies, cytoplasmic — common finding of eosinophilic inclusions in the cytoplasm of hepatocytes; increased with age

Inflammation (hepatitis) — very common finding (CD-1; 2000 males 19.3%, 2000 females 9.3%); up to 50% of CD-1 mice have small foci of both acute and chronic inflammatory cells scattered in the liver; small aggregates of lymphoid cells are common, 20% incidence was observed in 274 C57BL/6 female mice; larger foci are associated with coagulative necrosis which may be related to *Bacillus piliformis* (Tyzzer's disease) or mouse hepatitis virus occur in up to 5% of CD-1 mice of some laboratories; acute, chronic, and necrotic hepatitis can result from *Helicobacter hepaticus* infections

Karyomegaly — common finding in hepatocytes of aged mice; usually associated with anisokaryosis, polykarya, and cytoplasmic invagination into the nucleus (inclusions)

Necrosis — in addition to the necrosis associated with inflammation, necrotic lesions characterized by fibrous repair, round cell infiltration, oval cell proliferation, and usually hemosiderin deposition occur occasionally in untreated mice; individual cell necrosis of single or small aggregates of hepatocytes is a sporadic finding

Necrosis, hepatocellular (hepatocytic) — focal necrosis of unknown cause occasionally occurs in weanling mice; incidence < 2% reported in 445 B6C3F$_1$ males and females (CD-1; 2000 males 3.5%, 2000 females 9.7%)

Pigmentation — lipofuscin (ceroid) and hemosiderin are occasionally present in Kupffer cells

Telangiectasis (*see* Angiectasis)

Tumors — frequency varies greatly within strains and between strains; hepatocellular tumors can increase after infection by *Helicobacter hepaticus*

Hemangioma (angioma, hemangioendothelioma) — low incidence, 2–4% of CD-1 mice (CD-1; 891 males 1.5%, and 890 females 0.5%)

Hemangiosarcoma (angiosarcoma, hemangioendotheliosarcoma) — low incidence, < 0.4% in CD-1 mice (CD-1; four in 891 males 0.5%, and one in 890 females 0.1%)

Hepatoblastoma — rare finding; often associated with hepatocellular carcinomas; may be undifferentiated variant of hepatocellular carcinoma

Hepatocellular adenoma — very common
(CD-1; males 31%, females 3.5%)
(CD-1 2000 males 5.2%, 2000 females 1.7%)
(B6C3F$_1$; males 10%, females 4%)
(B6C3F$_1$; 2334 males 10.3%, 2469 females 4%)

Hepatocellular carcinoma (adenocarcinoma)
(CD-1; males 13%; females 0.5%)
(CD-1; 2000 males 4.4%, 2000 females < 1%)
(B6C3F$_1$; males 21%, females 5%)
(B6C3F$_1$; 2334 males 21.3%, 2469 females 4.1%)

Leukemia, myelogenous (myeloid, granulocytic) — often involve mainly liver and spleen in RF strain

Malignant lymphoma — lymphomas are commonly perivascular, either around portal triads or central veins

Metastatic tumors — common site for secondary and metastatic malignant tumors, especially lymphoreticular neoplasms

Bile ducts

Cholangiofibrosis (adenofibrosis) — uncommon finding; characterized by excessive proliferation of fibrous tissue and bile ducts

Inflammation (cholangitis) — occasional finding of acute inflammatory cells increases with age; frequently accompany bile duct hyperplasia and peritubular fibrosis

Hyperplasia — common in old mice accompanied by peritubular fibrosis and inflammatory cells

Tumors — very rare in mice

Cholangioma — one reported in CD-1 mice

Cholangiosarcoma — one reported in CD-1 mice

Lung

Abscess — occasional finding, usually in aged animals; result from local or systemic infections

Bronchiectasis — dilatation of bronchi or bronchioles usually results from infections with chronic inflammation; may be accompanied by squamous metaplasia

Bronchopneumonia — occasional finding in old mice; frequent in younger animals on gavage experiments (RF; 427 females 9.4%)

Congestion — frequent finding associated with agonal changes related to the mode of death; marked in animals found dead; accompanied by edema in cardiac failure

Chronic venous congestion — occasional finding associated with thrombosis of the left atrium; accompanied by alveolar septa thickening and fibrosis (fibrosing alveolitis or interstitial pneumonia)

Crystal pneumonitis — sporadic focal accumulations of eosinophilic crystals in terminal airways and alveolar sacs in some strains, especially C57BL

Degeneration, hyaline — eosinophilic droplets are commonly present in bronchiolar epithelial cells of aged $B6C3F_1$ mice

Edema — sporadic accompanying cardiac failure

Fibrosis — occasionally found as focal lesions in association with chronic inflammation; diffuse segmental fibrosis (fibrosing alveolitis) secondary to chronic venous congestion

Hemorrhage — frequent finding associated with agonal changes related to the mode of death or method of sacrifice

Hyperplasia, alveolar epithelium, focal (adenomatous hyperplasia, pulmonary adenomatosis, alveolar cell hyperplasia, epithelialization) — frequent finding, usually multicentric, increases with increased age

Hyperplasia, alveolar macrophage (foam cells, histiocytosis, lipidosis) — occasional finding of collections of foamy alveolar macrophages in older mice which may be associated with chronic or granulomatous inflammation and cholesterol clefts

Hyperplasia, goblet cell — hypersecretion by mucous cells of the bronchial epithelium associated with chronic inflammation

Hyperplasia, lymphoid — accumulations of lymphoid cells are often located in the visceral pleura within septal clefts; increased lymphoid cells are common in association with inflammation and respiratory infections

Inflammation, acute and chronic (alveolitis, bronchitis, bronchopneumonia, pneumonia) — very common to have small foci of inflammatory cells, predominantly lymphocytes in occasional alveoli or around bronchioles and small vessels; especially common in females

(C57BL/6; 274 females 51%)

(C3H; 298 males 4%)

Inflammation, granulomatous (granuloma) — occasional finding resulting from infections, inhaled foreign bodies, and aggregates of alveolar (foamy) macrophages with cholesterol deposits

Metaplasia, squamous cell — common in bronchi in association with chronic inflammation

Tumors

Alveolar/bronchiolar adenoma and carcinoma — very common with more in males than females; at 18–24 months, 25–30% in CD-1 males

Alveolar/bronchiolar adenoma
(CD-1; 891 males 15%, 890 females 14%)
(B6C3F$_1$; 2328 males 12.1%, 2388 females 5.5%)
Alveolar/bronchiolar carcinoma
(CD-1; 891 males 19%, 890 females 12.1%)
(B6C3F$_1$; 2328 males 5.1%, 2388 females 2%)
Squamous cell carcinoma — very rare
Hemangiosarcoma (hemangioendothelioma) — very rare
Malignant lymphoma — commonly involves lung around the bronchi, bronchioles, and blood vessels
Metastatic tumors — common site for metastatic malignant tumors especially liver, up to 5% of hepatocellular carcinomas, and mammary gland adenocarcinomas
Lymph node (unspecified, NOS): mandibular and mesenteric are most frequently examined
Amyloidosis — common especially in mesenteric lymph nodes (see Kidney) (CD-1; 2000 males 18.1%, 2000 females 18.1%)
Arteritis (CD-1; 2000 males 0.3%, 2000 females 0.3%)
Atrophy — common in aged mice
Congestion — common especially in mesenteric lymph nodes
Extramedullary hematopoiesis — usually occurs in association with leukemoid reactions and myeloid hyperplasia (see Bone Marrow); frequent in mice
Hemorrhage — frequent
Hyperplasia, lymphoid, (follicular hyperplasia) — common; usually associated with an active inflammatory lesion elsewhere in the body; nonneoplastic proliferation of lymphocytes accompanied by plasma cells and other inflammatory cell types (CD-1; 2000 males 15.3%, 2000 females 15.3%)
Hyperplasia, histiocytic — a form of lymphoid hyperplasia in which histiocytes are predominant cell type
Hyperplasia, plasma cell — common especially in mesenteric and cervical lymph nodes
Inflammation (lymphadenitis) (CD-1; 2000 males 1.2%, 2000 females 1.2%)
Lymphadenomegaly (mesenteric disease) — sporadic in aging mice of various strains, especially C3H; characterized by atrophy of lymphoid tissue and congestion of sinuses
Sinus histiocytosis — common finding in which the sinuses contain active histiocytes and numerous free macrophages
Tumors
Lymphoreticular neoplasms have a high spontaneous incidence in mice
Hemangiomas and hemangiosarcomas — low incidence (CD-1; 2000 males 0.7%, 2000 females 0.7%)
Hemangioma (angioma, hemangioendothelioma) — (B6C3F$_1$; two in 3807 males < 0.1%, and two in 3789 females < 0.1%)
Hemangiosarcoma (angiosarcoma, hemangioendotheliosarcoma) — (B6C3F$_1$; 3807 males 0.2%, one in 3789 females < 0.1%)
Histiocytic sarcoma (reticulum cell sarcoma, Type A) — rare before 12 months; common especially after 18 months of age; frequently the mesenteric lymph node appears to be site of origin; may occur early as single lesions in the mesenteric lymph node, other lymph nodes, Peyer's patches, liver, and spleen; thymus may be involved secondarily; frequently involve the uterus, vagina, and liver; and less often bone marrow, lungs, pancreas, dermis, mesentery, kidney, and epididymis
(RF; reticulum cell sarcoma, 427 females 56.2%)
(CD-1; 2000 males 2.5%, 2000 females 2.5%)

Leukemia, myelogenous (myeloid, granulocytic) — often secondarily involve lymph nodes

(RF; 427 females 0.9%)

(CD-1; 2000 males 3%, 2000 females 3%)

(B6C3F$_1$; 2343 males 0.7%, 2486 females 2.1%)

Leukemia, lymphatic (lymphocytic, lymphoblastic) — malignant lymphomas that have disseminated into the peripheral blood

Malignant lymphoma (lymphosarcoma) — lymphomas have been classified several ways, both on site of primary involvement or organ distribution and cell type; thymic lymphomas reportedly arise in the thymus of some strains of mice such as RF, then primarily involve the mediastinal organs, with subsequent spread to other organs, including the lungs, heart, liver, spleen, ovaries, uterus, and peripheral lymph nodes (also *see* Thymus) (RF; thymic lymphoma, 427 females 4.0%)

Nonthymic lymphoma (lymphosarcoma) reportedly arise as primary neoplasms in one or more lymph nodes, with spread to the spleen and liver; rare or little involvement of the thymus, lung, and heart; and occasional involvement of the ovary, uterus, kidney, and blood in some strains of mice such as RF (RF; nonthymic lymphoma, 427 females 7.0%)

Lymphoma, lymphocytic (small cell lymphoma): occur most commonly in spleen, lymph nodes, thymus, liver, pancreas, lungs, and bone marrow; if bone marrow involvement is extensive, becomes leukemic

Lymphoma, pleomorphic (follicular center cell lymphoma: reticulum cell sarcoma, type B) — rare before 12 months; frequent after 18 months in CD-1 mice; usually arise in Peyer's patches of small intestine, in mesenteric lymph nodes, or in the spleen; also involve other lymph nodes, liver, and bone marrow

Lymphoma, undifferentiated (lymphoblastic lymphoma, immunoblastic lymphoma, follicular center cell lymphoma; reticulum cell sarcoma, type B)

Lymphoma, mixed type

Malignant lymphoma (lymphosarcoma), all types

(CD-1; 2000 males 5.7%, 2000 females 5.7%)

(CD-1; 891 males 8.0%, 890 females 22.0%)

(B6C3F$_1$; 2343 males 12.0%, 2486 females 25.1%)

Mast cell tumor (mastocytoma) — rare; usually involve liver, spleen, kidneys, and bone marrow

(CD-1; two in 891 males 0.2%, none, 890 females)

Mast cell tumor, benign (B6C3F$_1$; none, 3766 males, one in 3751 females < 0.1%)

Mast cell tumor, malignant (B6C3F$_1$; one in 3766 males < 0.1%, none, 3751 females)

Plasma cell tumor (plasmacytoma, plasma cell lymphoma) — very low incidence in several strains; occur in lymph nodes, spleen, liver and bone marrow

Mammary gland

Cystic change (duct ectasia) — frequent finding often in the absence of hyperplasia in aged mice; incidence as high as 75% in CD-1 mice

Hyperplasia of duct epithelium and/or alveoli — common but less than duct ectasia in CD-1 mice

Inflammation (mastitis) — foci of inflammatory cells are an occasional finding. More severe inflammation including abscesses are usually associated with skin wounds or tumors.

Tumors

Incidence varies with strain; CD-1 strain has a low spontaneous incidence of mammary tumors, 5–7%.

Adenoma — rare in CD-1 and B6C3F$_1$ mice
(CD-1; one in 891 males 0.1%, 890 females 1.0%)
(B6C3F$_1$; none, 2343 males, 2486 females 0.3%)
(B6C3F$_1$; three in 2522 females 0.1%)

Adenoacanthoma — a malignant tumor consisting of both glandular and squamous cell differentiation; rare in CD-1 mice

Adenocarcinoma — low incidence
(CD-1; none, 891 males, 890 females 6.3%)
(B6C3F$_1$; none, 2343 males, 2486 females 1.6%)
(B6C3F$_1$; 2522 females 0.6%)

Fibroadenoma — rare; none in CD-1 mice (B6C3F$_1$; three in 2522 females 0.1%)

Myoepithelioma — infrequent in most strains, but more common in BALB mice, especially females
(B6C3F$_1$; one in 2522 females < 0.1%)

Mediastinum

Ectopic thyroid tissue

Mesentery

Ectopic pancreatic tissue

Fat necrosis — localized death of fat tissue which may be accompanied by encompassing fibrosis and mineralization

Inflammation (peritonitis) — small aggregates of lymphoid cells are common

Mouth (*see* Oral cavity)

Muscle (*see* Skeletal muscle)

Nose (nasal sinuses)

Degeneration, hyaline — eosinophilic droplets are commonly present in cells of the respiratory epithelium of some strains such as C57BL and B6C3F$_1$ mice

Inflammation (rhinitis, sinusitis) — acute and chronic inflammations are common and associated with respiratory tract infections and inhaled foreign materials

Hyperplasia, lymphoid — common finding in the nasolacrimal duct

Tumors — very rare; squamous cell carcinoma (CD-1; none, 891 males, one in 890 females 0.1%)

Oral cavity (gingiva, nasopharynx, oropharynx, palate, pharynx)

Inflammation — sporadic small focal aggregates of mononuclear inflammatory cells dispersed throughout the subepithelial tissues.

Tumors — rare; squamous cell papilloma (CD-1; one in 891 males 0.1%, none, 890 females)

Ovary

Angiectasis (angiectasia) — common in CD-1 mice

Amyloidosis — common, associated with systemic amyloidosis (*see* Kidney)

Atrophy — high incidence in aged mice

Cyst, all types — common in CD-1 mice
Dilatation of ovarian bursa — most frequent type
Hemorrhagic — occasional
Epidermoid — occasional

Extramedullary hematopoiesis — usually occurs in association with leukemoid reactions and myeloid hyperplasia (*see* Bone marrow); common in CD-1 mice

Interstitial cell hyperplasia — must be differentiated from relative increase associated with atrophy.

Pigmentation, ceroid (lipofuscin) — common in CD-1 mice

Tubular hyperplasia

Tumors

    Adenoma

    (CD-1; 10 in 890 females 1.1%)

    (B6C3F$_1$; 1 in 246 females 0.4%)

    Cystadenoma — low incidence

    (CD-1; 1000 females 2.5%)

    (B6C3F$_1$; 3 in 246 females 1.2%)

    Adenoma, tubular (B6C3F$_1$; 2167 females 0.9%)

    Adenocarcinoma, tubular (B6C3F$_1$; none in 2167 females)

    Papilloma (CD-1; 1 in 890 females 0.1%)

    Dysgerminoma — very rare, none CD-1 mice

    Granulosa cell tumors (included thecoma and luteoma)

    Low incidence (3.2% in CD-1 mice)

    (B6C3F$_1$; 2 in 2167 females 0.1%)

    Granulosa cell tumor

    (CD-1; 500 females 1.0%)

    (CD-1; 2 in 890 females 0.2%)

    Granulosa cell tumor, malignant

    (CD-1; 1 in 500 females 0.2%)

    (CD-1; 1 in 890 females 0.1%)

    Luteoma

    (CD-1; 500 females 1.8%)

    (CD-1; 6 in 890 females 0.7%)

    Theca cell tumor (thecoma)

    (CD-1; 1 in 500 females 0.2%)

    (CD-1; 4 in 890 females 0.5%)

    Hemangioma (angioma, hemangioendothelioma) — occasional finding in CD-1 and
        B6C3F$_1$

        (CD-1; 4 in 890 females 0.5%)

    Hemangiosarcoma (angiosarcoma, hemangioendotheliosarcoma) — occasional finding
        (CD-1; 1 in 890 females 0.1%)

    Ovarian yolk sac carcinoma — rare (B6C3F$_1$; none in 2390 females)

    Sertoli cell tumor — rare

    Teratoma — very low incidence

    (B6C3F$_1$; 1 in 246 females 0.4%)

    (B6C3F$_1$; 41,000 females 0.2%)

Oviducts

    Lesions are often associated with changes in ovary or uterus

    Dilatation — occasional finding

    Inflammation — usually associated with ovarian or peritoneal inflammation

    Tumor

        Papilloma — very low incidence (CD-1; one in 890 females 0.1%)

        Leiomyoma — very low incidence (CD-1; one in 890 females 0.1%)

Pancreas

    Amyloidosis — common site (*see* Kidney)

    Arteritis — frequent finding of fibrinoid necrosis and inflammation which can result in
        hemorrhage

    Atrophy — common focal finding having lobular pattern with various severities and du-
        rations, often accompanied by inflammation

    Cystic degeneration — occasional foci which resemble ballooning (cystic) degeneration
        common in rat livers

Dilated ducts — sporadic finding of unknown origin

Fibrosis, interstitial, diffuse — occasional finding in aged mice

Inflammation (pancreatitis) — frequent in aged mice (CD-1; 2000 males 2.8%, 2000 females 6.7%); small aggregates of lymphoid cells are common; 20% incidence was observed in 274 C57BL/6 female mice; chronic inflammatory cells are often adjacent to blood vessels or ducts, may be associated with focal acinar atrophy; acute necrotizing pancreatitis can result from virus infections, for example, reovirus and encephalomyocarditis virus as well as septicemic infections

Edema, interstitial, diffuse — common finding in aging mice usually associated with cardiac failure or severe renal disease and as an agonal change

Tumors — uncommon in mice

    Adenoma, acinar cell — very rare

    (CD-1; one in 891 males 0.1%, none in 890 females)

    (B6C3F$_1$; none, 2543 males, one in 2522 females < 0.1%)

    Adenocarcinoma, acinar cell — very rare (B6C3F$_1$; none in 2543 males, none in 2522 females)

    Cystadenoma — very rare (B6C3F$_1$; none in 2543 males, none in 2522 females)

Parathyroid gland

    Amyloidosis — common *(see* Kidney); incidence 10–40% in CD-1 mice

    Cyst — occasionally present

    Hyperplasia — uncommon; bilateral hyperplasia usually accompanies chronic renal disease (CD-1; 2000 males < 1%, 2000 females < 1%)

    Pigmentation, melanin (melanosis) — common in pigmented strains, such as C57BL

    Thymic rests

    Tumors

        Adenoma — very rare < 1% in mice (CD-1; none, 891 males, one in 890 females 0.1%)

Penis

    Inflammation — incidence variable; wounds are common

    The ulceration and abscess formation of the perineal region which accompany urethral plugs in obstructive uropathy may involve the penis and preputial glands *(see* Urethra)

Pericardium

    Inflammation — associated with inflammation of adjacent cardiac and mediastinal tissues

    Tumors — associated with neoplasia of adjacent tissues

Peripheral nerve (peripheral nervous system)

    Few lesions are observed in mice

    Degeneration — sporadic finding in ageing mice consisting of vacuoles containing cellular debris and a few macrophages

    Demyelination (segmental, Wallerian, distal axonopathy) — degenerative lesions involving the cell body, axon, and myelin sheath (Schwann cells) in various patterns; special stains and neuropathologic techniques are needed

    Tumors — the terminology and classification of peripheral nerve tumors is complex and confusing.

        Neurofibroma (perineural fibroma) — rare

        Neurofibrosarcomas are reported in skin and large intestine of B6C3F$_1$ mice, < 0.1%

        Schwannoma, benign or malignant (neurinoma, neurilemmoma, neurolemma, neurofibroma, neurofibrosarcoma) — some of these tumors were previously termed reticulum cell sarcoma, type A; sites of predilection: uterus, epididymis, and spinal nerve roots

        Ganglioneuroma — rare tumor, more often observed in the adrenal gland than the spinal ganglia

Peritoneum

    Extramedullary hematopoiesis — usually occurs in the perirenal fat associated with leukemoid reactions and myeloid hyperplasia (*see* Bone marrow)

    Inflammation — associated with inflammation of adjacent abdominal organs and tissues

    Necrosis, fat (B6C3F$_1$; 2543 males 1.3%, 2522 females 1.1%)

    Tumors — most often are secondary and associated with neoplasia of abdominal organs

        Mesothelioma (mesenchymal sarcoma)

            (CD-1; none in 891 males, one in 890 females, 0.1%)

            (B6C3F$_1$, three in 2343 males 0.1%, and none in 2486 females)

Pharynx (*see* Oral cavity)

Pituitary gland

    Cyst, simple — common; usually in pars distalis

    Extramedullary hematopoiesis — usually occurs in association with leukemoid reactions and myeloid hyperplasia (*see* Bone marrow)

    Hyperplasia, focal — low incidence, 1–2% CD-1 mice (CD-1; 2000 males < 1%, 2000 females < 1%)

    Tumors

        Adenoma, pars distalis — low incidence

            (RF; 427 females 1.4%)

            (CD-1; two in 891 males 0.2%, 890 females 4.7%)

            (CD-1; 2000 males < 1%, 2000 females 1%)

            (B6C3F$_1$; 1903 males 0.6%, 2051 females 7.9%)

        Carcinoma (adenocarcinoma), pars distalis

            (CD-1; two in 891 males 0.2% and two in 890 females 0.2%)

            (CD-1; 2000 males none, 2000 females < 1%)

            (B6C3F$_1$; one in 1903 males 0.1%, 2051 females 0.4%)

Pleura

    Usually pleural lesions are the result of changes in the underlying lung or adjacent mediastinum and thorax; neoplastic lesions usually result from systemic or multifocal tumors in the lungs

    Tumors

        Mesothelioma (mesenchymal sarcoma) — very rare (CD-1; one reported in an untreated female)

        Alveolar/bronchiolar (adeno) carcinomas (typically) and mammary gland (adeno) carcinomas (less often) invade the pleura from the lungs

        Malignant fibrous histiocytosis, malignant histiocytoma, and malignant lymphoma — occasionally involve the pleura

Preputial gland

    Atrophy — minor degrees are common in aged mice

    Cysts — minor degrees are common in aged mice

    Enlargement — frequently observed grossly

    Hyperplasia, squamous cells of duct epithelium — often accompanies suppurative inflammation orabscess

    Inflammation (adenitis): acute and chronic — common (up to 10%, CD-1 mice); often result after wounds from fighting; ulceration and abscess formation of the perineal region including the preputial glands accompany urethral plugs in obstructive uropathy (*see* Urethra)

    Tumors

        Adenoma — uncommon finding

        (CD-1; one in 891 males 0.1%)

(B6C3F$_1$; two in 2343 males 0.1%)

Carcinoma — very rare (B6C3F$_1$; one in 2855 males < 0.1%)

Myoepithelioma — infrequent in most strains, but more common in BALB mice

Prostate

 Atrophy — associated with simple squamous epithelium and dilatation

 Dilatation (ectasis) — usually associated with atrophy

 Hyperplasia, epithelial — occasional

 Inflammation (prostatitis)

  Chronic — frequently present in interstitial tissues

  Suppurative — usually associated with inflammation of seminal vesicles, coagulation glands, urinary bladder or kidneys (pyelonephritis)

 Tumors

  Adenoma — none in CD-1 mice

  Adenocarcinoma — very rare (CD-1; one in 891 males 0.1%)

Salivary gland (sublingual, mucous; parotid, serous; submandibular or submaxillary, mixed)

 Atrophy — occasional finding, usually lobular distribution in CD-1 mice

 Hyperplasia, lymphoid — aggregates of lymphoid cells tend to accumulate around ducts

 Inflammation (adenitis) — common finding of small foci of lymphocytes and plasmocytes

 Tumors

  Adenoma — uncommon finding

  Adenoma, parotid gland (CD-1; none, 891 males, two in 890 females 0.2%)

  Adenoma, submaxillary gland (CD-1; two in 891 males 0.2%, none, 890 females)

  Adenocarcinoma — very rare; none reported in more than 10,000 CD-1 and B6C3F$_1$ mice

  Myoepithelioma — infrequent in most strains, but more common in BALB mice, especially females

Seminal vesicles

 Dilatation, cystic — common

 Inflammation

  Chronic — common in interstitium

  Suppurative — usually associated with prostate, urinary bladder, or kidney inflammation (pyelonephritis)

 Tumors

  Adenoma — uncommon finding (CD-1; one in 891 males 0.1%)

  Adenocarcinoma — uncommon finding (CD-1; one in 891 males 0.1%)

  Granular cell tumor — very rare

Skeletal muscle

 Atrophy — occasional focal finding in aged mice

 Inflammation, chronic (myositis) — sporadic foci of lymphoid cells in CD-1 mice

 Tumors

  Rhabdomyosarcoma — very rare in mice (B6C3F$_1$; 2343 males 0.5%, two in 2486 females 0.1%)

Skin

 Amyloidosis — low incidence, usually with systemic amyloidosis (*see* Kidney)

 Epidermoid cyst — low incidence

 Hair loss (alopecia) — incidence variable, frequently physiological, but may be due to a variety of causes, including hair chewing or vices, genetics, mites, and local or systemic disease; patchy hair loss is common

 Inflammation (dermatitis) — incidence variable, frequently present; especially associated with fighting and wounds of ears, feet, penis, and tail

Tumors, Epidermal

    Basal cell tumors, All types (B6C3F$_1$; two in 2343 males 0.1%, 2486 females 0.2%)

    Basal cell carcinoma — low incidence < 1% CD-1 (CD-1; none, 891 males, one in 890 females 0.1%)

    Keratoacanthoma — low incidence
        (CD-1; one in 891 males 0.1%, and one in 890 females 0.1%)
        (B6C3F$_1$; 2343 males none, 2486 females none)

    Lymphoma — incidence variable, usually associated with multiple organ involvement

    Sebaceous adenoma — very low incidence

    Sebaceous carcinoma — very low incidence

    Squamous cell papilloma — very low incidence CD-1
        (CD-1; two in 891 males 0.2%, none, 890 females)
        (B6C3F$_1$; three in 2343 males 0.1%, 2486 females 0.2%)

    Squamous cell carcinoma — very low incidence
        (CD-1; 891 males 0.2%, 890 females 0.7%)
        (B6C3F$_1$; 2343 males 0.2%, 2486 females 0.2%)

Tumors, subcutaneous tissue

    Angioma (hemangioma, hemangioendothelioma) — low incidence CD-1 (CD-1; 891 males 0.5%, 890 females 0.9%)

    Angiosarcoma (hemangiosarcoma, hemangioendotheliosarcoma) — very low incidence CD-1
    (CD-1; 891 males 0.3%, 890 females 0.8%)

    Fibroma — very low incidence < 1% CD-1 (CD-1; one in 891 males 0.1%, and three in 890 females 0.3%)

    (Neuro) fibroma (B6C3F$_1$; 2343 males 1.2%, one in 2486 females < 0.1%)

    Fibrosarcoma — low incidence < 2% CD-1 (CD-1; 891 males 1.7%, 890 females 0.9%)

    (Neuro) fibrosarcoma (B6C3F$_1$; 2343 males 2.8%, 2486 females 0.8%)

    Fibrous histiocytoma — low incidence 4% CD-1 (CD-1; 891 males 0.3%, 890 females 0.5%)

    Leiomyoma — none in CD-1

    Leiomyosarcoma (CD-1; none, 891 males, one in 890 females 0.1%)

    Lipoma — very low incidence CD-1

    Liposarcoma — very low incidence CD-1 (CD-1; none, 891 males, 890 females 0.8%)

    Sarcoma, undifferentiated (sarcoma, NOS) — very low incidence CD-1 (B6C3F$_1$; 2343 males 1.7%, 2486 females 0.7%)

Spinal cord (*see* Brain)

    Neuroaxonal dystrophy — occasional finding in which terminal axons, especially in the nucleus gracilis, are swollen in aged mice

    Squamous epithelial cyst — uncommon finding

    Tumors — rare (*see* Brain)

Spleen

    Amyloidosis — frequent in CD-1 mice (*see* Kidney) (CD-1; 2000 males 11.6%, 2000 females 11.6%)

    Atrophy — lymphocyte depletion is common in aged mice

    Extramedullary hematopoiesis — minimal to moderate degrees are considered to be normal; marked or severe degree is abnormal; usually occurs associated with leukemoid reactions and myeloid hyperplasia (*see* Bone marrow) (CD-1; 2000 males 7.6%, 2000 females 7.6%)

Fibrosis — rare

Hyperplasia, erythroid — increased erythroid precursors are associated with anemia and extensive neoplasia

Hyperplasia, lymphoid — low incidence, usually in females
  (C57BL/6; 274 female mice 5%)
  (CD-1; 2000 males 13.9%, 2000 females 13.9%)

Hyperplasia, megakaryocytic — usually accompanies myeloid hyperplasia

Hyperplasia, myeloid (leukemoid reaction) — increased immature granulocytic precursors associated with systemic inflammatory conditions (*see* Bone marrow)

Pigmentation, hemosiderin — hemosiderin is normal in moderate numbers of macrophages in mice; increased hemosiderin is associated with some forms of anemia, hemolysis, and increased erythrocyte destruction

Pigmentation, lipofuscin — occurs in some strains

Pigmentation, melanin (melanosis) — commonly affects the splenic capsule and trabeculae in pigmented strains, such as C57BL; must be differentiated from hemosiderin

Tumors

  Hemangioma (angioma, hemangioendothelioma)
    (CD-1; 891 males 0.2%, 890 females 0.1%)
    (CD-1; 2000 males 0.4%, 2000 females 0.4%)
    (B6C3F$_1$; 3766 males 0.1%, 3751 females 0.2%)

  Hemangiosarcoma (angiosarcoma, hemangioendotheliosarcoma)
    (CD-1; 2000 males 0.6%, 2000 females 0.6%)
    (B6C3F$_1$; 3766 males 2.1%, 3751 females 1.0%)

  Histiocytic sarcoma (reticulum cell sarcoma, type A) — rare before 12 months; common especially after 18 months of age; frequently involve the uterus, vagina, and liver; and less often bone marrow, lungs, pancreas, dermis, mesentery, kidney, and epididymis (RF; reticulum cell sarcoma, 427 females 56.2%)
    (CD-1; 2000 males 1.2%, 2000 females 1.2%)

  Leukemia, myelogenous (myeloid, granulocytic) — often primarily involves liver and spleen in RF strain; must be differentiated from leukemoid reaction and myeloid hyperplasia
    (CD-1; 2000 males 1.9%, 2000 females 1.9%)
    (B6C3F$_1$; Systemic, 2343 males 0.7%, and 2486 females 2.1%)

  Leukemia, lymphatic (lymphocytic, lymphoblastic) — malignant lymphomas that have disseminated into the peripheral blood

  Lymphoid tumors — frequently involve the spleen (*see* Lymph node)
    (RF; thymic lymphoma, 427 females 4.0%)
    (RF; nonthymic lymphoma, 427 females 7.0%)

  Malignant lymphoma (lymphosarcoma), all types
    (C57BL/6; two in 274 female mice 0.7%)
    (CD-1; 2000 males 5.3%, 2000 females 5.3%)

  Mast cell tumor, malignant (B6C3F$_1$, one in 3766 males < 0.1%, none, 3751 females)

  Plasma cell tumor, malignant (B6C3F$_1$; none, 3766 males, one in 3751 females < 0.1%)

Stomach (glandular)

  Amyloidosis — common; begins basally (*see* Kidney)

  Arteritis — sporadic finding

  Cysts — very common to have intramucosal cysts; when large cyst walls often undergo squamous metaplasia

  Erosion (*see* Ulcer) (CD- 1; 2000 males < 1%, 2000 females < 1 %)

Degeneration, hyaline — eosinophilic droplets are commonly present in epithelial cells
of aged B6C3F$_1$ mice
Diverticulum — rare finding
Gastric hepatocytes — uncommon lesions in CD-1 and B6C3F$_1$ aged mice
Glandular hyperplasia (adenomatous hyperplasia, hypertrophic gastritis, proliferative
gastritis) — frequent finding, up to 20% of CD-1 mice; lower in B6C3F$_1$; occasional
finding of glandular elements in the submucosa
(CD-1; 2000 males 2.6%, 2000 females 2.8%)
(B6C3F$_1$; 2543 males 0.8%, 2522 females 0.7%)
Inflammation (gastritis) — acute and chronic active inflammation are common findings,
often accompanying erosions or ulcerations; scattered inflammatory cells can occur in
the mucosa without ulceration or necrosis; occasionally crypts contain leukocytes
(crypt abscess); chronic inflammation with lymphoid cells is occasionally observed in
the submucosa
(CD-1; 2000 males 2%, 2000 females 2%)
(B6C3F$_1$; 2543 males 1.8%, 2522 females 1.9%)
Mineralization (calcification) — focal aggregates of calcium are found in the gastric glandular epithelium; metastatic calcification occurs in the glandular mucosa in association
with severe renal disease and parathyroid hyperplasia; dystrophic calcification also occurs in the smooth muscles
(CD-1; 2000 males < 1%, 2000 females < 1%)
Necrosis — superficial necrosis (erosion) and deep necrosis (ulceration) are occasional
findings (*see* Ulcer) (CD-1; 2000 males 1%, 2000 females < 1%)
Ulcer — erosions and ulcers (focal necrosis) are sporadic low-incidence findings which
can result from a variety of causes accompanied by acute or chronic active inflamma-
tion (acute or chronic necrotizing inflammation) (CD-1; 2000 males < 1%, 2000 fe-
males < 1%)
Tumors — rare in CD-1 and B6C3F$_1$ mice
Adenoma — low incidence
(CD-1; one in 891 males 0.1%, none, 890 females)
(B6C3F$_1$; one in 3807 males < 0.1%, and one in 3789 females < 0.1%)
Adenocarcinoma — low incidence, < 0.1%
(B6C3F$_1$; one in 2543 males < 0.1%, and one in 2522 females < 0.1%)
(B6C3F$_1$; one in 3807 males < 0.1%, and one in 3789 females < 0.1%)
Adenomatous polyp — very low incidence (B6C3F$_1$; two in 2543 males < 0.1%, and
one in 2522 females < 0.1%)
Neuroendocrine cell tumors (gastric carcinoid, APUDoma) — rare in mice (B6C3F$_1$;
one, malignant, in 3807 males < 0.1%, and one, malignant, in 3789 females < 0.1%)
Stomach (nonglandular) (*see* Forestomach)
Subcutaneous tissue (*see* Skin)
Testes
Atrophy of seminiferous tubules — common finding; occurs in a variety of patterns and
frequencies; may be associated with a relative increase in Sertoli cell numbers (CD-1;
2000 males 2.7%)
Degeneration of seminiferous tubules — low incidence (B6C3F$_1$; 2543 males 1.5%)
Edema — must be differentiated from a common artifact resembling central edema
Inflammation, spermatic granulomas — occasional
Interstitial (Leydig) cell hyperplasia — diffuse hyperplasia, commonly accompanies at-
rophy; focal hyperplasia must be differentiated from adenoma
Mineralization, focal — common

       Periarteritis — occasional

         Fibrinoid arteriopathy — occasional

         Amyloidosis — occasional (*see* Kidney)

       Tumors

         Embryonal carcinoma — rare (B6C3F$_1$; two in 2543 males < 0. 1%)

         Interstitial (Leydig) cell tumors, all types

            (CD-1; eight in 891 males 0.9%)

            (CD-1; 2000 males < 1%)

            (B6C3F$_1$; 2543 males 0.3%)

         Interstitial (Leydig) cell adenoma — low incidence, 1–4% in CD-1 mice; less in B6C3F$_1$

         Interstitial (Leydig) cell carcinoma — very rare

         Papillary adenoma (CD-1; one in 891 males 0.1%)

         Seminoma — very rare

            (B6C3F$_1$; one in 244 males 0.4%)

            (B6C3F$_1$; one in 2543 males < 0.1%)

         Sertoli cell tumor — very rare

         Stromal tumor (CD-1; one in 891 males 0.1%)

         Teratoma — very rare

Thymus

       Amyloidosis (*see* Kidney) (CD-1; 2000 males 0.4%, 2000 females 0.4%)

       Atrophy — normal involution begins at sexual maturity; atrophy is associated with stress and infections

       (CD-1; 2000 males 1.7%, 2000 females 1.7%)

       Cyst — frequent finding in both cortex and medulla (CD-1; 2000 males 0.6%, 2000 females 0.6%)

       Ectopic parathyroid tissue — sporadic finding

       Hyperplasia, lymphoid — frequent finding especially in female mice after 6 months of age (CD-1; 2000 males 19%, 2000 females 19%)

       Tumors

         Histiocytic sarcoma (reticulum cell sarcoma, type A) — (CD-1; 2000 males 0.9%, 2000 females 0.9%)

         Leukemia, myelogenous (myeloid, granulocytic) (CD-1; 2000 males 1.4%, 2000 females1.4%)

         Malignant lymphoma (lymphosarcoma), all types — frequently involves thymus

            (CD-1; 2000 males 0.4%, 2000 females 0.4%)

            (CD-1; 891 males 0.6%, 890 females 0.6%)

            Thymic lymphomas reportedly arise in the thymus of some strains of mice such as RF, then predominantly involve the mediastinal organs, lungs, and heart, with subsequent spread to other organs, including the liver, spleen, ovaries, uterus, and peripheral lymph nodes (also *see* Lymph node)

         Thymoma — rare tumors composed of a mixture of epithelial and lymphoid elements

            (CD-1; 2000 males < 0.1%, 2000 females < 0.1%)

            (CD-1; one in 891 males 0.1%, none in 890 females)

Thyroid gland

       Amyloidosis — common; incidence 10–40% CD-1 mice (*see* Kidney)

       Cyst — common; often lined by ciliated or squamous cells; pharyngobrachialis duct remnant (ciliated lining); ultimobranchial duct remnant (squamous lining)

       Thymic rests

       Hyperplasia, C-cell (CD-1; 2000 males < 0.1%, 2000 females < 0.1%)

       Hyperplasia, follicular cell

Tumors

    Adenoma, C-cell — very low incidence
        (CD-1; 2000 males < 0.1%, 2000 females < 0.1%)
        (B6C3F$_1$; none in 2178 males, two in 2203 females 0.1%)

    Adenocarcinoma, C-cell — very low incidence
        (CD-1; 2000 males < 0.1%, none in 2000 females)
        (B6C3F$_1$; none in 2178 males, none in 2203 females)

    Adenoma, follicular cell — very low incidence, 1% or less in CD-1 mice
        (CD-1; 891 males 0.9%, 890 females 0.7%)
        (B6C3F$_1$; 2178 males 1%, 2203 females 1.8%)

    Adenocarcinoma, follicular cell (B6C3F$_1$; 2178 males 0.2%, 2203 females 0.3%)

Tongue

    Inflammation — sporadic; often associated with mineralization

    Mineralization — foci of calcification in muscles adjacent to lamina propria with concurrent granulomatous inflammation (*see* Heart)

    Tumors — rare; squamous cell carcinomas reported in B6C3F$_1$

Tooth

    Dysplasia

    Malocclusion — acquired and genetic predisposition

Trachea

    Calcification — occasional finding in tracheal cartilage

    Inflammation, acute and chronic (tracheitis) — frequent finding of small foci of inflammatory cell infiltrates; low incidence (up to 10%, CD-1 mice) sporadic finding resulting from infections caused by gavage accidents

    Osseous metaplasia — occasional finding in tracheal cartilage

    Tumors — none reported in CD-1 mice

Urinary bladder

    Inflammation, acute and chronic (cystitis) — aggregates of lymphoid cells are common, especially in the submucosa; approximately 10% of CD-1 mice; more severe inflammation is usually associated with inflammation of the prostate or pyelonephritis (CD-1; 2000 males 6.1%, 2000 females 12.9%)

    Dilatation — frequently observed at necropsy; important only in obstructive uropathy (*see* Urethra)

    Hyperplasia, urothelial (epithelial) — uncommon; usually associated with cystitis or calculi (CD-1; none, 2000 males, 2000 females < 0.1%)

    Tumors

        Transitional cell papilloma — very rare in mice (B6C3F$_1$; two in 3807 males < 0.1%, none, 3789 females)

        Transitional cell carcinoma — very rare in mice (CD-1; one in 891 males 0.1%, none in 890 females)

Ureter (*see* Kidney)

Urethra

    Mucous plugs — common

    Obstructive uropathy (urologic syndrome, obstructive genitourinary disease, dysuria) — a condition affecting male mice with a high mortality rate, 30–40%, which is often associated with mucous plugs, and urinary bladders distended with urine

Uterus

    Angiectasis, myometrial — common

    Adenomyosis-low incidence (1–3%, CD-1 mice)

    Hyperplasia, cystic endometrial — very common (> 50% of CD-1 mice)

Hyperplasia, stromal cell — usually associated with cystic endometrial hyperplasia

Hydrometra — common

Metaplasia, squamous — usually associated with pyometra

Mucometra — common finding characterized by dilatation of the uterine horns containing excessive mucinous contents; small amounts are normal during parts of the estrus cycle

Pyometra (suppurative inflammation) — occasional

Tumors

    Adenoma — low incidence (CD-1; five in 890 females 0.6%)

    Adenocarcinoma — very low incidence (CD-1; two in 890 females 0.2%)

    Choriocarcinoma — very rare

    Hemangioma (angioma, hemangioendothelioma) — low incidence, 1–2% in CD-1 mice (CD-1; eight in 890 females 0.9%)

    Hemangiosarcoma (angiosarcoma, hemangioendotheliosarcoma) — occasional finding (CD-1; one in 890 females 0.1%)

    Leiomyoma — low incidence, 1–2% in CD-1 mice (CD-1; twenty-one in 890 females 2.4%)

    Leiomyosarcoma — low incidence, 1–2% in CD-1 mice (CD-1; twelve in 890 females 1.4%)

    Papilloma (CD-1; five in 890 females 0.6%)

    Uterine stromal cell polyp — low incidence (B6C3F$_1$; 2360 females 0.9%)

    Uterine stromal cell sarcoma (endometrial sarcoma) — low incidence, 2%, CD-1 mice (CD-1; two in 890 females 0.2%)
    (B6C3F$_1$; 2360 females 0.6%)

    Yolk sac carcinoma — very rare (none in CD-1 mice) (B6C3F$_1$; none in 2445 females)

Vagina

    Inflammation — usually associated with changes of the uterus

    Tumors

        Adenocarcinoma — uncommon finding (B6C3F$_1$; one in 246 females 0.4%)

        Leiomyosarcoma — uncommon finding (CD-1; one in 890 females 0.1%)

Zymbal's gland (*see* Ear)

SECTION 4. HISTOPATHOLOGIC FINDINGS IN CONTROL LABORATORY RATS[10,11,13,18,19,21–25,27–29,32–46]

Adrenal gland, cortex

    Accessory cortical nodule — ancillary cortical tissue surrounded by a fibrous capsule

    Amyloidosis — very rare observation in Fischer 344 rats

    Angiectasis (telangiectasis) — common (Sprague-Dawley; 2000 males 4.6%, 2000 females 28.3%)

    Atrophy, brown (pigmentation, brown degeneration, ceroid deposition, hemosiderin) — uncommon in rat; usually associated with severe diffuse atrophy or focal compression by space-occupying lesion

    Atrophy, diffuse — usually related to increased adrenocortical steroids, uncommon finding

    Congestion — common finding; usually incidental

    Cortical changes, focal (cytoplasmic alterations)

        Basophilic cell foci — commonly seen in zona fasciculata of aged rats

        Clear cell foci — commonly seen in zona glomerulosa of aged rats

        Eosinophilic cell foci — commonly seen in zona fasciculata of aged rats

Mixed cell foci — commonly seen in zona glomerulosa of aged rats

Cystic degeneration (cystic change, peliosis) — similar to cystic change in the liver, especially reported in old breeder female rats; appear to start as foci of large eosinophilic cells (focal cortical hypertrophy) which degenerate to form cysts (Sprague-Dawley; 578 males 23.4%, 585 females 82.7%)

Extramedullary hematopoiesis — occasional finding

Fatty change, diffuse — commonly seen as cytoplasmic vacuolation of the adrenal cortical cells

Hemosiderosis — small amounts of iron-positive pigment can be observed occasionally in the deep cortex

Hemorrhage — common finding; usually incidental or accompanying cystic degeneration, inflammation, or necrosis

Hyperplasia, diffuse (lipid depletion) — lipid depletion occurs under various conditions; primarily affects zona fasciculata characterized by cells with dense eosinophilic cytoplasm; may be associated with increased adrenal weight

Hyperplasia, focal — common finding (Sprague-Dawley; 578 males 11.1%, 585 females 12.0%)

Inflammation, focal, acute — occasionally nonspecific accompaniment to several generalized inflammatory disease

Necrosis, focal — common finding; often accompanying cystic degeneration or inflammation

Osseous metaplasia — rare finding in Fischer 344 rat

Pigmentation (*see* Atrophy, brown)

Tumors

  Cortical adenoma — low incidence
    (Fischer 344/N; 1915 males 1.2%, 1968 females 2.8%)
    (Sprague-Dawley; 578 males 1.6%, 585 females 4.6%)

  Cortical carcinoma (adenocarcinoma) — low incidence
    (Fischer 344/N; 1915 males 0.1%, 1968 females 0.2%)
    (Sprague-Dawley; 578 males 1.0%, 585 females 0.5%)

Adrenal gland, medulla

Hyperplasia, focal — small foci are common which must be differentiated from pheochromocytomas (Sprague-Dawley; 578 males 30.3%, 585 females 16.9%)

Hypertrophy

Tumors

  Ganglioneuroma — very low incidence (Fischer 344/N; 1915 males 0.3%, 1968 females 0.2%)

  Pheochromocytoma, all types — very common, especially in Long-Evans strain, less in Sprague-Dawley (Fischer 344/N; 1915 males 25.5%, 1968 females 5%)

  Pheochromocytoma, benign (Sprague-Dawley; 578 males 19.0%, 585 females 5.3%)

  Pheochromocytoma, malignant (Sprague-Dawley; 578 males 1.9%, 585 females 0.9%)

Blood vessels

Angiectasis (ectasia) — common finding in endocrine organs, especially pituitary and adrenal glands with hyperplasia and neoplasia, less frequent in the ovaries

Arteriosclerosis — a variety of nonspecific changes occur in arteries including intimal plaque formation, medial degeneration (mucoid degeneration), hyaline degeneration, medial hypertrophy, and mineralization (calcification); involve aorta, iliac, renal, carotid, and cerebral arteries; incidence and severity appear to vary with strain, not reported in Fischer 344 rats

Arteritis (polyarteritis nodosa, periarteritis, perivasculitis) — frequent finding, most often in medium arteries of testes, pancreas, mesentery, and occasionally heart, ovary, uterus, brain, adrenal, and liver; characterized by inflammatory infiltrates of all layers of the vessel wall and necrosis (fibrinoid necrosis, necrotizing inflammation); incidence may be reduced by food restriction; incidence influenced by strain

(Fischer 344/N; males 1.8%, females 0.9%)

(Long-Evans; males 4.5%, females 2.6%)

(Wistar; males 9.1%, females 4.2%)

(August; males 45.4%, females 43.0%)

Atherosclerosis is not reported as a spontaneous lesion in laboratory rats

Hemorrhage — occasional spontaneous finding in several organs, particularly the thymus, lymph nodes, and lungs; often agonal change or associated with necropsy technique

Hypertrophy, medial — major pulmonary arteries of the aged Sprague-Dawley rat frequently have medial hypertrophy; other strains appear to have a low incidence

Mineralization — commonly observed associated with arteriosclerosis; isolated subendothelial deposits of calcium salts are sometimes seen in the pulmonary arteries of aged rats

Thrombosis — occasional finding in the pulmonary and hepatic veins

Tumors

Hemangioma (angioma, hemangioendothelioma), all sites — very low incidence (Fischer 344/N; two reported in 1936 males, 0.1%, and three reported in 1983 females, 0.2%)

Hemangiosarcoma (angiosarcoma, hemangioendotheliosarcoma), all sites — low incidence (Fischer 344/N; 1936 males 0.5%, 1983 females 0.3%)

Hemangiopericytoma — very rare (Fischer 344/N; less than 10 in 50,000 rats < 0.1%)

Paraganglioma, aortic body — rare in most strains, except female WAG/Rij rat 12%

Paraganglioma, retroperitoneal (near kidney) (Fischer 344/N; one reported in 1936 males 0.1%; and one reported in 1983 females 0.1%)

Bone

Cysts — solitary bone cysts are observed sporadically

Degeneration, mucinous or chondromucinous, cystic — a common lesion of cartilage, especially in the sternum but also other sites involving articular and growth plate cartilage

Exostosis — hyperplasia associated with trauma, fractures, degenerative disease, and chronic infections

Fracture callus — common in ribs and extremities, especially feet and tail from restraining or fighting

Inflammation (osteomyelitis) — most common in bones of jaw, legs, feet, and tail associated with trauma or spread of infections from adjacent abscesses or ulcered tumors

Necrosis, aseptic — also termed mucinous degeneration; may occur in the ossified menisci as ghostlike areas of bone

Osteodystrophy, fibrous (osteitis fibrosis, osteitis fibrosa) — sporadic finding associated with hyperparathyroidism and severe renal disease; unusually high in OFA-ICO strain of rat

Osteochondrosis — developmental defect of endochondral ossification involving the femur and humerus reported in Sprague-Dawley

Osteophytes (chondro-osseous outgrowths, spondylosis) — observed on vertebrae, primarily the ventral aspect in males; reported in Fischer 344 and other strains

Osteopetrosis (osteosclerosis, hyperostosis) — thickening of trabeculae or plates of bone, most often detected in calvaria of skull, nasal turbinates, and spongy bone of femur

Tumors — occasional finding especially osteosarcomas

Chordoma — uncommon malignant neoplasm arising in the vertebral column from embryonic notochord

Osteoma, all sites — very low incidence (Fischer 344/N; two reported in 1949 males 0.1%)

Osteosarcoma, all sites — very low incidence (Fischer 344/N; 1936 males 0.4%, 1983 females 0.4%)

Chondrosarcoma, all sites — very low incidence (Fischer 344/N; one reported in 1949 males 0.1%, and one reported in 1950 females 0.1%)

Hemangiosarcoma, vertebra (Fischer 344/N; one reported in 1936 males, 0.1%)

Hemangiosarcoma, pelvis (Fischer 344/N; one reported in 1983 females, 0.1%)

Bone marrow

Atrophy (hypoplasia, aplasia, panmyelopathy) — sporadic finding in aged rats in which hematopoietic cells are replaced fat (adipose) cells

Fibrosis — occasional small foci in the marrow space

Hyperplasia — the bone marrow of the rat is normally very cellular and with a few scattered fat cells fills the marrow cavity; under various stimuli, the marrow reacts by completely filling the cavity with normal hematopoietic cells; the most common responses consist predominantly of erythroid and myeloid cells; less commonly eosinophils, basophils, or megakaryocytes

Hyperplasia, erythroid — associated with anemia and increased red cell destruction

Hyperplasia, histiocytic, focal — proliferation of histiocytes in foci surrounded by inflammatory cells

Hyperplasia, megakaryocytic — associated with increased platelet consumption

Hyperplasia, myeloid (leukemoid reaction) — associated with neutrophilia in the peripheral blood; severe myeloid hyperplasia which commonly accompanies extensive necrosis or systemic infections must be differentiated from leukemia

Hyperplasia, plasma cell — commonly observed; may be accompanied by increased numbers of mast cells

Hyperplasia, stromal cell — occasional small focal lesions of adventitial reticular cells

Inflammation, granulomatous — occasional focal lesions observed in young adult and aged rats characterized by aggregates of macrophages or histiocytes; may be same as lesion termed histiocytic hyperplasia

Tumors

Myelogenous leukemia (granulocytic leukemia) — (Sprague-Dawley; 585 males 0.3%, 585 females 0.2%)

Mononuclear cell leukemia (large granular lymphocytic leukemia, monocytic leukemia, lymphosarcoma) — appears to arise in the spleen and secondarily involve the bone marrow and lymph nodes; common in Fischer 344 rats (Fischer 344/N; 1936 males 33.6%, 1983 females 20.2%); incidence is reportedly decreased in males by gavage with corn oil vehicle (Fischer 344/N; 1949 males 17.1%, 1950 females 19.3%)

Brain and meninges (central nervous system)

Atrophy, focal (compression) — common finding in rats with expanding pituitary adenomas, particularly if more than 0.5 cm in diameter; commonly associated with hydrocephalus

Chromatolysis — occasional finding characterized by dispersion and dissolution of Nissl substance.

Dark cells — common finding; foci of neurons which appear shrunken and basophilic without changes in the surrounding parenchyma or glial cell are regarded as artifacts

Edema — sometimes associated with tumors, especially pituitary adenomas

Gitter cells — microglial macrophages usually associated with myelin breakdown

Hemorrhage — common finding occurring from various causes, such as vascular changes associated with pituitary adenomas, leukemia, gliomas, and infarcts

Hydrocephalus — uncommon finding sometimes associated with compression by large pituitary adenomas

Infarction — uncommon focal finding as a result of vascular blockage, usually observed as a healing area of chronic inflammation with lipid and hemosiderin in macrophages

Inflammation — uncommon in laboratory rats unless extensive bacterial respiratory infections are present; occasional finding of small foci of chronic inflammatory cells, lymphocytes, and plasma cells in the brain and meninges or spontaneous arteritis of the cerebral arteries; chronic encephalitis associated with *Toxoplasma gondii* or focal granulomatous inflammation in the absence of necrosis associated with *Encephalitozoon (Nosema) cuniculi* may be observed in apparently normal rats

Malacia — necrosis of neural tissues with loss of architecture, breakdown of myelin or neuropil, and accumulation of foamy macrophages (Gitter cells)

Mineralization, cerebral — common, rounded or irregular basophilic bodies or concretions are found occasionally in rat brains, but sometimes reach incidences of up to 20%

Necrosis — ischemic neuronal injury, occasional finding of shrunken, hyaline, densely eosinophilic cell bodies and small, basophilic nuclei which results from a variety of causes including ischemia, anoxia, seizures, epilepsy, and some metabolic disturbances (*see* Malacia)

Pigmentation

    Lipofuscin (ceroid pigment) — periodic acid-Schiff (PAS) reagent-positive and acid-fast pigment is found in cerebral neurons with increasing age.

    Hemosiderin (Perl's-positive iron pigment) — found in macrophages associated with focal infarcts, hemorrhage, inflammation, or around expanding neoplasms

    Melanin — commonly seen in the meninges and the pituitary gland of pigmented strains of rats of all ages

    Vacuolation (vacuolar degeneration, vacuolar encephalopathy) — vacuoles are a frequent finding associated with a variety of causes including artifacts, intramyelinic edema, spongy degeneration, spongiform encephalopathies, uremia, and increasing age

Tumors

    Central nervous system tumors are uncommon in most rats; incidences at 26 months of age were males 1.0% and females 0.8% and at 34 months in life span studies were males 2.9% and females 2.2%

    Astrocytoma (astrocytic glioma, glioblastoma multiform) — low incidence
      (Fischer 344/N; 1928 males 0.5%, 1969 females 0.9%)
      (Sprague-Dawley; 585 males 0.7%, 585 females 0.5%)

    Ependymoma — very low incidence (Fischer 344/N, two reported in 1943 males 0.1%, and one reported in 1946 females 0.1%)

    Ependymoblastoma — very low incidence (Sprague-Dawley; one reported in 585 males 0.2%)

    Glioma, all types (Fischer 344/N; two reported in 1928 males 0.1%, and one reported in 1969 females 0.1%)

    Glioma, malignant (Sprague-Dawley; one reported in 585 males 0.2%)

    Granular cell tumors — common in cranial cavity of several rat strains; most are benign; very low incidence
      (Fischer 344/N; 1928 males 0.2%, 1946 females 0.3%)
      (Sprague-Dawley; one reported in 585 males 0.2%)

    Hemangioma (angioma, hemangioendothelioma) (Fischer 344/N; one reported in 1969 females 0.1%)

    Lymphoreticular tumors (lymphoma, malignant reticulosis, lymphoreticulosis, reticulum cell sarcoma, microglioma, gliomatosis) — uncommon mesenchymal tumors with unclear relationship to undifferentiated gliomas

Medulloblastoma — very low incidence
(Fischer 344/N; one reported in 1928 males 0.1%, and one reported in 1969 females
0.1%)
(Sprague-Dawley; one reported in 585 males 0.2%)
Meningioma — commonest tumor in central nervous system of some rat colonies
with syncytial and fibroblastic types; very low incidence (Fischer 344/N; two
reported in 1928 males 0.1%, and two reported in 1969 females 0.1%)
Oligodendroglia — very low incidence
(Fischer 344/N; two reported in 1928 males 0.1%, and three reported in 1969 fe-
males 0.2%)
(Sprague-Dawley; one reported in 585 males 0.2%)
Clitoral gland
Atrophy — occasional finding involving the acinar epithelium in aging rats
Cyst — minor cystic changes commonly accompany atrophy
Degeneration, cystic — common finding in aged males; combination of changes includ-
ing atrophy of acinar cells, fibrosis, distention of ducts by secreted material and limited
degrees of inflammation
Enlargement — frequently observed grossly
Hyperplasia, focal — occasional finding of the acinar epithelium in aging rats; sometimes
cystic
Hyperplasia, squamous cells of duct epithelium — often accompanies suppurative in-
flammation or abscess
Inflammation (adenitis) — occasional finding, especially suppurative inflammation or
abscesses
Tumors — usually arise from acinar or ductal epithelium
Adenoma — low incidence (Fischer 344/N; 1983 females 2.8%)
Carcinoma — low incidence (Fischer 344/N; 1983 females 3.0%)
Squamous cell papilloma (Fischer 344/N; one reported in 1950 females 0.1%)
Coagulating gland
Inflammation, chronic — common incidental focal finding of lymphocytic infiltrations
Inflammation, suppurative — usually associated with prostatic, urinary bladder or kidney
inflammation.
Tumors — none reported in 51,230 Fischer 344/N rats
Ductus (vas) deferens (*see* Epididymis)
Ear
External ear (pinna, auricle) and auditory canal
Auricular chondropathy (proliferative chondritis) — nodular lesions characterized by
granulomatous inflammation and chondrolysis with regenerative hyperplasia and
fibrosis; occurrence strain related; most frequent in Sprague-Dawley and
fawn-hooded rats; not observed in Fischer 344/N
Foreign body — cerumen, food, and other debris commonly are found in the external
auditory meatus.
Inflammation, chronic — frequent finding as result of wounds or trauma (*see* Skin
for additional lesions)
Inflammation, granulomatous (granulomas) — occasionally present in wall of auditory
canal
Tumors (same as skin) — occasionally observed
Neural crest tumors — resemble neurofibromas, neurofibrosarcomas, schwanno-
mas, fibromas and fibrosarcomas (Fischer 344/N; 1936 males 0.1 %, 1983 females 0.1 %)

Nerve sheath tumor, benign (schwannoma) (Sprague-Dawley; two reported in 585 males 0.3%)

Nerve sheath tumor, malignant (schwannoma) (Sprague-Dawley; one reported in 585 females 0.2%)

Middle ear — inflammation (otitis media) is occasional finding, often associated with sinus and upper respiratory tract infections; tympanic cavity usually contains purulent exudate

Inner ear — inflammation (otitis interna) extending from middle ear; can result in encephalitis and lost of balance or circling behavior

Zymbal's gland (auditory sebaceous glands) — holocrine glands at the base of the ear

Tumors — commonly observed in aged rats; have squamous, sebaceous, or mixed patterns

Adenoma, sebaceous — very low incidence

(Fischer 344/N; two reported in 1949 males 0.1%)

(Sprague-Dawley; one reported in 585 males 0.2%)

Adenocarcinoma, sebaceous — very low incidence (Sprague-Dawley; one of 585 males, 0.2% and one of 585 females 0.2%)

Carcinoma, sebaceous — low incidence (Fischer 344/N; 1936 males 1.4%; 1983 females 0.7%)

Squamous cell papilloma (Fischer 344/N; two reported in 1936 males 0.1%)

Epididymis

Changes commonly observed are secondary to testicular atrophy and include: lack or diminished spermatozoal contents, intraepithelial cyst formation, and tubular debris.

Inflammation, granulomatous (spermatic granuloma) — common

Tumors — very low incidence:

Hemangioma (angioma, hemangioendothelioma) (Fischer 344/N, one reported in 1936 males 0.1%)

Sarcoma (Fischer 344/N; two reported in 1949 males 0.1%)

Esophagus

Impaction — sporadic finding of distention with food and debris in some colonies; seldom seen in Sprague-Dawley

Inflammation — common in association with gavage injuries during dosing; severity and frequency range from small foci of macrophages to large areas of necrosis and abscess formation; perforations, can lead to extensive inflammation of subcutis or pleura; myositis, usual occurrence 2–6%

Tumors — very low incidence: squamous cell carcinomas have been reported (Fischer 344/N; one reported in 1850 males 0.1%; and one reported in 1836 females 0.1 %)

Eye

Cataract — common lens finding in aged rats

Chromodacryorrhea — excessive red secretions of apparently normal lacrimal and Harderian glands, which may be mistaken for blood, increased secretions are associated with stress

Coloboma — a congenital defect due to persistence of choroid tissue with protrusion of the retina into the optic nerve sheath.

Corneal dystrophy (hyalinization or mineralization) — low frequency findings in rats which are poorly defined, including hyalinization or mineralization (calcification) in Bowman's membrane or the anterior corneal stromal subepithelial mineralization in diabetic rats, and thickening of Descemet's membrane.

Inflammation, conjunctiva (conjunctivitis) — mild nonspecific inflammation is common; severe inflammation is most commonly associated with infections caused by the sialodacryoadenitis virus

Inflammation, cornea (keratitis) — usually is associated with inflammation of the con-junctiva; minimal infiltrates by inflammatory cells and edema can result from mild abrasions, slight trauma, or drying (epithelial desiccation)

Inflammation, periorbital (periorbititis) — usually is associated with trauma during blood sampling of the orbital sinus

Retinal atrophy — frequent finding from a variety of causes including age, strain, ambient light exposure, temperature, nutrition, and retinal inflammation with glaucoma. The retina of the albino rat is particularly sensitive to the effects of high light intensity which results in bilateral atrophy.

Retinal folds or rosettes — infolding of all retinal layers is occasionally seen, presumably having congenital origin or associated with acquired retinal detachment

Synechia — adhesion or attachment of the iris margin to the anterior cortex of the lens or the corneal endothelium; may occur as a congenital condition or follow inflammation in the anterior chamber.

Tumors — intraocular tumors are very rare in rats

    Glioma (Fischer 344/N; one reported in 1949 males 0.1%)

    Leiomyosarcoma (Sprague-Dawley; one reported in 585 males 0.2%)

    Squamous cell carcinoma of the conjunctiva is occasionally seen in aged rats (Fischer 344/N; one reported in 1936 males 0.1%)

Forestomach (stomach, nonglandular)

Erosion (*see* Ulcer and Necrosis)

Diverticulum — rare finding

Dysplasia — often associated with hyperplasia

Ulcer — erosions and ulcers (focal necrosis) with accompanying inflammation of the squamous mucosa are very common lesions; vary in severity; severe ulceration is ac-companied by acute and chronic inflammation, penetration of the inflammatory chang-es into the stomach wall, and in some animals, peritonitis

Hyperkeratosis — associated with hyperplasia

Hyperplasia, squamous (acanthosis, hyperkeratosis, parakeratosis) — most proliferative or hyperplastic changes of the squamous mucosa are reactive, focal, and associated with gastric inflammation; occasionally the entire forestomach is affected; focal hyper-plasia commonly involves the junction with the glandular stomach; may have exten-sive dysplasia

Inflammation (gastritis) — common finding often associated with erosion or ulceration; vary from focal acute or chronic inflammation to perforation of the stomach wall

Necrosis — superficial necrosis (erosion) and deep necrosis (ulceration) are common findings (*see* Ulcer)

Tumors — squamous cell tumors are uncommon

    Squamous papillomas — low incidence (Sprague-Dawley; 583 males 0.2%, 585 females 0.3%) (Fischer 344/N: 1912 males 0.2%, 1955 females 0.3%); incidence after gavage with corn oil vehicle
    (Fischer 344/N; 1924 males 0.3%, 1936 females 0.4%)

    Squamous carcinomas — very low incidence (Fischer 344/N; two reported in 1912 males 0.1%;and one reported in 1955 females 0.1%)

    Leiomyosarcoma — very low incidence (Fischer 344/N; one reported in 1912 males 0.1%)

Harderian gland — well developed in rats

Chromodacryorrhea — excessive red secretions of apparently normal Harderian glands which may be mistaken for blood; increases associated with stress

Atrophy, focal or diffuse, (glandular ectasia) — common finding; consists of cystic dila-tation of glandular lumens

Cysts — occasional finding

Hyperplasia, focal — occasional finding of small, noncompressive lesions with both cellular hyperplasia and hypertrophy

Inflammation — common finding; focal glandular atrophy, fibrosis and chronic inflammatory cells or necrosis can be result of orbital bleeding; severe inflammation with necrosis and squamous metaplasia is most commonly associated with infections caused by the sialodacryoadenitis virus

Tumors — uncommon but occasionally seen in aged rats

Adenoma — very low incidence

(Fischer 344/N; one reported in 1936 males 0.1%, and two reported in 1950 females 0.1%)

(Sprague-Dawley; one reported in 390 males < 0.1%)

Adenocarcinoma — very rare; none reported in the Fischer 344/N or Sprague-Dawley rat studies

Heart

Atrial thrombosis — sporadic finding in the right atrium (Sprague-Dawley; 2000 males < 1%, 2000 females < 1%)

Degeneration, myocardial — occasional finding in aged rats associated with necrosis or metaplasia

Degeneration, valvular — frequent finding in aged rats characterized by myxomatous or basophilic changes

Fibrosis — usually associated with necrosis (Sprague-Dawley; 2000 males 15.0%, 2000 females 5.8%)

Fibrosis, subendocardial — proliferation of mesenchymal cells, fibroblasts, in the subendocardium primarily involving of the left ventricle which increases with age

Hypertrophy, myocardial — usually a diffuse change which may require weights of the total heart and the individual ventricles as well as measurement of the thicknesses of the chamber walls for characterization; focal hypertrophy can be observed in areas of inflammation and fibrosis

Inflammation (myocarditis) — usually incidental focal small aggregates of inflammatory cells and fibrosis or in association with necrosis and infectious diseases; usual occurrence in young rats 2–7% (Sprague-Dawley; 2000 males 13.8%, 2000 females 9.5%)

Inflammation, valvular (endocarditis) — sporadic finding often found associated with suppurative inflammation elsewhere in the body, such as the feet (pododermatitis)

Necrosis, myocardial (focal necrosis; acute, necrotizing inflammation; acute focal inflammation; focal subacute or chronic inflammation; acute focal inflammation; focal subacute or chronic inflammation; focal fibrosis) — a frequent localized lesion accompanied by inflammatory cells and fibrosis occurs in aged rats; usually present in the inner region or subendocardial zone and papillary muscles of the left ventricle, possibly related to local ischemia; also, can result from bacterial infections

Metaplasia, cartilaginous and osseous — common finding in aged rats occurring in areas of myocardial degeneration

Pigmentation — pigment-laden macrophages and mononuclear cells with fibrosis indicate old myocardial injury

Tumors — spontaneous primary cardiac neoplasms are rare; mesenchymal, spindle-cell tumors are most common

Hemangioma (angioma, hemangioendothelioma) — very rare (Fischer 344/N; none in 1932 males and 1972 females)

Hemangiosarcoma (angiosarcoma, hemangioendotheliosarcoma) — very low incidence (Fischer 344/N; two reported in 1932 males 0.1%, and one reported in 1972 females 0.1%)

Anitschkow cell sarcoma — very rare (Fischer 344/N; none in 1932 males and 1972 females)

Atriocaval mesothelioma — very rare (Fischer 344/N; one reported in 1972 females 0.1%)

Fibrosarcoma — very rare (Fischer 344/N; one reported in 1947 males, 0.1%)

Malignant schwannoma — very low incidence (Fischer 344/N; 1932 males 0.1%, 1972 females 0.2%)

Neurofibrosarcoma — very rare (Fischer 344/N: one reported in 1972 females, 0.1%)

Rhabdomyosarcoma — very rare (Fischer 344/N; none in 1932 males and 1972 females)

Sarcoma, unspecified — very rare (Fischer 344/N; one reported in 1932 males, 0.1%)

Intestines, unspecified (NOS)

Arteritis — occasional finding in mesenteric and pancreatic arteries usually associated with polyarteritis

Atrophy — loss, shortening, stunting, or atrophy of the small intestine villi result from several causes including hormonal factors, reduced food intake or starvation; focal atrophy of the large intestine mucosa occurs occasionally in colon without other apparent lesions

Congestion — mucosal blood vessels become congested secondary to inflammation and occur as agonal changes

Dilatation — frequent finding in animals found dead, most commonly from bacterial gas production

Dilatation of the jejunum, ileum, or cecum — associated with paralytic ileus; can be a delayed response to intraperitoneal administration of an anesthetic agent such as chloral hydrate; must be differentiated from Tyzzer's disease megaloileitis

Diverticulum or pouch of small intestine — persistence of fetal yolk sac attachment in Sprague-Dawley; herniation along the mesenteric attachment in Fischer 344 rat

Ectopic pancreatic tissue — sporadic finding in the duodenum and jejunum

Fibrosis — occasional finding in the colon mucosa

Hyperplasia and hypertrophy — focal reactive hyperplasia or hypertrophy of the intestinal epithelium occurs around areas of inflammation, ulceration, and heavy parasitic infestation; mucosal hypertrophy of both the large and small intestine occurs under some physiological conditions such as lactation (Sprague-Dawley; 2000 males 1.5%, 2000 females 1.6%)

Hyperplasia, lymphoid — occasional finding of nonneoplastic proliferation of cells, predominantly lymphocytes, resulting from inflammation and other immunological stimulation; normal lymphoid follicles have prominent germinal centers in the gastrointestinal tract of rats; therefore, hyperplasia should be reserved for significant increases

Inflammation, large (colitis) — nonspecific inflammation is common; unless definite evidence of active inflammation is present, a slight increase in inflammatory cells in the lamina propria would be considered within normal limits; acute inflammation, ulceration, and necrosis (necrotizing inflammation) can occur in Tyzzer's disease, salmonellosis, and other bacterial infections.

Inflammation, small (duodenitis, jejunitis, ileitis) — uncommon finding in most laboratory colonies; can be result of several bacterial and parasitic infections as well as nonspecific stress; vary in type, severity, and duration including erosion, ulceration, necrosis, acute and chronic active inflammation, fibrosis, reactive lymphoid hyperplasia, reactive epithelial hyperplasia, lymph node inflammation, and peritonitis

Mineralization (calcification) — foci associated with inflammation and necrosis occur sporadically in the muscularis externa

Metazoan parasites

Protozoa — *Giardia muris*, *Hexamitis muris*, *Trichomonas* species occur in the small intestine usually with no apparent effect

Nematodiasis — pin worms (*Syphacia muris*) are common findings in the cecum and colon of rats with no inflammation; usual occurrence in young rats 3–8%

Tumors, large intestines, unspecified (NOS)

Adenoma (adenomatous polyp, villous adenoma) — very low incidence

(Fischer 344/N; two reported in 1949 males 0.1%)

(Sprague-Dawley; one reported in 576 females 0.2%)

Adenocarcinoma — very low incidence

(Fischer 344/N; two reported in 1936 males 0.1%)

(Sprague-Dawley; one reported in 569 males 0.2%)

Fibroma — very low incidence (Fischer 344/N; one reported in 1936 males 0.1%)

Fibrosarcoma — uncommon finding (Fischer 344/N; one reported in 1949 males 0.1%)

Lipoma — very low incidence (Fischer 344/N; one reported in 1950 females 0.1%)

Malignant schwannoma — very low incidence (Fischer 344/N; one reported in 1936 males 0. 1%)

Rhabdomyosarcoma (anus) — (Sprague-Dawley; one reported in 585 males 0.2%)

Tumors, small intestines, unspecified (NOS)

Adenoma (adenomatous polyp) — very low incidence (Fischer 344/N; one reported in 1887 males 0.1%)

Adenocarcinoma — very low incidence

(Fischer 344/N; seven reported in 1865 males 0.4%)

(Sprague-Dawley; one reported in 556 females 0.2%)

Fibrosarcoma — uncommon finding (Fischer 344/N; one reported in 1865 males, 0.1%; and one reported in 1939 females 0.2%)

Hemangioma — very rare (Fischer 344/N; one reported in a female rat < 0.1%)

Hemangiosarcoma — uncommon finding (Fischer 344/N; one reported in 1353 males 0.7%)

Leiomyoma — very low incidence (Fischer 344/N; one reported in 1865 males 0.1%)

Leiomyosarcoma — uncommon finding

(Fischer 344/N; three reported in 1865 males 0.2%; and two reported in 1939 females 0.1%)

(Sprague-Dawley; 556 males 0.4%, 556 females 0.4%)

Malignant lymphoma — occasionally seem to arise from gastrointestinal lymphoid tissue (Peyer's patches)

Malignant Schwannoma — very low incidence (Fischer 344/N; one reported in 1914 females 0.1%)

Sarcoma, unspecified — uncommon finding

(Fischer 344/N; one reported in 1865 males 0.1%; and one reported in 1939 females 0.1%)

(Sprague-Dawley; one reported in 556 females 0.2%)

Islets, pancreatic (Islets of Langerhans; pancreas, endocrine)

Atrophy, beta cell — diabetes mellitus is generally very rare in rats; genetically spontaneous occurrence in some strains, for example BB rat

Inflammation — spontaneous inflammation of the pancreas usually spares the islets; occasional mononuclear cells, focal chronic inflammation, can be observed in islets of aged rats

Hyperplasia — commonly aging rats develop large islets; size seems to be influenced by *ad libitum* feeding, obesity, and repeated breeding; characterized by several multilobular or multinodular large and pleomorphic islets (Sprague-Dawley, 583 males 5.5%; 585 females 3.9%)

Tumors

> Islet cell adenoma — low incidence
>> (Fischer 344/N; 1868 males 3.2%, 1934 females 1.0%)
>> (Sprague-Dawley; 583 males 7.5%, 585 females 3.9%)
>
> Islet cell carcinoma — low incidence
>> (Fischer 344/N; 1868 males 2.1%, 1934 females 0.3%)
>> (Sprague-Dawley; 583 males 1.9%, 585 females 1.0%)

Joints

Ankylosis — fusion of the joint with immobility resulting from chronic inflammation

Degeneration, mucinous or chondromucinous, cystic — a common lesion of cartilage, especially in the sternum, but also other sites involving articular and growth plate cartilage

Inflammation (arthritis) — sporadic lesions, usually adjacent to wounds or septic foci

Osteoarthritis (osteoarthrosis, degenerative joint disease) — a complex of lesions characterized by erosion of the articular cartilage, degeneration, and inflammation

Tumors

> Synovial sarcoma (Fischer 344/N; one reported in 1936 males 0.1%; and one reported in 1950 females 0.1%)

Kidney

Bowman's capsule changes (*see* Metaplasia)

Cysts — common finding associated with dilatation of tubules which may occur individually; but usually accompany renal nephritis and nephrosis

Endstage — marked or severe glomerular, tubular, and interstitial changes with inflammation

Extramedullary hematopoiesis — sporadically observed in adult rats at times of increased demand for bone marrow activity

Glomerulonephritis and glomerulosclerosis — usually associated with nephropathy *(see* Nephropathy)

Hydronephrosis (pelvis dilatation) — common finding; has both acquired and hereditary causes; usual occurrence in young rats 10%

Hyperplasia, pelvis — focal thickening of the urinary epithelium accompanies mineralization and pelvic inflammation

Hyperplasia, tubular epithelium, focal — occasional finding (Sprague-Dawley; 585 males 0.2%, none, in 584 females)

Inclusions, tubular (protein absorption or hyaline droplets) — hyaline droplets, P.A.S.-positive, occur occasionally in the cytoplasm of renal tubular cells of apparently normal kidneys from males; usual occurrence in young males 15%

Infarction — occasional finding resulting from metastatic tumors, septic thrombosis, or advanced mononuclear cell leukemia

Inflammation (nephritis, pyelonephritis) — a variety of inflammatory changes involve various portions of the kidney of rats; the most important inflammatory findings are associated with nephropathy *(see* Nephropathy); changes of the pelvis are often associated with mineralization, hydronephrosis, and pyelonephritis; acute pyelonephritis is usually associated with ascending lower urinary tract infections and uncommon in most research laboratories; embolic suppurative nephritis is infrequent

Inflammation, chronic — common finding of small lymphoid aggregates in interstitial tissues and in the renal pelvis beneath the transitional epithelium; usual occurrence in young rats, males 12%, females 7%

Metaplasia, Bowman's capsule — lining of the capsule by high cuboidal epithelium resembling the proximal tubule; also termed hyperplasia and adenomatoid transformation

Mineralization (calcification, calcium deposits, lithiasis, nephrocalcinosis) — mineral deposits are common in the urinary bladder, renal pelvis, and renal tubules; mineral deposits may be seen in the renal papilla and pelvic mucous membrane which are often accompanied by focal fibrosis; granuloma formation, and ulceration or hyperplasia of the overlying transitional epithelium; intratubular deposits consist generally of small concretions in the lumens that are found commonly in females at the corticomedullary junction of otherwise normal kidneys; usually occurrence in young female rats 6% (Sprague-Dawley; 2000 males 3.5%; 2000 females 27%); mineralization of large arteries is the most common vascular lesion; associated with nephropathy

Nephropathy (chronic nephrosis, chronic nephritis, chronic progressive nephrosis, glomerulonephritis, glomerulonephrosis, glomerulonephropathy, glomerulosclerosis, glomerular hyalinosis) — very common and important renal disease in adult and aged rats; can be observed as early as 5 months; more frequent and severe in males than females; can become a problem in studies that exceed two years duration; strain differences have been observed; OFA-ICO rats more affected than Sprague-Dawley (Sprague-Dawley; 2000 males 56%; 2000 females 23.2%)
(Long-Evans; males 74%; females, 44%)

Pigmentation, tubular — iron-positive brownish pigment granules are commonly observed in the tubular epithelial cells of kidneys from rats older than one year of age

Pyelonephritis — sporadic finding usually associated with inflammation of the lower urinary tract; more frequent in males accompanying inflammation of the prostate, seminal vesicles, coagulation gland, and urinary bladder

Regeneration, tubular — a common finding, predominantly in males; often an early stage of progressive nephropathy; usual occurrence in young rats, males 32%, females 4% (Sprague-Dawley; 2000 males 15.5%; 2000 females 14.9%)

Tumors
    Leiomyosarcoma (Fischer 344/N; one reported in 1943 males 0.1%)
    Lipoma (lipomatous tumors, lipomatous hamartoma, angiolipoma, myolipoma, angiomyolipoma, hamartoma, mixed tumors) — very low incidence
        (Fischer 344/N; two reported in 1928 males 0.1 %; and one reported in 1944 females 0.1 %)
        (Sprague-Dawley; 585 males 0.5%, 584 females 0.3%)
    Liposarcoma (malignant mixed tumors)
        (Fischer 344/N; one reported in 1943 males 0.1%)
        (Sprague-Dawley; 585 males 0.7%, none in 584 females)
    Nephroblastoma — very low incidence
        (Fischer 344/N; one reported in 1928 males 0.1%)
        (Sprague-Dawley; none in 585 males, 584 females 0.2%)
    Polyp (Sprague-Dawley; one reported in 585 males 0.2%)
    Sarcoma, unspecified (Fischer 344/N; one reported in 1928 males 0.1%)
    Tubular cell adenoma — very low incidence
        (Fischer 344/N; 1928 males 0.4%, 1977 females 0.1%)
        (Sprague-Dawley; 585 males 0.2%, none in 584 females)
    Tubular cell adenocarcinoma — very low incidence
        (Fischer 344/N; three reported in 1928 males 0.2%; and two reported in 1977 females 0.1%)
        (Sprague-Dawley; 585 males 0.2%, none in 584 females)
    Transitional cell papilloma — very low incidence (Fischer 344/N; three reported in 1928 males 0.2%)

Transitional cell carcinoma — Very low incidence (Fischer 344/N; two reported in 1928 males 0.2%

Lacrimal Gland (*see* Harderian Gland)

Tumor

Adenoma — very low incidence (Fischer 344/N; one reported in 1983 females 0.1%)

Larynx (also *see* Trachea)

Calcification (mineralization), ossification — the laryngeal cartilage may become focally calcified or ossified at any age in the rat

Inflammation, acute or chronic (laryngitis) — frequent findings of small foci of inflammatory cell infiltrates; submucosal aggregates of lymphoid cells are common in untreated rats; may be involved as a part of a variety of either upper or lower respiratory tract infections

Metaplasia, squamous — the laryngeal mucosa of the rat is particularly sensitive to inhaled irritants and responds by undergoing squamous metaplasia

Liver

Angiectasis (peliosis hepatis, telangiectasis) — common finding especially in male Fischer 344 rats; widely dilated vascular spaces lined by normal appearing endothelium which results in blood filled cystic spaces and distortion of the sinusoids (Sprague-Dawley; 2000 males 13.1%; 2000 females 15.4%)

Atrophy, hepatocyte — occasional finding resulting from local anoxia as during angiectasis or centrilobular congestion in mononuclear cell leukemia and malnutrition

Congestion — dilatation of sinusoids is a common finding dependent on the mode of death and length of time before tissue fixation; frequently centrilobular and more pronounced after cardiac failure; simple periportal sinusoidal is characterized by dilated spaces conforming in position and shape to normal appearing sinusoids

Cirrhosis — unusual finding of regenerating nodules of hepatocytes within encircling bands of fibrous tissue and associated cell necrosis

Cytomegaly — common finding in hepatocytes of aged rats

Degeneration — occurs in a variety of forms associated with metabolic changes, necrosis, and inflammation

Degeneration, cystic, focal (spongiosis hepatis, cystic focus, focal cystic change) — common finding in aged rats in which multilocular cystic lesions contain a finely granular or flocculent eosinophilic material; the cystlike cavities are not lined by epithelial or endothelial cells and occasionally contain erythrocytes

Dilatation, sinusoidal (*see* Angiectasis and Congestion)

Enlargement (*see* Hepatocytic hypertrophy)

Extramedullary hematopoiesis — frequent finding as foci along sinusoids or around central veins and portal vessels

Clear cell change — diffuse clear cell change may be seen in nonfasting normal, well-fed rats associated with storage of glycogen; focal clear cell changes are a form of the cellular alterations

Fatty change (fatty metamorphosis, lipidosis) — fat vacuoles in individual hepatocytes occur spontaneously in random patterns and increase with age; in foci of cellular alteration, fatty changes are termed vacuolated; diffuse fatty changes occur occasionally in aged or sick animals or associated with severe or metastatic neoplasia (Sprague-Dawley; 2000 males 23.5%, 2000 females 16.9%)

Fibrosis — common finding associated with cirrhosis and a variety of degenerative, necrotic, and inflammatory lesions

Fibrosis, peribiliary — common in aging rats and often involves only a few portal triads

Hepatocytic cellular alteration, focal — frequent finding of foci from one to several lobules in diameter consisting of hepatocytes; identified as clear cell, eosinophilic, basophilic, vacuolated, and mixed cell foci
(Sprague-Dawley; 585 males 21.2%, 585 females 22.2%)
(Sprague-Dawley; 2000 males 23.4%, 2000 females 22.4%

Hepatodiaphragmatic nodule (HDN) — common developmental anomaly in Fischer (F344) strain (1–11%), rare in other strains; usually a rounded mass protruding from diaphragmatic surface of median lobe

Hyperplasia, hepatocellular (hyperplastic nodule) — occasional finding of focal areas from a few cells, to several larger than a lobule consisting of normal or hypertrophic hepatocytes, portal tracts, and bile ducts (Sprague-Dawley; 2000 males 26.2%, 2000 females 28.1%)

Hypertrophy, hepatocytic — the most common form is cytomegaly in aged rats; less common finding in aged rats associated with degeneration, necrosis, or inflammation

Inclusion bodies, intranuclear — uncommon finding in hepatocytes of aged rats resulting from invaginations of the cytoplasm

Inflammation (hepatitis) — very common incidental finding (Sprague-Dawley; 2000 males 6.2%, 2000 females 4.2%); up to 80% of young rats have small aggregates of lymphoid cells or chronic inflammation and granulomas scattered in the liver; larger foci are associated with coagulative necrosis which rarely may be related to *Bacillus piliformis* (Tyzzer's disease) or salmonellosis in laboratory rats; chronic inflammation must be distinguished from extramedullary hematopoiesis, leukemias, and lymphomas

Karyomegaly — common finding in hepatocytes of aged rats

Necrosis — sporadic finding usually associated with inflammation, neoplasia, or systemic disease (Sprague-Dawley; 2000 males 6.1%, 2000 females 5.4%); individual cell necrosis (apoptosis) of single or small aggregates of hepatocytes is a sporadic finding; massive necrosis (infarction) is usually a result of vascular occlusion

Parasites — *Cysticercus fasciolaris* is the larval stage of *Taenia taeniaeformis,* forms cystic cavities with dense fibrous walls attached to the liver, and can result in the formation of sarcoma

Peliosis hepatis (*see* Angiectasis)

Pigmentation — a variety of pigments occur in the liver; lipofuscin (ceroid) in hepatocytes, bile pigment in canaliculi and ducts, and hemosiderin in Kupffer cells

Spongiosis hepatis (*see* Degeneration, cystic)

Tumors — primary tumors have low frequency in rats

Hemangioma (angioma, hemangioendothelioma) — (Fischer 344/N; one reported in 3569 males < 0.1%)

Hemangiosarcoma (angiosarcoma, hemangioendotheliosarcoma) — occasional (Sprague-Dawley; none in 585 males, 585 females 0.3%)

Hepatoblastoma — rare finding, may be undifferentiated variant of hepatocellular carcinoma; often concurrent with other hepatocellular tumors

Hepatocellular adenoma (including neoplastic nodule) — low incidence
(Fischer 344/N; 1928 males 4.1%, 1979 females 2.3%)
(Sprague-Dawley; 585 males 4.6%, 585 females 5.8%)

Hepatocellular carcinoma — uncommon in Sprague-Dawley and Fischer 344 strains
(Fischer 344/N; 1928 males 1.0%, 1979 females 0.2%)
(Sprague-Dawley; 585 males 2.4%, 585 females 0.2%)

Histiocytic sarcoma (malignant histiocytoma) — low incidence; often involves the liver and sometimes the liver appears to be the primary site

Histiocytoma, fibrous (Fischer 344/N; one reported in 1350 males 0.07%; and one reported in 1351 females 0.07%)

Lipoma — very low incidence (Fischer 344/N; one reported in 1928 males 0.1%)

Neoplastic nodule — a term used by some pathologists which combined the benign hepatocellular proliferative lesions, hyperplasia and adenoma (*see* Hepatocellular adenoma)

Sarcomas — most nonvascular sarcomas are rare in the liver; the majority reported have been associated with the larval tapeworm, *C. fasciolaris*

Secondary tumors — a large variety of malignant tumors may metastasize or have multicentric involvement of the liver, especially leukemia and lymphoma

Bile ducts

Cholangiofibrosis (adenofibrosis) — characterized by excessive proliferation of fibrous tissue and bile ducts; uncommon in rats

Cholestasis — sporadic finding usually associated with inflammation of liver and bile ducts

Cyst — solitary and multiple cysts commonly occur in livers of aged rats

Fibrosis, focal (peribiliary fibrosis, peribiliary sclerosis) — common in aging rats; often involves only a few portal triads

Hyperplasia — common in old rats; may be cystic; often accompanied by peritubular fibrosis and inflammatory cells; reduced by food restriction

Inflammation (cholangitis) — occasional finding of acute inflammatory cells increases with age; increased by bile duct obstruction and cholestasis; frequently accompanies bile duct hyperplasia and peritubular fibrosis

Tumors — uncommon in rats

Cholangioma (bile duct adenoma) — uncommon

(Fischer 344/N; one reported in 1928 males 0.1%)

(Sprague-Dawley; 585 males 0.2%, 585 females 0.2%)

Cholangiocarcinoma — very low incidence

(Fischer 344/N; one reported in 1946 males 0.1%; and two reported in 1945 females, 0.1%)

(Sprague-Dawley; 585 males 0.2%, none in 585 females)

Cholangiosarcoma — none in 7137 Fischer 344/N or 1170 Sprague-Dawley rats

Lung

Abscess — occasional finding, usually in aged animals; result from local or systemic infections

Atelectasis — sporadic finding of collapsed alveoli resulting from obstructive bronchial disease or neoplasms

Bronchiectasis — dilatation of bronchi or bronchioles usually result from infections with chronic inflammation; may be accompanied by squamous metaplasia

Bronchopneumonia — occasional finding in aged rats; frequent in younger animals on gavage experiments

Congestion — frequent finding associated with agonal changes related to the mode of death; marked in animals found dead; accompanied by edema in cardiac failure

Chronic venous congestion — occasional finding associated with thrombosis of the left atrium; accompanied by alveolar septa thickening and fibrosis (fibrosing alveolitis or interstitial pneumonia)

Edema — sporadic accompanying cardiac failure

Emphysema — focal emphysema may be found associated with inflammation and fibrosis or spontaneously in certain susceptible animals

Fibrosis — occasionally found as focal lesions in association with chronic and granulomatous inflammation; diffuse segmental fibrosis (fibrosing alveolitis) secondary to
chronic venous congestion

Hemorrhage — frequent finding associated with agonal changes related to the mode of
death or method of sacrifice

Hyperplasia, alveolar epithelium, focal (adenomatous hyperplasia, pulmonary adenomatosis, alveolar cell hyperplasia, epithelialization) — frequent finding, usually multicentric, increases with increased age

Hyperplasia, alveolar macrophage (foam cells, histiocytosis, lipidosis) — common finding of collections of foamy alveolar macrophages in older rats which may be associated with chronic or granulomatous inflammation and cholesterol clefts, may have fine
particulate pigment; usual occurrences in young rats 16–20%

Hyperplasia, goblet cell — hypersecretion by mucous cells of the bronchial epithelium associated with chronic inflammation

Hyperplasia, lymphoid — small aggregates of lymphocytes occur around proximal parts
of major bronchi as part of the bronchial-associated lymphoid tissue; increased lymphoid cells are common in association with inflammation and after viral and mycoplasma respiratory tract infections

Inflammation, acute or chronic (alveolitis, bronchitis, bronchopneumonia, pneumonia) —
very common to have small aggregates of lymphoid cells around bronchioles and small
vessels; usual occurrence in young rats up to 56%; more extensive inflammation, alveolitis, bronchiolitis, or pneumonitis, occurs in young rats at rates of 18–20%

Inflammation, granulomatous (granuloma) — occasional finding resulting from infections, inhaled foreign bodies, and aggregates of alveolar (foamy) macrophages with
cholesterol deposits

Metaplasia, squamous cell — common in bronchi in association with chronic inflammation

Pigmentation — pigment-laden macrophages usually containing iron (hemosiderin) may
accumulate in the air spaces; may be associated with congestion and hemorrhage

Tumors — uncommon in most strains of rats

   Alveolar/bronchiolar adenoma — low incidence
     (Fischer 344/N; 1933 males 1.3%, 1974 females 0.8%)
     (Sprague-Dawley; 585 males 0.2%, none in 585 females)

   Alveolar/bronchiolar carcinoma (adenocarcinoma) — very low incidence
     (Fischer 344/N; 1933 males 1.0%, 1974 females 0.3%)
     (Sprague-Dawley; 585 males 0.2%, none in 585 females)

   Squamous cell carcinoma — very low incidence (Fischer 344/N; 1933 males 0.2%,
     1945 females, 0.1%)

   Hemangioma (angioma, hemangioendothelioma) — rare (Fischer 344/N; one reported
     in 3567 females, < 0.1%)

   Hemangiosarcoma (angiosarcoma, hemangioendothelioma) — (Fischer 344/N; one
     reported in 3566 males, < 0.1%)

   Malignant lymphoma — sometimes lung is primary site

   Metastatic tumors — common site for metastatic malignant tumors

Lymph node (unspecified, NOS) — mandibular and mesenteric are most frequently examined

   Atrophy (hypoplasia) — depletion of lymphoid cells is common in aged rats

   Congestion — common especially in mesenteric lymph nodes; can be related to the node
    of death; usually agonal origin

   Extramedullary hematopoiesis (myeloid metaplasia, granulocytic metaplasia) — ob-
    served during increased hematopoietic demand; predominantly myelocytic

Fibrosis — associated with healing of inflammation

Granuloma (*see* Inflammation)

Hemorrhage — frequent finding; can be related to the mode of death; usually agonal in origin

Hyperplasia — occasional finding of nonneoplastic proliferation of mixed cell types usually associated with active inflammatory lesions elsewhere in the body; consist of plasma cells, lymphocytes, macrophages, and other inflammatory cell types; usual occurrence in young rats of 26–40%

Hyperplasia, lymphoid (follicular hyperplasia) — a common focal nonneoplastic proliferation of cells, predominantly paracortical lymphocytes accompanied by sinusoidal macrophages; hyperplasia of the germinal centers is a common reactive response to inflammation and systemic infections (Sprague-Dawley; 4000 males and females 13%)

Hyperplasia, plasma cell — commonly observed in sinusoids accompanying lymphoid hyperplasia

Hyperplasia, reactive (*see* Hyperplasia, lymphoid)

Inflammation (adenitis) — occasional finding, both as primary sites and secondary sites (Sprague-Dawley; 4000 males and females 2.7%); cervical lymph nodes become involved in sialodacryoadenitis; mesenteric lymph nodes may develop acute, necrotizing or granulomatous inflammation from *Salmonella spp.* infections

Inflammation, granulomatous (granuloma) — small granulomas are common findings resulting from several causes including foreign materials and infections, but most often are aggregates of pigment or ceroid-laden macrophages

Pigmentation — pigments are common finding in histiocytes or macrophages; both ceroid and iron-positive pigments may be observed

Sinus histiocytosis — very common findings in which distended sinuses contain numerous histiocytes and free macrophages; leucocytes, lymphocytes, and plasma cells also may be present; macrophages filled with ceroid or lipochrome may be seen, particularly in the mesenteric lymph nodes

Telangiectasis — occasional finding of prominent dilated blood vessels (*see* Congestion)

Tumors — lymphoreticular neoplasms have a high spontaneous incidence in rats

    Hemangioma (angioma, hemangioendothelioma) — benign vascular lesions are occasionally observed; some are believed to be congenital malformations and not true neoplasms; true tumors are uncommon (Sprague-Dawley; two reported in 581 males 0.3%)

    Hemangiosarcoma (angiosarcoma, hemangioendothelioma) (Sprague-Dawley; three reported in 581 males 0.5%)

    Histiocytic sarcoma (malignant histiocytoma) — frequently involve the liver, lymph nodes, lung, spleen, mediastinum, retroperitoneum, and subcutis; sometimes infiltrates in lymphomatous pattern; most frequent in Sprague-Dawley, Osborne-Mendel, and Wistar strains; all sites and multiple organ involvement incidence:
(Fischer 344/N; four reported in 1353 males 0.3%)
(Sprague-Dawley; 585 males 2.6%, 585 females 1.2%)

    Lymphangiosarcoma
(Sprague-Dawley; one reported in 581 males 0.2%)
(Sprague-Dawley; 4000 males and females 0.5%)

    Leukemia — frequently occur in some strains; occasionally observed at less than 6 months of age

    Leukemia, granulocytic (myeloid leukemia) — relatively common in aged rats, can occur spontaneously in rats less than 6 months of age; white cell counts in peripheral blood are often very high; splenic involvement may result in very large sizes;

myelocytic type with neutrophils is most common; eosinophilic type is sometimes observed; granulocytic leukemia must be differentiated from leukemoid reactions associated with infections and large tumors; all sites and multiple organ involvement incidence:

(Fischer 344/N; one reported in 1353 males 0.7%)

(Sprague-Dawley; 585 males 0.3%, 585 females 0.2%)

(Sprague-Dawley; 4000 males and females 0.7%)

Leukemia, mononuclear cell (large granular lymphocytic leukemia, monocytic leukemia, lymphosarcoma) — appears to arise in the spleen and secondarily involve the liver, bone marrow, lymph nodes, adrenal gland, and kidneys; very common in Fischer 344 rats (Fischer 344/N; 1936 males 33.6%, 1983 females 20.2%); incidence is reportedly decreased in males by gavage with corn oil vehicle (Fischer 344/N; 1949 males 17.1%, 1950 females 19.3%); mononuclear cell leukemia somewhat different from that of Fischer 344 rats has been reported with diffuse infiltration of spleen, liver, and lung in Wistar-Furth, Wistar, and other strains

Leukemia, myeloblastic — less common form

Leukemia, lymphocytic — high absolute lymphocyte counts in the peripheral blood resulting from increased numbers of small lymphocytes; may have extensive visceral infiltration

Leukemia, lymphoblastic — large numbers of lymphoblasts in the peripheral blood

Leukemia, stem cell — reported in young Sprague-Dawley rats; primarily affects the bone marrow with secondary involvement of central nervous system

Lymphoma, malignant — a variety of cell types occur in rats; both as monomorphic and mixed forms

Lymphoma, lymphocytic (lymphosarcoma, lymphoplasmacytic lymphoma, small cell lymphoma) — lymphoma composed of well and intermediately differentiated lymphocytes

Lymphoma, lymphoblastic (lymphoblastic lymphosarcoma) — lymphoma composed of poorly differentiated lymphocytes

Lymphoma, large cell (reticulum cell sarcoma, immunoblastic lymphoma) — these lymphomas occur in lymph nodes, spleen, liver, and bone marrow; rarely occur in skin; sometimes arise as single masses (lymphosarcoma) in lung, lymph nodes of the abdominal cavity (mesenteric and ileocecal), and thymus

Lymphoma, malignant — all types, multiple organ involvement incidence

(Fischer 344/N; 1353 males 0.37%, 1351 females 0.22%)

(Sprague-Dawley; 585 males 1.2%, 585 females 0.7%)

Plasma cell sarcoma (plasmacytoma, plasma cell lymphoma) — very low incidence finding in Sprague-Dawley rats; usually considered a form of lymphoma

Metastatic tumors — occasional; particularly malignant epithelial tumors in adjacent or lymphatic drainage areas

Mammary gland

Cystic change (cystic degeneration, duct ectasia) — frequent finding of cystic dilatation of ducts or ductules in the absence of hyperplasia in aged rats

Fibrosis — usually associated with fibroadenomas; occurs occasionally as small foci surrounding otherwise normal ducts and acini

Galactocele — common finding; characterized by prominent cystic dilatation of ducts and large cyst-like structures; rupture of the cystic lesions results in inflammation

Hyperplasia of duct epithelium and acini — common finding; hyperplasia of acinar epithelium (adenosis) and ductular epithelium can be pronounced; cystic hyperplasia has both epithelial hyperplasia and cystic change (Sprague-Dawley; one reported in 585 females 1.5%)

Inflammation (mastitis) — foci of inflammatory cells are an occasional finding; more severe inflammation including abscesses are usually associated with ruptured cysts and tumors

Tumors

Incidence varies with strain, diet, and housing; food restriction reduces the spontaneous mammary tumor incidence; the Sprague-Dawley strain females have a high spontaneous incidence of tumors; occasionally tumors are found before 6 months of age and in males

Adenoma — low incidence; a variety of types occur, including tubular and cystic forms (Fischer 344/N; 1936 males 0.1%, 1983 females 0.9%)
(Sprague-Dawley 493 males 0.4%; 585 females 6.5%)

Adenoacanthoma — a malignant tumor consisting of both glandular and squamous cell differentiation; rare (Fischer 344/N; one reported in 3572 males < 0.1%)

Adenocarcinoma (carcinoma) — the most common form of malignant mammary tumor in Sprague-Dawley rats; can become very large with necrosis, ulceration, and inflammation, leading to leukocytosis or leukemoid reactions; have various patterns including cribriform, tubular, papillary, solid, and in multiple combinations from well-differentiated to anaplastic; sometimes squamous metaplasia is observed (adenosquamous carcinoma)
(Fischer 344/N; 1936 males 0.2%, 1983 females 2.6%)
(Sprague-Dawley 493 males 0.8%, 585 females 16.8%)

Carcinosarcoma — rare; characterized by proliferating and malignant infiltrative growth of both glandular and spindle cell or sarcomatous elements (none in the Fischer 344/N and Sprague-Dawley studies)

Fibroadenoma — common in female rats; composed of benign fibrous and glandular tissues (Fischer 344/N; 1936 males 2.6%, 1983 females 29%)
(Sprague-Dawley 493 males 1.2%, 585 females 31.3%)

Fibroma — uncommon finding; most are fibroadenomas with atrophic or minimal glandular tissue (Fischer 344/N; three reported in 3572 males < 0.1 %; and one reported in 3570 females < 0.1%)

Fibrosarcoma — uncommon finding (Fischer 344/N; two reported in 1351 females 0.15%)

Intraduct papilloma — occasional finding; benign papillary growths within ducts

Mediastinum

Ectopic thyroid tissue

Mesentery (*see* also Peritoneum)

Ectopic pancreatic tissue — sporadic finding

Fat necrosis — common finding in aged rats

Inflammation (peritonitis) — common finding of small aggregates of lymphoid cells

Tumors

Mesothelioma (Fischer 344/N; 1936 males 2.7%, 1983 females 0.1%)

Paraganglioma (*see* Blood Vessels) — (Fischer 344/N; one reported in 1936 males 0.1%; and one reported in 1983 females 0.1%)

Fibroma (Fischer 344/N; one reported in 1936 males 0.1 %; and two reported in 1983 females 0.1 %)

Fibrosarcoma (Fischer 344/N; one reported in 1936 males 0.1%; and two reported in 1950 females 0.1%)

Leiomyosarcoma (Fischer 344/N; one reported in 1983 females 0.1%)

Lipoma (Fischer 344/N; one reported in 1936 males 0.1%; and two reported in 1983 females 0.1%)

Liposarcoma (Fischer 344/N; one reported in 1949 males 0.1%; and one reported in 1950 females 0.1%)

Neurofibrosarcoma (Fischer 344/N; one reported in 1936 males 0.1%; and one reported in 1983 females 0.1%)

Sarcoma, unspecified (Fischer 344/N; 1936 males 0.2%, 1983 females 0.2%)

Mouth *(see* Oral cavity)

Muscle *(see* Skeletal muscle)

Nose (nasal cavities, nasal sinuses)

Inflammation (rhinitis, sinusitis) — both acute and chronic inflammations are common and associated with respiratory tract infections and inhaled foreign materials; submucosal aggregates of lymphoid cells are common in untreated rats

Tumors — very low incidence; no spontaneous nasal tumors were reported in more than 1170 Sprague-Dawley rats

Adenoma (Fischer 344/N; two reported in 1949 males 0.1%)

Squamous cell papilloma (Fischer 344/N; one reported in 1936 males 0.1%)

Squamous cell carcinoma (Fischer 344/N; one reported in 1936 males 0.1%)

Squamous cell carcinoma of nasolacrimal duct (Fischer 344/N; two reported in 1936 males 0.1%)

Oral cavity (gingiva, nasopharynx, oropharynx, palate, pharynx)

Inflammation — nonspecific foci of inflammatory cells are occasionally observed in subepithelial tissues.

Tumors — occasional findings in oral cavity

Squamous cell papilloma (Fischer 344/N; one reported in 1936 males 0.1%; and one reported in 1983 females 0.1%)

Incidence after gavage with corn oil vehicle (Fischer 344/N; 1949 males 0.3%, 1950 females 0.3%)

Squamous cell carcinoma — usually highly invasive; infiltrate the surrounding structures and occasionally metastasize to the lungs and lymph nodes (Fischer 344/N; one reported in 1936 males 0.1%; and one reported in 1983 females 0.1%)

Mesenchymal tumors — sporadic (Fischer 344/N; none in 1936 males and 1983 females)

Ovary

Angiectasis (angiectasia) — sporadic finding

Atrophy — high incidence of small ovaries with increased age; wide variation in the appearance of these ovaries in aged rats; usually have decreased numbers of ova; may be accompanied with simple cysts, stromal fibrosis, interstitial cell hyperplasia, or tubular structures containing Sertoli-like cells

Corpus luteum — normal corpora lutea can be large; must be differentiated from luteal granulosa cell tumor or luteoma

Cyst, all types — common with occurrence of several types

Dilatation of ovarian bursa is normal as during the estrus cycle, but may be mistaken for cysts

Follicular and luteal — common; appear to develop in rats when estrus cycle becomes irregular with age

Hemorrhagic or hematomas — occasional

Parovarian *(see* Oviduct)

Simple — cysts lined by simple cuboidal or tubular epithelium; common in mature and aged females

Hyaline degeneration — usually affects corpora lutea; may undergo mineralization

Hyperplasia, granulosa cell — occasional focal finding

Hyperplasia, interstitial cell — a common aging change; must be differentiated from the relative increase associated with atrophy

Hyperplasia, sertoliform (*see* Atrophy)

Hyperplasia, epithelial cell (tubular) — uncommon in Fischer 344 rat; must be differentiated from neoplasms

Ovotestes — rare dysgenic developmental abnormalities in which female rats possess bilateral ovarian tissue and nonfunctional testicular tissue and epididymides have been reported in Sprague-Dawley rats

Pigmentation, ceroid (lipofuscin) — common; hemosiderin may also be present, usually associated with vascular changes

Tumors, ovarian tumors are observed occasionally in aged rats; classification and histogenesis is often uncertain; terminology is sometimes imprecise and varies widely

Tumors — serosal or epithelial

    Cystadenoma — very low incidence (Fischer 344/N; one reported in 1928 females 0.1%)

    Tubular adenoma (Fischer 344/N; one reported in 1928 females 0.1%)

    Tubular adenocarcinoma — none in 3886 Fischer 344/N strain

    Adenocarcinoma and cystadenocarcinoma — rare in Fischer 344/N

    Carcinoma, unspecified (NOS) — (Fischer 344/N; two reported in 1928 females 0.1%)

    Tubulostromal adenoma and adenocarcinoma — rare

    Mesothelioma — rare in Fischer 344/N rat; arise within ovarian bursa

Tumors, sex cord

    Granulosa cell tumors (include thecoma and luteoma) — can vary from almost pure granulosa cell to pure theca cell tumors; predominantly benign and unilateral

    Granulosa cell tumors — most common ovarian neoplasms in Fischer 344/N strain (Fischer 344/N; in 1958 females; benign 0.7%; malignant 0.2%) (Sprague-Dawley; one reported in 572 females 0.2%)

    Thecoma (Fischer 344/N; three reported in 1928 females 0.2%)

    Luteoma (Fischer 344/N; two reported in 1958 females 0.1%)

    Sertoli/Leydig cell tumors (androblastoma, arrhenoblastoma) — rare in aged rats (Sprague-Dawley, one reported in 572 females, 0.2%)

    Sertoli cell tumor — rare (Fischer 344/N; one reported in 1958 females 0.1%)

    Gonadal stromal tumor (undifferentiated theca-granulosa cell tumors) — low incidence (Fischer 344/N; one reported in 1928 females 0.1%)

Tumors, germ cell

    Teratoma — rare; none in 25,000 Fischer 344/N rats; none reported in more than 1170 Sprague-Dawley rats

    Dysgerminoma — rare; none in 3886 Fischer 344/N rats; one reported in Wistar strain

    Choriocarcinoma — very rare; one reported in 25,000 Fischer 344/N rats

    Ovarian yolk sac carcinoma — very rare; a few have been reported in Fischer 344/N rats and other strains

Tumors, mesenchymal (connective) tissue

    Lipoma (Fischer 344/N; one reported in 1928 females 0.1%)

    Fibroma (Fischer 344/N; one reported in 1928 females 0.1%)

    Sarcoma (Fischer 344/N; one reported in 1958 females 0.1%)

    Metastatic tumors — sporadic findings usually associated with malignant tumors of the peritoneal cavity; the most common is malignant histiocytoma (histiocytic sarcoma)

Oviducts — lesions are often associated with changes in ovary or uterus

    Cysts — common finding in mature and aged rats; must be differentiated from normal dilatation of bursa during estrous cycle; parovarian cysts around the ovaries probably arise from remnants of the paramesonephric or mesonephric ducts

Dilatation — normal in mature rats (*see* Cysts)

Inflammation (salpingitis) — uncommon in rats, can result from mycoplasma infections

Tumor

Leiomyoma — very rare; none in 3933 Fischer 344/N and 585 Sprague-Dawley rats

Pancreas (pancreas, exocrine)

Arteritis (polyarteritis nodosa, periarteritis, perivasculitis) — occasional finding in aged rats (see Blood vessels); peritoneal inflammation and malignant neoplasms may result in thrombosis and arteritis

Atrophy — common finding usually accompanying inflammation; diffuse atrophy can result from a variety of other causes, including starvation, malnutrition, zinc or copper deficiencies, and protein deprivation; characterized by diffuse loss of exocrine tissue with a general absence of inflammation and replacement by fatty tissue

Cyst — cystic dilatation of the pancreatic duct occurs occasionally; often associated with dilated bile ducts or acute inflammation

Cytoplasmic vacuolization — common finding in aged rats, apparently due to presence of lipid droplets

Dilated ducts — occasional finding (*see* Cyst)

Edema, interstitial — sporadic finding usually associated with acute inflammation, cardiac failure or as an agonal change

Eosinophilic change, focal — small irregular nonneoplastic foci of acinar cells having increased cytoplasmic eosinophilia or decreased (usual) cytoplasmic basophilia; may affect parts of single or several lobules

Fibrosis, interstitial — usually associated with chronic inflammation (Sprague-Dawley; 2000 males 6.4%, 2000 females < 1%)

Hyperplasia, acinar, focal (hyperplastic nodules) — sporadic finding in untreated rats; usually small numbers and multiple (Sprague-Dawley; 583 males 0.3%, none in 585 females)

Hyperplasia, focal of pancreatic duct — occasional finding

Inflammation (pancreatitis) — (Sprague-Dawley; 2000 males 3.8%, 2000 females 2.8%); acute inflammation occurs spontaneously as a sporadic finding in rats with leukocytes in the ducts and ductules, focal acinar cell inflammation, congestion, and interstitial edema; the duct epithelium can become very hyperplastic; fat necrosis may occur; chronic inflammation (chronic relapsing pancreatitis) usually occurs associated with lobular atrophy; early focal mononuclear intralobular infiltrates; later acinar cell degeneration and necrosis may lead to cystic (microcystic changes) dilatation of ducts and ductules (ectasia); fibrosis of interstitium increased numbers of fat cells may replace one or more lobules incidence appears influenced by strain, infrequent in Sprague-Dawley, 40% in Long-Evans strain

Pigmentation — occasional finding, usually iron-positive, associated chronic inflammation; hemosiderin may occur around islets

Tumors — occasional in aged rats

Acinar cell adenoma — very low incidence (Sprague-Dawley; 583 males 0.7%, none in 585 females)

(Fischer 344/N; 1868 males 0.3%, 1934 females 0.2%); incidence was reportedly increased in males by gavage with corn oil vehicle)

(Fischer 344/N; 1865 males 5.4%, 1875 females 0.4%)

Acinar cell carcinoma (adenocarcinoma) — rare (Fischer 344/N; none in 1868 males and none in 1934 females); incidence was reportedly increased in males by gavage with corn oil vehicle

(Fischer 344/N; 1865 males 0.3%, none in 1875 females)

Benign mixed tumor — very low incidence (Fischer 344/N; one reported in 1865 males 0.1%)

Malignant mixed tumor — very low incidence (Fischer 344/N; one reported in 1868 males 0.1%)

Pancreatic duct adenoma — very low incidence (Fischer 344/N; one reported in 1868 males 0.1%)

Parathyroid gland

Cyst — occasionally present

Fibrosis, interstitial — occasional finding

Hyperplasia, focal — occasional, sometimes multiple finding
(Sprague-Dawley; 559 males 2.7%, 550 females 0.7%)
(Sprague-Dawley; 2000 males 14%, 2000 females 1.9%)

Hyperplasia, diffuse — frequently occurs secondary to severe renal disease, a common disease in aged rats; high incidence in OFA-ICO rat is associated with severe renal disease and results in fibrous osteodystrophy

Thymic rests

Tumors

Adenoma — low incidence
(Fischer 344/N; 1303 males 0.5%, 1328 females 0.2%)
(Sprague-Dawley; 559 males 2.7%, 550 females 0.7%)

Penis

Inflammation — incidence variable; wounds are common

Tumors: squamous cell carcinoma — two reported in 51,230 Fischer 344/N rats

Pericardium

Hyperplasia, papillomatous — a reactive hyperplasia which sometimes occurs with inflammation

Inflammation — associated with inflammation of adjacent cardiac and mediastinal tissues

Tumors — associated with neoplasia of adjacent tissues

Peripheral nerve (peripheral nervous system)

Radiculoneuropathy (radicular myelinopathy, degenerative myelopathy) — common degenerative finding in several rat strains associated with increased age; characterized by focal swelling of myelin sheaths or segmental demyelinization and macrophages; most commonly affects the sciatic and tibial nerves, also the lumbar and ventral spinal nerve roots, and may involve dorsal spinal roots and spinal cord.

Tumors

Schwann cell tumors (schwannoma, benign or malignant; neurinoma, neurilemmoma, neurolemma, neurofibroma, neurofibrosarcoma, nerve sheath tumor, cystic sarcoma) — most common peripheral nerve tumors in rats; a granular cell variant has also been described

Ganglioneuroma — rare tumor, more often observed in the adrenal gland than the spinal ganglia

Peritoneum

Usually peritoneal lesions are result of changes in the mesentery, underlying intestine, or adjacent peritoneal cavity (acute, chronic, granulomatous inflammation, fat necrosis, fibrosis) (*see* also Mesentery)

Hemorrhage (hemoperitoneum) — sporadic finding resulting from rupture of intraabdominal blood vessels

Hyperplasia, mesothelial — reactive hyperplasia of the mesothelium is common, can be marked, and must be differentiated from neoplasia

Tumors

Mesothelioma (mesenchymal sarcoma) — common in Sprague-Dawley and Fischer rats, especially adjacent to the testes
(Fischer 344/N; 1936 males 2.7%, 1983 females 0.1%)

(Sprague-Dawley; two reported in 585 males 0.3%)

Metastatic tumors — common, especially sarcomas such as histiocytic sarcoma (malignant histiocytoma) and lymphoma

Pharynx (*see* Oral cavity)

Pineal gland — normal gland may appear large and be mistaken for hyperplasia or a tumor Tumors have been reported but are very rare

Pituitary gland

Atrophy — occasional finding

Cyst, simple — occasional finding, thought to be remnants of hypophyseal cleft (Rathke's pouch); occurrence 3%

Fibrosis — marked increases in connective tissue are considered normal in aged rats; focal fibrosis sometimes associated with iron pigment suggests healed lesions

Hyperplasia, focal — common proliferative findings related to hormones, diet changes, stress, light exposure, and temperature effects; may precede neoplasia

(Sprague-Dawley; 579 males 16.1%, 581 females 6.4%)

(Sprague-Dawley; 2000 males 5.6%, 2000 females 4.8%)

Tumors

Adenoma — common in several strains; adenomas may show considerable cellular pleomorphism and nuclear atypia

Adenoma pars distalis

(Fischer 344/N; 1868 males 22.8%, 1934 females 45.2%)

(Sprague-Dawley; 579 males 62.2%, 581 females 84.7%)

(Sprague-Dawley; 2000 males 37.4%, 2000 females 63.4%)

Adenoma, pars intermedia (Fischer 344/N; 1868 males 0.2%, 1934 females 0.1%)

Carcinoma (adenocarcinoma) — very low incidence; diagnosis should be made only if clear infiltration of the surrounding brain is evident

Carcinoma, pars distalis

(Fischer 344/N; 1868 males 2.3%, 1934 females 3.7%)

(Sprague-Dawley; 2000 males 3.1%, 2000 females 6.4%)

Craniopharyngiomas, malignant — rare tumors composed of squamous epithelium

(Fischer 344/N; one reported in 1898 males 0.1%)

(Sprague-Dawley; 579 males 0.2%, none in 581 females)

Pituitary, pars nervosa: glioma (Fischer 344/N; two reported in 1934 females 0.1%)

Pleura

Usually pleural lesions are the result of changes in the underlying lung or adjacent mediastinum and thorax

Tumors, mesothelioma (mesenchymal sarcoma) — very rare in Sprague-Dawley and Fischer rats; in contrast to the peritoneal serosa, especially testes (*see* Peritoneum)

Prepuce — inflammation, sporadic

Tumors — very rare

Keratoacanthoma — two reported in 51,230 Fischer 344/N rats

Squamous cell carcinoma — four reported in 51,230 Fischer 344/N rats

Preputial gland

Atrophy — occasional finding involving the acinar epithelium in aging rats

Cyst — minor cystic changes commonly accompany atrophy

Degeneration, cystic — common finding in aged males, combination of changes including atrophy of acinar cells, fibrosis, distention of ducts by secreted material and limited degrees of inflammation

Enlargement — frequently observed grossly

Hyperplasia, focal — occasional finding of the acinar epithelium in aging rats; sometimes cystic

Hyperplasia, squamous cells of duct epithelium — often accompanies suppurative inflammation or abscess
Inflammation (adenitis) — common findings which increase with age; acute adenitis
   characterized by accumulations of neutrophils which vary in severity from minimal to
   ulceration and abscess formation; chronic adenitis consists of focal and diffuse infil-
   trations by lymphocytes and occasional plasma cells with various proportions of neu-
   trophils, macrophages, foreign body giant cells, and fibrosis
Tumors — usually arise from acinar or ductal epithelium
   Adenoma — low incidence (Fischer 344/N, 1936 males 3.8%)
   Carcinoma — low incidence (Fischer 344/N, 1936 males 3.2%)
Prostate gland
   Atrophy — characterized by simple squamous epithelium and dilatation with accumula-
      tion of protein aceous secretions
   Cyst, mucinous — associated with chronic inflammation can be mistaken for a carcinoma
   Dilatation (ectasis) — usually associated with atrophy
   Edema — observed in the interstitium associated with inflammation and may represent
      an agonal change
   Hyperplasia, epithelial — reactive hyperplasia is an occasional finding associated with in-
      flammation; focal hyperplasia of the acinar epithelium is common in aged Spra-
      gue-Dawley rats; groups of 60–70 reported with range of 0.0–43.3%
      (Sprague-Dawley; 580 males 9.7%) (Fischer 344/N; 1038 males 10.3%)
   Inflammation (prostatitis) — both acute and chronic inflammatory changes are frequently
      present in aged rats; associated with inflammation of coagulating glands, seminal ves-
      icles, bulbourethral glands, and preputial glands; leukocytic foci usually occur in 14%
      of young males (dorsal lobe, Fischer 344/N; 1383 males 70.4%; ventral lobe; Fischer
      344/N; 1038 males 9.4%)
      Suppurative — usually associated with inflammation of seminal vesicles, coagulation
         glands, urinary bladder or kidneys (pyelonephritis)
      Chronic — chronic inflammation, necrosis, and fibrosis commonly occur as small
         foci in aged rats, may be accompanied by mucinous cysts
   Squamous metaplasia — occasional finding accompanying chronic inflammation and ep-
      ithelial hyperplasia
   Tumors
      Adenoma — very low incidence
      (Fischer 344/N, 1862 males 0.6%)
      (Sprague-Dawley; one reported in 580 males 0.2%)
      Carcinomas (Adenocarcinoma) — occur occasionally in certain strains of aging rats,
         especially ACI/SegHap BR rats; rare in Fischer 344/N strain; actual incidences
         may be higher than historical data indicate because carcinomas are usually reported
         in the dorsal lobe which was not routinely examined histologically
         (Fischer 344/N; none reported in 3736 males; ten reported in 51,230 Fischer 344/N rats)
         (Sprague-Dawley; none reported in 580 males)
      Lipoma (Sprague-Dawley; one reported in 580 males 0.2%)
      Sarcoma — malignant histiocytomas and various soft tissue tumors occur occasionally
         in the tissues around and in the prostate (Fischer 344/N; one leiomyosarcoma and
         one sarcoma, unspecified, reported in 51,230 rats)
Salivary gland (sublingual, mucous; parotid, serous; submandibular or submaxillary,
   mixed)
   Atrophy — occasional finding, with loss of acinar tissues and dilatation of ducts lined
      by flat epithelium; glandular tissue may be replaced by fat; and mild chronic
      inflammation may be present

Calculi (concretion, mineralization) — mineral deposits are occasionally found within the ducts

Fibrosis — occasional finding associated with inflammation

Inflammation (adenitis) — acute inflammation of the salivary gland is usually associated with virus infections, the most common being sialodacryoadenitis virus which also affects the lacrimal and Harderian glands, rat parvovirus, and cytomegalovirus

Inflammation, focal — small foci of chronic inflammation and fibrosis are sporadic findings in otherwise normal salivary glands

Tumors — spontaneous tumors are very rare

Adenoma — low incidence

Incidence after gavage with corn oil vehicle (Fischer 344/N; one reported in 1914 males 0.1%; and three reported in 1934 females 0.2%)

Adenocarcinoma — very low incidence (Fischer 344/N; one reported in 1895 males 0.1%)

Carcinoma, primary (Sprague-Dawley; one reported in 582 males 0.2%)

Squamous cell carcinoma — rare primary tumor; must be distinguished from infiltrating carcinomas

Fibrosarcoma — very low incidence (Fischer 344/N; one reported in 1895 males 0.1%)

Sarcoma — very low incidence; the most common sarcoma in Sprague-Dawley rats is the undifferentiated, cystic sarcoma; also termed malignant schwannoma (Fischer 344/N; two reported in 1895 males 0.1%)

Seminal vesicles

Atrophy — common finding associated with diffuse testicular atrophy

Dilatation, cystic — common

Inflammation — common

Chronic — most common in interstitium

Suppurative — usually associated with prostate, testes, urinary bladder, or kidney inflammation (pyelonephritis)

Tumors

Adenoma — very low incidence (Fischer 344/N; one reported in 1949 males 0.1%)

Adenocarcinoma — very rare (Fischer 344/N; one reported in 51,230 rats)

Carcinosarcoma — very low incidence (Fischer 344/N; one reported in 1936 males 0.1%)

Skeletal muscle

Atrophy — occasional focal finding accompanied by inflammation in association with spontaneous degeneration of peripheral nerves in aged rats

Inflammation, chronic (myositis) — sporadic foci of lymphoid cells; sometimes associated with atrophy

Tumors — very infrequent in rats

Lipoma (Fischer 344/N; two reported in 1949 males 0.1%)

Liposarcoma (Fischer 344/N; one reported in 1936 males 0.1%; and one reported in 1983 females 0.1%)

Fibrosarcoma — very low incidence (Fischer 344/N; one reported in 1936 males 0.1%)

Neurofibrosarcoma — very low incidence (Fischer 344/N; one reported in 1936 males 0.1%)

Hemangiosarcoma — very low incidence (Fischer 344/N; one reported in 1950 females 0.1%)

Rhabdomyosarcoma — very low incidence; must be differentiated from histiocytic sarcoma

(Fischer 344/N; 1949 males 0.2%, 1983 females 0.1%)

(Sprague-Dawley; one reported in 584 females 0.2%)

Sarcoma, unspecified (NOS) (Fischer 344/N; two reported in 1949 males 0.1%)

Skin

Acanthosis (papillomatosis) — thickening of the squamous cell layers; sporadic finding, usually with inflammation

Alopecia (hair loss) — sporadic finding, usually associated with other conditions including vices; patchy hair loss is most common; usual occurrence in young rats, 5–9%

Atrophy — occasional finding of the epidermis, sebaceous glands, and hair follicles, possibly associated with nutritional or hormone factors

Edema — subcutaneous edema is occasionally observed as a result of a variety of causes including trauma, inflammation, nutritional imbalances, or an agonal change

Epidermal cyst (inclusion cyst) — occasional finding of squamous cysts filled with keratin; sometimes accompanied by granulomatous inflammation (Sprague-Dawley; 585 males 1.7%, 584 females 0.3%)

Epidermoid cyst — occasional finding of squamous cysts containing hair follicle and sebaceous gland epithelium; sometimes accompanied by granulomatous inflammation

Fat necrosis — sporadic finding in the subcutaneous tissue; usually follows trauma or inflammation and is accompanied by granulomatous inflammation with macrophages, foreign body giant cells, fatty acid and cholesterol crystals, necrosis, and fibrosis

Hyperkeratosis — thickening of the keratin (horny) layers; sporadic finding, usually with inflammation

Inflammation — sporadic findings; usually related to trauma of the jaw, legs, feet, and tail; vary in severity and duration including focal ulceration of the epidermis, acute or acute necrotizing to chronic inflammation of the dermis and subcutis, and sometimes formation of abscesses and fibrosis; usual occurrence in young rats, males 4%; females 4%

Necrosis — usually associated with inflammation and trauma

Necrosis, gangrenous — dry gangrene involving the tail (ring tail) is associated with low humidity environment

Polyp, fibroepithelial — benign tumor-like lesions consisting of a fibrovascular stroma covered by normal appearing epidermis; considered to be hyperplastic lesions

Tumors, epidermal

Apocrine adenocarcinoma (Sprague-Dawley; one reported in 585 males 0.2%)

Basal cell adenoma (tumors) — low incidence (Fischer 344/N; 1936 males 0.7% 1950 females 0.5%)

Basal cell carcinoma — low incidence
(Fischer 344/N; 1936 males 0.7%, 1983 females 0.3%)
(Sprague-Dawley; two reported in 585 males 0.3%; one reported in 584 females 0.2%)

Basal cell epithelioma (Sprague-Dawley; one reported in 585 males 0.2%)

Inverted papilloma — the inverted papilloma forms a shallow cavity or depression usually filled with keratin and may be a type of keratoacanthoma

Keratoacanthoma — low incidence; characterized by masses of basal and squamous cells with excessive keratin formation either within a crater or as one or more superficial projections
(Fischer 344/N; 1936 males 1.6%, 1983 females 0.3%)
(Sprague-Dawley; 585 males 7.9%, 584 females 0.7%)

Sebaceous gland adenoma — very low incidence (Sprague-Dawley; two reported in 585 males 0.3%)

Sebaceous gland carcinoma (adenocarcinoma) — (Sprague-Dawley; three reported in 584 females 0.5%)

Squamous cell carcinoma — low incidence
(Fischer 344/N; 1936 males 0.9%, 1983 females 0.3%)
(Sprague-Dawley; 585 males 0.9%, 584 females 0.5%)

Squamous cell papilloma — low incidence
(Fischer 344/N; 1936 males 1.4%, 1983 females 0.3%)
(Sprague-Dawley; 585 males 2.1%, none in 584 females)
Trichoepithelioma
(Fischer 344/N; 1936 males 0.3%, 1983 females 0.1%)
Tumors, subcutaneous tissue
Hemangioma (angioma, hemangioendothelioma) — very rare; some are believed to be congenital vascular malformations, not true neoplasms (Fischer 344/N; two reported in 1949 males 0.1%)
Hemangiosarcoma (angiosarcoma, hemangioendotheliosarcoma) — very low incidence (Fischer 344/N; one reported in 1936 males 0.1%, and one reported in 1983 females 0.1%)
(Sprague-Dawley; one reported in 585 males 0.2%)
Cystic sarcoma (*see* Nerve sheath tumor, malignant) — undifferentiated sarcomas with a distinctive cystic appearance are occasionally observed in the subcutaneous tissue, salivary gland, uterus, mesentery, retroperitoneal tissues, and female genital tract; also termed malignant schwannoma
Dermatofibroma — superficial benign fibrous histiocytoma
Fibroma — low incidence
(Fischer 344/N; 1936 males 5.2%, 1983 females 1.3%)
(Sprague-Dawley; 585 males 1.9%, 584 females 0.3%)
Fibrosarcoma — low incidence
(Fischer 344/N; 1936 males 1.3%, 1983 females 1.1%)
(Sprague-Dawley; 585 males 1.2%, 584 females 0.3%)
Fibrous histiocytoma, malignant (malignant histiocytosis, extraskeletal giant cell tumor, fibrous histiocytoma, histiocytoma, one type of histiocytic sarcoma) (Fischer 344/N; 1936 males 0.2%, 1983 females 0.1%)
Hemangiopericytoma — very low incidence (Sprague-Dawley; one reported in 584 females, 0.2%)
Hibernoma (brown fat tumor) — very rare (Sprague-Dawley; one has been reported)
Histiocytic sarcoma — rare in Fischer 344/N
Lipoma — low incidence
(Fischer 344/N; 1936 males 0.4%, 1983 females 0.1%)
(Sprague-Dawley; 585 males 1.2%, 584 females 0.7%)
Liposarcoma — very low incidence; may have features of a malignant hibernoma
(Sprague-Dawley; one reported in 584 females 0.2%)
Lymphosarcoma (epitheliotropic lymphoma) — rare
Myxoma and myxosarcoma — very rare; existence is debated; usually considered as a form of fibroma or as undifferentiated sarcomas
Nerve sheath tumor, malignant (malignant schwannoma, neurilemoma, cystic sarcoma)
(Fischer 344/N; 1936 males 0.3%, 1983 females 0.2%)
(Sprague-Dawley; two reported in 585 males 0.3%; two reported in 584 females 0.3%)
Neurofibroma — low incidence (Fischer 344/N; two reported in 1936 males 0.1%)
Neurofibrosarcoma — very low incidence (Fischer 344/N; 1936 males 0.4%, 1983 females 0.3%)
Sarcoma, unspecified (undifferentiated sarcoma, sarcoma, NOS; mesenchymoma; *see* Cystic sarcoma)
(Fischer 344/N; 1936 males 0.5%, 1983 females 0.3%)
(Sprague-Dawley; one reported in 584 females 0.2%)

Spinal cord (also *see* Brain)

   Cysts, epidermal — occasional congenital finding has been reported in 2.5% of CDF strain rats with lower frequencies in Lewis and Wistar HH stains

   Radiculoneuropathy (radicular myelinopathy, degenerative myelopathy) — degeneration of the peripheral and spinal nerves in aged rats, may be accompanied by degeneration in the spinal cord and cauda equina; characterized by demyelinization, swelling of axon sheaths and astrocytes, infiltration by macrophages, and, in advanced cases, mineralization

   Pigmentation, lipofuscin — accumulates in neurons of aged rats as normal aging change

   Tumors — rare (*see* Brain)

      Astrocytoma, malignant — (Sprague-Dawley; two reported in 585 females 0.3%)

      Oligodendroglioma, malignant — (Sprague-Dawley; one reported in 585 females 0.2%)

      Malignant schwannoma (Fischer 344/N; one reported in 1936 males 0.1%)

Spleen

   Angiectasis — vascular dilatation usually focal and associated with fibrosis or scarring; sporadic

   Atrophy — lymphocyte depletion is common in aged rats; may occur as a nonspecific reaction to stress or severe weight loss

   Congestion — common finding; may be agonal related to the mode of death

   Extramedullary hematopoiesis — only occurs in rats when under various stimuli when additional hematopoiesis is required; frequently observed in female rats having mammary gland fibroadenomas, especially if large and ulcerated (Sprague-Dawley; 4000 males and females 6%)

   Fibrosis — occasional finding of increased collagenous connective tissue

   Hamartoma (*see* Nodular hyperplasia)

   Inflammation — rare; usually associated with inflammation extending from adjacent abdominal organs and peritoneum

   Hyperplasia, erythroid — increased erythroid precursors are associated with anemia, hemorrhage, or erythrocytic destruction

   Hyperplasia, lymphoid — low incidence, usually associated with systemic stimuli (Sprague-Dawley; 4000 males and females 6.2%)

   Hyperplasia, myeloid — increased immature granulocytic precursors associated with systemic inflammatory conditions

   Hyperplasia, nodular — occasional finding of well-defined, round, pale, or white nodules composed of a mixed population of mature lymphoid cells; may be hamartomas; must be differentiated from malignant lymphoma

   Hyperplasia, stromal — proliferation of mesenchymal cells associated with splenic trabeculae and marginal zones

   Pigmentation — iron-positive pigment (hemosiderin) is a normal finding in aged rats; in young rats, hemosiderin is generally more prominent in females than males; increased hemosiderin is associated with some forms of anemia, hemolysis, and increased erythrocyte destruction; lipofuscin or ceroid pigmentation occurs in some strains, including Fischer 344/N

   Mineralization — sometimes observed with necrosis; may be confused with pigmentation

   Tumors — blood vessel tumors and sarcomas are most common

      Hemangioma (angioma, hemangioendothelioma) — rare
         (Fischer 344/N; one reported in 1906 males 0.1%)
         (Sprague-Dawley; one reported in 585 males 0.2%)

      Hemangiosarcoma (angiosarcoma, hemangioendothelioma) — low incidence
         (Fischer 344/N; 1906 males 0.3%, 1961 females 0.1%)

(Sprague-Dawley; two reported in 585 males 0.3%)

Fibroma — low incidence (Fischer 344/N; one reported in 1906 males 0.1%)

Fibrosarcoma — low incidence (Fischer 344/N; one reported in 1348 males 0.07%)

Fibrous histiocytoma — low incidence (Fischer 344/N; one reported in 1348 males 0.07%)

Histiocytic sarcoma (malignant histiocytoma) — (Sprague-Dawley; 4000 males and females 0.2%)

Leiomyoma — very rare (Fischer 344/N; one reported in 1906 males 0.1%)

Leiomyosarcoma (Fischer 344/N; two reported in 1348 males 0.15%, and one reported in 1961 females 0.1%)

Leukemia, myelogenous (myeloid or granulocytic) (also *see* Lymph node) (Sprague-Dawley; 585 males 0.3%, 585 females 0.2%) (Sprague-Dawley; 4000 males and females 0.8%)

Leukemia, mononuclear cell (large granular lymphocytic leukemia, monocytic leukemia, lymphosarcoma) — appears to arise in the spleen and secondarily involve the bone marrow and lymph nodes; common in Fischer 344 rats (Fischer 344/N; 1936 males 33.6%, 1983 females 20.2%); incidence reportedly is decreased in males by gavage with corn oil vehicle (Fischer 344/N; 1949 males 17.1%, 1950 females 19.3%)

Lipoma (Fischer 344/N; one reported in 279 males 0.36%)

Lymphosarcoma (malignant lymphoma) — frequently involves the spleen as well as lymph nodes; uncommon in Fischer 344/N strain (also *see* Lymph node) (Sprague-Dawley; 4000 males and females 0.5%)

Sarcoma, unspecified (NOS) — low incidence (Fischer 344/N; 1906 males 0.4%, 1961 females 0.1%)

Stomach (glandular)

Atrophy — focal atrophy with fibrosis and dilatation of the gastric glands is occasionally observed in aged rats and has been reported to be very common in some Sprague-Dawley colonies

Congestion — common finding resulting as an agonal change or accompanying inflammation

Cyst — common to have cystic dilatation of glands accompanied by atrophy, chronic inflammation, hyperplasia, or mineralization (calcification)

Ectopic pancreatic tissue — sporadic finding

Erosion (*see* Ulcer)

Diverticulum — rare finding

Hyperplasia, glandular (adenomatous hyperplasia, hypertrophy, hypertrophic gastritis, proliferative gastritis, hyperplastic gastropathy) — occasional finding in aged rats of hyperplastic and cystic glands; thickened lamina propria, focal chronic inflammation, and dilated submucosal blood vessels (Sprague-Dawley; 2000 males 1.3%, 2000 females 1%)

Inflammation (gastritis) — acute and chronic active inflammation are common findings, often accompanying erosions or ulcerations; scattered inflammatory cells can occur in the mucosa without ulceration or necrosis; occasionally crypts contain leukocytes (crypt abscess); chronic inflammation with lymphoid cells is occasionally observed in the submucosa (Sprague-Dawley; 2000 males 1.2%, 2000 females 1.2%)

Mineralization (calcification) — focal aggregates of calcium are found in the gastric glandular epithelium; metastatic calcification occurs in the glandular mucosa associated with severe renal disease and parathyroid hyperplasia; dystrophic calcification also occurs in the smooth muscles (Sprague-Dawley; 2000 males 3.4%, 2000 females 1%)

Necrosis — superficial necrosis (erosion) and deep necrosis (ulceration) are common findings (*see* Ulcer); (Sprague-Dawley; 2000 males 4.2%, 2000 females 4%)

Ulcer — erosions and ulcers (focal necrosis) are sporadic low-incidence findings which can result from a variety of causes including cold, restraint, stress, shock, vascular occlusion, and feeding schedule; accompanied by acute or chronic active inflammation (acute or chronic necrotizing inflammation) (Sprague-Dawley; 2000 males 6.5%, 2000 females 5%)

Tumors — rare in rats

Adenoma — very rare (Fischer 344/N; none in 1912 males and 1955 females)

Adenocarcinoma (carcinoma) — very low incidence (Fischer 344/N; one reported in 1912 males 0.1%)

Fibrosarcoma — very low incidence (Fischer 344/N; one reported in 1924 males 0.1%)

Neurofibrosarcoma — very low incidence (Fischer 344/N; one reported in 1912 males 0.1%)

Sarcoma — very low incidence (Fischer 344/N; one reported in 1955 females 0.1%)

Stomach (nonglandular) (*see* Forestomach)

Subcutaneous tissue (*see* Skin)

Testes

Arteritis (periarteritis, polyarteritis nodosa) — occasional finding; usually in association with other organs

Atrophy of seminiferous tubules — common finding occurs in a variety of patterns and frequencies; may be associated with a relative increase in Sertoli cell numbers; may be observed at the first year of life; usual incidence rate in young males is 2%; pressure atrophy is often observed adjacent to large tumors, especially interstitial cell tumors such as in Fischer (F344) rats (Sprague-Dawley; 2000 males 12.3%)

Atrophy, focal — atrophy associated with aging usually begins as a focal lesion and may involve one or both testes; term focal may be used for lesions affecting less than 50% of the seminiferous tubules of the testis

Atrophy, diffuse — usually affects most or the whole of one or both testes; term may be used for lesions affecting 50% or more of the seminiferous tubules; often leaving only Sertoli cells in the tubules; tubules are usually smaller with thin walls; giant cells are associated with degenerated epithelium; mineralized deposits may be present

Degeneration, cystic — an age-related change characterized by the presence of fluid-filled cystic spaces; usually associated with focal atrophy

Dilatation — atrophy must be differentiated from simple dilatation of the seminiferous tubules

Edema — must be differentiated from a common artifact resembling central edema

Inflammation, spermatic granulomas — occasional

Interstitial (Leydig) cell hyperplasia — common finding especially in strains with high frequencies of interstitial cell tumors; may precede tumor formation; usually associated with testicular atrophy
(Sprague-Dawley; 580 males 3.4%)

Mineralization, focal — common

Necrosis, hemorrhagic, focal — reported as a result of parvovirus infections in adult rats.

Tumors

Adenomatoid tumor (mesothelioma) — rare tumor observed in epididymis, capsule, or spermatic cord of Sprague-Dawley rats (Sprague-Dawley; two malignant mesotheliomas reported in 585 males 0.3%) (*see* Peritoneum)

Hemangioma (angioma, hemangioendothelioma) — uncommon (Fischer 344/N; none reported in 1910 males)

Interstitial (Leydig) cell adenoma — most common testicular tumor; often bilateral, incidence increases with age; high incidence in several rat strains, especially in Fischer (F344)

(Fischer 344/N; 1910 males 87.8%)

(Sprague-Dawley; 585 males 6.5%)

(Sprague-Dawley; 2000 males 6.7%)

Interstitial (Leydig) cell carcinoma — uncommon to very low incidence depending on criteria used for diagnosis; up to 10% of interstitial cell tumors

(Fischer 344/N; one reported in 1350 males 0.07%)

(Sprague-Dawley; one reported in 585 males 0.2%)

Leukemias and lymphomas — occasionally infiltrate the testes

Malignant histiocytoma (histiocytic sarcoma) — occasional finding

Seminoma — very rare (Fischer 344/N; none reported in 1910 males)

Sertoli cell tumor — very rare (Fischer 344/N; none reported in 1910 males)

Teratoma — very rare (Fischer 344/N; none reported in 1910 males)

Thymus

Atrophy — normal physiological depletion of lymphocytes (involution) and proliferation of epithelial cells begins at sexual maturity and proceeds under the influence of sex and strain; the atrophy is accelerated by various infections and other diseases, stress, and trauma; as the lymphoid tissue of the cortex decreases, the Hassall's corpuscles become more prominent (Sprague-Dawley; 4000 males and females 10.7%)

Cyst — sporadic findings in both cortex and medulla; some cysts can be large and lined by columnar or flattened, squamous epithelium; some are derived from remnants of branchial endoderm, the thymopharyngeal duct (Sprague-Dawley; 4000 males and females 1.7%)

Ectopic parathyroid tissue — uncommon finding within the thymic capsule

Hyperplasia, cystic (cystic change, epithelial hyperplasia) — Hassall's corpuscles sometimes become cystic and hyperplastic; more common in Sprague-Dawley females

Hyperplasia, lymphoid — rare finding in rats (Sprague-Dawley; 4000 males and females 1.4%)

Hyperplasia, tubular (epithelial hyperplasia) — frequent finding especially in rats older than 2 years of age, especially Fischer 344/N

Tumors

Histiocytic sarcoma (malignant histiocytoma) (Sprague-Dawley; 4000 males and females 0.3%)

Leukemia, myelogenous (myeloid or granulocytic) (Sprague-Dawley; 4000 males and females 0.3%)

Lymphosarcoma — rare tumors in Fischer 344/N rats which arise in the thymus and extend into adjacent mediastinal tissues without splenic involvement (Sprague-Dawley; 4000 males and females 0.4%)

Thymoma — rare tumors composed of epithelial cells with various amounts of lymphoid cells; often large tumors resembling adenocarcinomas; may be infiltrative in the mediastinum (Fischer 344/N; 1484 males 0.2%, 1597 females 0.1%)

Thymoma, benign — (Sprague-Dawley; 530 males 0.4%, 537 females 0.6%)

Thyroid gland

Amyloidosis — very rare observation in rats; usually associated with C-cell (medullary) carcinomas

Cyst — common finding; usually arise from ultimobranchial duct remnants; single large follicles are normal in mature rats and should not be designated as cysts

Thymic rests — ectopic thymus occurs in 2–3% of young rats

Hyperplasia, C-cell, focal — common (frequent in Long-Evans strain)

(Sprague-Dawley; 583 males 8.6%, 581 females 13.3%)

(Sprague-Dawley; 2000 males 6.2%, 2000 females 7.8%)

Hyperplasia, follicular cell, focal — common (Sprague-Dawley; 583 males 1.9%, 581 females 0.5%)

Inflammation — focal acute inflammation and chronic inflammation are occasionally observed; chronic lymphocytic thyroiditis is sometimes reported in some strains

Pigmentation (hemosiderosis) — iron-positive pigment can be observed occasionally, usually in the large dilated follicles.

Tumors

C-cell tumors — common finding (Fischer 344/N; 1904 males 12%, 1938 females 11%)

C-cell adenoma — low incidence
(Fischer 344/N; 1904 males 7.7%, 1938 females 8.0%)
(Sprague-Dawley; 583 males 6.5%, 581 females 5.9%)
(Sprague-Dawley; 2000 males 3.5%, 2000 females 2.9%)

C-cell (medullary) carcinoma (adenocarcinoma)
(Fischer 344/N; 1904 males 3.8%, 1938 females 3.4%)
(Sprague-Dawley; 583 males 1.9%, 581 females 0.5%)
(Sprague-Dawley; 2000 males 2.8%, 2000 females 2.4%)

Follicular cell adenoma — low incidence
(Fischer 344/N; 1904 males 0.7%, 1938 females 0.6%)
(Sprague-Dawley; 583 males 3.9%, 581 females 1.5%)

Follicular cell adenocarcinoma (carcinoma) — very low incidence
(Fischer 344/N; 1904 males 0.5%, 1938 females 0.4%)
(Sprague-Dawley; 583 males 2.2%, 581 females 1.4%)

Tongue

Inflammation — uncommon

Tumors

Squamous cell papilloma (Fischer 344/N; 3572 males 0.3%, 3570 females 0.4%)

Squamous cell carcinoma (Fischer 344/N; one reported in 3572 males 0.03%)

Schwann cell tumors (schwannoma, benign or malignant; nerve sheath tumor, malignant) (Sprague-Dawley; one reported in 525 males 0.2%)

Tooth

Dysplasia

Malocclusion — acquired and genetic predisposition

Tumors — very low incidence

Odontoma (Fischer 344/N; two reported in 1936 males 0.1%)

Trachea

Inflammation, acute or chronic (tracheitis) — frequent findings of small foci of inflammatory cell infiltrates; submucosal aggregates of lymphoid cells are common; may be involved as a part of a variety of either upper or lower respiratory tract infections

Tumors: Adenocarcinoma (Fischer 344/N; one reported in 1934 males 0.1%)

Ureter (*see* Kidney)

Urethra

Inflammation, acute or chronic (urethritis) — sporadic; most inflammation in rats is usually associated with inflammation of the bladder and prostate, or pyelonephritis

Mucous plugs — occasional (*see* Urinary bladder)

Tumors — rare

Transitional cell carcinoma (adenocarcinoma) (Fischer 344/N; one reported in 1936 males 0.1%)

Urinary bladder

Inflammation, acute or chronic (cystitis) — sporadic; infiltrations of small numbers of inflammatory cells are common; most inflammation in rats is usually associated with inflammation of the prostate or pyelonephritis; the brown Norway rat (BN/Bi) has usually high frequency, probably secondary to ureteric or bladder tumors or urolithiasis (Sprague-Dawley; 2000 males 2.5%, 2000 females 0.7%)

Dilatation — frequently observed at necropsy; important only if obstruction is present

Hyperplasia, urothelial — focal (nodular) or diffuse; uncommon; usually a reactive response of the transitional cell epithelium associated with chronic inflammation or calculi; hyperplasia, especially papillary, must be differentiated from neoplasia (Sprague-Dawley; 2000 males 2.8%, 2000 females 0.7%)

Metaplasia, squamous — occasionally observed associated with chronic inflammation in aged rats; reported to occur as a result of vitamin A-deficient diets

Mineralization (calcification, calculi, stones) — calculi are usually a sporadic finding; some strains have higher frequencies than others which may relate to diet and metabolism; calculi have been reported to be related to increased tumor incidences

Mucous plugs — mucinous, hyaline amorphous or proteinaceous material occasionally present; usually considered incidental finding unless there is evidence of urinary obstruction; must be differentiated from calculi; other small rounded eosinophilic (proteinaceous) droplets may be observed in normal bladders which seem to arise from the urothelium

Tumors — spontaneous occurrence is very low

    Polyp (Sprague-Dawley; one reported in 581 females 0.2%)

    Transitional cell papilloma — very low incidence (Fischer 344/N; 1858 males 0.2%, 1932 females 0.2%)

    Transitional cell carcinoma (adenocarcinoma) — very low incidence (Fischer 344/N; two reported in 1891 males 0.1%; and one reported in 1932 females 0.1%)

    (Sprague-Dawley; 581 males 0.2%, 581 females 0.2%)

Uterus

Adenomyosis — rare finding of endometrial glands within the myometrium of aged rats

Atrophy — thinning of the endometrium and myometrium increases with age

Cysts (cystic change) — cystic dilated glands are common in the endometrium

Dilatation — common; uterine horns normally become distended with intraluminal fluid including mucus during the estrous cycle (proestrus); usual incidence is 14% in young female rats; must be differentiated from hydrometra

Fibrosis — increased amounts of collagen in endometrium and myometrium; accompanies cystic endometrial hyperplasia

Hydrometra — common; excessive dilatation of the uterus in aged rats

Hyperplasia, cystic endometrial — regularly results after prolonged estrogen exposure as occurs with ovarian follicular cysts and granulosa cell tumors

Hyperplasia and hypertrophy, stromal cell — usually associated with cystic endometrial hyperplasia

Hypertrophy, portio vaginalis uteri or cervical — sporadic finding in old rats which could be misinterpreted as a leiomyoma or fibroma

Inflammation (acute endometritis, chronic endometritis, myometritis, pyometra) — inflammation is sporadic in the endometrium; often occurs in association with vaginal inflammation; usually accompanies obstructive or neoplastic lesions; most inflammatory changes are associated with bacterial or mycoplasma infections

Metaplasia, squamous — usually associated with pyometra

Polyps, inflammatory — focal hyperplasia resulting from inflammation; must be differentiated from benign neoplastic polyps

Pyometra — suppurative inflammation (*see* Inflammation)

Tumors — occasional finding in aged rats

    Adenoma (polypoid adenoma or glandular polyp) — very low incidence
        (Fischer 344/N; 1966 females 0.2%)

    Adenocarcinoma — not common; usually polypoid
        (Fischer 344/N; 1966 females 0.4%)
        (Sprague-Dawley; one reported in 572 females 0.2%)

    Endometrial stromal polyp — common benign tumor in uterine horns; can be predominantly stromal, glandular or mixed; some polyps are probably not true neoplasms, but focal hyperplasia
        (Fischer 344/N; 1966 females 21.4%)
        (Sprague-Dawley; one reported in 572 females 0.2%)

    Endometrial stromal sarcoma — common malignant tumor
        (Fischer 344/N; 1966 females 1.1%)
        (Sprague-Dawley; one reported in 572 females 0.2%)

    Fibroma — occasional finding; must be differentiated from leiomyoma
        (Fischer 344/N; three reported in 1934 females 0.2%)
        (Sprague-Dawley; one fibroma of cervix reported in 261 females 0.4%)

    Fibrosarcoma — occasional finding; must be differentiated from leiomyosarcoma

    Granular cell tumor (Fischer 344/N; one reported in 1934 females 0.1%)

    Hemangioma (angioma, hemangioendothelioma)
        (Fischer 344/N; two reported in 1966 females 0.1%)
        (Sprague-Dawley; one of cervix reported in 261 females 0.4%)

    Hemangiosarcoma (angiosarcoma, hemangioendotheliosarcoma) — rare (Fischer 344/N; none reported in 1966 females)

    Leiomyoma — occasional tumors which may extend into the vagina; low incidence
        (Fischer 344/N; three reported in 1966 females 0.2%)
        (Sprague-Dawley; two reported in 584 females 0.3%)

    Leiomyosarcoma — low incidence
        (Fischer 344/N; four reported in 1966 females 0.2%)
        (Sprague-Dawley; one reported in 584 females 0.2%)
        (Sprague-Dawley; one of cervix reported in 261 females 0.4%)

    Lipoma — occasional tumors in Sprague-Dawley rats

    Malignant schwannoma (*see* Sarcoma, cystic) (Fischer 344/N; two reported in 1966 females 0.1%)

    Sarcoma, cystic — undifferentiated sarcoma with cystic areas which resembles cystic sarcoma of subcutis; also considered to be a form of malignant schwannoma

    Sarcoma, unspecified (NOS) (Fischer 344/N; three reported in 1966 females 0.2%)

    Squamous cell carcinoma
        (Fischer 344/N; two reported in 1966 females 0.1%)
        (Sprague-Dawley; two reported in 584 females 0.3%)

Vagina

    Inflammation, suppurative — occasional finding which is usually associated with changes of the uterus; must be differentiated from normal cyclical changes of metestrus and diestrus

    Dilatation (imperforate vagina) — occasional finding with massive cystic dilatation which may be mistaken for a cyst

    Fibrosis — increased deposition of collagen reported in the walls with increasing age

    Tumors

        Fibroma
            (Fischer 344/N; one reported in 1950 females 0.1%)

(Sprague-Dawley; one reported in 520 females 0.2%)
Granular cell tumor (Fischer 344/N; one reported in 1983 females 0.1%)
Leiomyosarcoma (Fischer 344/N; one reported in 1950 females 0.1%)
Sarcoma (Fischer 344/N; one reported in 1983 females 0.1%)
Squamous cell carcinoma — occasional finding in aged Sprague-Dawley rats (Sprague-Dawley; two reported in 520 females 0.4%)
Squamous cell papilloma (Fischer 344/N; one reported in 1950 females 0.1%)
Zymbal's gland (*see* Ear)

SECTION 5. GROSS AND HISTOPATHOLOGICAL FINDINGS IN CONTROL LABORATORY DOGS[47–79]

The dog preferred for regulatory toxicity studies is the beagle. These animals are bred for laboratory use, have known parentage, are generally free of disease, have a convenient size, and are easy to handle. The following findings are primarily reported for the laboratory beagle.

Adrenal gland, cortex
    The width of the various zones in the cortex can vary considerably. The zona glomerulosa may be thin or appear to be absent in places. Occasionally, medulla cells can be observed in the cortex.
    Degeneration — fatty degeneration was reported. This degeneration must be distinguished from normal variation in vacuolation.
    Inflammation — focal inflammation occurs infrequently. Mild focal inflammation was reported in 5 (8%) of 647 dogs.
    Hyperplasia — focal cortical or nodular hyperplasia was reported in 19 (3%) of 647 dogs.
    Vacuolation of cortical cells varies greatly from animal to animal.
Adrenal gland, medulla
    Occasionally cortical cells can be observed in the medulla.
Aorta (*see* Blood vessel)
Artery (*see* Blood vessel)
Blood
    Anemia is an absolute decrease in the packed cell volume, hemoglobin concentration, and red blood cell count. The clinical signs of anemia include pale mucous membranes, weakness, fatigue, labored breathing upon exertion, rapid heart rate, and altered heart sound such as a murmur. Hemolytic diseases result in anemia accompanied by icterus (jaundice), a yellowish pigmentation of the mucous membranes associated with deposition of bile pigment, especially bilirubin. Anemia with icterus can follow extensive hemorrhage or excessive lysis of red blood cells (hemolysis).
    Bacteremia — a persistent presence of bacteria in the blood is associated with canine brucellosis (*Brucella canis*).
Blood vessel (major)
    Collection of blood samples from the cephalic vein very rarely results in sufficient injury to cause lesions.
    Congenital patent ductus arteriosus was observed grossly in 1 (0.1%) of 1000 dogs.
    Degeneration, aorta — focal medial degeneration was reported in 1 (0.1%) of 647 dogs.
    Inflammation (arteritis) occurred in 2% of young beagles. Extramural periarteritis of the coronary artery was reported in 1 (0.1%) of 647 dogs.
    Mineralization of the aorta occurred occasionally in the aortic media near the base of the heart in 2–3% of young beagles.

Bone

    Fractures of ribs are unusual gross findings and were observed grossly in 1 (0.1%) of 1000 dogs.

    Chondrodystrophy of costochondral junction was reported in 1 (0.1%) of 647 dogs.

Brain

    Degeneration — degenerating axis cylinders may be observed as spherical, eosinophilic granular structures in the medulla oblongata, pons, or anterior cervical spinal cord, most common in the gracilis tract and nucleus. These structures apparently have no neurological or pathological significance.

    Gliosis — focal proliferation or small subependymal collections of glial cells are observed usually around the anterior parts of the lateral ventricles. Hemorrhage is occasionally seen in brains of untreated laboratory dogs. Brain hemorrhage was reported in 2 of 37 (5%) untreated beagle dogs.

    Hydrocephalus is characterized by dilatation of the ventricles or subarachnoid space as a result of abnormal accumulation of cerebrospinal (CSF) fluid. When the dilatation is limited to the ventricles, the usual form, it is termed internal hydrocephalus. When it affects the subarachnoid space, it is termed external hydrocephalus. When both locations are affected, it is termed communicating hydrocephalus. Extensive dilatation of the lateral ventricles may be found during trimming of brains from dogs that showed no neurological signs. It is the most frequently reported lesion of the nervous system of dogs, is probably congenital in origin, and is common in laboratory beagles. Hydrocephalus was observed grossly in 14 (1%) of 1000 dogs. A sponge-like alteration has been reported in the brain tissue adjacent to ventricular hydrocephalus.

    Inflammation (encephalitis, meningitis, meningoencephalitis) — chronic focal meningitis is common. It occurred in 44 (7%) of 630 dogs on 33 studies. Focal encephalitis is uncommon and was reported in 5 (0.8%) of 630 dogs.

    Inflammation, granulomatous — *Toxocara* granulomas have been reported in the brain.

Ear — middle and inner ears are not routinely examined during toxicology studies; therefore, spontaneous lesions in untreated control beagles were not reported in the literature reviewed. Lesions of the external ear or pinna are reported under skin.

Epididymis

    Inclusion bodies — intranuclear, eosinophilic, and periodic acid-Schiff positive inclusions are normal findings in the epididymal epithelium of dogs, and have unknown significance.

    Pigment — normal epididymal cells have granular, yellow to yellow-brown pigment.

    Inflammation (epididymitis) — epididymitis is uncommon. It was reported in 1 (0.3%) of 326 males. Lymphocytic epididymitis is characterized by infiltrates of lymphocytes. These lesions are usually associated with lymphocytic orchitis and thyroiditis in laboratory beagles. Inflammation can also be the result of canine brucellosis *(Brucella canis)*. *(See* Testes.)

    Inflammation, granulomatous — spermatogenic granulomas (spermatocele granulomas) result from injury to epididyimal tubules containing sperm.

Esophagus

    Dilatation — megaesophagus is characterized by a grossly dilated and flaccid esophagus. This is a congenital condition that can result from a persistent right aortic arch, or more commonly the result of an apparent neuromuscular developmental disorder.

    Dilatation, esophageal gland ducts — slightly dilated ducts may be seen in an otherwise-normal esophagus.

    Hypertrophy — swollen and thickened walls often associated with reflux esophagitis.

Inflammation (esophagitis) — an erosive and ulcerative esophagitis can result from repeated reflux of stomach contents.

Eye — microscopic lesions of eyes in laboratory dogs are uncommon. No microscopic lesions were observed in 630 beagles. However, ophthalmoscopic and slit-lamp biomicroscopic examinations reveal a variety of changes in laboratory beagles. Persistent hyaloid vessel remnants, vitreous floaters, vitreous filaments, atapetal fundi, tigroid fundi, tapetal hyperreflectivity, and old hemorrhage or scars have been reported in the eyes of beagles between 6 and 12 months of age.

Anemia results in pale mucous membranes. (*See* Blood.)

Blood vessels — hyaloid artery remnants persisted in 142 (26.7%) of 532 dogs examined. This is not considered to be a pathologic finding. The hyaloid artery usually regresses shortly after birth, but at times fails to regress and remains attached to the posterior lens capsule.

Gland of the third eyelid — adjacent to the third eyelid is a compound alveolar gland that may become neoplastic in older dogs, resulting in a red growth protruding from under the third eyelid at the medial canthus of the eye.

Protrusion or prolapse of the third eyelid occurs in young beagles. This is often associated with inflammation of the bulbar conjunctiva and superficial glandular tissue. The ducts of the gland may become dilated and contain leukocytes. The conjunctival tissue is usually hyperplastic.

Lymphoid cell infiltration of the third eyelid and gland has been reported.

Icterus (jaundice) is yellowish pigmentation of the mucous membranes associated with deposition of bile pigment, especially bilirubin. Icterus can be the result of extensive hemorrhage, lysis of red blood cells (hemolysis), gallbladder or bile duct obstruction, and liver diseases affecting the bile ducts.

Inflammation, conjunctiva — conjunctivitis associated with saw dust bedding and dust occurred in 4% of young beagles.

Inflammation, granulomatous — *Toxocara* granulomas have been reported in the retina and choroids of young beagles.

Eye, cornea

Opacities — corneal opacities were observed from 3 to 8 years of age.

Inflammation (keratitis) has been reported in beagles between 6 and 12 months of age, and at 8 years of age. Superficial keratitis or focal corneal opacities were observed in 35 (6.6%) of 532 dogs examined.

Eye, lens

Prominent posterior lens sutures were the only ophthalmoscopic change reported in 86 laboratory beagles less than 3 years of age. From 3 to 8 years, prominent posterior lens sutures, nuclear opacities, and capsular (anterior, posterior, and peripheral) opacities were observed. Other studies of beagles between 6 and 12 months of age reported additional findings of posterior cortical opacities, posterior polar opacities, lenticular sheen, vacuoles in the cortex, and zones of discontinuity.

Lenticular sheen — a yellowish sheen is observed when light is reflected as fluorescence from the lens media during ophthalmoscopic examinations. This is usually associated with senile or aging changes in the lens; however, it can occur in younger animals. Lenticular sheen was observed in 120 (22.6%) of 532 dogs examined.

Posterior cortical opacities or water clefts associated with the posterior Y sutures were observed in 54 (10.1%) of 532 dogs examined. These opacities are believed to be due to a greater proportion of water content in the cortex.

Zones of discontinuity are the result of refractive changes in normal stratification of the lens, and may be related to metabolic disturbances in lens fiber growth. They have been considered to be presenile changes, and occurred in 32 (6.0%) of 532 dogs examined.

Eye, retina

Atrophy — thinning and absence of tapetal cells. (*See* Pigment.)

Degeneration, cystoid — peripheral retinal cystoid degeneration consists of single or multiple microcysts within the retina at, or near the ora serrata. Although a common change in older beagles, it occurs in younger animals. At 8 years of age, this lesion had an 85% incidence rate.

Dysplasia — focal retinal dysplasia occurs occasionally and includes retinal folds, retinal rosettes, focal absence of retinal cells, and blending of nuclear layers.

Fibrosis — scarring of the retinal was observed at 8 years of age.

Mineralization — calcified bodies occur between the epithelial layer and the choroid.

Pigmentation — pigment cells have been observed in the rod and cone layer. Pigment clumps are normal findings in tapetum lucidum that are characterized by focal pigmentation of the retinal pigment epithelium overlaying the tapetum. Tigroid fundi represent a form of pigment hypoplasia in the retinal pigmented epithelium. This absence of pigment allows the choroidal vessels to be seen as irregular networks of orange-red broad ribbons. In atapetal fundi, the tapetum lucidum is missing. Other tapetal aberrations include focal or linear areas of hyperreflectivity, old focal hemorrhages or scars. Tapetal aberrations and pigment clumps were observed in 25 (4.7%) of 532 dogs examined. The pigmentation findings are considered structural variants of basically normal eyes.

Eye, vitreous

Vitreous floaters or asteroid bodies are small relucent bodies that are composed of calcium salts suspended in normal vitreous. These bodies move when the eye moves. Vitreous filaments result from vitreous hemorrhage, or remnants of the posterior vascular capsule that are observed as strands of fibrinous residues. Vitreous floaters and filaments occurred in 53 (10.0%) of 532 dogs examined.

Gallbladder

Hyperplasia — cystic mucinous hyperplasia at early stages may be present.

Lymphoid foci — individual lymphoid follicles may be prominent.

Gallstones — fine brown or black crystalline gallstones were reported.

Heart

A variety of congenital and acquired findings involve the heart of laboratory beagles.

Congenital findings included pulmonary stenosis, patent ductus arteriosus, and valvular telangiectasis. Pulmonary stenosis was observed grossly in 1 (0.1%) of 1000 dogs.

Degeneration — degenerative changes of the myocardium must be interpreted with caution because many artifacts result from handling and contraction of myofibrils during fixation.

Fatty infiltration of the myocardium was reported in 13 of 37 (35%) untreated beagle dogs.

Fibrosis is a component of chronic inflammation, occurs throughout the heart, and may be associated with mineralization (calcification). Fibrosis of the myocardium may be a healed lesion of parvovirus infection. Focal myocardial fibrosis and mineralization was reported in 2 (0.1%) (< 1%) of 647 dogs.

Hemorrhage — post mortem imbibition of blood pigments can stain the intima of both the heart and blood vessels to grossly resemble hemorrhage.

Inflammation, chronic — chronic valvular fibrosis was observed grossly in 27 (3%) of 1000 dogs. Chronic focal pericarditis was reported in 1 (0.1%) of 647 dogs.

Inflammation, granulomatous — *Toxocara* granulomas have been reported in the myocardium. Granulomas were reported in 2 (0.3%) of 647 dogs.

Inflammation, myocardium — myocarditis is infrequent. Focal myocarditis was reported in 4 (0.6%) of 647 dogs. Parvovirus causes myocarditis in puppies and recently weaned dogs, but is largely controlled by vaccination. Healed lesions may be present in older dogs.

Inflammation, coronary artery — periarteritis has been reported.

Leukocyte foci were observed within the myocardium in 1% of young beagles.

Valvular angiectasis (telangiectasis, hematocyst, congenital hematoma) is occasionally observed involving atrioventricular valves, usually the right. They appear grossly as small blood cysts, and consist microscopically of blood-filled endothelial-lined spaces. Valvular telangiectasis was observed grossly in 4 (0.4%) of 1000 dogs.

Valvular endocardiosis is considered the most frequent incidental finding in the heart and is characterized by swollen, soft, and glistening septal cusps of the right atrioventricular valve.

Nematodes (heartworms, *Dirofilaria immitis*) — heartworms were not reported in laboratory beagles, but are reported in experimental dogs from other sources. Heartworm microfilaria are transmitted by infected mosquitoes and are a risk to dog colonies. Infected dogs with early or moderate disease tire quickly during exercise. In advanced disease, the lungs can have large emboli, thrombi, and pneumonia; the right heart is enlarged with large adult nematodes. Clinical signs are consistent with right heart failure.

Intestine

Congestion — mucosal blood vessels are commonly congested as result of digestive processes, but can be secondary to inflammation, and occur as agonal changes.

Cysts — mucoepithelial cysts of the small intestine have been reported.

Diverticulum — Meckel's diverticulum, a congenital defect in the small intestine has been reported.

Hernia — intestines can protrude through congenital defects in the abdominal wall. Congenital hernias involving intestines were observed grossly in 5 (0.5%) of 1000 dogs.

Hyperplasia, lymphoid — mild hyperplasia of individual or aggregates of lymph follicles may be seen in the lamina propria of untreated animals. These hyperplastic follicles usually correlate with the presence of nodules observed at necropsy.

Inflammation, large intestine (cecitis; colitis) — mild focal cecitis or colitis was reported in 25 (4%) of 647 dogs.

Inflammation, granulomatous — granulomas were observed in the large intestine of 1–3%, and in the small intestine of 2–4% of young beagles. Small intestine granulomas were reported in 6 (0.9%) of 647 dogs. *Toxocara* granulomas have been reported in the intestine.

Inflammation, small intestine (enteritis) — catarrhal enteritis is common. It was reported in 148 (23%) of 647 dogs.

Parvovirus causes acute enteritis in weaned dogs, but is largely controlled by vaccination.

Intussusceptions have been observed in laboratory dogs. One dog was affected grossly in 1000 (0.1%) dogs.

Metazoan parasites

Protozoa — Giardiasis (*Giardia* sp.) is important in young dogs. The disease can result in intermittent or chronic diarrhea, which may persist for several months accompanied by malabsorption of nutrients with reduced growth rate, weight loss, dull hair coat, and other clinical signs.

Coccidiosis (*Isospora spp.*) in young dogs can result in diarrhea and dehydration. Infections with *Isospora bigemina* can cause intestinal hemorrhage.

Nematodes (roundworms: nematodiasis) — nematodes are common, and occurred in
23–28% of young beagles. Most were observed in the small intestine. Usually they
were ascarids.

Ancylostomiasis (*Ancylostoma* spp.) Hookworms usually affect young dogs and can
result in pale oral membranes, anemia, and reduced growth rate. If the infection is
heavy, black tarry feces can be observed. Ancylostomiasis was reported in 1 (3%)
of 37 untreated beagle dogs.

Ascariasis — the common large roundworms of dogs belong to the genera, *Toxocara*
spp. A few ascarids (*Toxocara canis* or *Toxascaris leonina*) are often observed in
small numbers free in the small intestine lumen of laboratory dogs. Ascarids were
observed grossly in 165 (17%) of 1000 dogs.[50] Ascarids were reported in 2 of 37
(5%) untreated beagle dogs.

Toxocara canis larvae migrate through the liver and lungs before reaching the small
intestines. When migrating larvae die or molt, they can incite chronic or granulomatous inflammation (granulomas) characterized by the presence of eosinophils.
Some larvae reach other tissues where they can cause additional inflammatory lesions. The most common sites for granulomas are the mesenteric lymph nodes and
lungs; other sites include the renal cortex.

Strongyloides (*Strongyloides sterocoralis*) — strongyloides are small thread-like nematodes found in the small intestines. They were reported in 9 (1%) of 647 dogs.

Trichuriasis — the whipworm of the dog, *Trichuris vulpis*, is uncommon in laboratory
beagles. They are found in the cecum and colon. Trichuriasis was reported in 7 of
37 (19%) in a colony of beagle dogs.

Tapeworms — cestodes are uncommon, and were observed grossly in 8 (0.8%) of 1000
dogs. The most common tapeworm is the "cucumber seed" *Dipylidium caninum*,
which is usually asymptomatic, but can result in diarrhea and anal pruritus.

Kidney

Agenesis — unilateral renal agenesis is a congenital failure of one kidney to develop. It
is not detected during routine physical examinations, but occasionally occurs in laboratory beagles. The ureter may be missing. The developed kidney is usually about
twice normal size. Unilateral renal agenesis was observed grossly in 4 (0.4%) of 1000
dogs.

Hydronephrosis occurs occasionally in dogs. It was observed grossly in 7 (0.7%) of 1000
dogs.

Inclusions, Intranuclear — rectangular or cubic acidophilic inclusions are frequent findings in the nuclei of renal tubular epithelial cells of dogs. These crystalline acidophilic
intranuclear inclusions are commonly observed in nuclei of cells lining proximal and
distal tubules. They are identical in appearance to those seen in hepatocytes.

Inflammation (nephritis) — focal nonspecific inflammation is common, and can occur as
leukocyte foci, or be the result of bacterial emboli. Leukocyte foci occurred in 1–4%
of young beagles. Minor focal nonspecific inflammation was reported in 76 (12%) of
647 dogs. Focal embolic nephritis was observed in one of the 647 dogs.

Inflammation, glomerulus (glomerulitis, glomerulonephritis, glomerulosclerosis) —
glomerulonephritis is characterized by inflammation involving the glomeruli. Glomerulitis and glomerulonephritis were reported in 2 (0.3%) of 647 dogs. Glomerulosclerosis — a progressive lesion of the glomerulus that has also been termed progressive
intercapillary glomerulosclerosis is seen as early as 6 months of age. It is characterized
by thickened basement membranes and increased mesangial matrix. Local or diffuse

mesangial proliferation and thickened, wrinkled glomerular basement membranes are not usual findings in clinically healthy laboratory beagles. Periglomerular sclerosis may also be present. The severity of intercapillary sclerosis increases with time, and intermittent or persistent proteinuria may occur.

Inflammation, granulomatous — cortical *Toxocara* granulomas are common, and were reported in 4% of young beagles. Granulomas were reported in 11 (2%) of 647 dogs. Cortical granulomas were reported in 2 of 37 (5%) untreated beagle dogs.

Inflammation, interstitium (chronic interstitial nephritis) — interstitial nephritis was observed in 6% of young beagles. Chronic interstitial nephritis was reported in 6 (0.9%) of 647 dogs.

Inflammation, pelvis (pyelitis, pyelonephritis) — pyelitis was observed in 4–7% of young beagles. Pyelonephritis is a nephritis that results from inflammation arising in the pelvis that spreads upwards to involve the medulla and, subsequently, the cortex. Pyelitis or pyelonephritis was reported in 12 (2%) of 647 dogs.

Lipidosis, glomerular — occasionally, one or more lobes of the glomerulus will be filled by large foam cells, which react positively when stained for fat. This lesion has unknown significance.

Mineralization (calcification) is very common, and occurred in 69–74% of young beagles. Mineralization usually occurs as microcalculi, small foci of basophilic deposits in collecting tubules of the renal medulla or papilla in almost 50% of both sexes. Microcalculi were reported in 312 (48%) of 647 dogs. Renal collecting tubule calcification was reported in 6 of 37 (16%) untreated beagle dogs.

Tumors — a renal cell carcinoma was observed grossly in 1 (0.1%) of 1000 dogs.

Liver

Gross and microscopic findings are very frequently reported in the liver.

Cysts — subcapsular cysts have been observed in untreated dogs.

Fatty change (fatty degeneration, fatty metamorphosis, lipidosis) — focal fatty change was observed grossly in 78 (8%) of 1000 dogs. Focal cytoplasmic vacuolization of hepatocytes can occur adjacent to the base of the hepatic ligaments. (*See* Tension lipidosis.)

Hepatocyte cytoplasmic vacuolation — this can result from normal storage of glycogen. Large amounts of glycogen are expected after a meal; however, extensive cytoplasmic vacuolation from glycogen can be present after fasting overnight.

Hepatocyte vacuolar degeneration — this may be a form of fatty change.

Hyperplasia, bile duct — hyperplasia occurs with, and without, portal inflammation. Focal bile duct hyperplasia was uncommon. It was reported in 2 (0.3%) of 647 dogs.

Inclusions, intracytoplasmic — acidophilic globular inclusions occur in the cytoplasm of hepatocytes of dogs. They stain positive with periodic acid-Schiff (PAS) reagents, but are not glycogen. They consist of proteinaceous material and bound lipids.

Inclusions, intranuclear — rectangular, cubic, or rhomboid acidophilic (hyaline) inclusions are frequent findings in the nuclei of hepatocytes of dogs. They are commonly termed acidophilic intranuclear inclusions, and appear to be composed of protein. They were reported in 2 (0.3%) of 647 dogs.

Inflammation, bile duct (cholangitis) — cholangitis is usually associated with necrosis or other inflammation of the liver parenchyma, and was not reported as a primary finding in control beagles.

Inflammation, veins — eosinophilic phlebitis and periphlebitis are suggestive of a hypersensitivity reaction to migrating parasites. Focal phlebitis was very common, and occurred in 409 (63%) of 647 dogs.

Inflammation, portal — mild portal inflammation with, and without, bile duct hyperplasia is common. It was reported in 50 (8%) of 647 dogs.

Inflammation, granulomatous — microgranulomas are the most common lesion observed microscopically in the liver of young beagles. These lesions consist of small focal collections of histiocytes (macrophages or mononuclear cells), lymphocytes, an occasional neutrophil, and a few degenerate hepatocytes. Their cause is unknown but some may be related to parasite migration, especially *Toxocara spp.* Granulomas were observed in 2–4% of young beagles. They were reported in 23 (4%) of 647 dogs.

Leukocyte foci are very common, and occurred in 47–60% of young beagles.

Lipidosis (*see* Fatty change)

Necrosis — hepatocyte necrosis is observed in several forms, and is associated with several degenerative and inflammatory lesions. Focal necrosis and inflammation was very common in the liver. They were reported in 423 (65%) of 647 dogs.

Pigmentation — small brown pigment granules are seen in both hepatocytes and Kupffer cells. The pigment is usually either lipofuscin, or hemosiderin, or both. Individual hepatocytes and Kupffer cells may have both pigments. Bile pigments may be present if biliary stasis is present.

Tension lipidosis — focal subcapsular lipidosis and necrosis seen near the hilus at the base of hepatic ligaments result from tension on the liver capsule and anoxia of adjacent hepatocytes.

Lung

Inflammation is very common in the lungs, and occurs in a large variety of forms including perivasculitis, peribronchiolitis, pleuritis, subpleural fibrosis, endobronchiolitis, bronchopneumonia, interstitial pneumonia, and various granulomas. Most of the pulmonary pathology observed in untreated laboratory beagles has been associated with infections by lungworms, the nematode *Filaroides hirthi*.[58] Some inflammatory lesions may be due to inhaled sawdust bedding. Gavage accidents resulting in lung lesions are very rare in dogs.

Anthracosis (*see* Pigmentation)

Atelectasis — collapsed alveoli are usually associated with inflammation, or pressure from fluid in the thorax.

Bronchopneumonia (*see* Inflammation, bronchi)

Congestion — active congestion is usually a component of inflammation, but also occurs with poor circulation from heart diseases and during agonal events. Pulmonary hyperemia was reported in 2 of 37 (5%) untreated beagle dogs.

Emphysema — distended or ruptured alveoli are uncommon.

Helminthiasis (*see* Nematodes)

Hemorrhage in the lung is an uncommon finding. Pulmonary hemorrhage was reported in one of 37 (3%) untreated beagle dogs.[54]

Hyperemia (*see* Congestion)

Inflammation, alveoli (alveolitis) — fibrosing alveolitis, a fibrous thickening of the alveolar walls, occurred in 1–3% of young beagles.

Inflammation, interstitium (pneumonitis, interstitial pneumonia) — interstitial pneumonia is common, and occurred in 22–28% of young beagles. Focal interstitial pneumonia was reported in 111 (17%) of the 647 dogs. Granulomatous pneumonitis was reported in 13 of 37 (35%) untreated beagle dogs.

Inflammation, bronchi and bronchioles — bronchopneumonia is unusual in laboratory dogs because of vaccination programs against canine distemper. Canine distemper is a virus that predisposes dogs to bacteria, which can cause pneumonia. Bronchopneumonia was reported in 3 of 37 (8%) untreated beagle dogs. Bronchopneumonia caused by *Mycoplasma* spp. has been reported. Localized bronchitis and bronchiolitis occurred in 2–8% of young beagles. Perivasculitis and peribronchiolitis were reported in 329

(51%) of 647 dogs. Subpleural fibrosis and endobronchiolitis occurred in 139 (21%) of the 647 dogs. Pleuritis was reported in 1 (3%) untreated beagle dogs.

Inflammation, granulomatous — granulomas are common. Granulomas were reported in 6–7% of young beagles and in 75 (12%) of 647 dogs on 39 studies. Both lungworms and migrating nematode larvae cause granulomas in the lungs. Granulomas are frequently observed as small tan, green, or gray subpleural nodules that are associated with the lung worm, *Filaroides hirthi*. *Toxocara* granulomas have also been reported. Vascular microgranulomas may result following emboli from intravenous injection sites. They were reported in 8 (1%) of the 647 dogs. Cholesterinic granulomas occur less frequently. One dog of the 647 had a cholesterinic granuloma. Granulomatous pneumonitis was reported in 13 of 37 (35%) untreated beagle dogs.

Leukocyte foci are common, and occurred in 17–18% of young beagles.

Nematodes (nematodiasis) — living nematodes were observed in 2–6% of young beagles. *See* Inflammation, granulomatous above.

Pigmentation (anthracosis) is unusual because most laboratory dogs are not exposed to dusty environments. Anthracosis was reported in 19 of 37 (51%) untreated beagle dogs from one colony.

Lymph node (unspecified, NOS)

Mandibular, mesenteric, and medial retropharyngeal lymph nodes are the most frequently processed for histopathology.

Congestion of the mesenteric lymph nodes is common, and can have a normal physiological origin. Congestion must be distinguished from hemorrhage.

Hyperplasia, lymphoid — non-neoplastic proliferation of lymphoid cells is frequently observed resulting in increased numbers of lymphocytes and related cells.

Hyperplasia is usually associated with inflammation and infections. It must be distinguished from early neoplastic lesions.

Plasmacytosis — a prominent increase in plasma cells has been reported.

Inflammation (lymphadenitis) — generalized lymphadenitis is associated with canine brucellosis (*Brucella canis*).

Inflammation, granulomatous — granulomas are most common in the mesenteric lymph nodes. They are often the result *Toxocara*. They were observed in 21–27% of young beagles, and in 16 (2%) of 647 dogs from 39 studies.

Tumors — lymphosarcoma affecting the lymph nodes has been reported in beagles less than one year of age.

Mammary gland

Hyperplasia — mammary nodules rarely occur in non-treated, control, female dogs. In a 7-year study, 40 mammary nodules were palpated in 7 of 18 control bitches. Most were transient observations. At the time of necropsy, nine were present in six animals. Five of the nine nodules were lobular or intraductal hyperplasia. Two were benign mixed mammary tumors. The other two were non-mammary lesions. In another 4-year study, nodules were palpable in 4 of 20 control bitches between 21 and 24 months, but none were present at necropsy.

Inflammation (mastitis) is rare; one animal (< 1%) with mastitis was reported in 321 female beagles.

Tumors — neoplasms of mammary glands are unusual in beagles less than seven year of age. During life-span observations of 1343 beagles, 476 (70.8%) of 672 females and 2 (0.3%) of 671 males had one or more mammary neoplasms. Classification and detailed descriptions of canine mammary tumors can be found in Moulton.

Benign mixed mammary tumors were observed in 2 (11%) of 18 control female beagles during a 7-year study.

Mouth (*see* Oral cavity)

Nerve (*see* Peripheral nerve)

Oral cavity (palate, nasopharynx)

 Papillomas (warts) are benign epithelial tumors caused by papovavirus that are usually observed in young dogs, and can spontaneously disappear. Oral papillomas may be found on the lips, inside the cheeks, and on the tongue, palate, and pharynx. The gums are usually not affected. Oral papillomas were observed grossly in 2 (0.2%) of 1000 dogs.

Oral mucosa

 Anemia results in pale mucous membranes. (*See* Blood)

 Icterus (jaundice) is yellowish pigmentation of the mucous membranes associated with deposition of bile pigment, especially bilirubin. Icterus can be the result of extensive hemorrhage, lysis of red blood cells (hemolysis), gallbladder or bile duct obstruction, and liver diseases affecting the bile ducts.

Ovary

 Cyst — clear cysts are occasionally observed in the vicinity of the ovary in young adult beagles. These have been reported as paraovarian cysts. This is not a specific diagnosis. Paraovarian cysts were observed grossly in 2 (0.4%) of 499 females.

Pancreas

 Degeneration — cytologic alteration has been reported in acinar and islets cells. Edema was reported.

 Infiltrates — various types of leukocytes have been observed infiltrating the pancreatic tissues.

 Inclusions, intracytoplasmic — ovoid acidophilic inclusions often containing basophilic particles in clear spaces may occur in acinar cells of dogs. These inclusions are ultrastructurally similar to dense ribosomal autophagic vacuoles.

 Inflammation (pancreatitis) — chronic focal pancreatitis was reported in 8 (1.2%) of 647 dogs.

 Inflammation, granulomatous — *Toxocara* granulomas have been reported in the pancreas. (*See* Liver)

Parathyroid gland

 Cysts are uncommon in the parathyroid. Small cysts may be found within or near the parathyroid apparently arising from the duct connecting the thymus and parathyroid primordia. They are usually multiloculated, lined by cuboidal to columnar epithelium, often ciliated, and contain densely eosinophilic material. Cysts occurred in 1% of young beagles.

 Hyperplasia of the parathyroid cells was reported in 7 (1%) of 647 dogs.

Penis

 Inflammation of glans penis (balanitis) — mild inflammation of the glans penis, and prepuce (balanoposthitis), is common in dogs.

Peripheral nerve

 Renaut bodies are normal structures within nerves that could be mistaken for nerve infarction or necrotizing angiopathic neuropathy. They appear as cylindrical, loosely textured, whorled, cell-sparse structures in nerves.

 Degeneration — spontaneous degenerative lesions of the peripheral nerve may be seen in the beagle. While commonly considered an aging change, occasionally "digestion chambers" and "myelin bubbles" are seen in the sciatic nerves of young beagles.[7]

 Pharynx (*see* Oral cavity)

Pituitary gland

 Cysts are very frequently observed in the pituitary. Most of these are remnants of the craniopharyngeal duct, and are located at the periphery of the pars tuberalis and distalis.

Usually the cysts are microscopic, lined by ciliated cuboidal to columnar epithelium, and contain mucin. Cysts occurred in 24–26% of young beagles, and in 44 (7%) of 647 dogs. Pituitary cysts were reported in 3 of 37 (8%) untreated beagle dogs.

Inflammation, Granulomatous — granulomas have been reported associated with *Toxocara*. Granuloma was reported in 1 (0.1%) of 647 dogs.

Prepuce

Inflammation (posthitis) — mild inflammation of the prepuce accompanied by inflammation of the glans penis (balanoposthitis) is common in dogs. It can result in a slight mucopurulent preputial discharge.

Prostate

Atrophy — atrophy of the epithelium has been associated with chronic inflammation. It was reported in 7 (2%) of 326 males.

Hyperplasia, cystic — focal cystic hyperplasia was reported in 15 (5%) of 326 dogs.

Lymphoid or leukocyte foci occurred in 12% of young beagles.[49] (*See* Inflammation, lymphocytic.)

Inflammation (prostatitis) — subclinical prostatitis is common in the dog. The inflammation is usually minimal in young adult beagles. Prostatitis was reported in 12% of young beagles, and in 124 (38%) of 326 dogs from 39 studies. Some prostatitis may result from catheterization during collection of urine.

Inflammation, lymphocytic — lymphocytic prostatitis may consist of minor lymphocytic infiltrates (foci), up to large lymphoid aggregates with germinal centers. Large lesions are accompanied by interstitial fibrosis and epithelial atrophy (chronic prostatitis). Inflammation can also be the result of canine brucellosis (*Brucella canis*).

Salivary gland

Inflammation (sialoadenitis) is not usual. Mild focal sialoadenitis was reported in 35 (5%) of 647 dogs.

Skeletal muscle

Hernias are congenital weaknesses in the abdominal wall, usually located in the umbilical area, and contain only omental fat. These are infrequent findings. Congenital hernias involving intestines were observed grossly in 5 (0.5%) of 1000 dogs.

Inflammation, granulomatous — granulomas of *Toxocara* sp. occur in skeletal muscle, but are unusual findings.

Skin

Skin lesions are quite common as a result of abrasions from concrete surfaces and caging, as well as from bite wounds caused by fighting.

Terminology for dermatohistopathology often uses a specialized vocabulary. Diagnostic criteria and illustrations of skin findings for laboratory dogs are well described by Hargis, Muller, and Yager and Scott.

Alopecia is commonly observed in laboratory dogs from a variety of causes; although some cases have unknown cause, most occur as complete, partial, diffuse, or circumscribed loss of hair without other skin changes over bony pressure points such as the elbow and hock. Alopecia that occurs as circumscribed, erythematous, and scaly areas near the eyes, at the commissures of the lips, around the mouth, or on the forelegs is often the result of demodectic mange mites. *Demodex canis* or *follicularum* is a normal resident of the skin, inhabits the hair follicles and sebaceous glands, and is estimated to be present in 80% of animals in some colonies. Demodectic mites were reported in 1 (0.1%) of 647 dogs on 39 studies.

Callus (callosity) — this is a localized hyperkeratotic lesion from continued trauma of the skin over the bony pressure points where alopecia occurs. These areas may become ulcerated and infected resulting in pressure point granulomas.

Dermatosis — ear margin lesions observed as multiple irregular, soft, tan nodules on the margins of the pinnae characterized by hyperkeratosis and parakeratosis.

Furunculosis — extensive areas of inflammation are often the result of a penetrating or perforating folliculitis, and can result from large demodectic mite populations.

Hyperkeratosis — increased amounts of keratin were not recorded as a primary finding.

Inflammation, skin (dermatitis) — dermatitis was observed in 4–7% of young beagles.

Inflammation, hair follicle (folliculitis) — folliculitis and perifolliculitis are often associated with demodectic mites.

Parakeratosis — a form of hyperkeratosis with cell nuclei in the accumulated keratin was not recorded as a primary finding.

Tumors — neoplasia in the dog is most common between ages 6 and 14 years; however, tumors do occur in younger animals. A detailed description of canine tumors can be found in Muller and Moulton.

Skin tumors reported in beagles less than 2 years of age are rare.

Histiocytoma was reported in 1 (0.1%) of 647 dogs.

Mast cell sarcoma and Sarcoma, unspecified have also been reported.

Spinal cord

Degeneration — degenerating axis cylinders may be observed as spherical, eosinophilic granular structures in the medulla oblongata, pons, or anterior cervical spinal cord, most common in the gracilis tract and nucleus. These structures apparently have no neurological or pathological significance.

Inflammation (myelitis) — focal myelitis has been observed in the spinal cords of 2 (0.3%) of 647 dogs.

Inflammation, granulomatous — *Toxocara* granulomas have been reported in the spinal cord (cauda equina).

Spleen

Accessory spleens are occasionally observed in the gastrosplenic omentum. They can be congenital, but many appear to be acquired through traumatic rupture of the spleen. Accessory spleens were observed grossly in 1 (0.1%) of 1000 dogs. Angiectasis (telangiectasis) is localized dilatation of blood vessels that are observed as dark red blebs around the margin of the spleen. They consist of blood-filled sinusoids that fail to empty during the splenic contraction associated with exsanguinations. They occurred in 7–14% of young beagles.

Congestion (hyperemia) is commonly observed grossly, especially following euthanasia with barbiturates. It must be distinguished from active congestion associated with inflammation and secondary congestion associated with poor blood circulation. Splenic hyperemia was reported in one of 37 (3%) untreated beagle dogs.

Extramedullary hematopoiesis — the production of blood cells in the splenic pulp, especially the erythroid series, is uncommon in adult dogs. Splenic extramedullary hematopoiesis was reported in 3 of 37 (8%) untreated beagle dogs.

Fibrosis — the proliferation of fibrous connective tissue usually accompanies inflammation. Splenic fibrosis was reported in 1 (3%) of 37 untreated beagle dogs.

Hemorrhage — because of the blood flow and abdominal location, hemorrhage is common in the spleen. Hemorrhage must be distinguished from congestion. Splenic hemorrhage was reported in 1 (3%) of 37 untreated beagle dogs.

Hematomas are localized areas of hemorrhage, and are infrequently observed. They were observed grossly in 2 (0.2%) of 1000 dogs.

Siderotic or siderofibrotic nodules can be small, localized, and nodular thickened areas on the capsular surface, larger irregular encrustations covering of extensive areas of the capsule, or nodules in the pulp. They are grossly yellow to grayish brown, and commonly occur around the margin of spleens, or at the attachment of the gastrosplenic omentum in older dogs. Siderofibrotic nodules were observed grossly in 90 (9%) of 1000 dogs. They have also been termed Gandy-Gamna bodies. Microscopically, they consist of fibrotic foci that are often calcified, and contain brown pigment (hemosiderin) and yellow pigment (hematoidin). They probably are the end result of hemorrhage and thrombosis.

Hemosiderosis — deposition of iron-containing pigment associated with the breakdown of red blood cells in splenic tissues is commonly associated with siderotic nodules.

Splenic hemosiderosis was reported in 17 of 37 (46%) untreated beagle dogs.

Hyperplasia, lymphoid — these are non-neoplastic proliferations of lymphoid cells, which result in increased numbers of lymphocytes and related cells, and can cause enlargement of the spleen. Hyperplasia is usually associated with inflammation and infections. It must be distinguished from early neoplastic lesions.

Inflammation, granulomatous — granulomas have been associated with *Toxocara,* and were observed in 21–27% of young beagles.

Reticulosis — this is a form of lymphoid hyperplasia with a predominance of reticuloendothelial or histiocytic cells.

Lymphosarcoma affecting the spleen and lymph nodes has been reported in beagles less than one year of age.

Stomach

Atrophy — atrophy of parietal cells may be associated with gastric spirillum-like bacteria.

Dilatation — dilatation of gastric glands may be associated with gastric spirillum-like bacteria.

Hyperplasia, lymphoid — lymphoreticular hyperplasia may be associated with large numbers of gastric spirillum-like bacteria that are commonly found within the lumen of gastric glands and in the intracellular canaliculi of parietal cells.

Inflammation (gastritis) — chronic gastritis is common in laboratory dogs, and was reported in 58 (9%) of 647 dogs.

Inflammation, granulomatous — granulomas were reported in 1 (0.1%) of 647 dogs.

Lymphoid foci — lymphoid nodules or follicles are commonly present within the lamina propria, especially in the pyloric region.

Mineralization occurs as basophilic granules in the middle fundic mucosa in both sexes, and affected 7–10% of young beagles.

Testes

Atrophy — focal atrophy of seminiferous tubules occurred in 5% of young beagles, and in 11 (3%) of 326 males.

Degeneration — testicular degeneration is frequently observed in adult dogs, and may be focal or diffuse, unilateral or bilateral. Early lesions consist of a loss of germ cells that can appear as individual degenerated cells, or as multinucleated giant cells. As degeneration progresses, more germinal cells are lost resulting in almost empty tubules lined by sustentacular (Sertoli) cells. Intratubular giant cells are observed in seminiferous tubules of 9 (3%) of 326 untreated young beagles.

Hyperplasia, interstitial cell — interstitial cell hyperplasia is rare in untreated beagles. It was reported in 1 (0.3%) of 326 dogs.

Inflammation (orchitis) — lymphocytic orchitis is characterized by diffuse, aggregated, or nodular infiltrates of lymphocytes. Germinal centers may be present. These lesions are usually associated with lymphocytic thyroiditis in laboratory beagles, and are commonly accompanied by focal or diffuse degeneration and atrophy of seminiferous tubules. The epididymis may be involved. Inflammation can also be the result of canine brucellosis (*Brucella canis*).

Thymus — the amount of thymus varies considerably in short-term toxicology studies. Involution begins prior to sexual maturity.

    Atrophy is uncommon in untreated beagles, and must be distinguished from involution.

    Ectopic thyroid occurred in 1% of young beagles.

    Cysts occurred in 1% of young beagles.

Thyroid gland

    Atrophy — follicular atrophy has been observed. Idiopathic thyroid atrophy is a progressive loss of follicular epithelium, with replacement by adipose cells. The lobes are affected unequally and if severely affected, may be difficult to find at necropsy. Parafollicular cells are unaffected, and can be seen in the adipose tissue.

    Ectopic thymus occurred in 1–2% of young beagles.

    Cysts — cysts are common findings. Ultimobranchial duct cysts are the most frequently observed in the thyroid, arise from remnants of the ultimobranchial body, and have a keratinized squamous epithelial lining. Cysts of the thyroid were observed in 1–2% of young beagles.

    Hyperplasia, C-cell (parafollicular cells) — the numbers of C-cells in young beagles varies widely with occasionally focal increases. C-cell hyperplasia occurred in 8–9% of young beagles.

    Hyperplasia, follicular cell — follicular cell hyperplasia was reported infrequently.

    Hyperplasia, lymphoid — lymphoid hyperplasia occurred in 2% of young beagles.

    Inflammation — lymphocytic and unspecified thyroiditis have been reported in beagles. Lymphocytic thyroiditis appears to be immunologically mediated, and have a familial occurrence in beagles. The lesions consist of multifocal to diffuse infiltrates of lymphocytes, plasma cells, and macrophages. Lymphoid nodules may be present. The thyroid follicles are usually small, and may contain degenerate follicle cells, lymphocytes, and plasma cells. Thyroiditis was reported in 3 of 37 (8%) untreated beagle dogs.

    Inflammation, granulomatous — granulomas associated with *Toxocara* have been reported.

    Metaplasia, squamous — focal squamous metaplasia has been reported.

Tongue

    Inflammation (glossitis) occurred in 1–2% of young beagles.

    Inflammation, granulomatous — granulomatous inflammation can be associated with fragments of sawdust bedding embedded in the tongue.

    Papillomas (warts) are benign epithelial tumors caused by papovavirus that usually are observed in young dogs, and can spontaneously disappear. *See* Oral cavity.

Tooth

    Minor dental abnormalities are frequently observed. They can include missing permanent teeth (usually upper and lower premolars), retained deciduous teeth (usually canine), imperfect apposition, dental plaque (soft masses of bacteria and food), and dental calculus or tartar (mineralized plaque, usually discolored, most abundant next to orifices of salivary ducts).

    Inflammation (gingivitis) is usually associated with plaque or tartar.

Trachea

    Inflammation (tracheitis) — chronic tracheitis was reported in 11 (2%) of 647 dogs on 39 studies.

Urinary bladder

    Inflammation (cystitis) — cystitis occurs infrequently in untreated beagles, predominantly in males. Some cystitis may result from catheterization during collection of urine. Cystitis was reported in 27, 23 males and 4 females, (4%) of 647 dogs.

Arteritis and periarteritis were present in 10 of 59 dogs with detrusor myopathy. Both sexes were equally affected.

Mineralization — calculi were observed grossly in the urinary bladder lumen of 5 (0.5%) of 1000 dogs. Calcification of the round ligament of the bladder, a remnant of the umbilical artery of the fetus, is an incidental finding in young beagles.

Myopathy — detrusor myopathy is characterized by degenerative lesions in the urinary bladder muscle tunic, and was present in 59 of 449 (13%) young beagle dogs. Arteritis and periarteritis were frequently present. Both sexes were equally affected.

Urethra

Congestion of the mucosal wall can be prominent at necropsy. This normal physiological filling of capillaries and veins can be confused with hemorrhage.

Mineralization — urethral calculi are unusual, and were observed grossly in 1 (0.1%) of 1000 dogs.

Uterus

Cyst — myometrial cysts have been reported in young beagles. One dog was affected in 499 females (0.2%).

Distension (dilatation) occurred in 11% of young beagles.

Inflammation (endometritis) — endometritis associated with canine brucellosis (*Brucella canis*) can result in abortion in the third trimester of pregnancy.

Zygomatic (orbital or dorsal buccal) gland is a salivary gland located at the apex of the orbit of the eye. It sometimes becomes abscessed, and can cause the eye to protrude.

Organs or tissues that had no reported spontaneous lesions in the available references included anal gland, anal sac, bone marrow, circumanal glands, clitoris, ductus deferens, ear, lacrimal gland, larynx, mesentery, nose, oviduct, pancreatic islets, ureter, and vagina. The dog does not have seminal vesicles or bulbourethral glands.

Comments: For a general review of disease problems of laboratory dogs, especially those from random sources and those conditioned for research, refer to Ringler and Peter. Pick and Eubanks reported gross and microscopic findings for 49 random source dogs in North Carolina. This is not a comprehensive presentation of all pathology findings for dogs used in toxicology studies. Additional information and more detailed descriptions of canine diseases, parasitology, and pathology are available in a number of veterinary medical texts. See Aiello, Bonagura, Carter, Hettinger and Feldman, Jones, Jubb, Muller, Summer, and Urquhart.

REFERENCES

1. Sanders, B. J., *Animal Histology Procedures of the Pathological Technology Section of the National Cancer Institute,* HEW Publication No. (NIH) 72-275 Superintendent of Documents, U. S. Government Printing Office, Washington, D.C., 1972.

2. Luna, L. G., Ed., *Manual of Histologic Staining Methods of the Armed Forces Institute of Pathology,* 3rd edition, McGraw-Hill, New York, 1968, chap. 1.

3. Luna, L. G., *Histopathologic Methods and Color Atlas of Special Stains and Tissue Artifacts,* American Histolabs, Inc., Gaitheresberg, MD, 1992.

4. Sheehan, D. C. and Hrapchak, B. B., *Theory and Practice of Histotechnology,* 2nd ed., C. V. Mosby, Saint Louis, MO, 1980.

5. Hardisty, J. F. and Eustis, S. L., Toxicological pathology: a critical stage in study interpretation, in *Progress in Predictive Toxicology,* Clayson, D. B., Munro, I. C., Shubik, P., and Swenberg, J. A., Eds., Elsevier, New York, 1990, 41.

6. World Health Organization, *Principles and Methods for Evaluating the Toxicity of Chemicals. Part 1,* Environmental Health Criteria 6, World Health Organization, Geneva, 1978, 192.

7. Hardisty, J. F. and Boorman, G. A., National toxicology program pathology quality assurance procedures, in *Managing Conduct and Data Quality of Toxicology Studies,* Hoover, K. B., Baldwin, J. K., Velner, A. F.,Whitmirem, C. E., Davies, C. L., and Bristol, D. W., Eds., Princeton Scientific, Princeton, NJ, 1986, 263.

8. Haseman, J. K., Arnold, J., and Eustis, S. L., Tumor incidences in Fischer 344 rats: NTP historical data, in *Pathology of the Fischer Rat,* Boorman, G. A., Eustis, S. L., Elwell, M. R., Montgomery, C. A., and MacKenzie, W. F., Academic Press, New York, 1990, 555.

9. Seaman, W. J., *Postmortem Change in the Rat: A Histologic Characterization,* Iowa State University Press, Ames, IA, 1987.

10. Benirschke, K., Garner, F. M., and Jones, T. C., Eds., *Pathology of Laboratory Animals,* vols. I and II, Springer-Verlag, New York, 1978.

11. Bhatt, P. N., Jacoby, R. O., Morse, H. C., and New, A. E., *Viral and Mycoplasmal Infections of Laboratory Rodents,* Academic Press, New York, 1986.

12. Clapp, N. K., *An Atlas of RF Mouse Pathology: Disease Descriptions and Incidences,* Technical Information Center, Office of Information Services, United States Atomic Energy Commission, Oak Ridge, TN, 1973.

13. Cotchin, E. and Roe, F. J. C., *Pathology of Laboratory Rats and Mice,* Blackwell Scientific, Oxford, 1967.

14. Faccini, J. M., Abbott, D. P., and Paulus, G. J. J., *Mouse Histopathology,* Elsevier, New York, 1990.

15. Firth, C. H. and Ward, J. M., *Color Atlas of Neoplastic and Non-neoplastic Lesions of Aging Mice,* Elsevier, New York, 1988.

16. Firth, C. H., Pattengale, P. K., and Ward, J. M., *Color Atlas of Hematopoietic Pathology of Mice,* Toxicologic Pathology Associates, Little Rock, AK, 1985.

17. Foster, H. L., Small, J. D., and Fox, J. G., *The Mouse in Biomedical Research,* vols. I, II, III, and IV, Academic Press, New York, 1982, 1983.

18. Fox, J. G., Cohen, B. J., and Loew, F. M., Eds. *Laboratory Animal Medicine,* Academic Press, New York, 1984.

19. Glaister, J. R., *Principles of Toxicological Pathology,* Taylor & Francis, Philadelphia, PA, 1986.

20. Goodman, D. G. and Strandberg, J. D., Neoplasms of the female reproductive tract, in *The Mouse in Biomedical Research, IV. Experimental Biology and Oncology,* Foster, H. L., Small, J. D., Fox, J. G., Eds., Academic Press, New York, 1982, 397.

21. Haseman, J. K., Huff, J., and Boorman, G. A., Use of historical control data in carcinogenicity studies in rodents, *Toxicol. Pathol.,* 12, 126, 1984.

22. Hall, W. C., Ganaway, J. R., Rao, G. N., Peters, R. L., Allen, A. M., Luczak, J. W., Sandberg, E. M., and Quigley, B. H., Histopathologic observations in weanling B6C3F1 mice and F344/N rats and their adult parental strains, *Toxicol. Pathol.,* 20, 146, 1992.

23. Harkness, J. E. and Wagner, J. E., *The Biology and Medicine of Rabbits and Rodents,* Lea and Febiger, Philadelphia, PA, 1989.

24. Hollander, C. F., Delort, P., and Duprat, P., Toxicology in the older age group, in *Progress in Predictive Toxicology,* Clayson, D. B., Munro, I. C., Shubik, P., and Swenberg, J. A., Eds., Elsevier, New York, 1990, 113.

25. Jones, T. C., Mohr, U., and Hunt, R. D., Eds., *Monographs on Pathology of Laboratory Animals,* Springer-Verlag, New York, series sponsored by International Life Sciences Institute: *Endocrine System,* 1983; *Digestive System,* 1985; *Respiratory System,* 1985; *Urinary System,* 1986; *Genital System,* 1987; *Nervous System,* 1988; *Integument and Mammary Glands,* 1989; *Hematopoietic System,* 1990; *Cardiovascular and Musculoskeletal System,* 1991; *Eye and Ear,* 1991.

26. Maita, K., Hirano, M., Harada, T., Mitsumori, K., Yoshida, A., Takahashi, K., Nagashima, M., Kitazawa, T., Enomoto, A., Inui, K., and Shirasu, Y., Mortality, major cause of moribundity, and spontaneous tumors in CD-1 mice, *Toxicol. Pathol.,* 16, 340, 1988.

27. Percy, D. H. and Barthold, S. W., *Pathology of Laboratory Rodents and Rabbits,* Iowa State University Press, Ames, IA, 1993.

28. Ribelin, W. E. and McCoy, J. R., *The Pathology of Laboratory Animals,* Charles C. Thomas, Springfield, IL, 1965.

29. Squire, R. A., Goodman, D. G., Valerio, M. G., Fredrickson, T., Strandberg, J. D., Levitt, M. H., Lingeman, C. H., Harshbarger, J. C., and Dawe, C. J., Tumors, in *Pathology of Laboratory Animals,* vol. II, Benirschke, K., Garner, F. M., and Jones, T. C., Eds., Springer-Verlag, New York, 1978, 1051.

30. Tamano, S., Hagiwara, A., Shibata, M., Karuta, Y., Fukushima, S., and Ito, N., Spontaneous tumors in aging (C57BL/6N × C3H/HeN) F1 (B6C3F1) mice, *Toxicol. Pathol.,* 16, 321, 1988.

31. Ward, J. M., Goodman, D. G., Squire, R. A., Chu, K. C., and Linhart, M. S., Neoplastic and non-neoplastic lesions in aging (C57BL/6N × C3H/HeN)F1 (B6C3F1) mice, *J. Natl. Cancer Inst.,* 63, 849, 1979.

32. Baker, H. J., Lindsey, J. R., and Weisbroth, S. H., Eds., *The Laboratory Rat. I. Biology and Diseases,* Academic Press, New York, 1979.

33. Boorman, G. A., Eustis, S. L., Elwell, M. R., Montgomery, C. A. Jr., and MacKenzie, W. F., Eds., *Pathology of the Fischer Rat,* Academic Press, New York, 1990.

34. Burek, J. D., *Pathology of the Aging Rats,* CRC Press, Boca Raton, FL, 1978.

35. Coleman, G. L., Barthold, S. W., Osbaldiston, G. W., Foster, S. J., and Jonas, A. M., Pathological changes during aging in barrier-reared Fischer 344 male rats, *J. Gerontol.,* 32, 258, 1977.

36. Goodman, D. G., Ward, J. M., Squire, R. H., Chu, K. C., and Linhart, M. S., Neoplasms and nonneoplastic lesions in aging F344 rats, *Toxicol. Appl. Pharmacol.,* 48, 237, 1979.

37. Greaves, P. and Faccini, J. M., *Rat Histopathology,* Elsevier, New York, 1984.

38. Haseman, J. K., Huff, J. E., Rao, G. N., Arnold, J. E., Boorman, G. A., and McConnell, E. E., Neoplasms observed in untreated and corn oil gavage control groups of F344/N rats and (C57BL/6N × C3H/HeN)F1 (B6C3F1) mice, *J. Natl. Cancer Inst.,* 75, 975, 1985.

39. Jacobs, B. B. and Huseby, R. A., Neoplasms occurring in aged Fischer rats with special reference to testicular, uterine, and thyroid tumors, *J. Nat. Cancer Inst.,* 39, 303, 1967.

40. McMartin, D. N., Sahota, P. S., Gunson, D. E., Han Hsu, H., and Spaet, R. H., Neoplasms and related proliferative lesions in control Sprague-Dawley rats from carcinogenicity studies. Historical data and diagnostic considerations, *Toxicol. Pathol.,* 20, 212, 1992.

41. Mohr, U., Dungworth, D. L., and Capen, C. C., Eds., *Pathobiology of the Aging Rat,* vols. 1 and 2, International Life Sciences Institute, Washington, D.C., 1992, 1993.

42. Sacksteder, M. R., Occurrence of spontaneous tumors in the germ-free F334 rat, *J. Natl. Cancer Inst.,* 57, 1371, 1976.

43. Sass, B., Rabstein, L. S., Madison, R., Nims, R. M., Peters, R. L., and Kelloff, G. J., Incidence of spontaneous neoplasms in F334 rats throughout the natural life-span, *J. Natl. Cancer Inst.,* 54, 1449, 1975.

44. Sher, S. P., Jensen, R. D., and Bokelman, D. L., Spontaneous tumors in control F334 and Charles River-CD rats and Charles River-CD1 and B6C3F1 mice, *Toxicol. Lett.,* 11, 103, 1982.

45. Solleveld, H. A., Haseman, J. K., and McConnell, E. E., Natural history of body weight gain, survival, and neoplasia in the F344 rat, *J. Natl. Cancer Inst.,* 72, 929, 1984.

46. Stinson, S. F., Schuller, H. M., and Resznik, G., *Atlas of Tumor Pathology of the Fischer Rat,* CRC Press, Boca Raton, FL, 1989.

47. Fritz, T. E., Semen, R. C., Poole, C. M., and Norris, W. P., Studies on the spontaneous disease and pathology in the experimental beagle, *Argonne Natl. Lab. Biol. Med. Res. Div. Ann. Rep.,* ANL-7278, 114–115, 1966.

48. Fritz, T. E., Semen, R. C., and Norris, W. P., Studies on the spontaneous disease and pathology in the experimental beagle colony, *Argonne Natl. Lab. Biol. Med. Res. Div. Ann. Rep.,* ANL-7409 (283–284), 1967.

49. Glaister, J. R., *Principles of Toxicological Pathology,* Taylor & Francis, Philadelphia, PA, 1986.

50. Hottendorf, G. H. and Hirth, R. S., Lesions of spontaneous subclinical disease in beagle dogs, *Vet. Pathol.,* 11, 240–258, 1974.

51. Maita, K., Masuda, H., and Suzuki, Y., Spontaneous lesions detected in the beagles used in toxicity studies, *Exp. Anim.,* 26, 161–167, 1977.

52. Oghiso, Y., Fukuda, S., and Hda, H., Histopathologic studies on distribution of spontaneous lesions and age changes in the beagle, *Jpn. J. Vet. Sci.,* 44, 941–950, 1982.

53. Thomassen, R. W., The dog: pathology, in *Animal Models in Toxicology,* Gad, S. C. and Chengelis, C. P. Marcel Dekker, New York, 1992, pp. 600–674.

54. Pick, J. R. and Eubanks, J. W., A clinicopathologic study of heterogeneous and homogenous dog populations in North Carolina, *Laboratory Animal Care,* 15 (1), 11–17, 1965.

55. Barron, C. N. and Saunders, L. Z., Visceral larva migrans in the dog, *Pathol. Vet.,* 3, 315, 1966.

56. Schiavo, D. M. and Field, W. E., The incidence of ocular defects in a closed colony of beagle dogs, *Laboratory Animal Science,* 24, 51–56, 1974.

57. Heywood, R., Hepworth, P. L., and Van Abbe, N. J., Age changes in the eyes of the beagle dog, *J. Small Anim. Pract.,* 17, 171–177, 1976.

58. Hirth, R. S. and Hottendorf, G. H., Lesions produced by a new lungworm in beagle dogs, *Vet. Pathol.,* 10, 385–407, 1973.

59. Kirchner, B. K., Port, C. D., Magoc, T. J., Sidor, M. A., and Ruben, Z., Spontaneous bronchopneumonia in laboratory dogs infected with untyped *Mycoplasma* spp., *Laboratory Animal Science,* 40, 625–628, 1990.

60. Giles, R. C., Kwapien, R. P., Geil, R. G., and Casey, H. W., Mammary nodules in beagle dogs administered investigational oral contraceptive steroids, *J. Natl. Cancer Inst.,* 60(6), 1351–64, 1978.

61. Nelson, L. W., Weikel, J. H., Jr., and Reno, F. E., Mammary nodules in dogs during four years' treatment with megestrol acetate or chlormadinone acetate, *J. Natl. Cancer Inst.,* 51(4), 1303–11, 1973.

62. Benjamin, S. A., Lee, A. C., and Saunders, W. J., Classification and behavior of canine mammary epithelial neoplasms based on life-span observations in beagles, *Vet. Pathol.,* 36, 423–436, 1999.

63. Moulton, J. E., *Tumors in Domestic Animals* University of California Press, Los Angeles, 1990.

64. Hartman, H. A., Robinson, R. L., and Visscher, G. E., Naturally occurring intracytoplasmic eosinophilic inclusions in the canine exocrine pancreas, *Vet. Pathol.,* 12, 210–219, 1975.

65. Hargis, A. M., Integument system, in *Special Veterinary Pathology,* Thomson, R. G. Decker, Philadelphia, 1988, pp. 1–68.

66. Muller, G. H., Scott, D. W., Miller, W. H., and Griffin C. E., *Muller and Kirk's Small Animal Dermatology,* 5th ed., Saunders, Philadelphia, 1995.

67. Yager, J. A. and Scott, D. W., The skin and appendages, in *Pathology of Domestic Animals,* Jubb, K. V. F., Kennedy, P. C., and Palmer, N., Academic Press, San Diego, 1985, pp. 407–549.

68. Fritz, T. E., Lombard, L. S., Tyler, S. A., and Norris, W. P., Pathology and familial incidence of orchitis and its relationship to thyroiditis in a closed beagle colony, *Exp. Molec. Pathol.,* 24, 142–158, 1976.

69. Cain, G. R., Tsai, K., Pulley, L. T., and Taylor, M., Detrusor myopathy in young beagle dogs, *Toxicol. Pathol.,* 28(4), 565–7, 2000.

70. Ringler, D. F. and Peter, G. K., Dogs and cats as laboratory animals, in *Laboratory Animal Medicine,* Fox, J. G., Cohen, B. J., and Loew, F. M., Academic Press, New York, 1984, pp. 241–271.

71. Aiello, S. E. a. M., A, *The Merck Veterinary Manual,* 8th ed., Merck & Co., Whitehouse Station, NJ, 1998.

72. Bonagura, J. D. and Kirk, R. W., *Kirk's Current Veterinary Therapy XII: Small Animal Practice* Saunders, Philadelphia, 1995.

73. Bonagura, J. D., *Kirk's Current Veterinary Therapy XIII Small Animal Practice,* Saunders, Philadelphia, 2000.

74. Carter, G. R., *Microbial Diseases: A Veterinarian's Guide to Laboratory Diagnosis,* 1st ed. Iowa State University Press, Ames, Iowa, 1993.

75. Ettinger, S. J. and Feldman, E. C., *Textbook of Veterinary Internal Medicine: Diseases of the Dog and Cat,* 4th ed., Saunders, Philadelphia, 1995.

76. Jones, C. T., Hunt, R. D., and King, N. W., *Veterinary Pathology,* 6th ed., Williams & Wilkins, Baltimore, 1997.

77. Jubb, K. V. F., Kennedy, P. C., and Palmer, N., *Pathology of Domestic Animals,* 4th ed., Academic Press, San Diego, 1993.

78. Summer, B. A., Cummings, J. F., and DeLahunta, A., *Veterinary Neuropathology,* Mosby, St. Louis, 1995.

79. Urquhart, G. M., Armour, J., Duncan, J. L., Dunn, A. M., and Jennings, F. W., *Veterinary Parasitology,* 2nd ed., Blackwell Science, Cambridge, MA, 1996.

80. Haseman, J. K., Elwell, M. R., and Hailey, J. R., Neoplasm incidences in B6C3F$_1$ mice: NTP historical data, in *Pathology of the Laboratory Mouse,* Manonpot, R. R., Boorman, G. A., and Gaul, B., Cache River Press, Vienna, IL, 1999, 679–689.

Note: National Toxicology Program Historical Data for Neoplastic Lesions in Control Fischer F344/N Rats and B6C3F Mice are available at http://ehis.niehs.nih.gov (subscription resource).

18 Animal Clinical Pathology

Barry S. Levine, D.Sc., D.A.B.T.

CONTENTS

0-8493-0370-2/02/$0.00+$1.50
© 2002 by CRC Press LLC

SECTION 1. BLOOD VOLUMES

The volume of blood in healthy mammals is relatively constant and typically represents about 5 to 9% of body weight, depending on species.[1] Blood volumes of ≈1% of body weight can be collected during the course of a study, (i.e., ≈2.5 ml for a 250 g rat); however, this may cause minimal to moderate stress and/or result in a mild compensatory response by the bone marrow. For frequent periodic sampling, e.g., once weekly, blood volumes of ≈0.5–0.75 ml can be collected from a 250–300 g rat without any untoward effects. Somewhat larger volumes, e.g., ≈1.5–2.0 ml, can be obtained routinely from this size animal on a monthly basis. At necropsy, about 50% of an animal's total blood volume can be obtained using suitable techniques as subsequently discussed. Approximate blood volumes for typical species used in toxicology research are shown in Table 18.1.

TABLE 18.1
Approximate Blood Volumes in Animals Typically Used in Nonclinical Toxicology Research[a]

Species	Typical Body Weight (kg)	Total Volume (ml)	Weekly Sampling	Monthly Sampling	At Necropsy
Mouse	0.03	2	0.075	0.2	1
Rat	0.3	20	1	2	10
Dog	12.0	1000	50	100	400
Monkey[b]	3.0	200	10	20	100
Rabbit	3.0	200	10	20	100

Columns header note: Blood Volume (ml) spans Total Volume, Weekly Sampling, Monthly Sampling.

[a] Modified from Loeb and Quimby[8] and Levine.[10]

[b] Rhesus or cynomolgus.

SECTION 2. BLOOD SAMPLING TECHNIQUES

Numerous sampling techniques are available to collect blood samples in toxicology research. Table 18.2 contains those procedures which are used most typically. Terminal sample procedures listed are usually utilized only when a nonterminal sample procedure would not provide sufficient quantities of blood.

Collection of blood samples from the orbital sinus of rodents is well documented and has been described by several authors.[2,3] The technique is rapid for experienced technicians; however, proficiency can be slow due to the nature of the procedure. One disadvantage is the inability to collect samples by this technique for use in coagulation studies.[4] The orbital sinus procedure results in mild tissue damage releasing tissue thromboplastin, which results in prolonged prothrombin times.

Blood sampling from the jugular vein of rats has recently become popular and has been described by Meeks.[5] The procedure can be performed with or without anesthesia and does not produce physical trauma, such as that encountered in the orbital sinus technique. It is quite rapid and Meeks[5] indicates that two experienced people can collect blood samples from rats at a rate of 1 every 30 seconds. Blood samples can also be obtained from the tail vein of rodents by tail tip transection or tail vein venipuncture. The former procedure may result in somewhat diluted samples, i.e., blood samples contaminated with tissue fluids. Although cardiac puncture has been successfully used to collect blood samples in some laboratories, the associated risks, including blood leakage into the pericardial sac, tend to outweigh any potential advantage over other, more accepted procedures.

Blood collection procedures in canines are typically limited to the cephalic and jugular veins. Although the jugular vein technique may require more training (by technicians and dogs) than sampling from the cephalic vein, the ability to sample repetitively from the jugular vein of dogs suggests that this procedure is more advantageous. This is especially critical in pharmacokinetics studies in which rapid and very repetitive sampling is required. In addition, repetitive sampling from the cephalic vein of dogs, especially by inexperienced technicians, often results in localized tissue damage. Alternatively, a cephalic vein catheter, protected from self-withdrawal, can be used.

For the measurement of routine clinical chemistry tests, venous blood samples typically are collected. If blood gases are to be measured, e.g., PO_2, PCO_2, bicarbonate concentration and pH, arterial samples are preferred; however, venous samples will provide reliable data.[6]

TABLE 18.2
Blood Sampling Techniques Used
in Nonclinical Toxicology Research

Species	Technique
Mouse	Orbital sinus
	Cardiac puncture
Rat	Orbital sinus
	Jugular vein
	Cardiac puncture
	Tail vein
	Aorta (terminal sample)
	Vena cava (terminal sample)
Dog	Jugular vein
	Cephalic vein
Monkey[a]	Femoral vein/artery
	Cephalic vein
Rabbit	Jugular vein
	Marginal ear vein
	Cardiac puncture

[a] Rhesus or cynomolgus.

SECTION 3. BLOOD SAMPLE REQUIREMENTS FOR CLINICAL PATHOLOGY TESTS

Most current clinical chemistry and hematology instruments require relatively small samples for analysis. In hematology testing, a 20–50 µl sample (depending on the instrument) obtained with a suitable anticoagulant such as the potassium salt of EDTA is sufficient to measure directly the following parameters: white blood cell (WBC) count, red blood cell (RBC) count, hemoglobin concentration, mean corpuscular volume (MCV) and platelet count. From these measurements, the following variables can be calculated: hematocrit (packed cell volume), mean corpuscular hemoglobin (MCH), and mean corpuscular hemoglobin concentration (MCHC). Many modern instruments can also directly measure mean platelet volume (MPV).

In addition to the above-described hematology tests, a WBC differential and a reticulocyte count each require about 50 μl, when assessed from separate blood smears with appropriate stains. A few instruments recently adopted for animal clinical pathology studies can measure these parameters directly; however, their cost, in addition to other factors, has not resulted in their routine use. Thus, a hematology sample of ≈300–400 μl collected in Microtainer® tubes coated with K+-EDTA is typically sufficient to measure routine hematologic variables necessary for nonclinical toxicity evaluations.

Additional hematology assays, which may be required in selected nonclinical toxicology studies, include methemoglobin, carboxyhemoglobin, fibrinogen, prothrombin time (PT), and activated partial thromboplastin time (APTT). The first two can be measured with a co-oximeter and can utilize the K+-EDTA sample mentioned previously. Since methemoglobin, the oxidized form of hemoglobin, is somewhat unstable because the blood enzyme methemoglobin reductase will reduce it back to hemoglobin, these samples should be collected on ice and assayed within 1 hour. PT and APTT should be measured from blood samples collected with citrate as the anticoagulant. Because the ratio of the citrate anticoagulant to blood sample is critical, exactly 1 ml of citrated blood must be obtained for coagulation tests using a tuberculin syringe prefilled with 0.1 ml of citrate solution. Larger samples can be collected in Vacutainer® tubes which automatically fill to a predetermined volume, e.g., 2.0 ml (0.2 ml liquid sodium citrate and 1.8 ml blood). Methemoglobin analysis by co-oximetry typically requires less than 100 μl.

When modern instrumentation is used, the volume of serum/plasma required for routine clinical chemistry assays is relatively small, e.g., 5–30 μl per test. Thus, the measurement of approximately 15–20 clinical chemistry parameters usually requires about 400–500 μl of serum/plasma. This, in turn, typically requires about 1.0–1.2 ml whole blood. To account for possible repeat analysis, poor serum yield, etc., approximately 1.5–1.8 ml of blood is routinely collected for a typical battery of hematology and clinical chemistry tests exclusive of coagulation assays (i.e., PT, APTT, and fibrinogen) and methemoglobin analysis.

SECTION 4. CLINICAL CHEMISTRY PARAMETERS

The development of clinical chemistry tests as diagnostic tools in nonclinical toxicology research is based on their use in disease diagnosis in clinical medicine. Thus, many of the routine tests are virtually identical with measurements performed in human clinical laboratories. Fortunately, many of the diagnostic tests adapted from human medicine are appropriate for identifying organ system damage in animals exposed to toxic doses of drugs and other chemicals. Certain clinical chemistry tests, however, are not appropriate, e.g., uric acid levels in laboratory animals. This analyte, typically used to assess renal function in humans, is rapidly converted to allantoin in animals (except for dalmatian dogs), which is not suitable for routine assay. It should be noted that commercial clinical chemistry reagents currently used in animal testing are for assay of human analytes. Thus, optical conditions for measurement of laboratory animal analytes may not be met by these reagents. The reader should consult other textbooks for an in-depth discussion on the significance of altered clinical chemistry measurements with regard to the diagnosis of disease, including those which are chemically induced.[7,8]

In 1992, a joint task force of the American Association for Clinical Chemistry's Division of Animal Clinical Chemistry (AACC-DACC) and the American Society for Veterinary Clinical Pathology (ASVCP) published clinical pathology testing recommendations in animals used in nonclinical toxicity testing programs.[9] These expert recommendations provided a standardized approach to the harmonization of clinical pathology testing in laboratory animals used in nonclinical toxicology research. The paper suggests general and specific approaches, and typical clinical chemistry tests which fulfill these testing requirements are summarized in Table 18.3.

The primary function of serum/plasma clinical chemistry testing in nonclinical safety assessment testing is to determine potential target organs of toxicity and the associated time course of that damage without the need of biopsy or necropsy samples. Histopathology studies typically performed at the end of a study support clinical pathology findings. In certain instances, the measurement of increased levels of certain analytes, e.g., enzymes, does not always indicate the specific target organ which is affected. Several organs contain reasonably high levels of the same enzyme, but in different isozyme forms. Thus, without suitable isozyme analysis, the assignment of specific organs at risk is sometimes fraught with uncertainty. Examples include lactate dehydrogenase (liver, muscle, heart), aspartate animotransferase (liver, muscle, RBCs), and creatine phosphokinase (liver, muscle).

Serum corticosteroid levels are not typically measured in safety assessment studies, but can be useful when drug-induced stress occurs or a debilitating condition is seen. Effects secondary to elevated corticosteroid levels include leukocytosis and thymic lymphocyte depletion.

TABLE 18.3
Routine Clinical Chemistry Testing Recommendations in Nonclinical Safety Assessment Studies[a]

Core Battery

Albumin	Glucose
Calcium	Phosphorus, inorganic
Chloride	Protein, total
Creatinine	Potassium
Cholesterol, total	Sodium
Globulin	Urea nitrogen

Hepatocellular Health	**Hepatobiliary Health**
(Minimum of two tests), e.g.,	(Minimum of two tests), e.g.,
Alanine aminotransferase	Alkaline phosphatase
Aspartate animotransferase	Gamma glutamyltransferase
Sorbitol dehydrogenase	5′-Nucleotidase
Total bile acids	Total bile acids

[a] Modified from Weingand et al.[9]

SECTION 5. HEMATOLOGY PARAMETERS

As described previously for clinical chemistry tests, hematology measurements in nonclinical toxicology research are also based on human diagnostic disease procedures. Hematology assays give vital information regarding the status of bone marrow activity, as well as potential intravascular effects, e.g., hemolysis. Hematology measurements and their significance in diagnostic veterinary medicine and nonclinical toxicology research are detailed in several textbooks that are beyond the scope of this chapter.[10,11]

The advent of hematology instrumentation has resulted in significantly greater accuracy and precision over manual methods. Many hematology instruments currently used in animal research can be adjusted for species differences in erythrocyte size. This allows for the determination of an accurate RBC count and subsequent calculations of packed cell volume (hematocrit), mean corpuscular hemoglobin, and mean corpuscular hemoglobin concentration. Although WBC differential counts are routinely determined in the laboratory as a percent of total WBCs, they must be multiplied by the total WBC count to result in quantitatively meaningful data, i.e., absolute differential WBC counts.[9] Leukocytes are classified by function into lymphocytes, neutrophils, eosinophils, basophils and monocytes. Lymphocytes and neutrophils predominate, with one cell type typically seen in greater numbers, depending on the species as follows: lymphocytes (rats, mice, rabbits); neutrophils (dogs); mixed (monkeys).

The AACC-DACC/ASVCP Joint Task Force publication described previously also includes hematology recommendations in nonclinical toxicology testing.[9] Those recommendations are shown in Table 4. However, other tests may be appropriate depending on the type of agent under investigation. These include but are not limited to the following: methemoglobin levels, RBCs with Heinz bodies, RBCs with Howell-Jolly bodies, and fibrinogen levels.

TABLE 18.4
Routine Hematology Testing Recommendations in Nonclinical Safety Assessment Studies[a]

Parameters

Activated partial thromboplastin time	Mean corpuscular hemoglobin
Erythrocyte count	Mean corpuscular hemoglobin concentration
Hematocrit	Mean corpuscular volume
Hemoglobin	Platelet count
Leukocyte count, total	Prothrombin time
Leukocyte count, differential	Reticulocyte count[b]

[a] Adopted from Weingand et al.[9]
[b] Slides should be prepared, but only evaluated if signs of anemia are present.

SECTION 6. URINALYSIS PARAMETERS

Urinalysis measurements are primarily concerned with renal function and can aid in the identification of chemically induced nephrotoxicity. The method of urine sample collection can alter the urinalysis, and a fresh sample may be preferred if urine volume is not necessary. This can be obtained directly from the bladder at necropsy or by physically manipulating the animal. If a timed (e.g., 16–24 h) urine volume is necessary, it may be useful to collect the sample into a cooled vessel or into one which contains a preservative.

The previously described AACC-DACC/ASVCP Joint Task Force publication includes recommendations for the conduct of urinalysis in safety assessment studies, which are shown in Table 18.5.[9] Urinalysis measurements are typically of limited usefulness and may only be appropriate if kidney toxicity is suspected from preliminary studies. Refer to Chapter 10 for detailed information on renal function parameters for various rat strains and Table 33.15 for other species.

TABLE 18.5
Routine Urinalysis Testing Recommendations in Nonclinical Safety Assessment Studies[a]

Recommended

Specific gravity
Volume (timed, 16–24 h)

TABLE 18.5 *(Continued)*
Routine Urinalysis Testing Recommendations in Nonclinical Safety Assessment Studies[a]

	Recommended
Optional	
Semiquantitative (reagent strips), e.g., microscopic examination of spun sediment	Bilirubin, glucose, ketones, occult blood, pH, protein, urobilinogen, etc.

[a] Adapted from Weingand et al.[9]

SECTION 7. REFERENCE VALUES

Although concurrent control animals should always be included in any aspect of toxicology research, the availability of in-house historical control clinical pathology data is often useful in data interpretation. Laboratories actively engaged in nonclinical toxicology research should therefore establish in-house reference ranges during the early phase of their testing programs. Although helpful for comparative purposes, control animal data from the literature as well as from other laboratories are inappropriate for use as in-house historical control databases. Clinical pathology test values are affected by numerous variables, as summarized in Table 18.6.

In an attempt to present "typical" control animal clinical pathology ranges, literature data in addition to unpublished observations have been used. The ranges presented are approximate and are shown for mean values, not for individual data points. Thus, estimates of variability within a given set of experimental measurements are not presented. These data sets were obtained under many different experimental conditions, e.g., source of animals, diet, fasted or nonfasted, caging conditions, environmental conditions, blood collection site, anesthetic, instrumentation, etc. The reader is directed to consult the references provided for specific details.

As mentioned previously, urinalysis measurements are usually of limited usefulness, unless kidney toxicity is evident. In general, semiquantitative measurements using reagent strips as shown in Table 18.5 typically yield negative to trace results in all species, whereas microscopic examination of a spun sediment yields negative to occasional quantities of cells, casts, crystals, bacteria, etc. In laboratory animals, urinary specific gravity usually ranges from ≈1.000 to ≈1.060, whereas pH typically ranges from 6 to 9.

Reference value data are presented in Tables 18.7 through 18.13 (clinical chemistry) and Tables 18.14 through 18.20 (hematology). Tables have been arranged by species, strain, and age. Generally, sex effects are either minimal or not apparent in laboratory animal clinical pathology measurements. Where significant differences do exist, e.g., serum alkaline phosphatase, cholesterol, protein and triglyceride levels, and leukocyte counts, both ranges are shown.

TABLE 18.6
Factors that can Affect Clinical Chemistry and Hematology Test Measurements

Biologic	**Methodologic**
Species	Blood collection site
Sex	Anesthetic use
Age	Instrumentation
Fasting conditions	Assay conditions, i.e., temperature, substrate concentration, etc.
Diet	

TABLE 18.7
Mean Control Ranges of Typical Serum Clinical Chemistry Measurements in CD® Rats[a]

Parameter	10–12 Weeks Old	18–20 Weeks Old	32–34 Weeks Old	58–60 Weeks Old	84–86 Weeks Old	108–110 Weeks Old
Alanine aminotransferase (ALT) (IU/l)	10–40	10–50	10–50	20–60	20–60	20–60
Albumin (g/dl)	3.4–4.1 (M) 3.5–4.5 (F)	3.3–4.2 (M) 3.5–4.7 (F)	3.5–4.0 (M) 4.0–5.0 (F)	3.0–3.8 (M) 3.5–4.5 (F)	3.0–4.0 (M) 3.7–4.5 (F)	2.7–3.5 (M) 3.3–3.7 (F)
Albumin/globulin ratio	1.0–1.5	1.0–1.5	1.0–1.5	0.75–1.75	0.75–1.75	0.75–1.5
Alkaline phosphatase (IU/l)	140–300 (M) 80–100 (F)	50–150 (M) 25–150 (F)	50–150 (M) 25–100 (F)	50–150 (M) 25–100 (F)	50–150 (M) 25–100 (F)	50–100 (M) 25–100 (F)
Aspartate aminotransferase (AST) (IU/l)	45–90	45–100	45–120	60–120	75–150	75–150
Bile acids, total (umol/l)	20–60	20–60	—b	—	—	—
Bilirubin, total (mg/dl)	0.2–0.4	0.1–0.5	0.1–0.5	0.1–0.5	0.1–0.5	0.1–0.4
Calcium (mg/dl)	9.8–12.0	9.8–12.0	9.8–12.0	9.8–12.0	9.8–12.0	9.8–12.0
Chloride (mEq/l)	97–105	97–105	95–105	97–105	97–105	95–105
Cholesterol, total (mg/dl)	50–85	50–100	70–140	60–150	130–180 (M) 100–150 (F)	130–180 (M) 90–150 (F)
Creatine kinase (CK) (IU/l)	50–400	50–300	50–500	—	—	—
Creatinine (mg/dl)	0.3–0.8	0.3–0.9	0.3–1.0	0.4–0.8	0.4–0.8	0.4–1.3
Gamma glutamyltransferase (γGT) (IU/l)	0–2	0–2	0–3	0–5	0–7	0–5
Globulin (g/dl)	2.5–4.0	2.5–4.0	2.0–4.5	2.0–4.5	2.0–4.5	2.0–4.5
Glucose (mg/dl)	90–175	100–175	100–200	100–200	100–175	100–175
Lactate dehydrogenase (LDH) (IU/l)	50–400	50–400	50–500	—	—	—
Phosphorus, inorganic (mg/dl)	7.0–10.0	4.0–8.5	4.0–8.0	3.5–7.0	3.5–8.0	4.0–7.0
Potassium (mEq/l)	5.5–8.0	4.0–7.0	4.0–7.0	4.0–7.0	3.5–6.0	3.5–6.0
Protein, total (g/dl)	6.2–7.6 (M) 6.3–8.2 (F)	6.2–7.8 (M) 6.5–8.5 (F)	6.2–8.0 (M) 7.0–9.0 (F)	6.0–8.0 (M) 6.5–8.5 (F)	6.3–7.6 (M) 6.7–8.0 (F)	5.7–6.5 (M) 6.3–7.1 (F)
Sodium (mEq/l)	140–153	140–153	140–153	140–153	140–153	140–145
Sorbitol dehydrogenase (SDH) (IU/l)	10–30	10–30	10–30	—	—	—
Triglycerides (mg/dl)	50–125	50–200	50–200	50–300	75–400	50–300
Urea nitrogen (BUN) (mg/dl)	12–18	12–20	12–20	12–18	12–18	12–30

[a] Modified from Levine[10] and Charles River Laboratories.[13]
[b] — = data unavailable.

TABLE 18.8
Mean Control Ranges of Typical Serum Clinical Chemistry Measurements in F-344 Rats[a]

Parameter	12–14 Weeks Old	18–20 Weeks Old	32–34 Weeks Old	58–60 Weeks Old	84–86 Weeks Old	110–112 Weeks Old
Alanine aminotransferase (ALT) (IU/l)	25–45	30–62	20–40	56–100 (M), 33–65 (F)	41–80 (M), 32–50 (F)	25–60
Albumin (g/dl)	3.8–4.7	3.0–5.0	4.0–5.0	3.8–5.0	3.8–5.0	3.5–5.0
Albumin/globulin ratio	1.5–2.3	1.1–2.5	1.5–2.0	1.4–1.9	1.4–2.0	1.2–1.8
Alkaline phosphatase (IU/l)	200–300 (M), 150–250 (F)	58–154 (M), 45–120 (F)	45–80	31–68	—[b]	—
Aspartate aminotransferase (AST) (IU/l)	50–90	50–100	—	—	—	—
Bile acids, total (umol/l)	10–50	—	—	—	—	—
Bilirubin, total (mg/dl)		0.1–0.5	0.1–0.4	0.1–0.5	0.1–0.5	0.1–0.4
Calcium (mg/dl)		9.5–12.0	9.5–11.2	9.5–11.5	9.5–11.5	9.8–11.7
Chloride (mEq/l)		97–115	98–110	100–112	97–100	104–113
Cholesterol, total (mg/dl)	70–110 (M), 90–135 (F)	50–80 (M), 80–120 (F)	50–80 (M), 85–130 (F)	68–125 (M), 110–150 (F)	100–120	125–175
Creatine kinase (CK) (IU/l)	60–300	100–400	300–700	300–500	100–500	100–400
Creatinine (mg/dl)	0.5–1.0	0.4–0.8	—	—	—	—
Globulin (g/dl)	1.5–2.5	1.2–2.8	2.0–3.0	2.3–3.5	2.0–3.0	2.2–3.2
Glucose (mg/dl)	100–180	90–170	80–130	90–140	90–140	90–140
Lactate dehydrogenase (LDH) (IU/l)	500–800	500–800	—	—	—	—
Phosphorus, inorganic (mg/dl)		3.9–7.3	400–800	150–400	—	—
Potassium (mEq/l)		3.6–5.9	4.0–5.7	4.1–5.5	4.0–5.2	4.0–5.1
Protein, total (g/dl)	6.0–7.2	5.7–7.6	6.2–7.5	6.5–7.6	6.0–7.8	6.1–8.0
Sodium (mEq/l)	140–155	140–155	142–158	142–156	138–149	138–146
Sorbitol dehydrogenase (SDH) (IU/l)	15–60	5–25	5–35	—	—	—
Triglycerides (mg/dl)	100–400 (M), 25–130 (F)	75–150 (M), 35–70 (F)	125–190 (M), 30–70 (F)	90–175 (M), 40–85 (F)	110–240 (M), 60–145 (F)	80–220
Urea nitrogen (BUN) (mg/dl)	15–25	10–26	12–24	10–20	10–20	12–25

[a] Modified from Levine,[10] NIEHS,[14] and Burns et al.[15]

[b] — = Data unavailable.

TABLE 18.9
Mean Control Ranges of Typical Serum Clinical Chemistry Measurements in B6C3F$_1$ Mice[a]

Parameter	12–14 Weeks Old	18–20 Weeks Old	32–34 Weeks Old	58–60 Weeks Old	84–86 Weeks Old	110–112 Weeks Old
Alanine aminotransferase (ALT) (IU/l)	20–50	25–100	22–90	20–50	23–60	23–60
Albumin (g/dl)	2.3–4.4	2.5–4.2	2.7–3.8	3.0–4.0	3.0–3.9	3.0–4.1
Albumin/globulin ratio	1.0–2.0	0.8–2.0	1.2–1.9	1.3–1.9	1.3–2.0	1.3–2.0
Alkaline phosphatase (IU/l)	30–80 (M) 40–140 (F)	20–55 (M) 45–85 (F)	—[b]	—	—	—
Aspartate aminotransferase (AST) (IU/l)	40–110	64–180	—	—	—	—
Bilirubin, total (mg/dl)	—	0.1–0.5	0.1–0.5	0.1–0.5	0.1–0.5	0.1–0.5
Calcium (mg/dl)	—	8.2–11.8	—	—	—	—
Chloride (mEq/l)	—	110–128	—	—	—	—
Cholesterol, total (mg/dl)	90–160	80–130	85–150	80–150	90–160	90–175
Creatine kinase (CK) (IU/l)	50–300	—	—	—	—	—
Creatinine (mg/dl)	0.3–0.8	0.2–0.8	—	—	—	—
Globulin (g/dl)	1.5–2.5	1.0–2.7	1.6–2.4	1.8–3.1	1.6–3.0	1.8–3.0
Glucose (mg/dl)	125–200	81–165	115–170	115–170	115–170	115–170
Phosphorus, inorganic (mg/dl)	—	3.6–7.3	—	—	—	—
Potassium (mEq/l)	4.5–5.5	4.0–6.0	4.2–6.2	4.8–6.5	4.8–6.6	5.4–6.5
Sodium (mEq/l)	—	147–163	—	—	—	—
Sorbitol dehydrogenase (SDH) (IU/l)	15–50	18–57	—	—	—	—
Triglycerides (mg/dl)	75–175	75–130	100–173	90–190	110–160	90–175
Urea nitrogen (BUN) (mg/dl)	15–35	12–34	12–27	12–24	10–24	15–28

[a] Modified from Levine[10] and NIEHS.[14]
[b] — = Data unavailable.

TABLE 18.10
Mean Control Ranges of Typical Serum Clinical Chemistry Measurements in CD-1 and BALB/c Mice[a]

Parameter	<1-Year-Old CD-1	>1-Year-Old CD-1	1–3-Month-Old BALB/c	6–12-Month-Old BALB/c
Alanine aminotransferase (ALT) (IU/l)	30–250 (M)	20–200 (M)	—[b]	—
	30–100 (F)	20–80 (F)	—	—
Albumin (g/dl)	—	—	1.6–2.6	1.3–2.6
Albumin/globulin ratio	—	—	—	—
Alkaline phosphatase (IU/l)	30–70	20–75	75–275	47–102
Aspartate aminotransferase (AST) (IU/l)	75–300	75–300	40–140	70–110
Bilirubin, total (mg/dl)	0.2–0.8	0.2–0.8	0.5–1.2	0.4–1.0
Calcium (mg/dl)	8.5–11.5	6.7–11.5	7.8–10.8	6.5–9.6
Chloride (mEq/l)	110–125	110–135	—	—
Cholesterol, total (mg/dl)	90–170 (M)	60–170 (M)	165–295	100–300
	60–125 (F)	50–100 (F)		
Creatine kinase (CK) (IU/l)	—	—	—	—
Creatinine (mg/dl)	0.3–1.0	0.2–2.0	—	—
Globulin (g/dl)	—	—	—	—
Glucose (mg/dl)	75–175	60–150	75–150	40–160
Phosphorus, inorganic (mg/dl)	7.5–11.0	6.0–10.0	4.5–8.9	4.7–7.2
Potassium (mEq/l)	6.5–9.0	6.6–9.0	—	—
Protein, total (g/dl)	4.5–6.0	3.5–5.6	4.4–6.0	4.4–6.4
Sodium (mEq/l)	145–160	155–170	—	—
Triglycerides (mg/dl)	60–140 (M)	40–150 (M)	—	—
	50–100 (F)	25–75 (F)		
Urea Nitrogen (BUN) (mg/dl)	20–40	20–70	10–30	10–30

[a] Modified from Frith et al.[16] and Wolford et al.[17]
[b] — = Data unavailable.

TABLE 18.11
Mean Control Ranges of Typical Serum Clinical Chemistry Measurements in Beagle Dogs[a]

Parameter	6–8 Months Old[b]	9–11 Months Old	12–14 Months Old	15–18 Months Old	19–30 Months Old
Alanine aminotransferase (ALT) (IU/l)	20–40	20–40	20–40	20–40	20–40
Albumin (g/dl)	2.5–3.5	2.5–3.5	2.5–3.5	2.5–4.0	2.7–4.5
Albumin/Globulin ratio	0.8–1.5	0.8–1.5	0.8–1.5	0.8–2.0	0.8–2.0
Alkaline phosphatase (IU/l)	120–160 (M) 100–130 (F)	70–120 (M) 60–100 (F)	50–100	35–100	35–100
Aspartate aminotransferase (AST) (IU/l)	30–45	30–50	25–50	25–50	25–50
Bilirubin, total (mg/dl)	0.1–0.7	0.1–0.7	0.1–0.7	0.1–0.3	0.1–0.3
Calcium (mg/dl)	9.0–11.5	9.0–11.5	9.0–11.5	10.0–11.3	10.0–11.5
Chloride (mEq/l)	100–115	100–115	100–115	105–119	105–115
Cholesterol, total (mg/dl)	150–250	125–250	125–250	125–250	125–225
Creatine kinase (CK) (IU/l)	100–400	100–400	100–400	—	—
Creatinine (mg/dl)	0.5–0.8	0.7–0.9	0.7–0.9	—	—
Gamma glutamyltransferase (γGT) (IU/l)	0–5	0–5	0–5	—	—
Globulin (g/dl)	2.5–3.5	2.5–3.5	2.5–3.5	2.5–3.5	2.5–3.5
Glucose (mg/dl)	100–130	100–130	100–130	70–110	70–110
Haptoglobin (mg/dl)	50–200	50–150	25–100	—	—
Lactate dehydrogenase (LDH) (IU/l)	30–100	30–100	30–100	—	—
Phosphorus, inorganic (mg/dl)	6.0–9.0	4.0–6.0	3.0–5.0	3.0–5.0	3.0–4.7
Potassium (mEq/l)	4.2–5.0	4.2–5.0	4.2–5.0	4.1–5.1	4.2–5.2
Protein, total (g/dl)	5.5–6.5	5.5–6.5	5.5–6.5	5.5–6.5	5.7–6.6
Sodium (mEq/l)	143–147	143–147	143–147	143–153	143–153
Triglycerides (mg/dl)	30–60	30–75	30–75	—	—
Urea nitrogen (BUN) (mg/dl)	10–20	10–20	10–20	10–20	10–20

[a] Modified from Levine,[10] Clarke et al.,[18] Pickrell et al.,[19] and Kaspar and Norris.[20]

[b] Mo = month; — = Data unavailable.

TABLE 18.12
Mean Control Ranges of Typical Serum Clinical Chemistry Measurements in Nonhuman Primates[a]

Parameter	3–7-Year-Old Cynomolgus	1–2-Year-Old Rhesus	3–7-Year-Old Rhesus	<1.5-Year-Old Marmoset	>1.5-Year-Old Marmoset	1–5-Year-Old Baboon	6–15-Year-Old Baboon
Alanine aminotransferase (ALT) (IU/l)	20–60	20–50	15–40	45–75	40–70	15–50	20–50
Albumin (g/dl)	3.5–4.8	3.0–4.5	3.2–4.5	3.5–5.8	3.5–5.8	3.1–4.5	2.0–4.5
Albumin/Globulin ratio	1.0–1.5	1.0–1.5	1.0–1.5	1.0–1.5	1.0–1.5	1.0–1.5	1.0–1.5
Alkaline phosphatase (IU/l))	300–800 (M) 200–500 (F)	200–600	70–300	100–250	35–80	200–1000	100–200
Amylase (IU/l)	200–500	—[b]	—	1000–2000	500–1500	200–400	200–500
Aspartate aminotransferase (AST) (IU/l)	25–60	25–60	15–70	100–200	100–200	18–35	20–35
Bilirubin, total (mg/dl)	0.3–0.8	0.1–0.8	0.1–0.6	0.1–0.9	0.1–0.9	0.3–0.7	0.3–0.5
Calcium (mg/dl)	9.0–11.0	8.2–10.5	8.5–10.3	8.1–12.4	8.5–11.7	8.0–9.5	7.5–10.0
Chloride (mEq/l)	100–115	103–115	97–110	80–110	93–119	105–115	100–110
Cholesterol, total (mg/dl)	90–160	90–160	90–170	90–210	105–230	75–200	70–125
Creatine kinase (CK) (IU/l)	140–200	200–1000	200–600	—	—	—	—
Creatinine (mg/dl)	0.7–1.2	0.5–0.9	0.7–1.2	0.2–1.0	0.2–1.0	0.8–1.2	1.0–1.8
Gamma glutamyltransferase (γGT) (IU/l)	40–90	—	10–60	—	—	—	—
Globulin (g/dl)	3.0–4.5	3.0–4.0	3.0–4.0	2.5–4.0	3.5–4.0	2.5–4.0	2.5–4.5
Glucose (mg/dl)	50–100	50–100	41–80	180–275	130–240	50–125	50–140
Lactate dehydrogenase (LDH) (IU/l)	300–600	130–600	125–600	125–500	100–350	100–400	100–350
Phosphorus, inorganic (mg/dl)	4.0–7.0	3.2–5.0	3.0–5.3	5.5–9.8	4.0–7.5	4.7–7.5	1.3–4.5
Potassium (mEq/l)	3.0–4.5	3.0–4.2	3.1–4.1	3.5–5.0	3.0–4.8	3.2–4.3	3.7–4.8
Protein, total (g/dl)	7.0–9.0	6.7–8.0	7.0–8.3	5.5–7.5	6.0–8.0	6.0–8.0	6.0–7.5
Sodium (mEq/l)	140–153	144–150	142–148	150–170	150–170	142–158	142–158
Triglycerides (mg/dl)	30–70	50–200	50–200	75–200	75–200	25–60	30–125
Urea nitrogen (BUN) (mg/dl)	15–25	14–26	14–25	17–35	15–32	10–25	10–25

a Modified from Clark et al.,[17] Levine,[10] Kapeghian et al.,[21] Davy et al.,[22] Yarbrough et al.,[23] and Hack and Gleiser[24]

b — = Data unavailable.

TABLE 18.13
Mean Control Ranges of Typical Serum Clinical Chemistry Measurements in New Zealand White Rabbits[a]

Parameter	15–20 Weeks Old	25–40 Weeks Old	1–2 Years Old
Alanine aminotransferase (ALT) (IU/l)	25–70	25–70	25–70
Albumin (g/dl)	3.8–5.0	3.5–4.7	3.0–4.5
Albumin/globulin ratio	2.0–3.0	2.0–3.0	2.0–3.0
Alkaline phosphatase (IU/l)	50–120	40–120	15–90
Aspartate aminotransferase (AST) (IU/l)	20–50	10–35	10–30
Bilirubin, total (mg/dl)	0.1–0.5	0.1–0.5	0.2–0.6
Calcium (mg/dl)	12.0–14.0	11.0–14.0	12.0–15.0
Chloride (mEq/l)	97–110	96–108	100–110
Cholesterol, total (mg/dl)	20–60	20–60	20–60
Creatine kinase (CK) (IU/l)	200–800	200–1000	200–1000
Creatinine (mg/dl)	1.0–1.6	0.8–1.6	0.8–1.7
Gamma glutamyltransferase (γ GT) (IU/l)	—[b]	0–10	0–6
Globulin (g/dl)	1.4–1.9	1.5–2.2	1.5–2.5
Glucose (mg/dl)	100–160	100–175	80–140
Lactate dehydrogenase (LDH) (IU/l)	50–200	50–200	35–125
Phosphous, inorganic (mg/dl)	4.6–7.2	4.0–7.0	3.0–5.0
Potassium (mEq/l)	4.0–5.2	4.0–5.0	3.3–4.5
Protein, total (g/dl)	5.4–6.6	5.5–7.0	5.5–7.5
Sodium (mEq/l)	132–144	132–145	132–150
Urea nitrogen (BUN) (mg/dl)	10–20	12–22	12–25

[a] Modified from Levine,[10] Hewett et al.,[25] and Yu et al.[26]
[b] — = Data unavailable.

TABLE 18.14
Mean Control Ranges of Typical Hematology Measurements in CD® Rats[a]

Parameters	10–12 Weeks Old	18–20 Weeks Old	32–34 Weeks Old	58–60 Weeks Old	84–86 Weeks Old	108–110 Weeks Old
Activated partial thromboplastin time (sec)	14.0–20.0 (M), 12.0–18.0 (F)	14.0–20.0 (M), 13.0–18.0 (F)	14.0–17.0 (M), 13.0–16.0 (F)	16.0–19.0 (M), 15.0–18.0 (F)	—[b]	—
Erythrocyte count (10^6/mm^3)	6.8–8.5 (M), 7.0–8.2 (F)	7.0–9.8 (M), 6.5–9.2 (F)	7.0–9.6 (M), 6.5–8.8 (F)	7.0–9.2(M), 6.5–8.5 (F)	7.0–9.2 (M), 6.0–8.5 (F)	6.2–8.2 (M), 5.8–8.0 (F)
Fibrinogen (mg/dl)		200–300 (M), 130–190 (F)				
Hematocrit(%)	40.0–48.0	36.0–52.0	36.0–50.0	38.0–48.0	38.0–50.0	35.0–45.0
Hemoglobin (g/dl)	14.0–17.0	14.0–17.0	14.0–17.0	14.0–17.0	14.0–17.0	12.0–15.0
Leukocyte count, total (10^3/mm^3)	6.0–18.0 (M), 4.0–14.0 (F)	6.0–19.0 (M), 5.0–14.0 (F)	6.0–18.0 (M), 4.0–11.0 (F)	5.0–15.0 (M), 3.0–9.0 (F)	10.0–15.0 (M), 6.0–10.0 (F)	5.0–18.0(M), 3.0–12.0 (F)
Mean corpuscular hemoglobin (pg)	19.0–22.0	16.0–20.0	17.0–21.0	16.0–21.0	16.0–20.0	16.0–20.0
Mean corpuscular hemoglobin conc. (g/dl)	33.0–38.0	31.0–38.0	31.0–38.0	32.0–38.0	31.0–36.0	31.0–36.0
Mean corpuscular volume (fl)	53.0–63.0	50.0–60.0	45.0–60.0	46.0–58.0	48.0–56.0	50.0–63.0
Methemoglobin (% Hgb)	0.4–1.2	0.4–1.2	0.4–1.2	—	—	—
Platelet count (10^3/mm^3)	900–1300	800–1200	700–1200	700–1200	700–1200	700–1200
Prothrombin time (sec)	9.0–14.0	9.0–14.0	10.0–14.0	10.0–14.0	—	—
Reticulocyte count (% RBC)	0.2–1.0	0.2–0.8	0.2–0.8	—	—	—

[a] Modified from Levine[10] and Charles River Laboratories.[27]
[b] — = Data not available.

TABLE 18.15

Mean Control Ranges of Typical Hematology Measurements in F-344 Rats[a]

Parameters	10–12 Weeks Old	18–20 Weeks Old	32–34 Weeks Old	58–60 Weeks Old	84–86 Weeks Old	108–110 Weeks Old
Erythrocyte count (10^6/mm^3)	7.2–8.6	7.0–10.0	8.5–9.6	7.2–9.5	7.5–9.8	6.5–9.6
Hematocrit (%)	39.5–45.5	42.0–50.0	41.4–46.7	40.0–46.6	40.3–45.5	40.0–48.5
Hemoglobin (g/dl)	15.0–17.0	15.0–17.3	15.0–17.8	15.7–17.5	15.5–17.6	13.0–18.5
Leukocyte count, total (10^3/mm^3)	7.1–13.5 (M)	6.5–10.7 (M)	6.5–8.7 (M)	5.8–9.0 (M)	5.7–8.5 (M)	5.0–15.0 (M)
	5.4–11.7 (F)	4.5–7.0 (F)	4.4–6.5 (F)	4.5–6.2 (F)	3.2–6.0 (F)	3.5–8.0 (F)
Mean corpuscular hemoglobin (pg)	18.5–21.0	17.5–20.8	18.5–21.0	18.1–20.7	18.0–20.5	18.5–22.0
Mean corpuscular hemoglobin conc. (g/dl)	36.6–39.6	35.3–39.2	37.8–40.0	36.9–40.5	37.0–40.6	36.3–40.9
Mean corpuscular volume (fl)	48.0–58.0	48.3–56.1	48.0–56.0	47.0–56.0	47.0–56.0	50.0–58.0
Methemoglobin (% Hgb)	—[b]	0–3.0	0–4.0	0–2.5	0–2.7	0–2.0
Platelet count (10^3/mm^3)	400–750	350–700	400–870	450–700	450–700	200–450
Reticulocyte count (% RBC)	1.0–2.0	0.7–2.0	0.8–2.0	0.8–2.0	0.3–1.5	0.5–2.5

[a] Modified, from Levine[10] and NIEHS.[14]

[b] — = Data not available.

TABLE 18.16
Mean Control Ranges of Typical Hematology Measurements in B6C3F$_1$ Mice[a]

Parameters	12–14 Weeks Old	18–20 Weeks Old	32–34 Weeks Old	58–60 Weeks Old	84–86 Weeks Old	110—112 Weeks Old
Erythrocyte count (10^6/mm^3)	9.0–10.2	7.5–10.5	8.0–10.4	8.0–10.0	8.6–10.4	7.7–10.4
Hematocrit (%)	44.1–49.5	36.0–48.6	40.8–46.6	38.5–45.5	40.0–46.9	36.0–43.5
Hemoglobin (g/dl)	15.0–17.1	13.1–16.5	15.2–18.2	14.5–17.9	15.0–18.2	13.0–16.8
Leukocyte count, total (10^3/mm^3)	3.0–7.8 (M)	5.5–10.9 (M)	6.1–13.3 (M)	6.1–13.2 (M)	7.0–13.4 (M)	5.0–16.5 (M)
	2.5–5.0 (F)	3.2–5.2 (F)	4.2–9.3 (F)	4.6–10.5 (F)	3.9–7.9 (F)	4.2–8.8 (F)
Mean corpuscular hemoglobin (pg)	16.6–18.8	16.9–20.2	16.4–18.9	15.8–18.0	15.9–18.3	15.7–18.7
Mean corpuscular hemoglobin conc. (g/dl)	34.6–38.4	34.6–40.4	37.1–41.2	36.5–39.0	36.2–39.4	35.7–38.8
Mean corpuscular volume (fl)	44.0–52.0	45.4–53.6	44.0–48.0	42.0–47.0	42.0–48.0	46.0–50.0
Methemoglobin (% Hgb)	—[b]	0–3.0	0–2.5	0–1.5	0–0.9	0–1.0
Platelet count (10^3/mm^3)	700–1100	500–1000	800–1200	700–1200	400–1100	400–800
Reticulocyte count (% RBC)	0.5–2.0	1.0–3.9	0.4–2.8	0.4–1.6	0.2–2.3	0.5–2.5

[a] Modified, from Levine[10] and NIEHS.[14]
[b] — = Data not available.

TABLE 18.17
Mean Control Ranges of Typical Hematology Measurements in CD-1 and BALB/c Mice[a]

Parameters	1–3-Month-Old BALB/c	6–12-Month-Old BALB/c	<1–Year-Old CD-1	>1–Year-Old CD-1
Erythrocyte count (10⁶/mm³)	8.5–10.5	8.8–10.6	8.0–10.0	6.0–9.0
Hematocrit (%)	42.5–47.9	38.3–46.9	36.9–46.9	28.2–41.1
Hemoglobin (g/dl)	14.5–16.8	14.2–17.0	13.6–16.8	10.4–14.9
Leukocyte count, total (10³/mm³)	2.0–5.7	2.0–5.0	4.0–12.0 (M)	3.4–17.0 (M)
			3.5–9.7 (F)	2.4–13.4 (F)
Mean corpuscular hemoglobin (pg)	15.8–18.4	15.1–17.5	16.1–18.6	15.1–18.4
Mean corpuscular hemoglobin concentration (g/dl)	34.2–38.1	35.1–40.6	34.8–38.2	34.6–37.6
Mean corpuscular volume (fl)	46.3–50.3	40.9–45.9	44.5–49.7	41.3–51.1
Platelet count (10³/mm³)	—[b]	—	700–1400	700–1500
Reticulocyte count (% RBC)	—	—	1.6–3.7	1.7–5.0

[a] Modified from Frith et al.[16] and Wolford et al.[17]

[b] — = Data not available.

TABLE 18.18
Mean Control Ranges of Typical Hematology Measurements in Beagle Dogs[a]

Parameters	6–8 Months Old[b]	9–11 Months Old	12–14 Months Old	15–18 Months Old	19–30 Months Old
Activated partial thromboplastin time (sec)	9.0–13.0	9.0–13.0	9.0–13.0	9.0–13.0	9.0–13.0
Erythrocyte count (10⁶/mm³)	6.0–7.3	6.2–8.0	6.2–8.2	5.8–7.3	5.8–7.3
Fibrinogen (mg/dl)	150–300	100–200	—[b]	—	—
Hematocrit (%)	41.5–49.0	44.3–54.9	46.0–54.6	42.5–55.0	42.0–52.0
Hemoglobin (g/dl)	14.5–17.3	15.8–18.0	16.0–18.8	13.0–19.0	13.0–19.0
Leukocyte count, total (10³/mm³)	5.5–14.0	6.8–13.6	5.7–15.5	5.0–15.0	6.0–18.0
Mean corpuscular hemoglobin (pg)	21.5–25.1	21.6–24.9	22.0–25.2	22.5–26.0	23.0–26.0
Mean corpuscular hemoglobin conc. (g/dl)	33.0–37.0	33.0–36.4	34.0–36.0	30.0–34.0	30.0–34.0
Mean corpuscular volume (fl)	65.0–71.0	64.0–73.0	64.0–72.0	65.0–78.0	65.0–78.0
Methemoglobin (% Hgb)	0–2.0	0–1.5	0–1.5	—	—
Platelet count (10³/mm³)	150–400	150–400	150–400	150–400	150–400
Prothrombin time (sec)	6.2–8.4	6.8–8.4	6.2–8.8	6.5–9.0	6.5–9.0
Reticulocyte count (% RBC)	0–0.7	0–0.7	0–0.7	0–0.7	0–0.7

[a] Modified from Levine,[10] Bulgin et al.,[28] and Jordan[29]

[b] — = Data not available.

TABLE 18.19
Mean Control Ranges of Typical Hematology Measurements in Nonhuman Primates[a]

Parameters	3–7-Year-Old Cynomolgus	1–2-Year-Old Rhesus	3–7-Year-Old Rhesus	<1.5-Year-Old Marmoset	>1.5-Year-Old Marmoset	1–5-Year-Old Baboon	6–15-Year-Old Baboon
Activated partial thromboplastin time (sec)	15.5–22.7	15.0–22.0	15.0–22.0	—[b]	—	—	30–60
Erythrocyte count (10^6/mm^3)	4.5–7.2	4.4–5.8	4.2–6.2	4.2–6.2	4.6–6.8	4.2–5.7	4.0–5.3
Hematocrit (%)	31.5–37.9	31.5–39.2	29.3–39.0	30.0–42.1	37.7–47.5	31.0–43.0	34.0–42.0
Hemoglobin (g/dl)	10.4–12.4	10.8–13.5	9.8–13.1	12.6–15.0	13.5–16.8	10.8–13.5	10.3–13.1
Leukocyte count, total (10^3/mm^3)	5.3–13.4	4.5–13.3	4.3–12.2	5.5–13.0	4.6–11.3	4.9–13.0	4.8–13.9
Mean corpuscular hemoglobin (pg)	18.9–22.3	19.8–24.8	19.6–23.2	24.0–30.5	23.0–29.0	22.0–27.0	22.0–28.0
Mean corpuscular hemoglobin conc. (g/dl)	32.0–35.6	31.3–35.5	31.7–37.5	32.1–42.6	32.2–42.5	28.0–34.0	30.0–35.0
Mean corpuscular volume (fl)	57.1–63.9	66.0–74.0	56.0–70.0	66.0–76.0	68.0–77.0	63.0–80.0	75.0–91.0
Platelet count (10^3/mm^3)	150–400	200–600	200–500	200–500	200–500	200–500	200–500
Prothrombin time (sec)	11.5–14.0	9.9–12.2	11.2–14.4	—	—	—	9.0–13.0
Reticulocyte count (% RBC)	0–0.5	0–1.4	0–1.5	0–5.0	0–4.7	0–2.3	0–1.9

[a] Modified from Levine,[10] Kapeghian and Verlangieri,[21] Yarbrough et al.,[23] and Hack and Gleiser.[24]
[b] — = Data not available.

TABLE 18.20
Mean Control Ranges of Typical Hematology Measurements in New Zealand White Rabbits[a]

Parameters	15–20 Weeks Old	25–40 Weeks Old	1–2 Years Old
Activated partial thromboplastin time (sec)	11.7–14.5	11.3–14.9	10.5–15.8
Erythrocyte count (10^6/mm³)	5.5–7.0	4.8–6.7	4.9–7.0
Fibrinogen (mg/dl)	125–300	125–300	125–400
Hematocrit (%)	37.0–44.5	37.0–44.5	37.5–44.7
Hemoglobin (g/dl)	12.0–14.7	10.9–14.4	10.5–14.8
Leukocyte count, total (10^3/mm³)	5.4–11.9	3.6–7.9	4.8–13.5
Mean corpuscular hemoglobin (pg)	20.2–23.0	21.8–24.5	20.4–23.4
Mean corpuscular hemoglobin conc. (g/dl)	32.3–34.9	32.2–34.8	30.0–34.1
Mean corpuscular volume (fl)	61.4–68.6	64.8–69.5	64.8–72.0
Platelet count (10^3/mm³)	175–500	175–500	200–500
Reticulocyte count (% RBC)	0–2.0	0–2.0	0–3.0
Prothrombin time (sec)	8.2–9.8	8.0–10.0	8.0–10.3

[a] Modified from Levine,[10] Jain,[11] and Hewett et al.[25]

SECTION 8. GLOSSARY

Activated partial thromboplastin time A measure of the relative activity of factors in the intrinsic clotting sequence and the common pathway necessary in normal blood coagulation.

Acute phase proteins A diverse group of proteins, primarily synthesized in the liver, whose blood levels can rise in response to tissue injury.

Alanine aminotransferase (ALT) An enzyme, primarily of liver origin, whose blood levels can rise in response to hepatocellular injury. Also known as SGPT (Serum Glutamic Pyruvic Transaminase).

Albumin The most abundant blood protein synthesized by the liver.

Albumin/globulin (A:G) ratio The ratio of the two major classes of blood proteins, which may decrease after chronic hepatocellular toxicity.

Alkaline phosphatase An enzyme whose blood levels can rise in response to hepatobiliary disease or increased osteoblastic (bone cell) activity. Serum alkaline phosphatase activity can decrease in fasted rats because the intestinal isozyme is an important component of serum enzyme activity.

Anemia Any conditions in which RBC count, hemoglobin concentration, and hematocrit are reduced.

Anisocytosis Variations in the size of red blood cells.

Aspartate aminotransferase (AST) An enzyme whose blood levels can rise in response to hepatotoxicity, muscle damage, or hemolysis. Also known as SGOT (Serum Glutamic Oxaloacetic Transaminase).

Azotemia An increase in serum urea nitrogen and/or creatinine levels.

Bile acids Endstage metabolites of cholesterol metabolism, which are secreted into bile. Levels may be elevated in hepatobiliary disease.

Bilirubin Metabolic product of hemoglobin.

Calcium Divalent cation necessary in many fundamental biologic processes.

Chloride Monovalent anion which in concert with sodium regulates water distribution, maintenance of osmotic pressure, and acid-base equilibrium.

Cholesterol A precursor to steroid hormones and bile acids, whose blood concentration may be altered in response to certain physiologic changes.

Creatine kinase (CK) An enzyme that is concentrated in skeletal muscle, brain, and heart tissue.

Creatinine The end product of creatine metabolism in muscle. Elevated blood levels can indicate renal (glomerular) injury.

Erythrocyte Mature red blood cell.

Erythropoiesis The formation of red blood cells.

Fibrinogen A glycoprotein that is involved in the formation of fibrin.

Gamma glutamyltransferase (γ GT) An enzyme of liver origin, whose blood concentration can be elevated in hepatobiliary disease.

Globulin A group of blood proteins synthesized by lymphatic tissue and in the liver.

Glucose A carbohydrate that provides a major energy source.

Haptoglobin One of the acute phase proteins secreted by the liver. Blood haptoglobin also binds to free plasma hemoglobin.

Hematocrit Packed (red) cell volume.

Hemoglobin A red blood cell hemoprotein that carries oxygen.

Hemolysis The destruction of red blood cells resulting in liberation of hemoglobin into plasma.

Hypokalemia Decrease in serum potassium concentration.

Icteric Relating to a jaundiced condition, typically as a result of elevated serum bilirubin levels.

Lactate dehydrogenase An enzyme found in several organs, including liver, kidney, heart, and skeletal muscle.

Leukocyte White blood cell.

Leukocytopenia Decrease in the number of white blood cells per unit volume.

Leukocytosis Increase in the number of white blood cells per unit volume.

Mean corpuscular hemoglobin The average amount of hemoglobin per red blood cell.

Mean corpuscular hemoglobin concentration The average hemoglobin concentration per red blood cell.

Mean corpuscular volume The average size of a red blood cell.

Methemoglobin Oxidized hemoglobin incapable of carrying oxygen.

Myeloid:erythroid (M:E) ratio The ratio of WBC to RBC precursors in the bone marrow.

5'-Nucleotidase An enzyme of liver origin, whose blood concentration can be elevated in hepatobiliary disease.

Packed cell volume The percent of blood that contains RBC components; synonymous with hematocrit.

Phosphorus, inorganic An anion that is concerned with intermediary metabolism and energy production.

Platelets Cytoplasmic fragments of bone marrow megakaryocytes that are necessary to maintain hemostasis.

Poikilocytosis Variations in the shape of red blood cells.

Polychromasia Increased basophilic staining of erythrocytes due to increased numbers of young or degenerating cells.

Polycythemia An increase in the number of red blood cells.

Potassium A cation that regulates intracellular osmotic pressure.

Prothrombin time A measure of the relative activity of factors in the extrinsic clotting sequence and the common pathway necessary in normal blood coagulation.

Reticulocyte An immature (polychromatic) erythrocyte.

Reticulocytosis Increased numbers of reticulocytes in the circulation, typically seen in response to regenerative anemia.

Sodium Monovalent cation that, in concert with chloride, regulates water distribution, maintenance of osmotic pressure, and acid-base equilibrium.

Sorbitol dehydrogenase (SDH) An enzyme of liver origin, whose blood concentration rises in response to hepatocellular injury.

Triglycerides Synthesized primarily in the liver and intestine; the major form of lipid storage.

Urea nitrogen (BUN) The endproduct of protein catabolism. Blood levels can rise after renal (glomerular) injury.

REFERENCES

1. Altman, P. L. and Dittmer, D. S., *Biology Data Book,* Federation of American Societies for Experimental Biology, Bethesda, MD, 1974.
2. Midgalof, B. H., Methods for obtaining drug time course data from individual small laboratory animals: serial microblood sampling and assay, *Drug Metab. Rev.,* 5, 295, 1976.
3. Sorg, D. A. and Buckner, B., A simple method of obtaining venous blood from small laboratory animals, *Soc. Exp. Biol. Med. Proc.,* 115, 1131, 1964.
4. Dameron, G. W., Weingand, K. W., Duderstadt, J. M., Odioso, L. W., Dierckman, T. A., Schwecke, W., and Baran, K., Effect of bleeding site on clinical laboratory testing of rats: orbital venous plexus versus posterior vena cava, *Lab. Anim. Sci.,* 42, 299, 1992.
5. Meeks, R. G., The rat, in *The Clinical Chemistry of Laboratory Animals,* Loeb, W. F. and Quimby, F. W., Eds., Pergamon Press, New York, 1989, chap. 2.
6. Riley, J. H. and Cornelius, L. M., Electrolytes, blood gases, and acid base balance, in *The Clinical Chemistry of Laboratory Animals,* Loeb, W. F. and Quimby, F. W., Eds., Pergamon Press, New York, 1989, chap. 5.
7. Kaneko, J. J., *Clinical Biochemistry of Domestic Animals,* Academic Press, San Diego, 1989.
8. Loeb, W. F. and Quimby, F. W., *The Clinical Chemistry of Laboratory Animals,* Pergamon Press, New York, 1989.
9. Weingand, K., Bloom, J., Carakostas, M., Hall, R., Helfrich, M., Latimer, K., Levine, B. S., Neptun, D., Rebar, A., Stitzel, K., and Troup, K., Clinical pathology testing recommendations for nonclinical toxicity and safety studies, *Toxicol. Pathol.,* 20, 539, 1992.
10. Levine, B. S., unpublished data, 1979–1993.
11. Suber, R. L., Clinical pathology for toxicologists, in *Principles and Methods of Toxicology,* Hayes, A. W., Ed., Raven Press, New York, 1989, chap. 16.
12. Jain, N. C., *Schalm's Veterinary Hematology,* Lea & Febiger, Philadelphia, 1986.
13. Charles River Laboratories, Serum chemistry parameters for the Crl:CD®BR rat, Wilmington, MA, 1993.
14. NIEHS, A summary of control values for F344 rats and B6C3F1 mice in 13 week subchronic studies, Program Resources, Research Triangle Park, NC, 1985.
15. Burns, K. F., Timmons, E. H., and Poiley, S. M., Serum chemistry and hematological values for axenic (germfree) and environmentally associated inbred rats, *Lab. Anim. Sci.,* 21, 415, 1971.
16. Frith, C. H., Suber, R. L., and Umholtz, R., Hematologic and clinical chemistry findings in control BALB/c and C57BL/6 mice, *Lab. Anim. Sci.,* 30, 835, 1980.
17. Wolford, S. T., Schroer, R. A., Gohs, F. X., Gallo, P. P., Brodeck, M., Falk, H. B., and Ruhren, R. J., Reference range data base for serum chemistry and hematology values in laboratory animals, *Toxicol. Environ. Health,* 18, 161, 1986.
18. Clarke, D., Tupari, G., Walker, R., and Smith, G., Stability of serum biochemical variables from Beagle dogs and Cynomolgus monkeys, *Am. Assoc. Clin. Chem. Special Issue* 17, October 1992.
19. Pickrell, J. A., Schluter, S. J., Belasich, J. J., Stewart, E. V., Meyer, J., Hubbs, C. H., and Jones, R. K., Relationship of age of normal dogs to blood serum constituents and reliability of measured single values, *Am. J. Vet. Res.,* 35, 897, 1974.
20. Kaspar, L. V. and Norris, W. P., Serum chemistry values of normal dogs (Beagles): associations with age, sex, and family line, *Lab. Anim. Sci.,* 27, 980, 1977.
21. Kapeghian, L. C. and Verlangieri, A. J., Effects of primaquine on serum biochemical and hematological parameters in anesthetized *Macaca fasicularis, J. Med. Primatol.,* 13, 97, 1984.
22. Davy, C. W., Jackson, M. R., and Walker, S., Reference intervals for some clinical chemical parameters in the marmoset (*Callithrix Jacchus*): effect of age and sex, *Lab. Anim.,* 18, 135, 1984.

23. Yarbrough, L. W., Tollett, J. L., Montrey, R. D., and Beattie, R. J., Serum biochemical, hematological and body measurement data for common marmosets (*Callithrix Jacchus*), *Lab. Anim. Sci.,* 34, 276, 1984.

24. Hack, C. A. and Gleiser, C. A., Hematologic and serum chemical reference values for adult and juvenile Baboons *(Papio* sp. *), Lab. Anim. Sci.,* 32, 502, 1982.

25. Hewett, C. D., Innes, D. J., Savory, J., and Wills, M. R., Normal biochemical and hematological values in New Zealand White rabbits, *Clin. Chem.,* 35, 1777, 1989.

26. Yu, L., Pragay, D. A., Chang, D., and Wicher, K., Biochemical parameters of normal rabbit serum, *Clin. Biochem.,* 12, 83, 1979.

27. Charles River Laboratories, Hematology parameters for the Crl:CD®BR rat, Wilmington, MA, 1993.

28. Bulgin, M. S., Munn, S. L., and Gee, S., Hematologic changes to 4 $^1/_2$ years of age in clinically normal Beagle dogs, *J. Am. Vet. Med. Assoc.,* 157, 1004, 1970.

29. Jordan, J. E., Normal laboratory values in Beagle dogs at twelve to eighteen months of age, *Am. J. Vet. Res.,* 38, 509, Ic7.

ADDITIONAL RELATED INFORMATION

TABLE 18.21
Normal Human Laboratory Values[a]

Blood, Plasma or Serum

Determination	Reference Value	
	Conventional Units	SI Units
Ammonia (NH₃)-diffusion	20–120 mcg/dl	12–70 mcmol/L
Ammonia Nitrogen	15–45 μg/dl	11–32 μmol/L
Amylase	35–118 IU/L	0.58–1.97 mckat/L
Anion Gap (Na⁺-[Cl⁻ + HCO₃⁻]) (P)	7–16 mEq/L	7–16 mmol/L
Antinuclear antibodies	negative at 1:10 dilution of serum	negative at 1:10 dilution of serum
Antithrombin III (AT III)	80–120 U/dl	800–1200 U/L
Bicarbonate: Arterial	21–28 mEq/L	21–28 mmol/L
Venous	22–29 mEq/L	22–29 mmol/L
Bilirubin: Conjugated (direct)	≤ 0.2 mg/dl	≤ 4 mcmol/L
Total	0.1–1 mg/dl	2–18 mcmol/L
Calcitonin	< 100 pg/ml	<100 ng/L
Calcium: Total	8.6–10.3 mg/dl	2.2–2.74 mmol/L
Ionized	4.4–5.1 mg/dl	1–1.3 mmol/L
Carbon dioxide content (plasma)	21–32 mmol/L	21–32 mmol/L
Carcinoembryonic antigen	< 3 ng/ml	< 3 mcg/L
Chloride	95–110 mEq/L	95–110 mmol/L
Coagulation screen:		
Bleeding time	3–9.5 min	180–570 sec
Prothrombin time	10–13 sec	10–13 sec
Partial thromboplastin time (activated)	22–37 sec	22–37 sec
Protein C	0.7–1.4 μ/ml	700–1400 U/ml
Protein S	0.7–1.4 μ/ml	700–1400 U/ml
Copper, total	70–160 mcg/dl	11–25 mcmol/L
Corticotropin (ACTH adrenocorticotropic hormone) — 0800 h	<60 pg/ml	<13.2 pmol/L
Cortisol: 0800 h	5–30 mcg/dl	138–810 nmol/L
1800 h	2–15 mcg/dl	50–410 nmol/L
2000 h	≤50% of 0800 h	≤50% of 0800 h
Creatine kinase: Female	20–170 IU/L	0.33–2.83 mckat/L
Male	30–220 IU/L	0.5–3.67 mckat/L
Creatine kinase isoenzymes, MB fraction	0–12 IU/L	0–0.2 mckat/L
Creatine	0.5–1.7 mg/dl	44–150 mcmol/L
Fibrinogen (coagulation factor 1)	150–360 mg/dl	1.5–3.6 g/L
Follicle-stimulating hormone (FSH)		
Female	2–13 mlU/ml	2–13 IU/L
Midcycle	5–22 mlU/ml	5–22 IU/L
Male	1–8 mlU/ml	1–8 IU/L
Glucose, fasting	65–115 mg/dl	3.6–6.3 mmol/L

Glucose Tolerance Test (Oral)

	mg/dL		mmol/L	
	Normal	*Diabetic*	*Normal*	*Diabetic*
Fasting	70–105	>140	3.9–5.8	>7.8
60 min	120–170	≥200	6.7–9.4	≥11.1
90 min	100–140	≥200	5.6–7.8	≥11.1
120 min	70–120	≥140	3.9–6.7	≥7.8

TABLE 18.21 *(Continued)*
Normal Human Laboratory Values[a]

Blood, Plasma or Serum

Determination		Reference Value	
		Conventional Units	**SI Units**
(γ)-Glutamyltransferase (GGT):	Male	9–50 units/L	9–50 units/L
	Female	8–40 units/L	8–40 units/L
Haptoglobin		44–303 mg/dl	0.44–3.03 g/L
Hematologic tests:			
Fibrinogen		200–400 mg/dl	2–4 g/L
Hematocrit (Hct),	female	36%–44.6%	0.36–0.446 fraction of 1
	male	40.7%–50.3%	0.4–0.503 fraction of 1
Hemoglobin A$_{1C}$		5.3%–7.5% of total Hgb	0.053–0.075
Hemoglobin (Hb),	female	12.1–15.3 g/dl	121–153 g/L
	male	13.8–17.5 g/dl	138–175 g/L
Leukocyte count (WBC)		3800–9800/mcl	3.8–9.8×10^9/L
Erythrocyte count (RBC), female		3.5–5×10^6/mcl	3.5–5×10^{12}/L
	male	4.3–5.9×10^6/mcl	4.3–5.9×10^{12}/L
Mean corpuscular volume (MCV)		80–97.6 mcm^3	80–97.6 fl
Mean corpuscular hemoglobin (MCH)		27–33 pg/cell	1.66–2.09 fmol/cell
Mean corpuscular hemoglobin concentration (MCHC)		33–36 g/dl	20.3–22 mmol/L
Erythrocyte sedimentation rate (sedrate, ESR)		≤30 mm/h	≤30 mm/h
Erythrocyte enzymes: Glucose-6-phosphate dehydroge nase (G-6-PD)		250–5000 units/10^6 cells	250–5000 mcunits/cell
Ferritin		10–383 ng/ml	23–862 pmol/L
Folic acid: normal		> 3.1–12.4 ng/ml	7–28.1 nmol/L
Platelet count		150–450×10^3/mcl	150–450×10^9/L
Reticulocytes		0.5%–1.5% of erythrocytes	0.005–0.015
Vitamin B$_{12}$		223–1132 pg/ml	165–835 pmol/L
Iron: Female		30–160 mcg/dl	5.4–31.3 mcmol/L
Male		45–160 mcg/dl	8.1–31.3 mcmol/L
Iron binding capacity		220–420 mcg/dl	39.4–75.2mcmol/L
Isocitrate. Dehydrogenase		1.2–7 units/L	1.2–7 units/L

NORMAL HUMAN LABORATORY VALUES
Blood, Plasma or Serum

Determination	Reference Value	
	Conventional Units	**SI Units**
Isoenzymes		
Fraction 1	14%–26% of total	0.14–0.26 fraction of total
Fraction 2	29%–39% of total	0.29–0.39 fraction of total
Fraction 3	20%–26% of total	0.20–0.26 fraction of total
Fraction 4	8%–16% of total	0.08–0.16 fraction of total
Fraction 5	6%–16% of total	0.06–0.16 fraction of total
Lactate dehydrogenase	100–250 IU/L	1.67–4.17 mckat/L
Lactic acid (lactate)	6–19 mg/dl	0.7–2.1 mmol/L
Lead	≤50 mcg/dl	≤2.41 mcmol/L

TABLE 18.21 *(Continued)*
Normal Human Laboratory Values[a]

NORMAL HUMAN LABORATORY VALUES
Blood, Plasma or Serum

Determination	Reference Value	
	Conventional Units	SI Units
Lipase	10–150 units/L	10–150 units/L
Lipids:		
Total Cholesterol		
Desirable	<200 mg/dl	<5.2 mmol/L
Borderline-high	200–239 mg/dl	<5.2–6.2 mmol/L
High	>239 mg/dl	>6.2 mmol/L
LDL		
Desirable	<130 mg/dl	<3.36 mmol/L
Borderline-high	130–159 mg/dl	3.36–4.11 mmol/L
High	>159 mg/dl	>4.11 mmol/L
HDL (low)	<35 mg/dl	<0.91 mmol/L
Triglycerides		
Desirable	<200 mg/dl	<2.26 mmol/L
Borderline-high	200–400 mg/dl	2.26–4.52 mmol/L
High	400–1000 mg/dl	4.52–11.3 mmol/L
Very high	>1000 mg/dl	>11.3 mmol/L
Magnesium	1.3–2.2 mEqL	0.65–1.1 mmol/L
Osmolality	280–300 mOsm/kg	280–300 mmol/kg
Oxygen saturation (arterial)	94%–100%	0.94–1 fraction of 1
PCO_2, arterial	35–45 mm Hg	4.7–6 kPa
PH, arterial	7.35–7.45	7.35–7.45
PO_2, arterial: Breathing room air[1]	80–105 mm Hg	10.6–14 kPa
On 100% O_2	>500 mm Hg	
Phosphatase (acid), total at 37°C	0.13–0.63 IU/L	2.2–10.5 IU/L or 2.2–10.5 mckat/L
Phosphatase alkaline[2]	20–130 IU/L	20–130 IU/L or 0.33–2.17 mckat/L
Phosphorus, inorganic[3] (phosphate)	2.5–5 mg/dl	0.8–1.6 mmol/L
Potassium	3.5–5 mEq/L	3.5–5 mmol/L
Progesterone		
Female	0.1–1.5 ng/ml	0.32–4.8 nmol/L
Follicular phase	0.1–1.5 ng/ml	0.32–4.8 nmol/L
Luteal phase	2.5–28 ng/ml	8–89 nmol/L
Male	<0.5 ng/ml	<1.6 nmol/L
Prolactin	1.4–24.2 ng/ml	1.4–24.2 mcg/L
Prostate specific antigen	0–4 ng/ml	0–4 ng/ml
Protein: Total	6–8 g/dl	60–80 g/L
Albumin	3.6–5 g/dl	36–50 g/L
Globulin	2.3–3.5 g/dl	23–35 g/L
Rheumatoid factor	<60 IU/ml	<60 kIU/L
Sodium	135–147 mEq/L	135–147 mmol/L
Testosterone: Female	6–86 ng/dl	0.21–3 nmol/L
Male	270–1070 ng/dl	9.3–37 nmol/L
Thyroid Hormone Function Tests:		
Thyroid-stimulating hormone (TSH)	0.35–6.2 mcU/ml	0.35–6.2 mU/L
Thyroxine-binding globulin capacity	10–26 mcg/dl	100–260 mcg/L

TABLE 18.21 *(Continued)*
Normal Human Laboratory Values[a]

NORMAL HUMAN LABORATORY VALUES

Blood, Plasma or Serum

Determination	Reference Value: Conventional Units	Reference Value: SI Units
Total triiodothyronine (T_3)	75–220 ng/dl	1.2–3.4 nmol/L
Total thyroxine by RIA (T_4)	4–11 mcg/dl	51–142 nmol/L
T_3 resin uptake	25%–38%	0.25–0.38 fraction of 1
Transaminase, AST (aspartate aminotransferase, SGOT)	11–47 IU/L	0.18–0.78 mckat/L
Transaminase, ALT (alanine aminotrans ferase, SGPT)	7–53 IU/L	0.12–0.88 mckat/L
Transferrin	220–400 mg/dL	2.20–4.00 g/L
Urea nitrogen (BUN)	8–25 mg/dl	2.9–8.9 mmol/L
Uric acid	3–8 mg/dl	179–476 mcmol/L
Vitamin A (retinol)	15–60 mcg/dl	0.52–2.09 mcmol/L
Zinc	50–150 mcg/dl	7.7–23 mcmol/L

[1] Age dependent
[2] Infants and adolescents up to 104 U/L
[3] Infants in the first year up to 6 mg/dl

Urine

Determination	Reference Value: Conventional Units	Reference Value: SI Units
Calcium[1]	50–250 mcg/day	1.25–6.25 mmol/day
Catecholamines: Epinephrine	<20 mcg/day	<109 nmol/day
Norepinephrine	<100 mcg/day	<590 nmol/day
Catecholamines, 24-h	<110 µg	<650 nmol
Copper[1]	15–60 mcg/day	0.24–0.95 mcmol/day
Creatinine: Child	8–22 mg/kg	71–195 µmol/kg
Adolescent	8–30 mg/kg	71–265 µmol/kg
Female	0.6–1.5 g/day	5.3–13.3 mmol/day
Male	0.8–1.8 g/day	7.1–15.9 mmol/day
pH	4.5–8	4.5–8
Phosphate[1]	0.9–1.3 g/day	29–42 mmol/day
Potassium[1]	25–100 mEq/day	25–100 mmol/day
Protein		
Total	1–14 mg/dL	10–140 mg/L
At rest	50–80 mg/day	50–80 mg/day
Protein, quantitative	<150 mg/day	<0.15 g/day
Sodium[1]	100–250 mEq/day	100–250 mmol/day
Specific Gravity, random	1.002–1.030	1.002–1.030
Uric Acid, 24-h	250–750 mg	1.48–4.43 mmol

[1] Diet dependent.

[a] In the following tables, normal reference values for commonly requested laboratory tests are listed in traditional units and in SI units. The tables are a guideline only. Values are method dependent and "normal values" may vary between laboratories.

From © 2000 by Facts and Comparisons, reprinted with permission from *Drug Facts and Comparisons. 2000 Loose Leaf Edition,* St Louis, MO: Facts and Comparisons, a Wolters Kluwer Company.

TABLE 18.22
Erythrocyte Life Span in Various Animals[a]

Species	Mean Life Span[b] (days)
Man	117–127 (120)[c]
Dog	90–135
Cat	66–79
Pig	62–86
Rabbit	50–80
Guinea pig	70–90
Hamster	60–70
Rat	50–68 (60)[c]
Mouse	41–55

[a] Determined by use of isotopes.

[b] Range of means from various studies.

[c] Most often cited.

19 Metabolism and Toxicokinetics of Xenobiotics

Mohamed B. Abou-Donia, Ph.D., Eman M. Elmasry, Ph.D., and Aqel W. Abu-Qare, Ph.D.

CONTENTS

0-8493-0370-2/02/$0.00+$1.50
© 2002 by CRC Press LLC

SECTION 1. INTRODUCTION

Xenobiotics entering biological systems undergo the following processes: (1) absorption: oral, dermal, inhalation; (2) tissue distribution (disposition); (3) protein and tissue binding; (4) enzymatic and nonenzymatic chemical transformation; and (5) excretion.

Pharmacokinetics are defined as the rates of all metabolic processes related to the expression of pharmacology. Toxicokinetics are defined as the rates of all metabolic processes related to the expression of toxicologic end points.

The purpose of pharmacokinetics or toxicokinetics is (1) to allow predictions of body burdens, both time to maximum and amount; (2) to allow prediction of duration in body after exposure terminated; (3) to determine percent absorbed; and (4) to determine schedule of drug dosage.

SECTION 2. METABOLISM

A. ABSORPTION

For a xenobiotic to reach its site of action, it must pass across various membranes, i.e., cells of skin, cells of lung, gastrointestinal tract, erythrocyte membrane, etc.

1. Membrane Structure

    a. Phospolipid bilayer
    b. Embedded with proteins
    c. Contains various size pores

2. Mechanisms by Which Xenobiotics Pass Body Membranes

    a. Passive transport
       i. Simple diffusion
          (1) The mechanism by which most chemicals pass membranes
          (2) Nonsaturable process
          (3) Both lipid-soluble substances and lipid-insoluble molecules of small size (i.e., urea) may cross body membranes by simple diffusion
          (4) Many xenobiotics (weak organic acids and bases) exist in solution in both the ionized and un-ionized form; the ionized form is often unable to penetrate the cell membrane because of its low lipid solubility, whereas the un-ionized form may be lipid soluble enough to diffuse across cell membranes
          (5) The amount of weak organic acid or base in the un-ionized form is dependent on its association constant (pK_a) and the pH of the internal environment; this relationship is described by the Henderson–Hasselbalch equation:

$$\text{For acids } pK_a - pH = \log \frac{[\text{nonionized}]}{[\text{ionized}]}$$

$$\text{For bases } pK_a - pH = \log \frac{[\text{ionized}]}{[\text{nonionized}]}$$

For weak acids:

$$pK_a - pH = \log \frac{[\text{nonionized}]}{[\text{ionized}]}$$

Benzoic acid $pK_a \approx 4$

Stomach pH ≈ 2

$$4 - 2 = \log \frac{[\text{nonionized}]}{[\text{ionized}]}$$

$$2 = \log \frac{[\text{nonionized}]}{[\text{ionized}]}$$

$$100 = \frac{[\text{nonionized}]}{[\text{ionized}]}$$

Ratio favors absorption

For weak bases:

$$pK_a - pH = \log \frac{[\text{ionized}]}{[\text{nonionized}]}$$

Aniline $pK_a \approx 5$

Stomach pH ≈ 2

$$5 - 2 = \log \frac{[\text{ionized}]}{[\text{nonionized}]}$$

$$3 = \log \frac{[\text{ionized}]}{[\text{nonionized}]}$$

$$1000 = \frac{[\text{ionized}]}{[\text{nonionized}]}$$

Intestine pH $\approx$ 6

$$4 - 6 = \log \frac{[\text{nonionized}]}{[\text{ionized}]}$$

$$-2 = \log \frac{[\text{nonionized}]}{[\text{ionized}]}$$

$$\frac{1}{100} = \frac{[\text{nonionized}]}{[\text{ionized}]}$$

Intestine pH $\approx$ 6

$$5 - 6 = \log \frac{[\text{ionized}]}{[\text{nonionized}]}$$

$$-1 = \log \frac{[\text{ionized}]}{[\text{nonionized}]}$$

$$\frac{1}{10} = \frac{[\text{ionized}]}{[\text{nonionized}]}$$

Ratio favors absorption

TABLE 19.1
Calculation of the Extent of Ionization, Given pK$_a$ and pH

pK$_a$ – pH	Percent Ionized (if anion)	Percent Ionized (if cation)
–4	99.99	0.01
–3	99.94	0.10
–2	99.01	0.99
–1	90.91	9.09
0	50.00	50.00
1	9.09	90.01
2	0.99	99.01
3	0.10	99.94
4	0.01	99.99

TABLE 19.2
pK$_a$ Values for Some Weak Acids and Bases (at 25°C)

Weak Acids	pK$_a$	Weak Bases	pK$_a$
Salicylic acid	3.00	Reserpine	6.6
Acetylsalicylic acid	3.49	Codeine	7.9
Sulfadiazine	6.48	Quinine	8.4
Barbital	7.91	Procaine	8.8
Boric acid	9.24	Ephedrine	9.36
		Atropine	9.65

TABLE 19.3
Effect of pH on the Ionization of Salicylic Acid (pK$_a$ = 3)

pH	Non-Ionized
1	99.0
2	90.9
3	50.0
4	9.09
5	0.99
6	0.10

ii. Filtration — When water flows in bulk across a porous membrane, any solute that is small enough to pass through the pores flows with it. Pores in most cells are 4Å, endothelial cells of capillaries are 40 Å, and endothelial cells of glomerular membrane of the kidney are 100 Å.

b. Special transport — There are three types of special transport:

i. Active transport: Occurs when substances are moving against a concentration or electrochemical gradient and has the following characteristics:
(1) Compounds move against concentration or electrical gradient
(2) Can be saturated
(3) Selectivity for compounds of the same size
(4) Competitive inhibition among substances handled by the same mechanism
(5) Requires energy (metabolic inhibitors block transport process)

ii. Facilitated transport: Similar to active transport; however, in this type, chemicals do not move against a concentration gradient and do not require energy.

iii. Pinocytosis: Refers to the ability of cells to engulf small droplets

3. Absorption of Xenobiotic in the Body

a. Gastrointestinal tract

i. Lipid-soluble compounds (non-ionized) are more readily absorbed than water-soluble compounds (water soluble, ionized)
(1) Weak organic bases are in the non-ionized, lipid-soluble form in intestine and tend to be absorbed there
(2) Weak organic acids are in the non-ionized, lipid-soluble form in stomach and are absorbed there, but intestine is more important because of time and area of exposure

ii. In general, the absorption of chemicals from the gastrointestinal tract is by simple diffusion

iii. The following chemicals are absorbed through specialized transport systems: sugars, amino acids, pyrimidines, calcium, and sodium ions

iv. Almost everything is absorbed at least to a small extent

v. Blood flow rate and surface area are more important than pH for the absorption of weak acids

TABLE 19.4
Blood Flow Rate and Surface Area

Tissue	pH	Blood Flow Rate (l/min)	Surface Area (m²)
Stomach	1–3	0.15	1
Intestine	5–8	1.0	200

vi. Effect of digestive fluids on chemicals:
(1) Nitrites plus secondary amines form nitrosamines (carcinogens)
(2) Intestinal flora degrade DDT to DDE

vii. Dilution — Increases toxicity because of more rapid absorption from intestine

viii. Age — Newborn has poor intestinal barrier

ix. First pass — Chemical can be extracted and/or biotransformed by intestine or liver before it reaches systemic circulation; this may be a protective mechanism in toxicology but not desirable in pharmacology

    b. Lungs
       i. Aerosol deposition
          (1) Nasopharyngeal — 5 μm or larger
          (2) Tracheobronchiolar — 1 to 5 μm
          (3) Alveolar — 1 μm
      ii. Muscociliary transport
      iii. Anatomically good for absorption
          (1) Large surface area (50 to 100 m²)
          (2) Blood flow is high
          (3) Close to blood (10 μm)
      iv. Absorption of gases is dependent on solubility of gas in blood
          (1) Chloroform — High solubility in blood, all absorbed, respiration limited
          (2) Ethylene — Low solubility, small percentage is inhaled
    c. Skin
       i. Skin is a relatively good barrier
      ii. Absorption through follicles is rapid
      iii. Absorption transdermally is quantitatively important
      iv. With most compounds, the surface loss rate must exceed the absorption rate, for the latter is generally less than 50%
      v. Absorption by passive diffusion, e.g., high lipid solubility of a chemical should favor its absorption
      vi. Diffusion barrier is stratum barrier
      vii. Abrasion increased absorption
    d. Relative rates of absorption: intravenous injection > inhalation > intraperitoneal injection > oral > dermal

B. DISTRIBUTION

1. Factors Affecting Distribution of Chemicals

    a. Blood flow through the organ
    b. Passage across cell membranes
    c. Affinity of various tissues for the toxicant

2. Site of Concentration in Body Is Not Necessarily the Target Organ of Toxicity

3. Plasma Proteins as a Storage Depot For Toxicants

    a. Toxicants become biologically inactive when they bind to plasma proteins
    b. Bound toxicants cannot be filtered at the kidney
    c. A bound chemical can displace another
    d. The binding capacity of a protein is not unlimited; once it becomes saturated, a sudden increase in toxicity occurs with further absorption of toxicants
    e. The protein responsible for binding is usually albumin globulins although it may be very important in binding of some hormonal agents and pesticides

4. Fat as a Storage Depot

Non-ionized, lipid-soluble xenobiotics, i.e., DDT, tend to concentrate in adipose tissue.

5. **Bone as a Storage (Depot for lead, stratinum, and fluoride)**

6. **Cellular Binding**

This usually results from the affinity of a substance to some cellular component. An example is the high concentrations of alkaloids in the liver and muscle which are attributed to the affinity of these naturally occurring amines to nucleoproteins.

7. **Blood–Brain Barriers**

The brain is protected by a membrane called the blood–brain barrier, which can only be penetrated by lipid-soluble substances. After passing this barrier, a xenobiotic still has to penetrate the membranes of the brain.

8. **Placenta Barrier**

   a. Placenta is a poor barrier — virus (Rubella), cellular pathogens (syphilis), antibody, globulins, and erythrocytes are transported
   b. Transport is by diffusion

C. BINDING

Binding of xenobiotics to proteins and other micromolecules in the body significantly affects their distribution, metabolism, and elimination. Albumin is the major protein to which xenobiotics bind, followed by globulins. Both anions and cations bind to albumins. Bound chemicals may displace each other. Binding to plasma proteins renders them biologically inactive and less available for filtering by kidney. When plasma proteins become saturated, further absorption of toxicants may result in toxicity.

Some xenobiotics have greater affinity for body tissues than plasma proteins. Alkaloids, the naturally occurring amines, have a high affinity for nucleoproteins resulting in their high concentrations in the liver. Furthermore, some metals and organic amines are transferred to the liver after their initial binding to plasma. Bones and teeth act as depots for some inorganic ions such as fluoride, lead, and strontium as well as drugs such as tetracycline. On the other hand, liquid-soluble xenobiotics such as DDT and leptophos tend to concentrate in adipose tissue.

Lipid-soluble xenobiotics cross the placenta and are deposited in the fetus. This process takes place via passive diffusion. Organophosphorus insecticides, e.g., methamidophos, acephate, and chloropyrofos, cross the placenta in pregnants rats. Likewise virus (for example, rubella) bacteria (e.g., syphilis), antibodies, globulins, and erythrocytes can also cross the placenta.

D. EXCRETION — ROUTES AND MECHANISMS

1. Urine

Two major mechanisms are involved in the renal handling of xenobiotics: (1) glomerular filtration with variable tubular reabsorption and (2) tubular secretion (an active transport mechanism). Usually the xenobiotic is filtered from the blood through the highly porous glomeruli and is partially reabsorbed by the tubules, depending on its lipid solubility property. Lipid-soluble compounds are reabsorbed from the tubules by non-ionic diffusion. The tubular epithelium of the distal convoluted tubule is selectively permeable or more permeable to the un-ionized, lipid-soluble molecule than the less-lipid-soluble corresponding anion or cation. Generally xenobiotics that are bases are excreted to a greater extent if the urine is acid (as salts), whereas acid compounds are excreted more favorably if the urine is alkaline (as salts).

    a. Excretion into renal tubule
       i. Glomerular filtration
          (1) All water-soluble toxicants with molecular weight (MW) < 60,000 are filtered from the blood through the highly porous glomeruli
      ii. Passive tubular diffusion
          (1) If lipid insoluble
          (2) If weak acid or weak base:
              (a) Weak acidic chemicals excreted better in alkalinized urine
              (b) Weak basic chemicals excreted better in acidic urine
      iii. Active secretion
          (1) Carrier mediated, with two separate carriers:
              (a) Organic acids, e.g., p-aminohippurate
              (b) Organic bases, e.g., N-methylnicontinamide
          (2) Characteristic of carriers
              (a) Rate of excretion is not affected by binding to plasma proteins
              (b) Competition for excretion
    b. Passive tubular reabsorption; influenced by:
       i. Lipid solubility
      ii. pK_a
      iii. Tubular fluid pH
      iv. Tubular fluid volume

2. Bile

A xenobiotic in circulation enters the liver via the hepatic artery or through the lymph. The compound emerges from the liver (as such, or in a degraded state) with the bile, which passes down the bile duct into the gallbladder, which exists for bile storage. At intervals, bile leaves the gallbladder by the bile duct, which discharges into the duodenum. Some xenobiotics are recycled by reabsorption from the small intestine by the portal vein and then into the liver, which secretes again into the small intestine. Both circuits involve a gradual decrement via the feces.

    a. Classification of toxicants excreted into the bile:
       i. Class A: Bile/plasma concentration ratio = 1
          Examples: sodium, potassium, mercury, etc.
      ii. Class B: Bile/plasma concentration ratio > 1 (10 to 100)
          Examples: bile salt, lead, manganese, weak acids, etc.
      iii. Class C: Bile/plasma concentration ratio < 1
          Examples: inulin, albumin, iron, mercury etc.
    b. Mechanisms of excretion into the bile
       i. Diffusion
      ii. Carrier-mediated transport (Class B)
          (1) Organic acid — BSP (bromosulfthalein)
          (2) Organic base — PAEB (procain amide ethyl bromide)
          (3) Organic neutral — Ouabain
    c. Factors favoring biliary excretion of weak acids
       i. Molecular weight > 325
      ii. Two or more aromatic rings
      iii. The presence of polar groups
      iv. Highly protein-bound substances in plasma are readily transferable directly to the secreting cells
      v. Microsomal enzyme inducers enhance biliary secretion

d. Enterohepatic circulation — Cholestyramine enhances biliary excretion of kepone:
e. The following species do not have a gallbladder: rat, horse, and deer

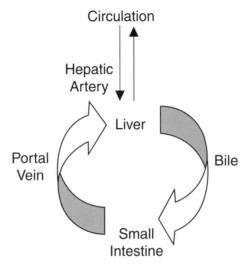

3. **Lung**

   a. Important for:
      i.   Substances that exist in gas phase at body temperature
      ii. Liquids
   b. Mechanisms for elimination–diffusion
   c. Rate of excretion
      i.   Low blood/gas solubility — rapid example, ethylene
      ii. High blood/gas solubility — slow example, chloroform

4. **Gastrointestinal Tract**

Sources of toxicants in feces

   a. Not completely absorbed after ingestion
   b. Excreted into bile
   c. Swallowed from respiratory tract
   d. Excreted in saliva, pancreatic, gastric, or intestinal secretions

5. **Cerebrospinal Fluid**

   a. With bulk flow of cerebrospinal fluid
   b. Diffusion from brain to blood
   c. Active transport at choroid plexus

6. **Milk**

   a. Lipid-soluble, non-ionized, non-protein-bound chemicals pass into milk by diffusion
   b. Toxic material may be passed from mother to nursing child
   c. Compounds may be passed from cows to humans
   d. Toxicants that have been detected in human and cow's milk: DDT, PCB (polychlorinated biphenyl), PBB (polybrominated biphenyls)

7. **Sweat and Saliva**

8. **Exhaled Air**

9. **Placental Transfer**

SECTION 3. METABOLIC BIOTRANSFORMATION OF XENOBIOTICS

Metabolic transformation of xenobiotics is the changes of these chemicals produced by biological environments. The alterations convert these chemicals into more polar and water-soluble derivatives that may be readily excreted. Xenobiotic-metabolizing enzymes occur in all tissues with the liver having the largest amount. The relative amounts of these enzymes in tissues are listed in Table 19.5.

TABLE 19.5
Tissues Localization of Xenobiotic-Metabolizing Enzymes

Relative Amount	Tissue
High	Liver
Medium	Lung, kidney, intestine
Low	Skin, tests, placenta, adrenals
Very low	Nervous system tissues

Metabolic biotransformation reactions of xenobiotics in biological systems are divided into two phases. Phase I reactions modify xenobiotics to undergo Phase II conjugation reactions. Phase I reactions are listed in Table 19.6. Phase I reactions introduce polar groups into the chemical that undergoes these reactions, including carboxyl, epoxide, hydroxyl, sulfhydryl, amine, hydroxyl amine, and imine. Some of the metabolites produced by reactions in this phase are more reactive than their parent compounds. This may result in covalent binding with critical targets leading to toxic reactions. On the other hand, most of these polar metabolites undergo conjugation through Phase II reactions listed in Table 19.6. These conjugated products are more polar and readily excreted via biliary or urinary routes. Phase II reactions result in the introduction of polar, acidic endogenous functional groups that usually render Phase II reactions products more polar, less lipid

TABLE 19.6
Metabolic Phase I and Phase II Reactions

Phase I	Phase II
Oxidation	Glucuronidation
Reduction	Glucosidation
Hydrolysis	Ethereal sulfation
Isomerization	Methylation
Others	Acetylation
	Amino acid conjugation
	Glutathione conjugation
	Fatty acid conjugation
	Condensation

soluble, more strongly acidic, and therefore more easily excreted. Metabolic pathways are affected by general factors such as the intrinsic properties of the chemical, dose, animal species, strain, sex, and age, as well as other environmental considerations.

SECTION 4. XENOBIOTIC-METABOLIZING REACTIONS: PHASE I

A. MICROSOMAL MIXED-FUNCTION OXIDASE (MFO, CYTOCHROME P-450)

The mixed-function oxidase enzyme system is an iron-containing porphyrin protein. The term *cytochrome P-450* is used because the reduced hemoprotein, with the iron moiety in its ferrous (Fe^{2+}) oxidation state, combines with carbon monoxide to form a ligand with a maximal absorbance at 450 nm. This property takes place only when the enzyme is intact and catalytically functional. When denatured, cytochrome P-450 loses its peak at 450 nm and produces only a 420-nm absorbance maximum. Notably, the nomenclature committee of the International Union of Biochemistry proposed the term *heme-thiolate protein* instead of *cytochrome* for P-450.

1. Isolation of MFO system

These enzymes are localized in the smooth endoplasmic reticulum of cells of most mammalian tissues. Homogenization of liver tissue followed by differential centrifugation separates the endoplasmic reticulum in the microsomal fraction. A 10% homogenate of liver in 0.25 M sucrose-10^{-3} M EDTA is prepared in a Waring blender at a full speed for 30 s. The homogenate is subjected to centrifugation of $600 \times g$ for 15 min to sediment nuclei, red cells, and cell debris. The supernatant is then centrifuged at $15,000 \times g$ for 30 min followed by centrifugation at $105,000 \times g$ for 60 min to sediment the microsomal fraction from the supernatant or soluble fraction. The microsomal fraction is heterogeneous in the following aspects: (a) morphologically, because it consists of different organelles; smooth endoplasmic reticulum, rough endoplasmic reticulum, ribosomes, and Glogi apparatus; (b) physiologically, because it performs various physiological functions; and (c) biochemically, because it contains many enzymes with diverse catalytic activities.

2. Classification of Cytochrome P-450

Early studies have demonstrated that cytochrome P-450 exists in more than one form. Thus, animal treatment with certain chemicals, e.g., 3-methyl cholanthrene and β-naphthoflavone, caused a shift in the spectral maximum of cytochrome P-450 to P-448. Recent studies isolated and characterized cytochrome P-450 isozymes. These isozymes differ in both the structure of the polypeptide chain and the specificity of the reaction they catalyze. The types and amounts of cytochrome P-450 vary with species, organ, age, health, sex, strain, and chemical exposure.

Cytochrome P-450 isozymes are grouped into families based on approximately 40% homology of amino acid sequence in any gene family. Gene families are further divided into subfamilies that are more than 59% identical. Gene families, 1, 2, 3, and 4 consist of hepatic and extrahepatic cytochrome P-450 isozymes involved in Phase I biotransformation reactions. Gene families 9, 17, 19 and 21 consist of extrahepatic cytochrome P-450s involved in steroid hormone biosynthesis.

A total of 221 cytochrome P-450 and 12 putative pseudogenes have been characterized. These genes belong to 31 eukaryotes (including 11 mammalian and 3 plant species) and 11 prokaryotes. Only 12 families exist in all mammals examined among 36 gene families described so far. The 12 mammalian families comprise 22 mammalian subfamilies. The recommended nomenclature for the gene and cDNA is as follows: the italicized root symbol *CYP* for human (*Cyp* for mouse), representing *cytochrome P*-450 is followed by an Arabic numeral denoting the family, a letter designating the subfamily, and an Arabic numeral representing the individual gene within the subfamily. A hyphen should precede the final number in mouse genes. If a gene is the only member

TABLE 19.7
Classification of Cytochrome P-450 Isozymes

Isozyme	Substrate
CYP1A1	7-Ethoxyresorufin, interferon
CYP1A2	Phenacetin, caffeine
CYP1B1	7-Ethoxyresorufin
CYP 2A1	Testosterone
CYP2A6	Coumarin
CYP2B1	Testosterone
CYP2B6	Coumarin
CYP2C8	Paclitaxel
CYP2C9	Diclofenac
CYP2C19	(*S*)-Mephenytoin
CYP2D6	Bufuralol
CYP2E1	*P*-Nitrophenol, chlorzoxazone
CYP3A4	6β-Testosterone
CYP3A5	6β-Testosterone
CYP3A7	6β-Testosterone
CYP4A11	Lauric acid

of a family, the subfamily letter and gene number are not included. Table 19.7 summarizes the classification of cytochrome P-450 gene families that are briefly described below.

a. The CYP1A subfamily is highly observed among mammalian species. CYP 1A1 retain activity toward polycyclic aromatic hydrocarbons and CYP1A2 retain activity toward aromatic and heterocyclic amines. In human, CYP1A1 is expressed only after exposure to inducers. Cigarette smoking has been shown to induce the CYP1A1 protein in placenta and in lung tissues. CYP1A2 is present in most human livers.

b. The CYP1B subfamily is recognized as being TCDD-inducible in human keratinocytes, but they may be present in other tissues after exposure to inducers.

c. The CYP2A subfamily: The CYP2A1 is expressed in the liver. Its role in the xenobiotic metabolism has not been extensively investigated. CYP2A6 is expressed in the liver that its hepatic level varies from very high to not detectable.

d. The CYP2B subfamily: CYP2B1 is expressed in liver and extrahepatic tissues. CYP2B6 is variably expressed in human liver specimen. It activates aflatoxin B_1.

e. The CYP2C subfamily enzymes are expressed in human liver and are present at lower levels in the small intestine. They comprise human CYP2C9, human CYP2C18, human CYP2C19, and rat CYP2C.

f. The CYP2D subfamily: Among them is CYP2D1, which is capable of metabolizing drugs such as bufuralol and debrisoquine in rat and human. CYP2D6 is responsible for a common genetic defect in the oxidation of many drugs. Quinidine is a potent inhibitor of this enzyme.

g. The CYP2E subfamily; CYP2E1 is constitutively expressed in human liver and subject to induction by a variety of mechanisms. It is capable of activating the procarcinogens *N*-nitrosodimethylamine and *N*-nitrosodiethylamine.

h. The CYP3A subfamily: CYP3A4 is the most abundant cytochrome P-450 in human liver. It plays an important role in the metabolism of drugs. CYP3A3 and CYP3A4 are similar in sequence and are expressed in livers of most adults. CYP3A5 is expressed in about 20% of human adult liver samples. CYP3A7 is expressed in human fetal liver and kidney samples.

i. The CYP4A subfamily: This subfamily has not been extensively studied in humans. It is catalyzed the ω-hydroxylation of lauric acid.

3. Mechanisms of Cytochrome P-450-Mediated Reactions

Cytochrome P-450 consists of (Figure 19.1)

a. Two flavoproteins (dehydrogenases), i.e., NADPH cytochrome P-450 reductase and NADH cytochrome b_5 reductase
b. Two hemoproteins, i.e., cytochrome P-450 and cytochrome b_5
c. Two pyridine nucleotides, i.e., NADH and NADPH

These enzymes are embedded in the phospholipid matrix of the endoplasmic reticulum. The phospholipids facilitate the interactions between the two enzymes. The flavoproteins function as dehydrogenases by transferring an electron from NADPH to cytochrome P-450 and from NADH to cytochrome b_5. The NADPH-cytochrome P-450 reductase donates the first of two electrons to cytochrome P-450, and cytochrome b_5 transfers the second electron to cytochrome P-450.

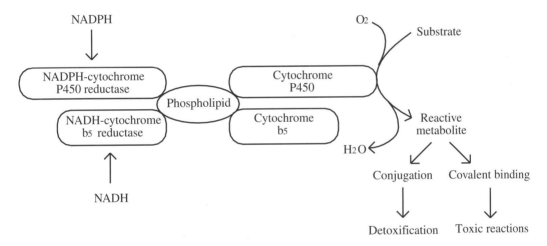

FIGURE 19.1 Scematic presentation of cytochrome P-450 components. (Modified after Spies and Gandolfi.)

4. Mechanism of Oxidation Reactions

Cytochrome P-450-mediated reactions require both NADPH and oxygen to oxidize a substrate (SH). This reaction follows the following steps.

Step 1: The substrate (SH) binds to the iron atom in the oxidized state (Fe^{3+}) at the active site of cytochrome P-450

$$P\text{-}450\text{---}Fe^{3+}$$
$$|$$
$$SH$$

Step 2: Cytochrome P-450–substrate complex is reduced with an electron transferred from NADPH cytochrome reductase.

$$\begin{array}{c} \text{P-450}\!-\!\text{Fe}^{2+} \\ | \\ \text{SH} \end{array}$$

Step 3: The reduced cytochrome P-450–substrate complex then binds to a molecular oxygen.

$$\begin{array}{ccc} \text{O}_2 & & \text{O}_{2-} \\ | & & | \\ \text{P-450}-\text{Fe}^{2+} & \rightleftharpoons & \text{P-450}-\text{Fe}^{3+} \\ | & & | \\ \text{SH} & & \text{SH} \end{array}$$

Step 4: The cytochrome P-450–substrate–oxygen complex is then reduced further by a second electron, possibly donated by:
   a. Cytochrome b_5 which received it from NADH by cytochrome b_5 reductase.
   b. NADH cytochrome b_5 reductase.

$$\begin{array}{c} \text{O}_{2=} \\ | \\ \text{P-450}\!-\!\text{Fe}^{3+} \\ | \\ \text{SH} \end{array}$$

Step 5: The cytochrome P-450–substrate–oxygen complex splits into:
   a. Water
   b. Oxidized substrate (SOH), and
   c. Oxidized form of cytochrome P-450 (P-450–Fe^{3+}).

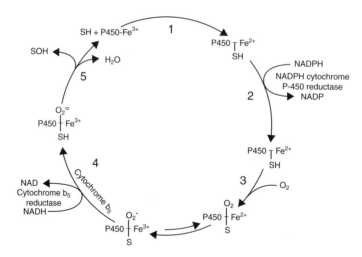

FIGURE 19.2 Schematic mechanism of cytochrome P-450-mediated oxidation.

The overall reaction is therefore presented by the following equation and Figure 19.2:

$$\text{SH} + \text{O}_2 + \text{NADPH} + \text{H}^+ \xrightarrow[\text{P450}]{\text{cytochrome}} \text{SOH} + \text{H}_2\text{O} + \text{NADP}^+$$

5. Cytochrome P-450-Mediated Reactions

Cytochrome P-450 enzymes mediate numerous reactions including the oxidative, peroxidative, reductive, and hydrolytic metabolism of endogenous substrates, e.g., steroids, bile acids, fatty acids, prostaglandins, leukotrienes, and biogenic amines. Also, the metabolism of many xenobiotics including drugs, industrial chemicals, pollutants, and natural products are metabolized with these enzymes.

a. Oxidation Reactions

    i. Aromatic hydroxylation — This reaction is common for aromatic ring-containing xenobiotics. For example, the carbamate insecticide carbaryl is oxidized to produce 4-hydroxy carbaryl.

| Carbaryl | 4-Hydryoxy carbaryl |

Another example is the oxidation of the local anesthetic drug lidocane to the 3-hydroxy derivative.

    ii. Aliphatic hydroxylation — Alkyl chains may be oxidized to form primary, secondary, or tertiary alcohols depending on the location of the oxidized carbon atom. Oxidation may occur at the ω, $\omega - 1$, or tertiary carbon atom.

        (1) ω-Oxidation. ω-Oxidation is a common oxidation reaction of aliphatic side chains as in barbitone.

| Barbitone | 5-Ethyl-5-hydroxyethyl barbituric acid |

Another example is the hydroxylation of a methyl group attached to aromatic or heterocyclic ring systems:

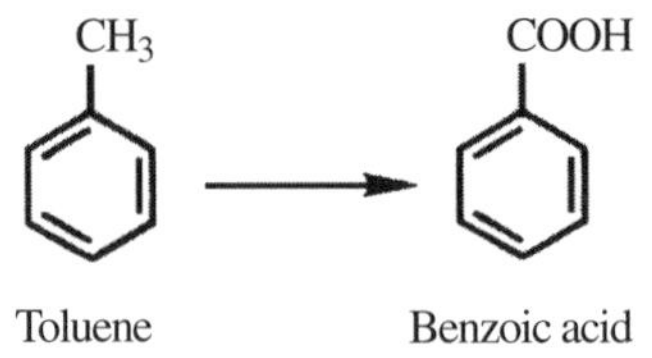

Toluene → Benzoic acid

(2) ω – 1 Oxidation. In addition to the oxidation of the terminal methyl group at the ω position, aliphatic chains are also oxidized at the ω – 1 methylene position. Examples are the hydroxylation of *n*-hexane to 2-hexanol and the oxidation of pentabarbitone.

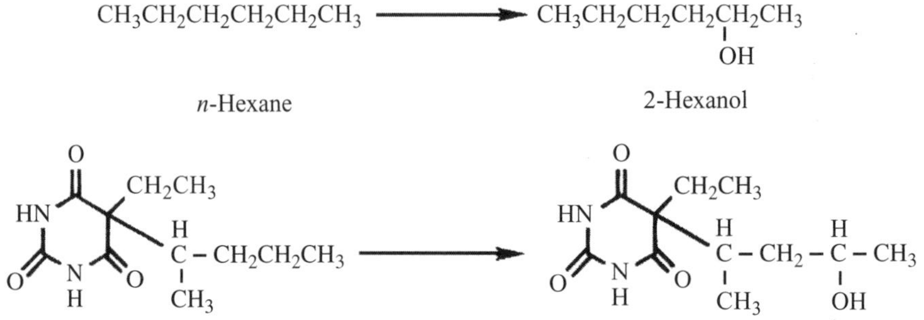

n-Hexane → 2-Hexanol

(3) Oxidation to tertiary alcohol. An example is the oxidation of amylobarbitone to produce the tertiary alcohol, 5-ethyl-5(3-hydroxyisomyl) barbituric acid.

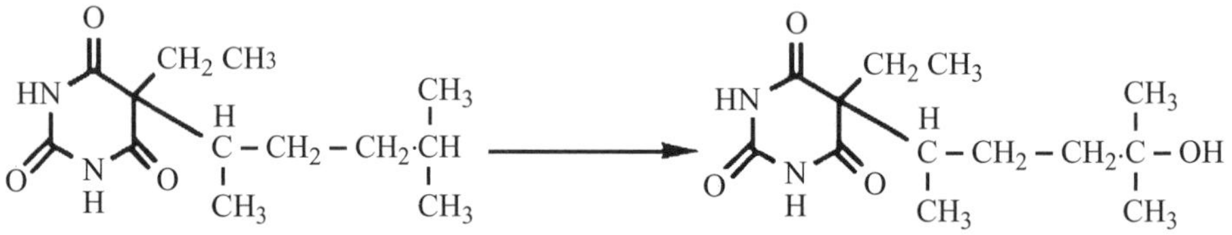

(4) Oxidation of the cycloalkane ring. Alcyclic compounds are hydroxylated to alcohols.

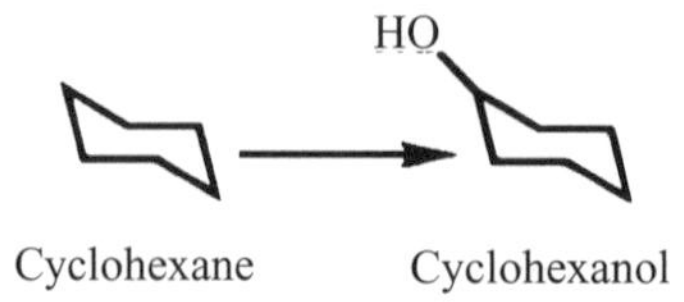

Cyclohexane   Cyclohexanol

The side methyl group of tri-*o*-cresyl phosphate (TOCP) is hydroxylated by cytochrome P-450 enzymes followed by cyclization to form *o*-tolyl saligenin cyclic phosphate.

TOCP

iii. Epoxidation — Although epoxides are usually unstable metabolites, some may be
stable enough to be isolated. Acrylamide undergoes epoxidation to form glycidamide

Acrylamide   Glycidamide

Epoxides are hydrolyzed by epoxide hydratase to form dihydrodiols. An example
is the peroxidation of benzo[a]pyrene (BP).

BP   BP-7,8-epoxide

BP-7,8-diol-9,10-epoxide   BP-7,8-diol

iv. Dealkylation — This reaction takes place with xenobiotics containing an alkoxy group, a secondary or tertiary amine, or an alkyl-substituted thiol. The alkyl group is removed as the corresponding aldehyde. Depending on the atom to which the alkyl group is attached, the reaction is known as *O*-, *N*-, or *S*-dealkylation.

(1) *O*-Dealkylation and *O*-dearylation — Codeine is *O*-demethylated to yield morphine. The reaction proceeds in two steps; first hydroxylation of methyl group on the oxygen, and second, the decomposition of hydroxylated intermediate (–O–CH$_2$OH).

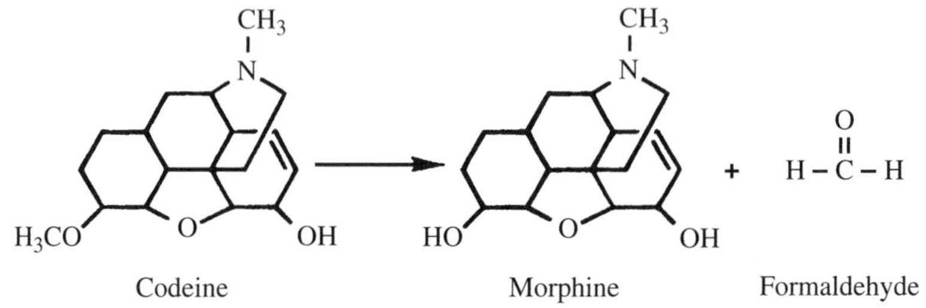

| Codeine | Morphine | Formaldehyde |

Oxidative deethylation reaction takes place in organophosphates, but not in Organopho-sphorothioate insecticides.

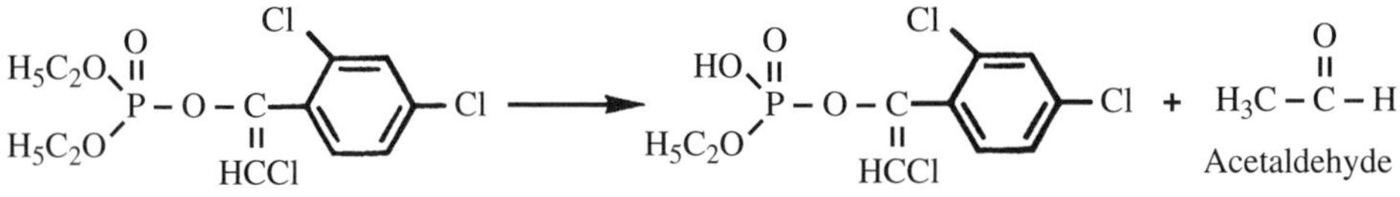

Acetaldehyde

EPN, a phenylphosphophonothioate insecticide, is dearylated to yield *p*-nitrophenol.

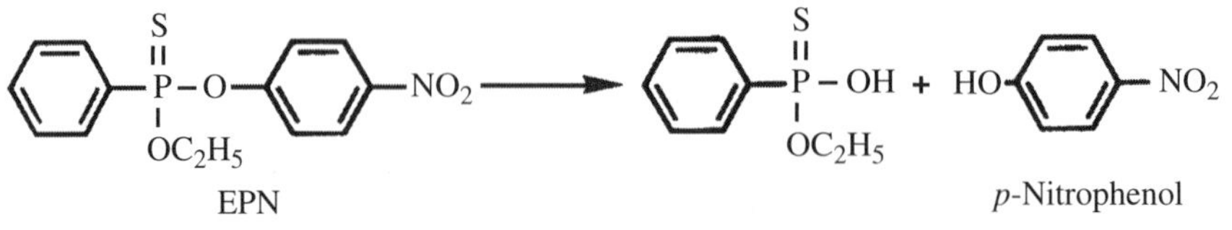

EPN *p*-Nitrophenol

(2) *N*-Dealkylation — This reaction proceeds in two steps similar to *O*-demethylation. An example is the *N*-demethylation of the carbamate insecticide Zectran.

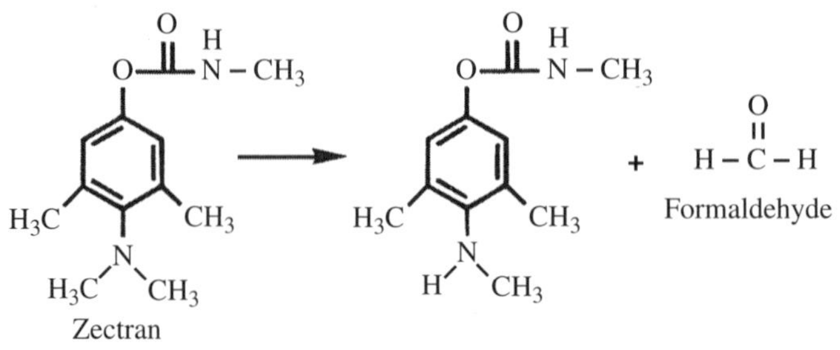

Formaldehyde

Zectran

Similarly, *N*-deethylation occurs with the insecticide phosphamidon.

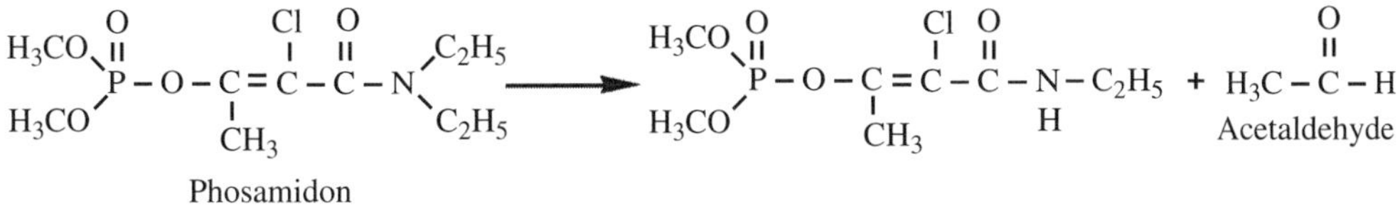

Phosamidon → + Acetaldehyde

Diazepam also undergoes *N*-demethylation with the loss of a methyl group as formaldehyde.

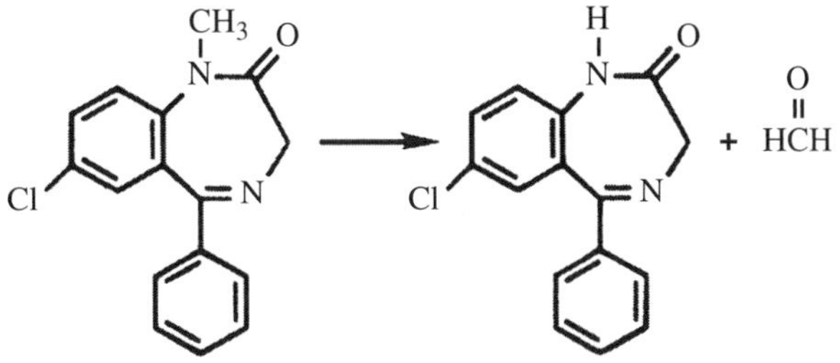

+ HCH

(3) *S*-Dealkylation — Mesurol, a carbamate insecticide, is *S*-dealkylated via microsomal cytochrome P-450 enzymes.

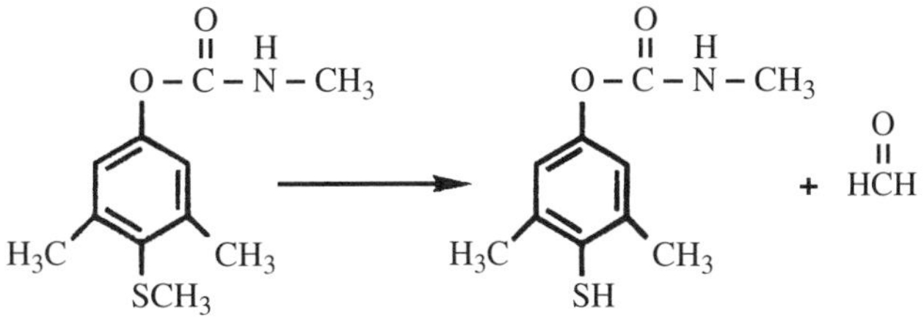

+ HCH

v. Oxidative deamination — some amines, e.g., amphetamines, undergo oxidative deamination to yield ammonia and a ketone. This reaction, which proceeds through an unstable intermediate, is different from monoamines (MAO)-mediated reactions.

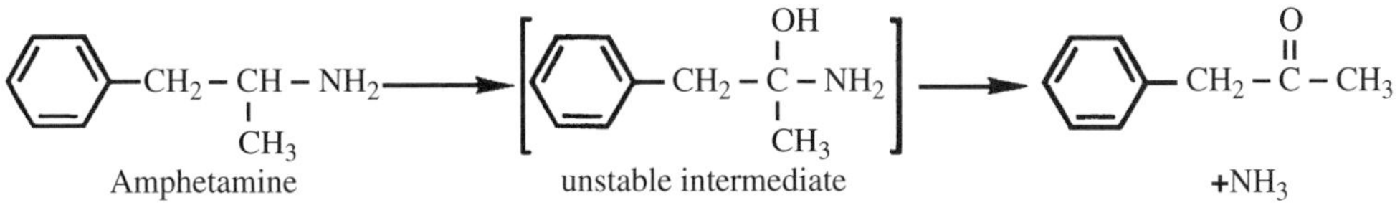

Amphetamine → unstable intermediate → +NH₃

vi. *N*-Oxidation — Cytochrome P-450-mediated *N*-oxidation may result in *N*-oxide as in 3-methylpyridine.

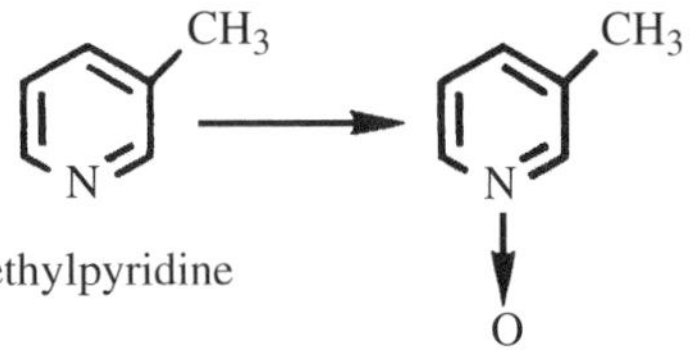

3-Methylpyridine

N-Oxidation of other compounds such as 2-acetylaminofluorine(2-AAF) yields a hydroxyl amine.

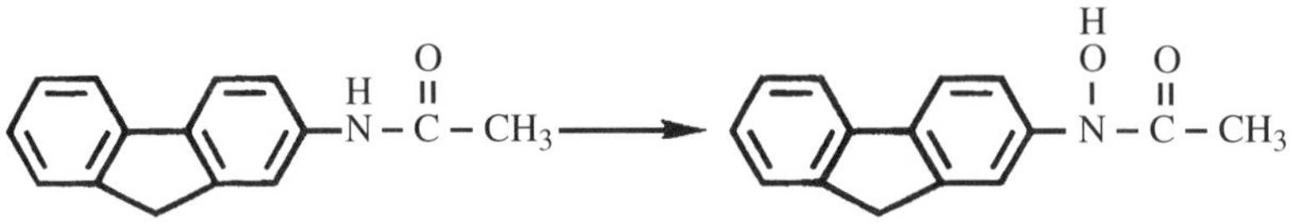

2-AAF

Notably, the hydroxyl amine of 2-AAF is considered active metabolite that is responsible for the carcinogenicity of 2-AAF.

vii. *S*-Oxidation — The insecticide disulfoton is oxidized to disulfoton sulfoxide, which is subsequently oxidized to disulfoton sulfone.

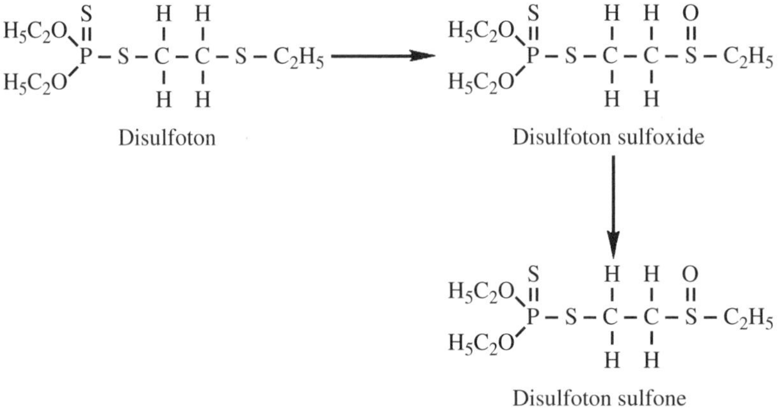

Disulfoton   Disulfoton sulfoxide

Disulfoton sulfone

Phenothiazines may also undergo *S*-oxidation to the sulfoxide derivative.

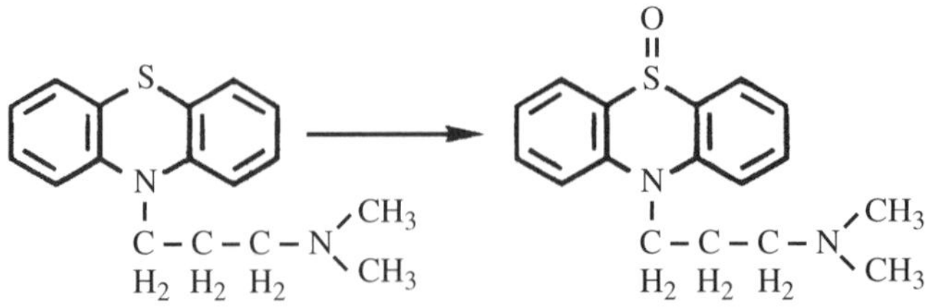

Chlorpromazine   Chlorpromazine sulfoxide

viii. Phosphorus oxidation — Trisubstituted phosphites are rapidly oxidized to the phosphate or the thiophosphate as in triphenyl phosphite and merphos, respectively.

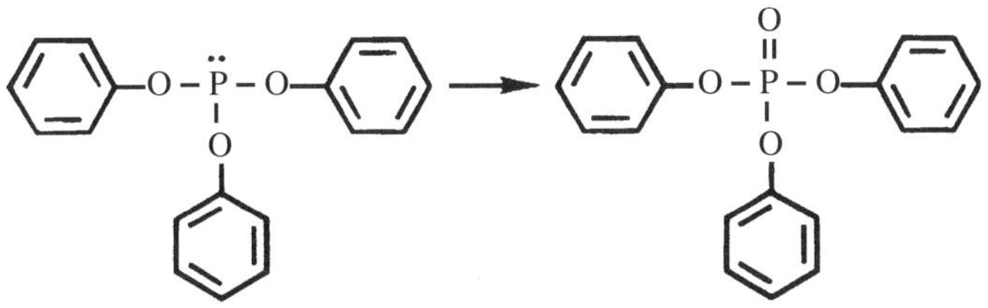

Triphenyl phosphite → Triphenyl phosphate

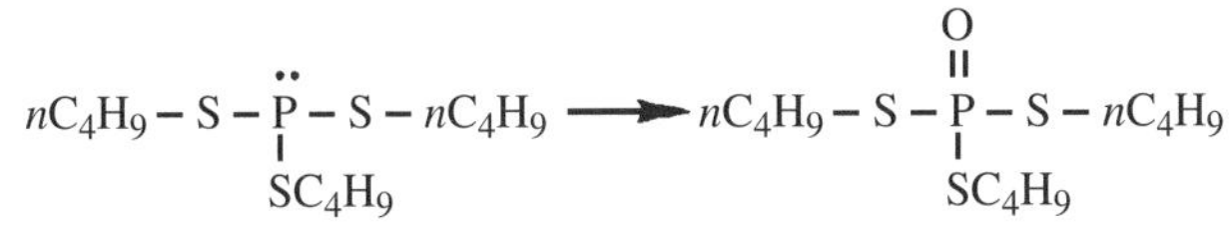

Merphos → DEF

ix. Oxidative desulfuration — Phosphorothioate insecticides are oxidized to phosphates with microsomal cytochrome P-450.

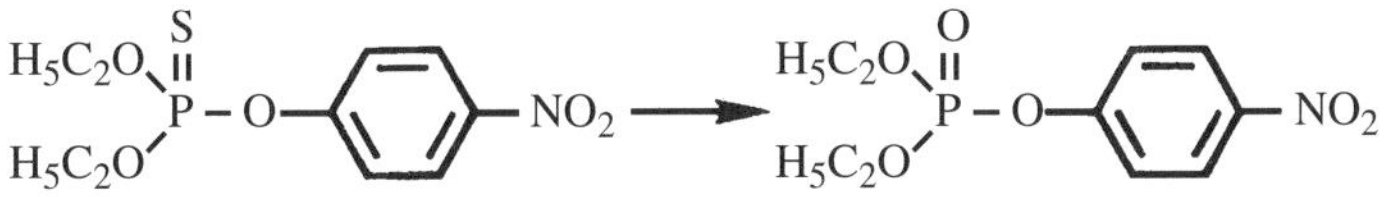

Parathion → Paraoxon

x. Dehalogenation — Halothane, a general anesthetic, undergoes dechlorination and debromination to yield the corresponding alcohol that is subsequently oxidized to an acid.

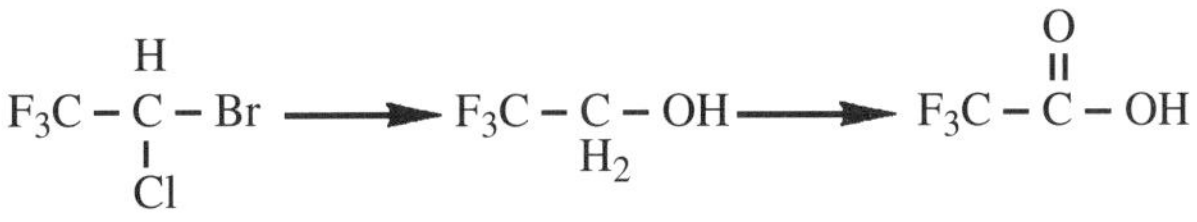

Halothane → Trifluoroethanol → Trifluoroacetic acid

Aromatic halogens are dehalogenated to yield phenols.

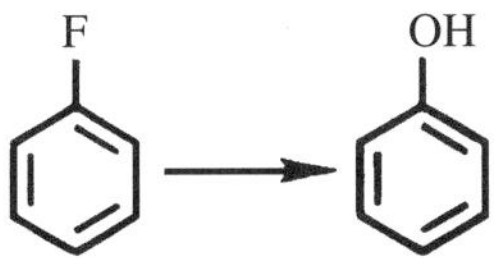

Fluorobenzene → Phenol

xi. Oxidation of aromatic methyl groups — The methyl group of fenitrothion is oxidized to a carboxyl by cytochrome P-450.

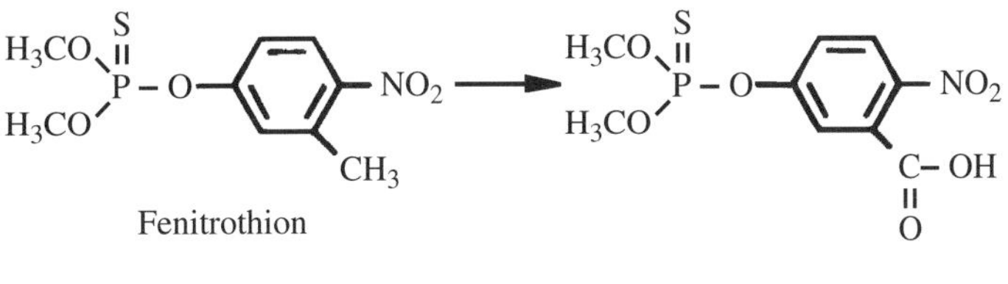

Fenitrothion

b. Reduction reactions
   i.   Azo reductions — Azo compounds, e.g., prontosil red, can undergo reductive metab-
        olism catalyzed by cytochrome P-450. This reaction resulted in the discovery of
        sulfonamides.

Prontosil red   Sulfonamid

   ii. Aromatic nitro reductions — The nitro group in chloramphenicol may be reduced
        via cytochrome P-450.

Chloramphenicol

The insecticide EPN undergoes cytochrome P-450-catalyzed reduction of its nitrio
group.

EPN   Amino EPN

   iii. Reductive dehalogenation — Halothane undergoes reductive defluorination via cyto-
        chrome p-450.

$$F_3C - \underset{\underset{Br}{|}}{\overset{\overset{H}{|}}{C}} - Cl \xrightarrow{-HF} F_2C = \underset{\underset{Br}{|}}{C} - Cl$$

6. Induction of Cytochrome P-450

Compounds that induce or inhibit the activity of xenobiotic-metabolizing enzymes may play a very
important role in the action of xenobiotics on the biological system. These chemicals constitute a
large number and include drugs, environmental pollutants, natural products, and pesticides.

a. Enzyme Induction

The induction of microsomal enzymes has been demonstrated in many species including humans.
Induction may require repeated or chronic exposure to a compound. Exposure may be classified
as acute, a single exposure; subacute, up to 14 days; subchronic, up to 90 days; chronic, up to
lifetime (18 months in mice or 2 years in rats). The enzymes induced include cytochrome P-450
monooxygenase system, glucuronyltransferase, UDP-glucose dehydrogenase, glutathionetrans-

---

TABLE 19.8
Microsomal Enzyme Induction[a]

Parameter	Phenobarbital	Polcyclic Hydrocarbons
Beginning of induction	8–12 h	3–6 h
Peak induction at	3–5 days	1–2 days
Duration of induction	5–7 days	5–12 days
Enlarged liver	+++	±
Protein synthesis	++++	+
Phospholipid synthesis	+++	−
Liver blood flow	++	−
Biliary flow	++	−
MFO components		
Cytochrome P-450	++	−
Cytochrome P-448	−	++
NADPH-cytochrome *c* reductase	++	−
Specific enzyme activity		
N-Demethylase	++	−
Aliphatic hydroxylase	++	−
Polycyclic hydrocarbon hydroxylase	+	++
Reductive dehalogenase	++	−
Epoxide hydrolase	++	+
β-Glucuronidase	++	+
Glutathione transferase	+	+

[a] Symbols: large increase, ++++; marked increase, +++; increase, ++; small increase, +; slight increase, ±; no effect, —.

Source: Modified after Sipes and Gandolfi, 1992.

---

ferase, esterases, microsomal ethanol oxidative system (MEOS), and steroid-metabolizing enzymes. There are three types of cytochrome P-450 inducers: (1) cytochrome P-450 inducers: typical inducer is phenobarbital; (2) cytochrome P-448 inducers: typical inducers are dioxin, 3-methyl cholanthrene, and β-naphthoflavone; (3) anabolic steroids, e.g., testosterone or methyltestosterone, enhance drug metabolism by a mechanism that is different from the other two groups of inducers.

Table 19.8 compares phenobarbital (PB) and 3-methyl cholanthrene (3-MC) induction of cytochrome P-450:

  i. They induce different spectral changes of CO-bound reduced cytochrome P-450. PB increases absorbance at 450 nm. 3-MC or β-naphthoflavone increase absorbance at 448 nm.

  ii PB causes proliferation of the smooth endoplasmic reticulum, whereas 3-MC does not.

  iii. PB induction is general, i.e., it induces many enzymes, whereas 3-MC or β-naphthoflavone are far more specific, i.e., induce a few enzymes.

  iv. PB also increases NADPH cytochrome P-450 reductase and RNA synthesis.

b. Mechanism of Cytochrome P-450 Induction

The genetic code incorporated in DNA molecules consists of pairs of bases arranged in triplets. The bases are the purine bases, adenine (A) and guanine (G); and the pyrimidine bases, thymidine (T) and cytosine (C). The basic mechanism on the transfer of the information encoded in DNA is shown in the following scheme:

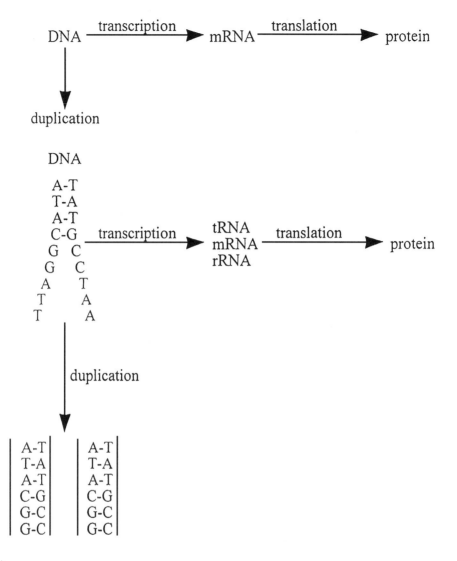

Induction:

    i. Is accompanied by an increase in messenger RNA (mRNA) synthesis.
   ii. Is accompanied by an increase in protein synthesis.
  iii. Can be blocked by actinomycin D, an mRNA *synthesis* inhibitor and other inhibitors such as cycloheximide and puromycin.
   iv. The data suggest that an *increase* in *de novo* synthesis of enzyme protein takes place.
   v. Increase in protein synthesis may result from a *genetic interaction* possibly in combination with a "repressor" gene to allow de-repression of the operator gene and hence the synthesis of mRNA.

B. REACTIONS OTHER THAN MICROSOMAL MIXED-FUNCTION OXIDASE

1. Oxidation Reactions

There are several enzymes in biologic systems that are not related to mixed-function oxidase and can catalyze xenobiotics. These enzymes are microsomal flavin-containing monooxygenase (FMO),

TABLE 19.9
Cytochrome P-450 and FMO

Parameter	P-450	FMO
Location	Microsomes	Microsomes
Cofactors	NADPH and O_2	NADPH, O_2, reductase
Inducers	Phenobarbital, 3-methylcholanthrene, ethanol	None
Substrates	Numerous	Few
Reactions	Oxidation, reduction	Oxidation
Oxidation	C, N, S, P	N, S, P

alcohol dehydrogenase, aldehyde dehydrogenase, xanthine oxidase, amine oxidases, aromatases, and alkylhydrazine oxidase.

a. *Flavin-containing monooxygenase* (FMO) is present in the microsomes and requires the following cofactors: NADPH, O_2, and reductase 14. It catalyzes oxygenation reactions of substrates containing N, S, or P atoms (i.e., no C oxidation). FMO catalyzes the oxidation of secondary and tertiary amines, hydrazines, sulfur, and phosphorus compounds (Table 19.9).

N-Oxidation

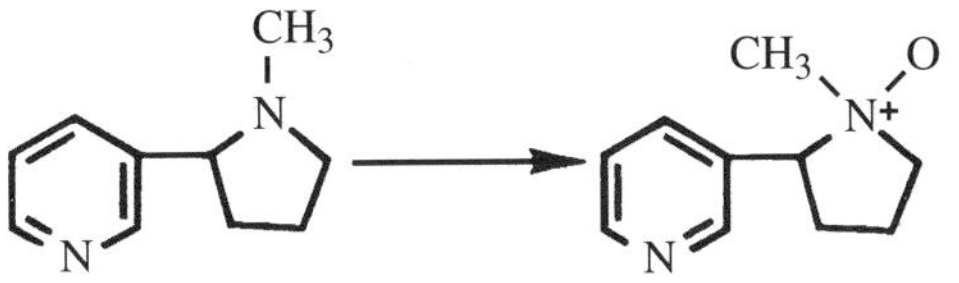

Nicotine

Secondary amines

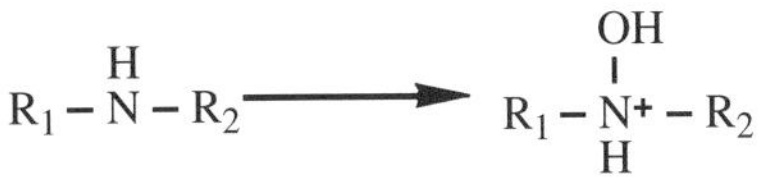

Hydroxylamine

Tertiary amines

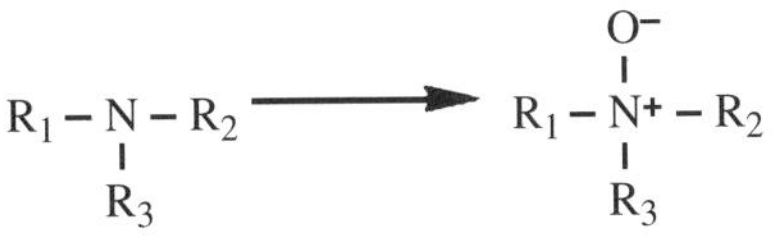

N-Oxide

Imines

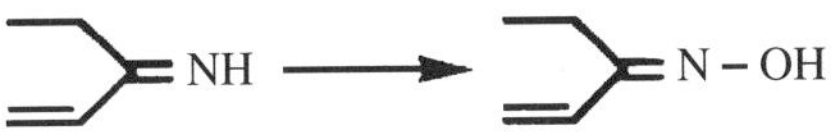

Hydrazines

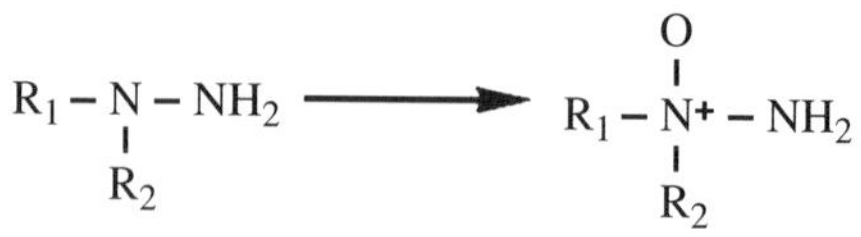

$$R_1 - \underset{\underset{R_2}{|}}{N} - NH_2 \longrightarrow R_1 - \underset{\underset{R_2}{|}}{\overset{\overset{O}{|}}{N^+}} - NH_2$$

S-Oxidation

Thiocarbamide

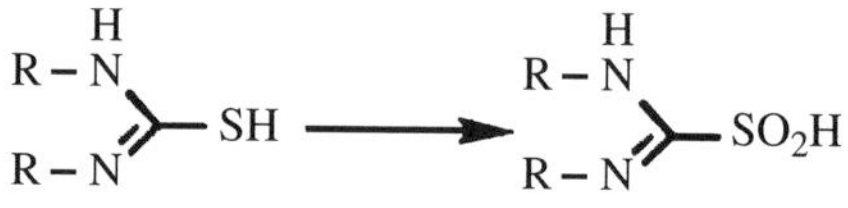

$$\underset{R-N}{\overset{R-\overset{H}{N}}{\diagup}}\!\!\!=\!\!\!\diagdown - SH \longrightarrow \underset{R-N}{\overset{R-\overset{H}{N}}{\diagup}}\!\!\!=\!\!\!\diagdown - SO_2H$$

Thioamide

$$R - \overset{\overset{S}{\|}}{C} - NH_2 \longrightarrow R - \overset{\overset{S=O}{\|}}{C} - NH_2$$

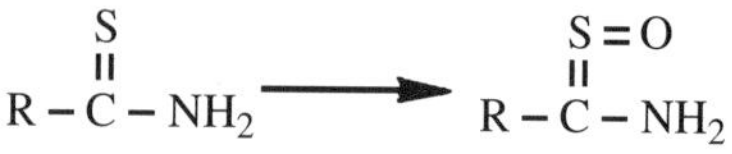

Thiol

$$RSH \longrightarrow RSO_2H$$

Aminothiol

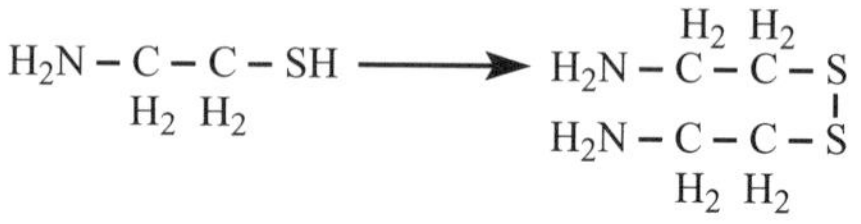

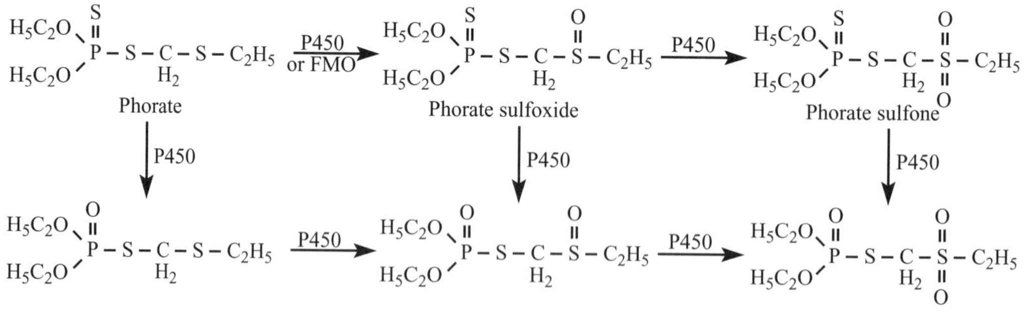

$$H_2N - C - C - SH \longrightarrow \begin{array}{c} \overset{H_2\ H_2}{H_2N - C - C - S} \\ | \\ H_2N - C - C - S \\ \overset{}{H_2\ H_2} \end{array}$$
$$\underset{H_2\ H_2}{}$$

b. *Microsomal ethanol-oxidizing system* (MEOS) is present in the microsomes of liver and requires O_2 and NADPH to oxidize ethanol. MEOS has a high K_m for ethanol, approximately 10 mM, and is responsible for 10 to 15% of its metabolism. It is inhibited by carbon monoxide, but unlike cytochrome P-450 is not inhibited by SKF 525-A or by pyrazole. MEOS activity, hepatic microsomal protein, smooth endoplasmic reticulum, and cytochrome P-450 are increased by prolonged ingestion of ethanol.

c. *Alcohol dehydrogenase* (ADH) is present in the cytosol (soluble fraction) of liver homogenate. This enzyme has a low K_m, for ethanol approximately 1.0 mM, and is responsible for 80 to 85% of its oxidation. ADH is not inducible by ethanol or other chemicals.

$$H_3C - CH_2 \cdot OH \xrightarrow[\text{NAD}^+ \qquad \text{NADH} + \text{H}^+]{\text{Alcohol dehydrogenase (Zn}^{2+}\text{)}} H_3C - \overset{\overset{\text{O}}{\|}}{C} - H$$

Ethanol   Acetaldehyde

d. *Aldehyde dehydrogenase*. Acetaldehyde, the oxidation product of ethanol, undergoes oxidation with acetaldehyde dehydrogenase to form acetic acid. Both enzymes use NAD$^+$ as a cofactor.

$$H_3C - \overset{\overset{\text{O}}{\|}}{C} - H \xrightarrow[\text{NAD}^+ \qquad \text{NADH} + \text{H}^+]{\text{Aldehyde dehydrogenase}} H_3C - \overset{\overset{\text{O}}{\|}}{C} - OH$$

Acetaldehyde   Acetic acid

e. *Peroxidase-catalase system,* which is present in peroxisomes in the liver, plays a minor role in the oxidative metabolism of ethanol.

f. *Xanthine oxidase* metabolizes xanthine and xanthine-containing drugs such as caffeine, theophylline, and theobromine to the corresponding uric acid derivative.

Theophylline   1,3-Dimethyluric acid

g. *Amine oxidases* are divided into two subclasses: monoamine oxidases and diamine oxidases:

i. *Monoamine oxidases* catalyze the oxidation of dietary exogenous amines, e.g., tyramine to the corresponding aldehyde.

$$R - CH_2 \cdot NH_2 \xrightarrow[\text{oxidase}]{\text{Monoamine}} R - \overset{\overset{\text{O}}{\|}}{CH}$$

This enzymatic system is found in mitochondria, at nerve endings, and in liver. This system does not oxidize amphetamines that are metabolized by the microsomal MFO system.

ii. *Diamine oxidase* mainly oxidizes endogenous substrates.

h. *Aromatases* are mitochondrial enzymes present in the liver and kidney. This system requires O_2 and FAD as cofactors. It converts cyclohexane carboxylic acid groups to benzoic acids after the conversion of the acid to the corresponding coenzyme A.

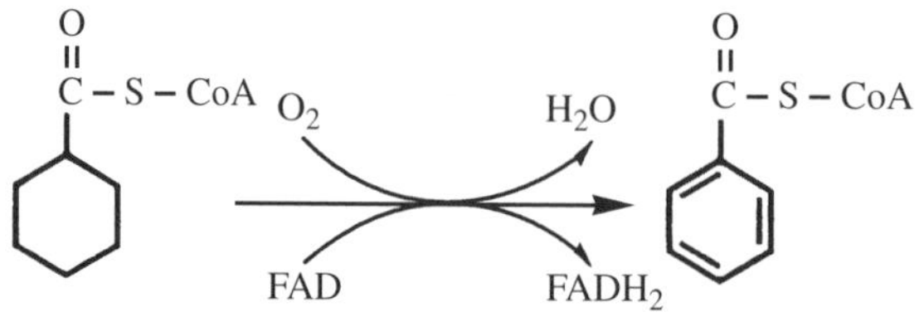

i. *Alkylhydrazine oxidase* is an enzyme that oxidizes alkylhydrazines followed by rearrangement and decomposition of the intermediate, e.g., the metabolism of carbidopa to 2-methyl-3', 4'- dihydroxyphenylpropionic acid.

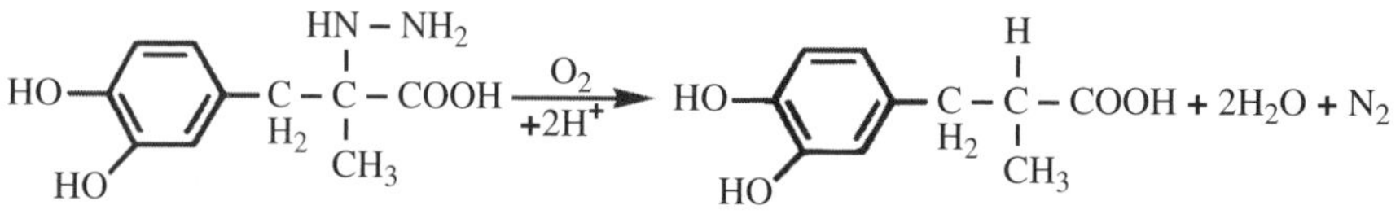

j. *Oxidative dehalogenation* results in the addition of an oxygen in the place of a halogen, such as the conversion of DDT to DDA.

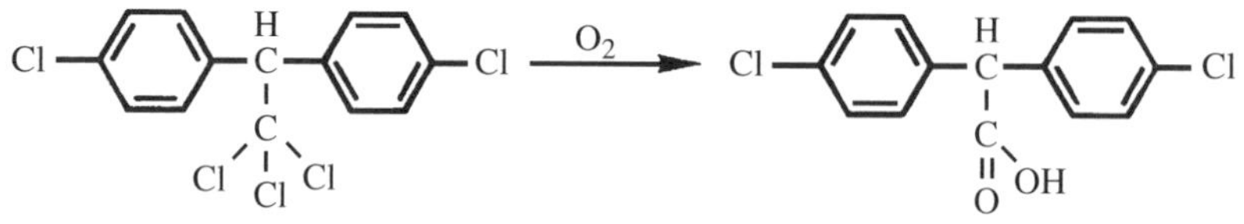

DDT   DDA

Other examples are the oxidative dehalogenations of halothane and DDT.

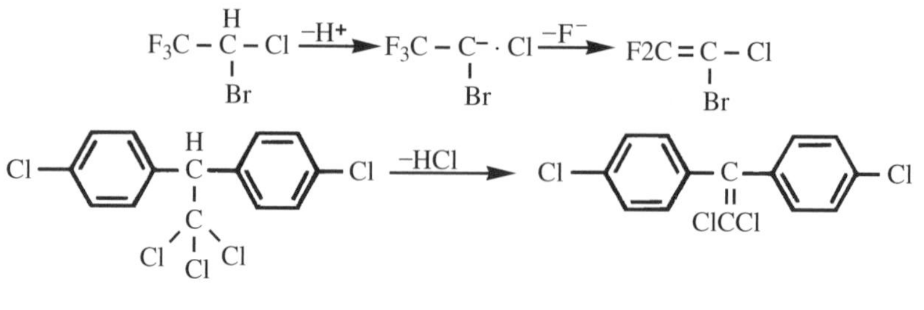

$$F_3C - \underset{\underset{Br}{|}}{\overset{\overset{H}{|}}{C}} - Cl \xrightarrow{-H^+} F_3C - \underset{\underset{Br}{|}}{\overset{}{C^-}} \cdot Cl \xrightarrow{-F^-} F2C = \underset{\underset{Br}{|}}{\overset{}{C}} - Cl$$

DDT   DDE

2. Reduction Reactions

These reactions NADPH, but unlike cytochrome P-450, they are generally inhibited by oxygen. The following compounds undergo reduction reactions: azo-compounds, nitro-compounds, epoxides, heterocyclic ring compounds, and halogenated hydrocarbons. Azo- and nitro-compound reduction may be catalyzed by cytochrome P-450, but can also be catalyzed by NADPH-cytochrome c reductase. Epoxides can be converted back to hydrocarbons. Also, some heterocyclic compounds may undergo ring cleavage by reduction. Such reactions may undergo rearrangement and hydrolysis.

DDT may undergo reductive dechlorination to form DDD.

3. Hydrolysis Reactions

Hydrolytic enzymes hydrolyze carboxylic acid esters, amides, carbamates, hydrazides, and phosphoric acid esters.

a. Xenobiotic Metabolizing Esterase

Esterases are distributed in the blood and tissues and catalyze the hydrolysis of a variety of esters. These enzymes do not have a well-defined role in the metabolism of either endogenous ester substrates or the metabolism of drugs and other foreign compounds. Most tissues are rich in esterases that have relatively broad structural requirements as far as these substrate specificities and inhibitor sensitivities.

Esterases play a very important role in the development of organophosphorus ester toxicity. This toxicity is dependent upon:

- The intrinsic toxicity of the organophosphorus ester
- The bioavailability or the concentration of the compound at the site of action

The bioavailability of the organophosphorus compounds at the neurotoxicity target is a function of:

- Route of entry of the chemical
- Sequestration and subsequent detoxification of organophosphorus compounds by binding or phosphorylation by blood proteins, such as albumin, serum ChE (B-esterase), or red blood cell ACHE. Protein-bound organophosphorus esters are secreted into the bile.
- Hydrolysis of organophosphorus esters by serum and hepatic A-esterases to water-soluble, less-toxic metabolites that are excreted in the urine. Hydrolysis is the most important route of the detoxification of organophosphorus esters.

Esterases in liver microsomes and cytosol as well as blood and tissues reduce the activity of many esters by acting as scavengers to sequester these esters or hydrolyze them. These enzymes have been classified according to their sensitivity to inhibition by organophosphorus compounds. Xenobiotic metabolizing esterases include:

i. *Red blood cell.* Acetylcholinesterase (RBC AChE, Ec 3.1.1.7) is similar to AChE in nervous system tissues; however, it has no known function in RBC. This enzyme inactivates organophosphorus esters either by binding and sequestering or by hydrolysis.

ii. *Plasma and tissues*

   (1) *A-Esterases.* These enzymes, which are resistant to inhibition by organophosphorus, include two subclasses of enzymes:

      (a) Arylesterase or aryl hydrolase, Are (EC 3.1.1.2), which is assayed using α-naphthylacetate and aromatic esters as substrates.

      (b) Paraoxonase or phosphoric triester hydrolase (EC 3.1.8.1) that is determined with paraoxon as a substrate. This enzyme is associated with high-density lipoproteins (HDL) in true serum.

   (2) *B-Esterases.* These enzymes are sensitive to inhibition by organophosphates. Two subclasses of enzymes belong to this class:

      (a) Cholinesterase (EC 3.1.1.8), which is also known as plasma or serum cholinesterase, nonspecific esterase, acylcholine acylhydrolase, cholinesterase II, and pseudocholinesterase, is an acidic glycoprotein with a molecular weight of 350 kDa and a half-life of 11 days. It is assayed by the use of the substrate butyrylthiocholine.

      (b) Carboxylesterase, which is also known as aliesterase, ALie (Ec 3.1.1.1.), is assayed using *p*-nitrophenyl acetate.

   (3) *C-Esterase*, which is also known as acetylesterase (EC 3.1.1.6), is resistant to inhibition by DFP but activated by *p*-chloromercuric benzoate and phenylmercuric acetate.

A-esterases and B-esterases including ChE activities vary widely within healthy populations and are influenced by both genetic and environmental factors, as well as diseased states. Variation in the activities of these enzymes may contribute to interindividual differences in susceptibility to organophosphorus compound toxicity.

iii. *Lymphocytes and tissues.* Neurotoxic esterase or neurotoxicity target esterase (NTE), which is present in lymphocytes and most tissues, is assayed using phenylvalerate as a substrate.[18] It is a good biomarker for organophosphorus ester-induced delayed neurotoxicity (OPIDN), which correlates well with its inhibition and aging. Organophosphorus compounds capable of producing OPIDN results in at least 70% inhibition of NTE. Like other nonspecific esterases, neither its natural biochemical nor physiological function is known.

b. Carboxylic Acid Esters

Hydrolysis of *carboxylic acid esters* is carried out by esterases present in plasma, e.g., pseudocholinesterases, or in the liver to produce carboxylic acid and alcohol.

c. Amide hydrolysis

The *amide hydrolysis* reaction is catalyzed by amidases to yield an amine and an acid.

d. Carbamates

Aromatic *carbamates* are hydrolyzed to yield phenols.

Baygon

e. Hydrazides

Isoniazid is hydrolyzed to isonicotinic acid and hydrazine.

Isoniazid   Isonicotinic acid

4. Hydration Reactions

Epoxide hydratase catalyzes the hydration of epoxides. This reaction involves the addition of a water molecule to produce the dihydrodiol.

Glycidamide   2,3-Dihydroxy propionamide

C. OTHER PHASE I REACTIONS

Cyclization

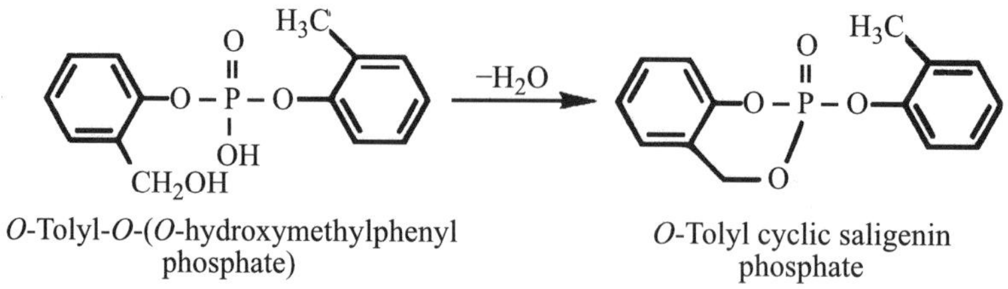

O-Tolyl-*O*-(*O*-hydroxymethylphenyl
phosphate)

O-Tolyl cyclic saligenin
phosphate

D. PROSTAGLANDIN ENDOPEROXIDE SYNTHETASE

The prostaglandin endoperoxide synthetase system involves two enzymes: fatty acid cyclooxygenase and hydroperoxidase. Fatty acid cyclooxygenase catalyzes bis-dioxygenation to produce the
hydroperoxy endoperoxide PGG_2.

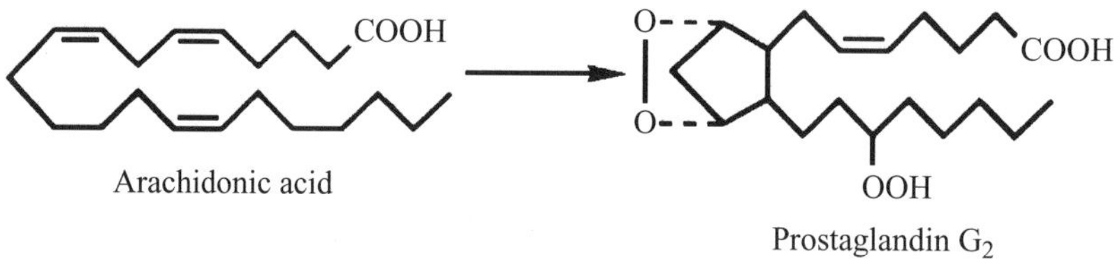

Arachidonic acid

Prostaglandin G_2

On the other hand, hydroxyperoxidase catalyzes the reduction of PGG_2 to PGH_2. This enzymatic
system metabolizes *N*-methyl carbamates that have a pair of electrons available for the last step of
the reaction in the presence of arachidonic acid, resulting in demethylation. Neither *S*- nor
O-demethylation takes place.

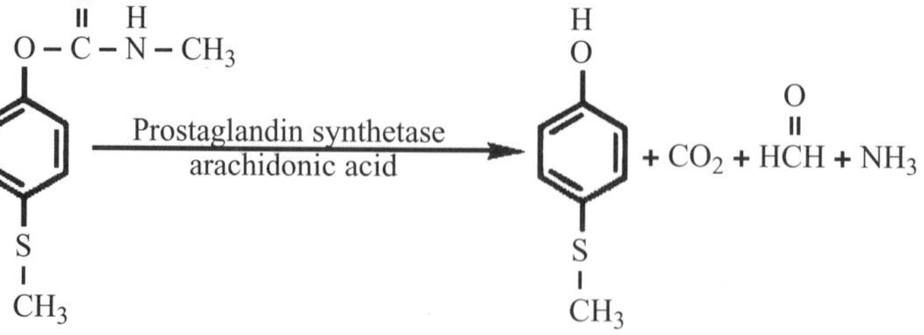

E. ENDOGENOUS METABOLISM BY PHASE I ENZYMES

Phase I enzymes carry out the metabolism of many endogenous substrates. Table 19.10 summarizes
these reactions.

TABLE 19.10
Endogenous Metabolism by Phase I Enzymes

Phase I Enzyme	Endogenous Substrate
Acetylcholinesterase	Acetylcholine
Diamine oxidase	Cadaverine
	Histamine
	Putrescine
Hydroxysteroid oxidoreductase	Steroids
Mixed-function oxidase	Fatty acids
	Leukotrienes
	Prostaglandins
	Steroids
	Sterols
	Thyroid hormones
	Vitamins
Monoamine oxidase	Monoamine neurotransmitters
Reductases	Steroids
Xanthine oxidase	Xanthines

SECTION 5. XENOBIOTIC-METABOLIZING REACTIONS: PHASE II

A xenobiotic is generally subjected to several competing reactions simultaneously. Also, some metabolic reactions proceed sequentially, and Phase I reactions, i.e., oxidation, reduction, and hydrolysis, are followed by Phase II or conjugation reactions of products. Phase II reactions involve the addition of a xenobiotic to endogenous groups that are generally polar and readily available *in vivo* (Table 19.11). This process renders the whole molecule more acidic, more polar, and less lipid soluble, thus facilitating elimination from the body. The conjugates formed are usually less toxic than their parent compounds; therefore, Phase II is considered a detoxification mechanism.

Conjugation requires: (1) ATP as a source of energy, (2) coenzymes, and (3) transferases. Conjugation reactions and transferases are listed in Table 19.12. The conjugation usually proceeds in two steps: (1) extramicrosomal synthesis of an acylcoenzyme and (2) the transfer of the acetyl moiety to the acylcone, which in some but not all cases is localized in microsomes.

All conjugation reactions require activated nucleotides as activated intermediates. There are two conjugation mechanisms: (1) activated conjugating agents:

$$\text{Conjugate agent} \xrightarrow{\text{ATP}} \text{activated conjugating agent} \xrightarrow{\text{Xenobiotic}} \text{Conjugate}$$

and (2) xenobiotic or its metabolite activated:

$$\text{Xenobiotic} \xrightarrow{\text{ATP}} \text{activated xenobiotic} \xrightarrow[\text{agent}]{\text{Conjugating}} \text{Conjugate}$$

Tissue and subcellular localization of conjugation reactions are listed in Table 19.13.

TABLE 19.11
Conjugation Reactions

Conjugating Chemical	Product
Glucuronic acid	Glucuronide
Sulfuric acid	Ethereal sulfate
Glycine	Hippuric acid
Glutamine[a]	Glutamine conjugate
Glutathione	Mercapturic acid
Methyl group	Methyl ether
Acetic acid	Acetyl ester
Thio group	Thiocyanate
Glucoside conjugation[b]	Glucoside
Ornithine conjugation[c]	Ornithine conjugate

[a] Occurs only in humans, apes, and new and old world monkeys.

[b] Occurs in insects.

[c] Occurs in certain birds.

TABLE 19.12
Conjugation Reactions, Transferase Enzymes, and Functional Groups

Reaction	Transferase	Functional Group
Glucuronidation	UDP-Glucuronyltransferase	–OH
		–COOH
		NH_2
		–SH
Glycosidation	UDP-Glycosyltransferase	–OH
		–COOH
		–SH
Sulfation	Sulfotransferase	–OH
		$-NH_2$
		$-SO_2NH_2$
Methylation	Methyltransferase	–OH
		$-NH_2$
Acetylation	Acetyltransferase	–OH
		$-NH_2$
		$-SO_2NH_2$
Amino acid conjugation		–COOH
Glutathione conjugation	Glutathione-S-transferase	Epoxide
		Organic halide
Fatty acid conjugation		–OH

TABLE 19.13
Tissue and Subcellular Localization of Conjugation Reactions

Conjugation Reaction	Intermediate Nucleotide	Localization	
		Tissue	**Subcellular**
a. Activated conjugation			
Glucuronidation	Uridine diphosphate Glucuronic acid	Liver, most tissue	Microsomes
Ethereal sulfation	Phosphadenosine Phosphosulfate	Liver, kidney, intestine	Supernatant
Methylation	S-Adenosylmethionine	Liver, many tissue	Microsomes, supernatant
Acetylation	Acetyl-CoA	Liver, other tissue	Supernatant
b. Activated xenobiotic			
Hippuric acid	Aryl-CoA	Liver, kidney	Mitochondria
Glutamine synthesis	Phenacetyl-CoA	Liver, kidney	Mitochondria

A. CONJUGATION WITH SUGARS

Conjugation with α-D-glucuronic acid to produce glucuronides is the most common sugar conjugation reaction. Other conjugations with sugars include conjugation with glucose, xylose, and ribose.

1. Glucuronidation

a. Mechanisms of the Reaction

i. Glucuronide formation is one of the most common routes of drug metabolism because of the availability of glucose.

ii. The reaction involves the condensation of D-glucuronic acid.

iii. This reaction requires the activation of glucuronic acid by the synthesis of uridine diphosphate glucuronic acid (UDPGA, "H" is α).

iv. Glucuronidation involves nucleophilic attack (SN_2) by the oxygen, sulfur, or nitrogen atom at C-1 carbon atom of the glucuronic acid moiety. Therefore, the H atom of glucuronic acid is inverted to a β-configuration when complexed with the xenobiotic compound.

$$\text{Glucose - 1 - phosphate} + \text{UTP} \xrightarrow{\text{Pyrophosphorylase}} \text{UDP - glucose} + \text{pyrophosphate}$$

$$\text{UDP - glucose - 2NAD}^+ + \text{H}_2\text{O} \xrightarrow{\text{UDP-dehydrogenase}} \underset{\text{(UDPGA)}}{\text{UDP - glucuronic acid}} + \text{NADH} + 2\text{H}^+$$

$$\text{UDPGA} + \text{R}_z\text{H} \xrightarrow[\text{(Liver, supernatant)}]{\text{Glucuronyl transferase}} \text{R}_z \text{ - glucuronic acid} + \text{UDP}$$

Where Z is

$$-\text{O}^-, \ -\overset{\overset{\textstyle O}{\|}}{\text{C}}-\text{O}^-, \ -\text{NH, or} -\text{S}$$

Table 19.14 lists various types of conjugation reactions.

TABLE 19.14
Types of Glucuronidation Reactions

Functional Group	Type of Chemical	Structure	Example
Hydroxyl	Phenol	ArOH	Morphine
	Enol	$-CH = COH$	4-Hydroxycoumarin
	Primary alcohol	$-CH_2OH$	Chloramphenicol
	Secondary alcohol	$\overset{\diagdown}{\underset{\diagup}{C}}H-OH$	*sec*-Butanol
	Tertiary alcohol	$-\overset{\mid}{\underset{\mid}{C}}-OH$	*tert*-Butanol
	Hydroxylamine	$Ar-\overset{\overset{O}{\parallel}}{C}-OH$	N-Hydroxy-N-2-fluorenylacetamide
Carboxyl	Aromatic acids		Salicylic acid
	Aliphatic acids	$-CH_2-\overset{\overset{O}{\parallel}}{C}-OH$	Indomethacin
Amino	Aromatic	$ArNH_2$	4,4'-Diaminodiphenylsulfone
	Carbamate	$-O\overset{\overset{O}{\parallel}}{C}-NH_2$	Meprobamate
Imino	Sulfonimide	$-\overset{\overset{O}{\parallel}}{\underset{\underset{O}{\parallel}}{S}}-NH-$	Sulfadimethoxine
	Heterocyclic	$\overset{\diagdown}{\underset{\diagup}{N}}H$	Sulfisoxazole
Sulfhydryl	Thiol	$-SH$	2-Mercaptobenzothiazole
	Carbodithioic	$-\overset{\overset{S}{\parallel}}{C}-SH$	Diethydithiocarbamic acid

b. Other Sugars

Unlike mammals, conjugation with glucose is most prevalent in insects. This reaction proceeds in an analogous fashion to glucuronide formation, but UDP-glucose is used instead of UDPGA, resulting in glucoside formation. Similarly, *O*-, *N*-, and *S*-glucosides may be formed. These reactions are also formed in plants. In some instances, UDP-xylose or UDP-ribose can be used to form xylosides or ribosides. An example of *N*-riboside formation is shown below:

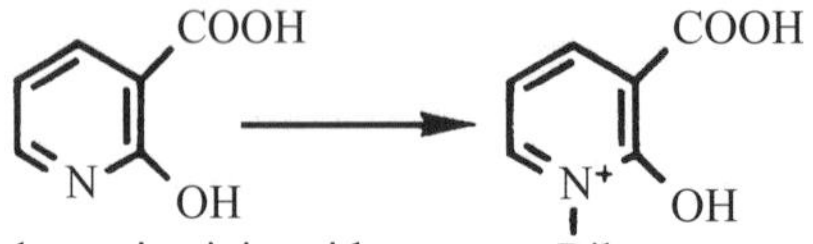

2-Hydroxynicotinic acid → (Ribose)

2. Substrates for the Reaction

a. O-Conjugation

i. Ether type — Alcohols and phenols form "ether type" glucuronides:

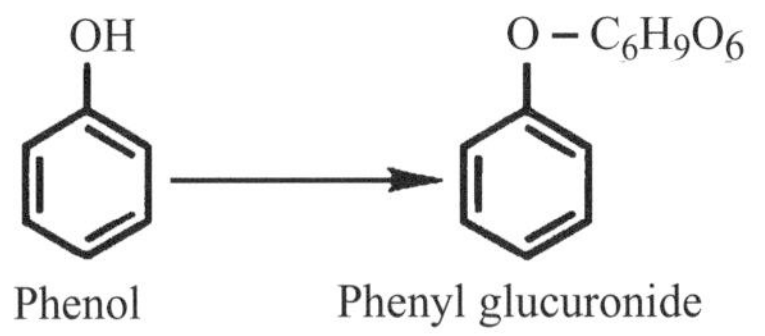

OH

Phenol

$O - C_6H_9O_6$

Phenyl glucuronide

ii. Ester type — Aromatic and some aliphatic carboxylic acids form "ester type" glucuronides:

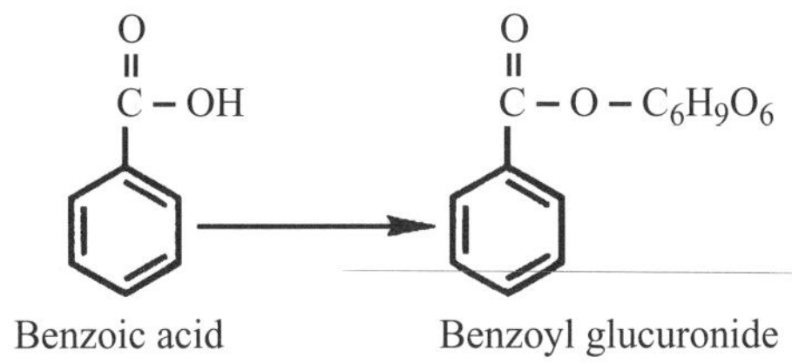

$$\overset{O}{\overset{\|}{C}} - OH$$

Benzoic acid

$$\overset{O}{\overset{\|}{C}} - O - C_6H_9O_6$$

Benzoyl glucuronide

b. N-Glucuronide

Amines, especially aromatic compounds, form N-glucuronides:

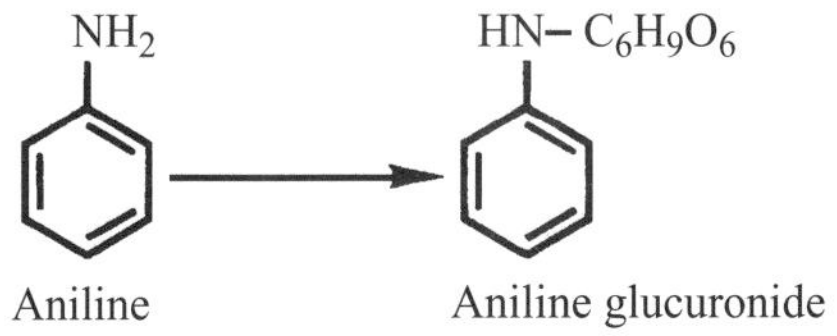

NH_2

Aniline

$HN- C_6H_9O_6$

Aniline glucuronide

Although conjugation generally decreases biological activity, including toxicity, occasionally there are exceptions. The N-hydroxyglucuronide is a more potent carcinogen than the parent compound acetylaminofluorene.

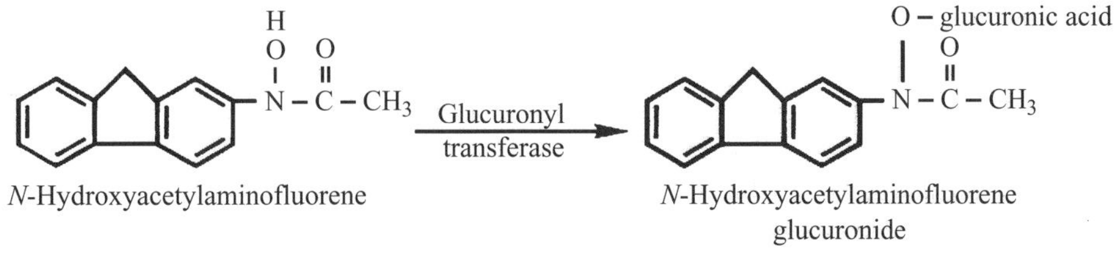

$$\overset{H}{\underset{|}{N}} \overset{O}{\underset{|}{C}} - CH_3$$

N-Hydroxyacetylaminofluorene

Glucuronyl
transferase

$$\overset{O - \text{glucuronic acid}}{\underset{|}{N}} \overset{O}{\underset{\|}{C}} - CH_3$$

N-Hydroxyacetylaminofluorene
glucuronide

c. S-Glucuronide

Certain thiol compounds form S-glucuronides:

Thiophenol   Phenol thioglucuronide

In addition, normally occurring substrates, such as steroids, thyroxin, and bilirubin, also conjugate with glucuronic acid.

3. Glucuronide Formation in Various Species

a. Glucuronidation takes place in most mammalian species with the exception of the cat.
b. The cat can synthesize UDPGA, but it lacks glucuronyltransferase.
c. Fish lack glucuronidaton because they are deficient in UDPGA.
d. In rats, males produce more glucuronides than females; this sex difference does not hold for humans, however.

4. Factors Affecting Glucuronide Formation

a. Inducers of drug metabolism increase the activity of glucuronyltransferase.
b. MFO inhibitors, such as SKF-525A, inhibit glucuronyl transferase activity *in vivo*.
c. Glucuronide formation is diminished during pregnancy. This may be explained by the increased levels of progesterone and pregnanediol, which inhibit transferase activity.
d. Patients with liver damage may have impaired glucuronide conjugation.
e. The newborn in humans and most species, except in the rat, has very low levels of glucuronyltransferase. In infants, the failure to conjugate chloramphenicol and its metabolites to nontoxic glucuronides results in the characteristic "gray baby" syndrome, characterized by cyanosis, cardiovascular toxicity, and death.

5. Excretion of Glucuronides

a. Urinary excretion
   i.   Glomerular filtration — High-molecular-weight conjugates, such as glucuronides of androsterone and pregnanediol, are eliminated by glomerular filtration alone.
   ii. Passive tubular diffusion — Lower-molecular-weight conjugates, i.e., phenols, are excreted by passive tubular diffusion.
   iii. Active secretion — This is a carrier-mediated, active transport process. Medium-molecular-weight glucuronides are frequently excreted by tubular secretion.
b. Bile excretion
   i.   Biliary excretion in the rat is preferred for compounds with molecular weight of 325, having one or more aromatic rings, and one or more hydroxyl groups. Thus, glucuronides of bilirubin, thyroxin, pregnanediol, morphine, and chloramphenicol are mostly excreted into the bile.
   ii. Glucuronides excreted via the bile in the gut (duodenum) may be hydrolyzed by β-glucuronidase (lysosomes). The free chemical may undergo absorption, transport to the liver, reconjugation, and re-excretion (interohepatic circulation).

6. Methods to Study Glucuronidation

a. It is possible to isolate glucuronides by precipitation from solutions followed by crystallization.

b. It is more customary to identify glucuronides by the use of β-glucuronidase enzyme. In these studies, radiolabeled xenobiotics are extracted with organic solvents followed by hydrolysis by incubation with β-glucuronidase. Glucuronides are then extracted with organic solvents.

B. SULFATION

Conjugation by sulfate is a very efficient pathway for eliminating xenobiotics through urine because the sulfate conjugates are completely ionized and highly water soluble. The major compounds that undergo sulfation reactions are alcohols, phenols, and arylamines. This reaction is catalyzed by the enzyme sulfotransferase.

TABLE 19.15
Sulfation Reactions

Compound	Enzyme	Tissue
Dimetranidazol	Alcohol sulfotransferase	Liver
Isoprenaline	Phenol sulfotransferase	Liver, kidney, gut
Oestrone	Steroid sulfotransferase	Liver
Paracetamol	Arylamine sulfotransferase	Liver

1. Mechanisms of the Reaction

The coenzyme participating in sulfuric acid conjugation is 3-phosphoadenosine-5-phosphosulfate, (PAPS). Sulfate conjugation reactions involve ATP and take place in the soluble fraction of cells.

$$SO_4^{2-} + ATP \xrightarrow{\text{ATP-sulfurylase}} \text{Adenosine - 5'- phosphosulfate (APS)} + \text{pyrophosphate}$$

$$APS + ATP \xrightarrow{\text{APS phosphokinase}} \text{3'- phosphoadenosine - 5'- phosphosulfate (PAPS)} + ADP$$

$$PAPS + RZH \xrightarrow{\text{Sulfokinase}} R - Z - SO_3H + \text{3'- phosphoadenosine - 5'- phosphate (PAP)}$$

where Z is O or NH.

2. SUBSTRATES FOR THE REACTION

a. Ethereal sulfates — Phenol and alcohols form "ethereal sulfates":

Phenol → Phenyl sulfate

b. Sulfamates — Aromatic amines form "*N*-sulfates" or sulfamates:

Endogenous sulfate conjugates include heparin, tyrosine sulfate, various sulfolipids, the sulfates of epinephrine, norepinephrine, progesterone, and estrone.

3. Factors Affecting Sulfate Conjugation

a. The total pool of sulfate is usually quite limited and can be readily exhausted; thus with increasing doses of a drug, conjugation with sulfate may become a zero-order reaction.
b. For this reason, conjugation with glucuronic acid is more predominant over that of sulfate.
c. Most species, including human's are able to make sulfate derivatives, although to a lesser extent in the pig and fish.
d. At birth, relatively little sulfokinase activity is present in many animals similar to that with glucuronyltransferase.
e. Sulfatases that can cleave the sulfate group from their derivatives are present in most species (liposomes).

4. Methods for Studying Sulfate Conjugation

a. Precipitation
b. Hydrolysis with sulfatases

C. METHYLATION

Methylation represents a relatively minor metabolic pathway for drugs. It differs from other conjugation reactions in that the products formed occasionally have extensive biological activity, e.g., epinephrine.

Norepinephrine   Epinephrine

TABLE 19.16
Methylation Reactions

Compound	Enzyme	Tissue
N-Acetylserotinin	Hydroxyndole O-methyltransferase	Pineal gland
Catechols	Catechol O-methyltransferase	Liver, kidney, skin, nervous tissue
Histamine	Imidazole N-methyltransferase	Liver
Noradrenaline	Phenylethanolamine N-methyltransferase	Adrenals

1. Mechanisms of the Reaction

$$\text{Methionine} + \text{ATP} \xrightarrow[\substack{\text{adenosine} \\ \text{transferase}}]{\text{Methionine}} \text{S - adenosylmethionine} + \text{pyrophosphate} + \text{phosphate}$$
(methyl donor)

$$s\text{ - Adenosylmethionine} + RZH \xrightarrow[\text{transferase}]{\text{Methyl}} RZCH_3 + S\text{ - adenosylhomocysteine}$$

Methyl transferases are localized in liver microsomes.

2. Substrates for the Reaction

a. *N*-Methylation

$$Norepinephrine \rightarrow Epinephrine \ (see \ above)$$

b. *O*-Methylation

c. *S*-Methylation

$$H_3C - CH_2 - SH \rightarrow H_3C - CH_2 - S - CH_3$$
Ethyl mercaptan

D. AMIDE SYNTHESIS

This reaction takes place in the mitochondria of liver and kidney cells. This reaction involves the condensation of an acid with an amine to form an amide. Two types of reactions will be considered.

a. Conjugation of carboxylic acid–containing drugs with endogenous amines (usually amino acids, e.g., glycine). The coenzyme participating in this reaction is acetyl coenzyme A.

a. Glycine
  (i) The formation of hippuric acid from benzoic acid and endogenous glycine was first demonstrated in the horse, and the name *hippuric acid* was chosen from the Greek word hippos for horse.
  (ii) For other acids, the ending "uric" still applies to the metabolite even though it has no relation to uric acid; thus, salicyluric acid is the glycine conjugate of salicylic acid.

Salicylic acid   Salicyluric acid

  (iii) The pool of endogenous glycine is limited, and hippuric acid formation may follow zero-order kinetics.
  (iv) Glycine conjugation may be impaired in certain cases of liver diseases, and hippuric acid formation after benzoic acid ingestion has been used as a test for liver function.
  (v) In the newborn and in elderly people, glycine is less available and hippuric acid formation is reduced.
b. Other amino acids
  (i) Glutamine — Conjugates acid drugs in certain primates
  (ii) Ornithine — Conjugation with ornithine takes place in reptiles and birds
2. Conjugation of amine drugs with endogenous carboxylic acids, e.g., acetic acid
  a. This takes place with aromatic primary amines, sulfonamides, and hydrazines.

Sulfanylamide

b. Phenols, alcohols, or thiols do not form acetyl derivatives.
c. The dog, unlike most mammalian species, is a poor acetylator.

d. Acetylation of isoniazid is genetically determined in humans. Slow acetylators have less *N*-acetyltransferase in their liver than rapid acetylators (inactivators).

e. Humans lack the ability to deacetylate acetylated aromatic amines, and the apparent rate of acetylation is relatively great.

E. Glutathione Conjugation (Mercapturic Acid Synthesis)

This reaction results in *N*-acetylcysteine (mercapturic acid conjugates) as follows:

1. An initial conjugation with glutathione (glutathione-*S*-transferase)
2. Cleavage of the glutamyl and glycinyl residues
3. Acetylation of the glycine moiety

The first step is catalyzed by glutathione-*S*-transferase that is primarily present in the soluble (cytosol) fraction of the cell, but is also found in the microsomes.

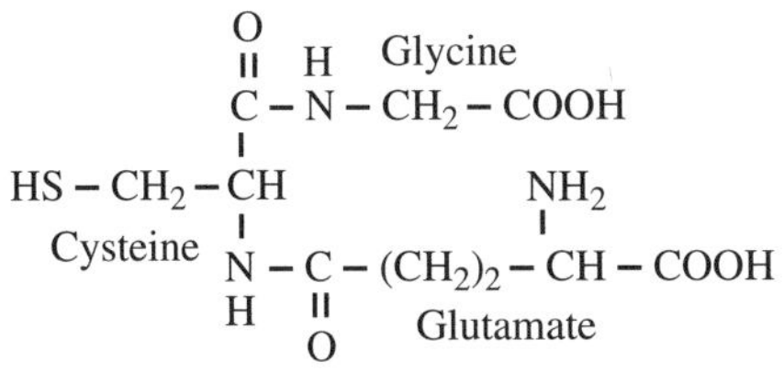

Glutathione

N-(*N-L*-γ-glutaryl-*L*-cysteinyl)glycine

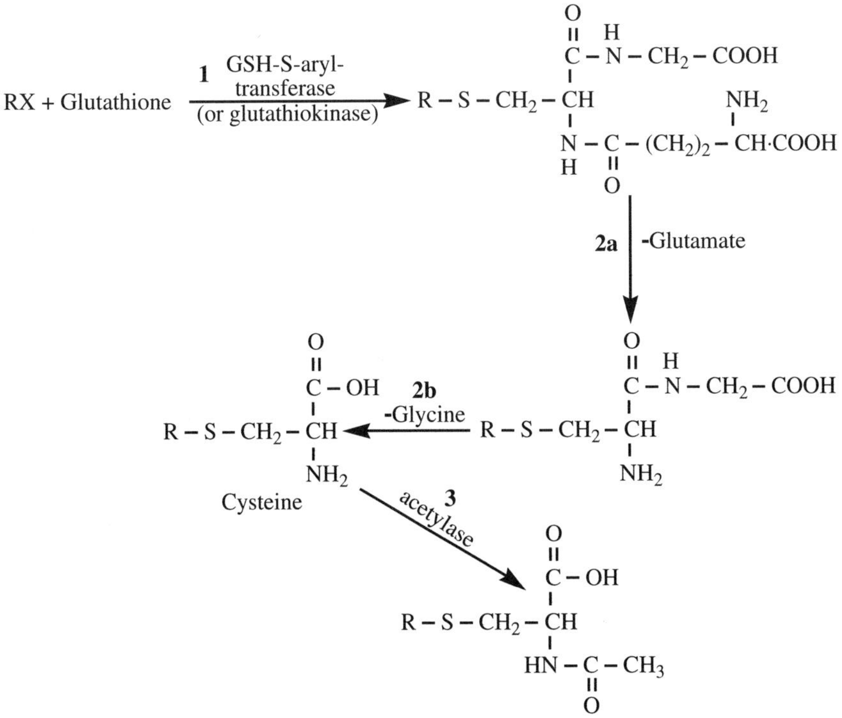

Mercapturic acid derivatives

Glutathione conjugation is a detoxification reaction because it masks reactive electrophiles. Examples:

1. Conjugation of benzene epoxide with glutathione and formation of phenyl mercapturate:

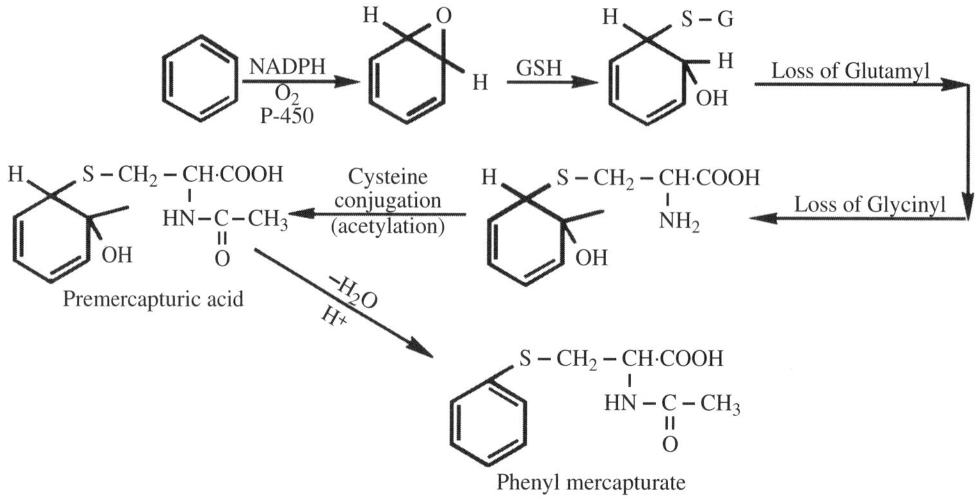

Premercapturic acid

Phenyl mercapturate

Xenobiotics subject to this reaction frequently contain an active halogen or a nitro group.

2. Conjugation of various epoxides with glutathione

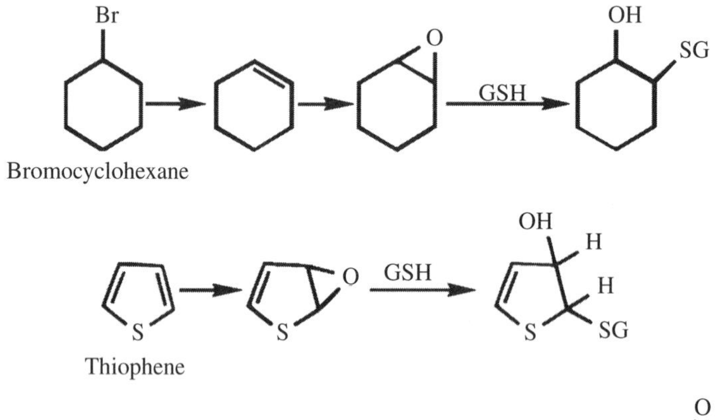

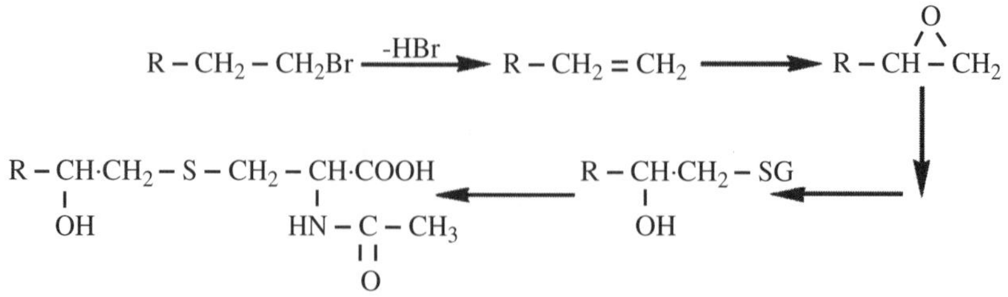

Bromocyclohexane

Thiophene

3. Displacement of aliphatic and aromatic halogens by glutathione

$$R - CH_2 - CH_2Br \xrightarrow{\text{GSH}} R - CH_2 - CH_2 - SG + HBr$$

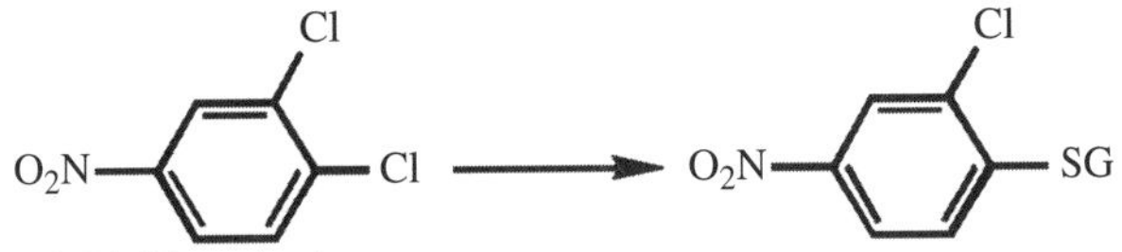

3, 4-Dichloronitrobenzene

4. Unsaturated aliphatic compounds with suitable electron-withdrawing groups. Chemicals such as diethyl maleate may react directly with glutathione *without* undergoing metabolic activation. Diethyl maleate may be used to deplete hepatic glutathione *in vivo* experimentally.

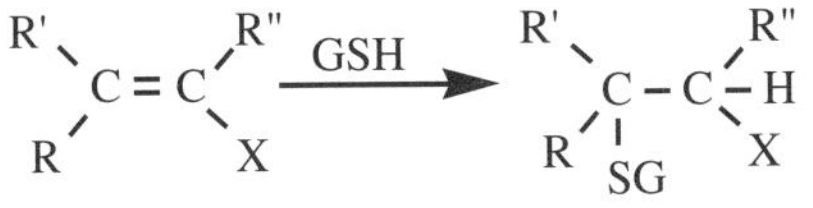

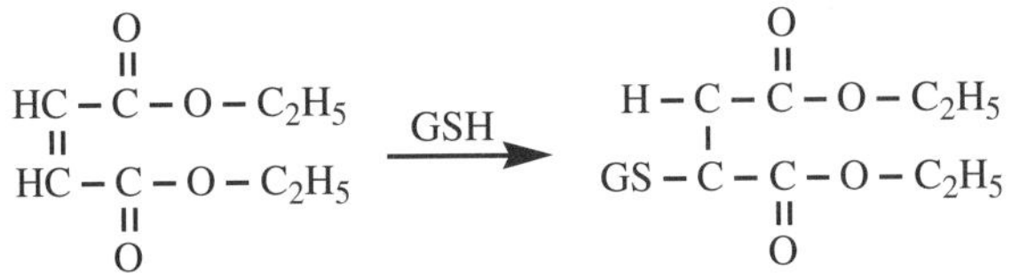

Diethyl maleate

F.   OTHER CONJUGATION REACTIONS

1.   Glucoside Conjugation

This reaction occurs in insects and plants where it replaces glucuronide conjugation. Ester and ether glucosides are formed:

$$ROH + UDP\text{-}glucose \xrightarrow[\text{transferase}]{\text{Glucose}} RO\text{-}\beta\text{-}glucoside + UDP$$

Mammals do not synthesize glucosides because they lack glucosyltransferase.

2.   Thiocyanates

$$CN^- + S_2O_2^= \xrightarrow[\text{(or Rhoduhase)}]{\overset{\text{Sulfur}}{\text{transferase}}} SCN^- + SO_3^=$$

Thiosulfate (endogenous)   Thiocyanate

a. Free cyanides or cyanides formed from nitriles or oximes from thiocyanates.
b. Sulfur transferase is found mainly in liver mitochondria.

G.   PHASE II METABOLISM OF ENDOGENOUS COMPOUNDS

Endogenous compounds undergo conjugation via Phase II metabolic pathways. Examples of these reactions are listed in Table 19.17.

TABLE 19.17
Phase II Metabolism of Endogenous Compounds

Conjugation Reaction	Substrates
Acetylation	Serotonin
Amino acid conjugation	Bile acid
Glucuronidation	Steroids
	Thyroxin
	Bilirubin
	Catecholamines
Glutathione conjugation	Arachidonic acid metabolites (leukotrienes)
Methylation	Biogenic amines
Sulfation	Carbohydrates
	Steroids

SECTION 6. TOXIC RESPONSES TO XENOBIOTICS

Xenobiotics may exert effects (pharmacological or toxic) at various leves: molecular, subcellular, cellular, tissue, and at the organism level.

A. MOLECULAR CHANGES

1. Interactions with nucleic acids, e.g., DNA, RNA, leading to irreversible conformational changes, and causing mutations or carcinogenesis.

$$\text{DNA} \xrightarrow{\text{transcription}} \text{mRNA} \xrightarrow{\text{translation}} \text{protein} \xrightarrow{\text{post-translation}} \text{e.g., P, Ca}^{2+}$$

2. Interactions with proteins, leading to denaturation, precipitation, allosteric effects (change in reactivity), or enzyme inhibition.

B. SUBCELLULAR CHANGES

1. Action on the permeability of cell membranes and disturbances of energy metabolism (ATPase), e.g., free radicals.
2. Decrease of the stability of lysosomal membranes resulting in the release of hydrolyses and leading to the disruption of the cell.

C. CELLULAR CHANGES

Action at the cellular level causes deranged reproduction, differentiation, and maturation resulting in teratogenesis.

D. ALLERGIC OR SENSITIZATION REACTIONS

Allergic reactions result from previous sensitization to a chemical. To produce an allergic reaction:

1. A chemical functions as a hapten:

$$\text{Hapten} + \text{protein} \rightarrow \text{antigen (or immunogen)}$$

2. Immune cells produce antibodies against the antigen:

$$\text{Antigen} + \text{lymphocyte} \rightarrow \text{antibody}$$

3. Subsequent exposure to the chemical yields an antigen, resulting in antigen–antibody interaction. This produces typical manifestions of allergy, e.g., dermatitis, itching, watery eyes, or bronchiolar constriction.

E. IDIOSYNCRASY

Genetically determined abnormal reactivity to drugs is known as idiosyncrasy. It is manifested as abnormal susceptibility to some drugs, proteins, or other agents that is characteristic of some individuals. Examples include reactions to isoniazid and succinylcholine.

1. Isoniazid

Isoniazid is used in chemotherapy for tuberculosis.

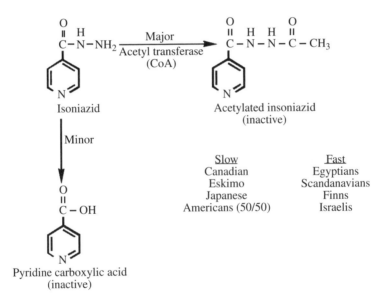

Both fast and slow acetylators have the same enzyme. Slow acetylators have less of the enzyme: less synthesis and/or more degradation of the enzyme.

2. Succinylcholine

$$\begin{array}{cccc} & \underset{|}{CH_3} & \underset{\|}{O} & \underset{\|}{O} & \underset{|}{CH_3} \\ CH_3 - \underset{|}{N^+} - CH_2 \cdot CH_2 \cdot O - C - CH_2 \cdot CH_2 \cdot C - O - CH_2 \cdot CH_2 \cdot \underset{|}{N^+} - CH_3 \\ & CH_3 & & & CH_3 \end{array}$$

a. Used in anesthesia as a neuromuscular blocking agent–depolarizing type
b. Used to produce muscle relaxation during surgery
c. Used because it has short duration due to its hydrolysis by plasma pseudocholine esterase or butyrylcholinesterase (BuChE)

d. Some individuals have "atypical" BuChE, which hydrolyzes succinylcholine at a slow rate resulting in a prolonged muscular relaxation and apnea (asphyxia) for several hours.

e. The "atypical" enzyme has 100-fold less affinity to succinylcholine.

SECTION 7. TOXICOKINETICS

Toxicokinetics is defined as the study of toxicant movement. It is concerned with the rates of all metabolic processes including absorption, distribution, biotransformation, binding, and elimination. Toxicokinetic studies are carried out by measuring the concentration of xenobiotics in various tissues and body fluids over time.

Toxicokinetic studies consider the body as a system of compartments. A compartment is defined by the organs, tissues, cells, and fluids that share similar rates of uptake and clearance of a xenobiotic. Chemicals equilibrate rapidly in the central compartment, which may include blood and tissue with profuse blood supply, e.g., liver, kidney, lung, and heart. On the other hand, slow-equilibrating compartments, known as peripheral compartments, may include tissues with poor blood supply, e.g., muscle, adipose tissues, and bones.

A. KINETIC ORDER OF ELIMINATION REACTION

The elimination of xenobiotics may follow a zero- or a first-order reaction.

1. Zero-order Process

Zero-order reactions are characterized by:

a. The processes of elimination are saturated.
b. Rate of elimination remains constant and is independent of concentration or amount of xenobiotics.
c. The drug is being cleared as fast as possible.
d. The biologic system is rate limiting.
e. The half-life ($t_{1/2}$) increases with dose.
f. A plot of drug concentration vs. time is linear.
g. Example: Ethanol. The body can metabolize 10 ml/h of ethanol, which is one beer or one mixed drink per hour. Thus, if a person drinks a six pack of beer (60 ml ethanol) in 1 h, the kinetics shown in Table 19.18 would occur.

TABLE 19.18
Ethanol Elimination from the Body

Ethanol	Time after Ethanol Consumption (h)						
	0	1	2	3	4	5	6
Ethanol eliminated (ml)	0	10	10	10	10	10	10
Ethanol remaining (ml)	60	50	40	30	20	10	0
Ethanol eliminated	0/60	10/60	10/50	10/40	10/30	10/20	10/10
(% of remaining)	0	17	20	25	33	50	100

2. First-Order Process

First-Order reactions are characterized by:

a. Rate of elimination of a chemical (dX/dt) from the body is directly proportional to the concentration (c) or amount (X) of chemical present at that time (t) shown in Equation 19.1:

$$\frac{dX}{dt} \propto X \text{ or } \frac{dX}{dt} = -aX \tag{19.1}$$

where a is a constant; the negative sign indicates that the xenobiotic is being lost from the body. Integration of Equation 19.1 and evaluation of the constant of integration at $t = 0$ where $X = X_0$ (the administered dose) yields equation 19.2.

$$X = X_0 e^{-at} \tag{19.2}$$

Equation 19.2 describes the content of the chemical (X) at time (t). Taking the natural logarithm of Equation 19.2 yields straight-line Equation 19.3.

$$\ln X = \ln X_0 e^{-at} \tag{19.3}$$

or

$$\log X = \log X_0 - \frac{kt}{2.303} \tag{19.4}$$

A plot of log X against time (t) gives a straight line with slope ($-a$) and ordinate intercept of log X_0. The slope (a) can be determined from the line that equals $k/2.303$, where k is the apparent first-order elimination rate constant for body content of the xenobiotic. It is easier, however, to determine (a) from the relationship:

$$k = \frac{0.693}{t_{1/2}} \tag{19.5}$$

then

$$slope = \frac{k}{2.303} = \frac{\log C_2 - \log C_1}{t_2 - t_1} \tag{19.6}$$

where C_1 and C_2 are plasma concentration at time t_1 and t_2, respectively; where $t_{1/2}$ is the biologic or elimination half-life of xenobiotic in the body and k is the fraction of dose eliminated per unit time.

b. In the first-order process, the chemical is rate limiting.
c. $T_{1/2}$ is independent of dose.
d. Most xenobiotics are handled by the body by first-order processes.
e. At high chemical concentrations, the biologic systems may become saturated and change from first-order to zero-order kinetics.
f. The elimination rate constant k is defined as the amount or concentration changes by some fraction per unit time. Thus, a k of 0.2/h for a xenobiotic means that 20% of the chemical is eliminated per hour. An example of a xenobiotic behaving according to first-order reaction is shown in Table 19.19.

TABLE 19.19
First-Order Process of a Xenobiotic

Xenobiotic	Time after Uptake, h								
	0	**1**	**2**	**3**	**4**	**5**	**6**	**7**	**8**
Chemical eliminated (mg)	0	20	16	12.8	10	8.2	6.6	5.2	4.2
Chemical remaining (mg)	100	80	64	51	41	33.0	26	21	16.8
Chemical eliminated (% of remaining)		20/100 20	16/80 20	12.8/63.8 20	10/51 20	8.1/41.2 20	6.6/32.6 20	5.2/26.2 20	4.3/21.0 20

3. Determination of the Kinetic Order

To determine whether the elimination process follows a zero- or first-order kinetic, the fraction of the chemical left in the body (fraction of dose) or plasma concentration is graphed at varying times of administration on rectilinear or semilog paper (Figure 19.3). Zero-order kinetic results in straight line on rectilinear paper and first-order are linear in semilog.

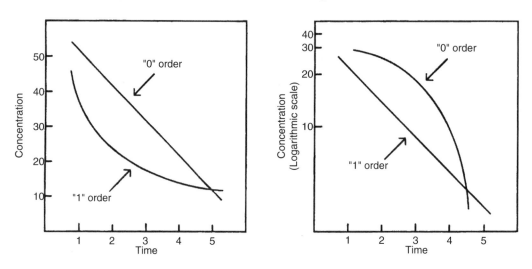

FIGURE 19.3 Determination of the kinetic order: "0" and "1" order.

B. Body Compartments

If a xenobiotic is present in the body in several tissues or organs, and if it passes from one location to another at different rates, then each location is considered a separate compartment for the xenobiotic.

1. One-Compartment Open-Model System

In this model, the body is considered as a single compartment in which the xenobiotic equilibrates instantaneously. In this instance, all body tissues and fluids are in rapid equilibrations within the blood, and the concentration of the xenobiotic is constant throughout.

Whereas the log fraction of xenobiotic in the body or its log concentration in the blood is plotted against time, a straight line is obtained indicating that its elimination process follows first-order kinetics (Figure 19.4). The reason xenobiotics are monoexponential or monophasic is that they equilibrate into tissues very quickly without siginificant storage or binding. In this model, the xenobiotic is eliminated from the body by apparent first-order kinetics, where the rate of elimination is proportional to its concentration in plasma at that time as described in Equation 19.7.

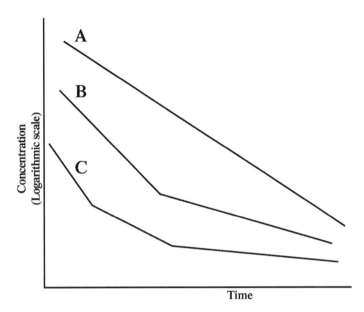

A. One-compartment open-model system

   $C_p = Be^{-\beta t}$

B. Two-compartment open-model system

   $C_p = Ae^{-\alpha t} + Be^{-\beta t}$

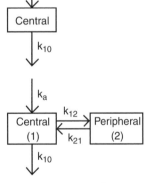

C. Three-compartment open-model system

   $C_p = Pe^{-\pi t} + Ae^{-\alpha t} + Be^{-\beta t}$

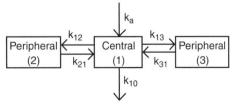

FIGURE 19.4 Xenobiotic plasma concentration (logarithmic scale) vs. time. (A) monoxponential, one-compartment; (B) biexponential, two-compartment; and (C) triexponential, three-compartment open-model system.

$$\frac{dC}{dt} = -kC \tag{19.7}$$

where c is the concentration of the chemical in the plasma at time t; k is the apparent first-order elimination rate constant for the xenobiotic; and the negative sign indicates that the chemical is being lost from the plasma. Integration of Equation 19.7 describes that the course of the xenobiotic concentration in plasma as shown in Equation 19.8.

$$C = C_0 e^{-kt} \tag{19.8}$$

or

$$\ln C = kt + \ln C_0 \tag{19.9}$$

or

$$\log C = -kt/2.303 + \log C_0 \tag{19.10}$$

where C_0 is the xenobiotic concentration in the plasma at time zero. A plot of $\log C$ vs. time yields a straight line with slope $= -k$ and intercept $= C_0$.

    a. Toxicokinetic parameters
        i. The *elimination half-life*, $t_{1/2}$, is the time required to decrease plasma concentration of a chemical to half of its original value, assuming that the chemical is eliminated by a first-order process. Its unit is time.

$$t_{1/2} = \frac{\ln 2}{k} = \frac{0.693}{k} = \frac{0.693 X V_d}{Cl} \tag{19.11}$$

          where (V_d) is the apparent volume of distribution and Cl is total clearance. Elimination half-life $(t_{1/2})$ is useful in determining the length of the period before multiple dosing would reach steady state. Table 19.20 demonstrates that it takes 4 to 5 half-life values to reach the steady state.

TABLE 19.20
Xenobiotic Steady State and Half-Life

Number of Half-Life	Xenobiotic Steady State (%)	Xenobiotic Left in Body (%)
1	50.00	50.00
2	75.00	25.00
3	87.50	12.50
4	93.75	6.25
5	96.87	3.13

        ii. The *apparent volume of distribution* (V_d) represents the relationship of concentration of chemical in plasma and amount in body. It is defined as the apparent volume to which the xenobiotic is distributed in the body.

$$V_d = \frac{\text{Amount of chemical in body}}{\text{Plasma concentration}} \tag{19.12}$$

To obtain V_d, plasma concentration at time zero intercept (C_0) is divided into applied dose (D_0) as described in Equation 19.13.

$$V_d = \frac{\text{Dose}}{C_0} \qquad (19.13)$$

V_d has a volume unit of milliliters or liters or adjusted for body weight, e.g., l/kg. The value of V_d gives some information about the xenobiotic in the body rather than representing a real body space. V_d increases as the distribution into the body increases. If a xenobiotic is not well distributed in the tissues, then its distribution is limited to plasma, extracellular fluid, or total body water, resulting in V_d values of 40, 170, and 580 ml/kg, respectively. On the other hand, if the chemical is thoroughly distributed or has a high affinity for a tissue such as fat or muscle, V_d may be more than 100 ml/kg. V_d also produces an indication of the fraction of the chemical that is available for elimination. A large V_d is an indication that the chemical is distributed extensively in the tissues, and therefore less of it will be available for excretion. A small V_d indicates less tissue distribution, and more of the chemical will be available for excretion. V_d may be calculated using equation 19.14:

$$V_d = \frac{D_{iv}}{\text{AUC} \cdot k} \qquad (19.14)$$

where D is the dose following an intravenous injection, AUC is the total area under plasma concentration vs. time course after a single dose. K is the elimination rate constant, which can be obtained from the equation: slope $= -k/2.303$. AUC can be obtained by (a) planimeter (rectilinear paper); (b) cut and weight (rectilinear paper); (c) trapezoidal rule.

$$A = {}_{1/2}(C_1 + C_2) \times (T_2 - T_1) \text{ etc.} + \frac{C*}{k} \qquad (19.15)$$

where $C*$ is the last plasma concentration time point. C_1 and C_2 are the plasma concentrations at t_1 and t_2, respectively.

iii. *Clearance (Cl)* is defined as the volume of the central compartment that is cleared of drug in unit time. Therefore, clearance measures the efficiency with which a chemical is eliminated from the body by all routes. Clearance may be determined by Equation 19.16.

$$Cl = V_d k = \frac{0.693}{t_{1/2}} V_d \qquad (19.16)$$

Clearance is usually calculated according to Equation 19.17.

$$Cl = \frac{\text{Dose}}{\text{AUC}} \qquad (19.17)$$

Total clearance includes clearance of all organs, e.g., liver (hepatic) clearance, (Cl_H) and kidney (renal) clearance (Cl_R). Clearance by any organ is determined by the blood flow through the organ, Q, and the extraction ratio, E, according to Equation 19.18.

$$Cl = QE \qquad (19.18)$$

E is determined by the in-flowing, C_{in}, and out-flowing, C_{out}, concentration of the xenobiotic (Equation 19.19).

$$E = \frac{C_{in} - C_{out}}{C_{in}} \qquad (19.19)$$

Renal clearance (Cl) may also be determined according to the following equation:

$$Cl = \frac{\text{urine flow} \times \text{concentration in urine}}{\text{plasma concentration}} = \text{ml} / \text{min} \qquad (19.20)$$

The maximum values for an organ clearance is that of its blood flow rate; thus, hepatic and renal clearance cannot exceed their blood flow rates of 1500 and 650 ml/min, respectively, in humans. High hepatic clearance results in "first-pass" effect, i.e., high biotransformation elimination of the chemical after oral administration, e.g., chlorpyrifos. Clearance unit is volume per time, e.g., ml/min or l/h, or expressed for body weight, e.g., l/h/kg. To determine clearance, urine should be collected over at least five elimination half-lives to maximize recovery of dose. Total (Cl) hepatic (Cl_H) and renal (Cl_R) clearance values are good indicators for the elimination processes of the xenobiotic and, consequently, its toxicity. High total and hepatic clearance values are consistent with high extraction values by the liver. This suggests that patients with liver diseases would have less total and hepatic clearances, resulting in high systematic availability and more toxicity. High renal clearance, e.g., 100 ml/min suggests that the xenobiotic will accumulate in patients with renal failure because less of the chemical will be eliminated via the kidney.

iv. *Bioavailability, F*, is the fraction of the dose that is absorbed into the systemic circulation. It is calculated as the ratio of AUCs obtained after dosing other than intravenous (IV) as compared to IV dosing according to Equation (19.21)

$$F = \frac{AUC_n \times Dose_{iv}}{AUC_{iv} \times Dose_n} \qquad (19.21)$$

n indicates dosing by a route other than IV dosing.

v. *Relative Residence (R_R)* of a xenobiotic in specific tissues is calculated according to Equation 19.22.

$$R_R = \frac{AUC_{organ}}{AUC_{plasma}} \qquad (19.22)$$

Thus, the R_R values reflect the relative accumulation of a xenobiotic in specific organ or the relative exposure of individual organs to the xenobiotic. The use of this parameter avoids the time-dependent changes in concentration ratios. R_R is a time-independent parameter and, assuming linear kinetics, it predicts the ratio of

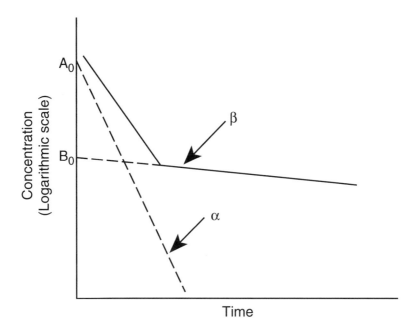

FIGURE 19.5 Biexponential decline of a xenobiotic concentration in plasma with time.

average concentrations of the xenobiotic in specific organs, $\overline{C}_{\text{organ}}$ to those in plasma $\overline{C}_{\text{plasma}}$, or

$$R_R = \frac{\overline{C}_{\text{organ}}}{\overline{C}_{\text{plasma}}} \tag{19.23}$$

2. Two-Compartment Open-Model System

After the introduction of xenobiotics into the central compartment, they undergo distribution in its highly perfused tissues. The concentration of some xenobiotic in these tissues, however, declines more rapidly during the distribution phase than during the postdistribution phase. The chemical eventually distributes to less perfused tissues, e.g., muscle, skin, and fat, known as peripheral compartments. The chemical concentrations in the peripheral compartments will reach a maximum and then begin to decline during the elimination phase. As a result, the plasma concentration of the xenobiotic rapidly declines biphasically and, in some cases, polyphasically. The early phase is associated with the distribution of the chemical into tissues, and the last phase is associated with the elimination of the chemical after the distribution phases have been completed. An equilibrium is attained, with time, between the concentration of the chemical in the central and peripheral compartments. Chemicals pass into and out of each compartment by a first-order process, and are eliminated only from the central compartment by a first-order process.

In the two-compartment open-model system (Figure 19.5), k_{12} is the rate constant for the movement of the xenobiotic from the central compartment (1) to the peripheral compartment (2), k_{21}, is the rate constant for the passage of the xenobiotic from the peripheral compartment back to the central compartment, and k_{10} is the rate constant of elimination from the central compartments. The time course of the xenobiotic concentration in the two-compartment open-model system is described by the following equation:

$$C_t = A_0 e^{-\alpha_t} + B_0 e^{-\beta_t} \tag{19.24}$$

C_t is plasma concentration of the chemical at time t. The rate constant for the first phase of the biphasic decline of the plasma chemical concentration is α (Figure 19.5). It is calculated by the method of residuals as follows: the straight line of the β-phase is extrapolated back to time zero. The extrapolated values are subtracted from the experimental values of the xenobiotic concentration and the resultant values are plotted on semilogarithmic paper. These rate constants are calculated as follows:

$$k_{21} = \frac{A\beta + B\alpha}{A + B} \tag{19.25}$$

$$k_{10} = \frac{\alpha B}{k_{21}} \tag{19.26}$$

$$k_{12} = (\alpha + \beta) - (k_{21} + k_{10}) \tag{19.27}$$

Then α is estimated from the slope of the secondary plot according to Equation 19.28.

$$\alpha = 2.303 \times \text{slope} \tag{19.28}$$

or from the half-time according to this relationship:

$$\alpha = 0.693/t_{1/2} \tag{19.29}$$

The rate constant for the second phase of the biexponential decline in the xenobiotic concentration is β. A_0 is the intercept of the straight line obtained after extrapolating the secondary plot back to time zero. B_0 is the intercept obtained by extrapolating the straight line associated with β back to time zero. α-Phase is the rapid phase of the biphasic decline of the xenobiotic concentration. It is described by Equation 19.30.

$$A = A_0 e^{-\alpha t} \tag{19.30}$$

β-phase is the slow phase of the biphasic decline of the chemical concentration. It is described by Equation 19.31.

$$B = B_0 e^{-\beta t} \tag{19.31}$$

$$\beta = \frac{0.693}{t_{1/2}} \tag{19.32}$$

Cl, total body clearance, $= \beta V_d$

$$Cl = \frac{DF}{\text{AUC}_{\text{plasma}}} \tag{19.33}$$

$$V_d = \frac{DF}{\beta(\text{AUC})_{\text{plasma}}} = \frac{Cl}{\beta} \tag{19.34}$$

where F is bioavailability.

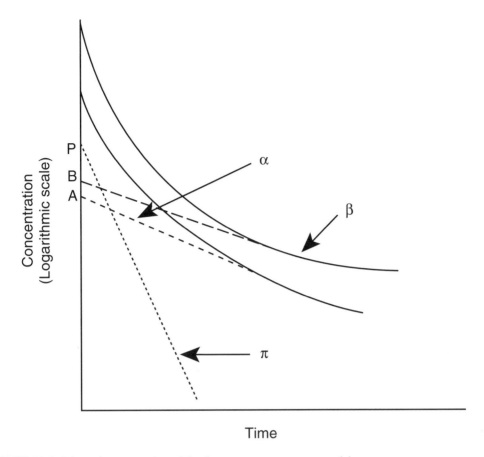

FIGURE 19.6 Schematic presentation of the three-compartment open-model system.

3. Three-Compartment Open-Model System

In this system, it is assumed that all processes are linear and that elimination occurs from the central compartment. The xenobiotic is introduced into the central compartment which is connected to two peripheral "shallow" and "deep" compartments. The central compartment is formed of the plasma and highly perfused nonfat tissues, such as blood cell, heart, lung, liver, kidney, and glands. The "shallow" peripheral compartment consists of poorly perfused tissues such as muscle, skin, and may include fatty tissues such as adipose tissues and bone marrow. The "deep" peripheral compartment contains tissues with negligible perfusion such as bone, teeth, cartilage, and hair. Figure 19.6 shows schematic representations of the body as a three-compartment open model with xenobiotic eliminations from the central component. The constants k_{12} and k_{21}, and k_{31} and k_{13} are the apparent first-order rate constants for intercompartmental transfer of the chemical between the shallow and central compartments, and deep and central compartments, respectively. The elimination rate constant from the central compartment is k_{10}. Figure 19.6 represents a three-compartment system for plasma concentration curve following rapid intravenous administration of a xenobiotic. The xenobiotic introduced into the central compartment is first rapidly distributed and equilibrated to well-perfused tissues, then slowly to tissues constituting the "shallow" compartment, and finally more slowly to the "deep" compartment. All processes are assessed to follow first-order kinetics. The plasma concentration curve appears triphasic and is described by Equation (19.35).

$$C_p = Pe^{-\pi t} + Ae^{-\alpha t} + B^{-Bt} \tag{19.35}$$

where C_p is the xenobiotic concentration in the central compartment at time t, and P, π, A, α, B, and β are constants. The values of the three hybrid rate constants, π, α, and β, reflect a rapid initial distribution of the chemical and a slower apparent elimination rate of the chemical from the body.

SECTION 8. TRANSPORTERS

Active transport of drugs, toxicants, and their metabolites plays an important role in therapeutic and toxic actions. Several transporters have been identified in the liver, kidney, intestine, and lung that transport various substances including sugars, amino acids, and peptides as well as drugs and pesticides.

A. *P*-GLYCOPROTEIN

P-glycoprotein (P-gp), an adenosine triphosphate (ATP)-dependent chemical transporter, is involved in the development of multidrug resistance in cancer chemotherapy and pesticide resistance. The presence of this protein, a member of the large ATP-binding cassette (ABC) transporter family, decreases intracellular accumulation of cytotoxic drugs, thereby increasing tumor cells despite the presence of otherwise toxic cellular drug levels. P-gp acts as a barrier to absorption of xenobiotics and assists in their removal. Thus, P-gp may diminish their absorption from the intestine and reduce oral bioavailability.

1. MDR Gene Family

P-gps belong to a gene family known as the multidrug resistance (MDR) genes. Human and other primates possess two members of the gene family, MDR1 and MDR2 (sometimes known as MDR3). On the other hand, mice, hamsters, and rats possess three members, i.e., mdr1a, mdr1b, and mdr2. These genes encode the drugs or phospholipid transporters listed in Table 19.21.

TABLE 19.21
P-gp Genes

Species	Drug Transporters		Phospholipid Translocators
Human	MDR1		MDR2, MDR3
Mouse	mdr3/mdr1a	mdr1/mdr1b	mdr2
Hamster	pgp1	pgp2	mdr3
Rat	mdr1a	mdr1b	mdr2

2. Structure and Function of *p*-Glycoprotein

MDR1 gene is 100 kb on chromosome 7, with 28 exons that are spliced into 4.5-kb mRNA. P-gp consists of 1280 amino acids within the amino and carboxy halves of the protein; each has six transmembrane domains and an ATP-binding region. Table 19.22 lists compounds that interact with P-gp. Increased expression of P-gp is associated with an MDR phenomenon in which cells become cross-resistant to structurally related chemicals. This MDR phenotype is confered to drug-sensitive cells by transfecting DNA isolated from drug-resistant cells.

TABLE 19.22
Representative P-gp Substrates

Anticancer Agents	Other
Actinomycin D	Celiprolo
Colchicine	Cortisol
Daunorubicin	Digoxin
Docetaxel	Diltiazem
Doxorubicin	Erythromycin
Etoposide	Estrogen glucuronide
Mitomycine C	Gramicidin D
Mitoxantrone C	Indinavir
Paclitaxel	Ivermectin
Teniposide	Loperimide
Topotecan	Morphine
Vinblasine	Nifedipine
Vincristine	Neflinavir
VP-16	Progestrone
	Rifampicin
	Saquinavir
	Terfenidine

3. Tissue Distribution of P-gp

P-gp is present in the epithelial cells lining the luminal surface of tissues associated with excretory or barrier functions, such as hepatic bile canalicular membrane, renal proximal tubule, villus-tip enterocyte in the small intestine, and the endothelial cells making up the blood–brain and blood–testes barriers. The extent of mRNA p-gp in tissues is listed in Table 19.23.

TABLE 19.23
Relative mRNA Expression of P-gp

Relative mRNA Expression	Tissue
High	Kidney, adrenal glands, liver, lung
Intermediate	Jejunum, colon, bone membrane, rectum
Low	Brain, prostate, muscle, skin, spleen, bone marrow

4. Significance of P-Glycoprotein in Pharmacokinetics of Drugs

P-gp facilitates the intestinal absorption of drugs and their excretion into bile. Coadministration of the P-gp inhibitors PSC833 or CsA with paclitaxel results in a tenfold increase in AUC. These results suggest the combined contribution of CYP3A inhibition in the intestine and liver in decreasing the oral bioavailability of substrate drugs. P-gp also decreases the oral bioavailbility of the HIV protease inhibitors indinavir, nelfinavir, and saquinavir, suggesting more effective therapeautic action of these drugs would result from coadministration with P-gp inhibitors.

Recently, a significant amount of drug metabolism has been shown to take place in the intestine mediated by CYP3A. Since more than 50% of the clinically important drugs are metabolized by CYP3A, its presence in the intestine suggests an important role in oral drug bioavailability. A striking overlap between the substrates for P-gp and CYP3A has been established. Compounds used to modify or reverse MDR include calcium-channel blockers (Verpamil, nifedipine), immunosuppressives (CsA, FK506), and antiarrhythmic drugs (quinidine and amidodarone). Table 19.24 shows a partial list of MDR reversal agents.

These compounds reverse P-gp by various mechanisms. Some reversal agents such as CsA, a substrate itself, act as a competitive inhibitor. Mechanisms of other agents are still unknown. Competition may result from binding at the same site. In summary, P-gp, a xenobiotic transporter that presents in the kidney, liver, intestine, blood, brain, and other epithelial tissues, plays a significant role in interactions between substrate chemicals and their subsequent bioavailability.

TABLE 19.24
Partial List of MDR Reversal Agents

Amidodarone	Quinidine
Cremophor EL	Quercetin
Cyclosporin A	Rapamycin
FK506	Reserpine
trans-Flupenthixol	Staurosporine
Genistein	Tamoxifen
Ketoconazole	TPGS
Progesterone	Trifluoroperizine
Verapamil	

---

5. P-Glycoprotein as an Absorption Barrier

Tumor necrosis factor (TNF-α) is a cytokine with antitumor activity against several cellular models. TNF- α-induced apoptosis seems to be mediated by a signaling pathway termed the sphingomyelin–ceramide pathway, which consists of the hydrolysis of sphingomyelin and the production of its breakdown product ceramide. The KGla cells, which are inherently resistant to TNF-α and do not produce ceramide upon cytokine stimulation, can be sensitized by the use of the P-gp inhibitor PSC833. Coincubation with 1μm of this cyclosporin derivative restored the apoptotic potential of 10 ng/ml TNF-α. This effect was associated with the restoration of ceramide generation (315%) and activation of neutral, but not acid, sphingomyelinase activity (143%). Furthermore, it has been demonstrated that treatment of KGla cells with 1 μm PSC833 led to a threefold increase in inner plasma membrane sphingomyelin content and basal neutral sphingomyelinase activity. These results support the hypothesis whereby resistance to TNF-α-mediated apoptosis of certain leukemic cells is linked to the disposability of the sphingomyelin pool. These data also suggest a role for P-gp in sphingomyelin transverse plasma membrane asymmetry.

Among the compounds endowed with the capacity to reverse the P-gp-mediated MDR of cancer cells, a powerful agent was found to be the cyclosporin D derivative SDZ PSC833. The brain penetration of SDZ PSC833 and its effect on the blood–brain barrier (BBB) permeability of an anticancer agent, vincristine, were assessed. At lower doses of SDZ PSC833 the brain penetration, defined as the brain-to-blood partition coefficient (K_p), was very low in spite of the high lipophilicity of this compound. At higher doses, however, the brain penetration of SDZ PSC833 proved to be linear in the dose range studied. These results demonstrated a dose-dependent brain passage of SDZ PSC833. The brain passage of cyclosporin A was also found to be dose-dependent. On the other hand, ten times higher doses of cyclosporin A were required to obtain the same K_p values recorded for SDZ PSC833. Moreover, the coadministration of SDZ PSC833 increased the brain penetration of cyclosporin A, whereas the latter did not modify that of SDZ PSC833. The increased effect of SDZ PSC833 is consistent with the hypothesis of a saturation of the P-gp pump present at the BBB. The involvement of P-gp in the brain passage of SDZ PSC833 could be of great significance for clinical application of the drug in the treatment of brain cancers when it is given in combination with anticancer agents.

Because the significance of P-gp in the *in vivo* secretion of beta blockers in intestinal epithelial cells is unclear, the secretory mechanism for beta blockers and other drugs has been evaluated. Uptake of the beta blockers acebutolol, celiprolol, nadolol, and timolol and the antiarrhythmic agent quinidine by the MDR leukemic cell line variant K562/ADM was significantly lower than that by drug-sensitive K562 cells, suggesting that these beta blockers are transported by P-gp out of cells. The reduced uptake of acebutolol by the drug-resistant K562/ADM cells was reversed by treating the cells with anti-P-gp monoclonal antibody, MRK16, whereas no such alteration in uptake was observed for drug-sensitive K562 cells. Acebutolol uptake by K562/ADM cells was, moreover, markedly enhanced, in a concentration-dependent manner, in the presence of the specific P-gp inhibitors MS-209 and cyclosporin. Caco-2 cells were used for evaluation of the role of P-gp in intestinal permeability to drugs *in vitro*. Basolateral-to-apical transport of acebutolol was twice that of transport in the reverse direction. A similar polarized flux was also observed in the transport of vinblastine, but not in that of acetamide or mannitol. When *in vivo* intestinal absorption was evaluated by the rat jejunal loop method, with simultaneous intravenous administration of a P-gp inhibitor, cyclosporin, intestinal absorption of both acebutolol and vinblastine increased 2.6- and 2.2-fold, respectively, but no such enhancement was observed in the absorption of acetamide. The effect of cyclosporin on the intestinal absorption of several drugs was further examined, and the extent of the contribution of P-gp as an absorption barrier to those drugs was evaluated. ATP depletion by occlusion of the superior mesenteric artery resulted in a clear increase in epithelial permeability to vinblastine, but not to 3-*O*-methylglucose or acetamide, indicating that vinblastine is secreted by ATP-dependent P-gp into the lumen. These findings demonstrate that P-gp plays a role as an absorption barrier by transporting several drugs from intestinal cells into the lumen.

6. P-Glycoproteins in Nonmammalians

Bacteria possess transmembrane transporters that confer resistance to toxic compounds. The short generation time and the ease of mutant selection and DNA manipulation associated with microorganisms offer great advantages over mammalian cells. Therefore, studies on multidrug transporters in microorganisms could yield valuable information about the general molecular mechanism and physiological role of these transport systems and their implications in human diseases.

Toxic compounds have always been part of the natural environment of microorganisms. The development of strategies for life in this habitat has been crucial for survival of the cell. As a result, microorganisms have developed versatile mechanisms to resist antibiotics and other cytotoxic drugs. Examples are the enzymatic degradation or inactivation of drugs. Some of these drug transporters are fairly specific for a given drug or class of drugs, but the so-called multidrug transporters have specificity for compounds with very different chemical structures and cellular targets. Also, microbial multidrug transporters may play a specific role in the transport of a common endogenous substrate, such as lipid; this remains to be established.

a. Bacteria

Using a prokaryote such as *Escherichia coli* to study mammalian P-gp has two advantages. First, if overexpression can be achieved, the purification of large amounts of P-gp for biochemical reconstitution and structural studies is possible, and could be achieved more rapidly than if carried out in animal cells. Earlier studies suggested that the glycosylation is dispensable for P-gp function, so that unglycosylated P-gp expressed in bacteria should be functional. Second, if even low-level expression of functional P-gp can be achieved in intact cells, the short generation time, ease of drug selection, and ease of plasmid manipulation associated with *E. coli* offer tremendous advantages. An example of a successful high-level overexpression of higher eukaryotic membrane proteins in *E. coli* was the 55-kDa bovine 17-α-hydroxylase cytochrome P-450 from microsomes, containing a single predicted transmembrane helix, expressed up to 16 mg/l of *E.coli* culture.

b. Yeast

Heterologous expression of P-gp in the yeast *Saccaromyces cerevisiae,* a simple eukaryote, has many of the same advantages of *E. coli.* The potential for overexpression is perhaps greater in yeast than in *E. coli* because of the presence of eukaryotic membrane biogenesis and trafficking machinery much more like that of the homologous P-gp system. The biochemical and bioenergetic characteristics of P-gp expressed in yeast have been extensively explored by Gros and co-workers in the last 4 years. Recently, Ruetz et al. used the NDH promoter, expressed mouse P-gp (mdr3), in inside-out plasma membrane vesicles and demonstrated ATP-dependent, osmotically sensitive transport of vinblastine and colchicine, which was inhibitable by verapamil. The transport properties of a variant of mouse P-gp (mdr3) bearing the (ser 939-Phe) mutation were quantitatively and qualitatively similar to those in animal cells. Unfortunately, the basal or drug-stimulated ATPase activities of P-gp could not be detected in this system.

REFERENCES

Abou-Donia, M. B., Pharmacokinetics of a neurotoxic oral dose of leptophos in hens, *Arch. Toxicol.,* 36, 103, 1976.

Abou-Donia, M. B., Metabolism and pharmacokinetics of a single oral dose of *O*-4-bromo-2,5-dichlorophenyl-*O*-methylphenylphosphonothioate (leptophos) in hens, *Toxicol. Appl. Pharmacol.,* 55, 131, 1980.

Abou-Donia, M. B., Disposition, metabolism, and toxicokinetics, in *Neurotoxicology,* Abou-Donia, M. B., Ed., CRC Press, Boca Raton, FL, 1992, 256.

Abou-Donia, M. B. and Nomeir, A. A., The role of pharmacokinetics and metabolism in species sensitivity of neurotoxic agents, *Fundam. Appl. Toxicol.,* 6, 190, 1986.

Abou-Donia, M. B., Nomeir, A. A., Bower, J. H., and Makkaway, H. A., Absorption, distribution, excretion, and metabolism of a single oral dose of [14C]tri-*o*-cresyl phosphate (TOCP) in the male rat, *Toxicology,* 65, 61, 1990.

Abu-Qare, A. W. and Abou-Donia, M. B., Urinary excretion of metabolites following a single dermal dose of [14C]methyl parathion in rats, *Toxicology,* 150, 119, 2000a.

Abu-Qare, A. W. and Abou-Donia, M. B., Simultaneous determination of pyridostigmine bromide, DEET (*N*, *N*-diethyl-*m*-toluamide), permethrin and metabolites in rat plasma and urine using high-performance liquid chromatography, *J. Chromatogr. B*, 749, 171, 2000b.

Abu-Qare, A. W., Abdel-Rahamn, A. A., Kishik, A., and Abou-Donia, M. B., Placental transfer and pharmacokinetics of a single dermal dose of [14C]methyl parathion in rats, *Toxicol. Sci.,* 53, 5, 2000a.

Abu-Qare, A. W., Brownie, C., and Abou-Donia, M. B. Placental transfer and pharmacokinetics of a single oral dose of [14C]*p*-nitrophenol in rats, *Arch. Toxicol,* 74, 188, 2000b.

Aldridge, W. N., Serum esterases. 1. Two types of esterases (A and B) hydrolysing *p*-nitrophenyl acetate, propionate and butyrate, and a method for their determination, *Biochem. J.,* 53, 110, 1953.

Ariyoshi, N., Oguri, K., Yoshimura, H., and Funae, Y., Metabolism of the highly persistent PCG congener, 2,4,5,2′,4′,5′-hexachlorobiphenyl, by human CYP2B6, *Biochem. Biophys. Res. Commun.* 212, 455–460, 1995.

Augustinsson, K. B., Multiple forms of esterases in vertebrate blood plasma, *Ann. N.Y. Acad. Sci.,* 94, 844, 1961.

Baker, K. J. and Bradley, S. E., Binding of sulfobromophthalein (BSP) sodium by plasma albumin. Its role in hepatic BSP extraction, *J. Clin. Invest.,* 45, 281, 1966.

Bakry, N. M., Salama, A. K., Aly, H. A., and Abou-Donia, M. B., Milk transfer, distribution, and metabolism of a single oral dose of [14CH3S] methamidophos in Sprague-Dawley rats, *Toxicologist,* 10, 346, 1990.

Baldwin, S. J. Bloomer, J. C., Smith, G. J., Ayrton, A. D., Clarke, S. E., and Chenery, R. J., Ketaconazole and sulphophenazole as the respective selective inhibitors of P4503a and 2C9, *Xenobiotica,* 25, 261–270, 1995.

Bergmann, E., Segal, R., and Rimon, S., A new type of esterase in hog-kidney extract, *Biochem. J.*, 67, 481, 1957.

Bloomer, J. C., Clarke, S. E., and Chenery, R. J., Determination of P4501A2 activity in human liver microsomes using [3-C-14-methyl] caffeine, *Xenobiotica* 25, 917–927, 1995.

Boyland, E., in *Concepts in Biochemical Pharamcology,* 2nd ed., Brondie, B. B. and Gillette, J. R., Eds., Springer-Verlag, Berlin, 1971, 584.

Brodie, B. B., in *Absorption and Distribution of Drugs,* Binns, T. E., Ed., Williams & Wilkins, Baltimore, 1964, 16.

Brodie, B. B. and Axelrod, J., The estimation of acetanilide and its metabolic products, aniline, *N*-acetyl-*p*-aminophenol and *p*-aminophenol (free and total conjugates) in biological fluids and tissues, *J. Pharmacol. Exp. Ther.,* 94, 22, 1948.

Carrington, C. D. and Abou-Donia, M. B., Variation between three strains of rats: inhibition of neurotoxic esterase and acetylcholinesterase by tri-*o*-cresyl phosphate, *J. Toxicol. Environ. Health*, 25, 259, 1988.

Chabra, R. S., Pohl, R. J., and Fouts, J. R., A comparative study of xenobiotic-metabolizing enzymes in liver and intestine of various species, *Drug Metab. Dispos.*, 2, 443, 1974.

Conney, A. H., Pharamcological implication of microsomal enzyme induction, *Pharmacol. Rev.*, 19, 317, 1967.

Crespi, C. L., Penman, B. W., Steimel, D. T., Smith, T., Yang, C. S., and Sutter, T. R. Development of a human lymphoblastoid cell line constitutively expressing human CYP1B1 cDNA: substrate specificity with model substitutes and promutagens, *Mutagenesis* 12, 83, 1997.

Dehal, S. S. and Kupfer, D., Metabolism of the proestrogenic pesticide methoxychlor by hepatic P450 monooxygenases in rats and humans. Dual pathways involving novel ortho ring-hydroxylation by CYP2B, *Drug Metab. Dispos*, 22, 937, 1994.

Delaporte, E., Cribb, A. E., and Renton, K, W., Interferon-mediated changes in the expression of CYP1A1 in human B lymphoblastoid (AHH-1 TK +/−) cells, *Can. J. Physiol. Pharmacol.*,73, 1692, 1995.

Dutton, G. J., in: *Concepts in Biochemical Pharmacology*, 2nd ed., Brodie, B. B. and Gillette, J. R., Eds., Springer-Verlag, Berlin, 1971, 378.

Elmasry, E. and Abou-Donia, M., Reversal of P-glycoprotein in an outer membrane permeability mutant of *Escherichia coli* by ascorbic acid, 2000, in press.

Elmasry, E. and Abou-Donia, M., Reversal of P-glycoprotein mediated multidrug resistance in *Escherichia coli* by chlorpromazine, *Bull. Fac. Sci. Zagazig Univ.*, 21(2), 18, 1999.

Feldman, R. J. and Maibach, H. I., Absorption of some organic compounds through the skin of man, *J. Invest. Dermatol.*, 54, 399, 1970.

Fitzsimmons, M. E. and Collins, J. M., Selective biotransformation of the human immuno-defeciency virus protease inhibitor saquinavir by human small-intestinal cytochrome P4503A4. Potential contribution to first pass metabolism, *Drug Metab. Dispos.*, 25, 256, 1997.

Fouts, J. R. and Brodie, B. B., The enzymatic reduction of chloramphenicol, *p*-nitrobenzoic acid, and other aromatic nitro compounds in mammals, *J. Pharamcol. Exp. Ther.*, 119, 197, 1957.

Gibson, J. E. and Becker, B. A., Demonstration of enhanced lethality of drugs in hypoexcretory animals, *J. Pharmacol. Sci.*, 56, 1503, 1976.

Gibson, G. G. and Skett, P., in *Introduction to Drug Metabolism*, 2nd ed., Gibson, G. G. and Skett, P., Eds., Blackie Academic and Professional, New York, 1994, 1.

Gillette, J. R., in *Pharmacology and Pharamcokinetics*, Toerell, T., Dedrick, R. L. and Condliffe, P. G., Eds., Plenum Press, New York, 1974, 209.

Gros, P., Neriah, Y., Croop, J., and Housman, D., Isolation and expression of a complementary DNA that confers multidrug resistance, *Nature* (London), 322, 728, 1986.

Guengerich, F. P., Human cytochrome P450 enzymes, *Life Sci.,* 50, 1471, 1992.

Johnson, M. K., Improved assay for neurotoxic esterase of screening organophosphates for delayed neurotoxicity potential, *Arch. Toxicol.*, 37, 113, 1977.

Kaminsky, L. S., Fasco, M. J., and Guengerich, F. P., Production and application of antibodies to rat liver cytochrome P450, *Methods Enzymol.*, 74, 262, 1981.

La Du, B. N., Mandel, G. H., and Way, E. L. in *Fundamental of Drug Metabolism and Drug Disposition*, Williams & Wilkins, Baltimore, 1972.

Lanning, C. L., Fine, R. L., Sachs, C. W., Rao, U. S., Corcoran, J. J., and Abou-Donia, M. B., Chlorpyrifos oxon interacts with the mammalian multidrug resistance protein, P-glycoprotein. *J. Toxicol. Environ. Health*, 47, 395, 1996.

Lemaire, M., Bruelisauer, A., Guntz, P., and Sato, H., Dose-dependent brain penetration of SDZ PSC 833, a novel multidrug resistance-reversing cyclosporin, in rats, *Cancer Chemothe. & Pharmacol.*, 38 (5), 481–486, 1996.

Levi, P. E. and Hodgson, E., in *Insecticide Action from Molecule to Organ*, Narahashi, T. and Chambers, J. E., Eds., Plenum Press, New York, 1989, 233.

Maibach, H. I., Feldman, R. J., Milby, T. H., and Serat, W. F., Regional variation in percutaneous penetration in man, *Arch. Environ. Health*, 23, 208, 1971.

Mason, H. S., Mechanism of oxygen metabolism, *Adv. Enzymol.*, 19, 79, 1957.

Milne, M. D., Schribner, B. N., and Craford, M. A., Non-toxic diffusion and excretion of weak acids and bases, *Am. S. Med.*, 24, 709, 1958.

Nakajima, M., Yamamoto, T., Nunoya, K. I., Yokoi, T., Nagashima, K., Inoue, K., Funae, Y., Shimada, N., Kamataki, T., and Kuroiwa, Y., Characterization of CYP2A6 involved in 3′-hydroxylation of cotinine in human liver microsomes, *J. Pharmacol. Exp. Ther.*, 277, 1010, 1996.

Nakamura, A., Hirota, T., Morino, A., Shimada, T., and Uematsu, T., Oxidation of risogladine by the CYP2C subfamily in the rat, dog, monkey, and man, *Xenobiotica,* 27, 995, 1997.

Nebert, D. W. and Gonzalez, F. J., P450 genes. Structure, evolution, and regulation, *Annu. Rev. Biochem.*, 56, 945, 1987.

Nelson, D. R., Kamataki, T., Waxman, D. J., Guengerich, F. P., Estabrook, R. W., Feyerisen, R., Gonzalez, F. J., Coon, M. J., Gunsalus, I. C., Gotoh, O., Okuda, K., and Nebert, D. W., The P450 superfamily: update on new suquences, gene mapping, accession numbers, early trivial names of enzymes., and nomenclature, *DNA Cell Biology.*, 122, 1, 1993.

Nomeir, A. A. and Abou-Donia, M. B., Disposition of tri-*o*-cresyl phosphate (TOCP) and its metabolites in various tissues of the male cat following a single dermal application of [14C]TOCP, *Drug Metab. Dispos.*, 12, 705, 1984.

Omura, T. and Sato, R., The carbon monoxide-binding pigment of liver microsomes, *J. Biol. Chem.*, 239, 2370, 1964.

Othman, M. A. and Abou-Donia, M. B., Pharmacokinetic profile of (±)-gossypol in male Sprague-Dawley rats following single intravenous and oral administration, *Proc. Soc. Exp. Biol. Med.*, 188, 17, 1988.

Rodrigues, A. D., and Roberts, E. M., The *in vitro* interaction dexmedetomidine with human liver microsomal cytochrome P4502D6 (CYP2D6). *Drug. Metab. Dispos.* 25, 651, 1997.

Roy, A. B., in *Concepts in Biochemical Pharmacology*, Vol 1., Brodie, B. B. and Gillette, J. R., Eds, Springer-Verlag, Berlin, 1971, 9.

Ruetz, S., Raymon, M., and Gros, P., Functional expression of P-glycoprotein encoded by the mouse and mdr3 gene in yeast cells, *Proc. Natl. Acad. Sci. USA,* 90, 11588, 1993.

Schanker, L. S., in *Concepts in Biochemical Pharmacology*, Vol 1., Brodie, B. B. and Gillette, J. R., Eds., Springer-Verlag, Berlin, 1971, 9.

Sipes, I. G. and Gandolfi, A. J., in *Casarett and Doul's Toxicology. The Basic Science of Poisons*, 3rd ed., Doul, J., Klassen, C. D., and Andur, M. O., Eds., Macmillian, New York, 1992, 88.

Smith, R. and John, L., in *The Excretory Function of Bile: The Elimination of Drugs and Toxic Substances in Bile*, John Wiley & Sons, New York, 1873, 3.

Sonnichsen, D. S., Liu, Q., Schuetz, E. G., Schuetz, J. D., Pappo, A., and Relling, M. V., Variability in human cytochrome P450 paclitaxel metabolism, *J. Pharmacol. Exp. Ther.*, 275, 566, 1995.

Suwita, E., Nomeir, A. A., and Abou-Donia, M. B., Disposition, pharmacokinetics, and metabolism of a dermal dose of [14C]2,5-hexanedione in hens, *Drug Metab. Dispos.*, 15, 779, 1987.

Terao, T., Hisanaga, E., Sai, Y., Tamai, I., and Tsuji, A., Active secretion of drugs from the small intestinal epithelium in rats by P-glycoprotein functioning as an absorption barrier, *J. Pharma. Pharmacol.*, 48 (10):, 1083–1089. 1996.

Waxman, D. J., Ko, A., and Walsh, C., Regioselectivity and stereoselectivity of androgen hydroxylation catalyzed by cytochrome P450 isozymes purified from phenobarbital-induced rat liver,. *J. Biol. Chem.*, 258, 11937, 1983.

Weber, W. W., in *Concepts in Biochemical Pharmacology*, Vol 1., Brodie, B. B. and Gillette, J. R., Eds., Springer-Verlag, Berlin, 1971, 564.

Weiner, I. M., in *Concepts in Biochemical Pharmacology*, Vol 1., Brodie, B. B., and Gillette, J. R., Eds., Springer-Verlag, Berlin, 1971, 328.

Williams, R. T., The influence of enterohepatic circulation on toxicity of drugs, *Ann. N.Y. Acad. Sci.*, 123, 110, 1965.

Zannoni, V. G., in *Fundamentals of Drug Metabolism and Drug Disposition*, Williams & Wilkins, Baltimore, 1972, 583.

Zerilli, A., Ratanasavanh, D., Lucas, D., Goasduff, T., Dreano, Y., Menard, C., Picart, D., and Berthou, F., Both cytochromes P450 2E1 and 3A are involved in the *O*-hydroxylation of p-nitrophenol, a catayltic activity known to be specific for P450 2E,. *Chem. Res. Toxicol.*, 10, 1205, 1997.

Ziegler, D. M., McKee, E. M., and Poulsen, L. L., Microsomal flavoproteincatalyzed *N*-oxidation of acrylamides, *Drug Metab. Dispos.*, 1, 314, 1973.

20 *In Vitro* Methods for the Prediction of Ocular and Dermal Toxicity

John W. Harbell, Ph.D. and Rodger D. Curren, Ph.D.

CONTENTS

SECTION 1. INTRODUCTION TO *IN VITRO* TOXICOLOGY

In vitro toxicity methods were first developed to examine the mechanisms underlying actions of chemicals on organs or tissues observed *in vivo*. They were used to isolate the presumed target cells or tissue from the external influences of surrounding tissues or organs. The test chemical could be delivered directly to cells and the changes in viability or other functional parameters measured. Since the gross effect on the tissue was known from *in vivo* studies, the *in vitro* model or models were designed to elucidate the possible mechanisms by which that change might be induced. As each test system might address only a subset of tissue targets, a battery of assays might be employed to screen for the mode of action for that chemical on the tissue in vivo. These *in vitro* studies were designed to explain the observed action *in vivo* rather than to predict future activities specifically. *In vitro* studies of this type remain a major part of cell and molecular biological research.

Increasingly, *in vitro* methods are being applied prospectively in many fields, including cancer biology, drug discovery, and toxicology. These studies are intended to predict the potential for action of the test material on the target tissue. Studies to assess potential action of the test chemical (efficacy or hazard) measure changes in the target cells under conditions of known *in vitro* exposure. Such exposure might not be achieved *in vivo* depending on the absorption, distribution, metabolism, and excretion of the chemical. Thus, the primary focus is on the action of individual chemicals/active ingredients under standardized conditions and/or assessment of their relative "potency" in a single cell type. The most common culture format for individual cell types is as a submerged cell monolayer attached to a plastic substrate (e.g., culture flask or multiwell plate).

Assessment of ocular and dermal toxicity has been a standard practice for many types of products. The development of *in vitro* assays to predict ocular and dermal toxicity has proved to be challenging. Even though the *in vivo* exposures are topical, the exposure kinetics may be quite complex. Therefore, topical application to tissues (natural or reconstructed) *in vitro* has proved to be the most useful methods of testing broad classes of chemicals. For predicting the ocular irritation potential of certain chemical/product classes, select monolayer cell culture systems have proved valuable. However, many other product classes are not amenable to these simpler systems and require a tissue-based assay system. These tissues may be short-term *ex vivo* organ cultures or engineered tissue constructs. More complex exposure kinetics, such as dermal penetration and subsequent action of topically applied formulations, require more complex systems that can model both the barrier properties of skin and provide the necessary target cells.

This chapter is divided into three parts. This first section, Tables 20.1 through 20.6, provides a general introduction to *in vitro* methods, measures of cellular function, assay end points, design considerations and controls. The second section, Tables 20.7 through 20.17, addresses current approaches to assessing ocular irritation potential of chemicals and formulations. The third section, Tables 20.18 through 20.26, focuses on systems to assess action on dermal tissue. Sample protocol summaries are provided to illustrate different types of assay for ocular and dermal activity. These protocols generally reflect the basic method, which may then be tailored to meet the user's specific needs. Sample data from several common *in vitro* methods are also provided. The historical positive control ranges come from the authors' laboratory. Positive controls are tested each time the assay is performed and these are used to judge the acceptability of that trial.

In vitro test systems include target cell cultures or tissues that are isolated and maintained in a supportive culture environment. These tissues may be either *ex vivo* or engineered tissue constructs. Influences of collateral tissues and/or the systemic environment are eliminated so that primary and secondary effects of the test substance can be more easily determined. Proper selection of the target cell(s)/tissue depends on the specific mode of action and exposure kinetics to be tested. A given cell/tissue test system will not necessarily possess all the possible targets on which a test chemical may act. Assay batteries may be employed to address a wider range of test article effects. Since cell/tissue homeostasis depends on the culture conditions, careful attention to all facets of test system maintenance and manipulation is essential. Maintenance of the required cell/tissue differentiation must be demonstrated for each test system.

Precise control of test article exposure dose and duration in the test system is a hallmark of *in vitro* systems. Modeling of complex tissue exposure may require specific equipment (e.g., perfusion devices) or test systems (e.g., skin models with barrier function). Prediction of the degree of toxicity to an *in vivo* tissue may require the careful modeling of the *in vivo* exposure conditions when designing *in vitro* systems. However, the *in vivo* exposure conditions are often poorly understood and potentially highly variable. Thus, the experimental design of the *in vitro* assay may only model a "best approximation" of the range of *in vivo* exposures. Once established, this assay design is uniformly applied to a range of test articles of similar chemical/product class.

Because the target cells/tissues are treated in isolation, the collateral changes that might be seen in the surrounding tissues *in vivo* will not be available to demonstrate the impact of the test article on the test system. For example, in the absence of a vascular system, edema and erythema end points will be meaningless in an *in vitro* skin model. Test article impact on cell culture systems may be manifested as cessation of cell replication, cell death, release of inflammatory mediators, or loss of differentiated cell function. Damage to isolated tissue systems may be assessed by similar measures as well as loss of epithelial barrier integrity and other measures of tissue degeneration. The mode of action of a given chemical/physical class of test articles may involve only a subset of these cellular changes *in vivo*. Determining the relevance of any of these changes to the action *in vivo* is part of the validation process.

By necessity, assessment of cell/tissue damage is generally made indirectly (e.g., by measuring an end point associated with normal cell function) and quantitatively on the treated population. Although cell death in cell culture may be detected by microscopic evaluation, such a process would be tedious and highly subjective. Understanding the impact on the population of treated cells requires methods that measure some aspect of normal cell function. The function may be continued cell replication (e.g., DNA synthesis, increased total cell number), cellular metabolic process (e.g., continued ATP synthesis, energy-dependent redox cycles), membrane integrity (e.g., loss of cytoplasmic contents), or some measure of differentiated cell function appropriate to the population under study. Isotope incorporation, vital dye uptake/metabolic conversion, and ELISA assays may be used to measure these functions on the populations. These end points lend themselves to objective scoring by spectrophotometric or other instruments, which helps speed the process and reduce the subjectivity of the assessment.

As the use of *in vitro* methods in predictive toxicology has grown, there is concurrent need to demonstrate the reproducibility and relevance (to the *in vivo* response) of the assay for its intended purpose. New assays go through a process of prevalidation,[1] where the transferability of the technology demonstrated, the study protocol is finalized, and the prediction model is developed. The prediction model is used to translate the data from the *in vitro* assay into terms that can be directly compared with the *in vivo* assay/response of interest. Validation of the assay then involves testing the appropriateness of the study protocol and prediction model across several laboratories with coded samples.[2,3] Good Laboratory Practices guidelines should be followed during this process to assure data integrity.[4] Mechanisms are now in place for the formal regulatory review of new methods in both Europe[5] and the United States.[6]

TABLE 20.1
Considerations in Selecting *In Vitro* Assays to Support Product Development Programs

Factors to Be Considered	Impact of Those Factors
Chemical Class of the Test Materials	
Alcohols	Not all *in vitro* systems have been characterized for their performance with a variety
Organics	of chemical classes. Carefully investigate individual *in vitro* systems to determine
Preservatives	with which chemical classes they are compatible.
Surfactants	
Physical Characteristics of the Test Material	
Solid/liquid	Solid or water insoluble materials should generally not be tested with a monolayer
Water soluble/insoluble	cell culture system since the test materials may not reach the target cells. Topical
Extremes of pH	application assays are preferred for such materials.
Highly reactive	Highly reactive materials may bind to constituents of the tissue culture medium and
Amount of material available	thus be unavailable to the target tissue. Dilution into buffered culture medium will
	reduce extremes of pH.
	Although *in vitro* tests generally require far less test material than do animal tests,
	there is still a considerable range of requirement among the *in vitro* systems. Some
	have been designed to use micro-quantities of materials.
Stage in Product Development	
Single (perhaps active) ingredient	Biological activity of single ingredients may be assessed in a variety of systems
Mixtures	including *ex vivo* tissues, tissue constructs, and monolayer culture systems. Water
Final formulation	solubility and the end point(s) of interest will guide selection.
	Depending on the target tissue, testing of mixtures and final formulations may
	require that the test system be able to model the expected exposure kinetics of the
	formulation as a whole. For example, dermal irritation studies may require a test
	system with a functional stratum corneum such as a tissue construct. In contrast,
	ocular irritation studies of surfactant formulations might well use *ex vivo* tissues,
	tissue constructs, and monolayer culture systems.
Expected Level of Toxicity	
Low	The dynamic range of response of the *in vitro* system should match the expected
Medium	level of toxicity of the test material. Some *in vitro* systems are designed to
High	differentiate between weakly reactive materials; more robust systems may be useful
	for highly toxic materials.
Expected Exposure to the Tissue of Interest	

TABLE 20.1 *(Continued)*
Considerations in Selecting *In Vitro* Assays to Support Product Development Programs

Factors to Be Considered	Impact of Those Factors
Incidental/accidental Short term or infrequent Leave-on vs. wash-off application Chronic application Use population (infants, adult, aged)	The exposure kinetics of the *in vitro* system can often be varied, and should closely match the expected *in vivo* exposures if an accurate estimate of toxicity is to be obtained.
	Resolution Required of the Test

Differentiate among similar test
  formulations
Separating highly toxic from non-
  toxic materials
	It may require a more sophisticated *in vitro* system to differentiate closely related materials than it would to place test materials into general classifications.

	Intended Use of the Data
Safety/efficacy screen Product development Formula optimization Claims support	The purpose of the testing should be matched to the test system; e.g., a simple, inexpensive *in vitro* model may be sufficient for use in screening, whereas a more sophisticated model might be necessary to characterize the effects of minor formulation changes.
	Resources Available
Funding Time Number of materials to be tested	Many *in vitro* tests can seem expensive if applied to a single test article, but are designed for easy batching of materials, which results in significant cost benefits.

TABLE 20.2
Measures of Normal Cell Function Often Used in *In Vitro* Toxicology Assays

Normal Cell Function	Assay End Points	Examples
Intact Cytoplasmic Membrane		
Permeability barrier	Exclusion of select dyes	Trypan Blue,[7] propidium iodide, ethidium bromide,[8] Calcein AM[9]
	Release of cytoplasmic contents	Lactate dehydrogenase release ^{51}Cr release[10]
Ion pumps and ion gradients	Changes in membrane potential	Patch-clamp membrane potentials[11]
	Ion-specific dyes (e.g., cytoplasmic Ca^{2+} gradient)	Fluo3-AM[9]
Membrane lipid integrity	Release of arachidonic acid metabolites (eicosanoids and leukotrienes)	ELISA–PGE_2[12]
Cellular Metabolism (continued regeneration of ATP/NADH)		
Production of CO_2/lactate	Rate of release of acidic metabolic by-products into the medium	Cytosensor™ microphysiometer[13,14]
Cellular ATP concentration	Concentration of ATP and/or ATP/ADP ratio in the population	Luciferin/Luciferase Assays[15]
Renewal of NADH/NADPH (cell/population redox potential)	Vital dye reduction (e.g., tetrazolium dyes)	MTT, XTT, Alamar Blue[16,17] Calcein AM
Maintenance of energy-dependent ion gradients	Assessment of the lysosomal H^+ ion gradient	Neutral Red Uptake[18,19]

TABLE 20.2 *(Continued)*
Measures of Normal Cell Function Often Used in *In Vitro* Toxicology Assays

Normal Cell Function	Assay End Points	Examples
	Mitochondrial H+ ion gradients	Rhodamine 123[20]
	Cell Replication	
Increase in cell number	Cell counts over time	Electronic cell counters
	Formation of cell colonies	Clonogenic assays[21]
	Increases in total protein	Kenacid blue or Coomassie blue[22]
	Increases in vital dye uptake/reduction	Neutral red, Tetrazolium dyes
Scheduled (S-phase) DNA synthesis	Incorporation of nucleotides	³H-thymidine[23,24]
		Bromodeoxyuridine
	S-phase specific proteins	ELISA, immunofluorescence, or fluorescent-activated cell sorter analysis
	Maintenance of Differentiated Function	
Normal cytoskeleton	Cell shape	Microscopic observation, immunofluorescence
Production of "marker" proteins	Constitute expression of appropriate membrane markers	ELISA, immunofluorescence, or fluorescent-activated cell sorter analysis
	Induction/release of protein products (e.g., collagen from fibroblasts)	ELISA

TABLE 20.3
Examples of Vital Dyes Used to Assess Cell Viability

Cell Function	Dye	Detection	Application	Notes
Membrane integrity	Trypan Blue[25]	Light microscopy (visible light)	Rapid screen for dead cells used in conjunction with manual cell counts	Will eventually penetrate cells if the incubation extends over 30 min
	Calcein-AM[9]	Fluorescence: Excitation/Emission 485–495/520–530 nm	Readily penetrates viable cells where AM is cleaved by esterases. Resulting dye is fluorescent and is retained by the intact cell.	Low background fluorescence from Calcein-AM
	Ethidium bromide[8]	Fluorescence: Excitation/Emission 510–520/595–605 nm	Stain DNA but do not pass through the intact cell membrane. Marker of dead cells. Often used in combination with Calcein-AM in "live/dead" stain combinations.	Generally not used alone since only dead cells are stained. Cells that have completely degenerated are lost from the count.
	Propidium iodide[8]	Fluorescence: Excitation/Emission 530–540/620–640 nm		
Cellular redox potential[26,27]	MTT 3-(4,5-dimethylthiazol-2-yl)-2,5-dephenyl tetrazolium bromide	Spectrophotometry: OD @ 540–570 nm	MTT is converted from the oxidized form to the reduced form by the NADH+dependent reaction catalyzed by cytoplasmic and microsomal associated enzymes. Upon reduction, dye turns from a yellow moderately water-soluble form to a blue/black insoluble form. The dye is then extracted from the cells or tissues and quantitated.	Little interference from oxidized dye. Good choice where nonspecific binding is expected (e.g., tissue constructs). Increased glycolytic activity will increase tetrazolium dye reduction. If present, reducing agents will reduce the dye and give a false indication of viability. Before testing, screen test chemicals for dye reduction if they will contact the dye.
	XTT sodium 2,3-bis(2-methoxy-4-nitro-5-sulfophenyl)-2H-tetrazolium-5-carboxanilide	Spectrophotometry: OD @ 540–570 nm	XTT is converted from the oxidized form to the reduced form by the NADH+dependent reaction catalyzed by cytoplasmic associated enzymes. Reduced XTT is water soluble so extraction is not needed.	Little interference from oxidized dye. Good choice where nonspecific binding is expected (e.g., tissue constructs). Increased glycolytic activity will increase tetrazolium dye reduction. If present, reducing agents will reduce the dye and give a false indication of viability. Before testing, screen test chemicals for dye reduction if they will contact the dye.

TABLE 20.3 (*Continued*)
Examples of Vital Dyes Used to Assess Cell Viability

Cell Function	Dye	Detection	Application	Notes
	WST-1	Spectrophotometric: OD @ 540–570 nm	Dye is converted from the oxidized form to the reduced form by the NADH⁺-dependent reaction catalyzed by plasma membrane-associated enzymes. Uses intermediate electron acceptor to pass through the plasma membrane. The reduced dye is water soluble so no extraction is needed.	Little interference from oxidized dye. Good choice where nonspecific binding is expected (e.g., tissue constructs). Increased glycolytic activity will increase tetrazolium dye reduction. If present, reducing agents will reduce the dye and give a false indication of viability. Before testing, screen test chemicals for dye reduction if they will contact the dye.
	Alamar Blue	Fluorescence: Excitation/Emission 530/590 nm	Alamar blue is converted from the oxidized form to the reduced form by the NADH⁺-dependent reaction catalyzed by cytoplasmic/membrane associated-enzymes. The reduced dye is water soluble so extraction is needed.	Little interference from oxidized dye. Good choice where nonspecific binding is expected (e.g., tissue constructs). Increased glycolytic activity will increase tetrazolium dye reduction. If present, reducing agents will reduce the dye and give a false indication of viability. Before testing, screen-test chemicals for dye reduction if they will contact the dye.
Energy-dependent ion gradients				
Lysosomal pH gradient[28,30]	Neutral red (3-amino-7-di methylamino-2-methylphenazine hydrochloride)	Spectrophotometric: OD @ 540–550 nm	At physiological pH, the uncharged dye passes through membranes. The dye develops a net charge at the lower pH of the lysosome and so does not readily pass out of the lysosome. The proton gradient across the lysosomal membrane is energy dependent. Dye must be extracted for spectrophotometric analysis.	Loss of this pH gradient, either through mortality/morbidity of the cell or permeation of the membrane, will release retained neutral red or prevent its accumulation. Nonspecific dye binding to test materials or tissue matrix will interfere with the assay. Not all cell types have sufficient lysosomal content for a strong signal.
Ca²⁺ gradients	Fluo-3 AM[9]	Fluorescence: Excitation/Emission 485/500–530 nm	Enters the cell where cleavage of the AM enhances retention. Fluorescence proportional to free Ca²⁺ bound to the dye.	Changes may be rapid and may require Ca²⁺ in the extracellular medium.
Energy-dependent esterases	Calcein-AM[9]	Fluorescence: Excitation/Emission 485–495/520–530 nm	Readily penetrates the viable cell where the AM cleavage by esterases is energy dependent. Resulting dye is fluorescent and is retained by the intact cell.	Low background fluorescence from Calcein-AM.

TABLE 20.4
Factors in the Design of Cell-Based Assays

Factors to be Considered	Impact of those Factors
Selection of the Target Cells	
Species Tissue/organ of interest Degree of differentiation required Normal Transformed/immortalized	Cells from the desired species and target tissue may not be available. A surrogate cell type or species may be sufficient. Normal cells may be required when differentiated function is assessed but may have a short life span in culture. Transformed/immortalized cells allow further characterization and more potential for genetic manipulation. A differentiated, often nondividing, cell type may be required to provide the normal xenobiotic biotransformation capabilities or desired cellular targets for the test chemical.
Cell Preparation and Maintenance	
The goal is to achieve a consistent starting population with the desired characteristics.	Procedures for maintaining stock cells include medium selection, initial seeding and refeeding, time/cell density for reseeding (passaging), and removal of the cells from the growth substrate.
Testing for adventitious agents	Cells should be free of bacteria (including mycoplasma), fungi, and other contaminants.
Selection of the Appropriate Substrate	
Plastic Protein substrate Semipermeable support Suspension	Most nontransformed cells are anchorage dependent. Cell adherence, polarization, and differentiation may be modulated by the substrate selected. Certain transformed or lymphocytic cell lines may grow well in suspension but can be difficult to manipulate in multiwell plates. Special techniques are needed to change the medium without losing cells.
Culture and Treatment Medium	
Serum-containing Serum-free Defined	Serum may bind the test material altering the effective exposure to the target cells. Serum may also complicate analysis of cell products. However, only a small fraction of available cell lines are adapted to serum-free medium.
Culture Format	
Dishes (treated petri dishes) Flasks Multiwell plates	Dishes and flasks are traditional vessels for maintaining stock cultures but may be cumbersome for assays with large numbers of replicate cultures. Multiwell plates are used to provide the required number of replicate cultures and facilitate handling and end point determination. When selecting a multiwell plate format, the required well surface/volume may be dictated by the assay end points planned.
Starting Cell Density	
Dividing Nondividing cells	Cell density should be high enough to provide strong end point signals. Densities of dividing cells should allow controls to remain in log-phase growth throughout the assay. Nondividing/differentiated cells (e.g., normal hepatocytes) may require high seeding densities to maintain their differentiated state.
Assay Dose Range and Test System Exposure	
Full range of doses to cover expected range of toxicity	Dose steps (e.g., half or quarter log) should be appropriately spaced to provide resolution among similar test materials and the steps should be similar for all materials being compared. The volume of medium and well as the test material concentration may impact the effective dose to the cells due to partitioning of lipophilic materials into the cell membrane or other tissue structures.
The duration of exposure	Exposure period may be modeled after expected *in vivo* exposure. Breakdown of the test material may reduce the effective exposure period.
"Expression" period before the end point assay(s) are performed	Manifestations of the action on the cells may not be immediate (e.g., antimetabolites) requiring hours or days before differences are observed.

TABLE 20.4
Factors in the Design of Cell-Based Assays

Factors to be Considered	Impact of those Factors
Examples of End Points in a Cytotoxicity Assay: Measuring Cell Death	
Measurements of the metabolic state	ATP concentration
	Neutral red–lysosomal sequestering
	Tetrazolium dye reduction
	Calcein AM cleavage
	Direct measurement (Cytosensor microphysiometer)
Measurements of membrane integrity	Trypan blue, calcein AM, or propidium iodide uptake
	"Live/dead" nuclear stains
	Cytoplasmic enzyme release (LDH)

TABLE 20.5
The Roles of the Negative Control, Positive Control, and Benchmark Materials[31]

Negative Control
- Provides the baseline values against which the test article and positive control treated cultures are compared
- May generate absolute values for the end point in the tissue that would be part of the acceptance criteria for the assay; these values would be expected to reflect normal constitution (e.g., number of cells) and function (e.g., metabolic state) of the cells or tissue

Positive Control
- Ensures the integrity of the test system and proper execution of the assay
- Needs to be included each time the assay is performed
- Provides one of the acceptance criteria for the assay
- Its use (concentration, exposure time, etc.) is consistent for each assay so that a historical range of responses can be generated; the response to the positive control in each assay trial is compared with the historical control range to determine that the trial is acceptable; independent of the type of unknown material being tested in the assay
- Should allow detection of over- *and* underresponse in an assay relative to its historical performance; positive controls that give only extreme responses are of little use

Benchmark(s)/Reference Materials
- Selected to match to the chemical/product type of the unknown(s) being tested
- Used to set upper and/or lower limits of response against which the unknown(s) are judged
- Should have an extensive *in vivo* database (e.g., clinical or other reference assay)
- Will change in an assay depending on the types of classes of materials being tested

TABLE 20.6
Laboratory Safety Requirements for the Use of Human Cells[32]

Precautions in a tissue culture laboratory using human tissue focus on:
- Concerns with human pathogens such as Hepatitis B, HIV, and other potentially unrecognized viruses
- Universal precautions and other legal requirements, as outlined by the Centers for Disease Control, which must be observed
- Documented sources of cells or tissues; certificate of test results should be available if commercial sources used
- Performing work in a biological safety cabinet (vertical laminar flow hood) to protect the operator and preserve the sterility of the test system
- Regular disinfection of surfaces to reduce contamination
- Sterilization of spent medium, plasticware, and cell cultures before disposal

Source: Centers for Disease Control.[32]

SECTION 2. ASSESSMENT OF OCULAR
IRRITATION POTENTIAL

Prediction of ocular irritation potential requires modeling both a target tissue and relevant exposure kinetics. This modeling is not necessarily a duplication of the *in vivo* condition but should be appropriate for the physicochemical class of the test material and potential modes of action on the tissue targets. Physicochemical properties, such as water solubility, impact the effective amount and duration of the exposure to the tissue. The test system must address the expected mode(s) of action, both in the end point(s) measured and the time course for that end point change to develop. For example, water-soluble surfactant materials might be expected to act rapidly on the cell membranes to produce cell lysis. Nonsurfactant perservatives might target cellular metabolic or replication functions and so require much more time to manifest their impact. Water-insoluble material may never reach the cells in a submerged test system and would require direct application to the tissue to model its *in vivo* exposure.

This section reviews a range of *in vitro* assays used to predict ocular irritation and discuss the selection process based on various applications. Assays may be divided into classes according to their exposure conditions, exposure kinetics, time to end point determination, and the end points themselves. For example, the Cytosensor™ Microphysiometer, Neutral Red Release, and Red Blood Cell Lysis assays are all based on short exposures to serial dilutions of the test article and immediate assessment of the cellular change (membrane damage). To this end, they are generally used to test surfactant materials as are the fluorescein leakage assays. The Neutral Red Uptake and SIRC assays use longer-term (24 h or greater) exposures of serial dilutions and so might be used where delayed damage is expected. The *ex vivo* models (bovine cornea and enucleated eye models) and three-dimensional engineered human tissue constructs allow direct application of the test material to the tissue, but differ considerably in the end points measured. These two types of models can be quite complementary in that they address different degrees of toxicity and end points. The human tissue constructs are able to resolve well in the very mild to moderate irritation range, while the *ex vivo* tissues can be used to address mild/moderate to severe materials. Used together, they can provide measures of cell death, corneal opacity, epithelial cell loss, and overall histological changes.

TABLE 20.7
Characteristics of Common *In Vitro* Assays for Ocular Irritation

Designation	General Description	Method of Applying Test Material
Bovine Corneal Opacity and Permeability (BCOP)[33,34]	Living bovine corneas treated with test material and changes in opacity and permeability are measured by instrument	Test materials applied neat or at end-use concentrations directly to the epithelial surface of the cornea
Chorioallantoic Membrane Vascular Assay (CAMVA)[35,36]	Chorioallantoic membrane of a fertilized chicken egg treated and scored for vascular constriction, hyperemia, and hemorrhage	Generally increasing dilutions of test material applied to the membrane of multiple eggs and damage to the membranes recorded; the dose effective in 50% of the eggs is calculated
Cytosensor Microphysiometer[13,14]	Cells held in a flow-through chamber with a sensor chip which measures pH; cells treated and changes in cellular metabolism (release of H+ ions) recorded in real time	Generally increasing concentrations of test material added to growth medium until a predetermined end point (decrease in metabolism) is reached
Enucleated Chicken or Rabbit Eye[37]	Isolated eyes treated topically and subsequently scored for opacity, corneal swelling, and fluorescein staining	Test materials applied neat or at end-use concentrations directly to the cornea
Fluorescein Leakage[38-40]	Target cells (primary or continuous) capable of forming tight junctions are grown in submerged monolayer or multilayered culture; medium may be removed for dosing	Either increasing dilutions of test material added to growth medium or cell surface for a set time, or a single concentration is added for varying times; end point is induction of permeability of the tissue to fluorescein
Hen's Egg Test Chorioallantoic Membrane (HETCAM)[41]	Chorioallantoic membrane of a chicken egg treated and scored for protein coagulation, hyperemia, and hemorrhage	Test materials applied neat or at in-use concentrations directly to the membrane and damage to the membrane recorded

Method		
IRRITECTION™ (EYTEX™)[42]	Precipitation/turbidity of protein in a nonviable commercially supplied matrix is the end point; meant to mimic opacity formation in the cornea	Either dilutions or neat test material added to a membrane bullet over a responding protein matrix
Neutral Red Release[29] Neutral Red Uptake[30]	Target cells (primary or continuous; fibroblasts or epithelial-like) grown in submerged monolayer culture in multiwell plates; exposures may be minutes (release) or days (uptake)	A range of test article dilutions prepared in growth medium to reach a predetermined end point (generally cytotoxicity)
Pollen Tube Growth[43]	Tobacco pollen allowed to germinate in the presence of test material	Dilutions of test material used; inhibition of pollen tube elongation is the end point
Red Blood Cell[44]	Red blood cells exposed to test material	Dilutions of test material used; lysis (release of hemoglobin) and hemoglobin denaturation monitored
SIRC[21]	Target cells (continuous cell line derived from rabbit cornea) grown in submerged culture at clonal densities and scored for reduction in colony formation	A range of test article dilutions prepared in growth medium to reach a predetermined end point (generally cytotoxicity)
Three-Dimensional Engineered Human Tissue Construct Assays[45–48]	Three-dimensional reconstructed tissue (often human) grown with top surface exposed to air; cell viability and inflammatory mediator release are common assay end points	Test materials applied neat or at end-use concentrations directly to the tissue construct and cell killing measured

TABLE 20.8
Assay Selection Considerations for *In Vitro* Ocular Irritation Testing: Impact of Water Solubility

Assay System Compatible with Water-Soluble Materials
• Bovine Corneal Opacity and Permeability Assay
• Three-Dimensional Engineered Human Tissue Construct Assays
• Fluorescein Leakage Assays
• Submerged Cell-Based Systems
  — Neutral Red Uptake/Release Assays
  — Cytosensor Microphysiometer
  — SIRC
  — Red Blood Cell Lysis
• CAM (Chorioallantoic membrane)-Based Systems
• IRRITECTION™

Assay System Applied to Hydrophobic Formulations
• Bovine Corneal Opacity and Permeability Assays
• Three-Dimensional Engineered Human Tissue Construct Assays
• Fluorescein Leakage Assays (limited)
• CAM-based Systems
• IRRITECTION™

Assay System Suitable for Undiluted Ingredients/Formulations
• Bovine Corneal Opacity and Permeability Assays
• Three-Dimensional Engineered Human Tissue Construct Assays
• HETCAM
• IRRITECTION™

TABLE 20.9
Advantages and Disadvantages of Dilution-Based Assays[a] for Ocular Irritation

Advantages	Disadvantages
Rapid to execute using multiwell plate formats	Cannot be used with water-insoluble materials
Most are machine scored based on dye incorporation/reduction	Dilution effects may mask toxicity of neat material (e.g., alcohols)
Generally very cost-effective — Multiple materials may be tested concurrently	Change in the physical form, e.g., solids to solutions, may impact exposure kinetics
Seem to work well with surfactants and surfactant-based formulations	Buffering effects of the medium may effect toxicity significantly
Often differentiate well between very mild materials	Possible reaction of the test material with the solvent/medium components

[a] Assays in which serial dilutions of the test material are applied to the test system, and the end point is the concentration of test material that causes a selected response.

TABLE 20.10
Advantages and Disadvantages of Topical Application Assays[a] for Ocular Irritation

Advantages	Disadvantages
• Material is tested in its "native" form, i.e., in the same form as an *in vivo* exposure • Exposure of the target tissue can be assured • In some models, exposure time can be selected to match expected *in vivo* exposure	• Test substrate can often be expensive • Exposure times may be inconveniently long, requiring work past the normal workday • Solid materials may require special handling to apply to the test system

[a] Assays in which only the neat or end-use concentration of test material is applied to the test system and the end point(s) depend on the dynamic range of the test system and/or exposure time vs. end point activity.

TABLE 20.11
Further Characterization of Common *In Vitro* Assays for Ocular Irritation

Test	End Point	*In Vivo* Tissue or Irritation Scale Modeled	Resources Needed	Skill Level
BCOP[33,34]	Opacity, permeability, opacity and permeability, histology	Draize maximum average score (MAS), cornea, cornea/conjunctiva?	Specialized equipment (opacity), spectrophotometer	General laboratory skills
CAMVA[35,36]	Vascular hemorrhage, constriction, and dilation	Draize MAS, conjunctiva	General laboratory equipment, shell-cutting tool	General laboratory skills with training for scoring lesions
Cytosensor microphysio-meter[13,14]	Cellular metabolism	Draize MAS	General tissue culture laboratory equipment, cytosensor (expensive)	Tissue culture skills
Enucleated Chicken/Rabbit Eye[37]	Opacity, corneal swelling, fluorescein staining, histology	Draize MAS, corneal damage	Specialized equipment, (expensive)	General laboratory skills
Fluorescein Leakage[38-40]	Increased epithelial permeability	Draize MAS, cojunctiva?, cornea	General tissue culture laboratory equipment, spectrophotometer	Tissue culture skills
HETCAM[41]	Vascular damage, coagulation	Draize MAS, conjunctiva	General laboratory equipment	General laboratory skills with training for scoring lesions
IRRITECTION (EYTEX)[42]	Precipitation	Draize MAS	Specialized equipment, multiwell plate reader	General laboratory skills
Neutral Red Release[29]	Cytotoxicity/ membrane damage	Draize MAS conjunctiva, corneal epithelium damage	General tissue culture laboratory equipment, 96-well plate reader	Tissue culture skills

TABLE 20.11 *(Continued)*
Further Characterization of Common *In Vitro* Assays for Ocular Irritation

Test	End Point	*In Vivo* Tissue or Irritation Scale Modeled	Resources Needed	Skill Level
Neutral Red Uptake[30]	Cytotoxicity	Draize MAS, conjunctiva, corneal epithelium damage	General tissue culture laboratory equipment, 96-well plate reader	Tissue culture skills
Pollen Tube Growth[43]	Cytotoxicity	Draize MAS	General laboratory equipment, spectrophotometer	General laboratory skills, source of pollen
Red Blood Cell[44]	Membrane lysis	Draize MAS	General laboratory equipment, spectrophotometer	General laboratory skills
SIRC[21]	Cytotoxicity	Draize MAS, conjunctiva	General tissue culture laboratory equipment	Tissue culture skills
Three-Dimensional Engineered Human Tissue Construct Assays[45-48]	Cytotoxicity	Draize MAS, corneal, conjunctival, and epithelium damage	General tissue culture laboratory equipment, spectrophotometer	Some tissue culture skills

TABLE 20.12
Sample Protocol Outline for the Neutral Red Release Assay

Theory
The rapid action of surface-active agents leads to loss of membrane integrity. Release of the neutral red dye from the lysosomes reflects the loss of their ion gradient and membrane integrity. Assay is appropriate only when rapid, generally membrane-associated toxicity, is the primary mechanism of toxicity (e.g., surfactants).[29,30]

Applications and Use
- The assay system may be used to predict ocular irritation of surfactant-based materials.
- The target cells are human epidermal keratinocytes.
- The test system uses a serum-free medium, which eliminates the possibility of serum protein and test article interaction.[49]
- Test is dilution based. Therefore, topical application cannot be modeled.
- The assay is best suited for water-soluble formulations.
- The neutral red release bioassay has been demonstrated in a multiassay system validation to be particularly effective at predicting ocular irritation due to surfactant formulations.
- The assay system has been demonstrated to be quite reproducible, and has provided a high level of resolution among similar formulations.

Experimental Procedure
Target Cell Preparation
- Frozen cells are thawed and cultured in KGM at $37 \pm 1°C$ in a humidified atmosphere containing $5 \pm 1\%$ CO_2.
- Cells are subcultured when the stock culture is 50 to 80% confluent.
- A cell suspension is prepared to yield 1.4×10^4 cells/ml.
- 250 μl (~3500 cells per well) of the cell suspension are added to designated wells of a 96-well bioassay plate.
- The cultures are incubated until the cells become 75 to 90% confluent (approximately 48 to 120 h) prior to test chemical dosing.

Sample and Positive Control Preparation

TABLE 20.12 *(Continued)*
Sample Protocol Outline for the Neutral Red Release Assay

- On the day of dosing, the test chemical is suspended in KGM (or another appropriate solvent).
- A total of eight dilutions of the test chemical are made for the dose range finding assay and a minimum of six doses for the definitive assay(s).
- Triton X-100 is used as the positive control. Four concentrations (10, 3.0, 1.0, and 0.3 mg/ml) are tested.

Assay Procedure
- Neutral Red Preloading: KGM is removed from the wells and 250 µl of neutral red solution (50 µg/ml) in KGM are added to each well. The plates are returned to the incubator for 3 h.
- The neutral red solution is removed and the cells re-fed with 125 µl of fresh KGM. Cells must be treated within 2 h after neutral red removal. This medium will be decanted immediately before dosing.
- 100 µl of test or control article dilutions are added to the appropriate wells *immediately* after the KGM is decanted.
- The plates are incubated for 5 min at room temperature.
- After incubation, the treatment solution is removed and the cultures are rinsed at least once with 125 µl of KGM.
- 200 µl of wash/fix solution are added to each well. After 2 min, the wash/fix is removed and 100 µl of neutral red solvent is added.
- The neutral red is extracted from the cultures for at least 20 min at room temperature while shaking.
- The absorbance of the neutral red at 540 to 550 nm (OD_{550}) is measured with a 96-well plate reader.

Data Evaluation
- The relative survival of each treatment group is determined by comparing the mean corrected OD_{550} of the test article-treated wells to the mean corrected OD_{550} of the negative control-treated wells.
- Dose–response curves may be plotted with the percent of control on the ordinate and log of the the test article doses on the abscissa.
- The NRR_{50} (the concentration of the test article that increases the release of preincorporated neutral red by 50%) is determined by interpolation from the dose–response curves.

TABLE 20.13
Sample Data for Personal Care Surfactant Formulations from the Neutral Red Release Assay

Test Article[a]	Neutral Red Release 50% (mg/ml) Mean ± SD[b]	Draize MAS (24-h score) Mean ± SD[c]
Polishing scrub	154 ± 48	1.0 ± 0
Eye makeup remover	43 ± 11	0.0 ± 0
Shampoo A	8.1 ± 1.4	1.3 ± 0.5
Shampoo B	4.7 ± 0.6	4 ± 4.1
Shampoo C	2.3 ± 0.3	15.2 ± 4.4
Shampoo D	2.7 ± 0.2	22.5 ± 13.1
Bubble bath	0.64 ± 0.1	39.7 ± 2.4
Historical positive control value:	0.2 ± 0.03	
Triton X-100	n = 82	

[a] Gettings et al.[50]
[b] Mean of three trials except positive control.
[c] Mean of six animals.

TABLE 20.14
Sample Protocol Outline for the Bovine Corneal Opacity and Permeability (BCOP) Assay

Theory

The potential ocular irritancy/toxicity of a test article as measured by the induction of either or both (1) corneal opacity, which may be caused by protein coagulation /cell precipitation, or the induction of stromal swelling; and (2) corneal permeability to fluorescein, reflecting a degradation/loss of the corneal epithelium. Histopathological changes may be used to assess depth of injury to the tissue.[34,51-53]

Applications and Use

- The BCOP model is a biologically complex *ex vivo* model with end points similar to many human corneal responses, yet is relatively inexpensive.
- Histological evaluation of the tissue can be performed to measure the depth of injury.
- BCOP is particularly suited for moderate to severely aggressive materials, where other models may not be suitable.
- Multiple end points allow the investigation of mechanisms of action.

Experimental Procedure

Bovine Cornea Preparation

- Bovine eyes are received from the abattoir shortly after the slaughter of the animal so the cells are still viable.
- The corneas are excised, mounted in the BCOP chambers, and allowed to equilibrate in MEM supplemented with 1% FBS and without phenol red (Complete MEM) for 1 h.

Sample and Positive Control Preparation

- The samples can be tested undiluted (neat) or at any concentration in a variety of solvents.
- Positive and negative controls are tested and are the basis for assay acceptance criteria, and reproducibility.
- Individual positive controls are used for the testing of either liquid or solid test materials. Ethanol at ~100% is used as the positive control for the liquid protocol and Imidazole at 20% in complete MEM for the solid protocol.

Assay Procedure

- The bovine eyes are harvested shortly after the animal is slaughtered, and shipped in cold HBSS supplemented with 1% penicillin/streptomycin.
- The bovine corneas are carefully checked for any damage (opacity, cuts, etc.) before being excised and mounted in the special BCOP chambers with complete MEM and incubated at 32°C for 1 h.
- After the 1 h incubation, an initial opacity for each cornea is read in an opacitometer and recorded.
- The corneas are divided into groups between three and six corneas per test article per exposure time and exposed to the test article at the concentration requested.
- A 750 µl aliquot of test material is exposed to the cornea. The material can be tested at any concentration and over a range of exposure times.
- The test article is rinsed from the cornea and opacities read and recorded before an additional 32°C incubation.
- Post-treatment incubation times may be varied to enhance postexposure expression of irritancy.
- A postincubation opacity reading is taken on each cornea and recorded.
- The initial opacity reading is subtracted from the postincubation opacity to calculate the final opacity reading.
- A permeability test is performed to measure the passage of fluorescein stain through the cornea. A medium sample is removed from the posterior end of the chamber and measured spectrophotometrically (490 nm) to determine the amount of fluorescein leakage (OD_{490}).
- Both opacity and permeability scores are used to calculate the final BCOP score.
- Corneas may also be fixed, sectioned, and examined in histopathology.

Data Evaluation

- Sina et al.[34] have proposed a scoring system integrating opacity and permeability: *in vitro* score = opacity + 15 × permeability
- 0 to 25 is considered a mild irritant, 25.1 to 55 is considered moderate, and 55.1 and above is considered severe.
- It is important to address the individual contributions of opacity and permeability relative to the chemical class tested.

TABLE 20.15
Sample Bovine Corneal Opacity and Permeability (BCOP) Assay Data

Chemical	Opacity[a]	Permeability (OD$_{490}$)	*In Vitro* Score[34]	Predicted Irritancy Class[34]
		Solvents		
Butanol	15.8	1.456	37.7	Moderate
Isopropanol	33.0	0.703	43.5	Moderate
Methyl ethyl ketone	72.3	0.059	73.2	Severe
Acetone	144.5	1.032	160.0	Severe
		Surfactants		
Polyglyceryl-12-laurate	0.3	0.005	0.4	Mild
Tween-20 (20%)	1.0	0.010	1.1	Mild
Adult shampoo (10%)	3.7	0.526	11.6	Moderate[b]
Sodium lauryl sulfate (10%)	6.1	1.712	31.8	Severe[b]
Alkyl dimethyl benzyl ammonium chloride	48.1	1.432	70.0	Severe
Decylisononyl dimethyl ammonium chloride	89.9	1.600	114.0	Severe
Benzalkonium chloride (10%)	120.9	2.640	160.5	Severe
Historical positive control range:	32.2 ± 5.3	1.319 ± 0.3	51.8 ± 6.6	Moderate
Ethanol (100%)	$n = 281$			
Historical positive control range:	84.0 ± 16.8	1.604 ± 0.5	108 ± 16.7	Severe
Imidazole (20% suspension)				
4-h exposure for solids	$n = 84$			

[a] A 10-min test article exposure with 120-min postexposure incubation.

[b] Anionic surfactants induce little increase in opacity relative to the damage caused. Permeability scores are used to predict damage.[51]

TABLE 20.16
Sample Protocol for the Topical Application Assay Using a Human Tissue Construct: EpiOcular™

Theory

Ocular irritancy of many classes of chemicals involves the cytotoxicity to cells of the eye. The prediction of ocular irritancy of a test article is determined by the exposure time of a test article required to reduce cell viability to 50% of control viability. Cell viability is measured by the NADH-dependent reduction of 3-[4,5-dimethylthiazol-2-yl]2,5-diphenyltetrazolium bromide (MTT) in the living cells and is expressed as relative viability of the treated to untreated (negative control) cultures.

Applications and Use

- Tissue constructs are particularly suited for very mild to moderately toxic materials.
- Test materials are applied topically at formulation strength.
- Both water-soluble and -insoluble formulations can be tested.
- Creams, pastes, highly viscous materials, and powders otherwise precluded from testing in other models are compatible with this system.
- Cells are of human origin and can be induced to express and release inflammatory mediators.

Experimental Procedure

Receipt and Preparation of Cultures

- Each culture is removed with sterile forceps from the agarose gel in the sterile shipping tray, inspected, and transferred to assay medium in a 6-well plate. The EpiOcular cultures will be incubated at 37 ± 1°C in a humidified atmosphere of 5 ± 1% CO_2 in air for at least 1 h prior to dosing.

TABLE 20.16 *(Continued)*
Sample Protocol for the Topical Application Assay Using a Human Tissue Construct: EpiOcular™

Assay Procedure

- The test chemicals/formulations may be tested neat or at end-use concentrations by topical application. Pastes and highly viscous materials may be "creamed" to effect application.
- The positive control is 0.3% Triton X-100 and is exposed for 15 and 45 min.
- The negative control is sterile, deionized water generally exposed concurrently with the longest and shortest exposure times of the test or positive control articles.
- 100 µl (liquids) or 30 mg (solids) of the test or control article are applied topically onto the tissue surface.
- The cultures are returned to the incubator for the appropriate exposure times. Generally, a minimum of four exposure times, ranging from 15 s to 240 min, is selected. For extremely mild materials routinely applied near the eyes, custom exposure times of up to 24 h may be selected.
- After the appropriate exposure time, the test articles are washed from the cultures using DPBS.
- The cultures are transferred to holding wells containing 5 ml of Assay Medium for a 10 to 20 min rinse soak.
- The cultures are transferred to wells containing 0.3 ml of MTT reagent (1 mg/ml) and incubated for 3 h.
- After incubation, the cultures are washed with DPBS and extracted in 2 ml of isopropanol for 2 h, with shaking.
- 200 µl of each extraction solution are transferred to a 96-well plate and the absorbance at 550 nm (OD_{550}) recorded.

Data Evaluation

- The relative survival is determined by comparing the mean corrected OD_{550} of the test article-treated wells to the mean corrected OD_{550} of the negative control wells.
- Exposure time response curves may be plotted with the percent of control on the ordinate and the test article exposure time on the abscissa.
- The ET_{50} (the time of exposure to the test article that reduces MTT conversion by 50%) is determined by interpolation from the exposure time response curves.
- Occasionally, a test article may directly reduce the MTT, giving erroneous results. A direct MTT reduction test is performed as a prescreen, and "killed tissue" controls may be assayed concurrently.
- **Interpretation:** Exposure response curves and ET_{50} values are compared between test formulations as well as benchmarks, where applicable. Several prediction models for interpreting data from a range of chemical classes are under development.

TABLE 20.17
Sample Data from the Topical Application Assay Using a Human Tissue Construct: EpiOcular™

Test Materials[a]	ET_{50} (min)[b]	Draize MMAS[c]
PPG-5 Ceteth-20	180	0.7
Polyoxyethylene[10] oleyl ether (10%)	240	9.6
Imidazolium compound (5%)	>240	1
Sodium linear alkylbenzene sulfonate	6.9	45
Adult shampoo	9	36
Disinfectant cleaner	5.6	40
Historical positive control range:	25.8 ± 5.3 min	
Triton X-100 (0.3%)	$n = 166$	

[a] Materials tested neat *in vivo* unless indicated.
[b] All materials tested at 20% of the indicated concentration that was used *in vivo*.[47]
[c] Draize modified maximum average scores taken 24 h or more after treatment.

SECTION 3. ASSESSMENT OF DERMAL IRRITATION POTENTIAL

Selection of the most appropriate dermal model depends on the question being asked and the cells/tissue available. Many models are used for both irritation and efficacy assessment. Often, the first step in assessing active ingredients may be to use a simple cell-based assay to identify hazard or effect, without regard to actual penetration and exposure in the skin. Most major cell types from human skin are available for cell-based studies. More complex exposure kinetics require *ex vivo* skin or three-dimensional engineered human skin construct model systems that provide both the barrier properties of skin and the necessary target cells, and offer a measure of the actual response expected in skin. Specialized assays using cell and tissue construct models have been developed for phototoxicity and corrosivity and have received a measure of regulatory approval.

Basic skin penetration studies may be performed with living or dead epidermis from humans or animals. Xenobiotic metabolism studies require live skin from the species of interest, although human skin constructs are being used for this purpose because of limited availability of fresh human skin. Although these constructs do not yet duplicate the barrier properties of adult human skin, they do provide reproducible target cells for metabolism studies.

TABLE 20.18
Cell/Tissue-Based Models for the Evaluation of Action on the Skin

Screening of individual chemicals/ingredients for toxicity or efficacy in monolayer culture systems:
- Models serve to assess the *potential* for the material to act on the target cells without regard to the actual exposure that might be achieved *in vivo*.
- The measurement is independent of penetration into skin since the cells are exposed directly in aqueous medium.
  - Model systems composed of monolayer cell cultures of individual cell types (e.g., keratinocytes, dermal fibroblasts, melanocytes, dendritic cells)
    - Test material prepared in aqueous medium and usually over a series of dilutions
      - Requires that ingredient be water miscible
      - Aqueous insoluble ingredients may be tested in a nontoxic solvent on a tissue construct
    - Assay end points may include:
      - Direct toxicity (immediate and delayed)
      - Induction/inhibition of inflammatory mediator expression
      - Phototoxicity
      - Inhibition of differentiated function (e.g., collagen synthesis/release)

Assessment of ingredients, mixtures, and formulations where the goal is to predict the action on skin *in vivo*:
- Action of the formulation/active ingredients is mediated by their ability to penetrate through the stratum corneum.
- Tissue constructs, with a functional stratum corneum, are the models of choice
  - Epidermal-only or epidermal/dermal "full-thickness" constructs
  - Allow direct application of the test material to the "dry" stratum corneum
  - Time to observed action depends on the penetration as well as the "innate" toxicity/potential activity of the material/formulation
- Applications
  - Direct toxicity (immediate and delayed)
  - Induction/inhibition of inflammatory mediator expression
  - Phototoxicity
  - Inhibition of differentiated function
  - Additional end points from specialized systems with multiple cells types:
    - Inhibition of melanin deposition in keratinocyte/melanocyte constructs
    - Epidermal–dermal cell interaction (e.g., balanced cytokine expression or induction of proteases)

TABLE 20.19
Examples of Monolayer Cell-Based Assay Systems for Assessing Action on the Skin

Cell Type	Culture System[a]	Applications	End Point(s)
Balb/c 3T3 fibroblasts (mouse)	Serum-containing medium	Phototoxicity	Neutral Red Uptake
Human keratinocytes	Serum-free medium derived from MCDB 153[30]	Direct cytotoxicity Phototoxicity	Neutral Red Uptake Neutral Red Uptake
	Serum-free medium derived from MCDB 153 without hydrocortisone[54]	Stimulation of expression/release of inflammatory mediators	ELISA: TNFα, IL-1α, IL-8
		Anti-inflammatory action-decreased expression/release of inflammatory mediators	ELISA: TNFα, IL-1α, IL-8
Human dermal fibroblasts	Serum-containing medium Ascorbic acid required	Direct cytotoxicity Suppression/stimulation of collagen synthesis	Tetrazolium dye reduction ELISA for procollagen c-peptide
Human melanocytes	Various media including low serum formulations	Melanin synthesis	Changes in tyrosinase activity
Human microvascular endothelial cells	Low serum medium	Proinflammatory responses	Upregulation of adhesion proteins
Human dendritic cells (from bone marrow stem cells)	Proprietary formulations that induce differentiation	Interaction with antigenic/sensitizing agents	Cytokine expression (e.g., IL-1β)

[a] See cell supplier literature for the recommended culture medium.

TABLE 20.20
Neutral Red Uptake Phototoxicity Assay in BALB/c 3T3 Mouse Fibroblasts

Theory

Cells are exposed to serial doses of the test article in the presence or absence of a nontoxic flux of UVA light. A phototoxin transfers light energy to the cells in a deleterious manner, leading to increased cytotoxicity relative to the doses of the test article alone. The uptake of neutral red dye (3-amino-7-dimethylamino-2-methylphenazine hydrochloride) by Balb/c 3T3 mouse fibroblast cell cultures is used to measure changes in cell viability relative to controls.[55-57]

Experimental Procedure

Target Cell Preparation
- Stock Balb/c 3T3 cell cultures are maintained at $37 \pm 1°C$ in a humidified atmosphere containing $5 \pm 1\%$ CO_2.
- Cells are subcultured when the stock culture is 50 to 80% confluent.
- A cell suspension is prepared to yield 1.0×10^5 cells/ml.
- 100 μl (~10,000 cells per well) of the cell suspension are added into the designated wells of the 96-well bioassay plate.
- The cultures are incubated for approximately 24 h.
- Since UV sensitivity of the cells increases with aging, cells are used at passage numbers <100. Stock cells are cultured in the absence of antibiotics and new stock cells are initiated from the frozen working bank every 3 months.

Sample and Positive Control Preparation (prepared the day of treatment)
- On the day of dosing, the test chemical is suspended in EBSS or HBSS ($2\times$ concentration). Intermediate solvents (DMSO or ethanol) may be used to prepare initial stock dilutions with subsequent dilution into the aqueous medium (final maximum solvent concentration of 1 or 0.5%, respectively).
- A total of eight dilutions of the test chemical is made for the dose range finding assay (100 μg/ml to 0.03 μg/ml in $^1/_2$ log increments) and a total of eight dilutions is made for the definitive assays based on the results of the dose range finding assay.
- Chlorpromazine is used as the positive control. Eight concentrations (100 to 1.77 μg/ml for the plate not exposed to UVA light (dark) and 9.96 to 0.176 μg/ml for the plate exposed to UVA light) are tested.

Assay Procedure
- At 24 h after seeding the cells into 96-well plates, the growth medium is removed, cells rinsed once with 125 μl EBSS or HBSS, and the appropriate wells are re-fed with 50 μl of the dosing vehicle (EBSS/HBSS). The outer wells are re-fed with 100 μl of isotonic solution to maintain the humidity.
- Two plates are designated for each test material: one plate for determination of cytotoxicity (dark) and the second plate for determination of phototoxicity (UVA); 50 μl of the test and control article dilutions are added to the appropriate wells yielding the final treatment dose. The cells are exposed to the test article dilutions for approximately 1 h.
- After the 1 h treatment, one plate is exposed to 1.7 ± 0.1 mW/cm^2 of UVA light and the second plate is placed in the dark at room temperature, both incubated for 50 ± 2 min. The plates are then rinsed at least once and re-fed with 100 μl of Assay Medium (growth medium supplemented with penicillin/streptomycin).
- Prior to the neutral red addition, the wells are evaluated microscopically for cytotoxicity.
- Approximately 24 h after the post-treatment incubation, the assay medium is removed from the wells and replaced with 100 μl of neutral red solution (50 μg/ml neutral red in assay medium). The 100 μl of isotonic solution is added to the blank wells (outer wells).
- The 96-well plates are returned to the incubator for 3 h to allow the neutral red uptake within the viable cells.
- After 3 h, the neutral red solution is removed and rinsed once with 250 μl EBSS or HBSS. Next, 100 μl of solvent (ethanol and acetic acid) is added.
- The neutral red is extracted from the cultures for at least 20 min at room temperature while shaking.
- The absorbance of the neutral red at 550 nm (OD_{550}) is measured with a 96-well plate reader.

Data Evaluation

- The relative survival of each treatment group is determined by comparing the mean corrected OD_{550} of the test article–treated wells to the mean corrected OD_{550} of the solvent control wells.
- Dose–response curves may be plotted with the percent of control on the ordinate and the test article doses on the abscissa.
- The IC_{50} (the concentration of the test article that inhibits the uptake of neutral red by 50%) is determined by interpolation from the dose–response curves.
- A Photo-Irritancy Factor (PIF) value and a Mean Photo Effect (MPE) value were calculated for each test article using the software program NRU-PIT2. The PIF is determined by comparing the IC_{50} without UVA (dark) with the IC_{50} with UVA to determine the "factor" difference. PIF = $IC_{50}(-UVA)/IC_{50}(+UVA)$. A PIF of >5 is indicative of phototoxic potential of the test material.
- The MPE measures the effect of UV exposure over a range of concentrations. A material is considered nonphototoxic if the MPE is <0.1 and phototoxic if the MPE is ≥ 0.1.

TABLE 20.21
**Sample Data from the Neutral Red Uptake Phototoxicity Assay in
BALB/c 3T3 Mouse Fibroblasts**

Test Articles[58] (Tetracycline Derivatives)	IC_{50} (µg/ml) (with UVA)	IC_{50} (µg/ml) (without UVA)	Photo Irritancy Factor[a]
Derivative A	>100	>100	none
Minocycline	58.2	>100	>1.7
Tetracycline	17.8	>100	>5.62
Doxycycline	3.24	74.9	23.0
Derivative D	0.33	>100	>305
Historical positive control range: Chlorpromazine in EBSS[b]	0.60 ± 0.35	9.57 ± 1.41	15.96
	$n = 14$		
Historical positive control range: Chlorpromazine in HBSS[b]	1.04 ± 0.33	26.34 ± 5.24	25.3
	$n = 21$		

[a] The ratio of the IC_{50} (without UVA)/IC_{50}(with UVA) where a value of 5 or greater is indicative of a phototoxin.
[b] EBSS (Earle's Balanced Salt Solution), HBSS (Hanks' Balanced Salt Solution).

TABLE 20.22
Examples of Tissue Models for Skin Studies

General Description	Applications	Examples of End Points Measured
	Excised Skin	
Human skin: Partial thickness, living or previously frozen[59]	Percutaneous absorption studies; live tissue allows assessment of biotransformation	Quantitative measurements of radiolabeled or nonlabeled materials in the receiver fluid
Full thickness, living	Cytotoxicity/irritancy/corrosion	Transepithelial resistance Transepithelial water loss Cell viability measured by vital dye reduction
	Regulation of inflammatory mediator (e.g., arachidonic acid products and cytokines)	ELISA or HPLC assays for arachidonic acid products RT-PCR for mRNA ELISA for protein products
	Biotransformation	Quantitative measurements of radiolabeled or nonlabeled materials in the receiver fluid
Porcine skin: Partial thickness, living or previously frozen	Percutaneous absorption studies.	Quantitative measurements of radiolabeled or nonlabeled materials in the receiver fluid
Rodent skin: Living or previously frozen[60]	Cytotoxicity/irritancy/corrosion	Transepithelial resistance Transepithelial water loss
	Tissue Constructs[61]	
EpiDerm™ Epidermal tissue only with a developed stratum corneum[62,63]	Cytotoxicity/irritancy/corrosion Phototoxicity Regulation of inflammatory mediator (e.g., arachidonic acid products and cytokines)	Cell viability measured by vital dye reduction ELISA or HPLC assays for arachidonic acid products RT-PCR for mRNA ELISA for protein products

TABLE 20.22 *(Continued)*
Examples of Tissue Models for Skin Studies

General Description	Applications	Examples of End Points Measured
EPISKIN™ Epidermal tissue only with a developed stratum corneum[64] (not commercially available)	Cytotoxicity/irritancy/corrosion	Cell viability measured by vital dye reduction
	Regulation of inflammatory mediator (e.g., arachidonic acid products and cytokines)	ELISA or HPLC assays for arachidonic acid products RT-PCR for mRNA ELISA for protein products
SkinEthic™ Epidermal tissue only with a developed stratum corneum[65]	Cytotoxicity/irritancy	Cell viability measured by vital dye reduction
	Regulation of inflammatory mediator (e.g., arachidonic acid products and cytokines)	ELISA or HPLC assays for arachidonic acid products RT-PCR for mRNA ELISA for protein products
TestSkin$_{II}$ Epidermal with a developed stratum corneum and dermal tissue (66)	Cytotoxicity/irritancy	Cell viability measured by vital dye reduction
	Regulation of inflammatory mediator (e.g., arachidonic acid products and cytokines)	ELISA or HPLC assays for arachidonic acid products RT-PCR for mRNA ELISA for protein products
	Interaction of epithelial and stromal cells	

TABLE 20.23
Sample Protocol for the Time Course Assay with EpiDerm™ Cultures: MTT End Point

Theory
For many classes of materials, irritancy/corrosivity is manifested in cell cytotoxicity and/or upregulation of inflammatory mediators. This assay evaluates the potential dermal irritancy of a test article as a function of the exposure time of a test article required to reduce cell viability to 50% of control viability to the EpiDerm™ construct. Cell viability is measured by the reduction of MTT and is expressed as a percentage relative to untreated (negative control) cultures. Cytokine expression may be combined with the cytotoxicity end point to refine the assay further.

Applications and Use
- The EpiDerm model is composed of human keratinocytes stratified into a three-dimensional epidermal structure consisting of several layers, including a functioning stratum corneum. Similar models may also be employed (see Table 20.22).
- The EpiDerm construct is suited to address the sensitivity range from very mild to severely aggressive, or corrosive, materials.
- Test materials are applied topically at formulation strength.
- Suited for both water-soluble and -insoluble formulations.
- Suitable for testing creams, pastes, highly viscous materials, and powders.
- Cells are of human origin and can be induced to express and generate inflammatory response cytokines.

Experimental Procedure
Receipt and Preparation of Cultures
- Each culture is removed with sterile forceps from the agarose gel in the shipping container, inspected, and transferred to a prelabeled six-well plate containing 0.9 ml of assay medium per well. The EpiDerm cultures are incubated at 37 ± 1°C in a humidified atmosphere of 5 ± 1% CO_2 in air for at least 1 h prior to dosing.

Assay Procedure
- The test materials are tested neat or at end-use concentrations by topical application to the stratum corneum. Pastes and highly viscous materials may be "creamed" to effect application.
- The positive control is 1.0% Triton X-100 and is exposed for 4 and 8 h.

TABLE 20.23 *(Continued)*
Sample Protocol for the Time Course Assay with EpiDerm™ Cultures: MTT End Point

- Positive controls for modeling inflammatory responses (e.g., croton oil, PMA) may be included.
- The negative control is sterile, deionized water generally exposed concurrently with the longest and shortest exposure times of the test or positive control articles.
- 100 μl (liquids) or 30 mg (solids) of the test or control article are applied topically onto the tissue surface.
- The cultures are returned to the incubator for the appropriate exposure times. Generally, a minimum of four exposure times, ranging from 30 min to 24 h, are selected. For addressing severely irritating or corrosive materials, exposure times of 3 to 60 min may be selected and the treatment volume reduced to 50 μl/tissue.
- After the appropriate exposure time, the test articles are rinsed from the cultures using DPBS without Ca^{2+} and Mg^{2+}.
- The cultures are transferred to wells containing 0.3 ml of MTT reagent (1 mg/ml) and incubated for 3 h.
- After incubation, the cultures are blotted on absorbent paper and extracted in 2 ml of isopropanol for 2 hours, while shaking.
- 200 μl of each extraction solution is transferred to a 96-well plate and the absorbance at 550 nm (OD_{550}) recorded.
- Medium samples may be collected and prepared for a variety of cytokine analyses to assess inflammatory responses.

Data Evaluation
- The relative survival is determined by comparing the mean corrected OD_{550} of the test article-treated wells to the mean corrected OD_{550} of the negative control–treated wells.
- Exposure time–response curves may be plotted with the percent of control on the ordinate and the test article exposure times on the abscissa.
- The ET_{50} (the time of exposure to the test article that reduces MTT conversion by 50%) is determined by interpolation from the exposure time–response curves.
- Occasionally, a test article may directly reduce the MTT giving erroneous results. A direct MTT reduction test is performed as a prescreen, and "killed tissue" controls may be assayed concurrently.
- *Interpretation:* Exposure response curves and ET_{50} values are compared between test formulations as well as benchmarks, if applicable.

TABLE 20.24
Sample Data from the Corrosivity and Irritancy Assays Using the Human Skin Construct EpiDerm™

Test Material Corrosivity Assay (50 μl treatment with 3-min exposure)[a]	Assay End Point Measure Percent viability compared with controls using MTT end point (<50% is corrosive) after a 3-min exposure	*In Vivo* Classification
Nitric acid	7.1	Corrosive
Potassium hydroxide (10%)	14.8	Corrosive
Acetic Acid (10%)	67.0	Noncorrosive
Oxalic Acid	92.6	Noncorrosive
Positive control: KOH (10%)	14.8 ± 6.6	
Irritancy Assay (100 μl treatment in time course studies)[b]	**ET_{50} (min)**	
1,1,1-Trichloroethane	27 min	Irritant
Sodium lauryl sulfate (20%)	50 min	Irritant
1,6-Dibromohexane	520 min	Mild irritant
3,3′-Dithiodipropionic acid	>1440 min	Nonirritant
Historical positive control range:		
Triton X-100 (1%)	329 ± 42 min	
	8 = 87	

[a] Data from Reference 63.
[b] Data from Reference 67.

TABLE 20.25
Assays for Skin Corrosion

Models	Basis of the Assay	End Point Measured	Scoring	Notes
		Nontissue Methods		
Corrositex™[a]	Penetration of the test material through a collagen biomatrix "biobarrier"	Color change in the chemical detection solution below the biobarrier	Time required to penetrate biobarrier	Generally applicable only to acids, acid derivatives, and bases; absence of a test article-induced color change in the chemical detection system precludes use of the assay
		Tissue-Based Methods		
EpiDerm[63]	Damage to cells in a three-dimensional artificial human skin construct after topical exposure to test materials	Number of viable cells as estimated by uptake and reduction of the dye MTT	Time required to reach 50% cell death	Applicable to most chemicals without regard to their physical state (solids or liquids) or water solubility
EPISKIN[69] (not commercially available)	Damage to cells in a three-dimensional artificial human skin construct after topical exposure to test materials	Number of viable cells as estimated by uptake and reduction of the dye MTT	Time required to reach 50% cell death	Applicable to most chemicals without regard to their physical state (solids or liquids) or water solubility
Rat Skin Transcutaneous Electrical Resistance[b]	Loss of normal stratum corneum integrity and barrier function after topical exposure to test material	Reduction in transcutaneous electrical resistance	Treatment time required to reduce transcutaneous electrical resistance below a predetermined threshold level	Applicable to most chemicals without regard to their physical state (solids or liquids) or water solubility

[a] Approved for use in the United States after review by ICCVAM and acceptance by several constituent regulatory agencies.
[b] Approved for use in the Europe an Union after validation by ECVAM and acceptance into Annex V test guidelines.

TABLE 20.26
Sample Protocol for the Corrositex Assay

Theory

Many corrosive materials act rapidly to break down tissue proteins as they penetrate through the skin. This assay evaluates the potential corrosivity of a test article as a function of the time required to penetrate through a calibrated protein biobarrier into a chemical detection system. The penetration time and acid/alkaline reserve potential of the test article are used in the prediction of corrosive potential.

Applications and Use

- The Corrositex assay is based on the time that is required for the test sample to pass through a biobarrier membrane and produce a change in the Chemical Detection System (CDS). The Corrositex biobarrier membrane consists of a reconstituted collagen matrix.
- The Corrositex assay has been approved by the U.S. Department of Transportation for testing potential corrosive materials and assigning United Nations packing group categories for certain chemical classes.
- Test materials are applied to the test system at formulation strength.
- The Corrositex assay system is limited to testing those materials that cause detectable pH changes in the CDS (i.e., acids, acid derivatives, and bases). Test materials must cause a color change in the CDS to be detected.
- The assay system is not suited for testing materials that cannot be detected in the CDS (i.e., neutral organics, some metals, etc.).

Experimental Procedure

Receipt and Preparation of Corrositex Biobarrier Membrane

- A qualification screen with the CDS is performed prior to biobarrier membrane preparation. The test article is added directly into a sample of the CDS solution to determine if a color change can be detected.
- A categorization screen is performed to categorize weak acids/bases and strong acids/bases.
- Weak acids and bases are assayed according to the 1 h protocol (Category 2); strong acids and bases are assayed according to the 4-h exposure protocol (Category 1).
- The biobarrier membrane is used no less than 8 h and no more than 7 days after preparation.

Assay Procedure

- The biobarriers are placed on the CDS solution tubes.
- The biobarrier membrane batch is qualified on each day of use by testing the positive control (NaOH). Results must fall within an acceptable range. A timer is started immediately.
- 500 μl (liquids) or 500 mg (solids) of test article are added to the biobarrier. A timer is started immediately.
- As soon as a color change is detected in the CDS, the elapsed detection time is recorded.
- Four replicate biobarrier membranes are treated with each test article.
- As soon as a color change is detected in each vial of the CDS, the elapsed detection times for each vial are recorded.
- Packing group assignments are made based upon the time required for the test article to break through the CDS and cause a color change.

Data Evaluation

Category	Time Required For Breakthrough to the CDS (Minutes)			
Category 1	0 to 3 min	>3 to 60 min	>60 to 240 min	>240 min
Category 2	0 to 3 min	>3 to 30 min	>30 to 60 min	>60 min
	Packing Group I	**Packing Group II**	**Packing Group III**	**Noncorrosive**

TABLE 20.27

Sample Data from the Corrositex Assay

| Test Material[a] | Category | Corrositex Results | | In Vivo Classification |
		Breakthrough Time (min)	*In Vitro* Classification	*In Vivo* Classification
Boron trifluoride-dihydrate	1	1.53	Packing Group I	Packing Group I
Phosphoric acid (85%)	1	10.96	Packing Group II	Packing Group II
Butyric acid	1	40.57	Packing Group II	Packing Group II
Ethanolamine	1	23.88	Packing Group II	Packing Group II
Sodium hydrogen fluoride	2	71.57	Noncorrosive	Noncorrosive
Calcium carbonate	2	>240	Noncorrosive	Noncorrosive
Sodium hypochlorite (5%)	2	>240	Noncorrosive	Noncorrosive
2-tert-Butylphenol	Not testable			Packing Group III
Isopropanol	Not testable			Noncorrosive
Historical positive control range:		11.97 ± 1.4		
Sodium hydroxide pellet		*n* = 113		

[a] Data from Reference 68.

REFERENCES

1. Curren, R. D., Southee, J. A., Spielmann, H., Liebsch, M., Fentem, J. H., and Balls, M., The role of prevalidation in the development, validation, and acceptance of alternative methods, *ATLA*, 23, 211–217, 1995.
2. Bruner, L. H., Carr, G. J., Chamberlain, M., and Curren, R. D., Validation of alternative methods for toxicity testing, *Toxicol. In Vitro,* 10, 479–501, 1996.
3. Bruner, L. H., Carr, G., Chamberlain, M., and Curren, R., No prediction model, no validation study, *ATLA*, 24, 139–142, 1996.
4. Cooper-Hannan, R., Harbell, J. W., Coecke, S., Balls, M., Bowe, G., Cervinka, M., Clothier, R., Hermann, F., Klahm, L. K., de Lange, J., Liebsch, M., and Vanparys, P., The principles of good laboratory practice: application to in vitro toxicology studies, *ATLA*, 27(4), 539–577, 1999.
5. Anonymous, ECVAM News and Views, *ATLA*, 22, 7–11, 1994.
6. Anonymous, Validation and Regulatory Acceptance of Toxicological Test Methods, National Institute of Health Publication 97-3981, Interagency Coordinating Committee on the Validation of Alternative Methods, National Institute of Environmental Health Sciences, Research Triangle Park, NC, 1997.
7. Ahmad, A. E., Aronson J., and Jacobs, S., Induction of oxidative stress and TNF-alpha secretion by dichloroacetonitrile, a water disinfectant by-product, as possible mediators of apoptosis or necrosis in a murine macrophase cell line (RAW), *Toxicol. In Vitro*, 14(3), 199–210, 2000.
8. Nieminen, A. L., Gores, G. J., Bond, J. M., Imberti, R., Herman, B., and Lemasters, J. J., A novel cytotoxicity screening assay using a multiwell fluorescence scanner, *Toxicol. Appl. Pharmacol.,* 115(2), 145–155, 1992.
9. Rhoads, L. S., Cook, J. R., Patrone L. M., and van Buskirk R. G., A human epidermal model can be assayed employing a multiple fluorescent endpoint assay and the Cytofluor 2300, *J. Toxicol. Cutaneous Ocular Toxicol.,* 12(2), 87–108, 1993.
10. Magoffin, D. A., Kushell, D. L., and Schlesinger, R. J., The chromium-51 release cytotoxicity test: comparison to the agar overlay and cell-growth inhibition tests, in *Cell-Culture Test Methods,* ASTM STP 810, Brown, S. A., Ed., American Society for Testing and Materials, Philadelphia, 1983, 94–101.
11. Bockman, C. S., Griffith, M., and Watsky, M. A., Properties of whole-cell ionic currents in cultured human corneal epithelial cells, *Invest. Ophthalmol. Vision Sci.,* 39(7), 1143–1151, 1998.
12. Buckman, S. Y., Gresham, A., Hale, P., Hruza, G., Anast, J., Masferrer, J., and Pentland, A. P., COX-2 expression is induced by UVB exposure in human skin: implications for the development of skin cancer, *Carcinogenesis,* 19(5), 723–729, 1998.

13. McConnell, H. M., Owicki, J. C., Parce, J. W., Miller, D. L., Baxter, G. T., Wada, H. G., and Pitchford, S., The Cytosensor microphysiometer: biological applications of silicon technology, *Science*, 257, 1906–1912, 1992.

14. Harbell, J. W., Osborne, R., Carr, G. J., and Peterson, A., Assessment of the Cytosensor microphysiometer in the COLIPA in vitro eye irritation validation study, *Toxicol. In Vitro*, 13, 313–323, 1999.

15. Masters, B. A., Palmoski, M. J., Flint, O. P., Gregg, R. E., Wang-Iverson, D., and Durham, S. K., *In vitro* myotoxicity of the 3-hydroxy-3-methylgluaryl coenzyme A reductase inhibitors, Parvastatin, Lovastatin, and Simvastatin, using neonatal rat skeletal myocytes, *Toxicol. Appl. Pharmacol.*, 131, 163–174, 1995.

16. Mosmann, T., Rapid colorimetric assay for cellular growth and survival: application to proliferation and cytotoxicity assays, *J. Immunol. Methods*, 65, 55–63, 1983.

17. Weislow, O. S., Kiser, R., Fine, D. L., Bader, J., Shoemaker, R. H., and Boyd, M. R., New soluble-formazan assay for HIV-1 cytopathic effects: application to high-flux screening of synthetic and natural products for AIDS-antiviral activity, *J. Natl. Cancer Inst.*, 81(8), 577–586, 1989.

18. Filman, D. J., Brawn R. J., and Dandliker, W. B., Intracellular supravital stain delocalization as an assay for antibody-dependent complement-mediated cell damage, *J. Immunol. Methods*, 6(3), 189–207, 1975.

19. Barstad, R., Cortesi, J., and Janus, J., Use of Clonetics' neutral red bioassay to optimize components of serum-free medium for normal human anchorage-dependent cells, *In Vitro Cell. Dev. Biol.*, 27(3), 160, 1991.

20. Jiang, T., Grant, R. L., and Acosta, D., A digitized fluorescence imaging study of intracellular free calcium, mitochondrial integrity and cytotoxicity in rat renal cells exposed to ionomycin, a calcium ionophore, *Toxicology*, 85(1), 41–65, 1993.

21. North-Root, H., Yackovich, F., Demetrulias, J., Gacula, M., Jr., and Heinze, J. E., Evaluation of an in vitro cell toxicity test using rabbit corneal cells to predict the eye irritation potential of surfactants, in *Safety Evaluation and Regulation of Chemicals*, Homburger, F., Ed., Karger, Basel, Switzerland, 1983, 259–269.

22. Pham, X. T. and Huff, J. W., Cytotoxicity evaluation of multipurpose contact lens solutions using an in vitro test battery, *CLAO J.*, 25(1), 28–35, 1999.

23. Livingston, R. B., Titus, G. A., and Heilbrun, L. K., *In vitro* effects on DNA synthesis as a predictor of biological effect from chemotherapy, *Cancer Res.*, 40, 2209–2212, 1980.

24. Harbell, J. W., Wallace, K. A., Curren, R. D., Naughton, G. K., and Triglia, D., A comparison of four measures of toxicity applied to human dermal fibroblasts grown in three dimensional culture on nylon mesh (Skin² Dermal Model), in *Alternative Methods Toxicol.*, Goldberg, A. M., Ed., Mary Ann Liebert, New York, 8, 301–309, 1991.

25. Lewis, R. W., McCall, J. C., and Botham, P. A., A comparison of two cytotoxicity tests for predicting the ocular irritancy of surfactants, *Toxicol. In Vitro*, 7, 155–158, 1993.

26. Berridge, M. V., Tan, A. S., McCoy, K. D., and Wang, R., The biochemical and cellular basis of cell proliferation assays that use tetrazolium salts, *Boehringer Mannheim Biochem.*, 4, 14–23, 1996.

27. Marshall, N. J., Goodwin, C. J., and Holt, S. J., A critical review of the use of microculture tetrazolium assays to measure cell growth and function, *Growth Regul.*, 5, 69–84, 1995.

28. Borenfreund, E. and Puerner, J. A., Toxicity determined *in vitro* by morphological alterations and neutral red absorption, *Toxicol. Lett.*, 24, 119–124, 1985.

29. Reader, S. J., Blackwell, V., O'Hara, R., Clothier, R. H., Griffin, G., and Balls, M., A vital dye release method for assessing the short term cytotoxic effects of chemicals and formulations, *ATLA*, 17, 28–37, 1989.

30. Harbell, J. W., Koontz, S. W., Lewis, R. W., Lovel, D., and Acosta, D., IRAG working Group 4: cell cytotoxicity assays, *Food Chem. Toxicol.*, 35, 79–126, 1997.

31. Harbell, J. W., Southee, J. A., and Curren, R. C., The path to regulatory acceptance of *in vitro* methods is paved with the strictest standards, in *Animal Alternatives, Welfare and Ethics*, van Zutphen, L. F. M. and Balls, M., Eds., Elsevier Science, Amsterdam, 1997, 1177–1181.

32. Centers for Disease Control, Biosafety in Microbiological and Biomedical Laboratories, 3rd ed., U. S. Government Printing Office, Washington, D. C., 1993.

33. Gautheron, P., Dukic, M., Alix, D., and Sina, J. F., Bovine corneal opacity and permeability test: an *in vitro* assay of ocular irritancy, *Fundam. Appl. Toxicol.*, 18, 442–449, 1992.

34. Sina, J. F., Galer, D. M., Sussman, R. G., Gautherone, P. D., Sargent, E. V., Leong, B., Shah, P. V., Curren, R. D., and Miller, K., A collaborative evaluation of seven alternatives to the Draize eye irritation test using pharmaceutical intermediates, *Fundam. Appl. Toxicol.*, 26, 20–31, 1995.

35. Bagley, D. M., Waters, D., and Kong, B. M., Development of a 10-day chorioallantoic membrane vascular assay as an alternative to the Draize rabbit eye irritation test, *Food Chem. Toxicol.*, 33(12), 1155–1160, 1994.

36. Bagley, D. M., Cervin, D., and Harbell, J. W., Assessment of the chorioallantoic membrane vascular assay (CAMVA) in the COLIPA *in vitro* eye irritation validation study, *Toxicol. In Vitro*, 13, 285–293, 1999.

37. Chamberlain, M., Gad, S. C., Gautherone P., and Prinsen, M. K., Organotypic models for the assessment/prediction of ocular irritation, *Food Chem. Toxicol.*, 35, 23–37, 1997.

38. Tchao, R., Trans-epithelial permeability of fluorescein *in vitro* as an assay to determine eye irritants, in *Alternative Methods in Toxicology*, Vol. 6, Goldberg, A. M., Ed., Mary Ann Liebert, New York, 1988, 271–283.

39. Shaw, A. J., Clothier, R. H., and Balls, M., Loss of trans-epithelial impermeability of a confluent monolayer of Madin-Darby canine kidney (MDCK) cells as a determinant of ocular irritancy potential, *ATLA*, 18, 145–151, 1990.

40. Kruszewski, F. H., Walker, T. L., Ward, S. L., and Dipasquale, L. C., Progress in the use of human ocular tissues for *in vitro* alternative methods, *Comments Toxicol.*, 5, 203–224, 1995.

41. Luepke, N. P. and Kemper F. H., HET-CAM: an alternative to the Draize eye test, *Food Chem. Toxicol.*, 24, 495–496, 1986.

42. Balls, M., Botham, P. A., Bruner, L. H., and Spielmann, H., The EC/HO international validation study on alternatives to the Draize eye irritation test, *Toxicol. In Vitro*, 9, 871–929, 1995.

43. Kristen, U. and Kappler, R., The pollen tube growth test, in *In Vitro Testing Protocols. Methods in Molecular Biology*, Vol. 43, O'Hare, S. and Atterwill, C. K., Humana Press, Totowa, NJ, 1995, 189–198.

44. Pape, W. J. W., Pfannenbecker, U., and Hoppe, U., Validation of the red blood cell test system as an *in vitro* assay for the rapid screening of irritation potential of surfactants, *Mol. Toxicol.*, 1, 525–536, 1987.

45. Osborne, R., Perkins, M. A., and Roberts, D. A., Development and intralaboratory evaluation of an *in vitro* human cell-based test to aid ocular irritancy assessments, *Fundam. Appl. Toxicol.*, 28, 139–153, 1995.

46. Stern, M., Klausner, M., Alvarado, R., Renskers, K., and Dickens, M., Evaluation of the EpiOcular™ tissue model as an alternative to the Draize eye irritation test, *Toxicol. In Vitro*, 12, 455–461, 1998.

47. Blazka, M. E., Harbell, J. W., Klauzner, M., Raabe, H., Kubilus, J., Hsia, F., Minerath, B., Kotler, M., and Bagley, D. M., Colgate-Palmolive's program to validate the EpiOcular™ human tissue construct model, *Toxicologist*, 54(1), 188, 2000.

48. Brantom, P. G., Bruner, L. H., Chamberlain, M., De Silva, O., Dupuis, J., Earl, L. K., Lovell, D. P., Pape, W. J. W., Uttley, M., Bagley, D. M., Baker, F. W., Bracher, M., Courtellemont, P., Declercq, L., Freeman, S., Steiling, W., Walker, A. P., Carr, G. J., Dami, N., Thomas, G., Harbell, J., Jones, P. A., Pfannenbecker, U., Southee, J. A., Tcheng, M., Argembeaux, H., Castelli, D., Clothier, R., Esdaile, D. J., Itigaki, H., Jung, K., Kasai, Y., Kojima, H., Kristen, U., Larnicol, M., Lewis, R. W., Marenus, K., Moreno, O., Peterson, A., Rasmussen, E. S., Robles, C., and Stern, M., A summary report of the COLIPA international validation study on alternatives to the Draize Rabbit Eye Irritation Test, *Toxicol. In Vitro*, 11, 141–179, 1997.

49. Shopsis, C. and Eng, B., *In vitro* ocular irritancy prediction: assays in serum-free medium correlate better with *in vivo* data, in *Alternative Methods in Toxicology*, Vol. 6, Goldberg, A. M., Ed., Mary Ann Liebert, New York, 1988, 253.

50. Gettings, S. D., Lordo, R. A., Hintze, K. L., Bagley, D. M., Casterton, P. L., Chudkowski, M., Curren, R. D., Demetrulias, J. L., DiPasquale, L. C., Earl, L. K., Feder, P. I., Galli, C. L., Glaza, S. M., Gordon, V. C., Janus, J., Kuntz, P. J., Marenus, K. D., Moral, J., Pape, W. J. W., Renskers, K. J., Rheins, L. A., Roddy, M. T., Rozen, M. G., Tedeschi, J. P., and Zyracki, J., The CTFA evaluation of alternatives program: an evaluation of *in vitro* alternatives to the Draize primary eye irritation test (Phase III). Surfactant-based formulations, *Food Chem. Toxicol.*, 34, 79–117, 1996.

51. Harbell, J. W. and Curren, R. D., The bovine corneal opacity and permeability assay: observations on assay performance, *In Vitro Mol. Toxicol.*, 11, 337–341, 1998.

52. Harbell, J., Raabe, H., Dobson, T., Evans, M., and Curren, R., Histopathology associated with opacity and permeability changes in bovine corneas *in vitro, ATLA*, 27, 347, 1999.

53. Curren, R. D., Evans, M. G., Raabe, H. A., Ruppalt, R. R., and Harbell, J. W., An histological analysis of damage to bovine corneas *in vitro* by selected ocular toxicants, *Toxicologist*, 54(1), 188, 2000.

54. Wilmer, J. L., Burleson, F. G., Kayama, F., Kanno, J., and Luster, M. I., Cytokine induction in human epidermal keratinocytes exposed to contact irritants and its relation to chemical-induced inflammation in mouse skin, *J. Invest. Dermatol.*, 102, 915–922, 1994.

55. Spielmann, H., Balls, M., Dupuis, J., Pape, W. J., Pechovitch, G., de Silva, O., Holzhütter, H. G., Clothier, R., Desolle, P., Gerberick, F., Liebsch, M., Potthast, J. M., Csato, M., Sladowski, D., Steiling, W., and Brantom, P., The international EU/COLIPA In Vitro Phototoxicity Validation Study: Results of Phase II (blind trial). Part 1: The 3T3 NRU Phototoxicity Test, *Toxicol. In Vitro*, 12, 305–327, 1998.

56. Holzhütter, H. G., A general measure of the *in vitro* phototoxicity derived from pairs of dose response curves and its use for predicting *in vivo* phototoxicity of chemicals, *ATLA*, 25, 445–462, 1997.

57. Spielmann, H., Balls, M., Dupuis, J., Pape, W. J., de Silva, O., Holzhütter, H. G., Gerberick, F., Liebsch, M., Lovell, W. W., and Pfannenbecker, U., A study on UV filter chemicals from Annex VII of European Union Directive 76/768/EEC, in the *In Vitro* 3T3 Phototoxicity Test, *ATLA*, 26, 679–708, 1998.

58. Zerler, B., Roemer, E., Raabe, H, Reeves, A., and Harbell, J. W., Evaluation of the phototoxic potential of chemically modified tetracyclines using the 3T3 Neutral Red Assay, *ATLA*, 27, 107, 1999.

59. Bronaugh, R. L. and Collier, S. W., *In vitro* methods for measuring skin permeation, in *Skin Permeation Fundamentals and Applications*, Zatz, J. L., Ed., Allured Publishing Corporation, Wheaton, IL, 1993, 93–111.

60. Heylings, J. R., Clowes, H. M., Trebilcock, K. L., and Hughes, L., Prediction of skin irritation potential using the skin integrity function test (SIFT), Kosmetica Speciale Dermatologia, May 2001.

61. van de Sandt, J., Roguet, R., Cohen, C., Esdaile, D., Ponec, M., Corsini, E., Barker, C., Fusenig, N., Liebsch, M., Benford, D., de Brugerolle de Fraissinette, A., and Fartasch, M., The use of human keratinocytes and human skin models for predicting skin irritation. The report and recommendations of ECVAM workshop 38, *ATLA*, 27, 723–743, 1999.

62. Koschier, F. J., Roth, R. N., Wallace, K. A., Curren, R. D., and Harbell, J. W., A comparison of three dimensional human skin models to evaluate the dermal irritation of selected petroleum products, *In Vitro Toxicol.*, 10(4), 391–406, 1997.

63. Liebsch, M., Traue, D., Barrabas, C., Spielmann, H., Uphill, P., Wilkins, S., McPherson, J. P., Wiemann, C., Kaufmann, T., Remmele, M., and Holzhütter, H-G., The ECVAM prevalidation study on the use of EpiDerm for skin corrosivity testing, *ATLA*, 28, 371–401, 2000.

64. Roguet, R., Cohen, C., Robles, C., Courtellemont, P., Tolle, M., Guillot, J. P., and Pouradier Duteil, X., An interlaboratory study of the reproducibility and relevance of Episkin™, a reconstructed human epidermis, in the assessment of cosmetics irritancy, *Toxicol. In Vitro*, 12, 295–304, 1998.

65. Osborne, S., Mayer, F. K., Spake, A., Rosdy, M., De Wever, B., Ettlin, R. A., and Cordier, A., Predictivity of an *in vitro* model for acute and chronic skin irritation (SkinEthic) applied to the testing of topical vehicles, *Cell Biol. Toxicol.*, 15, 121–135, 1999.

66. Medina, J., de Brugerolle de Fraissinette, A., Chibout, S. D., Kolopp, M., Kammermann, R., Burtin, P., Ebelin, M. E., and Cordier A., Use of human skin equivalent Apligraf for *in vitro* assessment of cumulative skin irritation potential of topical products, *Toxicol. Appl. Pharmacol.*, 164, 38–45, 2000.

67. Fentem, J. H., Briggs, D., Chesné, C., Elliott, G. R., Harbell, J. W., Heylings, J. R., Portes, P., Roguet, R., Van De Sandt, J. J. M., and Botham, P. A., A prevalidation study on *in vitro* tests for acute skin irritation: results and evaluation by the management team, *Toxicol. In Vitro*, 15, 57–93, 2001.

68. Anonymous, Corrostitex: An *In vitro* Test Method for Assessing Dermal Corrosivity Potential of Chemicals, National Institute of Health Publication 99-4495, Interagency Coordinating Committee on the Validation of Alternative Methods, National Institute of Environmental Health Sciences, Research Triangle Park, NC, 1999.

69. Fentem, J. H., Archer, G. E. B., Balls, M., Botham, P. A., Curren, R. D., Earl, L. K., Esdaile, D. J., Holzhütter, H. -G., and Liebsch, M., The ECVAM international validation study on *in vitro* tests for skin corrosivity. 2. Results and evaluation by the management team, *Toxicol. In Vitro*, 12, 483–524, 1998.

21 Ecotoxicology

David J. Hoffman, Ph.D., Barnett A. Rattner, Ph.D.,
G. Allen Burton, Jr., Ph.D., and Daniel R. Lavoie, M.S.

CONTENTS

SECTION 1. INTRODUCTION AND HISTORICAL OVERVIEW

The term *ecotoxicology* was first designated by Truhaut in 1969 as a natural extension of toxicology to include the ecological effects of pollutants.[1] Ecotoxicology employs ecological parameters to assess toxicity. In the broadest sense, ecotoxicology has been described as toxicity testing on one or more components of any ecosystem as described by Cairns.[2] The definition of ecotoxicology

TABLE 21.1
Historical Overview: First Observations of Ecotoxic Effects of Different Classes of Environmental Contaminants

Date	Contaminant(s)	Effects
1850s	Industrial revolution; soot from coal burning	Industrial melanism of moths
1863	Industrial wastewater	Toxicity to aquatic organisms, first acute toxicity tests
1874	Spent lead shot	Ingestion resulted in death of waterfowl and pheasants
1887	Industrial wastewater	Zones of pollution in rivers established by species tolerance
	Arsenic emissions from metal smelters	Death of fallow deer and foxes
1907	Crude oil spill	Death of thousands of puffins
1924	Lead and zinc mine runoff	Toxicity of metal ions to fish
1927	Hydrogen sulfide fumes in oil field	Large die-off of both wild birds and mammals
1950s	DDT and organochlorines	Decline in American robins linked to DDT use for Dutch Elm disease; eggshell thinning in bald eagles, osprey, and brown pelicans linked to DDT; fish-eating mammals at risk
1960s	Anticholinesterase pesticides	Die-offs of wild birds, mammals, and other vertebrate species
1970s	Mixtures of toxic wastes including dioxins at hazardous waste sites	Human, aquatic, and wildlife health at risk
1980s	Agricultural drain water containing selenium and other contaminants	Multiple malformations and impaired reproduction in aquatic birds in central California
1986	Radioactive substances from Chernobyl nuclear power station	Worst nuclear incident in peacetime, affecting a wide variety of organisms and ecosystems

Derived from Hoffman et al.[3]

can be further expanded as the science of predicting effects of potentially toxic agents on natural ecosystems and nontarget species. Historically, as shown in Table 21.1, some of the earliest observations of anthropogenic ecotoxic effects such as industrial melanism of moths date back to the industrial revolution of the 1850s.[3] In the field of aquatic toxicology, Forbes[4] recognized the significance of the presence or absence of species and communities within an aquatic ecosystem, and reported approaches for classifying rivers into zones of pollution based on species tolerance. During the same era, some of the earliest acute aquatic toxicity tests were first performed by Penny and Adams (1863)[5] and Weigelt, Saare, and Schwab (1885)[6] who were concerned with toxic chemicals in industrial wastewater. It was recognized that the presence or absence of species (especially populations or communities) living in a given aquatic ecosystem provides a more sensitive and reliable indicator of the suitability of environmental conditions than do chemical and physical measurements alone.

In the field of terrestrial toxicology, reports of anthropogenic contaminants affecting free-ranging wildlife included cases of arsenic pollution and smoke stack emission toxicity. One early report described the death of fallow deer (*Dama dama*) due to arsenic emissions from a silver foundry in Germany in 1887. Another report described hydrogen sulfide fumes in the vicinity of a Texas oil field that resulted in a large die-off of many species of wild birds and mammals,[7] thus affecting multiple species within an ecosystem. With the advent of modern pesticides, most notably the introduction of DDT in 1943, a marked decline in the population of American robins (*Turdus migratorius*) was linked to DDT spraying against Dutch Elm disease by the early 1950s. It soon became evident that ecosystems with bald eagles (*Haliaeetus leucocephalus*), osprey (*Pandion haliaetus*), brown pelicans (*Pelecanus occidentalis*), and populations of fish-eating mammals were at risk.[8,9] More recently, mortality of multiple species of vertebrates has occurred as a consequence of exposure to anticholinesterase pesticides.[10,11]

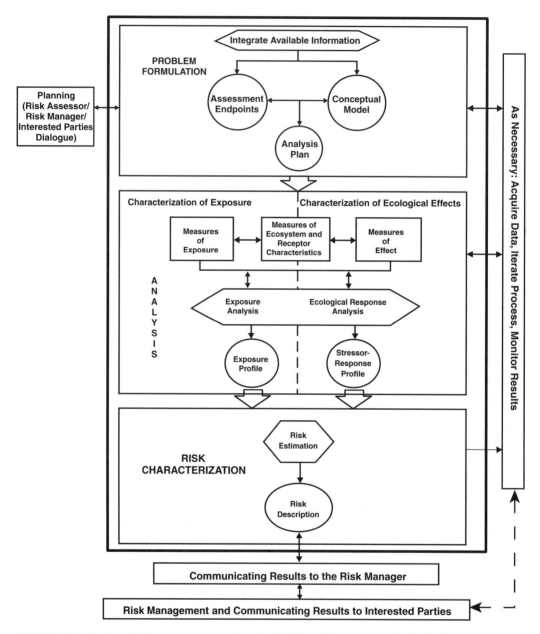

FIGURE 21.1 Ecological risk assessment examines the likelihood that adverse ecological effects are occurring as a result of exposure to one or more stressors. This process examines data, information, assumptions, and uncertainties in order to understand and predict the relationship between chemical, physical, or biological stressors and ecological effects. (Adapted from U.S. Environmental Protection Agency.[12])

An important tool of modern ecotoxicology is ecological risk assessment (ERA), which examines the likelihood that adverse ecological effects are occurring as a result of exposure to one or more stressors[12] as shown in Figure 21.1. This process examines data, information, assumptions, and uncertainties in order to understand and predict the relationship between chemical, physical, or biological stressors and ecological effects. The two major elements of this process include characterization of exposure and characterization of effects, and help focus problem formulation, analysis, and risk characterization. The overall effort expended in conducting an ERA should be consistent with the perceived magnitude of the problem. Results of an ERA, along with social, economic, political, and legal issues, can be used by professionals such as natural resource managers and risk managers as part of a cost–benefit analysis. In addition, results of an ERA can identify alternative chemicals or processes to mitigate risk.

The body of this chapter is presented in four sections including aquatic toxicity testing, wildlife toxicity testing, bioindicators used in aquatic and terrestrial monitoring, and classes of major environmental contaminants and their effects.

SECTION 2. AQUATIC TOXICITY TESTING

There have been a large number of aquatic toxicity test methods developed during the past two decades (Tables 21.2 through 21.4). During the past 10 years, methods for sediment toxicity testing have also increased dramatically (Table 21.5). Most of the standardized test methods have been developed by three North American entities: the U.S. Environmental Protection Agency (EPA), the American Society for Testing and Materials (ASTM), and Environment Canada (EC). In Europe, the Organisation of Economic Cooperation and Development (OECD), European Economic Community (EEC), and International Standards Organisation (ISO) have been the leading standards development organizations. In addition, some European countries, such as the Netherlands and Germany, have developed test methods that may be appropriate for use. Tables 21.2 through 21.5 list the available test methods that are currently available; however, the reader should verify whether new or revised methods have been published because the science of ecotoxicology is a rapidly developing field. Table 21.6 lists some useful Web sites to assist the reader in finding the most recent methods.

It is of interest that many of the laboratory toxicity test methods are quite similar in their basic experimental design. Most are conducted for 2 to 14 days, in static or static-renewal systems, which assess survival, growth, or reproduction as measurement end points. The freshwater test methods utilize laboratory-cultured test organisms of known quality and health, whereas the marine test methods often must use field-collected organisms from presumably clean reference areas. Most of the test organisms are available from commercial suppliers. The primary differences among the test methods are that they are species specific for different geographic areas or regulatory programs, which may dictate the need for species-specific feeding, culturing, testing, and end-point measurement requirements. In addition, the required quality assurance/quality control requirements may vary between protocols and standards-setting organizations. In addition to laboratory toxicity test methods, there has been a significant increase in the use of *in situ* (field-based) toxicity testing. (See the recent review by Chappie and Burton.[13]) *In situ* toxicity testing here is defined as exposure of test organisms in confined chambers in the field, followed by measurement of typical toxicity or bioaccumulation test end points. Many of these methods, particularly for marine systems, have involved deployment of bivalves or fish for determining bioaccumulation and exposure by measuring tissue residues or biomarkers, respectively. The *in situ* approaches provide unique information on receiving water conditions, not possible in laboratory methods. *In situ* exposures are more realistic than laboratory tests, as water/sediment quality conditions and interacting factors such as suspended solids, temperature, and light will occur naturally. In addition, possible alterations in contaminant bioavailability are less likely to occur as a result of sampling, handling, and manipulation effects required for laboratory testing.

TABLE 21.2
Summary of Published EPA, ASTM, and EC Methods for Conducting Aquatic Toxicity Tests

Agency	Test Description	Reference ID
EPA	Methods for Acute Toxicity Tests with Fish, Macroinvertebrates, and Amphibians	EPA-660/3-75-009
	Methods for Measuring the Acute Toxicity of Effluents and Receiving Waters to Freshwater and Marine Organisms	EPA/600/4-90/027F
	Short-Term Methods for Estimating the Chronic Toxicity of Effluents and Receiving Waters to Freshwater Organisms	EPA/600/4-91/002
	Short-Term Methods for Estimating the Chronic Toxicity of Effluents and Receiving Waters to Marine and Estuarine Organisms	EPA/600/R-95/136
	Methods Guidance and Recommendations for Whole Effluent Toxicity (WET) Testing (40 CFR Part 136)	EPA/821/B-00/004
	Methods for Aquatic Toxicity Identification Evaluations: Phase I. Toxicity Characterization Procedures	EPA-600/6-91/003
	Methods for Aquatic Toxicity Identification Evaluations: Phase II. Toxicity Identification Procedures for Samples Exhibiting Acute and Chronic Toxicity	EPA-600/R-92/060
	Methods for Aquatic Toxicity Identification Evaluations: Phase III. Toxicity Confirmation Procedures for Samples Exhibiting Acute and Chronic Toxicity	EPA-600/R-92/061
	Toxicity Identification Evaluation: Characterization of Chronically Toxic Effluents, Phase I	EPA-600/6-91/005F
ASTM	Practice for Algal Growth Potential Testing with *Selenastrum capricornutum*	ASTM D 3978-80
	Practice for Conducting Static Acute Toxicity Tests on Wastewaters with *Daphnia* (discontinued 1990)	ASTM D 4229-84
	Guide for Conducting Static Acute Toxicity Tests Starting with Embryos of Four Species of Saltwater Bivalve Mollusks	ASTM E 724-89
	Guide for Conducting Acute Toxicity Tests Starting with Fishes, Macroinvertebrates, and Amphibians	ASTM E 729-88
	Practice for Conducting Bioconcentration Tests with Fishes and Saltwater Bivalve Mollusks	ASTM E 1022-84
	Guide for Assessing the Hazard of a Material to Aquatic Organisms and Their Uses	ASTM E 1023-84
	Guide for Conducting Life Cycle Toxicity Tests with Saltwater Mysids	ASTM E 1191-90
	Guide for Conducting Acute Toxicity Tests on Aqueous Effluents with Fishes, Macroinvertebrates, and Amphibians	ASTM E 1192-88
	Guide for Conducting Renewal Life Cycle Toxicity Tests with *Daphnia magna*	ASTM E 1193-87
	Practice for Using Brine Shrimp Nauplii as Food for Test Animals in Aquatic Toxicology	ASTM E 1203-87
	Guide for Conducting Static 96-h Toxicity Tests with Microalgae	ASTM E 1218-90
	Guide for Conducting Early Life-Stage Toxicity Tests with Fishes	ASTM E 1241-92
	Practice for Using Octanol-Water Partition Coefficient to Estimate Median Lethal Concentration for Fishes Due to Narcosis	ASTM E 1242-88
	Guide for Conducting Three-Brood, Renewal Toxicity Tests with *Ceriodaphnia dubia*	ASTM E 1295-89
	Guide for Conducting Static Acute Aquatic Toxicity Screening Tests with Mosquito, *Wyeomyia smithii* (*Coquillett*)	ASTM E 1365-90
	Practice for Standardized Aquatic Microcosm: Fresh Water	ASTM E 1366-91
	Guide for Conducting Static Toxicity Tests with *Lemna gibba*	ASTM E 1415-91
	Guide for Conducting the Frog Embryo Teratogenesis Assay — *Xenopus* (FETAX)	ASTM E 1439-91
	Guide for Acute Toxicity Tests with the Rotifer *Brachionus*	ASTM E 1440-91
	Guide for Conducting Static and Flow-through Acute Toxicity Tests with Mysids from the West Coast of the United States	ASTM E 1463-92
EC	Acute Lethality Test Using Rainbow Trout	EPS 1/RM/9
	Acute Lethality Test Using Threespine Stickleback	EPS 1/RM/10
	Acute Lethality Test Using *Daphnia* spp.	EPS 1/RM/11
	Test of Reproduction and Survival Using the Cladoceran *Ceriodaphnia dubia*	EPS 1/RM/21

TABLE 21.2 *(Continued)*
Summary of Published EPA, ASTM, and EC Methods for Conducting Aquatic Toxicity Tests

Agency	Test Description	Reference ID
	Test of Larval Growth and Survival Using Fathead Minnows	EPS 1/RM/22
	Toxicity Test Using Luminescent Bacteria (*Photobacterium phosphoreum*)	EPS 1/RM/24
	Growth Inhibition Test Using the Freshwater Alga (*Selenastrum capricornutum*)	EPS 1/RM/25
	Fertilization Assay with Echinoids (Sea Urchin and Sand Dollars)	EPS 1/RM/27
	Toxicity Testing Using Early Life Stages of Salmonid Fish (Rainbow Trout), second edition	EPS 1/RM/28
	Test for Measuring the Inhibition of Growth Using the Freshwater Macrophyte *Lemna minor*	EPS 1/RM/37
	Reference Method for Determining Acute Lethality of Effluents to Rainbow Trout	EPS 1/RM/13

TABLE 21.3
Aquatic Toxicity Tests Required by the EPA for the Development of Water Quality Criteria

Type of Testing	Recommended Aquatic Tests
Acute toxicity tests	Eight different families must be tested for both freshwater and marine species (16 acute tests): Freshwater: 1. A species in Family Salmonidae 2. A species in another family of Class Osteichthyes 3. A species in another family of Phylum Chordata 4. A plankton species in Class Crustacea 5. A benthic species in Class Crustacea 6. A species in Class Insecta 7. A species in a phylum other than Chordata or Arthropoda 8. A species in another order of Insecta or another phylum Marine: 1. Two families in Phylum Chordata 2. A family in a phylum other than Arthropoda or Chordata 3. Either Family Mysidae or Penaeidae 4. Three other families not in Phylum Chordata (may include Mysidae of Penaeidae, whichever was not used above) 5. Any other family
Chronic toxicity tests	Three chronic or partial life cycle studies are required: One invertebrate and one fish One freshwater and one marine species
Plant testing	At least one algal or vascular plant test must be performed with a freshwater and marine species
Bioconcentration testing	At least one bioconcentration study with an appropriate freshwater and saltwater species is required

TABLE 21.4
Summary of the Aquatic Toxicity Test Requirements by Regulatory Guidelines

Regulatory Guidelines	Type of Testing Required
Clean Water Act (CWA)	Aquatic Tests for the Protection of Surface Waters
EPA NPDES Regulations	Effluent Biomonitoring Studies
	Toxicity Identification and Reduction Evaluations
Water Quality Standards	Aquatic Test for the Development of Water Quality Criteria (WQC)
Toxic Substances Control Act (TSCA)	Industrial and Specialty Chemicals: Aquatic Assessments
Premanufacture Notification, PMN	Algae, daphnid and other fish species
Section Four Test Rule	Data set requirements may include mulitple acutes with fish, algae, and invertebrates, freshwater and marine; followed by one to three chronic or partial life-cycle studies; a sediment study with midge and a bioconcentration study may be required if low $K_{ow} > 3.0$
TSCA Aquatic Test Guidelines Number:	
795.120	*Hyalella azteca* flow-through acute
797.1050	Algal toxicity test (*Selenastrum capricornutum*)
797.1160	Duckweed acute (*Lemna* sp.)
797.1300	*Daphnia magna* acute test
797.1310	Gammaraid acute test (*Gammarus* sp.)
797.1330	*Daphnia magna* chronic test
797.1400	Fish acute test (freshwater and marine)
797.1520	Fish bioconcentration test (bluegill, fathead minnow, rainbow trout)
797.1600	Fish early life stage test (fathead minnow, rainbow trout, sheephead minnow)
797.1800	Oyster shell deposition test
797.1830	Oyster bioconcentration study
797.1930	Mysid shrimp acute test
797.1950	Mysid shrimp chronic test
797.1970	Penaeid shrimp acute test
Adams et al. (1985)[57]	Midge partial life cycle test with sediments
Federal Insecticide, Fungicide and Rodenticide Act (FIFRA)	
Subdivision E Wildlife and Aquatic Organisms (Aquatic Test Guideline Number):	
72-1	Acute test for freshwater fish
72-2	Acute test for freshwater invertebrates
72-3	Acute test for estuarine and marine organisms
72-4a	Fish early life stage study
72-4b	Aquatic invertebrate life cycle studies
72-5	Life cycle test if fish
72-6	Aquatic organism accumulation tests
72-7	Simulated or actual field tests for aquatic organisms (mesocosms)
Food and Drug Administration (FDA)	New Drug Environmental Assessments
Environmental Effects test number:	
4.01	Algal test
4.08	*Daphnia magna* acute toxicity
4.09	*Daphnia magna* chronic toxicity
4.10	*Hyalella azteca* acute toxicity
4.11	Freshwater fish acute toxicity
4.12	Earthworm subacute toxicity

TABLE 21.4 *(Continued)*
Summary of the Aquatic Toxicity Test Requirements by Regulatory Guidelines

Regulatory Guidelines	Type of Testing Required
Organisation of Economic Cooperation and Development (OECD) and European Economic Community (EEC)	European Community Aquatic Testing Requirements
Aquatic Effects Testing;	
201	Algal growth inhibition test
202	*Daphnia magna* acute immobilization test and reproduction test
C2	Acute toxicity in *Daphnia magna*
203	Fish, acute toxicity test
204	Fish, prolonged toxicity test: 14-day study
210	Fish, early life-stage toxicity test
211	*Daphia magna* reproduction test
212	Fish, short-term toxicity test on embryo and sac-fry stages
215	Fish, juvenile growth test
305	Bioconcentration: flow-through fish test

TABLE 21.5
Summary of Published EPA, ASTM, and EC Methods for Conducting Sediment Toxicity Tests

Agency	Test Description	Reference ID
EPA	Methods for Measuring the Toxicity and Bioaccumulation of Sediment-Associated Contaminants with Freshwater Invertebrates	EPA/600/R-99/064
ASTM	Guide for Conducting 10-day Static Sediment Toxicity Tests with Marine and Estuarine Amphipods	ASTM E 1367-92
	Guide for Conducting Sediment Toxicity Tests with Freshwater Invertebrates	ASTM E 1383-93a
	Guide for Collection, Storage, Characterization, and Manipulation of Sediments for Toxicological Testing	ASTM E 1391-90
	Guide for Conducting Biological Tests with Sediment	ASTM E 1525-93
	Standard Test Methods for Measuring the Toxicity of Sediment-Associated Contaminants with Freshwater Invertebrates	ASTM E 1706-95b
	Standard Guide for Conducting Sediment Toxicity Tests with Marine and Estaurine Ploychaetous Annelids	ASTM E 1611
	Standard Guide for Determination of Bioaccumulation of Sediment-Associated Contaminants by Benthic Invertebrates	ASTM E 1688-97a
EC	Acute Test for Sediment Toxicity Using Marine and Estuarine Amphipods	EPS 1/RM/26
	Test for Survival and Growth in Sediment Using Freshwater Midge Larvae *Chironomus tentans* or *riparius*	EPS 1/RM/32
	Test for Survival and Growth in Sediment Using Freshwater Amphipod *Hyalella azteca*	EPS 1/RM/33
	Test for Survival and Growth for Sediment Using a Marine Ploychaete Worm	EPS 1/RM/**
	Reference Method for Determining Acute Lethality of Sediments to Estuarine or Marine Amphipods	EPS 1/RM/35
	Reference Method for Determining Sediment Toxicity Using Luminescent Bacteria	EPS 1/RM/**

TABLE 21.6
Useful Internet Web Sites for Standardized Toxicity Test Methods

Organisation of Economic Cooperation and Development (OECD)
  Main Web site: www.oecd.org/
  Guidelines for the Testing of Chemicals: www.oecd.ehs/test/testlist.htm

U.S. Environmental Protection Agency (U.S. EPA)
  Main Web site: www.epa.gov/
  Index to EPA Test Methods: www.epa.gov/epahome/index/

American Society for Testing and Materials (ASTM)
  Main Web site: www.astm.org/
  Search for test methods: www.astm.org/cgi-bin/SoftCart.exe/STORE/store.htm?E+mystore

U.S. Geologic Survey (USGC) Columbia Environmental Research Center (CERC): related Toxicity Test Method information
  Main Web site: www.cerc.usgs.gov/
  Sediment methods: www.cerc.usgs.gov/pubs/sedtox/index.htm

International Organisation for Standardization (ISO)
  Main Web site: www.iso.ch/
  International Standards: www.iso.ch/cate/cat.html

SECTION 3. WILDLIFE TOXICITY TESTING

Avian toxicity testing protocols were first utilized by the U.S. Fish and Wildlife Service as a consequence of wildlife losses in the 1950s because of the increased use of DDT and other pesticides. The first testing protocols focused on single-dose acute oral toxicities with lethality as the major end point; Table 21.7 shows acute avian sensitivities to certain organophosphorus pesticides of widely variable mammalian toxicity.[14] Further protocol development resulted in subacute 5-day dietary tests, which, along with the single acute oral dose tests, are currently required by the EPA for regulatory purposes under the Federal Insecticide, Fungicide, and Rodenticide Act (FIFRA) in support of pesticide registration and also under the Toxic Substances Control Act (TSCA) (Table 21.8). Figure 21.2 summarizes the protocols used in avian toxicity testing, including acute, subacute, subchronic, chronic, developmental, field, and behavioral tests of avian wildlife toxicity.[15] The avian subchronic dietary toxicity test was developed as an extension of the subacute test as a precursor to full-scale reproductive studies, but is not routinely required for regulatory purposes. Subchronic testing has been applied to compare the sublethal effects of different chemical forms including hepatotoxicity, and to study delayed neurotoxicity of certain organophosphorus insecticides. Avian chronic toxicity tests are designed with reproduction as the primary end point and are required for both waterfowl and upland gamebirds during chemical registration (see Avian reproduction test in Table 21.8). Persistent chemicals such as chlorinated hydrocarbons require relatively long-term exposures (at least 10 weeks) in advance of breeding, whereas shorter-term exposures may be utilized for less-persistent chemicals such as organophosphorus insecticides. Avian terrestrial field studies are basically of two types: (1) screening studies to ascertain whether impacts are occurring, and (2) definitive studies to estimate the magnitude.

Single-dose avian embryotoxicity and teratogenicity tests were developed, in part, to assess the potential contaminant hazard of external exposure of birds' eggs. Results of these tests with multiple species and chemicals have revealed differential toxicities of a spectrum of chemicals and sensitivities among species.[16] Table 21.9 summarizes the effects of herbicides applied by this exposure route. Developmental toxicity testing has also focused on the vulnerability of "neonatal" nestling altricial birds, as shown in kestrels and starlings, following oral ingestion of a variety of environmental contaminants (Table 21.10).[15]

Additionally, behavioral testing in field and pen studies has documented aberrations in wildlife behavior such as changes in nest attentiveness, brood behavior, and increased vulnerability to predation. Response time to maternal call, avoidance of fright stimulus, tests of operant learning ability, as well as time–activity budgets, have been successfully applied to laboratory studies.

Laboratory studies with environmental contaminants and mammalian wildlife have been limited compared with avian studies. Mammalian toxicity data of EPA FIFRA (Tier 1) has consisted largely of laboratory rat data for pesticide registration, whereas Tier 2 testing requires a dietary LC_{50} or acute oral LD_{50} study with a nonendangered representative species likely to be exposed, quite often a microtine rodent (see Table 21.8). Regulatory test guidelines for other terrestrial organisms including insects, plants, microbes, and earthworms are summarized in Table 21.8.

TABLE 21.7
Acute Avian Toxicity Testing of Organophosphorus Pesticides of Widely Variable Mammalian Toxicity

	Single-Dose Oral LD_{50}		
Pesticide	Rat[a]	Pheasant[b]	Blackbird[c]
Phorate	2	7	1
Azinphos-methyl	13	75	8
Ethion	65	1297	45
Dimethoate	215	20	7
Fenitrothion	740	26	25
Temephos	8600	35	42

[a] Sherman strain male laboratory rats, 3 months old, $n = 50$ to 60 per test.
[b] Farm-reared male and female ring-necked pheasants, 3 to 4 months old, $n = 8$ to 29 per test.
[c] Wild-captured pen-conditioned male and female red-winged blackbirds, adult, $n = 8$ to 28 per test.

Source: Adapted from Hill.[14]

TABLE 21.8
Summary of Ecological Effects Test Guidelines for Terrestrial Wildlife and Other Terrestrial Organisms

OPPTS[a] No.	Name of Test	OTS[b]	OPP[c]	OECD[d]	EPA Pub. No.
	Terrestrial Wildlife Tests				
850.2100	Avian acute oral toxicity test	797.2175	71-1	None	712-C-96-139
850.2200	Avian dietary toxicity test	797.2050	71-2	205	712-C-96-140
850.2300	Avian reproduction test	797.2130, .2150	71-4	206	712-C-96-141
850.2400	Wild mammal acute toxicity	None	71-3	None	712-C-96-142
850.2450	Terrestrial (soil-core) microcosm test	797.3775	None	None	712-C-96-143
850.2500	Field testing for terrestrial wildlife	None	71-5	None	712-C-96-144
	Beneficial Insects and Invertebrates Tests				
850.3020	Honeybee acute contact toxicity	None	141-1	None	712-C-96-147
850.3030	Honeybee toxicity of residues on foliage	None	141-2	None	712-C-96-148
850.3040	Field testing for pollinators	None	141-5	None	712-C-96-150

TABLE 21.8 *(Continued)*
Summary of Ecological Effects Test Guidelines for Terrestrial Wildlife and Other Terrestrial Organisms

Nontarget Plants Tests (except aquatic)					
850.4000	Background — nontarget plant testing	None	120-1	None	712-C-96-151
850.4025	Target area phytotoxicity	None	121-1	None	712-C-96-152
850.4100	Terrestrial plant toxicity, Tier I (seedling emergence)	None	122-1	None	712-C-96-153
850.4150	Terrestrial plant toxicity, Tier I (vegetative vigor)	None	122-1	None	712-C-96-163
850.4200	Seed germination/root elongation toxicity test	797.2750	122-1	None	712-C-96-154
850.4225	Seedling emergence, Tier II	797.2750	123-1	None	712-C-96-363
850.4230	Early seedling growth toxicity test	797.2800	123-1	None	712-C-96-347
850.4250	Vegetative vigor, Tier II	797.2750	123-1	None	712-C-96-364
850.4300	Terrestrial plants field study, Tier III	None	124-1	None	712-C-96-155
850.4600	Rhizobium-legume toxicity	797.2900	None	None	712-C-96-158
850.4800	Plant uptake and translocation test	797.2850	None	None	712-C-96-159
Toxicity to Microorganisms Tests					
850.5100	Soil microbial community toxicity test	797.3700	None	None	712-C-96-161
Chemical Specific Tests					
850.6200	Earthworm subchronic toxicity test	795.150	None	207	712-C-96-167
850.6800	Modified activated sludge, respiration inhibition test for sparingly soluble chemicals	795.170	None	209	712-C-96-168
Field Test Data Reporting					
850.7100	Data reporting for environmental chemistry methods	None	None	None	712-C-96-348

[a] Office of Pollution Prevention and Toxics.
[b] Office of Toxic Substances (for TSCA).
[c] Office of Pesticide Programs (for FIFRA).
[d] Organisation for Economic Cooperation and Development.

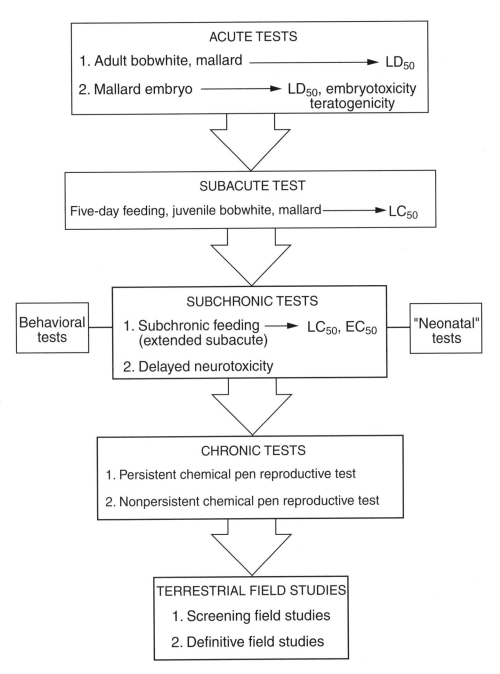

FIGURE 21.2 Protocols used in avian toxicity testing, which include acute, subacute, subchronic, chronic, developmental, field, and behavioral tests. The avian subchronic dietary toxicity test was developed as an extension of the subacute test as a precursor to full-scale reproductive studies, but is not routinely required for regulatory purposes. Avian chronic toxicity tests are designed with reproduction as the primary end point and are required for both waterfowl and upland gamebirds during chemical registration. (Adapted from Hoffman, D.J., Wildlife toxicity testing, in *Handbook of Ecotoxicology*, Hoffman.[15])

TABLE 21.9

Toxicity Testing of Herbicides by Application to Bird Eggs[a]

Herbicide Formulation	Species	Effects
Amitrole (Amitrol T®)	Mallard	LC_{50} = 211 g/l; stunted growth
Atrazine (Aatrex® 4L)	Mallard	LC_{50} > 479 g/l; not teratogenic
Bromoyxnil + MCPA (Bronate®)	Mallard	LC_{50} = 9 g/l; eye defects; edema; stunted growth
2,4-D (isoctyl ester)	Chicken, ring-necked pheasant	No apparent effects at 6 g/l
2,4-D (unspecified formulation)	Chicken, Japanese quail, gray partridge	Abnormal gonads; stunted growth; fused vertebrae at 3.75 ml/l
2,4-D (Hedonal®)	Japanese quail	No apparent effects at 4 l/ha (conc. was 500 g/l)
2,4-D (U-46-D-Fluid)	Ring-necked pheasant, Japanese quail	Decreased hatching at 30× normal application, not teratogenic
2,4-D (Esteron® 99)	Chicken	No apparent effects at 15 g/l
2,4-D (butyl ester)	Chicken	LD_{50} = 5 mg/egg; motor dysfunction; altered brain biochemistry
2,4-D (dimethylamine salt)	Mallard	LC_{50} = 230 g/l; not teratogenic
Dalapon (Dowpon® M)	Mallard	LC_{50} > 449 g/l; not teratogenic
Dicamba (Banvel®)	Mallard	LC_{50} > 240 g/l; eye defects; stunted growth
Fosamine ammonium (Krenite®)	Northern bobwhite, mallards	More reduced hatching in mallards than bobwhite at 65 g/l; not highly teratogenic
Glyphosate (Roundup®)	Mallard	LC_{50} = 213 g/l; not teratogenic
Methyldiclofop (Hoelon® 3EC)	Mallard	LC_{50} = 12 g/l; eye defects
Paraquat	Chicken, Japanese quail	4 g/l caused mortality and defects of the lung
Paraquat (Gramoxone®)	Japanese quail	0.5 g/l decreased hatching success
Paraquat (Ortho® paraquat CL)	Mallard	LC_{50} = 1.8 g/l; brain defects; edema; stunted growth
Pichloram (Tordon® 10K)	Mallard	LC_{50} = 120 g/l; stunted growth
Prometron (Pramitol® 25E)	Mallard	LC_{50} = 46 g/l; edema; stunted growth
Propanil (Stampede® 3E)	Mallard	LC_{50} = 8 g/l; limb and neck defects
2,4,5-T (unspecified formulation)	Chicken	4 g/l caused embryonic mortality; growth inhibition; abnormal gonads
2,4,5-T (Tormona® 80)	Japanese quail, ring-necked pheasant	Decreased hatching at 30× normal application; not teratogenic
2,4,5-T (Esteron® 245)	Chicken	No effects apparent at 15 g/l
2,4,5-T (isoctyl ester)	Mallard	LC_{50} = 127 g/l; not teratogenic
Trifluralin (Treflan®)	Mallard	LC_{50} = 2 g/l; bill defects, stunted growth
Trifluralin (Treflan®)	Northern bobwhite	Hatching success not affected but hatching weight lower at 38 g/l; decreased ratios of muscle and liver DNA to protein

[a] Herbicides were applied by immersion or spraying of eggs in these studies.

Source: Adapted from Hoffman.[16]

TABLE 21.10

"Neonatal" Toxicity Testing of Environmental Contaminants in Nestling Birds

Species	Exposure Method	Chemical	Observation Period	Effects
American kestrel	Daily oral	Lead, metallic	Days 1–10	525 mg/kg, high mortality; 125 mg/kg, reduced growth; 25 mg/kg, altered physiology
	Daily oral	Paraquat	Days 1–10	60 mg/kg, high mortality; 10–25 mg/kg, reduced growth, altered physiology

TABLE 21.10 *(Continued)*
"Neonatal" Toxicity Testing of Environmental Contaminants in Nestling Birds

	Daily oral	Bifenox	Days 1–10	500 mg/kg, high mortality, 250 mg/kg, reduced growth, altered physiology
	Daily oral	Nitrofen	Days 1–10	500 mg/kg, complete mortality; 250 mg/kg, reduced growth; 50 mg/kg, altered physiology
	Daily oral	Oxyfluorfen	Days 1–10	500 mg/kg, few effects
European starling	Single oral (day 5 or 15)	Dicrotophos	24 h postdose	Day 5 LD_{50} = 4.9 mg/kg; day 15 LD_{50} = 9.0 mg/kg; reduced growth, brain cholinesterase
	Single oral	Diazinon	24 h postdose	Day 1 LD_{50} =13 mg/kg; fledgling LD_{50} = 145 mg/kg
Herring gull	Single oral (3–4 weeks old)	Crude oil	For 9 days	0.3 mg/kg reduced growth, altered physiology
Black guillemot	Single oral	Crude oil (weathered)	For 22 days	0.1–0.2 ml reduced growth, altered physiology

Source: Adapted from Hoffman.[15]

SECTION 4. BIOMARKERS USED IN AQUATIC AND TERRESTRIAL MONITORING

Measures of exposure and effect may be quantified at a variety of levels of biological organization (molecular, cellular, organ system, organismal, population, and even biotic community). There have been efforts to classify toxicological measures with terminology linking them to levels of biological organization. The term *biomarker* has been used most broadly to encompass "any biological response to an environmental chemical at or below the level of the individual demonstrating a departure from the normal status." This definition encompasses biochemical, physiological, histological, morphological, and behavioral measurements. This is the most generally accepted definition, and will be used in this chapter. Ideally, all such response end points are contaminant dose– and exposure time–dependent phenomena. Population level effects are referred to as "bioindicator" responses, and changes at the community and ecosystem level are categorized as "ecological indicators."

Biomarkers may be used to assess chemical exposure and the cumulative, adverse effects of toxicants on biota *in situ*.[17] Biomarkers in ecological risk assessment have been used to assess ecosystem integrity (Figure 21.3). Biomarkers also play an important role in the evaluation of the effectiveness of remedial action to alleviate pollution.

When selecting appropriate biomarkers for such studies, there are many important factors that must be accounted for since they can affect the outcome, including species sensitivity, physiological condition, behavioral traits, and the time, rate, and frequency of chemical exposure to the ecosytem. As well as the ability to measure direct toxicological effects of chemical exposure, equally important are indirect effects (Figure 21.4). For example, for many avian species the reproductive season corresponds with peaks in invertebrate populations, which also occurs at the same time insects with insecticides are treated or unwanted vegetation may be sprayed with herbicides. All of these factors may impair the chance of successful reproduction and growth of young by decreasing the food supply, as well as decreasing important ground cover in nesting areas, thus increasing the likelihood of exposure to predators.[11]

Of the hundreds of potential biomarker end points that have been used in laboratory studies, few have gained widespread application in ecotoxicological "field" investigations. Table 21.11 summarizes ones used successfully in field studies. At the molecular level of organization, these include inhibition of esterases, porphyria, adduct formation (DNA and hemoglobin), cytochrome P-450 induction, inhibition of delta-aminolevulinic acid dehydratase, oxidative stress (shifts in ratios of oxidized:reduced glutathione concentration and associated enzymes), alterations in concentrations of hormones, metallothionein,, and increased activities of plasma/serum enzymes released as a consequence of cellular damage.[18] At the cellular and tissue level, substantial literature exists describing contaminant-linked histopathology, cytogenetic and cytotoxic end points, as well as an emerging literature on immunological end points. A few remarkable organ-system and whole-animal end points (e.g., gross anomalies such as bird deformity, teratogenesis, eggshell abnormalities, and behavior) have been linked to contaminant exposure. Many of these end points are sensitive, precise and specific "indicators of exposure" to various contaminants, although even fewer end points have well-documented association with population-level effects in wildlife. Select reviews on the use of biomarkers in ecotoxicology include those by Hugget et al.,[19] Fossi and Leonzio,[20] and Melancon.[21]

THE USE OF BIOMARKERS TO ASSESS ECOSYSTEM INTEGRITY

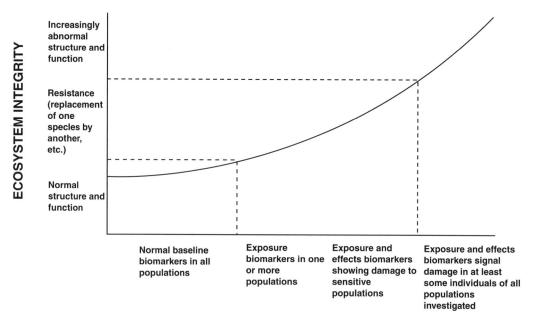

FIGURE 21.3 Biomarkers in ecological risk assessment have been used to help assess ecosystem integrity through association with such changes as replacement of sensitive species by more tolerant species, followed by eventual disruption of structure and function of the ecosystem. (From Depledge, M.H. and Fossi, M.C., *Ecotoxicology* 3, 161–172, 1994. With permission.)

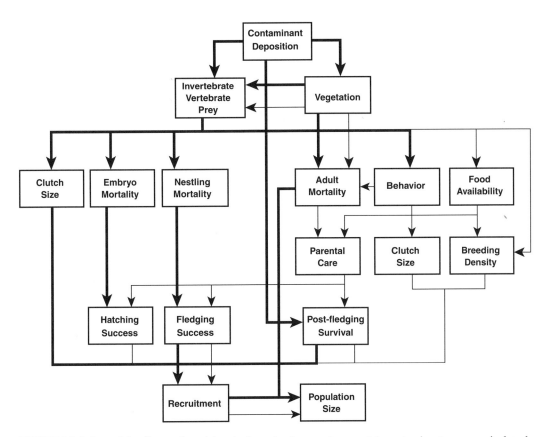

FIGURE 21.4 Potential effects of agrichemicals and other environmental contaminants on survival and reproduction of wild birds. Indirect effects, such as changes in invertebrate prey populations and vegetation, are as equally important as ones that measure direct toxicological effects of chemical exposure. All of these factors may impair the chance of successful reproduction and growth of young birds by decreasing the food supply and important ground cover vegetation in nesting areas. (Adapted from Grue et al.[11])

TABLE 21.11
Biomarkers for Environmental Monitoring

Biomarker	Biological Response	Pollutant[a]	Invasive Techniques	Nondestructive Techniques	Temporal Occurrence[b]	Reliability Index[c]
Esterases	Enzymer inhibition	Organophosphates and carbamates	Brain	Blood	Early	S, D, P
Porphyrins	Metabolic disorder	Toxic metals, PHAHs	Liver	Blood, excreta, feathers	Middle	S, D, P
Cytochrome P-450	Enzyme induction	PAHs, PHAHs	Liver	Skin, mucosa, blood	Early	S, D
Blood chemistry	Various enzymes	Toxic metals, PHAHs, organophosphates		Blood	Middle	S, D
Retinols	Retinol changes	PHAHs	Liver	Blood	Early	S
Thyroid function	Thyroid function alteration	PHAHs	Thyroid	Blood	Middle	S
delta-Aminolevulinic acid dehydratase	Inhibition	Toxic metals		Blood	Early	S, D, P
Immunotoxicology	Various	Toxic metals, PAHs, PHAHs, organophosphates	Lymphatic cells	Blood	Middle late	S
Hemoglobin adducts	Adducts	PAHs, PHAHs		Blood	Early	S, D
Stress proteins	Protein induction	Toxic metals, PHAHs		Blood	Early	S
DNA strand breakage	Strand breaks	PAHs, PHAHs	Several tissues	Blood, skin	Early	S
Adducts	Adducts	PAHs, PHAHs	Several tissues	Blood, skin	Early	S,D,P
Sister chromatid exchange	Chromosome	PAHs, PHAHs	Several tissues	Blood	Middle Late	S,D,P

[a] Pollutants: PAHs = polynuclear aromatic hydrocarbons; PHAHs = polyhalogenated aromatic hydrocarbons.
[b] Temporal occurrences: early — hours to days; middle — days to weeks/months; late — weeks/months to years.
[c] Reliability Index: S = signal of potential problem; D = definitive indicator of type or class of pollutant; P = predictive indicator of a long-term adverse effect.

Source: Adapted from Fossi et al.[18]

SECTION 5. CONTAMINANT EFFECTS

Table 21.12 lists the principal contaminants for which critical concentrations and diagnostic guidelines have been established for wild terrestrial vertebrates.[22]

TABLE 21.12
Principal Contaminants for Which Critical Concentrations and Diagnostic Guidelines Have Been Established for Wild Terrestrial Vertebrates

Organochlorine Pesticides
  Chlordecone
  p,p'-DDE
  Dicofol
  Dieldrin
  Endrin
  Heptachlor epoxide
  Hexachlorobenzene
  Hexachlorocyclohexane
  Methoxychlor
  Mirex
  Oxychlordane
  Toxaphene
Organophosphorus and Carbamate Pesticides

Polychlorinated biphenyls
  Total aroclors
  Coplanar congeners
Dioxins
Dibenzofurans
Petroleum hydrocarbons
  Crude oils
  Oil fractions
Metals, Metalloids, and Trace Elements
  Cadmium
  Fluoride
  Lead
  Mercury
  Selenium

Source: Adapted from Rattner et al.[22]

A. HEAVY METALS

1. Lead

Lead exposure in birds results from direct consumption of spent lead shot, consumption of shot or bullet fragments in food items, ingestion of lead fishing sinkers, and lead-based paints, and environmental contamination of urban and industrial areas. Lead-poisoning mortality has occurred in waterfowl and at least 30 species of birds other than waterfowl. Despite restrictions on the use of lead shot for hunting waterfowl and coots in the United States, lead shot and other lead-containing ammunition continue to be used for hunting many wild species.[23] Ingestion of merely one number 4 lead shot (about 230 mg lead) can be lethal to waterfowl under certain conditions. Lead exposure criteria include presence of lead shot in gizzards, lead residues in body tissues, and blood enzyme measurements as illustrated in Table 21.13. Tissue lead concentrations corresponding to background contamination, subclinical poisoning, clinical poisoning, and severe clinical poisoning[24] are presented in Table 21.14. Considerable toxicity data exist for Falconiformes, Columbiformes, and Galliformes, allowing categorization of lead residues according to the increasing severity of effects: (1) subclinical, the range of residues associated with physiological effects only; (2) toxic, the approximate threshold concentration consistent with the development of clinical signs of lead toxicosis; and (3) compatible with death, the approximate threshold concentration associated with mortality in field or laboratory cases of lead poisoning (Table 21.15). [25]

TABLE 21.13
Some Criteria for Determining Lead Problem Areas for Waterfowl

Endpoint/Measurement	Samples Required	Examination Process	Evaluation of Data
Mortality	Whole carcasses	Postmortem examination and laboratory assays, including microbiology and toxicology	Diagnosis of lead poisoning as a cause of mortality depends on a combination of pathological findings supported by appropriate toxicological results; liver is most often used for chemical analysis; lead values of 8 μg/g (wet weight) and above are consistent with lead intoxication when supported by pathology
Lead concentrations in body tissues	Liver, kidney, and blood	Liver and kidney are removed from dead birds; chemical analysis is usually by atomic absorption spectrophotometry	Values indicate the amount of lead present; concentrations of 2 μg/g or greater for liver and 0.2 μg/g or greater for blood should be considered elevated; these data must be supported by pathological findings before confidence can be placed in a lead poisoning diagnosis
Lead shot in gizzard samples	Intact gizzards	Examination of gizzard contents for presence or absence of lead shot	Presence of lead shot reflects exposure just prior to sampling and constitutes an index for lead poisoning risk; shot ingestion may be independent of cause of death, particularly if dissolution and absorption have not occurred; one or more ingested shot in 5% or more of gizzards examined is the threshold criteria for potential problem areas
Measurement of delta-aminolevulinic acid dehydratase (delta-ALAD) in soft tissues	Blood, brain, or liver	Red blood cells examined most often; analysis is usually by spectrophotometry	Inhibition of delta-ALAD is a sensitive indicator of lead exposure; suppression below normal values can occur within 24 h of lead absorption; recovery of delta-ALAD requires a month or more; the degree of suppression is directly correlated with blood lead levels
Measurement of protoporphyrin IX concentration in blood	Drop of blood	Fluorometric measurement of red blood cells	Concentration of protoporphyrin IX results from lead inhibition of heme synthetase, an enzyme responsible for incorporation of iron into protoporphyrin IX; values above 40 μg/dl indicate exposure to lead; recovery to normal levels occurs within a month following exposure; high values are correlated with body function impairment and reflect toxicity
Amount of lead shot in environment	Substrate samples	Soil and bottom samples taken at predetermined depths	The amount of shot present represents the potential for lead shot ingestion, but variables influence its probability of occurrence
Hunting pressure	Information on hunter-use days or birds shot per unit area	Calculation of relative amounts of lead shot deposited	Provides an index of potential lead shot availability to waterfowl; many variables impact the probability of lead shot ingestion and subsequent intoxication

Source: Adapted from Interpretation of Criteria Commonly Used to Determine Lead Poisoning Problem Areas, U.S. Department of the Interior, Fish and Wildlife Service, Fish and Wildlife Leaflet 2. Washington, D.C., 1985.[23]

TABLE 21.14
Tissue Lead Concentration Thresholds of Lead
Exposure and Poisoning in Waterfowl

Tissue Lead	Threshold Concentration
Blood (µg/dl)	>20 (elevated)
	>40 (indicative of poisoning)
	>50 (acute toxicity)
Liver (ppm of wet weight)	>2 (elevated)
	>6 (indicative of poisoning)
	>6–20 (acute exposure and absorption)
	>7 (poisoning)
	>8 (consistent with signs of poisoning)
	>12.5 (poisoning)
Bone (ppm of dry weight)	>20 (excessive exposure and absorption)

Source: Adapted from Pain.[24]

TABLE 21.15
Interpretation of Tissue Lead Residues (ppm
wet weight) in Falconiformes, Columbiformes,
and Galliformes[a]

Order	Blood	Liver	Kidney
Falconiformes			
Subclinical	0.2–1.5	2–4	2–5
Toxic	>1	>3	>3
Compatible with death	>5	>5	>5
Columbiformes			
Subclinical	0.2–2.5	2–6	2–20
Toxic	>2	>6	>15
Compatible with Death	>10	>20	>40
Galliformes			
Subclinical	0.2–3	2–6	2–20
Toxic	>5	>6	>15
Compatible with Death	>10	>15	>50

[a] Subclinical = physiological effects, e.g., ALAD depression, only, with no overt clinical signs; toxic = clinical signs, such as muscle wasting, green diarrhea, weakness, anemia, muscular incoordination; Compatible with death = residues associated with mortality in field reports of lead poisoning or in experimental dosing studies.

Source: Adapted from Franson.[25]

2. Methylmercury

Recent reports of high mercury concentrations in fish, particularly in newly flooded reservoirs and in low-alkalinity lakes have renewed concerns about mercury in the environment.[26] Neurotoxicity seems to be the most probable chronic response of wild adult fish to dietary methylmercury, even though other effects have been observed in laboratory studies. In the brain, concentrations of 7 μg/g wet weight or greater probably cause severe, potentially lethal effects. In mercury-sensitive species, such as the walleye, brain tissue concentrations of 3 μg/g wet weight or greater probably indicate significant toxic effects (Table 21.16). For axial muscle tissue, field studies indicate that residues of 6 to 20 μg/g wet weight are associated with toxicity. Sublethal and lethal effects on fish embryos are associated with mercury residues in eggs that are much lower than (perhaps 1 to 10% of) the residues associated with toxicity in adult fish. In birds and mammals, methylmercury is primarily neurotoxic, damaging the central nervous system. For some species of birds, such as mallards, adverse effects on reproduction have been associated with 3 mg of Hg/kg of diet (Table 21.17).[27] Additional interpretation on mercury poisoning in wildlife is provided by Heinz.[28]

TABLE 21.16
Total Mercury Concentrations in Tissues of Fish Exhibiting Symptoms of Methylmercury Toxicity

Type of Study and Species of Fish	Location or Mode and Duration of Exposure	Hg Concentration (μg/g wet weight)				Toxic Effect(s)[a]
		Brain	Liver	Muscle	Whole Body	
		Laboratory Studies				
Walleye	Diet (42–63 d)	3–6	6–14	5–8	—	Onset of mortality
						Fish emaciated
						(–) locomotor activity
						(–) coordination
						(–) appetite
	Diet (240–314 d)	15–40	18–50	15–45	—	(+) mortality
Rainbow trout	Diet (105 d)	—	—	12–23	—	(–) growth
	Diet (84 d)	—	—	—	30–35	Darkened skin
						Lethargic behavior
	Diet (84 d)	—	—	—	10–30	(–) appetite
						(–) growth
	Diet (270 d)	16–30	26–68	20–28	19	(–) appetite
						(–) activity
						(–) visual acuity
						(–) growth
						Darkened skin
						Loss of equilibrium
	Water (4 μg/l)[b] (30–98 d)	7–32	32–114	9–52	—	Death, preceded by (–) appetite and (–) activity
	Water (9 μg/l)[b] (12–33 d)	—	—	—	4–27	Death, preceded by (–) appetite and (–) activity
Brook trout	Water (2.9 μg/l)[b] (273 d)	42	58	24	24	Mortality, preceded by loss of appetite, muscle spasms, and deformities
	Water (0.93 μg/l)[b] (273 d)	17	24	10	5–7	(+) mortality
						(–) growth
						Sluggish behavior

TABLE 21.16 *(Continued)*
Total Mercury Concentrations in Tissues of Fish Exhibiting Symptoms of Methylmercury Toxicity

Type of Study and Species of Fish	Location or Mode and Duration of Exposure	Hg Concentration (µg/g wet weight)				Toxic Effect(s)[a]
		Brain	Liver	Muscle	Whole Body	
						Deformities
	Water (0.27 µg/l)[b] (273 d)	5	8	5	3	None observed
	Field Studies					
Nibea schlegeli	Minamata Bay	—	—	8–15	—	Fish enfeebled
Latcolabrax japonicus	Minamata Bay	—	—	17	—	Fish enfeebled
Sparus macrocephalus	Minamata Bay	—	—	24	—	Fish enfeebled
Scomberomorus niphonicus	Minamata Bay	—	15	9	—	Fish enfeebled
Striped mullet *Mugil cephalus*	Minamata Bay	—	—	11	—	Fish enfeebled
Cardinalfish *Apogon* sp.	Minamata Bay	—	—	19	—	Fish enfeebled
Northern pike	Clay Lake, Ontario	—	—	6–16	—	Fish emaciated, with biochemical symptoms of starvation and (–) immunity

[a] An increase is indicated by (+); a decrease is indicated by (–).

[b] Concentration of mercury in water, administered as methylmercuric chloride.

Source: Adapted from Wiener and Spry.[26]

TABLE 21.17
Lethality of Mercury to Birds

Species	Form of Mercury	Exposure	Concentration (mg Hg/kg body weight)	Effects
Chukar (*Alectoris chukar*)	Ethyl	Acute oral	26.9	LD_{50}
Mallard (*Anas platyrhynchos*)	Methyl	Acute oral	2.2–23.5	LD_{50}
	Ethyl	Acute oral	75.7	LD_{50}
	Phenyl	Acute oral	524.7	LD_{50}
Northern bobwhite (*Colinus virginianus*)	Methyl	Acute oral	23.8	LD_{50}
Coturnix (*Coturnix japonica*)	Methyl	Acute oral	11.0–33.7	LD_{50}
	Inorganic	Acute oral	26.0–54.0	LD_{50}
	Ethyl	Acute oral	21.4	LD_{50}
	Inorganic	Acute oral	31.1	LD_{50}
Rock dove (*Columba livia*)	Ethyl	Acute oral	22.8	LD_{50}
Fulvous whistling duck (*Dendrocygna bicolor*)	Methyl	Acute oral	37.8	LD_{50}
Chicken (*Gallus domesticus*)	Phenyl	Acute oral	60.0	LD_{50}

TABLE 21.17 *(Continued)*
Lethality of Mercury to Birds

Species	Form of Mercury	Exposure	Concentration (mg Hg/kg body weight)	Effects
House sparrow (*Passer domesticus*)	Methyl	Acute oral	12.6–37.8	LD_{50}
Gray partridge (*Perdix perdix*)	Ethyl	Acute oral	17.6	LD_{50}
Ring-necked pheasant (*Phasianus colchicus*)	Ethyl	Acute oral	11.5	LD_{50}
	Methyl	Acute oral	11.5–26.8	LD_{50}
	Phenyl	Acute oral	65.0–101.0	LD_{50}
Prairie chicken (*Tympanuchus cupido*)	Ethyl	Acute oral	11.5	LD_{50}
Mallard, hens	Methyl	Dietary (mg Hg/kg diet), for two reproductive seasons	3.0	Reduced duckling survival
Coturnix	Inorganic	Dietary, hatch to 9 weeks	32.0	LD_{0}
	Inorganic	Dietary, 5 d +7 d observation period	2956–5086	LD_{50}
	Inorganic in dry salt	Dietary, 28 d	500	LD_{86}
	Inorganic in ethanol, methanol, or water	Dietary, 28 d	500	LD_{55}
	Inorganic in caseinpremix	Dietary, 28 d	500	LD_{33}
	Methyl	Dietary, hatch to 9 weeks	4.0	LD_{0}
	Methyl	Dietary, 5 d	8.0	Some deaths
	Methyl	Dietary, 5 d +7 d observation period	31.0–47.0	LD_{50}
Zebra finch (*Poephila guttata*)	Methyl	Dietary, 77 days	2.5	LD_{50}
	Methyl	Dietary, 77 days	5.0	LD_{25}
Ring-necked pheasant	Ethyl	Dietary, 70 days	4.2	LD_{0}
	Ethyl	Dietary, 70 days	12.5	LD_{50}
	Ethyl	Dietary, 28 days	37.4	LD_{50}
	Ethyl	Dietary, 15 days	112.0	LD_{50}
Birds, 4 spp.	Methyl	Dietary, 6–11 d	40.0	LD_{33}
Birds, 3 spp.	Methyl	Dietary, 35 d	33.0	LD_{8} to LD_{90}

Source: Adapted from Eisler.[27]

3. Cadmium

Increased cadmium in the terrestrial habitats of small mammals is derived from a variety of anthropogenic sources including atmospheric deposition, the application of phosphatic fertilizers and sewage sludge to land, and disused mine waste. Field studies have shown that cadmium, whether derived from the atmosphere or soil, is commonly found in most biotic components within a terrestrial ecosystem. The concentrations of cadmium measured in wild small mammals caught in contaminated sites are elevated in many tissues and organs, but most of the body burden is in the kidney and liver (Table 21.18).[29] Kidney concentrations ranged from 2 to 90 mg of cadmium/kg of dry weight in mice and voles and were two to eight times the corresponding liver value. In shrews, liver values were usually higher, at 200 to 600 mg of cadmium/kg of dry weight as against kidney concentrations of 100 to 250 mg of cadmium/kg. Using response criteria similar to those for human cadmium exposure and using primarily laboratory experiments with rats and mice, it has been suggested that 100 mg of cadmium/kg of wet weight or 350 mg of cadmium/kg of dry weight could be considered as the critical kidney concentration on a whole-organ basis.

TABLE 21.18
Kidney and Liver Cadmium Concentrations in Species of Small Mammals from Contaminated Habitats

Species	Contaminated Site	Kidney Conc. (mg/kg dry wt)	Liver Conc. (mg/kg dry wt)	Ratio Kidney/Liver
Bank vole (*Clethrionomys glareolus*)	Dulowa Forest, Poland	29.6	12.8	2.3
	Y Fan, Pb/Zn mine, Wales	16.8	5.1	3.3
Wood mouse (*Apodemus sylvaticus*)	Smelter waste, Wales	18.0	5.5	3.3
	Minera, Pb/Zn mine, Wales	39.7	9.8	4.1
	Y Fan, Pb/Zn mine, Wales	10.3	2.49	4.1
	Cu/Cd refinery, England	41.7	18.2	2.3
	Fluorspar waste, England	1.78	0.71	2.5
Short-tailed field vole (*Microtus agretis*)	Y Fan, Pb/Zn mine, Wales	8.91	1.06	8.4
	Cu/Cd refinery, England	88.8	22.7	3.9
	Fluorspar waste, England	5.3	1.8	2.9
	Budel, The Netherlands	2.7	0.57	4.7
Meadow vole (*Microtus pennsylvanicus*)	Sludge-treated fields, USA	23[a]	7.9[a]	2.9
White-footed mouse (*Peromyscus leucopus*)	Wastewater-irrigated site, USA	2.3[a]	0.5[a]	5.0
Common shrew (*Sorex araneus*)	Cu/Cd refinery, England	253	578	0.43
	Fluorspar waste, England	158	236	0.67
	(Oct.–Nov.) Budel, The Netherlands	126	180	0.7
	(Feb.–Mar.) Budel, The Netherlands	200	268	0.75
European mole (*Talpa europea*)	Budel, The Netherlands	224	227	0.99

[a] Values changed from wet weight (dry weight = wet weight × 3.5).

Source: Adapted from Cooke.[29]

B. Selenium

Agricultural drain water, sewage sludge, fly ash from coal-fired power plants, and mining of phosphates and metal ores contribute to the selenium (Se) burden in the aquatic environment. Once in aquatic systems, selenium is readily taken up from solution by food-chain organisms and can quickly reach concentrations that are toxic to the fish and wildlife that consume them.[30] Selenium transferred to the eggs of fish from parents can result in edema, hemorrhaging, spinal deformities, and death of embryos. Reproductive success is more sensitive to selenium toxicity than are the growth and survival of juvenile and adult fish. Waterborne selenium concentrations of 2 µg/l or greater (on a total recoverable basis in 0.45-µm filtered samples) should be considered hazardous to the health and long-term survival of fish and wildlife populations because of the high potential for food-chain bioaccumulation, dietary toxicity, and reproductive effects. The dietary toxicity threshold for fish is 3 µg/g. Thresholds for tissue concentrations that affect the health and reproductive success of freshwater and anadromous fish are as follows: whole-body, 4 µg/g; skeletal muscle (skinless fillets), 8 µg/g; liver, 12 µg/g; and ovaries and eggs, 10 µg/g (Table 21.19).

In birds, historically, plant-derived Se in excess of 4 ppm in the diet of chickens was found to impair reproductive success and to be teratogenic.[31] In more recent years, adverse effects of Se in wild aquatic birds has been documented as a consequence of pollution of the aquatic environment by subsurface agricultural drain water and other sources.[32] Selenomethionine is a form of Se that wild aquatic birds are most likely exposed to since the toxic thresholds in eggs for decreased hatching success and teratogenicity from laboratory studies with mallards are very close to those derived from field studies.[33] Biological and physiological effects observed have included avian mortality, impaired reproduction and teratogenesis, and histopathological lesions with alterations in hepatic glutathione (Table 21.20).[34-42]

TABLE 21.19

Toxic Effects Thresholds for Selenium Concentrations in Water, Food Chain Organisms, and Fish Tissues

Selenium Source	Selenium Concentration[a]	Effect
Water		
Inorganic selenium	2 µg/l	Food chain bioaccumulation and reproductive failure in fish and wildlife
Organic selenium	<1 µg/l	Food chain bioaccumulation and reproductive failure in fish and wildlife
Food-chain organisms	3 µg/g	Reproductive failure in fish and wildlife
Fish tissues		
Whole body	4 µg/g	Mortality of juveniles and reproductive failure
Skeletal muscle (skinless fillets)	8 µg/g	Reproductive failure
Liver	12 µg/g	Reproductive failure
Ovary and eggs	10 µg/g	Reproductive failure

[a] Selenium concentrations in parts per billion for water; parts per million (µg/g) on a dry weight basis for food-chain organisms and fish tissues.

Source: Adapted from Lemly.[30]

TABLE 21.20
Laboratory Studies on Effects of Excess Selenium in Aquatic Birds

Species, Age	Form of Dietary Se (conc., ppm)	Observation Period	Effects	Ref.
Mallard, embryo	Sodium selenite (10)	Through hatching	0.5 ppm Se (ww) in eggs, edema and decreased hatching success, growth, plasma enzymes	34
	(25)		1.3 ppm Se (ww) in eggs, edema and decreased hatching success and growth, plasma chemistries	
	seleno-D,L-methionine (10)		4.6 ppm Se (ww) in eggs, malformations and decreased hatching, plasma chemistries	
Black-crowned night heron, embryo	seleno-D,L-methionine (10)	Through hatching	3.3 ppm Se (ww) in eggs, decreased growth, altered hepatic biochemistry	35
Mallard, duckling	Sodium selenite (10) (20) (40)	Day-old through 6 wks	5.0 ppm Se (ww) in liver, altered hepatic biochemistry; 3.2 ppm Se (ww) in liver, decreased growth, altered hepatic biochemistry; 2.8 ppm Se (ww) in liver, decreased survival and growth, plasma and hepatic biochemistries	36, 37
	seleno-D,L-methionine (10) (20) (40)	Day-old through 6 wks	4.8 ppm Se (ww) in liver, plasma and hepatic biochemistries; 26 ppm Se (ww) in liver, decreased growth, plasma and hepatic biochemistries; 68 ppm Se (ww) in liver, decreased survival and growth, altered plasma and hepatic biochemistries	36, 37
	seleno-D,L-methionine (15) (60)	4 wks	10.8, 11.6, 14.9 ppm Se (ww) in liver, decreased growth, altered plasma and hepatic biochemistries; 49, 56, 72 ppm Se (ww) in liver, decreased survival and growth, increased histopathological lesions, altered plasma and hepatic biochemistries	38–40
Mallard, adult	Sodium selenite in drinking water (3.5 mg/l)	12 wks	altered serum biochemistry	41
	Selenomethionine in drinking water (2.2 mg/l)	12 wks	5 ppm (ww) Se in liver, impaired immune function, increased serum ALT, and plasma GSH peroxidase activities	
Mallard, adult	seleno-D,L-methionine (2) (4) (8)	14 wks	2 ppm Se (ww) in liver, altered plasma biochemistry; 4 ppm Se (ww) in liver, altered plasma biochemistry; 12 ppm Se (ww) in liver, altered plasma and hepatic biochemistries	42

C. Pesticides

In the 1940s, use of the environmentally persistent lipophilic organochlorine pesticide DDT became widespread. "Long-term" dietary exposure (months to years) to this pesticide resulted in some direct mortality of juvenile and adult individuals. Its metabolite, p,p'-DDE, was readily transferred into the egg and caused the devastating population-level effects due to eggshell thinning, embryo mortality, and decreased reproductive success.[43] Table 21.21 presents residues of DDE in eggs of wild birds as related to eggshell thinning and reproductive success.

Organophosphorus and carbamate compounds are used extensively to control nuisance and disease-bearing insects and invertebrates, and even depredating vertebrate species. The mechanism of toxicity of these pesticides principally involves inhibition of esterase enzymes (particularly cholinesterases), resulting in the disruption of neural and end organ function, which can lead to death. Despite their short half-lives in the environment and in tissues of homeotherms, there is considerable documentation of unintentional exposure and poisoning of wildlife species ranging from loss of a few individuals to devastating effects on whole populations. In addition to esterase inhibition, numerous signs of intoxication have been documented in avian and mammalian wildlife.[9,10,44-46] Table 21.22 describes the physical signs and symptoms in vertebrates commonly associated with acute exposure to cholinesterase inhibitors. Although there is some evidence suggesting that birds are more sensitive to anticholinesterase pesticides than mammals, toxicity is not well correlated across these higher vertebrate taxonomic groups, as reviewed by Hill[47] and others. For example, red-winged blackbirds are clearly more sensitive than are rats to carbofuran, mexacarbate, dimethoate, and temephos, while in other instances they are equally sensitive or even more tolerant than are rats (Table 21.23). Pheasants, on the other hand, are much less sensitive than are rats to several commonly used cholinesterase-inhibiting pesticides (e.g., aldicarb, phorate, ethion, and methiocarb). Differences in sensitivity to anticholinesterase pesticides between birds and mammals are not readily explained by qualitative and/or quantitative differences in phase I and phase II metabolism. Rainbow trout and blue gill fish appear to be generally more tolerant than are birds and mammals, although the exposure route differs for aquatic vertebrates.

TABLE 21.21
Residues of DDE in Sample Eggs of Wild Birds Related to Eggshell Thinning and Reproductive Success

Species	DDE Conc. (μg/g wet weight) Associated with 20% Eggshell Thinning	Area[a]	Residues Detected (μg/g wet weight)	Young Produced per Active Nest[b]
Brown pelican (*Pelecanus occidentalis*)	8	SC[c]	<1.5	0.6 (FL),[d] 0.8 (EM)
		SC[c]	1.5–3	0.6 (FL),[d] 0.8 (EM)
		SC[c]	>3	0.0 (FL),[d] 0.6 (EM)
Great blue heron (*Ardea herodias*)	19	OR, WA	3	1.7–2.0
Black-crowned night heron (*Nycticorax nycticorax*)	54	US	<1	2.0
		US	1–4	1.7
		US	4–8	1.5
		US	8–12	1.1
		US	12–16	1.0
		US	16–25	0.8
		US	25–50	0.4
White-faced ibis (*Plegadis chihi*)	7	NV	<1	1.8
		NV	1–4	1.8
		NV	4–8	1.3
		NV	8–16	0.8
		NV	>16	0.6

TABLE 21.21 *(Continued)*
Residues of DDE in Sample Eggs of Wild Birds Related to Eggshell Thinning and Reproductive Success

Species	DDE Conc. (μg/g wet weight) Associated with 20% Eggshell Thinning	Area[a]	Residues Detected (μg/g wet weight)	Young Produced per Active Nest[b]
Osprey (*Pandion haliaetus*)	9–41	CT, NY	23[e,f,g]	0.0
		CT, NY	12[e,f,g]	1.0
		CT, NY	6[e,f,g]	2.1
		ID	14	0.0
		ID	6	1.6
Bald eagle (*Haliaeetus leucocephalus*)	60–110	US[g]	<2.2	1.0
		US[g]	2.2–3.5	1.0
		US[g]	3.6–6.2	0.5
		US[g]	6.3–11.9	0.3
		US[g]	>12	0.2
Merlin (*Falco columbarius*)	16	AB	11[e]	0.0
		AB	11[e]	1.0
		AB	6[e]	2.0
		AB	5[e]	3.0
		AB	6[e]	4.0
Peregrine falcon (*Falco peregrinus*)	15–22	AK	<15	1.8
		AK	15–30	2.0
		AK	>30	1.0
Prairie falcon (*Falco mexicanus*)	7	AB	2[e]	0.0
		AB	2[e]	1.0
		AB	2[e]	2.0
		AB	2[e]	3.0
		AB	1[e]	4.0

[a] CT, Conneticut; NY, New York; ID, Idaho; AK, Alaska; NV, Nevada; AB, Alberta and nearby areas; SC, South Carolina; US, Various locations within the United States.

[b] Young produced not adjusted for sample egg collected. Estimated mean or range of young normally fledged per nest: brown pelican, 1.1; great blue heron, 2.3; black-crowned night heron, 2.2–2.4; white-faced ibis, 1.4–3; osprey 1–2.1; bald eagle, 1.2–1.6; merlin, 3.6–4.0; peregrine falcon, 2–3.2; prairie falcon, 2.8.

[c] Sample egg either freshly laid or embryonated when collected.

[d] FL, freshly laid; EM, embryonated.

[e] Approximate adjustment from dry weight basis.

[f] Elevated levels (17 to 29 μg/g) of polychlorinated biphenyls also present.

[g] All or most eggs were collected after the fate of marked nests was determined. Production of young at each nest is based on 5-year mean.

Source: Adapted from Tables 7 and 10 in Blus.[43]

TABLE 21.22
Physical Signs and Symptoms in Vertebrates Commonly Associated with Acute Exposure to Cholinesterase Inhibitors

Sign/Symptom	Birds	Mammals	Humans
Ataraxia (induced tranquility)	✔	✔	
Ataxia	✔	✔	✔
Blindness	✔		
Blood pressure fluctuations			✔

TABLE 21.22 *(Continued)*
**Physical Signs and Symptoms in Vertebrates Commonly
Associated with Acute Exposure to Cholinesterase Inhibitors**

Convulsions	✔		✔
Cyanosis			✔
Defecation	✔		
Diarrhea	✔		✔
Dyspnea	✔	✔	✔
Epistaxis (bleeding from nares)	✔		
Exophthalmia	✔		
Fasciculation (uncoordinated muscle contraction)		✔	✔
Headaches			✔
Hyperexcitability	✔		
Incoordination	✔		
Intestinal cramps			✔
Lacrimation	✔		✔
Lethargy	✔	✔	✔
Miosis (contraction of pupils)	✔	✔	✔
Myasthenia (muscular weakness)	✔		
Mydriasis (dilation of pupils)	✔		
Nausea			✔
Nutation (nodding of the head)		✔	
Opisthotonos (head and limbs arched back)	✔		
Paresis	✔		
Phonation		✔	
Piloerection	✔		
Polydipsia (excessive thirst)	✔		
Ptosis (drooping of eyelid)	✔		
Pulomonary edema			✔
Salivation		✔	✔
Slurred speech	✔		✔
Spasmodic contraction of anal sphincter	✔		✔
Sweating			✔
Tachycardia		✔	✔
Tachypnea (rapid breathing)	✔	✔	
Tremors	✔	✔	✔
Urination			✔
Vomiting	✔		✔

Source: Adapted from Table 1 of Grue et al.[44]

TABLE 21.23
Acute Response and Toxicity Ranking of Some Anticholinesterase Pesticides in Fish, Birds, and Laboratory Rats

Pesticide	Rainbow Trout		Bluegill		Ring-Necked Pheasant		Red-Winged Blackbird		Laboratory Rat	
	Rank	LC_{50}[a]	Rank	LC_{50}[a]	Rank	LD_{50}[b,c]	Rank	LD_{50}[b,d]	Rank	LD_{50}[b,e]
Aldicarb	5	560	3	50	3	5.3	3	1.8	1	0.8
Phorate	2	13	1	2	4	7.1	2	1.0	2	2.3
Carbofuran	3	380	6	240	1	4.1	1	0.4	3	11

TABLE 21.23 *(Continued)*
Acute Response and Toxicity Ranking of Some Anticholinesterase Pesticides in Fish, Birds, and Laboratory Rats

Pesticide	Rainbow Trout		Bluegill		Ring-Necked Pheasant		Red-Winged Blackbird		Laboratory Rat	
	Rank	LC_{50}^{a}	Rank	LC_{50}^{a}	Rank	$LD_{50}^{b,c}$	Rank	$LD_{50}^{b,d}$	Rank	$LD_{50}^{b,e}$
Azinphos-methyl	1	4	2	22	7	75	6	8.5	4	13
Mexacarbate	10	12,000	10	22,900	2	4.6	7	10	5	37
Ethion	4	500	4	210	10	1297	9	45	6	65
Methiocarb	6	800	4	210	8	270	4	4.6	7	70
Dimethoate	9	6200	7	6000	5	20	5	6.6	8	215
Carbaryl	7	1950	8	6760	9	707	10	56	9	859
Temephos	8	3490	9	2180	6	35	8	42	10	8600

[a] LC_{50} = µg of active ingredient per liter of water calculated to kill 50% of test population during a standard 96-h exposure. Tests were conducted under static conditions.

[b] LD_{50} = mg of active ingredient per kilogram of body mass calculated to kill 50% of test population.

[c] Farm-reared male and female ring-necked pheasants; dosage by gelatin capsule.

[d] Wild-captured pen-conditioned male and female red-winged blackbirds; dosage by gavage in propylene glycol.

[e] Sherman strain male laboratory rats; dosage by gavage in peanut oil.

Source: Adapted from Hill.[47]

D. PCBs and Dioxins

Polychlorinated biphenyls (PCBs) and PCDDs are dispersed throughout the global ecosystem, are chemically stable, and bioaccumulate in animal tissues. Both are environmentally persistent, resisting bacterial and chemical breakdown, but are readily absorbed from water into the fats of plankton, thereby entering the aquatic food chain. Table 21.24 summarizes PCB concentrations that cause adverse effects in aquatic organisms based on laboratory studies.[48] This process continues as fish, and then pisciverous birds including gulls, cormorants, herons, and terns, accumulate progressively higher concentrations (biomagnification) of these compounds as they become deposited in the fat of the body while natural portions of food items are metabolized for energy or excreted. At the top of the aquatic food chain are bald eagles (*Haliaeetus leucocephalus*) and other raptors, which consume gulls and other fish-eating birds as well as fish. One of the most sensitive functional end points for PCB- and dioxin-mediated toxicity in birds appears to be reproductive impairment as associated with egg residues and as shown through controlled feeding studies (Table 21.25) as well as egg injection studies (Table 21.26).[49] The utility of egg injection studies for predicting potential embryotoxicity of PCBs and TCDD compares favorably with feeding studies. In instances where the same chemicals, Aroclors or TCDD, have been administered by both methods, egg concentrations and effects are quite similar. These studies have revealed the coplanar PCB congener 126 (3,3′, 4,4′,5-penta-CB) to be the most toxic of all PCB congeners to avian embryos. Several other recent reviews on the ecotoxicology of polyhalogenated aromatic hydrocarbons (PHAHs) include ones by Rice and O'Keefe[50] and by Giesy and Kannan [51]

TABLE 21.24
Summary of PCB Concentrations in Aquatic Organisms for Adverse Effects Based on Laboratory Studies[a]

Response	Algae, µg/l	Zooplankton, µg/l	Macroinvertebrates	Fish
Lethality	>0.5–1	>0.5	>25 mg/kg	>100 mg/kg
Growth	>0.5–1	>0.5	>25 mg/kg	>50 mg/kg
Reproduction	>0.5–1	>0.5	>25 mg/kg	
Female				>100 mg/kg
Progeny				>50 mg/kg
Behavior			>100 µg/l	>100 µg/l
Disease				mg/kg range
Cellular changes			Low mg/kg	High µg/kg to low mg/kg
Biochemical changes				High µg/kg to low mg/kg

[a] Estimates for algae include those for phytoplankton, and zooplankton estimates were primarily based on *Daphnia*. A maximum concentration of >100 mg/kg of PCBs in tissues was used because higher concentrations may have limited environmental relevance. Some threshold concentrations are expressed on a waterborne exposure basis, where estimates of tissue concentrations were poorly defined.

Source: Adapted from Niimi.[48]

TABLE 21.25
Reproductive Effects of Aroclors and Other PCB Mixtures in Birds

Species, Age	Conc. in Tissue (ppm wet wt)	Effect	Experimental Treatment
Chickens, laying hens	5 in eggs	Hatching reduced	Aroclor 1254 in diet, up to 50 ppm
	13.2 in eggs	Did not affect hatching	Aroclor 1254 in diet, 20 ppm
Chickens, white leghorn hens	Above 4 in eggs	Embryo mortality and teratogenic	Aroclor 1254 in drinking water at 50 ppm
	Less than 1 in eggs	Decreased hatching	Aroclor 1242 diet, up to 80 ppm
Chickens, fertile white leghorn eggs	10 in eggs	Embryonic mortality of 64%	Aroclor 1242 injected into air cell of eggs
Chickens, laying hens	23 in eggs	Decreased hatching	Aroclor 1248 in diet at 10 ppm
Chickens, fertile white leghorn eggs	5 in eggs	Hatching reduced to 17%	Aroclor 1248 injected into yolk sac
Chickens, fertile eggs	0.05 to 0.1 in eggs	Decreased gluconeogenic enzyme activity	Aroclor 1254 injected into air cell
Ringed turtledoves	16 in eggs, 5.5 in adult brain	Embryonic mortality; Decreased parental attentiveness	Aroclor 1254 in diet
	2.8 in brain	depletion of brain dopamine and norepinephrine	Aroclor 1254 in diet
Mallard hens	23 in eggs, 30 in 3-week-old ducklings and 55 in hens	No effects	Aroclor 1254 in diet at 25 ppm
	105 in eggs	Eggshell thickness decreased; hatching success not affected	Aroclor 1242 in diet
Screech owls	4 to 18 in eggs	No effects	Aroclor 1248 in diet at 3 ppm wet weight
Atlantic puffins	10 to 81 in eggs, 6 in adults	No effects detected	Aroclor 1254 dosed by implantation of 30–35 mg

Source: Adapted from Hoffman et al.[49]

TABLE 21.26
Egg Injection Studies with Planar PCBs and Dioxin

Species, Age	Compound, Conc.	Effect
Chicken, white leghorn embryo	2,3,7,8-TCDD[a]	
	10 ppt	Two-fold AHH* induction
	10–20 ppt	Onset of embryotoxicity
	40–50 ppt	Mortality, edema, surface hemorrhaging
	63 ppt	ED_{50} for AHH induction
	147 ppt	LD_{50} (air cell injection)
	115 ppt	LD_{50} (yolk sac injection)
	180 ppt	LD_{50} (air cell injection)
	240 ppt	LD_{50} (air cell injection)
	302 ppt	ED_{50} for AHH induction
	1 ppb	100% mortality
	3,3′,4,4′5-PeCB (PCB 126)	
	0.4 ppb	LD_{50} (air cell injection), day 4 through hatch
	3.1 ppb	LD_{50} (air cell injection), day 7 through 10
	3,3′4,4′-TeCB (PCB 77)	
	2.6 ppb	LD_{50} (air cell injection)
	8.6 ppb	LD_{50} (air cell injection)
	40 ppb	LD_{50} (air cell injection)
	2,3,3′4,4′-PeCB (PCB 105)	
	2,200 ppb	LD_{50} (air cell injection)
	2,3,3′4,4′5-HxCB (PCB 157)	
	2000 ppb	LD_{50} (air cell injection)
	1500 ppb	LD_{50} (air cell injection)
Pheasant, embryo	2,3,7,8-TCDD	
	1.4 ppb	LD_{50} (albumin)
	2.2 ppb	LD_{50} (yolk)
Bobwhite, embryo	3,3′,4,4′5-PeCB (PCB 126)	
	24 ppb	LD_{50} (air cell injection), through hatching
Common tern, embryo	3,3′,4,4′5-PeCB (PCB 126)	
	104 ppb	LD_{50} (air cell injection), through hatching
American kestrel, embryo	3,3′,4,4′5-PeCB (PCB 126)	
	65 ppb	LD_{50} (air cell injection), through hatching
Mallard, embryo; goldeneye, embryo	3,3′4,4′-TeCB (PCB 77)	
	5,000 ppb	No effects (air cell injection)

Source: Adapted from Hoffman et al.[49]
* Aryl hydrocarbon hydroxylase.

E. PAHs and Petroleum

Natural sources of polyaromatic hydrocarbons (PAHs) in the environment include forest and grass fires, oil seeps, volcanoes, and plants. Figure 21.5 shows natural and anthropogenic sources of PAHs, including petroleum spills and discharges, electric power generation, refuse incineration, home heating, and internal combustion engines. The primary mechanism for atmospheric contamination by PAHs is incomplete combustion of organic matter. Aquatic contamination by PAHs is caused by petroleum spills, discharges, and seepages, industrial and municipal wastewater, urban and suburban surface runoff, and atmospheric deposition. Sources of PAHs on land include natural fires, industrial activities, waste disposal and incineration, home heating, and automobile exhaust. Petroleum can cause environmental harm by toxic action, physical contact, chemical and physical changes within the soil or water medium, and habitat alteration (Table 21.27).[52] Oil spills have caused major changes in local plant and invertebrate populations lasting from several weeks to many years. Effects of oil spills on populations of mobile vertebrate species, such as fish, birds, and mammals, have been difficult to determine beyond the immediate losses in local populations. The induction of lesions and neoplasms in laboratory animals by metabolites of PAHs and observations of lesions and neoplasms in fish from PAH-contaminated sites indicate potential health problems for animals with cytochrome P-450 capable of metabolizing PAHs. Although evidence linking environmental PAHs to the incidence of cancerous neoplasms in wild animals is limited and primarily circumstantial, the growing quantities of PAHs entering the environment are a cause for concern. Reptiles and amphibians can be killed by petroleum, but available information is inadequate to evaluate properly the sensitivity of these organisms to petroleum or individual PAHs. Birds are often killed by oil spills, primarily because of plumage oiling and oil ingestion. Birds that spend much of their time on the water surface are the most vulnerable to spilled oil. Ingested oil can cause many sublethal effects, and transmittal to nests and eggs is highly embryotoxic. Mammals that rely on fur for insulation (polar bear, otters, fur seals, muskrat) are the most likely to die from oiling.

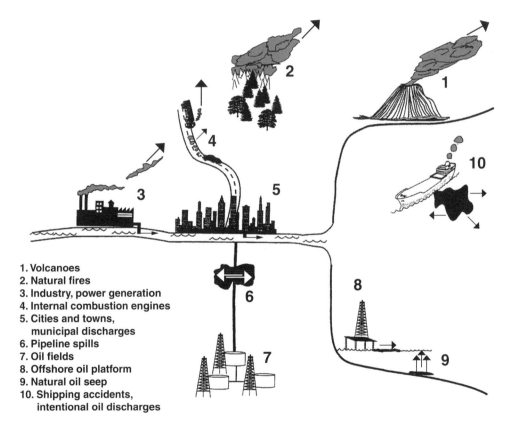

1. Volcanoes
2. Natural fires
3. Industry, power generation
4. Internal combustion engines
5. Cities and towns, municipal discharges
6. Pipeline spills
7. Oil fields
8. Offshore oil platform
9. Natural oil seep
10. Shipping accidents, intentional oil discharges

FIGURE 21.5 Sources of petroleum and PAHs in the environment. The primary mechanism for atmospheric contamination by PAHs is incomplete combustion of organic matter. Aquatic contamination by PAHs is caused by petroleum spills, discharges, and seepages, industrial and municipal wastewater, urban and suburban surface runoff, and atmospheric deposition. Sources of PAHs on land include natural fires, industrial activities, waste disposal and incineration, home heating, and automobile exhaust. (Adapted from Albers.[52])

TABLE 21.27
Effects of Petroleum and Individual PAHs on Living Organisms

Effects	Plant	Invertebrate	Fish	Reptile and Amphibian	Bird	Mammal
Individual Organisms						
Death	✔	✔	✔	✔	✔	✔
Impaired reproduction	✔	✔	✔	✔	✔	
Reduced growth and development	✔	✔	✔	✔	✔	
Impaired immune system						✔
Altered endocrine function			✔		✔	
Altered rate of photosynthesis	✔					
Malformations			✔		✔	
Tumors and lesions		✔	✔	✔		✔
Cancer			✔	✔		✔
Altered behavior		✔	✔	✔	✔	✔
Blood disorders		✔	✔	✔	✔	✔
Liver and kidney disorders			✔		✔	✔
Hypothermia					✔	✔
Inflammation of epithelial tissue					✔	✔
Altered respiration or heart rate		✔	✔	✔		
Impaired salt gland function				✔	✔	
Gill hyperplasia			✔			
Fin erosion			✔			
Groups of Organisms[a]						
Local population changes	✔	✔			✔	
Altered community structure	✔	✔			✔	
Biomass change	✔	✔				

[a] Populations of chlorophyllous and nonchlorophyllous plants (bacteria, filamentous fungi, yeast, microalgae) can increase or decrease in the presence of petroleum, whereas animal populations decrease.

Source: Adapted from Albers.[52]

F. RADIONUCLIDES

On a global basis, radiation from natural sources is a much greater contributor to radiation dose to living organisms than is radiation from anthropogenic sources. However, ionizing radiation can harm biological systems, causing a range of syndromes from prompt lethality to reduced vigor, shortened life span, diminished reproductive rate, and genetic transmission of radiation-altered genes that are most commonly recessive and usually disadvantageous. In general, more-primitive organisms are the most-radioresistant taxonomic groups and the more-advanced, complex organisms, such as mammals, are the most radiosensitive (Figure 21.6).[53] The early effects of exposure to ionizing radiation result primarily from cell death where dividing cells, frequently undergoing mitosis, are the most sensitive, and cells that do not divide are the most radioresistant. Thus, embryos and fetuses are particularly susceptible to ionizing radiation, and very young animals are consistently more radiosensitive than adults. Among birds, as in most other tested species, there is a direct relation between dose and mortality at single high doses of ionizing radiations (Table 21.28).[54] For any given total dose, the survival of a bird is higher if the dose is delivered at a lower rate or over a longer period of time and suggests that biological repair processes compensate for radiation-induced cellular and tissue damage over a prolonged period or at a comparatively low dose rate.[55]

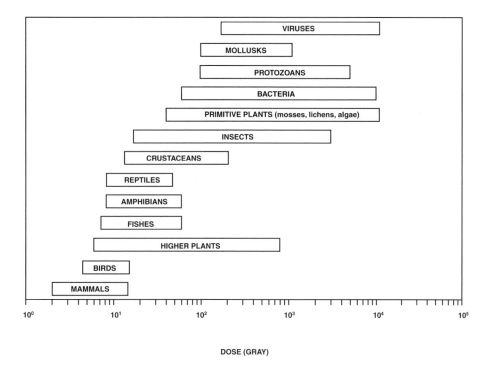

FIGURE 21.6 Ranges of acute lethal doses of radiation to various taxonomic groups. Dose of radiation is expressed in grays (Gy, where 1 Gy = 100 rad). In general, more primitive organisms are the most radioresistant taxonomic groups and more-advanced complex organisms, such as mammals, are the most radiosensitive. (Adapted from Talmage and Meyers-Schone.[53])

TABLE 21.28
Radiation Effects on Birds

Species	Dose/Exposure	Effects
Green-winged teal (*Anas carolinensis*)	4.8 Gy, single acute exposure	LD_{50}, 30 days postexposure
Northern shoveler (*Anas clypeata*)	8.9 Gy, single acute exposure	LD_{50}, 30 days postexposure
Blue-winged teal (*Anas discors*)	7.2 Gy, single acute exposure	LD_{50}, 30 days postexposure
Passerine species eggs	5–10 Gy, single acute exposure	LD_{100}
Passerine species nestlings	1 Gy daily	Growth retardation
Common quail (*Coturnix coturnix*) eggs	Exposed first 9 days of incubation, single acute exposure	
	5 Gy	Negligible effect on survival
	7 GY	Mortality > 50%
	9 GY	All dead before hatch
Chicken (*Gallus domesticus*) eggs	Exposed before incubation, single acute exposure, 0.05–2.1 GY	No adverse effects on embryonic development at 1.6 Gy and lower; at 2.1 Gy, adverse effects on development, survival, and body weight of hatched chicks
Chicks, age 15 days	2.1 GY	Reversible changes in blood chemistry within 60 days; no deaths
	6.6 GY	Irreversible and permanent damage to red blood cells, hemoglobin, and hematocrit; all dead within 7 days

TABLE 21.28 *(Continued)*
Radiation Effects on Birds

Species	Dose/Exposure	Effects
Laying hens	Fed diet containing 400 Bq of ^{137}Cs/kg ration for 4 weeks	Of total ^{137}Cs ingested, 3% was distributed in egg contents (29–33 Bq/kg egg; 2 Bq egg); 9% in muscle (171 Bq/kg FW*); and 81% in excreta
Broiler chickens	Fed diet containing 400 Bq of ^{137}Cs/kg ration for 40 days; some diets contained up to 5% bentonite	Feeding with bentonite reduced ^{137}Cs concentration in muscle by 32%, from 155 to 105 Bq/kg FW
Black-headed gull (*Larus ridibundus ridibundus*) eggs	9.6 GY over 20 days	LD$_{50}$
Great crested flycatcher (*Myiarchus crinitus*) nestlings	Single acute exposure > 8 Gy	All dead by fledging
Eastern bluebird (*Sialia sialis*) nestlings, age 2 days	Single acute exposure	
	3 GY	Reduced growth after 16 days
	3–5 GY	Reduced growth and shorter primary feathers at fledging
	4–12 Gy	Developed normally and fledged successfully
	5-6 Gy	LD$_{50}$, nestling to fledgling
	25 Gy	LD$_{50}$, 16 days postexposure
	30 Gy	All dead 4 days postexposure
Eastern bluebird eggs	Single acute exposure 6 Gy	All dead before hatch
European starling (*Sturnus vulgaris*)	Single exposure > 2 GY	Fatal
Tree swallow (*Tachycineta bicolor*)	0.006 mGy/h during breeding season equivalent to annual dose of about 50 mSv	No adverse effects on breeding performance of adults, or growth performance of nestlings
Tree swallow nestlings	0.9–4.5 Gy, single acute exposure	Adverse effects on growth, survival, or both
	1.0 Gy daily, chronic	Reduced hatch, depressed growth
House wren (*Troglodytes aedon*) fledglings	0.9 Gy, single acute exposure	Growth reduction

Source: Adapted from Eisler.[54]
* FW = Fresh weight.

G. SUMMARY OF STUDIES OF PERSISTENT ENVIRONMENTAL CONTAMINANTS IN TERRESTRIAL VERTEBRATES

Table 21.29 summarizes field studies of persistent environmental contaminants by species studied, contaminants detected, and locations.[56]

TABLE 21.29
Summary of Studies of Persistent Environmental Contaminants in Terrestrial Vertebrates

Species	Contaminants[a]	Area
Snapping turtle (*Chelydra serpentina*)	HM	New Jersey, Maryland
	OC, PCB	New York, New Jersey, Great Lakes, Canada
	Hg	Canada, Tennessee
	Pb	Missouri

TABLE 21.29 *(Continued)*
Summary of Studies of Persistent Environmental Contaminants in Terrestrial Vertebrates

Species	Contaminants[a]	Area
Diamondback terrapin (*Malaclemys terrapin*)	OC, PCB	Georgia
Brown pelican (*Pelecanus occidentalis*)	DDE	U.S., Mexico, Puerto Rico, Virgin Islands
	OC, PCB	Florida, South Carolina, California, Louisiana
	PCB	Georgia, Puerto Rico, Virgin Islands
	OC, PCB, HM	Texas, Southeastern U.S.
Double-crested cormorant (*Phalacrocorax auritus*)	DDE, PCB, Hg, Se	Florida
	OC, PCB, Hg	South Dakota
	OC, PCB	Texas, Canada, Mexico, Maine
	TEQ	Canada, Great Lakes
	HM	Washington, Canada
	OC, PCB, Hg	Great Lakes
	DDE, Hg	California
Anhinga (*Anhinga anhinga*)	OC, PCB, Hg	Eastern U.S.
Great blue heron (*Ardea herodias*)	OC, PCB, TEQ, HM	U.S.
	OC, PCB, TEQ	Canada
Snowy egret (*Egretta thula*)	DDE, PCB	Eastern U.S., Idaho
	PCB	Nevada
	OC, PCB, HM	San Francisco Bay, Texas
	HM	South Carolina, Florida
	Hg	New York
	OC	Florida
Tricolored heron (*Egretta tricolor*)	Hg	Florida
	DDE, PCB, HM	Texas
	OC, PCB	Eastern U.S.
Cattle egret (*Bubulcus ibis*)	OC, PCB	Baja, California
Black-crowned night heron (*Nycticorax nycticorax*)	OC, PCB, TEQ, HM	U.S.
	OC, PCB	Italy
White-faced ibis (*Plegadis chihi*)	OC	Texas
	DDE, Se, Hg	Nevada
Roseate spoonbill (*Ajaia ajaja*)	OC, PCB	Texas
Woodstork (*Mycteria americana*)	OC	Eastern U.S.
Black vulture (*Coragyps atratus*)	OC	Mexico
California condor (*Gymnogyps californianus*)	DDE, Pb	California
Greater snow goose (*Chen caerulescens atlantica*)	OC, PCB, Hg	Canada
Mute swan (*Cygnus olor*)	DDE	Scotland
	HM	Sweden, Chesapeake Bay
	Pb	UK
	DDE, PCB, HM	Denmark
Wood duck (*Aix sponsa*)	OC	Mississippi
Black duck (*Anas rubripes*)	OC, PCB, HM	Canada, Eastern U.S.
Canvasback duck (*Aythya valisineria*)	OC, PCB, Hg	North America
Greater scaup (*Aythya marila*)	DDE, PCB	Scotland, Finland, Northeastern U.S.
	HM	British Columbia, Chesapeake Bay, Northeastern U.S.
	PCB	Netherlands, Poland
	OC, HM	San Francisco Bay, Poland
	OC, PCB	New York, Michigan, Great Lakes
	Hg	Utah, Finland
Mergansers (*Mergus* spp.)	OC, PCB, Hg	U.S.

TABLE 21.29 *(Continued)*
Summary of Studies of Persistent Environmental Contaminants in Terrestrial Vertebrates

Species	Contaminants[a]	Area
Ruddy duck (*Oxyura jamaicansis*)	HM	Delaware River, Chesapeake Bay
	Se	California
Osprey (*Pandion haliaetus*)	OC, PCB, HM	U.S.
Mississippi kite (*Ictinia mississippiensis*)	OC	U.S.
Bald eagle (*Haliaeetus leucocephalus*)	OC, PCB, Hg, Pb	U.S., Canada
	TEQ	British Columbia
Fish eagle (*Haliaeetus vocifer*)	DDE	Zimbabwe
Spanish eagle (*Aquila adalberti*)	OC, PCB, HM	Spain
Red-tailed hawk (*Buteo jamaicensis*)	OC	Ohio
White-tailed eagle (*Haliaeetus albicilla*)	OC, PCB, Hg	Sweden
Peregrine falcon (*Falco peregrinus*)	OC, PCB, DDE	Worldwide
Prairie falcon (*Falco mexicanus*)	DDE	Colorado
Clapper rail (*Rallus longirostris*)	OC, PCB	New Jersey, South Carolina, Virginia
	OC, PCB, HM	Georgia, California
American oystercatcher (*Haematopus palliatus*)	DDE, PCB	South Carolina
Willet (*Catoptrophorus semipalmatus*)	OC, PCB, HM	Delaware Bay
	DDE, PCB, HM	Texas
Long-billed curlew (*Numenius americanus*)	OC, PCB	Oregon
Laughing gull (*Larus atricilla*)	OC, PCB, HM	Texas
	DDE, PCB	South Carolina
	HM	New York
	OC	Florida
Herring gull (*Larus argentatus*)	OC, PCB	Germany, Newfoundland
	Hg	Denmark, Ontario
	HM	UK, Germany, New York, New Jersey
	OC, PCB, TEQ, HM	Great Lakes, Canada
	DDE, PCB	Maine, Scotland, Portugal, Gibraltar, Finland, Canada, Virginia, Denmark, Crete, Cyprus
	OC, PCB, Flouride	Norway
Gull-billed tern (*Sterna nilotica*)	OC, PCB	South Carolina
Caspian tern (*Sterna caspia*)	OC, PCB	Southern California
Common tern (*Sterna hirundo*)	DDE, PCB, HM	Rhode Island
	OC, PCB, HM	Great Lakes, Eastern U.S., Canada
	TEQ	Netherlands, Massachusetts
	Hg	Germany
Forster's tern (*Sterna forsteri*)	PCB	Wisconsin
Black skimmer (*Rynchops niger*)	OC, PCB	Florida, South Carolina, Texas, Mexico
	HM	Florida, New York, New Jersey, Texas
Barn owl (*Tyto alba*)	OC, PCB	Chesapeake Bay
Great horned owl (*Bubo virginianus*)	OC	Ohio
Loggerhead shrike (*Lanius ludovicianus*)	DDE	Illinois
Tree swallow (*Tachycineta bicolor*)	OC, PCB	Colorado, Oregon, Wyoming, Montana, Idaho, Utah, South Dakota, New Mexico
	PCB, TEQ	Wisconsin, Michigan, New York
	PCB	Pennsylvania, Indiana, Maryland
	HM	New York, New Jersey, Canada
	Pb	Idaho
	DDE, PCB	Canada, Wisconsin
	OC, PCB, Hg	Great Lakes

TABLE 21.29 *(Continued)*
Summary of Studies of Persistent Environmental Contaminants in Terrestrial Vertebrates

Species	Contaminants[a]	Area
Mink (*Mustela vison*)	Hg	Georgia, Wisconsin River, Wisconsin, Connecticut, Massachusetts, Ontario, Manitoba, Southern Atlantic Coast
	OC, PCB	Canada, Maryland, Oregon, Great Lakes, New York, Connecticut, Massachusetts, Southern Atlantic Coast, Minnesota
	OC	Iowa
	HM	Virginia, Washington, Idaho, New York, Illinois, Minnesota, Canada
Muskrat (*Ondatra zibethicus*)	Se	New York
	HM	Pennsylvania, Missouri, Manitoba
	Hg	Tennessee
	OC, PCB, HM	Virginia
River otter (*Lontra canadensis*)	DDE, PCB, Hg	New York
	HM	Virginia
	OC, Cs, Hg	Georgia

[a] OC = organochlorine insecticides; PCB = polychlorinated biphenyls; HM = heavy metals; PCS = polychlorinated styrenes; TEQ = toxic equivalents.

Source: Adapted from Keith.[56]

REFERENCES

1. Moriarity, F., *Ecotoxicology, the Study of Pollutants in Ecosystems*, 2nd ed., Academic Press, San Diego, CA, 1988.
2. Cairns, J., Jr., Will the real ecotoxicologist please stand up? *Environ. Toxicol. Chem.,* 8, 843, 1989.
3. Hoffman, D. J., Rattner, B. A., Burton, G. A., Jr., and Cairns, J., Jr., Introduction, in *Handbook of Ecotoxicology*, Hoffman, D. J., Rattner, B. A., Burton, G. A. Jr., and Cairns, J. Jr., Eds., CRC Press, Boca Raton, FL, 1995, 1–10.
4. Forbes, S. A., The lake as a microcosm, *Bulletin of the Peoria Scientific Association*, 1887; reprinted in *Bull. Ill. State Natl. Hist. Sur.,* 15, 537–550, 1925.
5. Penny, C. and Adams, C., Fourth Report Royal Commission on Pollution in Scotland, *London,* 2, 377, 1863.
6. Weigelt, C., Saare, O., and Schwab, L., Die Schädigung van fischerei und fischzueht durch industrie und haus abwasser, *Arch. Hyg.*, 3, 39, 1885.
7. Newman, J. R., Effects of industrial air pollution on wildlife, *Biol. Conserv.,* 15, 181, 1979.
8. Carson, R., *Silent Spring*, Houghton Mifflin, Boston, 1962, 103.
9. Blus, L. J., Gish, C. D., Belisle, A. A., and Prouty, R. M., Logarithmic relationship of DDE residues to eggshell thinning, *Nature,* 235, 376, 1972.
10. Hill, E. F. and Fleming, W. J., Anticholinesterase poisoning of birds; field monitoring and diagnosis of acute poisoning, *Environ. Toxicol. Chem.,* 1, 27, 1982.
11. Grue, C. E., Fleming, W. J., Busby, D. G., and Hill, E. F., Assessing hazards of organophosphate pesticide to wildlife, *Trans. North Am. Wildl. Nat. Res. Conf.,* 48, 200, 1983.
12. U.S. Environmental Protection Agency, Guidelines for Ecological Risk Assessment, Washington, D.C., *Fed. Reg.,* 63(93), 26846–26924, 1998.
13. Chappie, D. J. and Burton, G. A., Jr., Applications of aquatic and sediment toxicity testing *in situ*, *Soil Sediment Contam.,* 9, 219–245, 2000.
14. Hill, E. F., Acute and subacute toxicology in evaluation of pesticide hazard to avian wildlife, in *Wildlife Toxicology and Population Modeling: Integrated Studies of Agroecosystems*, Kendall, R. J. and Lacher, T. E., Jr., Eds., Lewis Publishers/CRC Press, Boca Raton, FL, 1994, 2077–226.

15. Hoffman, D. J., Wildlife toxicity testing, in *Handbook of Ecotoxicology*, Hoffman, D. J., Rattner, B. A., Burton, G. A., Jr., and Cairns, J., Jr., Eds., Lewis Publishers/CRC Press, Boca Raton, FL, 1995, 47–69.

16. Hoffman, D. J., Measurements of toxicity and critical stages of development, in *Wildlife Toxicology and Population Modeling: Integrated Studies of Agroecosystems*, Kendall, R. J. and Lacher, T. E., Jr., Eds., Lewis Publishers/CRC Press, Boca Raton, FL, 1994, 47–67.

17. Depledge, M. H. and Fossi, M. C., The role of biomarkers in environmental assessment (2). Invertebrates, *Ecotoxicology*, 3, 161–172, 1994.

18. Fossi, M. C., Leonzio, C., and Peakall, D. B., The use of nondestructive biomarkers in the hazard assessments of vertebrate populations, in *Nondestructive Biomarkers in Vertebrates*, Fossi, M.C. and Leonzio, C., Eds., Lewis Publishers, Boca Raton, FL, 1994, 3–34.

19. Huggett, R. J., Kimerle, R. A., Mehrle, P. M., Jr., and Bergman, H. L., Biomarkers: biochemical, physiological, and histological markers of anthropogenic stress, *SETAC Special Publication Series*, Lewis Publishers, Boca Raton, FL, 1992, 347 pp.

20. Fossi, M. C. and Leonzio, C., Eds., *Nondestructive Biomarkers in Vertebrates*, Lewis Publishers, Boca Raton, FL, 1994, 345 pp.

21. Melancon, M. J., Bioindicators used in aquatic and terrestrial monitoring, in *Handbook of Ecotoxicology*, Hoffman, D. J., Rattner, B. A., Burton, G. A., Jr., and Cairns, J., Jr., Eds., Lewis Publishers/CRC Press, Boca Raton, FL, 1995, 220–240.

22. Rattner, B. A., Cohen, J. B., and Golden, N. H., Contaminant effect endpoints in terrestrial vertebrates at and above the level of the "individual," in *Environmental Contaminants and Terrestrial Vertebrates: Effects on Populations, Communities and Ecosystems*, Albers, P. H., Ed., SETAC Press, Pensacola, FL, 2000, 61–94.

23. Interpretation of Criteria Commonly Used to Determine Lead Poisoning Problem Areas, U.S. Department of the Interior, Fish and Wildlife Service, Fish and Wildlife Leaflet 2, Washington, D.C., 1985.

24. Pain, D. J., Lead in waterfowl, in *Environmental Contaminants in Wildlife: Interpreting Tissue Concentrations*, Beyer, W. N., Heinz, G. H., and Redmon-Norwood, A. W., Eds., Lewis Publishers/CRC Press, Boca Raton, FL, 1996, 251–264.

25. Franson, J. C., Interpretation of tissue lead residues in birds other than waterfowl, in *Environmental Contaminants in Wildlife: Interpreting Tissue Concentrations*, Beyer, W.N., Heinz, G.H., and Redmon-Norwood, A. W., Eds., Lewis Publishers/CRC Press, Boca Raton, FL, 1996, 265–280.

26. Wiener, J. G. and Spry, D. J., Toxilogical significance of mercury in freshwater fish, in *Environmental Contaminants in Wildlife: Interpreting Tissue Concentrations*, Beyer, W. N., Heinz, G. H., and Redmon-Norwood, A. W., Eds., Lewis Publishers/CRC Press, Boca Raton, FL, 1996, 297–340.

27. Eisler, R., *Handbook of Chemical Risk Assessment: Health Hazards to Humans, Plants, and Animals*, Vol. 1, Lewis Publishers/CRC Press, Boca Raton, FL, 2000, 313–411.

28. Heinz, G. H., Mercury poisoning in wildlife, in *Noninfectious Diseases of Wildlife*, Fairbrother, A., Locke, L. N., and Hoff, G. L., Eds., Iowa State University Press, Ames, 1996, 118–122.

29. Cooke, J. A. and Johnson, M. S., Cadmium in small mammals, in *Environmental Contaminants in Wildlife: Interpreting Tissue Concentrations*, Beyer, W.N., Heinz, G.H., and Redmon-Norwood, A.W., Eds., Lewis Publishers/CRC Press, Boca Raton, FL, 1996, 377–388.

30. Lemly, A .D., Selenium in aquatic organisms, in *Environmental Contaminants in Wildlife: Interpreting Tissue Concentrations*, Beyer, W. N., Heinz, G. H., and Redmon-Norwood, A. W., Eds., Lewis Publishers/CRC Press, Boca Raton, FL, 1996, 427–446.

31. Poley, W. E. and Moxon, A. L., Tolerance levels of seleniferous grains in laying rations, *Poult. Sci.*, 17, 72–76, 1938.

32. Ohlendorf, H. M., Bioaccumulation and effects of selenium in wildlife, in *Selenium in Agriculture and the Environment*, Jacobs, L. W., Ed., SSSA Special Publication 23, Soil Science Society of America, Madison, WI, 1989, 133-177.

33. Heinz, G. H., Selenium in birds, in *Environmental Contaminants in Wildlife*, Beyer, W. N., Heinz, G. H., and Redmon-Norwood, A. W., Eds., CRC Press, Boca Raton, FL, 1996, 447–458.

34. Hoffman, D. J. and Heinz, G. H.,Embryotoxic and teratogenic effects of selenium in the diet of mallards, *J. Toxicol. Environ. Health*, 24, 477–490, 1988.

35. Smith, G. J., Heinz, G. H., Hoffman, D. J., Spann, J. W., and Krynitsky, A. J., Reproduction in black-crowned night-herons fed selenium, *Lake Reservoir Manage.*, 4, 175–180, 1988.

36. Heinz, G. H., Hoffman, D. J., and Gold, L. G., Toxicity of organic and inorganic selenium to mallard ducklings, *Environ. Toxicol. Chem.*, 17, 561–568, 1988.

37. Hoffman, D. J., Heinz, G. H., and Krynitsky, A. J., Hepatic glutathione metabolism and lipid peroxidation in response to excess dietary selenomethionine and selenite in mallard ducklings, *J. Toxicol. Environ. Health,* 27, 263–271, 1989.

38. Hoffman, D. J., Sanderson, C. J., LeCaptain, L. J., Cromartie, E., and Pendleton, G. S., Interactive effects of arsenic, selenium, and dietary protein on survival, growth, and physiology in mallard ducklings, *Arch. Environ. Contam. Toxicol.*, 20, 288–294, 1992.

39. Hoffman, D. J., Sanderson, C. J., LeCaptain, L. J., Cromartie, E., and Pendleton, G. S., Interactive effects of boron, selenium and dietary protein on survival, growth, and physiology in mallard ducklings, *Arch. Environ. Contam. Toxicol.*, 20, 288–294, 1991.

40. Hoffman, D. J., Sanderson, C. J., LeCaptain, L. J., Cromartie, E., and Pendleton, G. S., Interactive effects of selenium, methionine and dietary protein on survival, growth, and physiology in mallard ducklings, *Arch. Environ. Contam. Toxicol.*, 23, 163–186, 1992.

41. Fairbrother, A. and Fowles, J., Subchronic effects of sodium selenite and selenomethionine on several immune functions in mallards, *Arch. Environ. Contam. Toxicol.*, 19, 836–844, 1990.

42. Hoffman, D. J., Heinz, G. H., LeCaptain, L. J., Bunck, C. M., and Green, D. E., Subchronic hepatotoxicity of selenomethionine in mallard ducks, *J. Toxicol. Environ. Health.*, 32, 449–464, 1991.

43. Blus, L. J., DDT, DDD, and DDE in birds, in *Environmental Contaminants in Wildlife*, Beyer, W.N., Heinz, G. H., and Redmon-Norwood, A. W., Eds., Lewis Publishers, Boca Raton, FL, 1996.

44. Grue, C. E., Hart, A. D. M., and Mineau, P., Biological consequences of depressed brain cholinesterase activity in wildlife, in *Cholinesterase-Inhibiting Insecticides: Their Impact on Wildlife and the Environment*, Mineau, P., Ed., Elsevier, New York, 1991, 157–158.

45. Hardy, A. R., Fletcher, M. R., and Stanley, P. I., Pesticides and wildlife: twenty years of vertebrate wildlife incident investigations by MAFF, *State Vet. J.*, 40, 182–192, 1986.

46. Mineau, P., Fletcher, M. R., Glasser, L. C., Thomas, N. J., Brassard, C., Wilson, L. K., Elliott, J. E., Lyon, L. A., Henny, C. J., Bollinger, T., and Porter, S. L., Poisoning of raptors with organophosphorus and carbamate pesticides with emphasis on Canada, U.S. and U.K., *J. Raptor Res.*, 33, 1–37, 1999.

47. Hill, E. F., Organophosphorus and carbamate pesticides, in *Handbook of Ecotoxicology*, Hoffman, D. J., Rattner, B. A., Burton, A. G., Jr., and Cairns, J., Jr., Eds., Lewis Publishers, Boca Raton, FL, 1995, 243–273.

48. Niimi, A. J., PCBs in aquatic organisms, in *Environmental Contaminants in Wildlife: Interpreting Tissue Concentrations*, Beyer, W. N., Heinz, G. H., and Redmon-Norwood, A. W., Eds., Lewis Publishers/CRC Press, Boca Raton, FL, 1996, 117–152.

49. Hoffman, D. J., Rice, C. P., and Kubiak, T. J., PCBs and dioxins in birds, in *Environmental Contaminants in Wildlife: Interpreting Tissue Concentrations*, Beyer, W. N., Heinz, G. H., and Redmon-Norwood, A. W., Eds., Lewis Publishers/CRC Press, Boca Raton, FL, 1996, 165–208.

50. Rice, C. P. and O'Keefe, P., Sources, pathways, and effects of PCBs, dioxins, and dibenzofurans, in *Handbook of Ecotoxicology*, Hoffman, D. J., Rattner, B. A., Burton, G. A., Jr., and Cairns, J., Jr., Eds., Lewis Publishers/CRC Press, Boca Raton, FL, 1995, 424–468.

51. Giesy, J. P. and Kannan, K., Dioxin-like and non-dioxin-like toxic effects of polychlorinated biphenyls (PCBs): implications for risk assessment, *Crit. Rev. Toxicol.*, 28(6), 511–569, 1998.

52. Albers, P. H., Petroleum and individual polycyclic aromatic hydrocarbons, in *Handbook of Ecotoxicology*, Hoffman, D. J., Rattner, B. A., Burton, G. A., Jr., and Cairns, J., Jr., Eds., Lewis Publishers,/CRC Press, Boca Raton, FL, 1995, 330–355.

53. Talmage, S. S. and Meyers-Schone, L., Nuclear and thermal, in *Handbook of Ecotoxicology*, Hoffman, D. J., Rattner, B. A., Burton, G. A., Jr., and Cairns, J., Jr., Eds., Lewis Publishers/CRC Press, Boca Raton, FL, 1995, 469–491.

54. Eisler, R., *Handbook of Chemical Risk Assessment: Health Hazards to Humans, Plants, and Animals*, Vol. 3, Lewis Publishers/CRC Press, Boca Raton, FL, 2000, 1707–1828.

55. Brisbin, I. L., Jr., Avian radioecology, in *Current Ornithology*, Vol. 8, Power, D. M., Ed., Plenum Press, New York, 1991, 69–140.

56. Keith, J. O., Residue analyses: how they were used to assess the hazards of contaminants to wildlife, in *Environmental Contaminants in Wildlife*, Beyer, W. N., Heinz, G. H., and Redmon-Norwood, A. W., Eds., Lewis Publishers, Boca Raton, FL, 1996.

57. Adams, W. J., Kimerle, R. A., and Mosher, R. G., An approach for assessing the environmental safety of chemicals sorbed to sediments, in *Aquatic Toxicology and Hazard Evaluation: Seventh Symposium,* Purdy, R. and Bahner, R. C., Eds., American Society for Testing and Materials, Philadelphia, 1985, 429–453.

ADDITIONAL RELATED INFORMATION*

A. Glossary of Ecotoxicological Terms

Bioaccumulation General term describing a process by which chemicals are taken up by aquatic organisms directly from water as well as from exposure through other routes, such as consumption of food and sediment containing chemicals.

Bioaccumulation Factor (BAF) The ratio of tissue chemical residue to chemical concentration in an external environmental phase (i.e., water, sediment, or food). BAF is measured as steady state in situations where organisms are exposed from multiple sources (i.e., water, sediment, and food), unless noted otherwise.

Biochemical oxygen demand (BOD) Sometimes called *biological oxygen demand,* a measure of the rate at which molecular oxygen is consumed by microorganisms during oxidation of organic matter. The standard test is the 5-day BOD test, in which the amount of dissolved oxygen required for oxidation over a 5-day period is measured. The results are measured in mg of oxygen/l (mg/l), or parts per million (ppm).

Bioconcentration A process by which there is a net accumulation of a chemical directly from water into aquatic organisms resulting from simultaneous uptake (e.g., by gill or epithelial tissue) and elimination.

Bioconcentration factor (BCF) A term describing the degree to which a chemical can be concentrated in the tissues of an organism in the aquatic environment as a result of exposure to waterborne chemical. At steady state during the uptake phase of a bioconcentration test, the BCF is a value that is equal to the concentration of a chemical in one or more tissues of the exposed aquatic organisms divided by the average exposure water concentration of the chemical in the test.

Biodegradation The transformation of a material resulting from the complex enzymatic action of microorganisms (e.g., bacteria, fungi). It usually leads to disappearance of the parent chemical structure and to the formation of smaller chemical species, some of which are used for cell anabolism. Although typically used with reference to microbial activity, it may also refer to general metabolic breakdown of a substance by any living organism.

Chemical oxygen demand (COD) COD is measured instead of BOD when organic materials are not easily degraded by microorganisms. Strong oxidizing agents (e.g., potassium permanganate) are used to enhance oxidation. COD values will be larger than BOD values.

EC_{50} (median effective concentration) The concentration of chemical in water to which test organisms are exposed that is estimated to be effective in producing some sublethal response in 50% of the test organisms. The EC_{50} is usually expressed as a time-dependent value (e.g., 24-h or 96-h EC_{50}). The sublethal response elicited from the test organisms as a result of exposure to the chemical must be clearly defined (e.g., test organisms may be immobilized, lose equilibrium, or undergo physiological or behavioral changes).

Fate Disposition of a material in various environmental compartments (e.g., soil or sediment, water, air, biota) as a result of transport, transformation, and degradation.

Flow-through system An exposure system for aquatic toxicity tests in which the test material solutions and control water flow into and out of test chambers on a once-through basis either intermittently or continuously.

LC_{50} (median lethal concentration) The concentration of chemical in water to which test organisms are exposed that is estimated to be lethal to 50% of the test organisms. The LC_{50} is often expressed as a time-dependent value (e.g., 24-h or 96 h LC_{50}).

---

* *Source:* Rand, G.M., Ed., *Fundamentals of Aquatic Toxicology,* 2nd ed., Taylor & Francis, Washington, D.C., 1995. With permission.

Life cycle study A chronic study in which all the significant life stages of an organism are exposed to a test material. Generally, a life cycle test involves an entire reproductive cycle of the organism.

Lowest observed effect concentration (LOEC) The lowest concentration of a chemical used in a toxicity test that has a statistically significant adverse effect on the exposed population of test organisms compared with the controls. Also called the lowest observed adverse effect level (LOAEL).

Maximum acceptable toxicant concentration (MATC) The hypothetical toxic threshold concentration lying in a range bounded at the lower end by the highest tested concentration having no observed effect (NOEC) and at the higher end by the lowest concentration having a statistically significant toxic effect (LOEC) in a life cycle (full chronic) or a partial life cycle (partial chronic) test. This can be represented by NOEC < MATC < LOEC.

No observed adverse effect level (NOAEL) *See* NOEC.

No observed effect concentration (NOEC) The highest concentration of chemical in a toxicity test at which no statistically significant adverse effect was observed on the exposed population when compared with the controls.

Octanol-water partition coefficient (K_{ow}) The ratio of the solubility of a chemical in *n*-ocatanol and water at steady state; also expressed as *P*. The logarithm of *P* or K_{ow} (i.e., log *P* or log K_{ow}) is used as an indication of the propensity of a chemical for bioconcentration by aquatic organisms.

Static system An exposure system for aquatic toxicity tests in which the test chambers contain still solutions of the test material or control water.

TLm or TL_{50} (median tolerance limit) The concentration of material in water at which 50% of the test organisms survive after a specified time of exposure. The TLm (or TL_{50}) is usually expressed as a time-dependent value (e.g., 24-h or 96 h TL_{50}).

22 Metal Toxicology

Akira Yasutake, Ph.D. and Kimiko Hirayama, Ph.D.

CONTENTS

0-8493-0370-2/02/$0.00+$1.50

ABBREVIATIONS

ALA δ-aminolevulinic acid
ALAD δ-aminolevulinic acid dehydratase
ALT alanine aminotransferase
AST aspartate aminotransferase
BUN blood urea nitrogen
Cat catalase
CNS central nervous system
D6PD glucose-6-phosphate dehydrogenase
DA dopamine
γ-GCS γ-glutamylcysteine synthetase
GFR glomerular filtration rate
GPx glutathione peroxidase
GSH reduced glutathione
GSR glutathione reductase
GSSG oxidized glutathione
γ-GTP γ-glutamyltranspeptidase
IgM immunoglobulin M
LDH lactate dehydrogenase
LPO lipid peroxide
MAO monoamineoxidase
MT metallothionein
NE norepinephrine
PAH p-aminohippurate
RBC erythrocytes
ZPP zinc protoporphyrin

SECTION 1. INTRODUCTION

The various toxic effects caused by a number of metals have been documented in experimental animals. The specific organ toxicity closely related to the tissue distribution has been documented for each metal. Since susceptibility to metal toxicity sometimes varies significantly between sex or strain, this information has also been cited. Here, the focus is on recent rodent data. Since the amount of data cited here may not be sufficient for some colleagues, previous publications[1,2] are recommended for additional information.

SECTION 2. ARSENIC

Arsenic (As) occurs in the environment in its inorganic and organic forms; the toxicity of the latter is very low. In a variety of inorganic arsenic compounds, arsenite (trivalent), arsenate (pentavalent), arsenic oxide, gallium arsenide, and arsine are mentioned in the literature. Toxic effects of arsenite and arsenate are shown in Table 22.1. The LD_{50} value for sodium arsenite ($NaAsO_2$) was shown as 6.7 mg As/kg in mice after subcutaneous (sc) injection.[6] Hyperglycemia and glucose intolerance were documented as acute effects of sodium arsenite in rats.[3] Oral exposure to arsenite using drinking water (100 ppm) for 4 to 11 days caused decreased acetylcholine esterase and sorbitol dehydrogenase activities in axons and increased leucine amino peptidase activity in glial cells.[4] Giving 0.5 to 10 ppm As-containing water for 3 weeks caused immunosuppressive effects in mice.[7] Fowler and Woods[8] observed mitochondria swelling and decreased monoamine oxidase activity in the liver of mice given water containing 40 or 85 ppm As as sodium arsenate for 6 weeks. Chronic exposure of rats to arsenite or arsenate in food up to 400 ppm caused reduced body weight and survival period and enlargement of common bile duct.[5] When $NaAsO_2$ was given to pregnant mice at dose levels of 40 (for oral, po) or 12 (for intraperitoneal, ip) mg As/kg, fetal death or resorption resulted.[9,10] Injection of arsenate (45 mg As/kg, ip) also caused fetal resorption.[11]

Gallium arsenide (GaAs) is an excellent semiconductor material used in microcircuits. Intratracheal injection of GaAs up to 200 mg/kg or oral administration of up to 2000 mg/kg caused pathological changes in lung and kidney,[14] inhibition of tissue δ-aminolevulinic acid dehydratase (ALAD) activities,[12,14] and increased urinary elimination of porphyrin and δ-aminolevulinic acid (ALA) (Table 22.2).[12-14] Acute fibrogenic responses of the lung were also documented in rats intratracheally injected with GaAs (100 mg/kg).[15] Sikorski et al.[16] found that female mice intratracheally treated by 50 to 200 mg GaAs/kg showed reduced IgM antibody response to sheep erythrocytes.

The LD_{50} value for arsenic oxide (As_2O_3) was shown to be 11.3 mg/kg after sc injection in mice.[17] Webb et al.[15] reported that As_2O_3 caused effects similar to GaAs in rat lung. Serial oral administration of As_2O_3 (3 mg/kg) for 10 days resulted in increased motor activity, whereas higher dose level (10 mg/kg × 10 days) brought about the reverse result.[18] Inhalation of As_2O_3 aerosol (270 to 940 μg As/m^3) for 3 h caused decreased pulmonary bacterial activity and increased infectious mortality in mice.[19] Arsine gas was documented to cause various hematological alterations in mice, such as decreased hematocrit, erythropoiesis, and hemolytic anemia.[20,21]

TABLE 22.1
Toxic Effects of Arsenate and Arsenite

Animal Strain, Sex, (Weight)[a]	Chemical	Dose (mg As/kg or ppm As)	Route	Effects	Ref.
Rats					
CD, M	$NaAsO_2$	5 or 10	ip	Hyperglycemia, glucose intolerance (1.5–3 h)	3
Wistar, M	$NaAsO_2$	100 ppm/water × 4–11 d		Axons: acetylcholine esterase, sorbitol dehydrogenase ↓ Glial cells: leucine amino peptidase ↑	4

TABLE 22.1 *(Continued)*
Toxic Effects of Arsenate and Arsenite

Animal Strain, Sex, (Weight)[a]	Chemical	Dose (mg As/kg or ppm As)	Route	Effects	Ref.
Osborne, M + F	NaAsO$_2$	125–400 ppm/food × 2 y		Body weight, survival ↓;	5
	Na$_2$HAsO$_4$	250–400 ppm/food × 2 y		enlargement of common bile duct	
Mice					
CD-1, M	NaAsO$_2$	6.7	sc	50% mortality	6
Swiss cross, M	NaAsO$_2$	0.5–10 ppm/water × 3 wk		Immunosuppressive effect	7
C57BL/6, ?, (10–15 g)	Na$_2$HAsO$_4$	40, 85 ppm/water × 6 wk		Liver: mitochondrial swelling, MAO ↑	8
CD-1, pregnant	NaAsO$_2$	40 or 45	po	Fetal death (max: G.D. 13 injection)	9
CD-1, pregnant	NaAsO$_2$	12 (G.D. 9 or 13)	ip	Fetal death, resorption (G.D. 13, 44–51%; G.D. 9, 73–95%)	10
Swiss, pregnant	Na$_2$HAsO$_4$	45	ip	Fetal abnormality, resorption (G.D. 8, injection)	11

[a] Data from adult animals, unless otherwise specified.
Note: G.D. = gestation day; MAO = monoamine oxidase.

TABLE 22.2
Toxic Effects of GaAs and As$_2$O$_3$

Animal Strain, Sex, (Age)[a]	Chemical	Dose (mg GaAs or As$_2$O$_3$/kg)	Route	Effects	Ref.
Rats					
?, M	GaAs	500–2000	po	Blood: ALAD, Zn-protoporphyrin ↑ Brain, liver: ALAD ↑	12
F344, M	GaAs	10, 30, 100	it	Lung weight, urinary porphyrin ↑	13
		1000	po	Urinary porphyrin ↑	
CD, M	GaAs	100, 200	it	Blood, liver, kidney: ALAD ↓ Urine: ALA ↑ Lung, kidney: pathological change	14
F344, M	GaAs	100	it	Lung: tissue weight, protein, DNA, 4-HyPro ↑; acute fibrogenic response	15
	As$_2$O$_3$	17	it	Lung: tissue weight protein, DNA, 4-HyPro ↑; acute fibrogenic response	
Mice					
B6C3F1, F	GaAs	50, 100, 200	it	Splenic accessory cell function ↓ IgM antibody response to sheep RBC ↓	16
NMRI, M	As$_2$O$_3$	11.3	sc	50% mortality (30 d)	
ddY, ?, (4 wk)	As$_2$O$_3$	3 × 10 d	po	Motor activity ↑	17
		10 × 10 d	po	Motor activity ↓ Brain: alteration in monoamine metabolite	18
CD-1, F, (4–5 wk)	As$_2$O$_3$ (aerosol)	270–940 μg As per m^3 × 3 h		Infectious mortality ↑ Bactericidal activity ↓	19

[a] Data from adult animals, unless otherwise specified.
Note: it = intratracheal.

SECTION 3. BERYLLIUM

Toxic effects of beryllium (Be) have been well investigated by the inhalation route, because most cases in humans occur via this route. The lung is the major target in beryllium inhalation (Table 22.3). Consecutive exposure for 14 days to 2.59 mg $Be/m^3 \times 2$ h as $BeSO_4$ caused 80% mortality in male rats.[22] Single (1-h) exposure to the same salt in a relatively higher dose (3.3 to 13 mg Be/m^3) resulted in pathological changes[23] or increase in lavage LDH and alkaline phosphatase activities.[24] Inhalation of beryllium oxide (0.45 mg Be/m^3 for 1 h) also caused similar effects.[25] Chronic exposure to a much lower dose caused lung tumor.[26] Intratracheal injection of beryllium was also effective for examination of pulmonary toxicity. Groth et al.[27] showed that beryllium (metal or passivated) and its alloy with high beryllium content could induce lung neoplasms in rats 16 to 19 months after intratracheal injection (>0.3 mg Be), but alloys containing a low amount (<4%) of beryllium failed. If rats were intravenously injected with $BeSO_4$, inhibitions of the hepatic enzyme inductions by the specific drugs were observed.[28] Vacher et al.[29] demonstrated that the toxic effect of the soluble salt of beryllium was much higher than that of insoluble salt after intravenous (iv) injection in mice. Mathur et al.[30] found that if nitrate salt (14.6 µg Be/kg, iv) was injected into pregnant rats on gestation day 11, all embryos were resorbed. However, no resorption occurred from its injection on other days.

TABLE 22.3
Pulmonary Toxicity of Beryllium Aerosol Inhalation or Intratracheal Injection

Animal Strain, Sex	Chemicals	Dose (mg $Be/m^3 \times$ h)	Duration of Exposure	Effect	Ref.
Rats					
F344, M	$BeSO_4$	2.59×2	14 d	80% mortality (15 d)	22
F344, M	$BeSO_4$	13×1		Pathological change (8 d)	23
F344, M	$BeSO_4$	3.3 or 7.2×1		Lavage LDH, alkaline phosphatase (21 d) ↑	24
F344, M	BeO	0.45×1		Lavage LDH, acid, and alkaline phosphatase ↑	25
?, M + F	$BeSO_4$	0.035×7	9 months (5 d/wk)	Tumor	26
Mice					
BALB/c, M	$BeSO_4$	13×1		Pathological change (5 d)	23
BALB/c, M	$BeSO_4$	7.2×1		Lavage LDH, alkaline phosphatase (21 d) ↑	24

SECTION 4. CADMIUM

Cadmium (Cd) damages various organs, such as liver, kidney, testis, bone, and lung of experimental animals. The organ toxicity varies widely depending on its chemical forms, administration routes, and dosing schedule.

A. ACUTE TOXICITY

When injected into animals as chloride or acetate, cadmium damages various tissues of liver, reproductive tissues, kidney, heart, brain, and immune systems in the acute phase, and sometimes has lethal effects (Table 22.4). Numerous investigators reported the lethal effect of a single injection of Cd in mice and rats. LD_{50} values showed a wide variation with the administration route. Oral administration yielded the highest LD_{50} value, followed by sc, ip, and iv injections.[50] The lethal response is higher in weanling animals than in adults.[42,56] In adult animals, it should be noted that susceptibility sometimes varies widely among strains. For example, more than 50% of male F344 rats died within 7 days following sc injection of 3.4 mg Cd/kg,[38] whereas male Wistar rats only showed chronic nephropathy or tumors with a slight shortening of life span after the same treatment.[81] Of course, similar variations should be considered between sexes or species. At an acute phase of cadmium injection, liver and testis damage was most frequently observed in adult animals, whereas damage to neural tissue was often observed in young animals.[40,41,45,46] Cd-induced liver damage is recognized by conventional markers, such as increased blood levels of hepatic enzymes[32,43,49] and morphological changes.[32,33,43] Less hepatic damage was apt to be caused in weanling rats than in adults.[43]

Similarly, the reproductive tissues of the liver show a very high susceptibility to cadmium acute toxicity. Testicular damage could be detected by hemorrhage,[39] decreased glutathione levels,[37] and pathological changes.[39,43] The testicular LPO level may not be a good indicator of Cd exposure because it tends to decrease after low-dose injection.[60] Laskey et al.[44] suggested that a decrease in serum testosterone levels induced by human chorionic gonadotropin (h-GC) was the most sensitive marker of cadmium toxicity. Maitani and Suzuki[58] reported alterations in essential metal levels of liver, testis, and kidney in five strains of $CdCl_2$-treated mice. Testis of young animals showed a higher susceptibility to Cd toxicity than that of adults.[61]

Since the placenta is one of the target organs of Cd toxicity, its injection in pregnant animals might cause adverse effects on the fetus via damage to the placenta (Table 22.5). High dosing-induced placental necrosis may result in fetal death.[63] Lower dosing leads to embryo malformation[65,70] and decreases in body weight,[68] DNA, and protein.[64, 67] Early death of offspring was also documented.[62]

TABLE 22.4
Acute Effects of Cadmium Toxicity

Animal Strain, Sex, (Age)[a]	Dose[b] (mg Cd/kg)	Route	Effects	Ref.
Rats				
Wistar, F	1.8	iv	LD_{50}	31
SD, M	3.9	iv	Liver lesions (1 h)	32
SD, M	2	iv	Liver: stress protein synthesis (2 h) ↑	33
SD, F	7	iv	55% mortality (96 h); ovary, liver: lesions	34
SD, M	6.6	sc	Testis: lesions	
SD, M	1.65	sc	Testis, epididymis: *in situ* pH (24 h) ↑	35
F344, M	2.24	sc	Testis: lesions (24 h)	36
SD, M	2.24 (acetate)	sc	Sertoli and Leydig cells: GP × ↑; GSR, GSH	37
F344, M	3.4	sc	>50% mortality (7 d)	38
Wistar, M	3.4	sc	Testis: hemorrhage (12 h)	39
LE, M + F, (5 d)	4	sc	Decreased motor activity (8–11 d)	40
SD, M, (4 d)	4	sc	Brain lesions, hyperactivity (4–18 d)	41
SD, M + F, (7 d)	6	sc	30% mortality (48 h)	42
SD, M + F, (28 d)	6	sc	4% mortality (48 h)	
SD, M	4	iv	Liver: lesions (10 h)	43
SD, M + F, (10 d)	4–6		No damage	
SD, M	8.3	sc	10% mortality	44
	0.18	sc	hGC-induced serum testosterone ↓	
?, (3 d)	2 × 3 (on 3, 10, and 17 d)	ip	Brain: hypomyelination (5 d)	45

TABLE 22.4 *(Continued)*
Acute Effects of Cadmium Toxicity

Animal Strain, Sex, (Age)[a]	Dose[b] (mg Cd/kg)	Route	Effects	Ref.
Wistar (d 19)	11.2 µg/fetus	ip	Hydrocephalus, brain necrosis	46
Wistar, M	2.6	ip	Heart: GSH, LPO, MT ↑	47
Wistar, F	64	po	22% mortality (96 h)	48
SD, M	75	po	Liver: MT induction; GSH (4 h) ↓	49
SD, M	3.35	iv	LD_{50} (14 d)	50
	3.55	ip	LD_{50} (14 d)	
	9.3	sc	LD_{50} (14 d)	
	225	po	LD_{50} (14 d)	
Mice				
Swiss-Webster, M	4	iv	60% mortality (14 d)	51
Swiss-Webster, M	0.2	ip	Liver: MT induction	52
CFLP, M	1	ip	Testis: pathological change (3 d)	53
ICR, F	1.2	ip	Blood: ALAD (1 d) ↑	54
ICR, M	5	ip	40% mortality (10 d)	55
	112	po	60% mortality (10 d)	
C57BL/6, M, (50 d)	4.08	ip	LD_{50} (7 d)	56
C57BL/6, M, (7 d)	1.65	ip	LD_{50} (7 d)	
C3H, F	2.8	sc	Sheep RBC-induced immune response ↓	57
5 strains, M	3.36	sc	Liver, testis: alterations in essential metal levels	58
CBA, M	53	po	11% mortality (10 d)	59

[a] Data from adult animals, unless otherwise specified.
[b] $CdCl_2$ was used, unless otherwise specified.

TABLE 22.5
Effects of Cadmium on Pregnant Animals

Animal Strain	Dose (mg Cd/kg or ppm Cd)	Injection Time (G.D.)[a]	Route	Effects	Ref.
Rats					
SD	2.1 × 4	8, 10, 12, 14	ip	Offspring: 75% mortality (12 d)	62
Wistar	4.5	18	sc	Placental necrosis (24 h) Fetal death	63
	1.25	12	iv	Fetus: DNA and protein synthesis ↓	64
	1.25	12	ip or iv	Fetus: skeletal malformation	65
	0.49 × 20	1–20	sc	Neonatal: thymus weight and liver Zn ↓	66
LE	4.9 × 4	12–15	sc	Fetal: lung DNA and protein ↓	67
SD	50, 100 ppm water × 15 d	6–20		Fetus: body weight and liver Zn ↓ Mother: body weight, serum ALAD, and alkaline phosphatase ↓	68
Wistar	60 ppm/ water × 20 d	1–20		Offspring: impaired movement	69
Mice					
CD-1	5.6	10	sc	Embryo: malformation	70

[a] G.D. = gestation day.

B. Subacute to Chronic Toxicities

Continuous exposure to Cd was carried out by repeated injection or by giving Cd-contaminated food or drinking water. Long-term treatment at low levels increases the damage to other organs, including the kidney (Table 22.6). Chronic and subchronic renal damage induced by cadmium salt was recognized by the pathological changes[71,72,77] or the appearance of abnormal urinary components.[74,78,82] Urinary B_2-microglobulin was reported to be an earlier marker than albumin.[82] Abnormalities of bone tissue were also documented as chronic effects of cadmium.[84,88] It should be noted that, particularly in a repeated injection experiment, Cd injection of even a sublethal dose induced metallothionein synthesis in the target organs, which lead to increased resistance to Cd (and other metal) toxicities.[52,90,91] Nishimura et al.[92] suggested urinary trehalase activity was a sensitive indicator for cadmium-induced chronic renal failure in rabbits.

When animals were exposed to aerosol of CdO or $CdCl_2$ or when the metal was instilled intratracheally, the lung primarily was damaged (Table 22.7). Increase in tissue weight[93,96,99] and various cytosolic enzyme activities[93,97] and decrease in mitochondrial enzymes[94,98] have been documented. Long-term treatment caused an increase in the connective-tissue components.[96]

Damage to the kidney in the acute phase of cadmium salt injection is very rare. However, when cadmium was injected as Cd-metallothionein or coinjected with an SH compound such as cysteine even via an alternative route, the kidney became a primary target organ (Table 22.8). The renal damage was detected, for example, in the case of chronic Cd toxicity. Suppression of PAH uptake by the renal slice prepared from the intoxicated rats was suggested to be a sensitive marker for Cd plus cysteine-induced nephrotoxicity.[109] Goering et al.[106] found induction of renal stress proteins at the initial phase of renal damage in rats treated by Cd-cysteine.

TABLE 22.6
Subacute to Chronic Effects of Cadmium

Animal Strain, Sex, (Weight)[a]	Dose (mg/kg or ppm Cd)	Route	Effects	Ref.
Rats				
SD, M	1.8×14 d	iv	Liver, kidney: pathological change	71
	$0.6 \times 2–6$ wk (5 d/wk)	sc	Kidney: membrane degeneration	72
	0.025×6 wk (5 d/wk)	po	Liver: cytochrome c-oxidase ↓	73
Wistar, M	1.5×26 d	sc	Urinary protein, AST, amino acids ↑	74
BN, F	0.49×3 wk (5 d/wk)	sc	S-phase thymocytes ↓	75
Lewis, F	0.49×3 wk (5 d/wk)	sc	G_2-phase thymocytes ↑	75
?, M, (40–50 g)	0.4×30 d	ip	Brain: SOD ↓; LPO ↑	76
SD, M	0.5×26 wk (6 d/wk)	sc	Liver damage (4 wk); renal damage (8 wk)	77
Wistar, F	0.4×13 wk (5 d/wk)	sc	Urinary protein, HyPro, HyLys ↑	78
	$6.12 \times 1–3$ months	po	Duodenum: Ca^{2+} transport ↓	79
Wistar, M	1.49×11 wk (5 d/wk)	sc	Intestinal mucosa: alkaline phosphatase ↓	80
	3.4×1		Chronic nephropathy, testicular tumors (90 wk)	81
SD, F	100 ppm/water $\times$ 7 months		Urine: transferrin, IgG, β_2-M, albumin ↑	82
Wistar, M	50 ppm/water $\times$ 10 months		Alteration in skeletal muscle ultrastructure	83
	50–100 ppm/food $\times$ 6–8 wk		Bone: pathological change; lysil oxidase ↓	84
	50 ppm/food $\times$ 52 wk		Bone: collagen cross-linking ↓	
LE, F	1 ppm/water $\times$ 18 months		Hypertension (2 months)	85
			Heart, liver, kidney: ATP ↓; ADP ↑	
SD, M	50 ppm/water $\times$ 30 d		Small intestine: hemoxygenase activity ↑	86
Mice				
C57BL/6, M	50–200 ppm/water $\times$ 3 wk		Proliferative response of spleen cell ↑	87
CF1, F	50 ppm/food $\times$ 252 d		Femur Ca levels ↓	88
QS, F	10, 100 ppm/water $\times$ 22 wk		Brain: degenerative damage in choroid plexus	89

[a] Data from adult animals, unless otherwise specified.

TABLE 22.7
Pulmonary Toxicity of Aerosol Inhalation or Intratracheal Injection of Cadmium

Animal Strain, Sex	Chemicals	Cd Level (mg/m³)	Exposure Time (h × days)	Effects on Lung	Ref.
Rats					
SD, M	CdO, CdCl₂	0.45–4.5	2 × 1	Tissue weight, GSR, GST, and G6PD ↑	93
	CdO	4.5	0.5 × 1	Monooxygenase and cytochrome P-450 ↓	94
Wistar, M	CdO	5	3 × 1	Nonprotein SH ↑	95
F344, F	CdCl₂	1	6 × 62	Tissue weight, elastin, collagen ↑	96
Lewis, M	CdO	1.6	3 × 20	G6PD, GSR, Cat, and GPx ↑	97
		8.4	3 × 1	Alkaline and acid phosphatase, LDH, and protein ↑	
CD-1, M	CdCl₂	0.85	2 × 1	Mitochondrial enzymes ↓	98
Wistar, M	CdO, CdCl₂	0.5–10 μg Cd/rat (it)		Tissue weight, lavage fluid cell number ↑	99
F344, F	CdCl₂	0.1, 0.4 mg Cd/kg (it)		HyPro ↑	100
Mice					
BALB/c, F	CdCl₂	4.9	1 × 1	Pathological change	101
	CdCl₂	4.9	1 × 1	Cell proliferation ↑	102

TABLE 22.8
Renal Toxicities by Cadmium-Metallothionein or Cadmium Plus Thiol Co-Injection

Animal Strain, Sex	Chemicals	Dose (mg Cd/kg)	Routes	Effects	Ref.
Rats					
SD, M	Cd-MT	0.3	ip	Pathological changes; PHA uptake by kidney slice ↓	103
Wistar, M	Cd-MT	0.4	sc	Ca²⁺ uptake by luminal and batholateral membrane vesicles ↓	104
	Cd + Cys	1.3–1.7	iv	Urinary protein, glucose, amino acids ↑	105
	Cd + Cys-peptide	0.51–0.64			
	Cd-MT	0.16–0.23			
SD, M	Cd + Cys	2	iv	Stress protein synthesis ↑	106
	CD + β-ME	1.68	ip	Urinary protein, amino acids ↑	107
Mice					
4 strains, M	Cd-MT	0.4–1.6	sc	Urinary glucose ↑	108
ICR, M	Cd + Cys	1.5	iv	Urinary glucose, protein ↑ PHA uptake by kidney slice ↓	109

SECTION 5. CHROMIUM

Trivalent chromium (Cr) is essential in animals including humans, whereas hexavalent chromium, which is easily absorbed from the gastrointestinal tract, is very toxic. Hepatic and renal damages have been reported in the acute phase of chromium parenteral injection at dose levels 7.9 to 15.8 mg Cr/kg in rats (Table 22.9).[110-113] Tsapakos et al.[109] detected DNA-protein cross-links in liver and kidney of Cr-injected rats, suggesting relationships to carcinogenicity and toxicity of Cr(VI). In the subacute to chronic phase, reproductive tissues were also affected. Serial ip injection of 1 to 4 mg Cr/kg as dichromate for 5 to 90 days caused pathological changes in testis cells or altered enzyme activities in rats.[114-116] Vyskocil et al.[117] showed that female rats manifested renal dysfunction after 6-month exposure to 25 ppm Cr (as chromate) in drinking water, but males did not. Increased DNA-protein cross-link was detected in lymphocytes and liver of rats given drinking water contaminated by 100 to 200 ppm Cr as chromate.[118] Chronic inhalation experiments of Cr aerosol were reported to cause adverse effects in the lung. Glaser and co-workers[119] found that although exposure to low Cr level caused activation of alveolar macrophages, high-level exposure inactivated it. They also showed that Cr_5O_{12} aerosol was much more toxic to lung and blood cells than $Na_2Cr_2O_7$ aerosol.[120] If pregnant mice were exposed to $K_2Cr_2O_7$ from drinking water containing 250 to 1000 ppm Cr throughout the gestation period, embryonic death and malformation of offspring occurred.[121]

TABLE 22.9
Toxic Effects of Hexavalent Chromium in Rats

Animal Strain, Sex (Age)[a]	Chemical	Dose (mg Cr/kg or ppm Cr)	Route	Effects	Ref.
Rats					
SD, M	$Na_2Cr_2O_7$	7.9, 19.8	ip	Liver, kidney: DNA-protein cross-links	110
	$Na_2Cr_2O_7$	10.5	ip	Liver: GSH ↑	111
Wistar, M	Na_2CrO_4	4.7 × 3	ip	Liver microsome: Cr(VI) reductase, cytochrome P-450, cytochrome b_5 ↓	112
SD, M	$Na_2Cr_2O_7$	7.9, 15.8	sc	Serum: BUN, lactate, glucose ↑; insulin ↓	113
Wistar, M	Na_2CrO_4	1, 2, or 4 × 5	ip	Testis: tissue weight, epididymal sperm number ↓; pathological change	114
ITRC, M, (weanling)	$K_2Cr_2O_7$	1–3 × 90	ip	Testis: pathological change; γ-GTP, LDH ↑; sorbitol dehydrogenase, G6PD ↓	115
Druckrey, M	$K_2Cr_2O_7$	2 × 15	ip	Testis: pathological change in epithelial cells	116
Wistar, M + F	Na_2CrO_4	25 ppm/water × 6 months		Female: urinary albumin, β_2-M ↑ Male: no change	117
F344, M	K_2CrO_4	100–200 ppm/water × 3–6 wk		Liver: DNA-protein cross-link	118

[a] Data from adult animals, unless otherwise specified.

SECTION 6. CISPLATIN

Cisplatin (CDDP; *cis*-diaminodichloroplatinum) is an effective anticancer drug widely used in cancer chemotherapy. However, it also acts as a nephrotoxin. The nephrotoxic actions of cisplatin have been well documented in laboratory animals (Table 22.10); 50% mortality was documented, for example, in rats (7.7 mg/kg, ip)[123] and mice (9.5 to 13.4 mg/kg, sc, iv).[142,143] Cisplatin-induced renal damage was detected in the form of increased BUN and serum creatinine levels, pathological change or decreased enzyme activities in the kidney, and alteration in urine constituents. Urinalysis was suggested to be a more sensitive method.[124] De Witt et al.[126] demonstrated that increase in the Ca^{2+} pump activity of the renal endoplasmic reticulum (ER) was the earlier marker, followed by renal failure in the cisplatin-treated rat. Litterst[125] showed that a high salt concentration of the vehicle markedly lowered the toxic effects of cisplatin in rat.

Cisplatin affects neural tissue, not only through its nephrotoxic action but also through glucose metabolism, testes, blood cells, and embryo. Neurotoxic action could be detected by pathological change,[132,133] electrophysiological methods[134] and abnormal behavior.[147] Goldstein and co-workers[135,136] demonstrated the increased plasma glucagon half-life and impaired glucose tolerance, which possibly lead to renal failure. Effects on rat testes were observed as decreased plasma testosterone levels[137] and functional and morphological alterations of Sertoli cells.[138] Reduction in reticulocytes was documented in cisplatin-treated mice.[145,146] Aggarwal and co-worker[140,141] found that embryonic resorption or death occurred in cisplatin-treated rats and mice. They suggested that the cisplatin-induced decreases of sex hormone levels are responsible for the embryonic toxicity.

TABLE 22.10
Toxic Effects of CDDP

Animal Strain, Sex, (Age)[a]	Dose (mg CDDP/kg)	Route	Effects	Ref.
Rats				
F344, M	6, 25	ip	GFR ↓; jejunal crypt cell survival (3–5 d) ↓	122
	0.5–12	ip	LD_{50}: 7.7 mg/kg; renal damage: BUN ↑; histology	123
	2.5–15	iv	Renal damage: urine analysis as sensitive method	124
SD, M	9	ip	Decreased toxicity (lethality) by high-salt vehicle	125
	5, 7.5	ip	Renal endoplasmic reticulum: Ca^{2+} pump activity, Ca^{2+} content (4–24 h) ↑	126
	7	iv	Renal cytochrome P-450, b_5, γ-GCS, γ-GTP (7 d) ↓	127
SD, ?	5	ip	Defect in papillary hypertonicity; damage at S_3 segment	128
Wistar, M	5	iv	Creatinine clearance ↓	129
	5	ip	Kidney, liver: LPO ↑ GPx, GST, Cat ↓; kidney SOD ↓	130
BN, M	3 × 3 (21-d interval)	ip	Kidney: cytochrome P-450, GSR, GST, GPx, GSH ↓; N-glucuronyl transferase, GSSG, LPO ↑	131
Wistar, (10 d)	5	sc	Brain: abnormal shape of the dendritic tree (24 h)	132
Wistar, F	2 × 9 (1 or 2/wk)	ip	Pathological change in spinal ganglia neuron and sciatic and peroneal nerve	133
	1 × 15 or 34 (2/wk)	ip	Sensory nerve condition velocities (48 h) ↓	134
	15	ip	Cisplatin-DNA binding in DRG satellite cells (6 h)	
F344, M	5	iv	Plasma glucagon half-life ↑; renal failure (96 h)	135
	5	iv	Impaired glucose tolerance (48 h)	136
Wistar, M	9	iv	Plasma testosterone, testis cytochrome P-450 (72 h) ↓	137
SD, M	2 × 5	ip	Leakage of the Sertoli cell tight junction (24 h); abnormal Sertoli cell secretory function	138
F344, M	5	iv	Intestinal epithelium (ileum): pathological change (24 h)	139
Wistar, pregnant		ip	Embryonic LD_{50}: G.D. 6, 2.88 mg/kg; G.D. 8, 1.28 mg/kg; G.D. 11, 1.0 mg/kg	140
	4, 7 (on G.D. 6)	ip	Serum: LH, progesterone, 20 α-hydroxysteroid dehydrogenase ↓; embryonal resorption	141
Mice				
BDF1, ?	9.5	sc	Plasma: BUN, CRT ↑; 50% mortality (30 d)	142
Swiss, M + F		iv	LD_{50}: M, 13.4 mg/kg; F, 12.32 mg/kg	143
Swiss, M	18, 20	ip	Decreased nephrotoxicity in high NaCl vehicle	125
B6D2F1, M	5 × 2 months (1 d/wk)	iv	Lesion in renal cortical tubules and bone marrow; circadian rhythm affected	144
B6C3F1, M + F	15.5	iv	Reticulocytes ↓	145
B6D2F1, M	6.5	iv	Immature WBC, PMN ↑; immature RBC ↓	146
CD1, M	10	ip	Tail flick temperature and distal sensory latency ↑	147
Swiss, pregnant	5.24	ip	Embryonic LD_{50} (day 8)	140

[a] Data from adult animals, unless otherwise specified.

Note: G.D. = gestation day.

SECTION 7. COBALT

Cobalt (Co) is an essential component of vitamin B_{12}. Its toxicity is summarized in Table 22.11. The increase of lysozyme level in lavage fluid was documented in rabbits exposed to $CoCl_2$ aerosol (0.5 mg Co/m^3 × 6 h/day) for a month.[156] Increased tissue weight and inflammatory response of the rat lung were documented in rat after intratracheal injection (10 mg Co/kg) of metallic Co dust.[148] Chronic exposure experiments using Co-contaminated food or water revealed testicular atrophy and reduced behavioral activity in rats[150] and abnormal testis morphology in mice.[154] Di Giulio et al.[149] indicated that consecutive ip injection of $CoCl_2$ (10 mg Co/kg) for 42 days caused increased hematocrit and hypertrophy of glomus cells in the rat carotid body. $CoCl_2$ treatment (10 to 20 mg Co/mg × 2, sc) caused a significant reduction in the hepatic P-450 levels of rats in the acute phase,[151] an effect much more prominent in Co-protoporphyrin-treated rats[153] and hamsters.[155] Since serial injection of 100 mg Co/kg as $CoCl_2$ in pregnant rats for 10 days caused no damage to the fetus,[152] embryo toxicity of $CoCl_2$ was considered to be very low.

TABLE 22.11
Toxic Effects of Cobalt in Experimental Animals

Animal Strain, Sex[a]	Compound	Dose (mg/kg or ppm Co)	Route	Effects	Ref.
Rats					
SD, F	Co (metal dust)	10	it	Lung: moderate inflammatory response, weight ↑	148
SD, M	$CoCl_2$	10 × 42	ip	Glomus cell hypertrophy; hematocrit ↑	149
	$CoCl_2$	20 × 69	Food	Testicular atrophy; slower lever press	150
	$CoCl_2$	10–20 × 2	sc	Liver: cytochrome P-450 (24 h) ↓	151
SD, pregnant	$CoCl_2$	100 × 10 (G.D. 6–15)	po	No fetotoxicity	152
SD, M	Co-protoporphyrin	0.88–3.5	sc	Liver: cytochrome P-450, cytochrome b_5, NADPH-P-450 reductase ↓	153
CD-1, M	$CoCl_2$	400 ppm/water × 13 wk		Pathological change in testis cells	154
Hamsters					
Syrian, M	Co-protoporphyrin	5.3	sc	Liver: cytochrome P-450 ↓	155

[a] Data from adult animals, unless otherwise specified.
Note: G.D. = gestation day.

SECTION 8. COPPER

Although copper (Cu) is an essential metal, its excessive intake has been shown to have a variety of toxic effects. Metabolism and pulmonary toxicity of intratracheally instilled $CuSO_4$ or CuO have been reported in rat at dose levels of 2.5 to 50 μg Cu/rat.[157, 158] The biochemical and elemental inflammatory indices in bronchoalveolar lavage fluid reached maximum values at 12 to 72 h after instillation of 5 μg Cu/rat. Toxic effects on liver or kidney have been reported in rats fed a diet containing 1500 ppm Cu as $CuSO_4$ for 15 or 16 weeks, respectively.[159,160] Hemolytic anemia has also been documented in rats after consecutive ip injection of Cu-nitrilotriacetate at a dose level of 4 to 7 mg Cu/kg.[161] Mascular mutant mouse, which has been proposed as an animal model of Menke's Kinky-hair disease, was reported to be sensitive to the acute hepatotoxic effects of Cu as compared with normal mice.[162] Clastogenic effects of Cu on the bone marrow chromosomes were shown in mice injected ip with $CuSO_4$ (1.1 to 6.6 mg/kg).[163]

SECTION 9. IRON

Despite its abundance and necessity in almost all living organisms, excess iron (Fe) causes various toxic effects if accumulated in human and animal tissues. The effects of iron overload in experimental animals vary among species, strains, and sex (Table 22.12). Since the liver is the major storage organ of the excess iron, hepatotoxicity is the most common finding in animals undergoing iron overload experiments. Hepatic fibrosis was induced in rats by feeding them an iron carbonyl-contaminated diet for as long as 8 months.[168,169] On the other hand, single dosing of iron dextran caused hepatic fibrosis in gerbils,[175] which were suggested to be a sensitive model for induction of hepatic fibrosis.

Cardiotoxicity is the other major effect of iron overload observed in humans, but no experimental model has been reported in mice or rats. Recently, Garthew et al.[174] demonstrated that repeated sc injection of gerbils with iron dextran resulted in hemochromatosis with a heart pathology similar to human cases.

Since iron has a catalytic action in reactive oxygen generation *in vivo*, a considerable part of its toxicity may be the oxidative damage caused. Several studies demonstrated elevated lipid peroxidation in the tissue of iron-overloaded animals.[164,165,170,171] The catalytic action of iron was also suggested to be involved in the carcinogenic action of polyhalogenated aromatic hydrocarbons.[176]

TABLE 22.12
Toxic Effects of Iron Overload in Experimental Animals

Animal Strain, Sex (Age)[a]	Fe-compound	Dose (mg/kg or ppm Fe)	Route	Effects	Ref.
Rats					
Wistar, M	Dextran	500 mg/kg	ip	Liver: chemiluminescence, LPO ↑; cytochrome P-450, SOD, Cat ↓	164
	Dextran	116 mg Fe per kg × 3 d	ip	Liver: dimethylhydrazine demethylase, UDP	165
Wistar, F	Carbonyl	25,000 ppm/food × 10 wk		Proliferative activity after a mitogenic stimulus ↓	166
Wistar, F, (4 wk)	Saccharate	5 mg Fe per kg × 12 wk	ip	Mesothelioma	167
SD, M	Carbonyl	20,000 ppm/food × 4–15 months		Hemochromatosis	168
	Carbonyl	25,000 ppm/food × 12 months		Hemochromatosis, hepatic fibrosis	169
	NTA	2 mg Fe per kg × 14 wk	ip	Liver mitochondria: LPO ↑	170
	Carbonyl	25,000 ppm Fe per food × 28–44 d		Liver mitochondria and microsome: LPO ↑	
	Sulfate	305 ppm Fe per food × 10 wk		Liver: LPO ↑; non-Se-GPx ↑	171
Mice					
SWR, M	Dextran	600 mg Fe per kg	sc	Porphyria (25 wk)	172
A/J, M + F	NTA	1.8–2.7 mg Fe per kg × 12 wk (6 d/wk)	ip	Nephrotoxicity, renal carcinoma	173
Gerbil					
Mongolian	Dextran	1000 mg Fe per kg × 7 wk (1 d/wk)	sc	Liver, heart: hemosiderosis, hemochromatosis (12 wk)	174

[a] Data from adult animals, unless otherwise specified.

SECTION 10. LEAD

Lead (Pb) may cause various adverse effects in experimental animals in both acute and chronic phases. Toxic effects of inorganic lead as related to hematopoietic, nervous, gastrointestinal, and renal systems, whereas those of organic lead are largely related to the nervous system. Although rats are the most frequently used animals in studies of metal toxicity, adult rats are relatively insensitive to lead toxicity,[177] whereas perinatal animals are very sensitive. Accordingly, numerous experimental studies have been carried out using young animals.

A. Inorganic Lead Toxicity

There are marked differences in LD_{50} values for lead toxicity among species, sex, and age (Table 22.13).[178-181] Acute lead encephalopathy occurs easily in young animals but only rarely in adults.[184,188] Kumar and Desiraju[184] reported that about 20% of rat pups orally administered lead acetate (0.4 g Pb/pup) for 10 to 11 days developed hind limb paralysis and died within 24 h.

The characteristic disturbances in the central nervous system (CNS) functions during chronic lead exposure (lead encephalopathy) have stimulated numerous behavioral, pathological, and neurochemical investigations (Table 22.14). CNS disturbance seems more apt to occur during development,[186,189] possibly due to high lead absorbability[193,194] and high susceptibility.[195] In the last decade, an increasing amount of evidence has accumulated to show that lead exposure, particularly in the perinatal period, disrupts the development of opioid peptide systems in the rat brain.[196] Disturbance of the peripheral nerve has been documented by histopathological[183] and electrophysiological methods.[197]

In the chronic phase, disturbances in hematological, nervous, and renal systems have been documented as lead toxicity in animals. Anemia is a common chronic systemic effect of lead, which is considered to be caused by a combined effect of the inhibition of hemoglobin (Hb) synthesis and shortened life span of circulating erythrocytes (RBC). Lead has been shown to interfere with heme biosynthesis even at a low level of exposure.[209] Inhibition of the heme biosynthetic enzyme δ-aminolevulinic acid dehydratase (ALAD) and elevation of free RBC and zinc protoporphyrin (ZPP) are the earliest effects, followed by increase in urinary δ-aminolevulinic acid (ALA) and coproporphyrin, and fall in Hb and hematocrit (Ht) level (Table 22.15). ALAD activity in RBC is shown to be the most sensitive indicator of lead exposure. Maes and Gerber[210] reported that when rats were severely intoxicated, marked shortening of RBC survival led to increased ALAD activity in circulating erythrocytes.

Kidney is also a target organ of chronic lead toxicity. A number of transient effects on renal function in experimental animals are consistent with pathological findings of reversible lesions.[211-214] Irreversible lesions such as interstitial fibrosis have also been documented in animals following long-term lead exposure.[214,215]

Studies during the last decade have shown that chronic and low-level lead exposure might induce subtle alterations in the immune systems of experimental animals. Enhanced host susceptibility to bacteria and viral infections[216-218] and increased growth and metastasis of implanted tumors[219,220] have also been reported. Other studies demonstrated the ability of lead to reduce the number of antibody-forming cells,[221] to suppress antibody synthesis,[222,223] and to diminish the phagocytic function of the reticuloendothelial systems.[223] Lead has also been shown to induce perivascular edema,[183] teratogenicity,[224] and testicular toxicity[225] in experimental animals.

TABLE 22.13
The LD_{50} of Lead Salts for Rats and Mice after Intraperitoneal Dose

Animal Strain	Sex	Age or Weight	Salt	LD_{50} (mg/kg)	Days	Ref.
Rats						
?	M	3 wk	Acetate	225	8	178
	F	3 wk		231	8	
	M	18 wk		170	8	
	F	18 wk		258	8	
SD	M	20 wk	Acetate	172	8	179
	F	20 wk		280	8	
Mice						
DBA/2	M	60–70 d	Nitrate	74	10	180
C57BL/6	M			102	10	
Swiss-Webster	M			148	10	
ICR	M	26 g	Acetate	278	8	181
	F	23 g		280	8	

TABLE 22.14
Neurobehavioral Effects of Lead

Animal Strain, Sex	Age or Weight	Salt	Dose	Route	Effects	Ref.
Rabbits						
NZ, M + F	Newborn	Nitrate	4.5–18 mg/pup × 30 d	po	Pathological changes in CNS	182
Rats						
Wistar, M	400 g	Carbonate	1000 mg/kg × 600 d	po	Histopathological changes in CNS	183
Wistar, M + F	Newborn	Acetate	400 mg Pb per kg × 60 d	po	Hind limb paralysis, brain edema and hemorrhages, biogenic amines and GABA/glutamate system changes	184
Wistar	Newborn	Acetate	45–180 mg Pb per kg × 19 d	po	Behavioral changes	185
Wistar, M	Perinatal	Acetate	750 ppm/food × 17 d	Maternal	Behavioral changes	186
SD, M	Newborn	Nitrate	10 mg/kg × 15 d	ip	Histopathological changes in CNS	187
LE, M + F	Newborn	Acetate	600 mg/kg × 10 or 30 d	po	Alteration in cerebellum development	188
	Newborn	Acetate	10–90 mg/kg × 19 d	po	Behavioral changes	189
ITRC, M	220–240 g	Acetate	5–12 mg/kg × 14 d	ip	Behavioral changes and alteration in biogenic amine levels	190
Mice						
HET, M	60 d, 1 year	Acetate	5000 ppm/water × 7 wk		Behavioral changes	191
BK/W, M + F	Perinatal	Acetate	2500 ppm/water	Maternal	Behavioral changes	192

TABLE 22.15
Hematopoietic Effects of Lead

Animal Strain, Sex	Age or Weight	Salt	Dose	Route	Effects	Ref.
Rabbits						
NZ, F	2.5–2.8 kg	Acetate	0.2 mg/kg × 48 d (3 d/wk)	sc	RBC: ALAD ↓; urinary ZPP ↑	198
			0.8–1.2 mg/kg × 97–181 d (3 d/wk)		RBC: ALAD ↓; urinary ZPP and ALA ↑	
NZ, M	90 d	Subacetate	5000 ppm/food × 90–120 d		Hb ↓; nephropathy	199
NZ, M + F	Newborn	Nitrate	4.5 mg/pup × 20 d		Ht ↓	
Rats						
SD, M + F	Perinatal	Acetate	2500 ppm Pb/water × 7 wk	Maternal	RBC, kidney: ALAD ↓; Ht ↓; urinary ALA ↑	200
Wistar, M + F	Newborn	Acetate	20,000 ppm/food × 20–22 d	Maternal	Brain, liver: ALAD ↓	201
Wistar, F	Pregnant	Acetate	500 ppm Pb/water × 3 wk		RBC: ALAD ↓	202
Wistar, M + F	Prenatal			Maternal	RBC: ALAD ↓; Hb ↓; Ht ↓	
Wistar, M	180–250 g	Acetate	500 ppm Pb/water × 30 d		Urinary ALA and CP ↑	203
CF, M	180–200 g	Acetate	8 mg PB per kg × 7 d	ip	RBC: ALAD ↓	204
?, M	160–180 g	Acetate	550 ppm Pb/water × 1–4 months		RBC: ALAD ↓; ZPP ↑; urinary ALA ↑	205
?, ?	Newborn	Acetate	10,000 ppm/water × 40–60 d	Maternal	ALAD: RBC, liver, kidney spleen ↓	206
					ALAS: spleen ↑; liver ↓	
					ALA: brain, spleen, kidney, urine ↑	
	40–60 d	Acetate	2 mg Pb per kg × 3	ip	ALAD: RBC, liver, kidney, spleen ↓	
					ALAS: liver, spleen ↑; kidney ↓	
					ALA: spleen, kidney, urine ↑	
?, M	150–170 d	Acetate	10 mg Pb per kg × 4 wk	po	RBC: ALAD ↓; ZPP ↑; urinary ALA ↑	207
Mice						
ddy, M + F	30–40 g	Acetate	500 ppm Pb/water × 30 d		Urinary ALA ↑	203
NMRI, M	20–25 g	Acetate	500–5000 ppm/water × 30 d or 500–2500 ppm/water × 90 d		RBC, liver, brain, bone marrow: ALAD ↓	208
		Acetate	0.1 mg/kg	iv	RBC, liver, brain, bone marrow: ALAD ↓	
DBA/2, M	60–70 d	Carbonate	4000 ppm/food × 12 d		Liver: ALAD ↓	180
C57BL/6, M						
Swiss-Webster, M					Liver: ALAD ↓; Ht ↓	

B. Organic Lead Toxicity

Triethyllead (TEL) and other organic lead compounds have been shown to affect preferentially the nervous system.[226] Degenerative changes have been observed in the cerebral cortex, cerebellum, and hippocampus of rabbits receiving lethal or near-lethal doses of tetraethyl lead.[227,228] Rats subjected to both acute and short-term repeated TEL exposure experienced alterations in reactivity, locomotor activity, and avoidance learning.[229,230] Moreover, organic lead has been shown to have several biochemical effects, including alteration of enkephalin levels,[231] dopaminergic processes,[232] and enhanced lipid peroxidation[233] in brain.

SECTION 11. MANGANESE

Manganese (Mn) is an essential metal, considered to have low toxicity. The chronic and subchronic effects on the neural tissues have been widely investigated (Table 22.16). Serial ip injection of 4 mg Mn/kg for 30 days caused reduced LPO[236] or increased norepinephrine (NE) levels[237] in rats. Exposure via drinking water containing 1000 ppm Mn for 14 days effected increases in brain dopamine (DA) and NE levels and activated behavior.[243] A 30-day exposure to the same level increased turnover rates of DA and NE.[242] Bonilla and Prasad[244] have shown significant decreases of the biogenic amines in several regions of the brain of rats given 100 or 1000 ppm Mn-containing water for 8 months. Komura and Sakamoto[250] have reported that effects of several Mn compounds (chloride, acetate, carbonate, and dioxide) on the brain biogenic amine levels in mice were different, within the highest toxicity shown by MnO_2. In addition to its neurotoxic effects, $MnCl_2$ was also documented to cause a pancreatitis-like reaction,[245] hepatic damage,[247] and reduced antibody production[249] in mice or rats. Rogers et al.[248] observed increases in the splenic natural killer cell activity and plasma interferon levels in three strains of mice.

Methylcyclopentadienyl manganese tricarbonyl (MMT) is used as an octane enhancer in unleaded gasoline. LD_{50} values of MMT after po and ip injections were determined in rats to be 50 mg/kg[254] and 12.1 to 23 mg/kg,[251,254] respectively (Table 22.17). Fishman et al.[256] showed the lethal effect of MMT was more potent in propyrene glycol vehicle than in corn oil vehicle. MMT affected lung tissue of experimental animals was detected as pathological change[253,254] and increased lavage protein levels.[252,255]

TABLE 22.16
Toxic Effects of Manganese Chloride

Animal Strain, Sex (Age)[a]	Dose (mg/kg or ppm Mn)	Route	Effects	Ref.
Rats				
SD, (3 d)	150 × 44		Striatum and hypothalamus: homovanillic acid (15–22 d) ↓	234
Wistar, M	10	ip	Brain, heart: cholin esterase, carboxylesterase ↓	235
ITRC, M, (30 d)	4 × 30	ip	Brain: LPO ↓	236
MRC, M	4 × 30	ip	Brain: NE ↑; serum: Tyr, Trp ↓	237
Wistar, M	2, 8 × 48 (2/wk)	ip	Motor nerve conduction velocity ↑	238
?, M, (3 wk)	50 μg/rat × 60	po	Brain: MAO activity ↑; morphological change (30 d)	239
SD, M, (20 d)	10,000 ppm/water × 60 d		Dorsal caudate putamen: DA ↑	240
SD, M	1000 ppm/water × 65 wk		High locomotor activity (5–6 wk)	241
SD, M, (50 g)	1000 ppm/water × 30 d		Brain: turnover rate of DA and NE ↑	242
ITRC, M	1000 ppm/water × 14 d		Brain: DA, NE ↑; SMA ↑; learning activity ↓	243
SD, M	100, 1000 ppm/water × 8 months		Brain: catecholamines, 5-HT, 5-HIAA ↓	244
	3 × 30	ip	Pancreatitis-like reaction	245
	100, 200	iv	Liver: cellular necrosis, cholestasis (12 h)	246
?, M	200 ppm/water × 10 wk		Liver: change in ultrastructure	247
Mice				
CBA, A, C57BL/6, M	40, 80	im	NK-cell activity ↑; plasma interferon ↑ Susceptibility: CBA, A > C57BL/6	248

TABLE 22.16 *(Continued)*
Toxic Effects of Manganese Chloride

Animal Strain, Sex (Age)[a]	Dose (mg/kg or ppm Mn)	Route	Effects	Ref.
CD-1, M	1, 3, 10 × 28	ip	Antibody production ↓	249
ddy, M	130 ppm/food × 1 yr		Alteration in brain biogenic amines	250
			Toxicity: $MnO_2 > MnCl_2$	

[a] Data from adult animals, unless otherwise specified.

TABLE 22.17
Toxic Effects of Methylcyclopentadienyl Manganese Tricarbonyl (MMT)

Animals Strain, Sex	Dose (mg MMT/kg)	Route	Effects	Ref.
Rats				
SD, M	6–37.4	ip	LD_{50}: 12.1 mg/kg (24 h)	251
	4	sc	Lung: lavage protein (24 h) ↑	252
S/A, F	5	ip	Lung cell damage	253
SD, M		po	LD_{50} (14 d): 50 mg/kg; pulmonary hemorrhagic edema	254
		ip	LD_{50} (14 d): 23 mg/kg	
	0.5–2.5	sc	Bronchoalveolar lavage protein ↑	255
Mice				
CD-1, M		ip	LD_{50} (2 h): 152 mg/kg (propyrene glycol vehicle), 999 mg/kg (corn oil vehicle)	256
BALB/c, F	120	ip	Lung cell damage	253
Hamster Syrian, F	180	ip	Lung cell damage	253

SECTION 12. MERCURY

In the terms of its toxicological properties, mercury (Hg) can be classified into metallic mercury, inorganic mercuric salt, and organic mercury. Among various inorganic and organic Hg compounds, the focus here is on the toxic actions of mercuric chloride ($HgCl_2$) and methylmercury (MeHg) for the latter two mercurial species.

Exposure to metallic mercury can take place by inhalation of Hg vapor. Since metallic mercury easily penetrates the blood–brain barrier, exposure to low-dose levels (<3 mg Hg/m³) disturbs the neural tissues and causes behavioral changes in young and adult rats.[257,258] Prenatal exposure to Hg vapor was found to cause similar effects in offspring after growing up.[259] An extremely high dose (30 g Hg/m³) for 2 h damaged lung tissue, resulting in a significant mortality.[260]

Inorganic mercuric mercury is well documented as a potent nephrotoxin. Numerous investigators have reported the acute and subacute toxic actions of $HgCl_2$ using various indicators (Table 22.18). The toxic effects could be detected by pathological change, enzyme activities and lipid peroxidation in the kidney, and alterations in urinary components. However, because of its poor absorbability by the gastrointestinal tract, the effective dose of this Hg species by oral administration is higher than by parenteral injection. Mortality within 7 days was documented in rats and mice with dose levels of 3.6 mg/kg or above via the sc or iv route.[261,274] It should be noticed that young rats hardly show nephrotoxic symptoms even after injection of dose levels toxic for adult rats.[261] Interestingly, $HgCl_2$, particularly at low dose, increases the renal GSH level.[275] Bernard et al.[272]

documented an increase in urinary albumin and beta-2-microglobulin in newborn rats by daily injection of dams during pregnancy with $HgCl_2$ (0.74 mg Hg/kg). Holt and Webb[271] found that variation of the LD_{50} value for a pregnant rat during the pregnancy was rather small (1.00 to 1.18 mg/kg) despite a drastic increase of body weight. In animals (sub)chronically treated by $HgCl_2$, the toxic effects were observed in other tissues (Table 22.19). Abnormalities of the epididymis,[277] heart,[279] and, in the case of young animals, the brain[278] have been documented in rats. In mice, disturbance of the immune system was reported.[281,282]

Among various organic Hg, toxicity of MeHg has been well investigated because of its natural occurrence and the history of Minamata disease. Acute and subacute toxic effects of MeHg after single and multiple injections were summarized in Tables 22.20 and 22.21. Although the LD_{50} values were reported to be around 10 mg Hg/kg (ip) in rats[283] and mice[291] after single injection, its variation should be considered between sexes and strains. Female mice showed higher resistance to MeHg acute toxicity than did males.[276,290] However, after serial injection of a sublethal dose, male C57BL/6 strain mice survived much longer than females.[306] Acute and subacute effects were observed not only in brain but also in liver and kidney. In the liver induction of protein synthesis,[284] mild glycogen accumulation,[304] and morphological changes[295] were observed. Nephrotoxic actions of MeHg in the acute phase were also documented,[276,288,301] although histochemical abnormality was very slight.[276] A significant decrease in serum albumin in mice was documented 24 h after 16 mg Hg/kg dosing.[307] It should be noted that, like $HgCl_2$, MeHg could also induce GSH synthesis in the kidney of rats and mice in the acute and subacute phases.[292,311]

MeHg exposure using contaminated food or water is a useful method particularly for a long-term exposure experiment. Table 22.22 summarized the toxic effects of MeHg from food and drinking water. Similar effects in the form of abnormalities in neural tissue and kidney were often observed as in repeated injection studies. Woods et al.[310] suggested urinary porphyrin might be a biomarker for renal damage induced by MeHg. From life-long exposure to MeHg, males manifested neurotoxic symptoms earlier than females in mice and rats.[312,316]

MeHg induced congenital abnormalities through prenatal exposure (Table 22.23). Effects could be documented as fetal death,[317,323] renal failure[319] and neural disorders detected by behavioral[320] and pathological methods.[318,321,322] It should be noted that the susceptibility of the fetus to MeHg toxicity varied with the time of exposure during the gestation period. For example, the induction rate of hydrocephalus in offspring of B10D2 strain mice was highest by injection on gestation day 15.[322] Similar variations were seen with other metals. Inouye and Kajiwara[324] observed abnormal morphology in the fetal brain of guinea pig, whose gestation period was much longer than in rats or mice, after a single injection of MeHg (7.5 mg Hg/animal) during pregnancy.

TABLE 22.18
Acute Effects of Mercuric Chloride

Animal Strain, Sex (Age)[a]	Dose (mg Hg/kg)	Route	Effects	Ref.
Rats				
SD, M + F, (1, 29 d)	3.7	sc	29 d: 20% mortality; kidney damage	261
			1 d: no effect	
SD, M	0.37	ip	Urine: glucose, maltase (24 h) ↑	262
	3	sc	Kidney damage: pathological (30 min), functional (6 h)	263
SD, F	11	sc	Renal cortex amino acids ↓	264
SD, M	1.1	ip	Kidney mitochondria: GSH ↓; H_2O_2 formation, LPO ↑	265
Wistar, M	1 × 2	ip	Urine: Ca^{2+}, Mg^{2+}, MT ↑	266
	1.5, 3	sc	Urine: alkaline phosphatase, LDH ↑	267
	3	sc	Kidney: LPO ↑; vitamin C, E ↓	268

TABLE 22.18 *(Continued)*
Acute Effects of Mercuric Chloride

Animal Strain, Sex (Age)[a]	Dose (mg Hg/kg)	Route	Effects	Ref.
	0.5, 1	ip	Urine: alkaline phosphatase ↑; pathological change	269
	4.4	sc	100% mortality (48 h)	270
Wistar, pregnant	0.79 (G.D. 8 or 16)	iv	Placental transport activity ↓	271
			LD_{50} (G.D. 8–19): 1.00–1.18 mg/kg	
SD, pregnant	1	sc	Dam and newborn: urinary β_2-M, albumin ↑	272
Mice				
?, M	0.5	ip	Kidney: ribosome disaggregation	273
ICR, M	3.6	iv	Urine: NAG, LDH ↑; 100% mortality (7 d)	274
NMRI, F	5–40	po	Renal GSH, GPx, protein: dose-dependent alteration; necrosis (>20 mg/kg)	275
C57BL/6, M + F	2, 4	iv	Urinary PSP excretion ↓; pathological change	276

[a] Data from adult animals, unless otherwise specified.
Note: G.D. = gestation day.

TABLE 22.19
Subchronic to Chronic Effects of Mercuric Chloride

Animal Strain, Sex (Age)[a]	Dose (mg/kg or ppm Hg)	Route	Effects	Ref.
Rat				
Charles Foster, M	0.037, 0.074 × 30	ip	Morphological change at epididymal epithelium; sperm count ↓	277
Wistar, (2 d)	3 × 59	po	Brain: NE, DA ↑; acetylcholine esterase ↓	278
SD, M	50 ppm/water × 320 d		Alteration in cardiovascular response to epinephrine and NE	279
Mice				
Swiss, F	6 × 10	po	Renal UDP-glucuronyltransferase ↑	280
STL/N, F	1.8 or 3.7 ppm/water × 10 wk		Autoimmunity, immune-complex disease	281
B6C3F1, M	3, 15, or 75 ppm/water × 7 wk		Bone marrow, thymus, and spleen: sugar metabolizing enzymes ↓	282

[a] Data from adult animals, unless otherwise specified.

TABLE 22.20
Toxic Effects by Single Methylmercury Injection

Animal Strain, Sex (Age)[a]	Dose (mg Hg/kg)	Route	Effects	Ref.
Rat				
SD, M	9.5	ip	LD_{50} (24 h)	283
	8–40	sc	Protein synthesis, RNA polymerase: liver ↑; brain ↓	284
Wistar, M	8	ip	Cerebellum: granule cell swelling (1–3 d)	285
SD, ?, (10–20 d)	8	ip	Brain: t-RNA amino acylation ↓	286
CD, M	4.65	ip	Cerebellum: reactive oxygen species ↑	287
Mice				
C57BL/6, M	0.93	ip	Cerebellum: reactive oxygen species ↑	287
Swiss OF1, M	74	po	Damage at renal proximal tubules	288
BALB/c, M + F, (2 d)	4	po	Cerebellum: mitotic arrest; cell number ↓	289
RF, M + F	30	po	Mortality (10 d): M > 70%; F 60%	290
ICR, M + F			Mortality (10 d): M > 70%; F 3%	
Swiss Webster, M	10.8	ip	LD_{50} (7 d)	291
C57BL/6, F	32	po	Kidney: γ-GCS activity, GSH ↑	292
	40	po	33% mortality (7 d)	276
C57BL/6, M	16	po	67% mortality (7 d)	
	8	po	Serum albumin (24 h) ↓	307

[a] Data from adult animals, unless otherwise specified.

TABLE 22.21
Toxic Effects of Multiple Methylmercury Injection

Animal Strain, Sex (Age)[a]	Dose (mg Hg/kg)	Route	Effects	Ref.
Rats				
Wistar, M	8 × 3	sc	MT induction in liver and kidney	293
	8 × 3	sc	Inflammation in kidney; urinary NE, DA (90 d) ↓	294
SD, M	8 × 4	sc	Ultrastructure change in liver	295
Wistar, M + F	8 × 5	po	Damage at cerebellar glandular layer and dorsal root ganglion (M < F, 10–12 d)	296
LE, M	6.4 × 5	sc	Impaired auditory function (6 –7 wk)	297
SD, M	6.4 × 6	po	Brain: general blood flow (at silent phase) ↓	298
Wistar, F	8 × 7	sc	Sciatic nerve: phosphorylation of specific proteins (15 d) ↓	299
SD, F	9.3 × 7	po	[14]Leu incorporation into cerebellar slice ↓	300
SD, M	0.8 × 20	ip	Kidney: lysosome and mitochondria dysfunction	301
Wistar, M	8 × 20	sc	Kidney, serum: LPO (2 d) ↑	302
SD, ?, (5 d)	5 × 10–27	sc	Neurological symptoms (23 d)	303
SD, M	0.8 × 8	sc	Liver: glycogen accumulation, SER proliferation (1–2 wk); pathological change (11 wk)	304
Mice				
ICR, F	10 × 5	sc	Brain: protein kinase C ↓	305
C57BL/6, M + F	4 × 49	po	50% mortality: C57BL/6 M, 45 d; F, 21 d	306
BALB/c, M + F			50% mortality: BALB/c M, 15 d; F, 17 d	

[a] Data from adult animals, unless otherwise specified.

TABLE 22.22
Effects of Methylmercury Exposure From Food or Drinking Water

Animal Strain, Sex (Age)[a]	Hg Level × Duration (ppm Hg)	Effect	Ref.
Rats			
SD (offspring)	3.9/food before mating, → gestation, → lactation, → 50 d postpartum	Cerebellar NE (50 d) ↑	308
Wistar, M	16/water × 95 d (2-d intervals)	Ataxia, Hg staining at CNS	309
F344, M	4.3/water × 2 wk, or 8.6/water × 1 wk	Urinary porphyrin (biomarker for renal damage) ↑	310
	4.3, 8.6/water × 4 wk	Kidney: GSH, γ-GCS ↑	311
SD, M + F	8/food × 130 wk	Ataxia (M, F); renal failure (M)	312
	1.6, 8/food × 130 wk	Pathological changes in spinal ganglion, spinal dorsal root, proximal tubules	313
Mice			
CBA, M	8–32/water × 2 wk	LPO in liver, kidney, brain ↑	314
BALB/c, F	10/water × 60–71 d 20/water × 20–75 d 40/water × 7 d	Ataxia	315
Swiss cross, M	0.5–10/water × 3 wk	Immunosuppressive effects	7
B6C3F1, M + F	8/food × 104 wk	Neurotoxic signs, chronic nephropathy (M > F)	316

[a] Data from adult animals, unless otherwise specified.

TABLE 22.23
Effect of Prenatal Exposure to Methylmercury

Animal Strain	Dose (mg/kg or ppm Hg)	Injection Time	Route	Effect	Ref.
Rats					
Wistar	8	18	ip	Fetal death (4 h)	317
SD	6.4	15	po	DA receptor density (14 d) ↑	318
SD	2.4 or 4.8 × 3	8, 10, 12	ip	Urine: γ-GTP, alkaline phosphatase, NAG (3 or 6 d) ↑	319
Wistar	0.01 or 0.05 × 4	6–9	po	Behavioral performance deficits (4 months)	320
Mice					
C57BL/6	3.2 × 3	14–16	ip	Abnormal neuronal migration at cortical layers II and III in newborn	321
B10D2, C57BL/10, DBA/2	8	15	po	Hydrocephalus in newborn: B10D2, 88%; C57BL/10, 54%; DBA/2, 0%	322
IVCS	3.2 or 6.4 ppm/food	−30–18		Litter size ↓; resorption, dead embryo ↑	323
Guinea pigs					
Hartley	7.5/animal	21, 28, 35, 42, or 49	po	Abnormal morphology in fetal brain	324

SECTION 13. NICKEL

Nickel (Ni) is considered to be an essential element in several animal species. Inhalation of nickel compounds causes lesions in the lung. Dunnick et al.[340] demonstrated that the lung toxicity and lethality in rats and mice of aerosols containing nickel sulfate and subsulfide depended on the solubilities of the salts. Parenteral injection of nickel salts affected various tissues in experimental animals (Table 22.24). Intraperitoneal injection of 6.75 mg Ni/kg as acetate to adult rats caused 57% mortality during the 14 days after injection.[329] Hogan[338] found LD_{50} values were higher in weanling mice than in adults. The acute effects of nickel toxicity proved to be increased tissue hemoxygenase activities,[325] hyperglycemia, [329,333] hepatic dysfunction,[331,335] and decreased natural killer cell activity.[328,337] The incidence of sarcoma was documented in nickel subsulfide-treated rats.[327] Nickel caused adverse effects also in embryos. LD_{50} values in rat embryos varied with the time of injection during the gestation period.[326] Smith et al.[334] reported that the lowest observed adverse effect level for pups was 10 ppm Ni in drinking water, which caused a significant number of embryo deaths in the second of two successive gestations.

TABLE 22.24
Toxic Effects of Nickel

Animal Strain, Sex (Age)[a]	Compound	Dose (mg/kg or ppm Ni)	Route	Effects	Ref.
Rats					
F344, M	$NiCl_2$	15	sc	Kidney, liver, lung, brain: hemeoxygenase (17 h) ↑	325
F344, pregnant	$NiCl_2$	16	im	Fetal death: 18.5–20% (G.D. 8 and 18) LD_{50} (dam, 14 d): 22 mg Ni/kg (G.D. 8); 16 mg Ni/kg (G.D. 18)	326
F344, M	Ni_3S_2	0.88	im	Sarcoma in 77% of rats (2 years)	327
F344, M + F	$NiCl_2$	10–20	im	NK-cell activity (24 h) ↓	328
F344, M	$Ni(OAc)_2$	6.75	ip	57% mortality (14 d)	329
		5.6	ip	Hyperglycemia, renal cytochrome P-450 ↓	
	$NiCl_2$	3.6–29	sc	Alveolar macrophage: cAMP ↑; 5′-nucleochidase (1–4 h) ↓; LPO (72 h) ↑	330
	$Ni(OAc)_2$	6.28	ip	Liver, kidney: LPO ↑; Cat, GPx, GSH, GSR (3 h) ↓ Serum: ALT, AST ↑	331
	$Ni(His)_2$	1.2	iv	Oxidative damage at DNA	332
Wistar, F	$NiCl_2$	4, 6	ip	Plasma: glucagon ↑; insulin ↓; hyperglycemia (1–4 h)	333
LE, pregnant	$NiCl_2$	10–250 ppm/water		Fetal death	334
Mice					
C57BL/6, M	$NiCl_2$	15	sc	Kidney: hemeoxygenase (17 h) ↑	325
	$Ni(OAc)_2$	10	ip	Liver: Cat, GSH, SOD, GST ↓; GSR, LPO ↑	335
C3H, M					
BALB/c, M					
B6C3F1, M	Ni_3S_2	2.85	it	50% mortality (14 d)	336
C57BL/6, M	$NiCl_2$	8.3	im	NK-cell activity ↓	337
CBA, M					

TABLE 22.24 *(Continued)*
Toxic Effects of Nickel

Animal Strain, Sex (Age)[a]	Compound	Dose (mg/kg or ppm Ni)	Route	Effects	Ref.
ICR, M + F, (3, 9, 14 wk)	Ni (OAc)$_2$		ip	LD_{50} (5 d): 3 wk M, 29.6; F, 32.2 (mg Ni/kg) 9 wk M, 16.6; F, 17.9 (mg Ni/kg) 14 wk M, 13.0; F, 15.9 (mg Ni/kg)	338
B6C3F1, F	NiSO$_4$	380–3800 ppm water × 180 d		Bone marrow cellularity ↓	339

[a] Data from adult animals, unless otherwise specified.

Note: G.D. = gestation day.

SECTION 14. SELENIUM

Selenium (Se) is one of the essential trace elements, and its deficiency has widely been documented in human and experimental animals. However, excess selenium also causes various adverse effects (Table 22.25). Mortality from selenium overload has been documented in mice and rats. Jacobs and Forst[343] showed that giving water containing 16 ppm Se (as Na$_2$SeO$_3$) to rats for 35 days caused a lethal effect of up to 80% mortality. They also found that susceptibility varied with sex and age. Mortalities in mice were documented from an experiment in which they were given water containing 64 ppm Se for 46 days.[346] Since selenium functions as a potent SH oxidizing reagent *in vivo*, decreased GSH and increased GSSG were documented in tissues of Na$_2$SeO$_3$-treated rats. David and Shearer[341] found that decreased lens GSH level was accompanied by cataract formation and increased insoluble protein levels in selenite-treated rats. LeBoeuf and Hoekstra[342] observed increased GSSG, GSR, and γ-GTP in the liver of Na$_2$SeO$_3$-treated rats. Watanabe and Suzuki[345] reported that selenite injection caused a transient hypothermia and cold-seeking behavior in mice. Inhalation of dimethylselenide gas up to 8000 ppm for 1 h caused alterations of DNA, RNA and protein levels in lung, liver, and spleen of rats, but no pathological change was observed.[347]

TABLE 22.25
Toxic Effects of Sodium Selenite

Animal Strain, Sex (Age)[a]	Dose (mg/kg or ppm Se)	Route	Effects	Ref.
Rats				
SD, M	1.6	sc	Lens: GSH, insoluble protein ↑; cataract formation (4 d)	341
	1.2 or 6 ppm/food × 6 wk	ip	Liver: GSSG, GSR, γ-GTP ↑	342
SD, M + F (5, 12 wk)	16 ppm/water × 35 d		Mortality: 5 wk M, 60%; F, 80%; 12 wk M, 0%; F, 20%; liver damage	343
Mice				
ICR, F	0.9 × 1–3 (2-d interval)	ip	WBC number (16 d) ↓	344
ICR, M	1.6–4.7	sc	Transient hypothermia, cold-seeking behavior (1 h)	345
Swiss, M + F (7, 18 wk)	64 ppm/water × 46 d		Mortality: 20% (7 wk, M, F); 80% (18 wk, M); 40% (18 wk, F); liver necrosis	346

[a] Data from adult animals, unless otherwise specified.

SECTION 15. THALLIUM

Soluble thallium (Tl) salts are easily absorbed from the gastrointestinal tract and are widely distributed among various tissues to cause adverse effects (Table 22.26). The LD_{50} value (4 days) was documented as 24.8 mg Tl/kg in TlOAc-injected (ip) male rats.[348] Around this dose level, increases in serotonin turnover rate and monoamine oxidase activity in the brain were observed within 24 h.[351] Peele et al.[349] showed that oral administration of Tl_2SO_4 caused flavor aversion effect in rats, whereas ip injection at the same dose level was much less effective. Decreased brain glutathione levels[350] or the increased spontaneous discharge rate of Purkinje neurons[352] were documented after serial injections of lower doses.

Woods and Fowler[353] observed dose-related ultrastructural changes in the liver with concomitant increases of mitochondrial membranous enzyme activities and decreases of microsomal enzyme activities after ip injection of $TlCl_3$. Effects on the kidney were reduced GFR, proteinuria, and pathological change in the loop of Henle in $TlSO_4$-treated female rats.[354] Effects on testes were reported in rats given drinking water containing 10 ppm Tl for 60 days.[355]

TABLE 22.26
Toxic Effects of Thallium on Rats

Strain, Sex	Chemicals	Dose (mg/kg or ppm Tl)	Route	Effect	Ref.
Wistar, M	TlOAc	16–54	ip	LD_{50} (4 d): 24.8 mg/kg	348
LE, M	Tl_2SO_4	1.7–13.6	po	Flavor aversion effect; ip less effective	349
Charles Foster, M	TlOAc	5 × 6	ip	Brain: GSH, R-SH ↓	350
Wistar, M	TlOAc	23 or 39	ip	Brain: serotonin turnover, MAO activity (24 h) ↑	351
SD, M	TlOAc	3.1 × 7	ip	Spontaneous discharge rate of Purkinje neurons ↑	352
	$TlCl_3$	50–200	ip	Liver: change in ultrastructure (16 h) Mitochondrial membrane enzyme ↑; microsome enzyme ↓	353
Wistar, F	Tl_2SO_4	3.4–13.6	ip	Kidney: GFR ↓; protein level ↑; pathological change in loop of Henle	354
Wistar, M	Tl_2SO_4	10 ppm/water × 60 d		Pathological change in Sertoli cells; spermatozoa motility, testicular β-glucuronidase ↓	355

SECTION 16. TIN

Oral toxicities of inorganic tin (Sn), including metallic Sn, are thought to be rather low because of poor gastrointestinal absorption. High dose exposure to inorganic Sn caused a decrease in weight gain and food intake as a result of damage of the gastrointestinal tract. de Groot et al.[356] reported hemoglobin levels proved to be the most sensitive parameter in rats fed $SnCl_2$-contaminated food above 1000 ppm. Macroscopic and microscopic examinations were reported in $SnCl_2$-fed rats.[357,358] Zareba and Chmielnicka[359] showed decreased ALAD activity after seven sc or ip injections of 2 mg Sn/kg as $SnCl_2$ in rats.

Toxicities of organic Sn compounds are much higher than those of inorganic compounds. Particularly, trialkylated Sn compounds are well known to penetrate and damage the brain tissue owing to high lipophilicity. Sublethal effects reported include abnormal behavior, such as hyperactivity, tremor, increase in hot plate or tail flick latency, disrupted learning, and flavor aversion (Table 22.27). Pathologically, lesions in the hippocampus were documented in trimethyltin-treated animals.[361,371] Triethyltin showed the highest toxicity, followed by trimethyl-, tripropyl-, and tributyltin.[371] Chang et al.[361] demonstrated mice had higher susceptibility to trimethyltin toxicity than had rats. In addition to neural tissue, inhibitions of protein phosphorylation and Ca^{2+}-ATPase activity in the heart[367] and natural killer cell activity[374] were documented.

In contrast to trialkylated tin compounds, triphenyltin (TPT) was shown to damage hepatic functions in adult rats after three consecutive ip injections of 0.34 mg Sn/kg.[376] Lehotzky et al.[377] found that when pregnant rats were treated by TPT (1.74 mg/kg/day) during gestation days 7 to 15, the surviving offspring showed hyperactivity. Bis(tributyltin)oxide (0.5 ml/kg, intramuscular injection) brought about liver damage[378] and corneal edema[379] in rats. Feeding on dioctyltin chloride (DOTC)-contaminated food (50 to 150 ppm) for several weeks caused thymus atrophy in rats.[380,381] Oral administration of DOTC (500 mg/kg) once a week for 8 weeks resulted in a suppressed anti-self RBC antibody response in mice.[382] Seinen et al.[381] compared the effectiveness of various dialkylated tin compounds, and found that dioctyl- and dibutyl-compounds were most effective, whereas dimethyltin had no effect on the thymus.

TABLE 22.27
Toxic Effects of Trialkyltin Compounds

Animal Strain, Sex (Age)[a]	Compound[b]	Dose (mg/kg or ppm Sn)	Route	Effects	Ref.
Rats					
LE, M	TMT	2.6×4	po	Hippocampus: Synapsin I $\downarrow$	360
SD and LE, M	TMT	4.5	po	Lesion in hippocampus, susceptibility: LE > SD	361
LE, M	TMT	3.6–5.1	po	Length of pyramidal cell line (30 d) $\downarrow$	362
	TMT	3.6–5.1	po	Disrupted learning and memory (21 d)	363
	TMT	2.9–5.1	po	Visual system dysfunction	364
	TMT	2.2 (EC_{50})	ip	Flavor aversion	365
	TET	1.0 (EC_{50})	ip		
F344, M	TMT	2.5	sc	Hot plate latency (21–28 d) $\uparrow$	366
	TET	1.12	sc	Hot plate latency $\uparrow$	
		1.68	sc	80% mortality	
SD, M	TMT	1.8×6	po	Heart: ^{45}Ca uptake by sarcoplasmic reticulum, Ca^{2+}-ATPase $\downarrow$; phosphorylation of specific protein $\downarrow$	367
	TET	0.87×6	po		
	TBT	1.2×6	po		
LE, M	TET	0.62×6	ip	Visual evoked potential $\downarrow$; CNS depression	368
F344, M	TET	0.21×14	sc	Latency in tail flick and hot plate $\uparrow$	369
LE, (3 d)	TMT	0.22×27	po	Hyperactivity; learning memory function (180–200 d) $\downarrow$	370
	TET	0.17×27	po		
LE, (newborn)	TMT	2	po	100% mortality (5–6 d)	371
	TET	1.3	po	100% mortality (6–10 d)	
	TPT	4.2	po	100% mortality (15–20 d)	
	TBT	10	po	100% mortality (5–8 d)	
	TMT	0.66×24	po	67% mortality	
Mice					
C57BL/6, M	TMT	2.2	ip	Hippocampus, front cortex; O_2-reactive species (48 h) $\uparrow$	372
	TMT	1.8	po	Hippocampus: lesions (48 h)	361
BALB/c, M	TMT	1.8	ip	SMA (24 h) $\downarrow$	373
ICR, M	TET	0.58 or 2.8	po	Anticonvulsant effect; interaction with adrenergic and GABAergic transmitter systems	374

TABLE 22.27 *(Continued)*
Toxic Effects of Trialkyltin Compounds

Animal Strain, Sex (Age)[a]	Compound[b]	Dose (mg/kg or ppm Sn)	Route	Effects	Ref.
C3H, M	TBT	3.6 or 36 ppm/water × 1 wk		NK-cell activity ↓	375

[a] Data from adult animals, unless otherwise specified.
[b] TMT = trimethyltin; TET = triethyltin; TPT = tripropyltin; TBT = tributyltin.

SECTION 17. ZINC

Zinc (Zn) is an essential metal and functions as a cofactor of various enzymes and insulin. Although zinc deficiency is well documented in humans and in animals, its toxic effects have also been reported in experimental animals. Young mice showed twofold higher LD_{50} values (115.2 mg Zn/kg) after ip injection of zinc acetate than did adults (44.4 to 50.4 mg Zn/kg).[383] In the case of subchronic oral toxicity, the most severe histological lesions were observed in the kidney.[384] Inhalation exposure (5 mg Zn/m^3 × 3 h) or intratracheal instillation (20 µg/rat) of ZnO has been demonstrated to cause functional, morphological, or biochemical changes in lungs of rats[385,386] and guinea pigs.[387]

REFERENCES

1. B. Venugopal and T.D. Luckey, Eds., *Metal Toxicity in Mammals,* Vol. 2. *Chemical Toxicity of Metals and Metalloids,* Plenum Press, New York, 1978.
2. L. Friberg, G.F. Nordberg, and V.B. Vouk, Eds., *Handbook of the Toxicology of Metals,* Vol. II, Elsevier Science Publishers, Amsterdam, 1986.
3. T. Ghafghazi, J.W. Ridlington, and B.A. Fowler, The effects of acute and subacute sodium arsenite administration on carbohydrate metabolism, *Toxicol. Appl. Pharmacol.,* 55, 126–130, 1980.
4. S. Valkonen, H. Savolainen, and J. Jarvisalo, Arsenic distribution and neurochemical effects in peroral sodium arsenite exposure of rats, *Bull. Environ. Contam. Toxicol.,* 30, 303–308, 1983.
5. W.R. Byron, G.W. Bierbower, J.B. Brouwer, and W.H. Hansen, Pathologic changes in rats and dogs from two-year feeding of sodium arsenite or sodium arsenate, *Toxicol. Appl. Pharmacol.,* 10, 132–147, 1967.
6. H.V. Aposhian, C.H. Tadlock, and T.E. Moon, Protection of mice against the lethal effects of sodium arsenite: a quantitative comparison of a number of chelating agents, *Toxicol. Appl. Pharmacol.,* 61, 385–392, 1981.
7. B.R. Blakley, C.S. Sisodia, and T.K. Mukkur, The effects of methylmercury, tetraethyl lead, and sodium arsenite on the humoral immune response in mice, *Toxicol. Appl. Pharmacol.,* 52, 245–254, 1980.
8. B.A. Fowler and J.S. Woods, The effects of prolonged oral arsenate exposure on liver mitochondria of mice: morphometric and biochemical studies, *Toxicol. Appl. Pharmacol.,* 50, 177–187, 1979.
9. M.N. Baxley, R.D. Hood, G.C. Vedel, W.P. Harrison, and G.M. Szczech, Prenatal toxicity of orally administered sodium arsenite in mice, *Bull. Environ. Contam. Toxicol.,* 26, 749–756, 1981.
10. R.D. Hood and G.C. Vedel-Macrander, Evaluation of the effect of BAL (2,3-dimercaptopropanol) on arsenite-induced teratogenesis in mice, *Toxicol. Appl. Pharmacol.,* 73, 1–7, 1984.
11. M.A. Bosque, J.L. Domingo, J.M. Llobet, and J. Corbella, Effects of meso-2,3-dimercaptosuccicic acid (DMSA) on the teratogenicity of sodium arsenate in mice, *Bull. Environ. Contam. Toxicol.,* 47, 682–688, 1991.

12. S.J.S. Flora and S.D. Gupta, Effect of single gallium arsenide exposure on some biochemical variables in porphyrin metabolism in rats, *J. Appl. Toxicol.*, 12, 333–334, 1992.

13. D.R. Webb, I.G. Sipes, and D.E. Carter, *In vitro* solubility and *in vivo* toxicity of gallium arsenide, *Toxicol. Appl. Pharmacol.*, 76, 96–104, 1984.

14. P.L. Goering, R.R. Maronpot, and B.A. Fowler, Effect of intratracheal gallium arsenide administration on δ-aminolevulinic acid dehydratase in rats: relationship to urinary excretion of aminolevulinic acid, *Toxicol. Appl. Pharmacol.*, 92, 179–193, 1988.

15. D.R. Webb, S.E. Wilson, and D.E. Carter, Comparative pulmonary toxicity of gallium arsenide, gallium (III) oxide, or arsenic (III) oxide intratracheally instilled into rats, *Toxicol. Appl. Pharmacol.*, 82, 405–416, 1986.

16. E.E. Sikorski, L.A. Burns, K.L. McCoy, M. Stern, and A.E. Munson, Suppression of splenic accessory cell function in mice exposed to gallium arsenide, *Toxicol. Appl. Pharmacol.*, 110, 143–156, 1991.

17. H. Kreppel, F.-X. Reichl, L. Szinicz, B. Fichtl, and W. Forth, Efficacy of various dithiol compounds in acute As_2O_3 poisoning in mice, *Arch. Toxicol.*, 64, 387–392, 1990.

18. T. Itoh, Y.F. Zhang, S. Murai, H. Saito, H. Nagahama, H. Miyate, Y. Saito, and E. Abe, The effect of arsenic trioxide on brain monoamine metabolism and locomotor activity of mice, *Toxicol. Lett.*, 54, 345–353, 1990.

19. C. Aranyi, J.N. Bradof, W.J. O'Shea, J.A. Graham, and F.J. Miller, Effects of arsenic trioxide inhalation exposure on pulmonary antibacterial defenses in mice, *J. Toxicol. Environ. Health*, 15, 163–172, 1985.

20. H.L. Hong, B.A. Fowler, and G.A. Boorman, Hematopoietic effects in mice exposed to arsine gas, *Toxicol. Appl. Pharmacol.*, 97, 173–182, 1989.

21. P.C. Blair, M.B. Thompson, M. Bechtold, R.E. Wilson, M.P. Moorman, and B.A. Fowler, Evidence for oxidative damage to red blood cells in mice induced by arsine gas, *Toxicology*, 63, 25–34, 1990.

22. L.E. Sendelbach and H.P. Witschi, Protection by parenteral iron administration against the inhalation toxicity of beryllium sulfate, *Toxicol. Lett.*, 35, 321–325, 1987.

23. L.E. Sendelbach, H.P. Witschi, and A.F. Tryka, Acute pulmonary toxicity of beryllium sulfate inhalation in rats and mice: cell kinetics and histopathology, *Toxicol. Appl. Pharmacol.*, 85, 248–256, 1986.

24. L.E. Sendelbach and H.P. Witschi, Bronchoalveolar lavage in rats and mice following beryllium sulfate inhalation, *Toxicol. Appl. Pharmacol.*, 90, 322–329, 1987.

25. B.A. Hart, A.G. Harmsen, R.B. Low, and R. Emerson, Biochemical, cytological, and histological alterations in rat lung following acute beryllium aerosol exposure, *Toxicol. Appl. Pharmacol.*, 75, 454–465, 1984.

26. D.H. Groth, Carcinogenicity of beryllium: review of the literature, *Environ. Res.*, 21, 56–62, 1980.

27. D.H. Groth, C. Kommineni, and G.R. Mackay, Carcinogenicity of beryllium hydroxide and alloys, *Environ. Res.*, 21, 63–84, 1980.

28. H.P. Witschi and P. Marchand, Interference of beryllium with enzyme induction in rat liver, *Toxicol. Appl. Pharmacol.*, 20, 565–572, 1971.

29. J. Vacher, R. Deraedt, and J. Benzoni, Compared effects of two beryllium salts (soluble and insoluble): toxicity and blockade of the reticuloendothelial system, *Toxicol. Appl. Pharmacol.*, 24, 497–506, 1973.

30. R. Mathur, S. Sharma, S. Mathur, and A.O. Prakash, Effect of beryllium nitrate on early and late pregnancy in rats, *Bull. Environ. Contam. Toxicol.*, 38, 73–77, 1987.

31. G.P. Samarawickrama and M. Webb, The acute toxicity and teratogenicity of cadmium in the pregnant rat, *J. Appl. Toxicol.*, 1, 264–269, 1981.

32. R.E. Dudley, D.J. Svoboda, and C.D. Klaassen, Acute exposure to cadmium causes severe liver injury in rats, *Toxicol. Appl. Pharmacol.*, 65, 302–313, 1982.

33. P.L. Goering, B.R. Fisher, and C.L. Kish, Stress protein synthesis induced in rat liver by cadmium precedes hepatotoxicity, *Toxicol. Appl. Pharmacol.*, 122, 139–148, 1993.

34. G. Lázár, D. Serra, and B. Tuchweber, Effect on cadmium toxicity of substances influencing reticuloendothelial activity, *Toxicol. Appl. Pharmacol.*, 29, 367–376, 1974.

35. C.R. Caflisch and T.D. DuBose, Jr., Cadmium-induced changes in luminal fluid pH in testis and epididymis of the rat *in vivo*, *J. Toxicol. Environ. Health*, 32, 49–57, 1991.

36. N. Shiraishi, R.A. Barter, H. Uno, and M.P. Waalkes, Effect of progesterone pretreatment on cadmium toxicity in the male Fischer (F344/NCr) rat, *Toxicol. Appl. Pharmacol.*, 118, 113–118, 1993.

37. A.-S. Chung and M.D. Maines, Differential effect of cadmium on GSH-peroxidase activity in the Leydig and the Sertori cells of rat testis: suppression by selenium and the possible relationship to heme concentration. *Biochem. Pharmacol.*, 36, 1367–1372, 1987.

38. N. Konishi, J.M. Ward, and M.P. Waalkes, Pancreatic hepatocytes in Fischer and Wister rats induced by repeated injections of cadmium chloride, *Toxicol. Appl. Pharmacol.,* 104, 149–156, 1990.

39. T. Koizumi and Z.G. Li, Role of oxidative stress in single-dose, cadmium-induced testicular cancer, *J. Toxicol. Environ. Health,* 37, 25–36, 1992.

40. P.H. Ruppert, K.F. Dean, and L.W. Reiter, Development of locomotor activity of rat pups exposed to heavy metals, *Toxicol. Appl. Pharmacol.,* 78, 69–77, 1985.

41. K.-L. Wong and C.D. Klaassen, Neurotoxic effects of cadmium in young rats, *Toxicol. Appl. Pharmacol.,* 63, 330–337, 1982.

42. J.U. Bell, Induction of hepatic metallothionein in the immature rat following administration of cadmium, *Toxicol. Appl. Pharmacol.,* 54, 148–155, 1980.

43. P.L. Goering and C.D. Klaassen, Resistance to cadmium-induced hepatotoxicity in immature rats, *Toxicol. Appl. Pharmacol.,* 74, 321–329, 1984.

44. J.W. Laskey, G.L. Rehnberg, S.C. Laws, and J.F. Hein, Reproductive effects of low acute doses of cadmium chloride in adult male rats, *Toxicol. Appl. Pharmacol.,* 73, 250–255, 1984.

45. S. Gulati, K.D. Gill, and R. Nath, Effect of cadmium on lipid composition of the weanling rat brain, *Acta Pharmacol. Toxicol.,* 59, 89–93, 1986.

46. T.E.K. White, R.B. Baggs, and R.K. Miller, Central nervous system lesions in the Wister rat fetus following direct fetal injections of cadmium, *Teratology,* 42, 7–13, 1990.

47. L. Yáñez, L. Carrizales, M.T. Zanatta, J.D.J. Mejía, L. Batres, and F. Díaz-Barriga, Arsenic-cadmium interaction in rats: toxic effects in the heart and tissue metal shifts, *Toxicology,* 67, 227–234, 1991.

48. L.G. Scharpf, Jr., F.J. Ramos, and I.D. Hill, Influence of nitrilotriacetate (NTA) on the toxicity, excretion and distribution of cadmium in female rats, *Toxicol. Appl. Pharmacol.,* 22, 186–192, 1972.

49. M. Shimizu and S. Morita, Effects of fasting on cadmium toxicity, glutathione metabolism, and metallothionein synthesis in rats, *Toxicol. Appl. Pharmacol.,* 103, 28–39, 1990.

50. F.N. Kotsonis and C.D. Klaassen, Toxicity and distribution of cadmium administered to rats at sublethal doses, *Toxicol. Appl. Pharmacol.,* 41, 667–680, 1977.

51. L.R. Cantilena, Jr. and C.D. Klaassen, Comparison of the effectiveness of several chelators after single administration on the toxicity, excretion, and distribution of cadmium, *Toxicol. Appl. Pharmacol.,* 58, 452–460, 1981.

52. G.S. Probst, W.F. Bousquet, and T.S. Miya, Correlation of hepatic metallothionein concentrations with acute cadmium toxicity in the mouse, *Toxicol. Appl. Pharmacol.,* 39, 61–69, 1977.

53. A. Selypes, P. Serényi, I. Boldog, F. Bokros, and S. Takács, Acute and "long-term" genotoxic effects of $CdCl_2$ on testes of mice, *J. Toxicol. Environ. Health,* 36, 401–409, 1992.

54. G.R. Hogan and S.L. Razniak, Split dose studies on the erythropoietic effects of cadmium, *Bull. Environ. Contam. Toxicol.,* 48, 857–864, 1992.

55. M.M. Jones, M.A. Basinger, R.J. Topping, G.R. Gale, S.G. Jones, and M.A. Holscher, Meso-2,3-dimercaptosuccinic acid and sodium *N*-benzyl-*N*-dithiocarboxy-D-glucamine as antagonists for cadmium intoxication, *Arch. Toxicol.,* 62, 29–36, 1988.

56. D.J. Thomas, R.A. Winchurch, and P.C. Huang, Ontogenic variation in acute lethality of cadmium in C57BL/6J mice, *Toxicology,* 47, 317–323, 1987.

57. R.L. Shippee, D.H. Burgess, R.P. Ciavarra, R.A. DiCapua, and P.E. Stake, Cadmium-induced suppression of the primary immune response and acute toxicity in mice: differential interaction of zinc, *Toxicol. Appl. Pharmacol.,* 71, 303–306, 1983.

58. T. Maitani and K.T. Suzuki, Effect of cadmium on essential metal concentrations in testis, liver and kidney of five inbred strains of mice, *Toxicology,* 42, 121–130, 1986.

59. O. Andersen, J.B. Nielsen, and P. Svendsen, Oral cadmium chloride intoxication in mice: effects of chelation, *Toxicology,* 52, 65–79, 1988.

60. D. Manca, A.C. Ricard, B. Trottier, and G. Chevalier, Studies on lipid peroxidation in rat tissues following administration of low and moderate doses of cadmium chloride, *Toxicology,* 67, 303–323, 1991.

61. J.W. Laskey, G.L. Rehnberg, S.C. Laws, and J.F. Hein, Age-related dose response of selected reproductive parameters to acute cadmium chloride exposure in the male Long-Evance rat, *J. Toxicol. Environ. Health,* 19, 393–401, 1986.

62. A.M. Saillenfait, J.P. Payan, M.T. Brondeau, D. Zissu, and J. de Ceaurriz, Changes on urinary proximal tubule parameters in neonatal rats exposed to cadmium chloride during pregnancy, *J. Appl. Toxicol.,* 11, 23–27, 1991.

63. A.A. Levin and R.K. Miller, Fetal toxicity of cadmium in the rat: decreased utero-placental blood flow, *Toxicol. Appl. Pharmacol.,* 58, 297–306, 1981.

64. D. Holt and M. Webb, Comparison of some biochemical effects of teratogenic doses of mercuric mercury and cadmium in the pregnant rat, *Arch. Toxicol.,* 58, 249–254, 1986.

65. D. Holt and M. Webb, Teratogenicity of ionic cadmium in the Wister rat, *Arch. Toxicol.,* 59, 443–447, 1987.

66. W.H. Roelfzema, A.M. Roelofsen, W. Leene, and J.H.J. Copius Peereboom-Stegeman, Effects of cadmium exposure during pregnancy on cadmium and zinc concentrations in neonatal liver and consequences for the offspring, *Arch. Toxicol.,* 63, 38–42, 1989.

67. G.P. Daston, Toxic effects of cadmium on the developing rat lung. II. Glycogen and phospholipid metabolism, *J. Toxicol. Environ. Health,* 9, 51–61, 1982.

68. T.L. Sorell and J.H. Graziano, Effect of oral cadmium exposure during pregnancy on maternal and fetal zinc metabolism in the rat, *Toxicol. Appl. Pharmacol.,* 102, 537–545, 1990.

69. B. Barański, Effect of maternal cadmium exposure on postnatal development and tissue cadmium, copper and zinc concentrations in rats, *Arch. Toxicol.,* 58, 255–260, 1986.

70. S.K. De, S.K. Dey, and G.K. Andrews, Cadmium teratogenicity and its relationship with metallothionein gene expression in midgestation mouse embryos, *Toxicology,* 64, 89–104, 1990.

71. O. Katsuta, H. Hiratsuka, J. Matsumoto, M. Tsuchitani, T. Umemura, and F. Marumo, Ovariectomy enhances cadmium-induced nephrotoxicity and hepatotoxicity in rats, *Toxicol. Appl. Pharmacol.,* 119, 267–274, 1993.

72. R.A. Goyer, C.R. Miller, S.-Y. Zhu, and W. Victery, Non-metallothionein-bound cadmium in the pathogenesis of cadmium nephrotoxicity in the rat, *Toxicol. Appl. Pharmacol.,* 101, 232–244, 1989.

73. L. Müller and N.H. Stacey, Subcellular toxicity of low level cadmium in rats: effect on cytochrome c oxidase, *Toxicology,* 51, 25–34, 1988.

74. S. Kojima, H. Ono, M. Kiyozumi, T. Honda, and A. Takadate, Effect of N-benzyl-D-glucamine dithiocarbamate on the renal toxicity produced by subacute exposure to cadmium in rats, *Toxicol. Appl. Pharmacol.,* 98, 39–48, 1989.

75. A.F.W. Morsert, W. Leene, C. De Groot, J.B.A. Kipp, M. Evers, A.M. Roelofsen, and K.S. Bosch, Differences in immunological susceptibility to cadmium toxicity between two rat strains as demonstrated with cell biological methods. Effect of cadmium on DNA synthesis of thymus lymphocytes, *Toxicology,* 48, 127–139, 1988.

76. G.S. Shukla, T. Hussain, and S.V. Chandra, Possible role of regional superoxide dismutase activity and lipid peroxide levels in cadmium neurotoxicity: *in vivo* and *in vitro* studies in growing rats. *Life Sci.,* 41, 2215–2221, 1987.

77. R.E. Dudley, L.M. Gammal, and C.D. Klaassen, Cadmium-induced hepatic and renal injury in chronically exposed rats: likely role of hepatic cadmium-metallothionein in nephrotoxicity, *Toxicol. Appl. Pharmacol.,* 77, 414–426, 1985.

78. Y. Nagai, M. Sato, and M. Sasaki, Effect of cadmium administration upon urinary excretion of hydroxylysine and hydroxyproline in the rat, *Toxicol. Appl. Pharmacol.,* 63, 188–193, 1982.

79. M. Ando and S. Matsui, Effect of cadmium on vitamin D-non-stimulated intestinal calcium absorption in rats, *Toxicology,* 45, 1–11, 1987.

80. I.G. O'Brien and L.J. King, The effect of chronic parenteral administration of cadmium on isoenzyme levels of alkaline phosphatase in intestinal mucosa, *Toxicology,* 56, 87–94, 1989.

81. M.P. Waalkes, R. Kovatch, and S. Rehm, Effect of chronic dietary zinc deficiency on cadmium toxicity and carcinogenesis in the male Wister [Hsd: (WI)BR] rat, *Toxicol. Appl. Pharmacol.,* 108, 448–456, 1991.

82. A. Cárdenas, A. Bernard, and R. Lauwerys, Incorporation of [^{35}S]sulfate into glomerular membranes of rats chronically exposed to cadmium and its relation with urinary glycosaminoglycans and proteinuria, *Toxicology,* 76, 219–231, 1992.

83. R. Toury, N. Stelly, E. Boissonneau, and Y. Dupuis, Degenerative processes in skeletal muscle of Cd^{2+}-treated rats and Cd^{2+} inhibition of mitochondrial Ca^{2+} transport, *Toxicol. Appl. Pharmacol.,* 77, 19–35, 1985.

84. H. Iguchi and S. Sano, Effect of cadmium on the bone collagen metabolism of rat, *Toxicol. Appl. Pharmacol.,* 62, 126–136, 1982.

85. S.J. Kopp, H.M. Perry, Jr., E.F. Perry, and M. Erlanger, Cardiac physiologic and tissue metabolic changes following chronic low-level cadmium and cadmium plus lead ingestion in the rat, *Toxicol. Appl. Pharmacol.*, 69, 149–160, 1983.

86. D.W. Rosenberg and A. Kappas, Induction of heme oxygenase in the small intestinal epithelium: a response to oral cadmium exposure, *Toxicology*, 67, 199–210, 1991.

87. B.A. Chowdhury, J.K. Friel, and R.K. Chandra, Cadmium-induced immunopathology is prevented by zinc administration in mice, *J. Nutr.*, 117, 1788–1794, 1987.

88. M.H. Bhattacharyya, B.D. Whelton, D.P. Peterson, B.A. Carnes, E.S. Moretti, J.M. Toomey, and L.L. Williams, Skeletal changes in multiparous mice fed a nutrient-sufficient diet containing cadmium, *Toxicology*, 50, 193–204, 1988.

89. A.A. Valois and W.S. Webster, The choroid plexus as a target site for cadmium toxicity following chronic exposure in the adult mouse: an ultrastructural study, *Toxicology*, 55, 193–205, 1989.

90. P.L. Goering and C.D. Klaassen, Altered subcellular distribution of cadmium following cadmium pretreatment: possible mechanism of tolerance to cadmium-induced lethality, *Toxicol. Appl. Pharmacol.*, 70, 195–203, 1983.

91. U. Wormser and I. Nir, Effect of age on cadmium-induced metallothionein synthesis in the rat, *Arch. Toxicol.*, 62, 392–394, 1988.

92. N. Nishimura, H. Oshima, and M. Nakano, Urinary trehalase as an early indicator of cadmium-induced renal tubular damage in rabbit, *Arch. Toxicol.*, 59, 255–260, 1986.

93. E.C. Grose, J.H. Richards, R.H. Jaskot, M.G. Ménache, J.A. Graham, and W.C. Dauterman, A comparative study of the effects of inhaled cadmium chloride and cadmium oxide: pulmonary response, *J. Toxicol. Environ. Health*, 21, 219–232, 1987.

94. M. Boisset and C. Boudene, Effect of a single exposure to cadmium oxide fumes on rat lung microsomal enzymes, *Toxicol. Appl. Pharmacol.*, 57, 335–345, 1981.

95. B.J. Buckley and D.J.P. Bassett, Glutathione redox status of control and cadmium oxide-exposed rat lungs during oxidant stress, *J. Toxicol. Environ. Health*, 22, 287–299, 1987.

96. R.S. Kutzman, R.T. Drew, R.N. Shiotsuka, and B.Y. Cockrell, Pulmonary changes resulting from subchronic exposure to cadmium chloride aerosol, *J. Toxicol. Environ. Health*, 17, 175–189, 1986.

97. B.A. Hart, G.W. Voss, and C.L. Willean, Pulmonary tolerance to cadmium following cadmium aerosol pretreatment, *Toxicol. Appl. Pharmacol.*, 101, 447–460, 1989.

98. P.V.V. Prasada Rao and D.E. Gardner, Effects of cadmium inhalation on mitochondrial enzymes in rat tissues, *J. Toxicol. Environ. Health*, 17, 191–199, 1986.

99. S. Hirano, N. Tsukamoto, S. Higo, and K.T. Suzuki, Toxicity of cadmium oxide instilled into the rat lung. II. Inflammatory responses in broncho-alveolar lavage fluid, *Toxicology*, 55, 25–35, 1989.

100. K.E. Driscoll, J.K. Maurer, J. Poynter, J. Higgins, T. Asquith, and N.S. Miller, Stimulation of rat alveolar macrophage fibronectin release in a cadmium chloride model of lung injury and fibrosis, *Toxicol. Appl. Pharmacol.*, 116, 30–37, 1992.

101. P.J. Hakkinen, C.C. Morse, F.M. Martin, W.E. Dalbey, W.M. Haschek, and H.R. Witschi, Potentiating effects of oxygen in lungs damaged by methylcyclopentadienyl manganese tricarbonyl, cadmium chloride, oleic acid, and antitumor drugs, *Toxicol. Appl. Pharmacol.*, 67, 55–69, 1983.

102. F.M. Martin and H.P. Witschi, Cadmium-induced lung injury: cell kinetics and long-term effects, *Toxicol. Appl. Pharmacol.*, 80, 215–227, 1985.

103. C.A.M. Suzuki and M.G. Cherian, Renal glutathione depletion and nephrotoxicity of cadmium-metallothionein in rats, *Toxicol. Appl. Pharmacol.*, 98, 544–552, 1989.

104. T. Jin, P. Leffler, and G.F. Nordberg, Cadmium-metallothionein nephrotoxicity in the rat: transient calcuria and proteinuria, *Toxicology*, 45, 307–317, 1987.

105. K.-S. Min, K. Kobayashi, S. Onosaka, N. Ohta, Y. Okada, and K. Tanaka, Tissue distribution of cadmium and nephropathy after administration of cadmium in several chemical forms, *Toxicol. Appl. Pharmacol.*, 86, 262–270, 1986.

106. P.L. Goering, C.L. Kish, and B.R. Fisher, Stress protein synthesis induced by cadmium-cysteine in rat kidney, *Toxicology*, 85, 25–39, 1993.

107. J.Y. Zhao, E.C. Foulkes, and M. Jones, Delayed nephrotoxic effects of cadmium and their reversibility by chelation, *Toxicology*, 64, 235–243, 1990.

108. L.E. Sendelbach, W.C. Kershaw, F. Cuppage, and C.D. Klaassen, Cd-metallothionein nephrotoxicity in inbred strains of mice, *J. Toxicol. Environ. Health*, 35, 115–126, 1992.

109. T. Maitani, A. Watahiki, and K.T. Suzuki, Acute renal dysfunction by cadmium injected with cysteine in relation to renal critical concentration of cadmium, *Arch. Toxicol.,* 58, 136–140, 1986.

110. M.J. Tsapakos, T.H. Hampton, and K.W, Jennette, The carcinogen chromate induces DNA cross-links in rat liver and kidney, *J. Biol. Chem.,* 256, 3623–3626, 1981.

111. A.M. Standeven and K.E. Wetterhahn, Possible role of glutathione in chromium (VI) metabolism and toxicity in rats. *Pharmacol. Toxicol.,* 69, 469–476, 1991.

112. A. Mikalsen, J. Alexander, R.A. Andersen, and M. Ingelman-Sundberg, Effect of *in vivo* chromate, acetone and combined treatment on rat liver *in vitro* microsomal chromium (VI) reductive activity and on cytochrome P450 expression, *Pharmacol. Toxicol.,* 68, 456–463, 1991.

113. E. Kim and K.J. Na, Effect of sodium dichromate on carbohydrate metabolism, *Toxicol. Appl. Pharmacol.,* 110, 251–258, 1991.

114. E. Ernst, Testicular toxicity following short-term exposure to tri- and hexavalent chromium: an experimental study in the rat, *Toxicol. Lett.,* 51, 269–275, 1990.

115. D.K. Saxena, R.C. Murthy, B. Lal, R.S. Srivastava, and S.V. Chandra, Effect of hexavalent chromium on testicular maturation in the rat, *Reprod. Toxicol.,* 4, 223–228, 1990.

116. R.C. Murthy, D.K. Saxena, S.K. Gupta, and S.V. Chandra, Ultrastructural observations in testicular tissue of chromium-treated rats, *Reprod. Toxicol.,* 5, 443–447, 1991.

117. A. Vyskočil, C. Viau, M. Čížková, and G. Truchon, Kidney function in male and female rats chronically exposed to potassium dichromate, *J. Appl. Toxicol.,* 13, 375–376, 1993.

118. T.P. Coogan, J. Motz, C.A. Snyder, K.S. Squibb, and M. Costa, Differential DNA-protein crosslinking in lymphocytes and liver following chronic drinking water exposure of rats to potassium chromate, *Toxicol. Appl. Pharmacol.,* 109, 60–72, 1991.

119. U. Glaser, D. Hochrainer, H. Klöppel, and H. Kuhnen, Low level chromium (VI) inhalation effects on alveolar macrophages and immune functions in Wistar rats, *Arch. Toxicol.,* 57, 250–256, 1985.

120. U. Glaser, D. Hochrainer, H. Klöppel, and H. Oldiges, Carcinogenicity of sodium dichromate and chromium (VI/III) oxide aerosols inhaled by male Wistar rats, *Toxicology,* 42, 219–232, 1986.

121. B. Trivedi, D.K. Saxena, R.C. Murthy, and S.V. Chandra, Embryotoxicity and fetotoxicity of orally administered hexavalent chromium in mice, *Reprod. Toxicol.,* 3, 275–278, 1989.

122. R.A. Newman, A.R. Khokhar, B.A. Sunderland, E.L. Travis, and R.E. Bulger, A comparison in rodents of renal and intestinal toxicity of cisplatin and a new water-soluble antitumor platinum complex: *N*-methyl-iminodiacetato-diaminocyclohexane platinum (II), *Toxicol. Appl. Pharmacol.,* 84, 454–463, 1986.

123. J.M. Ward and K.A. Fauvie, The nephrotoxic effects of *cis*-diammine-dichloroplatinum (II) (NSC-119875) in male F344 rats, *Toxicol. Appl. Pharmacol.,* 38, 535–547, 1976.

124. R.S. Goldstein, B. Noordewier, J.T. Bond, J.B. Hook, and G.H. Mayor, *cis*-Dichlorodiammineplatinum nephrotoxicity: time course and dose response of renal functional impairment, *Toxicol. Appl. Pharmacol.,* 60, 163–175, 1981.

125. C.L. Litterst, Alterations in the toxicity of *cis*-dichlorodiammineplatinum-II and in tissue localization of platinum as a function of NaCl concentration in the vehicle of administration, *Toxicol. Appl. Pharmacol.,* 61, 99–108, 1981.

126. L.M. De Witt, T.W. Jones, and L. Moore, Stimulation of the renal endoplasmic reticulum calcium pump: a possible biomarker for platinate toxicity, *Toxicol. Appl. Pharmacol.,* 92, 157–169, 1988.

127. R.D. Mayer and M.D. Maines, Promotion of *trans*-platinum *in vivo* effects on renal heme and hemoprotein metabolism by D,L-buthionine-*S,R*-sulfoximine: possible role of glutathione. *Biochem. Pharmacol.,* 39, 1565–1571, 1990.

128. R. Safirstein, P. Miller, S. Dikman, N. Lyman, and C. Shapiro, Cisplatin nephrotoxicity in rats: defect in papillary hypertonicity. *Am, J. Physiol.,* 241, F175–F185, 1981.

129. H.Th. Heidemann, St. Müller, L. Mertins, G. Stepan, K. Hoffmann, and the late E.E. Ohnhaus, Effect of aminophylline on cisplatin nephrotoxicity in the rat, *Br. J. Pharmacol.,* 97, 313–318, 1989.

130. Y. Sadzuka, T. Shoji, and Y. Takino, Mechanism of the increase in lipid peroxide induced by cisplatin in the kidneys of rats, *Toxicol. Lett.,* 62, 293–300, 1992.

131. G. Bompart and C. Orfila, Cisplatin nephrotoxicity in lead-pretreated rats: enzymatic and morphological studies, *Toxicol. Lett.,* 50, 237–247, 1990.

132. E. Scherini, Permanent alterations of the dendritic tree of cerebellar Purkinje neurons in the rat following postnatal exposure to *cis*-dichlorodiammineplatinum, *Acta Neuropathol.,* 81, 324–327, 1991.

133. G. Cavaletti, G. Tredici, P. Marmiroli, M.G. Petruccioli, I. Barajon, and D. Fabbrica, Morphometric study of the sensory neuron and peripheral nerve changes induced by chronic cisplatin (DDP) administration in rats, *Acta Neuropathol.*, 84, 364–371, 1992.

134. P.M.A.B. Terheggen, R.G. Van Der Hoop, B.G.J. Floot, and W.H. Gispen, Cellular distribution of *cis*-diamminedichloroplatinum (II)-DNA binding in rat dorsal root spinal ganglia: effect of the neuroprotecting peptide ORG.2766, *Toxicol. Appl. Pharmacol.*, 99, 334–343, 1989.

135. R.S. Goldstein, G.H. Mayor, R.L. Gingerich, J.B. Hook, B. Robinson, and J.T. Bond, Hyperglucagonemia following cisplatin treatment, *Toxicol. Appl. Pharmacol.*, 68, 250–259, 1983.

136. R.S. Goldstein, G.H. Mayor, R.L. Gingerich, J.B. Hook, R.W. Rosenbaum, and J.T. Bond, The effects of cisplatin and other divalent platinum compounds on glucose metabolism and pancreatic endocrine function, *Toxicol. Appl. Pharmacol.*, 69, 432–441, 1983.

137. H. Azouri, J.-M. Bidart, and C. Bohuon, *In vivo* toxicity of cisplatin and carboplatin on the Leydig cell function and effect of the human choriogonadotropin. *Biochem. Pharmacol.*, 38, 567–571, 1989.

138. L.M. Pogach, Y. Lee, S. Gould, W. Giglio, M. Meyenhofer, and H.F.S. Huang, Characterization of *cis*-platinum-induced Sertoli cell dysfunction in rodents, *Toxicol. Appl. Pharmacol.*, 98, 350–361, 1989.

139. D.D. Choie, D.S. Longnecker, and M.P. Copley, Cytotoxicity of cisplatin in rat intestine, *Toxicol. Appl. Pharmacol.*, 60, 354–359, 1981.

140. K.A. Keller and S.K. Aggarwal, Embryotoxicity of cisplatin in rats and mice, *Toxicol. Appl. Pharmacol.*, 69, 245–256, 1983.

141. M.L. Bajt and S.K. Aggarwal, An analysis of factors responsible for resorption of embryos in cisplatin-treated rats, *Toxicol. Appl. Pharmacol.*, 80, 97–107, 1985.

142. M. Satoh, A. Naganuma, and N. Imura, Deficiency of selenium intake enhances manifestation of renal toxicity of *cis*-diamminedichloroplatinum in mice, *Toxicol. Lett.*, 38, 155–160, 1987.

143. U. Schaeppi, I.A. Heyman, R.W. Fleischman, H. Rosenkrantz, V. Ilievski, R. Phelan, D.A. Cooney, and R.D. Davis, *cis*-Dichlorodiammineplatinum (II) (NSC-119 875): preclinical toxicologic evaluation of intravenous injection in dogs, monkeys and mice, *Toxicol. Appl. Pharmacol.*, 25, 230–241, 1973.

144. N.A. Boughattas, F. Lévi, C. Fournier, B. Hecquet, G. Lemaigre, A. Roulon, G. Mathé, and A. Reinberg, Stable circadian mechanisms of toxicity of two platinum analogs (cisplatin and carboplatin) despite repeated dosages in mice, *J. Pharmacol. Exp. Ther.*, 255, 672–679, 1990.

145. R. Lerza, G. Bogliolo, C. Muzzulini, and I. Pannacciulli, Failure of *N*-acetylcysteine to protect against *cis*-dichlorodiammine-platinum (II)-induced hematopoietic toxicity in mice. *Life Sci.*, 38, 1795–1800, 1986.

146. D. Wierda and M. Matamoros, Partial characterization of bone marrow hemopoiesis in mice after cisplatin administration, *Toxicol. Appl. Pharmacol.*, 75, 25–34, 1984.

147. S.C. Apfel, J.C. Arezzo, L.A. Lipson, and J.A. Kessler, Nerve growth factor prevents experimental cisplatin neuropathy. *Ann. Neurol.*, 31, 76–80, 1992.

148. G. Lasfargues, D. Lison, P. Maldague, and R. Lauwerys, Comparative study of the acute lung toxicity of pure cobalt powder and cobalt-tungsten carbide mixture in rat, *Toxicol. Appl. Pharmacol.*, 112, 41–50, 1992.

149. C. Di Giulio, P.G. Data, and S. Lahiri, Chronic cobalt causes hypertrophy of glomus cells in the rat carotid body, *Am. J. Physiol.*, 261, C102–C105, 1991.

150. J.R. Nation, A.E. Bourgeois, D.E. Clark, and M.F. Hare, The effects of chronic cobalt exposure on behavior and metallothionein levels in the adult rat, *Neurobehav. Toxicol. Teratol.*, 5, 9–15, 1983.

151. K.A. Suarez and P. Bhonsle, The relationship of cobaltous chloride-induced alterations of hepatic microsomal enzymes to altered carbon tetrachloride hepatotoxicity, *Toxicol. Appl. Pharmacol.*, 37, 23–27, 1976.

152. J.L. Paternain, J.L. Domingo, and J. Corbella, Developmental toxicity of cobalt in the rat, *J. Toxicol. Environ. Health*, 24, 193–200, 1988.

153. B.B. Muhoberac, T. Hanew, S. Halter, and S. Schenker, A model of cytochrome P-450-centered hepatic dysfunction in drug metabolism induced by cobalt-protoporphyrin administration, *Biochem. Pharmacol.*, 38, 4103–4113, 1989.

154. M.B. Anderson, N.G. Pedigo, R.P. Katz, and W.J. George, Histopathology of testes from mice chronically treated with cobalt, *Reprod. Toxicol.*, 6, 41–50, 1992.

155. S.M. Spaethe and D.J. Jollow, Effect of cobalt protoporphyrin on hepatic drug-metabolizing enzymes, *Biochem. Pharmacol.*, 38, 2027–2038, 1989.

156. M. Lundborg and P. Camner, Lysozyme levels in rabbit after inhalation of nickel, cadmium, cobalt, and copper chlorides, *Environ. Res.,* 34, 335–342, 1984.

157. S. Hirano, H. Ebihara, S. Sakai, N. Kodama, and K.T. Suzuki, Pulmonary clearance and toxicity of intratracheally instilled cupric oxide in rats, *Arch. Toxicol.,* 67, 312–317, 1993.

158. S. Hirano, S. Sakai, H. Ebihara, N. Kodama, and K.T. Suzuki, Metabolism and pulmonary toxicity of intratracheally instilled cupric sulfate in rats, *Toxicology,* 64, 223–233, 1990.

159. I.C. Fuentealba, R.W. Davis, M.E. Elmes, B. Jasani, and S. Haywood, Mechanisms of tolerance in the copper-loaded rat liver, *Exp. Mol. Pathol.,* 59, 71–84, 1993.

160. I.C. Fuentealba, S. Haywood, and J. Foster, Cellular mechanisms of toxicity and tolerance in the copper-loaded rat. III. Ultrastructural changes and copper localization in the kidney, *Br. J. Exp. Pathol.,* 70, 543–556, 1989.

161. S. Toyokuni, S. Okada, S. Hamazaki, M. Fujioka, J.-L. Li, and O. Midorikawa, Cirrhosis of the liver induced by cupric nitrilotriacetate in Wister rats, *Am. J. Pathol.,* 134, 1263–1274, 1989.

162. N. Shiraishi, T. Taguchi, and H. Kinebuchi, Copper-induced toxicity in macular mutant mouse: an animal model for Menkes' kidney-hair disease, *Toxicol. Appl. Pharmacol.,* 110, 89–96, 1991.

163. K. Agarwal, A. Sharma, and G. Talukder, Clastogenic effects of copper sulphate on the bone marrow chromosomes of mice *in vivo, Mutat. Res.,* 243, 1–6, 1990.

164. M. Galleano and S. Puntarulo, Hepatic chemiluminescence and lipid peroxidation in mild iron overload, *Toxicology,* 76, 27–38, 1992.

165. M. Younes, I. Eberhardt, and R. Lemoine, Effect of iron overload on spontaneous and xenobiotic-induced lipid peroxidation *in vivo, J. Appl. Toxicol.,* 9, 103–108, 1989.

166. A. Pietrangelo, A. Cossarizza, D. Monti, E. Ventura, and C. Franceschi, DNA repair in lymphocytes from humans and rats with chronic iron overload, *Biochem. Biophys. Res. Commun.,* 154, 698–704, 1988.

167. S. Okada, S. Hamazaki, S. Toyokuni, and O. Midorikawa, Induction of mesothelioma by intraperitoneal injections of ferric sacchrate in male Wister rats, *Br. J. Cancer,* 60, 708–711, 1989.

168. T.C. Iancu, R.J. Ward, and T.J. Peters, Ultrastructural observations in the carbonyl iron-fed rat, an animal model for hemochromatosis, *Virchows Arch. B.,* 53, 208–217, 1987.

169. C.H. Park, B.R. Bacon, G.M. Brittenham, and A.S. Tavill, Pathology of dietary carbonyl iron overload in rats, *Lab. Invest.,* 57, 555–563, 1987.

170. B.R. Bacon, A.S. Tavill, G.M. Brittenham, C.H. Park, and R.O. Recknagel, Hepatic lipid peroxidation *in vivo* in rats with chronic iron overload, *J. Clin. Invest.,* 71, 429–439, 1983.

171. L. Golberg, L.E. Martin, and A. Batchelor, Biochemical changes in the tissues of animals injected with iron. 3. Lipid peroxidation. *Biochem. J.,* 83, 201–298, 1961.

172. A.G. Smith and J.E. Francis, Genetic variation of iron-induced uroporphyria in mice, *Biochem. J.,* 291, 29–35, 1993.

173. J.-L. Li, S. Okada, S. Hamazaki, Y. Ebina, and O. Midorikawa, Subacute nephrotoxicity and induction of renal cell carcinoma in mice treated with ferric nitrilotriacetate, *Cancer Res.,* 47, 1867–1869, 1987.

174. P. Carthew, B.M. Dorman, R.E. Edwards, J.E. Francis, and A.G. Smith, A unique rodent model for both the cardiotoxic and hepatotoxic effects of prolonged iron overload, *Lab. Invest.,* 69, 217–222, 1993.

175. P. Garthew, R.E. Edwars, B.M. Dorman, and J.E. Francis, Rapid induction of hepatic fibrosis in the gerbil after the paretenal administration of iron-dextran complex, *Hepatology,* 13, 534–539, 1991.

176. A.G. Smith, J.R.P. Cabral, P. Carthew, J.E. Francis, and M.M. Manson, Carcinogenicity of iron in conjection with a chlorinated environmental chemical, hexachlorobenzene, in C57BL/10ScSn mice, *Int. J. Cancer,* 43, 492–496, 1989.

177. N.N. Scharding and F.W. Oehme, The use of animal models for comparative studies of lead poisoning, *Clin. Toxicol.,* 6, 419–424, 1973.

178. K. Kostial, T. Maljkovic, and S. Jugo, Lead acute toxicity in rats in relation to age and sex, *Arch. Toxicol.,* 31, 265–269, 1974.

179. G.R. Hogan, Effects of ovariectomy and orchiectomy on lead-induced mortality in rats, *Environ. Res.,* 21, 314–316, 1980.

180. B. Garbar and E. Wei, Lead toxicity in mice with genetically different levels of d-aminolevulic acid, *Bull. Environ. Contam. Toxicol.,* 9, 80–83, 1973.

181. G.R. Hogan, Variation of lead-induced lethality in estradiol-treated mice, *J. Toxicol. Environ. Health,* 9, 353–357, 1982.

182. A.V. Lorenzo, M. Gewirtz, and D. Averill, CNS lead toxicity in rabbit offspring, *Environ. Res.,* 17, 131–150, 1978.

183. K. Nagatoshi, Experimental chronic lead poisoning, *Fol. Psychiatr. Neurol. Jpn.,* 33, 123–131, 1979.

184. M.V.S. Kumar and T. Desiraju, Regional alterations of brain biogenic amines and GABA/glutamate levels in rats following chronic lead exposure during neonatal development, *Arch. Toxicol.,* 64, 305–314, 1990.

185. R. Kishi and E. Uchino, Effects of low lead exposure on neuro-behavioral function in the rat, *Arch. Environ. Health,* 38, 25–33, 1983.

186. L. Altman, F. Weinsberg, K. Sveinsson, H. Lilienthal, H. Wiegand, and G. Winneke, Impairment of long-term potentiation and learning following chronic lead exposure, *Toxicol. Lett.,* 66, 105–112, 1993.

187. R. Sundström, K. Müntzing, H. Kalimo, and P. Sourander, Changes in the integrity of the blood-brain barrier in suckling rats with low dose lead encephalopathy, *Acta Neuropathol.,* 68, 1–9, 1985.

188. D. Lorton and W.J. Anderson, The effects of postnatal lead toxicity on the development of cerebellum in rats, *Neurobehav. Toxicol. Teratol.,* 8, 51–59, 1986.

189. S.R. Overmann, Behavioral effects of symptomatic lead exposure during neonatal development in rats, *Toxicol. Appl. Pharmacol.,* 41, 459–471, 1977.

190. S.V. Chandra, M.M. Ali, D.K. Saxena, and R.C. Murthy, Behavioral and neurochemical changes in rats simultaneously exposed to manganese and lead, *Arch. Toxicol.,* 49, 49–56, 1981.

191. J. Deluca, P.J. Donovick, and R.G. Burright, Lead exposure, environmental temperature, nesting and consummatory behavior of adult mice of two ages, *Neurotoxicol. Teratol.,* 11, 7–11, 1989.

192. J.M. Donald, M.G. Cutler, and M.R. Moore, Effects of lead in the laboratory mouse development and social behavior after lifelong exposure to 12 µ*M* lead in drinking fluid, *Neuropharmacology,* 26, 391–399, 1987.

193. E.E. Aiegler, B.B. Edwards, R.L. Jensen, K.R. Mahaffer, and S.J. Fomon, Adsorption and retention of lead by infants, *Pediatr. Res.,* 12, 29–34, 1978.

194. H.M. Mykkanen, J.W.T. Dickerson, and M.C. Lancaster, Effects of age on the tissue distribution of lead in the rat, *Toxicol. Appl. Pharmacol.,* 51, 447–454, 1979.

195. D.R. Brown, Neonatal lead exposure in the rat: decreased learning as a function of age and blood concentrations, *Toxicol. Appl. Pharmacol.,* 32, 628–637, 1975.

196. I. Kitchen, Lead toxicity and alterations in opioid systems, *Neurotoxicology,* 14, 115–124, 1993.

197. K. Tokoyama and S. Araki, Alterations nerve conduction velocity in low and high lead exposure: an animal study, *Ind. Health,* 24, 67–74, 1986.

198. H.E. Falke and W.C.M. Zwennis, Toxicity of lead acetate to female rabbits after chronic subcutaneous administration. 1. Biochemical and clinical effects, *Arch. Toxicol.,* 64, 522–529, 1990.

199. G.M. Hass, D.V.L. Brown, R. Eisenstein, and A. Hemmens, Relations between lead poisoning in rabbit and man, *Am. J. Pathol.,* 45, 691–715, 1964.

200. A. Oskarsson, Effects of perinatal treatment with lead and disculfiram on ALAD activity in blood, liver and kidney and urinary ALA excretion in rats, *Pharmacol. Toxicol.,* 64, 344–348, 1989.

201. J.J. Barlow, J.K. Baruah, and A. Davison, δ-Aminolevulinic acid dehydratase activity and focal brain hemorrhages in lead-treated rats, *Acta Neuropathol.,* 39, 219–223, 1977.

202. M. Hayashi, Lead toxicity in the pregnant rat, *Environ. Res.,* 30, 152–160, 1983.

203. K. Tomokuni, M. Ichiba, and Y. Hirai, Species defference of urinary excretion of d-aminolevurinic acid and coproporphyrin in mice and rats exposed to lead, *Toxicol. Lett.,* 41, 255–259, 1988.

204. S.U. Rehman, Effects of zinc, copper, and lead toxicity on d-aminolevulinic acid dehydratase activity, *Bull. Environ. Contam. Toxicol.,* 33, 92–98, 1984.

205. S.K. Tandon and S.J.S. Flora, Dose and time effects of combine exposure to lead and ethanol on lead body burden and some neuronal, hepatic and haematopoietic biochemical induces in the rats, *J. Appl. Toxicol.,* 9, 347–352, 1989.

206. E.K. Silbergeld, R.E. Hruska, D. Bradly, Lamon, J.M., and B.C. Frykholm, Neurotoxic aspects of porphyrinopathies: lead and succinylacetone, *Environ. Res.,* 29, 459–471, 1982.

207. S.J.S. Flora, S. Singh, and S.K. Tandon, Chelation in metal intoxication XVIII: combined effects of thiamine and calcium disodium versenate on lead toxicity, *Life Sci.,* 38, 67–71, 1986.

208. E. Schlick, K. Mengel, and K.D. Friedberg, The effect of low lead doses in vitro and in vivo on the d-ala-d activity of erythrocytes, bone marrow cells, liver and brain of the mouse, *Arch. Toxicol.*, 53, 193–205, 1983.

209. S. Sassa, Toxic effects of lead, with particular reference to porphyrin and heme metabolism, in *Handbook of Experimental Pharmacology*, Vol. 44, Springer Verlag, Berlin, 1978, 333.

210. J. Maes and G.B. Gerber, Increased ALA dehydratase activity and spleen weight in lead-intoxicated rats. A consequence of increased blood cell destruction, *Experimentia*, 34, 381–382, 1978.

211. N. Karmakar, R. Saxena, and S. Ananda, Histopathological changes induced in rats tissues by oral intake of lead acetate, *Environ. Res.*, 41, 23–28, 1986.

212. B.A. Fowler, C.A. Kimmel, J.S. Woods, E.E. McConnell, and L.D. Grant, Chronic low level lead toxicity in the rat. III. An integrated assessment of long-term toxicity with special reference to the kidney, *Toxicol. Appl. Pharmacol.*, 56, 59–77, 1980.

213. B.J. Spit, A.A.E. Wibowo, V.J. Feron, and R.L. Zielhuis, Ultrasonic changes in the kidneys of rabbits treated with lead acetate, *Arch. Toxicol.*, 49, 85–91, 1981.

214. F. Khalil-Manesh, H.C. Gonic, A. Cohen, E. Bergamaschi, and A. Mutti, Experimental model of lead nephropathy. II. Effect of removal from lead exposure and chelation treatment with dimercaptosuccinic acid (DMSA), *Environ. Res.*, 58, 35–54, 1992.

215. R.A. Goyer, Lead toxicity: a problem in environmental pathology, *Am. J. Pathol.*, 64, 167–181, 1971.

216. F.E. Hemphill, M.L. Kaerberle, and W.B. Buck, Lead suppression of mouse resistance to *Salmonella typhimurium*, *Science*, 172, 1031–1033, 1971.

217. B.R. Blakley and D.L. Archer, The effect of lead acetate on the immune response in mice, *Toxicol. Appl. Pharmacol.*, 61, 18–26, 1981.

218. L.D. Koller, The immunotoxic effects of lead in lead-exposed laboratory animals. *Ann. N. Y. Acad. Sci.*, 587, 160–167, 1990.

219. N. Kobayashi and T. Okamoto, Effect of lead oxide on the induction of lung tumors in Syrian hamsters, *J. Natl. Cancer Inst.*, 52, 1605–1610, 1974.

220. N.I. Kerkvliet and L. Baecher-Steppan, Immunotoxicology studies on lead: effect of exposure on tumor growth and cell-mediated tumor immunity after synergic or allogenic stimulation, *Immunopharmacology*, 4, 213–224, 1982.

221. L.D. Koller and S. Kovacic, Decreased antibody response in mice exposed to lead, *Nature*, 250, 148–150, 1974.

222. L.D. Koller, J.H. Exon, and J.G. Roan, Humoral antibody response in mice after single dose exposure to lead or cadmium, *Proc. Soc. Exp. Biol. Med.*, 151, 339–342, 1976.

223. R.A. Trejo, N.R. DiLuzio, L.D. Loose, and E. Hoffman, Reticuloendothelial and hepatic alterations following lead acetate administration, *Exp. Mol. Pathol.*, 17, 145–158, 1972.

224. R.M. McClain and B.A. Becker, Teratogenicity, fetal toxicity, and placental transfer of lead nitrate in rats, *Toxicol. Appl. Pharmacol.*, 31, 72–78, 1975.

225. R.Z. Sokol and N. Berman, The effects of age exposure on lead-induced testicular toxicity, *Toxicology*, 69, 269–278, 1991.

226. T.J. Walsh and H.A. Tilson, Neurobehavioral toxicology of the organoleads, *Neurotoxicology*, 5, 67–86, 1984.

227. W.J. Niklowitz, Ultrastructural effects of acute teraethyllead poisoning on nerve cells of the rabbit brain, *Environ. Res.*, 8, 17–36, 1974.

228. W. Niklowitz, Neurofibrillary changes after acute experimental lead poisoning, *Neurology*, 25, 927–934, 1975.

229. H.A. Tilson, C.F. Mactutus, R. McLamb, and T.A. Burne, Characterization of triethyllead chloride neurotoxicity in adult rats, *Neurobehav. Toxicol. Teratol.*, 4, 671–681, 1982.

230. T.J. Walsh, R.L. McLamb, and H.A. Tilson, Organometal-induced antinociception: a time and dose-response comparison of triethyl and trimethyl lead and tin, *Toxicol. Appl. Pharmacol.*, 73, 295–299, 1984.

231. J.S. Hong, H.A. Tilson, P. Hudson, S.F. Ali, W.E. Wilson, and V. Hunter, Corelation of neurochemical and behavioral effects of triethyl lead chloride in rats, *Toxicol. Appl. Pharmacol.*, 69, 471–479, 1983.

232. T.J. Walsh, D.W. Schulz, H.A. Tilson, and D. Dehaven, Acute exposure to triethyl lead enhances the behavioral effects of dopaminergic agonists: involvement of brain dopamine in organolead neurotoxicity, *Brain Res.*, 363, 222–229, 1986.

233. S.F. Ali and S.C. Bondy, Triethyllead-induced peroxidative damage in various regions on the rat brain, *J. Toxicol. Environ. Health*, 26, 235–242, 1989.

234. K. Kristensson, H. Eriksson, B. Lundh, L.-O. Plantin, L. Wachtmeister, M.L. Azazi, C. Morath, and E. Heilbronn, Effects of manganese chloride on the rat developing nervous system, *Acta Pharmacol. Toxicol.*, 59, 345–348, 1986.

235. J.K. Malik and A.K. Srivastava, Studies on the interaction between manganese and fenitrothion in rats, *Toxicol. Lett.*, 36, 221–226, 1987.

236. G.S. Shukla and S.V. Chandra, Manganese toxicity: lipid peroxidation in rat brain, *Acta Pharmacol. Toxicol.*, 48, 95–100, 1981.

237. S.V. Chandra, G.S. Shukla, and R.C. Murthy, Effect of stress on the response of rat brain to manganese, *Toxicol. Appl. Pharmacol.*, 47, 603–608, 1979.

238. K. Teramoto, F. Wakitani, S. Horiguchi, T. Jo, T. Yamamoto, H. Mitsutake, and H. Nakaseko, Comparison of the neurotoxicity of several chemicals estimated by the peripheral nerve conduction velocity in rats, *Environ. Res.*, 62, 148–154, 1993.

239. S.V. Chandra and G.S. Shukla, Manganese encephalopathy in growing rats, *Environ. Res.*, 15, 28–37, 1978.

240. H. Eriksson, S. Lenngren, and E. Heilbronn, Effect of long-term administration of manganese on biogenic amine levels in discrete striatal regions of rat brain, *Arch. Toxicol.*, 59, 426–431, 1987.

241. J.P. Nachtman, R.E. Tubben, and R.L. Commissaris, Behavioral effects of chronic manganese administration in rats: locomotor activity studies, *Neurobehav. Toxicol. Teratol.*, 8, 711–715, 1986.

242. S.V. Chandra and G.S. Shukla, Effect of manganese on synthesis of brain catecholamines in growing rats, *Acta Pharmacol. Toxicol.*, 48, 349–354, 1981.

243. S.V. Chandra, M.M. Ali, D.K. Saxena, and R.C. Murthy, Behavioral and neurochemical changes in rats simultaneously exposed to manganese and lead, *Arch. Toxicol.*, 49, 49–56, 1981.

244. E. Bonilla and A.L.N. Prasad, Effects of chronic manganese intake on the levels of biogenic amines in rat brain regions, *Neurobehav. Toxicol. Teratol.*, 6, 341–344, 1984.

245. A.M. Scheuhammer, Chronic manganese exposure in rats: histological changes in the pancreas, *J. Toxicol. Environ. Health*, 12, 353–360, 1983.

246. C.L. Witzleben, P. Pitlick, J. Bergmeyer, and R. Benoit, A new experimental model of intrahepatic cholestasis, *Am. J. Pathol.*, 53, 409–423, 1968.

247. D. Wassermann and M. Wassermann, The ultrastructure of the liver cell in subacute manganese administration, *Environ. Res.*, 14, 379–390, 1977.

248. R.R. Rogers, R.J. Garner, M.M. Riddle, R.W. Luebke, and R.J. Smialowicz, Augmentation of murine natural killer cell activity by manganese chloride, *Toxicol. Appl. Pharmacol.*, 70, 7–17, 1983.

249. B. Srisuchart, M.J. Taylor, and R.P. Sharma, Alteration of humoral and cellular immunity in manganese chloride-treated mice, *J. Toxicol. Environ. Health*, 22, 91–99, 1987.

250. J. Komura and M. Sakamoto, Effects of manganese forms on biogenic amines in the brain and behavioral alterations in the mouse: long-term oral administration of several manganese compounds, *Environ. Res.*, 57, 34–44, 1992.

251. D.N. Cox, G.J. Traiger, S.P. Jacober, and R.P. Hanzlik, Comparison of the toxicity of methylcyclopentadienyl manganese tricarbonyl with that of its two major metabolites, *Toxicol. Lett.*, 39, 1–5, 1987.

252. P.A. McGinley, J.B. Morris, R.J. Clay, and G. Gianutsos, Disposition and toxicity of methylcyclopentadienyl manganese tricarbonyl in the rat, *Toxicol. Lett.*, 36, 137–145, 1987.

253. P.J. Hakkinen and W.M. Haschek, Pulmonary toxicity of methylcyclopentadienyl manganese tricarbonyl: nonciliated bronchiolar epithelial (Clara) cell necrosis and alveolar damage in the mouse, rat, and hamster, *Toxicol. Appl. Pharmacol.*, 65, 11–22, 1982.

254. R.P. Hanzlik, R. Stitt, and G.J. Traiger, Toxic effects of methylcyclopentadienyl manganese tricarbonyl (MMT) in rats: role of metabolism, *Toxicol. Appl. Pharmacol.*, 56, 353–360, 1980.

255. R.J. Clay and J.B. Morris, Comparative pneumotoxicity of cyclopentadienyl manganese tricarbonyl and methylcyclopentadienyl manganese tricarbonyl, *Toxicol. Appl. Pharmacol.*, 98, 434–443, 1989.

256. B.E. Fishman, P.A. McGinley, and G. Gianutsos, Neurotoxic effects of methylcyclopentadienyl manganese tricarbonyl (MMT) in the mouse: basis of MMT-induced seizure activity, *Toxicology*, 45, 193–201, 1987.

257. R. Kishi, K. Hashimoto, S. Shimizu, and M. Kobayashi, Behavioral changes and mercury concentrations in tissues of rats exposed to mercury vapor, *Toxicol. Appl. Pharmacol.*, 46, 555–566, 1978.

258. A. Fredriksson, L. Dahlgren, B. Danielsson, P. Eriksson, L. Dencker, and T. Archer, Behavioural effects of neonatal metallic mercury exposure in rats, *Toxicology,* 74, 151–160, 1992.

259. B.R.G. Danielsson, A. Fredriksson, L. Dahlgren, A.T. Gårdlund, L. Olsson, L. Dencker, and T. Archer, Behavioural effects of prenatal metallic mercury inhalation exposure in rats, *Neurotoxicol. Teratol.,* 15, 391–396, 1993.

260. F. Livardjani, M. Ledig, P. Kopp, M. Dahlet, M. Leroy, and A. Jaeger, Lung and blood superoxide dismutase activity in mercury vapor exposed rats: effect of N-acetylcysteine treatment, *Toxicology,* 66, 289–295, 1991.

261. G.P. Daston, R.J. Kavlock, E.H. Rogers, and B. Carver, Toxicity of mercuric chloride to the developing rat kidney. I. Postnatal ontogeny of renal sensitivity, *Toxicol. Appl. Pharmacol.,* 71, 24–41, 1983.

262. G.M. Kyle, R. Luthra, J.V. Bruckner, W.F. MacKenzie, and D. Acosta, Assessment of functional, morphological, and enzymatic tests for acute nephrotoxicity induced by mercuric chloride, *J. Toxicol. Environ. Health,* 12, 99–117, 1983.

263. E.M. McDowell, R.B. Nagle, R.C. Zalme, J.S. McNeil, W. Flamenbaum, and B.F. Trump, Studies on the pathophysiology of acute renal failure. I. Correlation of ultrastructure and function in the proximal tubule of the rat following administration of mercuric chloride, *Virchows Arch. B Cell Pathol.,* 22, 173–196, 1976.

264. M.-A. Duran, D. Spencer, M. Weise, N.O. Kronfol, R.F. Spencer, and D.E. Oken, Renal epithelial amino acid concentrations in mercury-induced and postischemic acute renal failure, *Toxicol. Appl. Pharmacol.,* 105, 183–194, 1990.

265. B.O. Lund, D.M. Miller, and J.S. Woods, Studies on Hg(II)-induced H_2O_2 formation and oxidative stress *in vivo* and *in vitro* in rat kidney mitochondria, *Biochem. Pharmacol.,* 45, 2017–2024, 1993.

266. X. Liu, T. Jin, and G.F. Nordberg, Increased urinary calcium and magnesium excretion in rats injected with mercuric chloride, *Pharmacol. Toxicol.,* 68, 254–259, 1991.

267. H. Fukino, M. Hirai, Y.M. Hsueh, S. Moriyasu, and Y. Yamane, Mechanism of protection by zinc against mercuric chloride toxicity in rats: effects of zinc and mercury on glutathione metabolism, *J. Toxicol. Environ. Health.,* 19, 75–89, 1986.

268. H. Fukino, M. Hirai, Y.M. Hsueh, and Y. Yamane, Effect of zinc pretreatment on mercuric chloride-induced lipid peroxidation in the rat kidney, *Toxicol. Appl. Pharmacol.,* 73, 395–401, 1984.

269. L. Magos, S. Sparrow, and R. Snowden, The comparative renotoxicology of phenylmercury and mercuric chloride, *Arch. Toxicol.,* 50, 133–139, 1982.

270. Y. Yamane and T. Koizumi, Protective effect of molybdenum on the acute toxicity of mercuric chloride, *Toxicol. Appl. Pharmacol.,* 65, 214–221, 1982.

271. D. Holt and M. Webb, The toxicity and teratogenicity of mercuric mercury in the pregnant rat, *Arch. Toxicol.,* 58, 243–248, 1986.

272. A.M. Bernard, C. Collette, and R. Lauwerys, Renal effects of in utero exposure to mercuric chloride in rats, *Arch. Toxicol.,* 66, 508–513, 1992.

273. D. Pezerovic, P. Narancsik, and S. Gamulin, Effects of mercury bichloride on mouse kidney polyribosome structure and function, *Arch. Toxicol.,* 48, 167–172, 1981.

274. T. Tanaka, A. Naganuma, and N. Imura, Role of γ-glutamyltranspeptidase in renal uptake and toxicity of inorganic mercury in mice, *Toxicology,* 60, 187–198, 1990.

275. J.B. Nielsen, H.R. Andersen, O. Andersen, and H. Starklint, Mercuric chloride-induced kidney damage in mice: time course and effect of dose, *J. Toxicol. Environ. Health,* 34, 469–483, 1991.

276. A. Yasutake, K. Hirayama, and M. Inouye, Sex difference in acute renal dysfunction induced by methylmercury in mice, *Renal Failure,* 12, 233–240, 1990.

277. A.R. Chowdhury, S. Makhija, K.D. Vachhrajani, and A.K. Gautam, Methylmercury- and mercuric chloride-induced alterations in rat epididymal sperm, *Toxicol. Lett.,* 47, 125–134, 1989.

278. M.K. Lakshmana, T. Desiraju, and T.R. Raju, Mercuric chloride-induced alterations of levels of noradrenaline, dopamine, serotonin and acetylcholine esterase activity in different regions of rat brain during postnatal development, *Arch. Toxicol.,* 67, 422–427, 1993.

279. M. Carmignani, V.N. Finelli, and P. Boscolo, Mechanisms in cardiovascular regulation following chronic exposure of male rats to inorganic mercury, *Toxicol. Appl. Pharmacol.,* 69, 442–450, 1983.

280. T.M.C. Tan, Y.M. Sin, and K.P. Wong, Mercury-induced UDP glucuronyltransferase (UDPGT) activity in mouse kidney, *Toxicology,* 64, 81–87, 1990.

281. P. Hultman and S. Eneström, Dose-response studies in murine mercury-induced autoimmunity and immune-complex disease, *Toxicol. Appl. Pharmacol.*, 113, 199–208, 1992.

282. M.P. Dieter, M.I. Luster, G.A. Boorman, C.W. Jameson, J.H. Dean, and J.W. Cox, Immunological and biochemical responses in mice treated with mercuric chloride, *Toxicol. Appl. Pharmacol.*, 68, 218–228, 1983.

283. B.B. Hoskins and E.W. Hupp, Methylmercury effects in rat, hamster, and squirrel monkey: lethality, symptoms, brain mercury, and amino acids, *Environ. Res.*, 15, 5–19, 1978.

284. S. Omata, H. Tsubaki, K. Sakimura, M. Sato, R. Yoshimura, E. Hirakawa, and H. Sugano, Stimulation of protein and RNA synthesis by methylmercury chloride in the liver of intact and adrenalectomized rats, *Arch. Toxicol.*, 47, 113–123, 1981.

285. T.L.M. Syversen, G. Totland, and P.R. Flood, Early morphological changes in rat cerebellum caused by a single dose of methylmercury, *Arch. Toxicol.*, 47, 101–111, 1981.

286. M.K. Cheung and M.A. Verity, Experimental methyl mercury neurotoxicity: locus of mercurial inhibition of brain protein synthesis *in vivo* and *in vitro*, *J. Neurochem.*, 44, 1799–1808, 1985.

287. S.F. Ali, C.P. Lebel, and S.C. Bondy, Reactive oxygen species formation as a biomarker of methylmercury and trimethyltin neurotoxicity, *Neurotoxicology*, 13, 637–648, 1992.

288. J. De Ceaurriz and M. Ban, Role of γ-glutamyltranspeptidase and β-lyase in the nephrotoxicity of hexachloro-1,3-butadiene and methyl mercury in mice, *Toxicol. Lett.*, 50, 249–256, 1990.

289. P.R. Sager, M. Aschner, and P.M. Rodier, Persistent, differential alterations in developing cerebellar cortex of male and female mice after methylmercury exposure, *Dev. Brain Res.*, 12, 1–11, 1984.

290. K. Nomiyama, K. Matsui, and H. Nomiyama, Effects of temperature and other factors on the toxicity of methylmercury in mice, *Toxicol. Appl. Pharmacol.*, 56, 392–398, 1980.

291. P. Salvaterra, E.J. Massaro, J.B. Morganti, and B.A. Lown, Time-dependent tissue/organ uptake and distribution of [203]Hg in mice exposed to multiple sublethal doses of methyl mercury, *Toxicol. Appl. Pharmacol.*, 32, 432–442, 1975.

292. A. Yasutake and K. Hirayama, Acute effects of methylmercury on hepatic and renal glutathione metabolisms in mice, *Arch. Toxicol.*, 68, 512–516, 1994.

293. M. Sato, H. Sugano, and Y. Takizawa, Effects of methylmercury on zinc-thionein levels of rat liver, *Arch. Toxicol.*, 47, 125–133, 1981.

294. M. Kabuto, Chronic effects of methylmercury on the urinary excretion of catecholamines and their responses to hypoglycemic stress, *Arch. Toxicol.*, 65, 164–167, 1991.

295. P.A. Desnoyers and L.W. Chang, Ultrastructual changes in rat hepatocytes following acute methyl mercury intoxication, *Environ. Res.*, 9, 224–239, 1975.

296. L. Magos, G.C. Peristianis, T.W. Clarkson, A. Brown, S. Preston, and R.T. Snowden, Comparative study of the sensitivity of male and female rats to methylmercury, *Arch. Toxicol.*, 48, 11–20, 1981.

297. M.-F. Wu, J.R. Ison, J.R. Wecker, and L.W. Lapham, Cutaneous and auditory function in rats following methyl mercury poisoning, *Toxicol. Appl. Pharmacol.*, 79, 377–388, 1985.

298. R.J. Hargreaves, B.P. Eley, S.R. Moorhouse, and D. Pelling, Regional cerebral glucose metabolism and blood flow during the silent phase of methylmercury neurotoxicity in rats, *J. Neurochem.*, 51, 1350–1355, 1988.

299. O. Kawamata, H. Kasama, S. Omata, and H. Sugano, Decrease in protein phosphorylation in central and peripheral nervous tissues of methylmercury-treated rat, *Arch. Toxicol.*, 59, 346–352, 1987.

300. M.A. Verity, W.J. Brown, M. Cheung, and G. Czer, Methyl mercury inhibition of synaptosome and brain slice protein synthesis: *in vivo* and *in vitro* studies, *J. Neurochem.*, 29, 673–679, 1977.

301. W.E. Stroo and J.B. Hook, Renal functional correlates of methyl mercury intoxication: interaction with acute mercuric chloride toxicity, *Toxicol. Appl. Pharmacol.*, 42, 399–410, 1977.

302. M. Yonaha, M. Saito, and M. Sagai, Stimulation of lipid peroxidation by methyl mercury in rats, *Life Sci.*, 32, 1507–1514, 1983.

303. J.R. O'Kusky and E.G. McGeer, Methylmercury-induced movement and postural disorders in developing rat: high-affinity uptake of choline, glutamate, and γ-aminobutyric acid in the cerebral cortex and caudate-putamen, *J. Neurochem.*, 53, 999–1006, 1989.

304. P.A. Desnoyers and L.W. Chang, Ultrastructual changes in the liver after chronic exposure to methylmercury, *Environ. Res.*, 10, 59–75, 1975.

305. K. Saijoh, T. Fukunaga, H. Katsuyama, M.J. Lee, and K. Sumino, Effects of methylmercury on protein kinase A and protein kinase C in the mouse brain, *Environ. Res.*, 63, 264–273, 1993.

306. A. Yasutake and K. Hirayama, Sex and strain differences of susceptibility to methylmercury toxicity in mice, *Toxicology,* 51, 47–55, 1988.

307. A. Yasutake, T. Adachi, K. Hirayama, and M. Inouye, Integrity of the blood-brain barrier system against methylmercury acute toxicity, *Jpn. J. Toxicol. Environ. Health*, 37, 355–362, 1991.

308. H. Lindström, J. Luthman, A. Oskarsson, J. Sundberg, and L. Olson, Effects of long-term treatment with methyl mercury on the developing rat brain, *Environ. Res.,* 56, 158–169, 1991.

309. B. Moller-Madsen and G. Danscher, Localization of mercury in CNS of the rat. IV. The effect of selenium on orally administered organic and inorganic mercury, *Toxicol. Appl. Pharmacol.,* 108, 457–473, 1991.

310. J.S. Woods, M.A. Bowers, and H.A. Davis, Urinary porphyrin profiles as biomarkers of trace metal exposure and toxicity: studies on urinary porphyrin excretion patterns in rats during prolonged exposure to methyl mercury, *Toxicol. Appl. Pharmacol.,* 110, 464–476, 1991.

311. J.S. Woods, H.A. Davis, and R.P. Baer, Enhancement of γ-glutamylcysteine synthetase mRNA in rat kidney by methyl mercury, *Arch. Biochem. Biophys.,* 296, 350–353, 1992.

312. K. Mitsumori, K. Takahashi, O. Matano, S. Goto, and Y. Shirasu, Chronic toxicity of methylmercury chloride in rats: clinical study and chemical analysis, *Jpn. J. Vet. Sci.,* 45, 747–757, 1983.

313. K. Mitsumori, K. Maita, and Y. Shirasu, Chronic toxicity of methylmercury chloride in rats: pathological study, *Jpn. J. Vet. Sci.,* 46, 549–557, 1984.

314. H.R. Andersen and O. Andersen, Effects of dietary α-tocopherol and β-carotene on lipid peroxidation induced by methyl mercuric chloride in mice. *Pharmacol. Toxicol.,* 73, 192–201, 1993.

315. S.G. Gilbert and J.P.J. Maurissen, Assessment of the effects of acrylamide, methylmercury, and 2,5-hexanedione on motor functions in mice, *J. Toxicol. Environ. Health,* 10, 31–41, 1982.

316. K. Mitsumori, M. Hirano, H. Ueda, K. Maita, and Y. Shirasu, Chronic toxicity and carcinogenicity of methylmercury chloride in B6C3F1 mice, *Fundam. Appl. Toxicol.,* 14, 179–190, 1990.

317. J.A.G. Geelen, J.A.M.A. Dormans, and A. Verhoef, The early effects of methylmercury on the developing rat brain, *Acta Neuropathol.,* 80, 432–438, 1990.

318. R. Cagiano, M.A. De Salvia, G. Renna, E. Tortella, D. Braghiroli, C. Parenti, P. Zanoli, M. Baraldi, Z. Annau, and V. Cuomo, Evidence that exposure to methyl mercury during gestation induces behavioral and neurochemical changes in offspring of rats, *Neurotoxicol. Teratol.,* 12, 23–28, 1990.

319. A.M. Saillenfait, M.T. Brondeau, D. Zissu, and J. De Ceaurriz, Effects of prenatal methylmercury exposure on urinary proximal tubular enzyme excretion in neonatal rats, *Toxicology,* 55, 153–160, 1989.

320. M. Bornhausen, H.R. Müsch, and H. Greim, Operant behavior performance changes in rats after prenatal methylmercury exposure, *Toxicol. Appl. Pharmacol.,* 56, 305–310, 1980.

321. N.H. Peckham and B.H. Choi, Abnormal neuronal distribution within the cerebral cortex after prenatal methylmercury intoxication, *Acta Neuropathol.,* 76, 222–226, 1988.

322. M. Inouye and Y. Kajiwara, Strain difference of the mouse in manifestation of hydrocephalus following prenatal methylmercury exposure, *Teratology,* 41, 205–210, 1990.

323. T. Nobunaga, H. Satoh, and T. Suzuki, Effects of sodium selenite on methylmercury embryotoxicity and teratogenicity in mice, *Toxicol. Appl. Pharmacol.,* 47, 79–88, 1979.

324. M. Inouye and Y. Kajiwara, Developmental disturbances of the fetal brain in guinea-pigs caused by methylmercury, *Arch. Toxicol.,* 62, 15–21, 1988.

325. F.W. Sunderman, Jr., M.C. Reid, L.M. Bibeau, and J.V. Linden, Nickel induction of microsomal heme oxygenase activity in rodents, *Toxicol. Appl. Pharmacol.,* 68, 87–95, 1983.

326. F.W. Sunderman, Jr., S.K. Shen, J.M. Mitchell, P.R. Allpass, and I. Damjanov, Embryotoxicity and fetal toxicity of nickel in rats, *Toxicol. Appl. Pharmacol.,* 43, 381–390, 1978.

327. F.W. Sunderman, Jr., K.S. Kasprzak, T.J. Lau, P.P. Minghetti, R.M. Maenza, N. Becker, C. Onkelinx, and P.J. Goldblatt, Effects of manganese on carcinogenicity and metabolism of nickel subsulfide, *Cancer Res.,* 36, 1790–1800, 1976.

328. R.J. Smialowicz, R.R. Rogers, D.G. Rowe, M.M. Riddle, and R.W. Luebke, The effects of nickel on immune function in the rat, *Toxicology,* 44, 271–281, 1987.

329. K.S. Kasprzak, M.P. Waalkes, and L.A. Poirier, Effects of magnesium acetate on the toxicity of nickelous acetate in rats, *Toxicology,* 42, 57–68, 1986.

330. F.W. Sunderman, Jr., S.M. Hopfer, S.-M. Lin, M.C. Plowman, T. Stojanovic, S.H-Y. Wong, O. Zaharia, and L. Ziebka, Toxicity to alveolar macrophages in rats following parenteral injection of nickel chloride, *Toxicol. Appl. Pharmacol.,* 100, 107–118, 1989.

331. M. Misra, R.E. Rodriguez, and K.S. Kasprzak, Nickel induced lipid peroxidation in the rat: correlation with nickel effect on antioxidant defense systems, *Toxicology,* 64, 1–17, 1990.

332. M. Misra, R. Olinski, M. Dizdaroglu, and K.S. Kasprzak, Enhancement by L-histidine of nickel (II)-induced DNA-protein cross-linking and oxidative DNA base damage in the rat kidney, *Chem. Res. Toxicol.,* 6, 33–37, 1993.

333. J. Cartana and L. Arola, Nickel-induced hyperglycaemia: the role of insulin and glucagon, *Toxicology,* 71, 181–192, 1992.

334. M.K. Smith, E.L. George, J.A. Stober, H.A. Feng, and G.L. Kimmel, Perinatal toxicity associated with nickel chloride exposure, *Environ. Res.,* 61, 200–211, 1993.

335. R.E. Rodriguez, M. Misra, S.L. North, and K.S. Kasprzak, Nickel-induced lipid peroxidation in the liver of different strains of mice and its relation to nickel effects on antioxidant systems, *Toxicol. Lett.,* 57, 269–281, 1991.

336. G.L. Fisher, C.E. Chrisp, and D.A. McNeill, Lifetime effects of intratracheally instilled nickel subsulfide on B6C3F$_1$ mice, *Environ. Res.,* 40, 313–320, 1986.

337. R.J. Smialowicz, R.R. Rogers, M.M. Riddle, R.J. Garner, D.G. Rowe, and R.W. Luebke, Immunologic effects of nickel. II. Suppression of natural killer cell activity, *Environ. Res.,* 36, 56–66, 1985.

338. G.R. Hogan, Nickel acetate-induced mortality in mice of different ages, *Bull. Environ. Contam. Toxicol.,* 34, 446–450, 1985.

339. M.P. Dieter, C.W. Jameson, A.N. Tucker, M.I. Luster, J.E. French, H.L. Hong, and G.A. Boorman, Evaluation of tissue disposition, myelopoietic, and immunologic responses in mice after long-term exposure to nickel sulfate in the drinking water, *J. Toxicol. Environ. Health,* 24, 357–372, 1988.

340. J.K. Dunnick, J.M. Benson, C.H. Hobbs, F.F. Hahn, Y.S. Cheng, and A.F. Edison, Comparative toxicity of nickel oxide, nickel sulfate hexahydrate, and nickel subsulfide after 12 days of inhalation exposure to F344/N rats and B6C3F$_1$ mice, *Toxicology,* 50, 145–156, 1988.

341. L.L. David and T.R. Shearer, State of sulfhydryl in selenite cataract, *Toxicol. Appl. Pharmacol.,* 74, 109–115, 1984.

342. R.A. LeBoeuf and W.G. Hoekstra, Adaptive changes in hepatic glutathione metabolism in response to excess selenium in rats, *J. Nutr.,* 113, 845–854, 1983.

343. M. Jacobs and C. Forst, Toxicological effects of sodium selenite in Sprague-Dawley rats, *J. Toxicol. Environ. Health,* 8, 575–585, 1981.

344. G.R. Hogan, Decreased levels of peripheral leukocytes following sodium selenite treatment in female mice, *Bull. Environ. Contam. Toxicol.,* 37, 175–179, 1986.

345. C. Watanabe and T. Suzuki, Sodium selenite-induced hypothermia in mice: indirect evidence for a neural effect, *Toxicol. Appl. Pharmacol.,* 86, 372–379, 1986.

346. M. Jacobs and C. Forst, Toxicological effects of sodium selenite in Swiss mice, *J. Toxicol. Environ. Health,* 8, 587–598, 1981.

347. M.A. Al-Bayati, O.G. Raabe, and S.V. Teague, Effect of inhaled dimethylselenide in the Fischer 344 male rat, *J. Toxicol Environ. Health,* 37, 549–557, 1992.

348. C. Rios and A. Monroy-Noyola, D-Penicillamine and Prussian blue as antidotes against thallium intoxication in rats, *Toxicology,* 74, 69–76, 1992.

349. D.B. Peele, R.C. MacPhail, and J.D. Farmer, Flavor aversions induced by thallium sulfate: importance of route of administration, *Neurobehav. Toxicol. Teratol.,* 8, 273–277, 1986.

350. M. Hasan and S.S. Haider, Acetyl-homocysteine thiolactone protects against some neurotoxic effects of thallium, *Neurotoxicology,* 10, 257–262, 1989.

351. L. Osorio-Rico, S. Galvan-Arzate, and C. Rios, Thallium increases monoamine oxidase activity and serotonin turnover rate in rat brain regions, *Neurotoxicol. Teratol.,* 17, 1–5, 1995.

352. J. Marwaha, R. Freedman, and B. Hoffer, Electrophysiological changes at a central noradrenergic synapse during thallium toxicosis, *Toxicol. Appl. Pharmacol.,* 56, 345–352, 1980.

353. J.S. Woods and B.A. Fowler, Alteration of hepatocellular structure and function by thallium chloride: ultrastructural, morphometric, and biochemical studies, *Toxicol. Appl. Pharmacol.,* 83, 218–229, 1986.

354. D. Appenroth, S. Gambaryan, K. Winnefeld, M. Leiterer, C. Fleck, and H. Braunlich, Functional and morphological aspects of thallium-induced nephrotoxicity in rats, *Toxicology,* 96, 203–215, 1995.

355. L.Formigli, R. Scelsi, P. Poggi, C. Gregotti, A.D. Nucci, E. Sabbioni, L. Gottardi, and L. Manzo, Thallium-induced testicular toxicity in the rat, *Environ. Res.,* 40, 531–539, 1986.

356. A.P. de Groot, V.J. Feron, and H.P. Til, Short-term toxicity studies on some salts and oxides of tin in rats, *Food Cosmet. Toxicol.,* 11, 19–30, 1973.

357. P.J.M. Janssen, M.C. Bosland, J.P. Van Hees, B.J. Spit, M.I. Willems, and C.F. Kuper, Effects of feeding stannous chloride on defferent parts of the gastrointestinal tract of the rat, *Toxicol. Appl. Pharmacol.,* 78, 19–28, 1985.

358. H.C. Dreef-van der Meulen, V.J. Feron, and H.P. Til, Pancreatic atrophy and other pathological changes in rats following the feeding of stannous chloride, *Pathol. Eur.,* 9, 185–192, 1974.

359. G. Zareba and J. Chmielnicka, Aminolevulinic acid dehydratase activity in the blood of rats exposed to tin and zinc, *Ecotoxicol. Environ. Saf.,* 9, 40–46, 1985.

360. G.J. Harry, J.F. Goodrum, M.R. Krigman, and P. Morell, The use of synapsin I as a biochemical marker for neuronal damage by trimethyltin. *Brain Res.,* 326, 9–18, 1985.

361. L.W. Chang, G.R. Wenger, D.E. McMillan, and R.S. Dyer, Species and strain comparison of acute neurotoxic effects of trimethyltin in mice and rats, *Neurobehav. Toxicol. Teratol.,* 5, 337–350, 1983.

362. R.S. Dyer, T.L. Deshields, and W.F. Wonderlin, Trimethyltin-induced changes in gross morphology of the hippocampus, *Neurobehav. Toxicol. Teratol.,* 4, 141–147, 1982.

363. T.J. Walsh, M. Gallagher, E. Bostock, and R.S. Dyer, Trimethyltin impairs retention of a passive avoidance task, *Neurobehav. Toxicol. Teratol.,* 4, 163–167, 1982.

364. R.S. Dyer, W.E. Howell, and W.F. Wonderlin, Visual system dysfunction following acute trimethyltin exposure in rats, *Neurobehav. Toxicol. Teratol.,* 4, 191–195, 1982.

365. R.C. MacPhail, Studies on the flavor aversions induced by trialkyltin compounds, *Neurobehav. Toxicol. Teratol.,* 4, 225–230, 1982.

366. T.J. Walsh, R.L. McLamb, and H.A. Tilson, Organometal-induced antinociception: a time- and dose-response comparison of triethyl and trimethyl lead and tin, *Toxicol. Appl. Pharmacol.,* 73, 295–299, 1984.

367. P.R.S. Kodavanti, J.A. Cameron, P.R. Yallapragada, P.J.S.Vig, and D. Desaiah, Inhibition of Ca^{2+} transport associated with cAMP-dependent protein phosphorylation in rat cardiac sarcoplasmic reticulum by triorganotins, *Arch. Toxicol.,* 65, 311–317, 1991.

368. R.S. Dyer and W.E. Howell, Acute triethyltin exposure: effects on the visual evoked potential and hippocampal afterdischarge, *Neurobehav. Toxicol. Teratol.,* 4, 259–266, 1982.

369. H.A. Tilson and T.A. Burne, Effects of triethyl tin on pain reactivity and neuromotor function of rats, *J. Toxicol. Environ. Health,* 8, 317–324, 1981.

370. D.B. Miller, D.A. Eckerman, M.R. Krigman, and L.D. Grant, Chronic neonatal organotin exposure alters radial-arm maze performance in adult rats, *Neurobehav. Toxicol. Teratol.,* 4, 185–190, 1982.

371. P. Mushak, M.R. Krigman, and R.B. Mailman, Comparative organotin toxicity in the developing rat: somatic and morphological changes and relationship to accumulation of total tin, *Neurobehav. Toxicol. Teratol.,* 4, 209–215, 1982.

372. C.P. LeBel, S.F. Ali, M. McKee, and S.C. Bondy, Organometal-induced increases in oxygen reactive species: the potential of 2′,7′-dichlorofluorescin diacetate as an index of neurotoxic damage, *Toxicol. Appl. Pharmacol.,* 104, 17–24, 1990.

373. G.R. Wenger, D.E. McMillan, and L.W. Chang, Behavioral toxicology of acute trimethyltin exposure in the mouse, *Neurobehav. Toxicol. Teratol.,* 4, 157–161, 1982.

374. D.A. Fox, Pharmacological and biochemical evaluation of triethyltin's anticonvulsant effects, *Neurobehav. Toxicol. Teratol.,* 4, 273–278, 1982.

375. M. Ghoneum, A.E. Hussein, G. Gill, and L.J. Alfred, Suppression of murine natural killer cell activity by tributyltin: *in vivo* and *in vitro* assessment, *Environ. Res.,* 52, 178–186, 1990.

376. A.D. Nucci, C. Gregotti, and L. Manzo, Triphenyl tin hepatotoxicity in rats, *Arch. Toxicol.,* 59, 402–405, 1986.

377. K. Lehotzky, J.M. Szeberenyi, Z. Gonda, F. Horkay, and A. Kiss, Effects of prenatal triphenyl-tin exposure on the development of behavior and conditioned learning in rat pups, *Neurobehav. Toxicol. Teratol.,* 4, 247–250, 1982.

378. M. Yoshizuka, K. Hara, N. Haramaki, M. Yokoyama, N. Mori, Y. Doi, A. Kawahara, and S. Fujimoto, Studies on the hepatotoxicity induced by bis (tributyltin) oxide, *Arch. Toxicol.,* 66, 182–187, 1992.

379. M. Yoshizuka, N. Haramaki, M. Yokoyama, K. Hara, A. Kawahara, Y. Umezu, H. Araki, N. Mori, and S. Fujimoto, Corneal edema induced by bis (ributyltin) oxide, *Arch. Toxicol.,* 65, 651–655, 1991.

380. W. Seinen and M.I. Willems, Toxicity of organotin compounds. I. Atrophy of thymus and thymus-dependent lymphoid tissue in rats fed di-*n*-octyltindichloride, *Toxicol. Appl. Pharmacol.*, 35, 63–75, 1976.

381. W. Seinen, J.G. Vos, I.V. Spanje, M. Snoek, R. Brands, and H. Hooykaas, Toxicity of organotin compounds. II. Comparative *in vivo* and *in vitro* studies with various organotin and organolead compounds in different animal species with special emphasis on lymphocyte cytotoxicity, *Toxicol. Appl. Pharmacol.*, 42, 197–212, 1977.

382. K. Miller, J. Maisey, and S. Nicklin, Effect of orally administered dioctyltin dichloride on murine immunocompetence, *Environ. Res.*, 39, 434–441, 1986.

383. G.R. Hogan, B.S. Cole, and J.M. Lovelace, Sex and age mortality responses in zinc acetate-treated mice, *Bull. Environ. Contam. Toxicol.*, 39, 156–161, 1987.

384. J.M. Llobet, J.L. Domingo, M.T. Colomina, E. Mayayo, and J. Corbella, Subchronic oral toxicity of zinc in rats, *Bull Environ. Contam. Toxicol.*, 41, 36–43, 1988.

385. G. Cosma, H. Fulton, T. Defeo, and T. Gordon, Rat lung metallothionein and heme oxygenase gene expression following ozone and zinc oxide exposure, *Toxicol. Appl. Pharmacol.*, 117, 75–80, 1992.

386. S. Hirano, S. Higo, N. Tsukamoto, E. Kobayashi, and K.T. Suzuki, Pulmonary clearance and toxicity of zinc oxide instilled into the rat lung, *Arch. Toxicol.*, 63, 336–342, 1989.

387. H.F. Lam, M.W. Conner, A.E. Rogers, S. Fitzgerald, and M.O. Amdur, Functional and morphologic changes in the lung of guinea pigs exposed to freshly generated ultrafine zinc oxide, *Toxicol. Appl. Pharmacol.*, 78, 29–38, 1985.

23 Human Clinical Toxicology

Jill Dolgin, Pharm. D., A.B.A.T

CONTENTS

SECTION 1. INTRODUCTION

Nearly two million human poisonings are reported to poison information centers each year; however, there are an estimated 2 to 3 million additional unreported exposures.[1] The purpose of this chapter is to review the epidemiological characteristics of human poisoning, clinical toxicology research designs, and general management techniques of the acutely poisoned patient. In addition, the role of the poison control centers in managing these patients and several contemporary issues in clinical toxicology are discussed.

Although several excellent texts contain valuable information on the toxicity and treatment of poisoned patients,[2,3] the most up-to-date information on both human and animal poisonings is provided by Poisindex® (MICROMEDEX, Medical Information Systems, Denver). It contains data on the chemical composition, toxicity, and the current medical management of more than 750,000 drugs, household chemicals, industrial and environmental toxins, and biologicals (including plant and animal toxins). Poisindex® also facilitates the identification of manufactured drugs by providing a description of the tablet/capsule shape, color, and the symbols imprinted on them. It also provides slang terminology, color, and shape for street drugs. Poisindex is edited and updated every 3 months.

Another valuable source of information is a regional poison control center. Currently there are more than 100 regional poison control centers located throughout the United States; 38 have been certified by the American Association of Poison Control Centers (AAPCC). (See Section 6.)

SECTION 2. CLINICAL RESEARCH DESIGN

Predicting the effects of toxic agents in animals are critical and mandatory facts of human risk management. The three main tasks of experimental animal studies in toxicology are listed in Table 23.1.[4]

Basic to understanding human toxicities is the assumption that information gained from animal models can be extrapolated to analogous human situations. This places great importance on the validations of extrapolations from animal data. However, extrapolation from an animal requires specification of the effects that will serve to test the validity of the model. A hierarchy of five criteria, shown in Table 23.2, can be used to determine the validity of animal models. Other relevant information, from epidemiology studies and clinical research, is then integrated with the animal data to make regulatory decisions regarding human safety.

The principle of research design in clinical toxicology involves assessing causation in disease-exposure associations, evaluating the appropriateness of the research design, and evaluating the validity of a particular research study.

The various research designs available to study clinical problems include the randomized clinical trial (RCT), cohort studies, case-control studies, cross-sectional studies, case series, and case reports.

The advantages and disadvantages of each method are beyond the scope of this chapter and are outlined in Chapter 24 and discussed in several excellent texts on epidemiology.[6,7]

TABLE 23.1
The Three Main Tasks of Experimental Toxicology

1. Spectrum of toxicity
   Detection of adverse effects of chemicals in selected laboratory animal species and description of the dose-effect relationship over a broad range of doses.
2. Extrapolation
   Prediction of adverse effects in other species, particularly in man.
3. Safety
   Prediction of safe levels of exposure in other species, particularly in man.

From Zbinden (1991).[4] Reprinted with permission.

TABLE 23.2
Five Criteria that Test the Validity of Animal Models

1. Face validity
   A model is superficially similar to the human condition.
2. Content validity
   Examining the characteristics shared in common by an animal model and the human condition it seeks to simulate, to determine whether the model represents the specific content which a study is designed to measure
3. Concurrent validity
   Multiple measures of toxic reactions within subjects can provide profiles distinctive to particular toxins or classes of toxins.
4. Construct validity
   Utilizing a theoretical model of the nature of living organisms and how they interact with their biosphere
5. Predictive validity
   Demonstration that extrapolation from animal models compares or can be predictive of human toxicity

From Russell (1991).[5] Reprinted with permission.

SECTION 3. EPIDEMIOLOGY OF POISONING

A. GENERAL CHARACTERISTICS

The AAPCC estimates that 4.4 million poisonings occurred nationwide in 1991. Of the 1.8 million exposures reported, 764 resulted in death.

Although nonpharmaceuticals were involved in more than 50% of all poisonings (Table 23.3), pharmaceuticals were most frequently involved in fatalities (Table 23.4).

Ingestion was the most common route of exposure (Table 23.5). Accidental exposures accounted for more than 87% of all poisonings (Table 23.6); they were most common in children younger than 6 years of age and in the elderly. Intentional exposures were most common in adolescents (>14 years of age) and the most frequent cause of death in the adult population (Tables 23.6 and 23.7). Most accidental poisonings involved only one substance; however, 50 to 60% of intentional poisonings in adults were poly-drug exposures (Table 23.8).

TABLE 23.3
Substances Most Frequently Involved in Human Exposure

Substance	No.	%[a]
Cleaning substances	191,830	10.4
Analgesics	183,013	10.0
Cosmetics	153,424	8.3
Plants	112,564	6.1
Cough and cold preparations	105,185	5.7
Bites/envenomations	76,941	4.2
Pesticides (includes rodenticides)	70,523	3.8
Topicals	69,096	3.8
Antimicrobials	64,805	3.5
Foreign bodies	64,472	3.5
Hydrocarbons	63,536	3.5
Sedatives/hypnotics/antipsychotics	58,450	3.2
Chemicals	53,666	2.9
Alcohols	50,296	2.7
Food poisoning	46,482	2.5
Vitamins	40,883	2.2

Note: Despite a high frequency of involvement, these substances are not necessarily the most toxic, but rather often represent only ready availability.

[a] Percentages are based on the total number of human exposures rather than the total number of substances.

From Litovitz et al., 1992.[1] Reprinted with permission.

TABLE 23.4

Categories with Largest Numbers of Deaths

Category	No.	% of All Exposures in Category
Analgesics	190	0.104
Antidepressants	188	0.525
Sedative/hypnotics	97	0.166
Stimulants and street drugs	90	0.434
Cardiovascular drugs	87	0.348
Alcohols	72	0.143
Gases and fumes	49	0.188
Asthma therapies	39	0.229
Chemicals	37	0.069
Hydrocarbons	36	0.057
Cleaning substances	26	0.014
Pesticides (including rodenticides)	18	0.026

From Litovitz et al., 1992.[1] Reprinted with permission.

TABLE 23.5

Distribution of Route of Exposure for Human Poison Exposure Cases and 764 Fatalities

Route	All Exposure Cases No.	All Exposure Cases %	Fatal Exposure Cases No.	Fatal Exposure Cases %
Ingestion	1,473,361	76.3	622	75.7
Dermal	143,196	7.4	8	1.0
Ophthalmic	119,027	6.2	2	0.2
Inhalation	107,634	5.6	116	14.1
Bites and stings	72,331	3.7	5	0.6
Parenteral	5,217	0.3	37	4.5
Other	4,917	0.3	3	0.4
Unknown	6,423	0.3	29	3.5
Total	1,932,106	100.0	822	100.0

Note: Multiple routes of exposure were observed in many poison exposure victims. Percentage is based on the total number of exposure mutes (1,932,106 for all patients, 822 for fatal cases) rather than the total number of human exposures (1,837,939) or fatalities (764).

From Litovitz, 1992.[1] Reprinted with permission.

TABLE 23.6
Distribution of Reason for Exposure by Age

Reason	>6 Years		6–12 Years		13–17 Years		18–64 Years		>64 Years		Unknown		Total	
	No.	%	No.	%	No.	%	No.	%	No.	%	No.	%	No.	%
Accidental	1,093,264	59.5	93,941	5.1	39,874	2.2	223,533	12.2	25,409	1.4	130,486	7.1	1,606,507	87.4
Intentional	2583	0.1	6391	0.3	40,286	2.2	114,451	6.2	3338	0.2	27,148	1.5	194,197	10.6
Adverse reaction	3437	0.2	1812	0.1	1598	0.1	14,361	0.8	1564	0.1	7272	0.4	30,044	1.6
Unknown	784	0.0	556	0.0	57	0.0	2877	0.2	419	0.0	1798	0.1	7191	0.4
Total	1,100,068	59.9	102,700	5.6	82,515	4.5	355,222	19.3	30,730	1.7	166,704	9.1	1,837,939	100.0

From Litovitz et al., 1992.[1] Reprinted with permission.

TABLE 23.7
Distribution of Reason for Exposure and Age for 764 Fatalities

Reason	<6 Years	6–12 Years	13–17 Years	>17 Years	Total
Accidental					
General	30	0	0	8	38
Environmental	6	3	1	20	30
Misuse	3	1	2	29	35
Occupational	0	0	0	12	12
Unknown	0	0	0	2	2
Total	39	4	3	71	117
Intentional					
Suicide	0	0	23	385	408
Misuse	1	0	0	24	25
Abuse	0	0	16	66	82
Unknown	0	0	5	56	61
Total	1	0	44	531	576
Adverse reaction	2	0	0	15	17
Unknown	2	0	1	51	54
Total	44	4	48	668	764

From Litovitz et al., 1992.[1] Reprinted with permission.

TABLE 23.8
**Number of Substances Involved in
Human Poison Exposure Cases**

No. of Substances	No. of Cases	% of Cases
1	1,666,684	90.7
2	92,378	5.0
3	67,662	3.7
4	5693	0.3
5	2294	0.1
6	935	0.1
7	476	0.0
8	219	0.0
9	136	0.0
≥10	391	0.0
Unknown	1071	0.1
Total	1,837,939	100.0

From Litovitz et al., 1992.[1] Reprinted with permission.

B. Pediatric Poisonings

According to the 1991 statistics, approximately 60% of exposures involved children younger than 6 years of age. The number of pediatric deaths due to poisonings increased from 25 deaths in 1990 to 44 deaths in 1991.

A 5-year (1985–1989) retrospective analysis of pediatric deaths was conducted to aid poison prevention and educational efforts, guide new product formulation and aversive agent use, reassess over-the-counter status for selected pharmaceuticals, and identify areas of research for the treatment of pediatric poisonings.[8] A hazard factor was devised to assess the risk of each agent to produce a major (residual disability) or life-threatening outcome when a child is involved in an overdose. This factor indicates a substance's relative pediatric hazard by evaluating its packaging, accessibility (as a reflection of common storage practices in the home), availability (as a reflection of marketing), formulation, and closure types. The hazard score ranking allows for a comparison among categories.

Of the 3.8 million pediatric exposures reported between 1985 and 1989, 2117 patients experienced a major outcome and 111 fatalities occurred. Table 23.9 shows the substance categories implicated in pediatric exposure calls, the total number of pediatric exposures that occurred in each category, the number of major effects, the number of fatal exposures, and the hazard factor. Tables 23.10 and 23.11 address unintentional pediatric ingestion fatalities reported to the AAPCC in 1983 through 1990. Iron supplements emerge as the single most frequent cause of unintentional death in pediatrics, representing more than 30% of all deaths.

The ingestion hazards parallel the substances required to have child-resistant closures by the Poison Prevention Packaging Act. This demonstrates, however, that the requirement of child-resistant closures does not render a product "child-proof." In 1989, King and Palmisana performed an epidemiological study to identify the risk factors responsible for the ineffectiveness of child-resistant closures. Although the Poison Prevention Packaging Act of 1970 has resulted in a 65% decline in the ingestion of products packaged in child-resistant containers, ingestion of prescription drugs by children has declined by only 36%. Reasons for these data include:

1. Availability of non-child-resistant packaging upon consumer request (i.e., consumer noncompliance)
2. Misuse of child-resistant closures by the consumer in the home
3. Transferring medicines from child-resistant packages to unsafe containers, or using no container at all
4. Unsafe storage practices, such as leaving containers within easy reach; and
5. Violations of the ACT by the dispensing pharmacist, physician, or Health Care Facility. Reprinted with permission (King and Palmisana, 1989).[9]

Pharmacies and health care facilities have also been shown to be noncompliant with the packaging act of 1970. Reports indicate that between 14% and 44% of pharmacies surveyed were in violation of federal packaging standards.

Table 23.12 demonstrates that 2 year olds accounted for the majority (53.7%) of ingestions of prescription drugs.[9] Table 23.13 demonstrates that in more than 75% of cases surveyed, non-child-resistant packages or no containers were involved in the ingestion.[9] Table 23.14 indicates the leading solid prescription drugs ingested that resulted in hospitalization.[9] Table 23.15 demonstrates that the owner of each prescription was able to be identified in 80% of the cases surveyed. Although parents' prescriptions accounted for 53.6% of the ingestions, nearly 30% involved grandparents' medications. [9] Noncompliance with child-resistant packaging was a major reason for the exposure as indicated in Table 23.16.[9]

Other barriers to pediatric poisonings include the use of warning stickers designed to deter children from getting into containers. However, studies have failed to demonstrate any benefit from their use and, in fact, the warning stickers may attract children who otherwise would have ignored the product.[10] Woolf and Lovejoy[10] discuss the epidemiology of drug overdose in children and the determinants that result in a high risk of drug poisoning in this group (Table 23.17).

TABLE 23.9
Reported Poison Exposures in Children Younger than 6 Years of Age, 1985 through 1989

Substance Categories and Subcategories[a]	Total Pediatric Exposures (1985–1989)	No. of Major Effects	No. of Deaths	Hazard Factor[b]
Nonpharmaceutical exposures				
Adhesives/glues	37,986	15	0	0.7
Alcohols	80,443	46	5	1.0
Ethanol (beverage)	2622	11	2	8.0[c]
Arts/crafts/office supplies	80,294	3	0	0.1
Auto/aircraft/boat products	12,019	11	4	2.0
Ethylene glycol	2321	4	1	3.5[c]
Methanol	1883	3	3	5.1[c]
Batteries	12,753	7	0	0.9
Bites/envenormations	48,821	100	0	3.3[c]
Copperhead	44	4	0	146.4[c]
Rattlesnake	125	19	0	244.8[c]
Unknown snake	651	10	0	24.7[c]
Other/unknown reptile	682	3	0	7.1[c]
Scorpion	1585	43	0	43.7[c]
Black widow spider	1240	4	0	5.2[c]
Brown recluse spider	455	2	0	7.1[c]
Building products	13,721	2	0	0.2
Chemicals	87,463	72	3	1.4[c]
Acid: hydrochloric	784	3	0	6.2[c]
Alkali	10,267	24	0	3.8[c]
Dioxin	11	1	0	146.4[c]
Ethylene glycol	1002	6	0	9.6[c]
Strychnine	32	1	0	50.3[c]
Cleaning substances	386,052	205	4	0.9
Acid: drain cleaner	208	6	0	46.5[c]
Acid: industrial cleaner	438	3	0	11.0[c]
Aklali: drain cleaner	1474	19	1	21.9[c]
Alkali: industrial cleaner	938	17	0	29.2[c]
Alkali: oven cleaner	4619	10	0	3.5[c]
Oven cleaner: other/unknown	224	4	0	28.8[c]
Cosmetics/personal care	395,985	57	3	0.2
Deodorizers (nonpersonal)	39,408	1	0	0.0
Dyes	10,369	0	0	0.0
Essential oils	6557	5	0	1.2
Fertilizers	23,581	1	0	0.1
Fire extinguishers	860	0	0	0.0
Food products/poisoning	49,500	7	0	0.2
Foreign bodies/toys	163,722	21	0	0.2
Fumes/gases/vapors	8436	55	21	14.5[c]
Carbon monoxide	3103	42	18	31.1[c]
Chlorine gas	2208	6	0	4.4[c]
Hydrogen sulfide	228	2	0	14.1[c]
Methane and natural gas	700	3	1	9.2[c]
Gas:other	1138	1	2	4.2[c]
Fungicides (nonmedicinal)	2714	1	0	0.6
Heavy metals	11,926	14	0	1.9[c]

TABLE 23.9 *(Continued)*
Reported Poison Exposures in Children Younger than 6 Years of Age, 1985 through 1989

Substance Categories and Subcategories[a]	Total Pediatric Exposures (1985–1989)	No. of Major Effects	No. of Deaths	Hazard Factor[b]
Other	1094	4	0	5.9[c]
Unknown	39	1	0	41.3[c]
Herbicides	6488	3	0	0.7
Paraquat	66	1	0	24.4[c]
Hydrocarbons	129,024	168	5	2.2[c]
Kerosene	10,751	51	2	7.9[c]
Lighter fluid/naphtha	8865	24	0	4.4[c]
Mineral seal oil	6564	13	0	3.2[c]
Insecticides/pesticides	100,105	122	6	2.1[c]
Chlorinated hydrocarbon alone	9694	29	0	4.8[c]
Organophosphate alone	16,560	56	2	5.6[c]
Organophosphate with other pesticide	1806	4	0	3.6[c]
Rotenone	284	2	0	11.3[c]
Lacrimators	4779	1	0	0.3
Matches/fireworks/explosive	11,655	1	0	0.1
Moth repellants	19,548	6	0	0.5
Mushrooms	32,724	9	0	0.4
Paints/stripping agents	47,114	10	0	0.3
Photographic products	2688	1	0	0.6
Plants	375,649	33	1	0.1
Polishes/waxes	12,249	4	0	0.5
Rodenticides	41,261	2	1	0.1
Sporting equipment	2134	0	4	3.0[c]
Gun bluing compound	100	0	3	48.3[c]
Swimming pool/aquarium	8067	1	0	0.2
Tobacco products	36,742	14	0	0.6
Unknown nondrug substance	20,318	14	0	1.1
Pharmaceutical exposures				
Analgesics	325,539	119	8	0.6
Acetaminophen with propoxyphene	2171	6	0	4.5[c]
Aspirin: unknown formulation	10,002	18	1	3.1[c]
Methadone	127	4	2	76.1[c]
Morphine	164	3	0	29.5[c]
Propoxyphene	514	1	1	6.3[c]
Other/unknown narcotic	732	4	0	8.8[c]
Anesthetics	14,025	17	4	2.4
Anticholinergic	6516	13	0	3.2[c]
Anticoagulants	1860	1	0	0.9
Anticonvulsants	9198	106	4	19.3[c]
Carbamazepine	4113	81	2	32.5[c]
Phenytoin	3619	19	2	9.3[c]
Valproic acid	1197	5	0	6.7[c]
Other anticonvulsant	54	1	0	29.8[c]
Antidepressants	12,003	125	7	17.7[c]
Arnitriptyline	2897	39	2	22.8[c]
Amoxapine	200	4	0	32.2[c]
Desipramine	935	13	3	27.6[c]
Doxepin	887	8	0	14.5[c]
Imipramine	2503	29	2	20.0[c]
Maprotiline	209	3	0	23.1[c]

TABLE 23.9 (Continued)
Reported Poison Exposures in Children Younger than 6 Years of Age, 1985 through 1989

Substance Categories and Subcategories[a]	Total Pediatric Exposures (1985–1989)	No. of Major Effects	No. of Deaths	Hazard Factor[b]
Nortriptyline	347	2	0	9.3[c]
Other cyclic antidepressant	179	2	0	18.0[c]
Unknown cyclic antidepressant	142	5	0	56.7[c]
Cyclic antidepressant with benzodiazepine	288	2	0	11.2[c]
Cyclic antidepressant with phenothiazine	832	10	0	19.4[c]
Lithium	1054	7	0	10.7[c]
Antihistamines	38,390	20	4	1.0
Antimicrobials	122,686	28	3	0.4
Antimalarials	204	2	2	31.6[c]
Isoniazid	219	3	0	22.1[c]
Rifampin	84	2	0	38.4[c]
Antineoplastics	570	0	1	2.8
Asthma therapies	20,502	43	3	3.6[c]
Aminophylline	8622	38	3	7.7[c]
Cardiovascular drugs	37,385	182	7	8.1[c]
Antiarrhythmics	1203	3	0	4.0[c]
Antihypertensives	8099	139	0	27.6[c]
Cardiac glycosides	3846	24	2	10.9[c]
Nitroprusside	47	1	1	68.5[c]
Cough/cold preparations	249,038	72	4	0.5
Diagnostic agents	697	1	0	2.3
Diuretics	11,175	8	0	1.2
Electrolytes/minerals	50,751	57	8	2.1[c]
Iron	11,234	52	7	8.5[c]
Eye/ear/nose/throat preparations	32,805	17	0	0.8
Glaucoma medications	74	1	0	21.8[c]
Gastrointestinal preparations	99,636	48	3	0.8
Antidiarrheals: diphenoxylate/atropine	2500	18	1	12.2[c]
Hormones and antagonists	6357	20	1	0.5[c]
Insulin	217	2	1	22.3[c]
Oral hypoglycemics	2609	11	0	6.8[c]
Miscellaneous drugs	17,650	10	2	1.1
Neuromuscular blocking agents	8	2	0	402.7[c]
Muscle relaxants	3165	7	0	3.6[c]
Methocarbamol	341	2	0	9.4[c]
Other	1012	3	0	4.8[c]
Sedative/hypnotics/antipsychotics	33,048	153	2	7.6[c]
Barbiturates: long acting	4475	37	0	13.3[c]
Barbiturates: short acting	1051	4	0	6.1[c]
Chloral hydrate	443	18	0	65.5[c]
Ethchlorvynol	81	1	0	19.9[c]
Glutethimide	30	2	0	107.4[c]
Methaqualone	66	1	0	24.4[c]
Phenothiazines	7451	57	2	12.8[c]
Other	330	2	0	9.8[c]
Serums, toxoids, vaccines	448	0	0	0.0
Stimulants/street drugs	21,260	84	1	6.4[c]
Amphetamines	6409	18	0	4.5[c]
Cocaine	546	20	0	59.0[c]
Lysergic acid diethylamide	117	2	0	27.5[c]

TABLE 23.9 *(Continued)*
Reported Poison Exposures in Children Younger than 6 Years of Age, 1985 through 1989

Substance Categories and Subcategories[a]	Total Pediatric Exposures (1985–1989)	No. of Major Effects	No. of Deaths	Hazard Factor[b]
Marijuana	694	3	0	7.0[c]
Mescaline/peyote	325	2	0	9.9[c]
Phencyclidine	177	30	0	273.0[c]
Topicals	175,378	55	2	0.5
Silver nitrate	44	1	0	36.6[c]
Miscellaneous veterinary	4630	0	0	0.0
Vitamins	145,872	33	1	0.4
Unknown drugs	21,020	38	0	2.9[c]
Total	3,852,618	2,270	122	1.0

[a] Subcategories with hazard factors ≥3 and statistical significance[a] are listed under each substance category.

[b] See text for explanation.

[c] $p < .05$, Fisher's Exact Test comparing each individual category (or subcategory) with all other cases.

From Litovitz and Manoguerra, 1992.[8] Reprinted with permission.

TABLE 23.10
Pediatric Pharmaceutical Ingestion Fatalities:
1983–1990

Substances Ingested	N	% Total (N-53)
Anticonvulsants	3	5.7
Antidepressants	10	18.9
Cardiovascular drugs	8	13.2
Iron supplements	16	30.2
Salicylates	6	11.3
Miscellaneous	11	20.7

From Litovitz and Manoguerra, 1992.[8] Modified with permission.

TABLE 23.11
Pediatric Nonpharmaceutical Ingestion Fatalities
1983–1990 (Total N = 44)

Substances	N	%
Pesticides	12	27.3
Hydrocarbons	12	27.3
Alcohols and glycols	7	15.9
Gun-bluing	4	9.1
Cleaning substances	3	6.8
Chemicals	3	6.8
Cosmetics and personal care products	2	4.5
Plants	1	2.3

From Litovitz and Manoguerra, 1992.[1] Modified with permission.

TABLE 23.12
Ingestions of Solid Prescription Drugs, by Age of Victim

Age Categories (months)	No.	(%)
Infant (< 12 mo)	1	(0.1)
1 (12–23)	205	(24.2)
2 (24–35)	456	(53.7)
3 (36–47)	124	(14.6)
4 (48–59)	37	(4.4)
5 (60–71)	25	(2.9)
Unknown	1	(0.1)
Total	849	(100.0)

From King and Palmisano, 1989.[9] Reprinted with permission.

TABLE 23.13
Ingestions of Solid Prescription Drugs, by Container Type

Container Type	No.[a]	(%)
Child-resistant	159	(24.1)
Non-child-resistant	268	(40.5)
No container	214	(32.4)
Other	20	(3.0)
Total	661	(100.0)

[a] Number reporting container type.

From King and Palmisano, 1989.[9] Reprinted with permission.

TABLE 23.14
Leading Solid Prescription Drugs Ingested, Resulting in Hospitalization

Prescription Drug	No. of Cases	No. Hospitalized (%)
Ferrous sulfate	32	12 (37.5)
Catapres (clonidine HCl)	26	12 (46.2)
Ativan (lorazepam)	22	3 (13.6)
Lanoxin (digoxin)	18	4 (22.2)
Lomotil (diphenoxylate/atropine)	11	7 (66.6)
Elavil (amitriptyline HCl)	10	7 (70.0)
Tylox (oxycodone/acetaminophen)	5	3 (60.0)

From King and Palmisano, 1989.[9] Reprinted with permission.

TABLE 23.15
Owner of Medication Ingested

Owner	No.	(%)	Cumulative %
Mother	294	(43.3)	43.3
Father	70	(10.3)	53.6
Grandmother	143	(21.0)	74.6
Grandfather	51	(7.5)	82.1
Sibling	10	(1.5)	83.6
Self	4	(0.6)	84.2
Dog	4	(0.6)	84.8
Other (neighbor, relative)	103	(15.2)	100.0
Total	679	(100.0)	

From King and Palmisano, 1989.[9] Reprinted with permission.

TABLE 23.16
Container Type and Ownership of Medication[a]

	Father	Mother	Grandfather	Grandmother	Totals
Child-resistant	13	82	7	27	129
No container	23	75	13	40	151
Non-child-resistant	25	79	25	56	185
Totals (%)	61 (13.1%)	236 (50.8%)	45 (9.7%)	123 (26.4%)	465
Total noncompliance (%)	48 (78.6%)	154 (65.3%)	38 (84.4%)	96 (78.0%)	
Parent's noncompliance	202 (68.0%)				
Grandparent's noncompliance			134 (79.8%)		

[a] Excludes other owners of medication (i.e., neighbor, aunt, sibling, other).

From King and Palmisano, 1989.[9] Reprinted with permission.

TABLE 23.17
Risk Factors Involved in Drug Poisoning in Children 0 to 17 Years

High-risk children
Sex/age difference
Developmental/behavioral determinants
Family determinants
Repetitive poisonings
Adolescent psychiatric illness
Intentional poisoning (Munchausen's Syndrome by Proxy)
Environmental determinants
   Locale and time of overdose
   Storage practices, child-resistant packaging
   Warning stickers
   Dispensing practices

From Woolf and Lovejoy, 1993.[10]

C. ADOLESCENT TOXIC EXPOSURES

Paulson (1988)[11] indicated that intentional poisonings in adolescents is one of the 10 leading causes of death and potentially productive years of life lost in the U.S. Alcohol use and abuse plays a large role in fatal injuries in this age group.

Approximately 8% of all intentional exposures resulting in death were in children aged 13 to 17 years as illustrated in Table 23.7. Drug-related fatalities by drug class among adolescents 11 to 17 years old reported to the AAPCC from 1989 to 1991 are listed in Table 23.18. Of 764 fatalities reported in 1991, 52 (6.8%) were in the adolescent age group; 92% were 13 to 17 years old.

TABLE 23.18

Drug-Related Fatalities by Drug Class among Adolescents 11 to 17 Years Old Reported to the American Association of Poison Control Centers in 1989, 1990, and 1991

Drug Class	1989	1990	1991	Totals
Cyclic antidepressants	13	7	11	31
Amitriptyline	1	3[a]	1	
Desipramine	4	2	7[b]	
Doxepine	1[c]	0	2	
Imipramine	5[d]	1	0	
Maprotaline	1	0	0	
Nortriptyline	1[e]	1	1	
Calcium channel blockers	2	2	3	7
Nifedipine	0	0	1	
Verapamil	2[f]	2[g]	2[h]	
Salicylates	1	0	5	6
Theophylline	3[i]	1	1	5
Propranolol	3	2[j]	1	5
Methamphetamine	1	0	0	1
Cocaine	0	0	1	1
Street drug (unknown type)	1	0	0	1
Paracetamol (acetaminophen)	1	0	2[k]	3
Carbamazepine	1[l]	0	0	1
Haloperidol	0	1	0	1
Glipizide + cyclobenzaprine	0	1	0	1
Isoniazid	0	0	1	1
Lidocaine (lignocaine)	0	1	0	1
Methocarbamol	0	0	1	1
Chlorpromazine	0	0	1	1
Temazepam	0	0	1	1
Colchicine/allopunnol/ibuprofen	0	0	1	1
Amfebutamone (bupropion) + lithium	0	1	0	1
Phenylpropanolamine/chlorphenamine	0	1	0	1
Paracetamol + doxylamine + detromethorphan + pseudoephedrine	0	1	0	1
Totals	26	18	29	72

[a] Ethanol also present in 1 case, thioridazine + alprazolam in another, methyldopa + perphenazine in the third case.
[b] Salicylate also present in 1 case.
[c] Verapamil + piroxicam also present.
[d] Tranylcypromine also present.
[e] Mesoridizine also present.
[f] Digoxin present in 1 case, meclizine present in the other.
[g] Propranolol also present in one case.
[h] Naproxen + propranolol also present in 1 case.
[i] Amoxicillin + cafalexin present in 1 case, ephedrine in another.
[j] Atenolol also present.
[k] Dextropropoxyphene also present in 1 case.
[l] Ampicillin + erythromycin also present.

From Woolf and Lovejoy, 1993.[10] Reprinted with permission.

D. POISONING IN THE ELDERLY

Poisoning in the elderly is a continuing public health problem. Accidental poisoning, due to dementia and confusion, improper use or storage of a product, and therapeutic errors account for the most exposures of patients >64 years of age.[12] However, approximately 11% were intentional with suicidal intent. The mortality rate from poisoning is much higher in the elderly than in other age groups. Of the 764 fatalities reported in 1991, 18% were ≥64 years old (Table 23.19).

Woolf et al.[13] analyzed poisoning-related hospitalization and mortality rates among older adults in Massachusetts from 1983 to 1985. The poisoning hospitalization rates and poisoning-related death rates are listed in Tables 23.20 and 23.21. Table 23.22 lists intentionality and agent of poisoning deaths for 152 of the 275 total deaths.

TABLE 23.19
Distribution of Age and Sex for 764 Fatalities

Age (yr)	Male	Female	Unknown	Total	%	Cumulative Total	Cumulative %
<1	1	4	0	5	0.7	5	0.7
1	9	8	0	17	2.2	22	2.9
2	8	5	0	13	1.7	35	4.6
3	4	1	0	5	0.7	40	5.2
4	1	0	0	1	0.1	41	5.4
5	2	1	0	3	0.4	44	5.8
6–12	2	2	0	4	0.5	48	6.3
13–19	37	27	0	54	8.4	112	14.7
20–29	67	52	0	119	15.6	231	30.2
30–39	98	81	0	179	23.4	410	53.7
40–49	50	64	0	114	14.9	524	68.6
50–59	36	31	0	67	8.8	591	77.4
60–69	34	21	0	55	7.2	646	84.6
70–79	24	29	0	53	6.9	699	91.5
80–89	14	19	0	33	4.3	732	95.8
90–99	6	5	0	11	1.4	743	97.3
Unknown adult	12	8	1	21	2.8	764	100.0
Total	405	358	1	764	100.0		

From Litovitz et al., 1992.[1] Reprinted with permission.

TABLE 23.20
Annualized Poisoning Hospitalization Rates and Relative Risks,[a] Massachusetts 1982–1985

Age Groups (years)	Males (Hosp/10^5/Yr)	RR[a] (95% CI)	Females (Hosp/10^5/Yr)	RR[a] (95% CI)
60–64	44	0.47 (0.40, 0.55)	58	0.47 (0.42, 0.53)
65–69	57	0.61 (0.52, 0.70)	64	0.52 (0.46, 0.58)
70–74	58	0.62 (0.52, 0.73)	74	0.60 (0.52, 0.67)
75–79	64	0.68 (0.56, 0.83)	91	0.73 (0.65, 0.83)
80–84	116	1.23 (1.01, 1.50)	102	0.82 (0.72, 0.95)
85	112	1.19 (0.94, 1.51)	96	0.77 (0.67, 0.89)
State average (all ages)	89		114	
State average (persons less than 60 years old)	94		124	

[a] RR = relative risk (age specific rate/state average rate, <60 yr). 95% confidence intervals in parentheses.

From Woolf et al., 1990.[13] Reprinted with permission.

TABLE 23.21
Annualized Poisoning-Related Death Rates and Relative Risks,[a] Massachusetts 1983–1985

Age Group (years)	Males (Deaths/10⁵/Yr)	RR[a] (95% Cl)	Females (Deaths/10⁵/Yr)	RR[a] (95% Cl)
	Males (Deaths/10^5/Yr)	RR[a] (95% Cl)	Females (Deaths/10^5/Yr)	RR[a] (95% Cl)
60–64	8.34	1.04 (0.73, 1.48)	6.62	1.74 (1.20, 2.22)
65–69	7.45	0.93 (0.62, 1.40)	7.04	1.85 (1.26, 2.70)
				1.49 (0.95, 2.34)
70–74	14.43	1.80 (1.27, 2.55)	5.68	
75–79	13.07	1.63 (1.04, 2.55)	7.79	2.04 (1.32, 3.15)
				1.59 (0.89, 2.84)
80–84	14.00	1.75 (0.99, 3.09)	6.07	
85+	20.54	2.56 (1.48, 4.44)	13.07	3.43 (2.28, 5.16)
State average (all ages)	9.37		5.16	
State average (persons <60 years old)	8.02		3.81	

[a] RR = relative risk (age specific rate/state average rate, <80 yr). 95% confidence intervals in parentheses.

From Woolf et al., 1990.[13] Reprinted with permission.

TABLE 23.22
Intentionality and Agent of Poisoning Deaths in Massachusetts Adults 60 Years and Older, 1983–1985[a]

	Sex	
	Male	Female
Circumstance/Intentionality	N = 78	N = 78
Accidental/unintentional		
Drugs	20	26
Carbon monoxide	5	5
Isopropanol	1	0
Benzene	1	0
Subtotal	27	31
Indeterminate		
Drugs	3	9
Suicide/Intentional		
Drugs	9	32
Carbon Monoxide	31	5
Corrosive	1	0
Carbon tetrachloride	1	0
Other agents	2	0
Subtotal	44	38

[a] Table includes only those deaths for which E-codes were available (152 out of 275 total deaths).

From Woolf et al., 1990.[13] Reprinted with permission.

SECTION 4. MANAGEMENT TRENDS

Table 23.23 outlines the frequency of initial decontamination procedures, measures used to enhance toxin elimination, and antidotes administered to patients reported to the 1991 AAPCC database. The use of Syrup of Ipecac as an initial method of gastrointestinal decontamination has declined in the emergency department setting. It is most often administered to the pediatric patient in a non-health care facility environment. This trend was reversed in adult patients (Table 23.24) Table 23.25 demonstrates a continued decline from 1983 to 1991 in the use of emesis induced by Syrup of Ipecac and an increase in the sole use of activated charcoal administration in the emergency department.

TABLE 23.23
Therapy Provided in Human Exposure Cases

Therapy	No.
Initial decontamination	
Dilution	653,687
Irrigation/washing	366,557
Activated charcoal	129,203
Cathartic	107,556
Ipepac syrup	95,124
Gastric lavage	58,677
Other emetic	4239
Measures to enhance elimination	
Alkalinization (with or without diuresis)	7092
Hemodialysis	692
Forced diuresis	500
Hemoperfusion (charcoal)	124
Exchange transfusion	106
Acidification (with or without diuresis)	99
Hemoperfusion (resin)	38
Peritoneal dialysis	11
Specific antidote administration	
Naloxone	7136
N-Acetylcysteine (oral)	7075
Atropine	923
Deferoxamine	901
Antivenim	579
Ethanol	540
Hydroxocobalamin	384
N-Acetylcysteine (IV)	250
Pralidoxime (2-PAM)	248
Fab fragments	241
Pyridoxine	227
Physostigmine	226
Dimercaprol (BAL)	146
Methylene blue	117
Cyanide antidote kit	99
EDTA	94
Penicillamine	86

From Litovitz et al., 1992.[1] Reprinted with permission.

TABLE 23.24
Ipecac Administration by Site and Age

Age (yr)	Non-Health Care Facility		Health Care Facility		Unknown		Total	
	No.	%	No.	%	No.	%	No.	%
<1	1,002	1.1	1,184	1.2	9	0.0	2,195	2.3
1	11,414	12.0	6,876	7.2	55	0.1	18,345	19.3
2	20,522	21.6	11,312	11.9	84	0.1	31,918	33.6
3	9,515	10.0	4,743	5.0	44	0.0	14,302	15.0
4	3,140	3.3	1,557	1.6	10	0.0	4,707	4.9
6–12	1,174	1.2	972	1.0	10	0.0	2,156	2.3
13–17	229	0.2	5,353	5.6	5	0.0	5,587	5.9
>17	782	0.8	12,907	13.6	24	0.0	13,713	14.4
Unknown	201	0.2	331	0.3	3	0.0	535	0.6
Total	49,062	51.6	45,814	48.2	248	0.3	95,124	100.0

From Litovitz et al., 1992.[1] Reprinted with permission.

TABLE 23.25
Decontamination Trends

Year	Human Exposures Reported	% of Exposures Involving Children <6 Years	Ipecac Administered (% of Exposures)	Activated Charcoal Administered (% of Exposures)
1983	251,012	64.0	13.4	4.0
1984	730,224	64.1	12.9	4.0
1985	900,513	63.4	15.0	4.6
1986	1,098,894	63.0	13.3	5.2
1987	1,166,940	62.3	10.1	5.2
1988	1,368,748	61.8	8.4	6.5
1989	1,581,540	61.1	7.0	6.4
1990	1,713,462	60.8	6.1	6.7
1991	1,837,939	59.9	5.2	7.0

From Litovitz et al., 1992.[1] Reprinted with permission.

SECTION 5. ROLE OF THE TOXICOLOGY LABORATORY

Toxicological testing or a "Tox Screen" of blood, urine, and gastric contents is frequently ordered for patients with suspected drug overdoses in the emergency department. Because 10 to 15 drugs account for more than 90% of all drug overdoses, most laboratories limit the number of drugs tested to the common drugs of abuse and other agents, such as over-the-counter analgesics (Table 23.26). Osterloh[14] reviewed and evaluated the circumstances, types of toxicological testing, utility, reliability, and application of the laboratory tests in the emergency evaluation of the overdosed patient. Table 23.27 lists the three types of medical testing, (monitoring, diagnostic, and screening), the prevalence of the test condition, and the primary attribute of the referred test.

Initial workup of an intoxicated patient always includes a history and physical examination as an assessment of their condition. During this initial evaluation, a preliminary toxicological diagnosis may be made based on a constellation of signs and symptoms (Tables 23.28 and 23.29). Drug and nondrug tests may be useful in the diagnosis. Examples of these tests are listed in Table 23.30. Comparison of toxicologic methods are outlined in Table 23.31.

A toxicology screen uses various methodologies to identify the drugs most frequently used or abused by the poisoned patient. The screens are usually focused on identifying the common drugs of abuse. Drug quantitation in serum is used to monitor the course of the patient, to diagnose whether toxicity is occurring, but not yet clinically apparent, to establish a prognosis, and determine whether extracorporeal methods of toxin elimination will be necessary. In the emergency setting there are relatively few toxins that require quantitation to have an impact on patient management. The toxins that require quantitation in emergency toxicology and the potential interferences in assays are listed in Table 23.32.

TABLE 23.26
Common Drugs Included on Most Toxicology Screens

Alcohols — Ethanol, methanol, isopropanol, acetone

Barbiturates/sedatives — Amobarbital, secobarbital, pentobarbital, butalbital, butabarbital, phenobarbital, glutethimide, ethchlorvynol, methaqualone

Antiepileptics — Phenytoin, carbamazepine, primadone, phenobarbital

Benzodiazepines — Chlordiazepoxide, diazepam, alprazolam, temazepam

Antihistamines — Diphenhydramine, chlorpheniramine, brompheniramine, tripelennamine, trihexiphenidyl, doxylamine, pyrilamine

Antidepressants — Amitriptyline, nortriptyline, doxepin, imipramine, desipramine, trazedone, amoxapine, maprotiline

Antipsychotics — Trifluoperazine, perphenazine, prochlorperazine, chlorpromazine

Stimulants — Amphetamine, methamphetamine, phenylpropanolamine, ephedrine, MDA, MDMA (other phenylethylamines), cocaine, phencyclicline

Narcotics analgesics — Heroin, morphine, codeine, oxycodone, hydrocodone, hydromorphone, meperidine, pentazocine, propoxyphene, methadone

Other analgesics — Salicylates, acetaminophen

Cardiovascular drugs — Lidocaine, propranolol, metoprolol, quinidine, procainamide, verapamil

Others — Theophylline, caffeine, nicotine, oral hypoglycemics, strychnine

From Osterloh, 1990.[14] Reprinted with permission.

TABLE 23.27
Types of Medical and Toxicological Test Situations

Type of Medical Testing	Preselection of Population	Prior Probability of Prevalence of Test Condition in Population Tested	Primary Attribute Required of Test	Clinical Example	Toxicological Example
Monitoring	Yes	85–100%	Precision	BP, T[Oa]	TDM[b]
Diagnostic	Yes	30–85%	Specificity	CPK-MB	Toxicology screen
Screening	No	0–30%	Sensitivity	PKU	Employee drug testing, Misapplication of "toxicology screen"

[a] Temperature.

[b] Therapeutic drug monitoring.

From Osterloh, 1990.[14] Reprinted with permission.

TABLE 23.28

Some Common Clinical Presentations and Differential Diagnoses in Overdose

Presentation	Toxicological Causes	Other Medical Examples
Asymptomatic with history	Almost any drug	Not applicable
Gastrointestinal complaints	Salicylate, theophylline, iron, colchicine quinidine, almost any drug	Food poisoning, allergy, ulcer, pancreatitis, obstruction, gallstones, genitourinary
Coma	Narcotics, sedatives, antipsychotics, alcohol, tricyclics, long-lasting benzodiazepines	Infectious and metabolic encephalopathy, trauma, anoxia, cerebrovascular accident, brain death
Seizures	Theophylline, tricyclics, isoniazid, stimulants, camphor, carbon monoxide, hypoglycemic agents, alcohol withdrawal	Idiopathic, arteriovenous malformation, tumor, trauma, hypoxia, febrile, inborn errors
Psychosis and altered mental status	Anticholinergics, stimulants, withdrawal	Psychiatric, infection, metabolic/inborn errors
Acidosis	Salicylate, ethanol, methanol, ethylene glycol, cyanide drugs causing seizures	Shock, diabetes, uremia, lactic acidosis
Respiratory depression (usually with coma)	Narcotics, sedatives, benzodiazepines	Cerebrovascular accident, metabolic coma, tumor
Pulmonary edema	Salicylates, narcotics, iron, paraquat (initially)	Heart failure, disseminated intravascular coagulation
Arrhythmias	Tricylics, quinidine, anticholinergics, β-blockers, digoxin, lithium, antipsychotics, organophosphates	Atherosclerotic heart disease
Hypotension	Narcotics, sedatives, tricyclics, antipsychotics, β-blockers, theophylline, iron	Heart failure, shock, hypovolemia, disseminated intravascular coagulation
Hypertension	Cocaine, amphetamines, cyanide, nicotine, clonidine (initially)	Essential, pheochromocytoma, carcinoid, hyperrenin states, renal failure
Ataxia	Antiepileptics, barbiturates, alcohol, lithium, organomercury	Cerebellar degeneration

From Osterloh, 1990.[14] Reprinted with permission.

TABLE 23.29

Toxicological Syndromes by Class of Drugs[a]

Narcotics

Heroin, morphine, codeine, oxycodone, hydromorphone, hydrocodenone, propoxyphene, pentazocine, meperidine, diphenoxylate, fentanyl and derivatives, buprenorphine, methadone

CNS depression (somnolent → coma)	If BP decreases, pulse does not increase
Slowed respiratory rate	Pinpoint pupils
T° normal or low	DTR usually decrease

Alcohols — Barbiturates

Ethanol, methanol, isopropanol, ethylene glycol, amo-, pento-, seco-, buta-, phenobarbital, butalbital, glutethimide, methaqualone, ethchlorvynol, phenytoin

CNS depression (stuporous → coma)	DTR decreases

TABLE 23.29 *(Continued)*
Toxicological Syndromes by Class of Drugs[a]

Ataxia

T° usually decreases

Metabolic acidosis with alcohols and ethylene glycol except isopropanol

If BP decreases, pulse may increase

Anticholinergics

Atropine, scopolamine, antihistamines, phenothiazines, tricyclics, quinidine, amantadine, jimson weed, mushrooms

Delirious

Increased pulse, increased T°

Skin flushed, warm, pink

Dry (no sweating)

Decreased bowel sounds

Urinary retention

Blurred vision

Arrhythmias, prolonged QT

Stimulants

Cocaine, amphetamines and derivatives (e.g., ice, MDA, MDMA, DOB), phencyclidine, lysergic acid, psilocybin

Acute psychosis (nonreality)

Increased pulse, increased BP, increased T°

Increased respiratory rate

Agitation

Increased muscle tone/activity

Dilated pupils

Sweating

Seizures

Antidepressants

Anticholinergic syndrome

Hypotension

Coma

Seizures

Sinus tachycardia (early)

Supraventricular tachycardia (early)

Widened QRS, QT

Ventricular arrhythmias

Benzodiazepines

CNS depression

Respiratory depression

BP, pulse, T° not greatly affected

DTR intact

Phenothiazines

Decreased BP, decreased T°

Rigidity, dystonias, torticollis

Pinpoint pupils

Anticholinergic syndrome (see above)

Seizures

Salicylates

Abdominal pain

Respiratory alkalosis (early)

Metabolic acidosis

Shock

Diaphoresis

Hypoglycemia

Theophylline

Tachycardia

Hypokalemia

Hypotension

Seizures

Iron

Abdominal pain

GI bleeding

Hypotension

Hypovolemia

Acidosis

Renal failure

Cardiovascular collapse

Lithium

Tremor

Chorea

Abdominal pain

Hyperreflexia

Rigidity

Seizures

Isoniazid

Metabolic acidosis

Seizures

Hepatitis

TABLE 23.29 *(Continued)*
Toxicological Syndromes by Class of Drugs[a]

Oral Hypoglycemics

Hypoglycemia	Diaphoresis
Coma	

Acetaminophen

Liver necrosis

β-blockers

Bradycardia	Hypotension with slowed cardiac conduction
Hyperglycemia	

[a] Abbreviations: CNS = central nervous system; BP = blood pressure; DTR = deep tendon reflexes; GI = gastrointestinal; QRS, QT = electrocardiogram parameters; MDA = methylenedioxy amphetamine; MDMA = 3,4-methylenedioxy methamphetamine; DOB = 4-bromo-2,5-dimethoxyamphetamine.

From Osterloh, 1990.[14] Reprinted with permission.

TABLE 23.30
Useful Laboratory Tests in Toxicological Diagnosis[a]

Classes of Drugs	Clinical and Laboratory Tests	Toxicological Procedures for Identification
Narcotics	IV Narcan, ABGs	IA, TLC, GC, GC-MS
Alcohols	Breath odor, osmolar gap	GC, EZ, IA
Sedatives	Calorics, ABGs	IA, TLC, HPLC, GC, GC-MS
Anticholinergics	EKG, CPK, K	TLC, GC, HPLC, GC-MS
Stimulants	CPK, K	IA, TLC, GC, GC-MS
Antipsychotics	EKG, ABGs	Spot, TLC, GC, HPLC, GC-MS
Tricyclics	EKG, ABGs	Spot, IA, TLC, CC, HPLC, CC-MS
β-Blockers	EKG	TLC, GC, HPLC
Oral hypoglycemics	Serum glucose	TLC, HPLC, GC
Specific Toxins		
Salicylates[b]	Anion gap, HCO$_3$ gap	Spot, SM, IA, HPLC, GC
Theophylline[b]	K, glucose	IA, HPLC, SM
Acetaminophen[b]	ALT, AST	TLC, IA, SM, HPLC
Methanol[b]	Anion and osmolar gaps	GLC
Ethylene glycol[b]	Anion and osmolar gaps	GLC
Lithium[b]	Serum creatinine	Flame, ISE
Iron[b]	WBC, serum glucose, serum iron	SM
Carbon monoxide	O$_2$ saturation gap	Co-oximeter, SM
Cyanide	A-V O$_2$ difference	SM
Nitrites	Brown blood	Co-oximeter, SM

[a] Abbreviations: EZ = enzymatic: SM = spectrometric; spot = chemical test; ISE = ion-selective electrode; flame = flame emission spectrometry: ABGs = arterial blood gases; K = potassium; CPK = creatinine phosphokinase; HCO$_3$ = bicarbonate; IA = immunoassays; TLC = thin-layer chromatography; GC, gas chromatography; HPLC, high-performance liquid chromatography; GC-MS, gas chromatography-mass spectrometry; EKG = electrocardiogram; WBC = white blood cell count; AST, ALT = liver enzyme tests; A-V = arterial-venous.

[b] Require quantitation for effective therapy. Concentration-effect relationships are known.

From Osterloh, 1990.[14] Modified with permission.

TABLE 23.31
Comparison of Generic Toxicological Method[a]

Method	Specificity	Sensitivity	Multidrug Drug Detection Possible	Quantitative Ability	Turnaround Time (HR)	Labor Intensive	Technical Expertise	Initial Capital Costs ($)*
Chemical-spot	+	+	No	No	<0.5	+	0	500
Spectrometric	+	+	No	Yes	<2	++	++	10,000
IA	++	++	Some	Some	<1	+	+	7000
TLC	++	+	Yes	No	2–4	+++	+++	1500
GC	++	++	Yes	Yes	<4	++	++	15,000
HPLC	++	++	Yes	Yes	<4	++	++	20,000
GC-MS	+++	+++	Yes	Yes	<8	+++	++++	65,000

[a] Abbreviations: IA = immunoassays; TLC = thin-layer chromatography; GC = gas chromatography; HPLC = high performance liquid chromatography; GC-MS = gas chromatography-mass spectrometry.

* Note: Costs in 1990, current costs will be higher.

From Osterloh, 1990.[14] Reprinted with permission.

TABLE 23.32
Potential Interferences for Quantitative Serum Drug Tests Used in Emergency Toxicology[a]

Drug	Generic Method	Interferences
Salicylate	SC	Phenothiazines,[c] ketosis,[c] acetaminophen, diflunisal, salicylamide, phenylketones, around 10% inc due to cross-reaction with accumulated salicylate metabolites in RF
	GC[b]	Methylsalicylate, eucalyptol, theophylline
	HPLC	Theophylline, antibiotics
Theophylline	SC[b]	Diazepam, caffeine, metabolites in RF
	HPLC	Acetazolamide, cephalosporin antibiotics, endogenous xanthines, and theo metabolites in RF (minor elevations)
	GC	Phenobarbital (rare)
	IA	Caffeine, cross-reaction with metabolites in RF
Acetaminophen	SC	Salicylate, salicylamide, methylsalicylate (salicylate from these sources will inc at 10% of salicylate value in µg/ml), phenols, bilirubin, RF itself (for each inc mg/dl creatinine inc 30 µg/ml acetaminophen)
	GC	Phenacetin
	HPLC	Cephalosporins, sulfonamides
	IA	Phenacetin
Ethanol	SC[b]	Other alcohols, ketones (for oxidation methods), isopropanol (for enzymatic methods)
	GC	Few
Isopropranol	GC	Skin disinfectant containing isopropanol during venipuncture
Iron	SC	Deferoxamine causes 15% lowering of TIBC, lavendertop Vacutainer contains EDTA, which binds iron (lowers iron)
Lithium	SC	Green-top (lithium heparin) Vacutainer specimen tube
Digoxin	IA	Endogenous digoxin-like natriuretic substances (around 1 ng/ml in newborns, RF, pregnancy, liver disease, volume loading), cross reaction with accumulated metabolites in RF (up to 2 ng/ml); oleander ingestion (glycosides may be detectable as digoxin)
Methemoglobin	SC	Sulfhemoglobin, methylene blue (15% unit increase after 2 mg/kg dose), hemoglobin regeneration is time dependent (in Vacutainer around 10%/h and rapid following methylene blue)
Osmolality		Lavender-top (EDTA) Vacutainer tube (15 mOsm) graytop (NaF/K oxalate) tube (150 mOsm) blue-top (citrate) tube (10 mOsm)
	VP	Methanol, ethanol, acetone contribution to osm gap are underestimated

[a] All interferences listed do not occur in one assay but have been reported individually as interfering in one or another method variation. Interferences listed cause increase in measured drug, unless otherwise indicated. Abbreviations: SC = spectrochemical; RF = renal failure; GC = gas chromatography; TLC = thin-layer chromatography; HPLC = high performance liquid chromatography; IA = immunoassay; inc = increase; VP = vapor pressure; OSM = osmolar.

[b] Uncommon methodology.

[c] More common in urine test.

From Osterloh, 1990.[14] Reprinted with permission.

TABLE 23.33
Site of Caller and Site of Exposure to Human Poison Exposures Cases

	Site of Caller (%)	Site of Exposure (%)
Residence	80.7	92.0
Workplace	1.5	2.5
Health care facility	15.6	0.6
School	0.7	0.9
Other	1.2	2.1
Unknown	0.4	1.8

From Litovitz et al., 1992.[1] Reprinted with permission.

SECTION 6. ROLE OF THE POISON CONTROL CENTER

Poison Control Centers have had and continue to have a vital role in the provision of poison information since their inception almost 40 years ago. The regional poison centers (listed in Table 23.38) that are members of, or are certified by, the American Association of Poison control Centers (AAPCC) serve several functions:

1. Provide expert information and consultation to the public and health professionals.
2. Provide public education programs in poison prevention, counseling, and management.
3. Provide regional professional education programs.
4. Interact with prehospital care providers, health care facilities, and analytical toxicology laboratories to improve the management of the poisoned patient.
5. Collect uniform data on poisonings and participate in nationwide sharing of data regarding poisonings.

Most of the calls received by poison centers are managed by poison information specialists who are either registered nurses, pharmacists, or other health-related professionals. Doctors of clinical pharmacy (Pharm.D.), clinical pharmacologists (Ph.D.), and/or physicians who have had special training and/or board certifications are employed by most centers as managing directors to oversee and assist the information specialists handle the exposure calls.

Table 23.33 provides data regarding the site of the caller and the site of human exposures reported to 73 regional poison control centers in 1991. Poison center call volumes are highest between 9:00 am and 11:90 pm with a peak call volume between 4:00 and 11:00 pm.

Tables 23.34 and 23.35 display symptom assessment and the subsequent site of management of the exposure cases. Importantly, more than two thirds of cases are managed in a non-health care facility suggesting that significant health care dollars are saved by using poison center services. Tables 23.36 and 23.37 depict medical outcome by reason and by age for exposures reported to AAPCC.

TABLE 23.34
Symptom Assessment at Time of Initial Call to Poison Center

Symptom Assessment	No.	%
Asymptomatic	1,159,054	63.1
Symptomatic, related to exposure	518,912	28.2
Symptomatic, unrelated to exposure	31,915	1.7
Symptomatic, unknown if related	89,008	4.8
Unknown	39,050	2.1
Total	1,837,939	100.0

From Litovitz et al., 1992.[1] Reprinted with permission.

TABLE 23.35
Management Site of Human Poison Exposure Cases

Site	No.	%
Nonhealth care facility	1,316,605	71.6
Health care facility		
Already there when poison center called	244,544	13.3
Referred by poison center	231,053	12.6
Other/unknown	45,737	2.5
Total	1,837,939	100.0

From Litovitz et al., 1992.[1] Reprinted with permission.

TABLE 23.36
Medical Outcome of Human Poison Exposure Cases by Patient Age

Outcome	<6 Years No.	%	6–12 Years No.	%	13–17 Years No.	%	>17 Years No.	%	Unknown No.	%	Total No.	%
No effect	388,537	21.1	21,437	1.2	15,177	0.8	62,663	3.4	2607	0.1	490,421	26.7
Minor effect	146,567	8.0	29,288	1.6	30,510	1.7	197,915	10.8	5257	0.3	409,537	22.3
Moderate effect	5645	0.3	1704	0.1	3920	0.2	29,785	1.6	559	0.0	41,613	2.3
Major effect	548	0.0	105	0.0	426	0.0	4677	0.3	56	0.0	5812	0.3
Death	44	0.0	4	0.0	48	0.0	668	0.0	0	0.0	764	0.0
Unknown, nontoxic[a]	467,021	25.4	34,773	1.9	15,318	0.8	96,793	5.230				
Unknown, potentially toxic[b]	74,112	4.0	12,221	0.7	14,927	0.8	109,541	6.0	5.925	0.3	216,726	11.8
Unrelated effect	16,611	0.9	3089	0.2	2098	0.1	24,664	1.3	458	0.0	46,920	2.6
Unknown	983	0.1	79	0.0	91	0.0	537	0.0	321	0.0	2011	0.1
Total	1,100,068	59.9	102,700	5.6	82,515	4.5	527,243	28.7	25,413	1.4	1,837,939	100.0

[a] No follow-up provided because exposure was assessed as nontoxic.

[b] Patient lost to follow-up. Exposure was assessed as potentially toxic.

From Litovitz et al., 1992.[1] Reprinted with permission.

TABLE 23.37

Distribution of Medical Outcome by Reason for Exposure for Human Poison Exposure Victims

Outcome	Accidental No	Accidental %	Intentional No	Intentional %	Adverse Reaction No	Adverse Reaction %	Unknown No	Unknown %	Total No	Total %
No effect	455,084	24.8	33,870	1.8	821	0.0	646	0.0	490,421	26.7
Minor effect	327,546	17.8	68,088	3.7	12,346	0.7	1557	0.1	409,537	22.3
Moderate effect	23,171	1.3	16,179	0.9	1685	0.1	578	0.0	41,613	2.3
Major effect	1438	0.1	4091	0.2	115	0.0	168	0.0	5812	0.3
Death	117	0.0	576	0.0	17	0.0	54	0.0	764	0.0
Unknown, nontoxic	600,723	32.7	17,120	0.9	5220	0.3	1072	0.1	624,135	34.0
Unknown, potentially toxic	157,834	8.6	50,755	2.8	5815	0.3	2322	0.1	216,726	11.8
Unrelated effect	38,921	2.1	3257	0.2	3989	0.2	753	0.0	46,920	2.6
Unknown	1673	0.1	261	0.0	36	0.0	41	0.0	2011	0.1
Total	1,606,507	87.4	194,197	10.6	30,044	1.6	7191	0.4	1,837,939	100.0

From Litovitz et al., 1992.[1] Reprinted with permission.

SECTION 7. CONTEMPORARY ISSUES

Under the leadership of AAPCC, many regional poison control centers have taken active roles in local and national lobbying efforts to enact legislation that could influence the number and severity of poisonings. The earlist efforts resulted in the Poison Prevention Packaging Act of 1970 requiring child-resistant closures on certain medications. Deaths due to accidental poisoning in children have been reduced by 70%; however, there still is a need for additional legislation for packaging additional substances.

Additional PCC legislative efforts include the following substances:

	Status	Local vs. National
Child-resistant packaging and reduction of ethanol content of mouthwashes	Passed	National effort
Removal of DEET (>50% concentration) from commercial use	Tabled	Local (New York State)
Addition of bittering agents (Bitrex) to selective poisons	Tabled (New York State)	National
Relabeling of over-the-counter iron supplements	Pending	National

Toxicologists are also starting to take an active role in the evaluation of prescription medications being considered for a switch to over-the-counter status.

Currently, poison centers nationwide rely on a variety of funding sources to stay in business including state funds, federal and state grants, and industrial and health care facility contracts. However, as cost-saving measures have become necessary, many public and privately operated agencies are cutting back financial support of poison control centers, resulting in poison control center closures or limiting their availability to less than 24 hours/day; leaving millions of people without access to poison control center services. Table 23.38 is an up-to-date list of poison control centers nationwide. Testimony before the congressional subcommittee on government operations has brought this problem to a federal level in an attempt to find alternative funding sources for all poison centers (March 15, 1994).

Poison centers have proven to be effective in reducing emergency room visits for suspected poisonings[15] and thus have proven their value in health care cost containment. It is estimated that for every dollar spent in operating a poison control center, a minimum of $7 is saved. In addition, poison control centers reduce unnecessary health care expenditures for poisonings and reduce the burden on our 911 systems and emergency transport services. It has been estimated that if there were no poison control center services, 70% of people would call 911 or an emergency medical service.[16] For example, in 1992 the six poison control centers in New York State treated more than 91,000 poisoning exposures safely and effectively at home, by telephone management. These clients were spared unnecessary visits to hospital emergency departments. In anticipation of changes in our national health system, federal funding would help ensure stable funds for poison control centers during this managed care era and assure that all Americans have easy access to immediate assistance in a poison emergency.

TABLE 23.38
Nationwide Poison Control Centers — Directory

Alabama
Alabama Poison Center
2503 Phoenix Drive
Tuscaloosa, AL 35405
Emergency Phone: (800) 462-0800 (AL only);
(205) 345-0600

Regional Poison Control Center
Children's Hospital
1600 7th Avenue South
Birmingham, AL 35233
Emergency Phone: (800) 292-6678 (AL only);
(205) 933-4050

Alaska
Anchorage Poison Control Center
3200 Providence Drive
P.O. Box 196604
Anchorage, AK 99519-6604
Emergency Phone: (800) 478-3193; (907) 261-3193

Arizona
Arizona Poison and Drug Information Center
Arizona Health Sciences Center, Room 1156
1501 North Campbell Avenue
Tucson, AZ 85724
Emergency Phone: (800) 362-0101 (AZ only);
(520) 626-6016

Samaritan Regional Poison Center
Good Samaritan Regional Medical Center
1111 E. McDowell — Ancillary 1
Phoenix, AZ 85006
Emergency Phone: (800) 362-0101 (AZ only);
(602) 253-3334

TABLE 23.38 *(Continued)*
Nationwide Poison Control Centers — Directory

Arkansas
Arkansas Poison and Drug Information Center
College of Pharmacy
University of Arkansas for Medical Sciences
4301 W. Markham, Mail Slot 522
Little Rock, AR 72205
Emergency Phone: (800) 376-4766
TDD/TTY: (800) 641-3805

California
California Poison Control System — Fresno/Madera Division
Valley Children's Hospital
9300 Valley Children's Place
Madera, CA 93638-8762
Emergency Phone: (800) 876-4766 (CA only)
TDD/TTY: (800) 972-3323

California Poison Control System — Sacramento Division
UC Davis Medical Center
2315 Stockton Boulevard
Sacramento, CA 95817
Emergency Phone: (800) 876-4766 (CA only)
TDD/TTY: (800) 972-3323

California Poison Control System — San Diego Division
University of CA, San Diego, Medical Center
200 West Arbor Drive
San Diego, CA 92103-8925
Emergency Phone: (800) 876-4766 (CA only)
TDD/TTY: (800) 972-3323

California Poison Control System — San Francisco Division
San Francisco General Hospital
1001 Potrero Avenue, Room 1E86
San Francisco, CA 94110
Emergency Phone: (800) 876-4766 (CA only)
TDD/TTY: (800) 876-4766

Colorado
Rocky Mountain Poison and Drug Center
1010 Yosemite Circle, Building 752
Denver, CO 80230-6800
Emergency Phone: (800) 332-3073 (CO only/outside metro area);
(303) 739-1123 (Denver metro)

Connecticut
Connecticut Poison Control Center
University of Connecticut Health Center
263 Farmington Avenue
Farmington, CT 06030-5365
Emergency Phone: (800) 343-2722 (CT only);
(860) 679-3456
TDD/TTY: (860) 679-4346

TABLE 23.38 *(Continued)*
Nationwide Poison Control Centers — Directory

Delaware
The Poison Control Center
3535 Market Street, Suite 985
Philadelphia, PA 19104-3309
Emergency Phone: (800) 722-7112; (215) 386-2100;
(215) 590-2100

District of Columbia
National Capital Poison Center
3201 New Mexico Avenue, NW, Suite 310
Washington, D.C. 20016
Emergency Phone: (202) 625-3333
TDD/TTY: (202) 362-8563 (TTY)

Florida
Florida Poison Information Center — Jacksonville
655 West Eighth Street
Jacksonville, FL 32209
Emergency Phone: (800) 282-3171 (FL only);
(904) 244-4480
TDD/TTY: (800) 282-3171 (FL only)

Florida Poison Information Center — Miami
University of Miami
Department of Pediatrics
Jackson Memorial Medical Center
P.O. Box 016960 (R-131)
Miami, FL 33101
Emergency Phone: (800) 282-3171 (FL only);
(305) 585-5253

Florida Poison Information Center — Tampa
Tampa General Hospital
P.O. Box 1289
Tampa, FL 33601
Emergency Phone: (800) 282-3171 (FL only);
(813) 253-4444

Georgia
Georgia Poison Center
Hughes Spalding Children's Hospital
Grady Health System
80 Butler Street, SE, P.O. Box 26066
Atlanta, GA 30335-3801
Emergency Phone: (800) 282-5846; (404) 616-9000
TDD/TTY: (404) 616-9287 (TDD)

Hawaii
Hawaii Poison Center
1319 Punahou Street
Honolulu, HI 96826
Emergency Phone: (808) 941-4411

TABLE 23.38 *(Continued)*
Nationwide Poison Control Centers — Directory

Idaho
Rocky Mountain Poison and Drug Center
1010 Yosemite Circle, Building 752
Denver, CO 80230-6800
Emergency Phone: (800) 860-0620 (ID only)

Illinois
Illinois Poison Center
222 S. Riverside Plaza
Suite 1900
Chicago, IL 60606
Emergency Phone: (800) 942-5969 (IL only)
TDD/TTY: (312) 906-6185

Indiana
Indiana Poison Center
Methodist Hospital
Clarian Health Partners
I-65 at 21st Street
Indianapolis, IN 46206-1367
Emergency Phone: (800) 382-9097 (IN only);
(317) 929-2323
TDD/TTY: (317) 929-2336 (TTY)

Iowa
Iowa Statewide Poison Control Center
St. Luke's Regional Medical Center
2720 Stone Park Boulevard
Sioux City, IA 51104
Emergency Phone: (800) 352-2222; (712) 277-2222

Kansas
Mid-America Poison Control Center
University of Kansas Medical Center
3901 Rainbow Blvd.
Room B-400
Kansas City, KS 66160-7231
Emergency Phone: (800) 332-6633 (KS only);
(913) 588-6633
TDD/TTY: (913) 588-6639 (TDD)

Kentucky
Kentucky Regional Poison Center
Medical Towers South
Suite 572
234 East Gray Street
Louisville, KY 40202
Emergency Phone: (800) 722-5725; (502) 589-8222

TABLE 23.38 *(Continued)*
Nationwide Poison Control Centers — Directory

Louisiana
Louisiana Drug and Poison Information Center
University of Louisiana at Monroe
College of Pharmacy
Sugar Hall
Monroe, LA 71209-6430
Emergency Phone: (800) 256-9822 (LA only)

Maine
Maine Poison Control Center
Maine Medical Center
22 Bramhall Street
Portland, ME 04102
Emergency Phone: (800) 442-6305 (ME only);
(207) 871-2950
TDD/TTY: (877) 299-4447 (ME only); (207) 871-2879

Maryland
Maryland Poison Center
University of MD at Baltimore
School of Pharmacy
20 North Pine Street, PH 772
Baltimore, MD 21201
Emergency Phone: (800) 492-2414 (MD only);
(410) 706-7701
TDD/TTY: (410) 706-1858 (TDD)

National Capital Poison Center
3201 New Mexico Avenue, NW
Suite 310
Washington, D.C. 20016
Emergency Phone: (202) 625-3333
TDD/TTY: (202) 362-8563 (TTY)

Massachusetts
Regional Center for Poison Control and Prevention
Serving Massachusetts and Rhode Island
300 Longwood Avenue
Boston, MA 02115
Emergency Phone: (800) 682-9211 (MA and RI only);
(617) 232-2120
TDD/TTY: (888) 244-5313

Michigan
Children's Hospital of Michigan
Regional Poison Control Center
4160 John R Harper Professional Office Building
Suite 616
Detroit, MI 48201
Emergency Phone: (800) 764-7661 (MI only);
(313) 745-5711
TDD/TTY: (800) 356-3232 (TDD)

TABLE 23.38 *(Continued)*
Nationwide Poison Control Centers — Directory

DeVos Children's Hospital
Regional Poison Center
1840 Wealthy S.E.
 Grand Rapids, MI 49506-2968
Emergency Phone: (800) 764-7661 (MI only)
TDD/TTY: (800) 356-3232 (TTY)

Minnesota

Hennepin Regional Poison Center
Hennepin County Medical Center
701 Park Avenue
Minneapolis, MN 55415
Emergency Phone: (800) 222-1222 (MN);
(800) POISON1 (SD only)
TDD/TTY: (612) 904-4691 (TTY)

Mississippi

Mississippi Regional Poison Control Center
University of Mississippi Medical Center
2500 N. State Street
Jackson, MS 39216
Emergency Phone: (601) 354-7660

Missouri

Cardinal Glennon Children's Hospital
Regional Poison Center
1465 S. Grand Blvd.
St. Louis, MO 63104
Emergency Phone: (800) 366-8888; (314) 772-5200

Montana

Rocky Mountain Poison and Drug Center
1010 Yosemite Circle, Building 752
Denver, CO 80230-6800
Emergency Phone: (800) 525-5042 (MT only)

Nebraska

The Poison Center
Children's Hospital
8301 Dodge Street
Omaha, NE 68114
Emergency Phone: (800) 955-9119 (NE and WY only);
(402) 955-5555

Nevada

Oregon Poison Center
Oregon Health Sciences University
3181 SW Sam Jackson Park Road, CB550
Portland, OR 97201
Emergency Phone: (503) 494-8968

TABLE 23.38 *(Continued)*
Nationwide Poison Control Centers — Directory

Rocky Mountain Poison and Drug Center
1010 Yosemite Circle
Building 752
Denver, CO 80230-6800
Emergency Phone: (800) 446-6179 (NV only)

New Hampshire
New Hampshire Poison Information Center
Dartmouth-Hitchcock Medical Center
One Medical Center Drive
Lebanon, NH 03756
Emergency Phone: (800) 562-8236 (NH only);
(603) 650-8000

New Jersey
New Jersey Poison Information and Education System
201 Lyons Avenue
Newark, NJ 07112
Emergency Phone: (800) POISON-1 (NJ only)
TDD/TTY: (973) 926-8008

New Mexico
New Mexico Poison and Drug Information Center
Health Science Center Library
Room 130
University of New Mexico
Albuquerque, NM 87131-1076
Emergency Phone: (800) 432-6866 (NM only);
(505) 272-2222

New York
Central New York Poison Center
750 East Adams Street
Syracuse, NY 13210
Emergency Phone: (800) 252-5655 (NY only);
(315) 476-4766

Finger Lakes Regional Poison and Drug Information Center
University of Rochester Medical Center
601 Elmwood Avenue, P.O. Box 321
Rochester, NY 14642
Emergency Phone: (800) 333-0542 (NY only);
(716) 275-3232
TDD/TTY: (716) 273-3854 (TTY)

Hudson Valley Regional Poison Center
Phelps Memorial Hospital Center
701 North Broadway
Sleepy Hollow, NY 10591
Emergency Phone: (800) 336-6997 (NY only);
(914) 366-3030

TABLE 23.38 *(Continued)*
Nationwide Poison Control Centers — Directory

Long Island Regional Poison and Drug Information Center
Winthrop University Hospital
259 First Street
Mineola, NY 11501
Emergency Phone: (516) 542-2323; (516) 663-2650
TDD/TTY: (516) 924-8811 (TDD Suffolk);
(516) 747-3323 (TDD Nassau)

New York City Poison Control Center
NYC Department of Health
455 First Avenue
Room 123, Box 81
New York, NY 10016
Emergency Phone: (800) 210-3985; (212) 340-4494;
(212) POI-SONS;(212) VEN-ENOS
TDD/TTY: (212) 689-9014 (TDD)

Western New York Regional Poison Control Center
Children's Hospital of Buffalo
219 Bryant Street
Buffalo, NY 14222
Emergency Phone: (800) 888-7655; (716) 878-7654

North Carolina
Carolinas Poison Center
Carolinas Medical Center
5000 Airport Center Parkway
Suite B
Charlotte, NC 28208
Emergency Phone: (800) 848-6946; (704) 355-4000

North Dakota
North Dakota Poison Information Center
Meritcare Medical Center
720 4th Street North
Fargo, ND 58122
Emergency Phone: (800) 732-2200 (ND, MN, SD only);
(701) 234-5575

Ohio
Central Ohio Poison Center
700 Children's Drive
Room L032
Columbus, OH 43205
Emergency Phone: (800) 682-7625 (OH only);
(800) 762-0727 (Dayton, OH only)
TDD/TTY: (614) 228-2272 (TTY)

TABLE 23.38 *(Continued)*
Nationwide Poison Control Centers — Directory

Cincinnati Drug and Poison Information Center
Regional Poison Control System
3333 Burnet Avenue
Vernon Place
3rd Floor
Cincinnati, OH 45229
Emergency Phone: (800) 872-5111 (OH only);
(513) 558-5111

Greater Cleveland Poison Control Center
11100 Euclid Avenue
Cleveland, OH 44106-6010
Emergency Phone: (888) 231-4455 (OH only);
(216) 231-4455

Oklahoma
Oklahoma Poison Control Center
Children's Hospital of Oklahoma
Room 3512
940 N.E. 13th Street
Oklahoma City, OK 73104
Emergency Phone: (800) 764-7661 (OK only);
(405) 271-5454
TDD/TTY: (405) 271-1122

Oregon
Oregon Poison Center
Oregon Health Sciences University
3181 SW Sam Jackson Park Road, CB550
Portland, OR 97201
Emergency Phone: (800) 452-7165 (OR only);
(503) 494-8968

Pennsylvania
Central Pennsylvania Poison Center
Pennsylvania State University
The Milton S. Hershey Medical Center
MC H043, PO Box 850
500 University Drive
Hershey, PA 17033-0850
Emergency Phone: (800) 521-6110; (717) 531-6111
TDD/TTY: (717) 531-8335 (TTY)

Pittsburgh Poison Center
Children's Hospital of Pittsburgh
3705 Fifth Avenue
Pittsburgh, PA 15213
Emergency Phone: (412) 681-6669

TABLE 23.38 *(Continued)*
Nationwide Poison Control Centers — Directory

The Poison Control Center
3535 Market Street
Suite 985
Philadelphia, PA 19104-3309
Emergency Phone: (800) 722-7112; (215) 386-2100;
(215) 590-2100

Rhode Island
Regional Center for Poison Control and Prevention
Serving Massachusetts and Rhode Island
300 Longwood Avenue
Boston, MA 02115
Emergency Phone: (800) 682-9211 (MA and RI only);
(617) 232-2120
TDD/TTY: (888) 244-5313

South Carolina
Palmetto Poison Center
College of Pharmacy
University of South Carolina
Columbia, SC 29208
Emergency Phone: (800) 922-1117 (SC only);
(803) 777-1117

South Dakota
Hennepin Regional Poison Center
Hennepin County Medical Center
701 Park Avenue
Minneapolis, MN 55415
Emergency Phone: (800) POISON1 (SD only);
(800) POISON1 (SD only)
TDD/TTY: (612) 904-4691 (TTY)

Tennessee
Middle Tennessee Poison Center
501 Oxford House
1161 21st Avenue South
Nashville, TN 37232-4632
Emergency Phone: (800) 288-9999 (TN only);
(615) 936-2034 (Greater Nashville)
TDD/TTY: (615) 936-2047 (TDD)

Southern Poison Center
875 Monroe Avenue
Suite 104
Memphis, TN 38163
Emergency Phone: (800) 288-9999 (TN only);
(901) 528-6048

TABLE 23.38 *(Continued)*
Nationwide Poison Control Centers — Directory

Texas

Central Texas Poison Center
Scott and White Memorial Hospital
2401 South 31st Street
Temple, TX 76508
Emergency Phone: (800) POISON-1(TX only);
(254) 724-7401

North Texas Poison Center
Texas Poison Center Network
Parkland Health and Hospital System
5201 Harry Hines Blvd.
P.O. Box 35926
Dallas, TX 75235
Emergency Phone: (800) 764-7661 (TX only)

South Texas Poison Center
The University of Texas Health Science Center — San Antonio
Department of Surgery
Mail Code 7849
7703 Floyd Curl Drive
San Antonio, TX 78229-3900
Emergency Phone: (800) 764-7661 (TX only)
TDD/TTY: (800) 764-7661 (TX only)

Southeast Texas Poison Center
The University of Texas Medical Branch
3.112 Trauma Building
Galveston, TX 77555-1175
Emergency Phone: (800) 764-7661 (TX only);
(409) 765-1420

Texas Panhandle Poison Center
1501 S. Coulter
Amarillo, TX 79106
Emergency Phone: (800) 764-7661 (TX only)

West Texas Regional Poison Center
Thomason Hospital
4815 Alameda Avenue
EI Paso, TX 79905
Emergency Phone: (800) 764-7661 (TX only)

Utah

Utah Poison Control Center
410 Chipeta Way, Suite 230
Salt Lake City, UT 84108
Emergency Phone: (800) 456-7707 (UT only);
(801) 581-2151

TABLE 23.38 *(Continued)*
Nationwide Poison Control Centers — Directory

Vermont
Vermont Poison Center
Fletcher Allen Health Care
111 Colchester Avenue
Burlington, VT 05401
Emergency Phone: (877) 658-3456 (toll free);
(802) 658-3456

Virginia
Blue Ridge Poison Center
University of Virginia Health System
PO Box 800774
Charlottesville, VA 22908-0774
Emergency Phone: (800) 451-1428 (VA only);
(804) 924-5543

National Capital Poison Center
3201 New Mexico Avenue, NW
Suite 310
Washington, D.C. 20016
Emergency Phone: (202) 625-3333
TDD/TTY: (202) 362-8563 (TTY)

Virginia Poison Center
Medical College of Virginia Hospitals
Virginia Commonwealth University
P.O. Box 980522
Richmond, VA 23298-0522
Emergency Phone: (800) 552-6337; (804) 828-9123

Washington
Washington Poison Center
155 NE 100th Street
Suite 400
Seattle, WA 98125-8012
Emergency Phone: (800) 732-6985 (WA only);
(206) 526-2121
TDD/TTY: (206) 517-2394 (TDD);
(800) 572-0638 (TDD WA only)

West Virginia
West Virginia Poison Center
3110 MacCorkle Ave, S.E.
Charleston, WV 25304
Emergency Phone: (800) 642-3625 (WV only)

Wisconsin
Children's Hospital of Wisconsin Poison Center
P.O. Box 1997
Milwaukee, WI 53201
Emergency Phone: (800) 815-8855 (WI only);
(414) 266-2222

TABLE 23.38 *(Continued)*
Nationwide Poison Control Centers — Directory

University of Wisconsin Hospital and Clinics
Poison Control Center
600 Highland Avenue, F6/133
Madison, WI 53792
Emergency Phone: (800) 815-8855 (WI only);
(608) 262-3702

Wyoming
The Poison Center
Children's Hospital
8301 Dodge Street
Omaha, NE 68114
Emergency Phone: (800) 955-9119 (NE and WY only);
(402) 955-5555

REFERENCES

1. Litovitz, T. et al., 1991 AAPCC Annual Report, *Am. J. Emerg. Med.,* 10, 452, 1992.
2. Goldfrank, L. et al., *Goldfran's Toxicologic Emergencies,* 5th ed., Appleton & Lange, Norwalk, CT, 1994.
3. Haddad, L. and Winchester, J., *Clinical Management of Poisoning & Drug Overdose,* 2nd ed., WB Saunders, Philadelphia, PA, 1990.
4. Zbinden G., Predictive value of animal studies in toxicology, *Regul. Toxicol. Pharmacol.,* 14, 167, 1991.
5. Russell, R., Essential roles for animal models in understanding human toxicities, *Neurosci. Biobehav. Rev.,* 15, 7, 1991.
6. Schlesselman, J.J., *Case Control Studies: Design, Conduct, Analysis,* Oxford University Press, New York, 1982.
7. Fletcher, R., *Clinical Epidemiology: The Essentials,* 2nd ed., Williams & Wilkins, Baltimore, MD, 1988.
8. Litovitz, T. and Manoguerra, A., Comparison of pediatric poisoning hazards: an analysis of 3.8 million exposure incidents. A report from the AAPCC, *Pediatrics,* 89, 999, 1992.
9. King, W. and Palmisano, P., Ingestion of prescription drugs by children: an epidemiologic study, *S. Med. J.,* 82, 1468, 1989.
10. Woolf, A. and Lovejoy, F., Epidemiology of drug overdose in children, *Drug Safety,* 9, 291, 1993.
11. Paulson, J.A., The epidemiology of injuries in adolescents, *Pediatr. Ann.,* 17, 84, 1988.
12. Klein-Schwartz, W. and Oderda, G., Poisoning in the elderly: Epidemiological, clinical and management considerations, *Drugs and Aging,* 1, 67, 1991.
13. Woolf, A. et al., Serious poisonings among older adults: a study of hospitalization and mortality rates in Massachusetts 1983–1985, *Am. J. Public Health,* 80, 867, 1990.
14. Osterloh, J., Utility and reliability of emergency toxicologic testing, *Emerg. Med. Clin. N. Am.,* 8, 693, 1990.
15. National Committee for Injury Prevention and Control, *Injury Prevention: Meeting the Challenge,* Education Development Center, Inc., Oxford University Press, 1989.
16. Annual Reports, New York State Regional Poison Control Centers.

24 Risk Assessment

Michael J. Derelanko, Ph.D, D.A.B.T., F.A.T.S

CONTENTS

SECTION 1. INTRODUCTION

The purpose of this chapter is to provide information to familiarize the reader with the basic concepts and process of risk assessment and to provide a handy and quick reference source for standard assumptions, terminology, equations, and values used in performing these assessments. Although the information presented in this chapter is generally representative of the risk assessment process as currently practiced by regulatory bodies such as the U.S. Environmental Protection Agency, risk assessment is an ever evolving discipline. As such, methods and procedures are often modified or replaced to reflect current scientific practice and theory.

There is little or no scientific evidence to support many of the concepts and assumptions on which the risk assessment process is based. Therefore, other approaches for assessing risk may be equally valid. Moreover, the likelihood that all individuals in all situations can fit into any standardized model is extremely remote. In practice, each risk assessment should ideally be unique and the use of standardized assumptions and values may not always be appropriate.

Risk assessment is an imprecise science. Many assumptions are made where actual data is not available or difficult to obtain. Many of the models are based on hypothetical mechanisms of toxicity which may not be scientifically valid. Because of these limitations, a great deal of uncertainty is inherent in the risk assessment process. Due to this uncertainty and the desire to protect human populations under a variety of exposure scenarios, risk assessments generally are conservative and overestimate risk.

This chapter is divided into 10 sections. Section 2 presents an overview of the risk assessment process and outlines some of the basic theoretical considerations and concepts that form the foundation on which the risk assessment process is based.

Section 3 deals with dose-response-relationships and their use in risk assessment. Section 4 covers basic terminology, methodology, and concepts of epidemiology. In addition, reference information is presented on causation and incidence of human cancer and reproductive and developmental effects. Section 5 contains relative risk tables useful for making risk comparisons. Standard reference values for use in interspecies extrapolation and exposure assessment are presented in Section 6. Section 7 provides a brief overview of physiologically based pharmacokinetic (PBPK) modeling and presents reference values for physiological and biochemical parameters used in these models. Equations for calculations commonly encountered in risk assessments can be found in Section 8. Section 9 presents toxicity classification schemes based on lethality and carcinogenicity. Section 10 provides a glossary of common risk assessment terms, acronyms, and abbreviations.

SECTION 2. RISK ASSESSMENT: INTRODUCTION AND OVERVIEW

With few exceptions such as veterinary and agricultural products, toxicology studies are not conducted solely to assess the toxic effects of chemicals in animals but to identify the effects which might occur in humans. Risk assessment is the process of evaluating the toxic properties of chemicals and the conditions of human exposure to ascertain the likelihood that humans will be adversely affected and to characterize the nature of the effects which may be experienced.

The risk assessment process, such as performed by the U.S. Environmental Protection Agency, can be divided into four steps: hazard identification, dose-response assessment, exposure assessment, and risk characterization (Figure 24.1). In hazard identification, a determination is made of whether a substance of concern, be it a pharmaceutical, industrial chemical, environmental pollutant, etc., can be linked to an adverse effect. Dose-response assessment establishes relationships between the magnitude of exposure and the occurrence of the adverse effect. The major activities of toxicologists are concentrated in these two steps. In exposure assessment, human exposure to the substance of concern is identified through characterization of the exposed population, routes of exposure, and magnitude of the exposure under various conditions. All the information derived in these three steps of the risk assessment process is used in the risk characterization step. In this fourth and final stage of the risk assessment process, a determination is made of the likelihood that humans may experience the identified adverse effect under actual or plausible hypothetical conditions of exposure.

Based on the risk characterization, the need for and the degree of risk management will be determined. A number of options are available to the risk manager, including education and communication of risk, exposure monitoring and controls, limitations in the use of the substance of concern or a total ban of the chemical. Risk management decisions are influenced by economic, political, and social concerns. Risk management is considered separately from the risk assessment process. Further discussion of risk management is beyond the scope of this book.

An overview of some of the major concepts that form the foundation of the risk assessment process, as well as assumptions and factors considered and/or used in risk assesment, is presented in the tables and figures of this section. A review of this information will provide a basic understanding of risk assessment. The reader should consult the cited references for more detailed information on the risk assessment process.

ELEMENTS OF RISK ASSESSMENT

HAZARD IDENTIFICTION

Does a Chemical of Concern Cause an Adverse Effect?

- Epidemiology
- Animal Studies
- Short Term Assays
- Structure/Activity Relationships

EXPOSURE ASSESSMENT

What Exposures are Exerienced or Anticipated Under Different Conditions?

- Identification of Exposed Populations
- Identification of Routes of Exposure
- Estimation of Degree of Exposure

DOSE-RESPONSE ASSESSMENT

How is the Identified Adverse Effect Influenced by the Level of Exposure?

- Quantitative Toxicity Information Collected
- Dose-Response Relationships Established
- Extrapolation of Animal Data to Humans

RISK CHARACTERIZATION

What is the Estimated Likelihood of the Adverse Effect Occurring in a Given Population?

- Estimation of the Potential for Adverse Health Effects to Occur
- Evaluation of Uncertainty
- Risk Information Summarized

FIGURE 24.1 The four major elements of risk assessment. *Hazard identification* — In this step, a determination is made of whether a chemical of concern is or is not causally linked to a particular health effect. Information can come from human and animal studies, *in vitro* assays, and through analogy to structurally similar chemicals. *Exposure assessment* — involves the characterization of the amount, frequency, and duration of human exposure. Determinations are made of the concentration of hazardous substances in media (i.e., air, water, soil, etc.), magnitude and pathways of exposure, environmental fate, and populations at risk. The purpose of this step is to provide a quantitative estimate of human exposure. *Dose-response assessment* — The relationship between the magnitude of exposure and the occurrence of the expected health effects is determined in this step. Information obtained from animal studies is extrapolated to humans. Generally, different assessments are performed for noncarcinogenic and carcinogenic materials. Along with hazard identification, the major activities of most toxicologists are focused on this portion of the risk assessment process. *Risk characterization* — In this final stage of the risk assessment process, information from the three previous steps are evaluated to produce a determination of the nature and magnitude of human risk. The risk assessment process is completed with a summary of the risk information. The information developed in the risk assessment process will be utilized in the *risk management process* in which decisions are made as to the need for, the degree of, and the steps to be taken to control exposures to the chemical of concern. (*Source:* U.S. Environmental Protection Agency, 1989,[1] National Research Council as, 1983.[2] Adapted from Hooper et al., 1992.[3])

TABLE 24.1
Hierarchy Data Selection for Risk Assessment

1. Human data *lifetime exposure* via the more appropriate route (inhalation or oral)
2. Human data *less than lifetime exposure* with lifetime observation (exposure via the more appropriate route)
3. Human data *less than lifetime exposure* with less-than-lifetime observation (exposure via the more appropriate route)
4. Human data *lifetime* exposure via the less appropriate route if reasonable toxicologically
5. Human data *less than lifetime exposure* with lifetime observation (exposure via the less appropriate route)
6. Human data *less than lifetime exposure* with less-than-lifetime observation (exposure via the less appropriate route)
7. Animal data the same sequence as for human data. Animal studies of less than 90 days of exposure and/or less than 18 months of observation from first exposure should not be used.

Adapted from Hallenback and Cunningham, *Quantitative Risk Assessment for Environmental and Occupational Health,* 1986.[4] With permission.

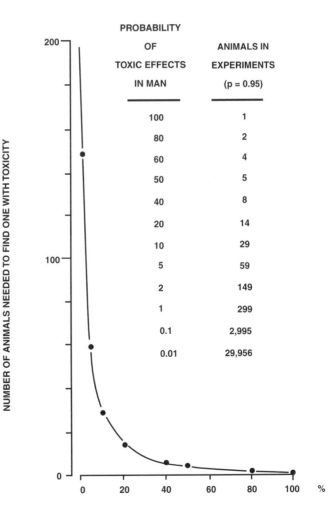

FIGURE 24.2 The interrelationship between the probability (percent) of a given toxic effect in humans and the number of animals required in a toxicology study to ensure that the same toxic effect can be observed. With a high incidence of occurrence in humans, few animals are needed, but because the incidence frequently is very low, then astronomical numbers of animals would be required to "guarantee" that the same effect would be observed. This relationship is usually cited as the reason for using unrealistically large dose levels in animal studies to increase the probability that toxic effects will be observed with relatively small numbers of animals. (Data derived from Zbinden, 1973[5] from Ecobichon, *The Basis of Toxicity Testing*, 1992.[6] With permission.)

PROBABILITY OF TOXICITY IN MAN

PROBABILITY OF TOXIC EFFECTS IN MAN	ANIMALS IN EXPERIMENTS (p = 0.95)
100	1
80	2
60	4
50	5
40	8
20	14
10	29
5	59
2	149
1	299
0.1	2,995
0.01	29,956

TABLE 24.2
Typical Factors Considered in a Risk Assessment

- Physical and chemical properties of the chemical
- Patterns of use
- Handling procedures
- Availability and reliability of control measures
- Source and route of exposure under ordinary and extraordinary conditions
- Potential for misuse
- Magnitude, duration, and frequency of exposure
- Nature of exposure (oral, dermal, inhalation)
- Physical nature of the exposure (solid, liquid, vapor, etc.)
- Influence of environmental conditions of exposure
- Population exposed
    Number
    Sex
    Health status
    Personal habits (e.g., smoking)
    Lifestyles (e.g., hobbies, activities)

Source: Ballantyne and Sullivan, 1992.[7] With permission.

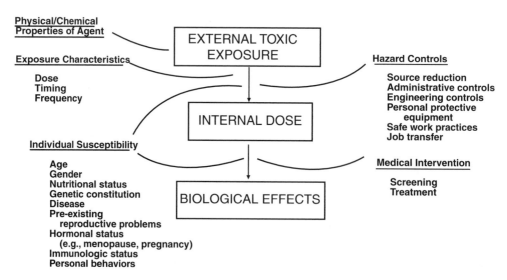

FIGURE 24.3 Factors that influence the risk posed to an individual by xenobiotic exposures. These factors as well as others should be considered in a well-conducted risk assessment. Historically, risk assessments have been based on external exposures which create large uncertainties in extrapolating animal data to humans. The use of internal dose can provide more accurate interspecies extrapolation resulting in a more realistic characterization of risk. (From Paul, *Occupational and Environmental Reproductive Hazards: A Guide for Clinicians*, 1993.[8] With permission.)

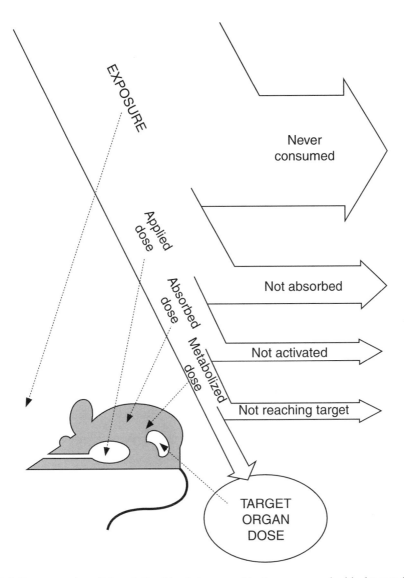

FIGURE 24.4 Representation of the relationships between ambient exposure and critical target dose and the progressive decrease in effective exposure due to various biological barriers. From *Low-Dose Extrapolation of Cancer Risks: Issues and Perspectives*[77]. Used with permission. © 1995 International Life Sciences Institute, Washington, D.C.

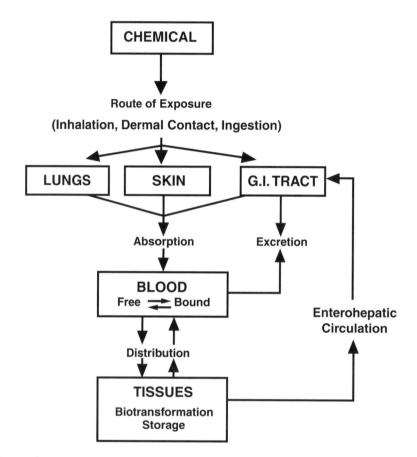

FIGURE 24.5 Diagrammatic representation of the possible pharmacokinetic fate of a chemical after exposure by inhalation, dermal contact, and ingestion. The lungs and skin also have enzyme systems capable of biotransformation (not shown). The fate of a chemical after exposure can vary considerably between species. Pharmacokinetic information is essential for accurate risk assessments. Such information can be obtained from animal studies/or physiologically based pharmacokinetic models (*see* Section 7). In the absence of such data, assumptions are often made that introduce a great degree of uncertainty into the risk assessment process. (Modified from Ballantyne and Sullivan, 1992.[7])

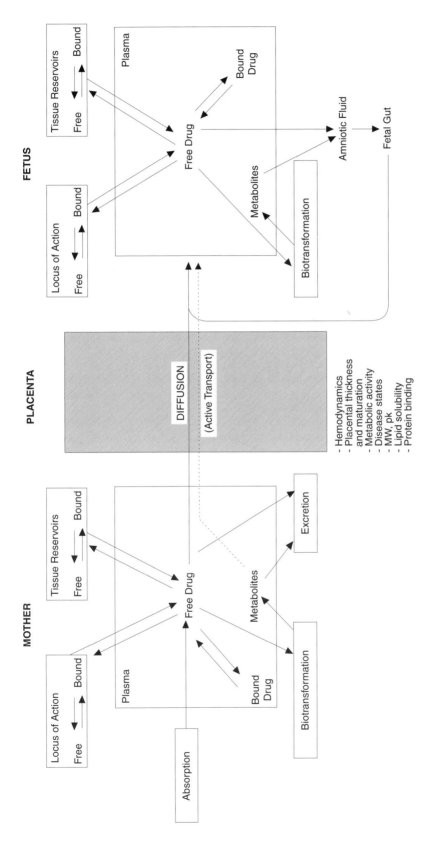

FIGURE 24.6 Maternal-placental-fetal pharmacokinetic relationships that can influence the risk posed by a reproductive toxin. (Adapted from Chow and Jewesson, 1985,[9] from McGuigan, *Hazardous Materials Toxicology: Clinical Principles of Environmental Health*, 1992.[10] With permission.)

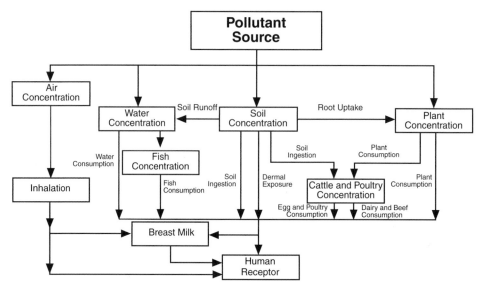

FIGURE 24.7 Diagrammatic representation of potential exposure pathways available to an environmental pollutant. Limitations in analytical methodology (e.g., sampling, analytical sensitivity, accuracy, etc.) used in measuring concentrations of chemicals in media (i.e., air, water) can introduce uncertainty into a risk assessment. Modeled data are often used in the absence of actual analytical measurements. Exposure estimates are generally based on standard exposure values (i.e., water consumption, soil ingestion) which can range from average to worst case (*see* Table 24.45). In general, the accuracy of an exposure assessment and subsequent risk characterization is only as good as the information from which it was made. (Modified from Lowe et al., *Health Effects of Municipal Waste Incineration*, 1991.[11])

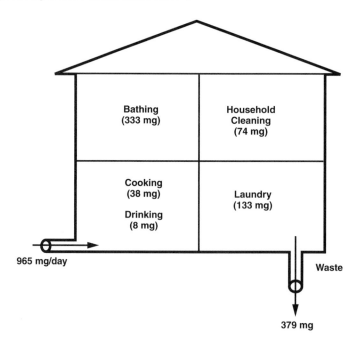

FIGURE 24.8 Example of the distribution of a contaminant present in household water at a concentration of 1 mg/liter based on household water use patterns. Presented as an example of the type of data generated in an exposure assessment. Such information is necessary to develop estimates of exposure (*see* Table 24.3). (Adapted from U.S. Environmental Protection Agency, 1984.[12])

TABLE 24.3
Comparative Assessment of Absorbed Dose from a Volatile Pollutant (100 μg/liter) in Drinking Water

	Absorbed Dose (Micrograms/Day)				
	Formula Fed Infant (4 kg)	Preteen (32 kg)	Adult Female (60 kg)	Adult Male[a] (70 kg)	Male[b] (70 kg)
Fluid ingestion	80	150	200	200	200
Inhalation of enriched indoor air	10	10	70	50	50
Inhalation of enclosed shower air	—	100	300	200	—
Dermal absorption bathing	0.02–0.06	—	—	—	2.5
Swimming	—	10–300	—	—	—
Total absorbed dose, μg/kg/day	20	10–20	10	7	4

[a] Showering adult male.

[b] Adult male that does not take showers.

From U.S. Environmental Protection Agency, 1984.[12]

TABLE 24.4
Typical Assumptions Made in a Risk Assessment of an Animal Carcinogen Water Pollutant

- National monitoring is representative of the existing exposure profile.
- The equivalent amount of toxicant per liter in water is transferred to a liter of air.
- 100% of the toxicant in water is released to the air.
- Everyone is exposed to the same level of the contaminant.
- The average human ingests 2 liters of drinking water per day and daily inhales an average of 20 m^3 of air.
- All of the ingested or inhaled toxicant is absorbed into the blood.
- Dermal exposure is insignificant compared with oral and inhalation exposures.
- The same effects observed in animals will occur in humans.
- The only difference between humans and animals is one of scale.
- There are no thresholds.
- Both benign and malignant tumors are indicative of cancer.
- The mathematical expression used to reflect the biological dose response is curvilinear at low doses.

Source: U.S. Environmental Protection Agency, 1984.[12]

TABLE 24.5
Major Factors that Influence a Risk Assessment

Factor	Effect
Low dose extrapolation	Can involve as many as 50 or more assumptions each of which introduce uncertainty. Often considered the greatest weakness in risk assessment.
Population variation	The use of standard exposure factors can underestimate actual risk to hypersensitive individuals. Addressing the risk assessment to the most sensitive individuals can overestimate risk to the population as a whole.
Exposure variation	The use of modeling and measurement techniques can provide exposure estimates that diverge widely from reality.
Environmental variation	Can affect actual exposures to a greater or lesser degree than assumed to exist.
Multiple exposures	Risk assessments generally deal with one contaminant for which additive, synergistic, and antagonistic effects are unaccounted. Can result in underestimate or overestimate of risk.
Species differences	It is generally assumed that humans are equivalent to the most sensitive species. Can overestimate or underestimate risk.
Dose based on body weight	Toxicity generally does not vary linearly with body weight but exponentially with body surface area.
Choice of dose levels	Use of unrealistically high dose levels can result in toxicity unlikely to occur at actual exposure levels. The number of animals being studied may be insufficient to detect toxicity at lower doses.
Uncertainty factors	The use of uncertainty factors in attempting to counter the potential uncertainty of a risk assessment can overestimate risk by several orders of magnitude.
Confidence intervals	The upper confidence interval does not represent the true likelihood of an event; can overestimate risk by an order of magnitude or more.
Statistics	Experimental data may be inadequate for statistical analysis. Statistical significance may not indicate biological significance, and a biologically significant effect may not be statistically significant. Statistical significance does not prove causality. Conversely, lack of statistical significance does not prove safety.

TABLE 24.6
Criteria Defining "High-Exposure" Chemicals

- Production greater than 100,000 kg
- More than 1000 workers exposed
- More than 100 workers exposed by inhalation to greater than 10 mg/kg/day
- More than 100 workers exposed by inhalation to 1–10 mg/day for more than 100 days/year
- More than 250 workers exposed by routine dermal contact for more than 100 days/year
- Presence of the chemical in any consumer product in which the physical state of the chemical in the product and the manner of use would make exposure likely
- More than 70 mg/year of exposure via surface water
- More than 70 mg/year of exposure via air
- More than 70 mg/year of exposure via groundwater
- More than 10,000 kg/year release to environmental media
- More than 1000 kg/year total release to surface water after calculated estimates of treatment

Source: U.S. Environmental Protection Agency, 1988.[13]

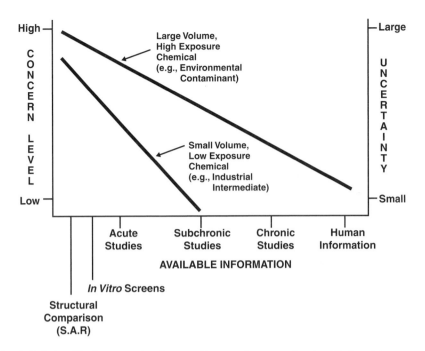

FIGURE 24.9 Relationship between the degree of uncertainty associated with the risk assessment of a chemical, the concern for human exposure, and the toxicological information available on the chemical. In practice, the larger the toxicological database available on a chemical of concern ("weight-of-evidence"), the greater the certainty (less uncertainty) that the estimated "safe" exposure level will be protective of individuals exposed to the chemical. Similarly, the concern that the risk assessment will underestimate the risk decreases with a larger toxicological database. Generally, less toxicological information will be required to reduce the concern level and uncertainty associated with a small volume, low-exposure chemical (for which the exposed population is well characterized and the exposures can be controlled) as compared with a large volume, high-exposure chemical.

TABLE 24.7
Factors that Influence Risk Management Decisions

Decreases Degree of Risk Management	Increases Degree of Risk Management
Risk assumed voluntarily	Risk borne involuntarily
No alternatives available	Safer alternatives available
Exposure is essential	Exposure considered a luxury
Exposure primarily occupational	Exposure nonoccupational
Exposure primarily to average individuals	Exposure involves hypersensitive individuals
Intended use can be reasonably guaranteed	Potential for misuse high
Toxic effects reversible	Toxic effects permanent
Toxic effects not inheritable	Toxic effects inheritable
Risk perceived acceptable	Risk perceived unacceptable

Adapted from Lowrance, *Of Acceptable Risk: Science and the Determination of Safety*, 1976.[15]

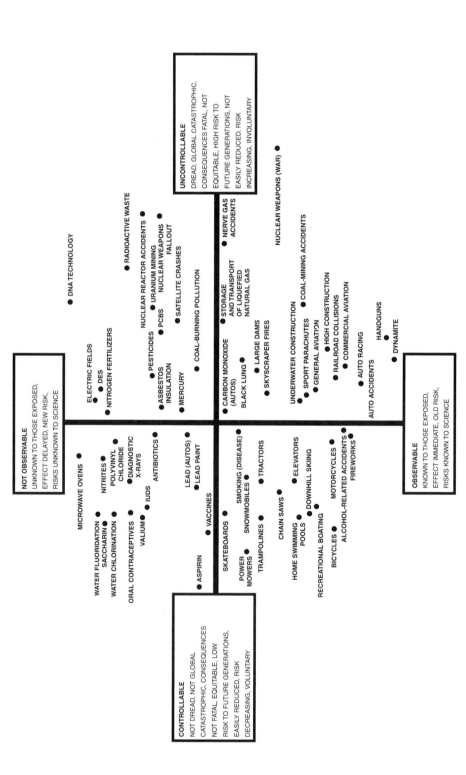

FIGURE 24.10 Graphic representation of risk perception which roughly corresponds to a hazard's "dreadfulness" and degree to which it is understood. Public concern increases above the horizontal axis and to the right of the vertical axis. Conversely, concern decreases below the horizontal axis and left of the vertical axis. Factors which impact on the perception of risk management decisions. (Illustration by J. Johnson. From Morgan, M.G., *Risk Analysis and Management*,[14] copyright © by Scientific American. All rights reserved.)

SECTION 3. DOSE-RESPONSE RELATIONSHIPS

The dose-response relationship forms the basis of the most fundamental concept of toxicology, that the toxicity of any material is defined by its dose-response curve; or, to paraphrase Paracelsus, "the dose makes the poison." Dose-response assessment is one of the four steps in the risk assessment process (see Figure 24.1).

The dose-response curve generally takes two forms: the first displays the distribution of an effect within a population as a function of changing exposure, and the second indicates the degree of change of an effect in an exposed individual of a population as a function of changing exposure. The demonstration of dose-response suggests causality.

The typical dose-response curve is sigmoidal, but can also be linear, concave, convex, or bimodal. The shape of the curve can offer clues to the mechanism of action of the toxin, indicate multiple toxic effects, and identify the existence and extent of sensitive subpopulations. Analysis of the dose-response curve can demonstrate average response, the degree of susceptibility within a population, and the range of exposure affecting hyperreactive individuals. The slope of the dose-response curve categorizes the potency of the toxin and indicates the magnitude of effect associated with incremental increases in exposure. The curve can display the degree of confidence (and conversely uncertainty) associated with the data. The reader should refer to general toxicology and pharmacology textbooks for a more detailed discussion of dose-response relationships.

The purpose of this section is to provide examples of some of the ways dose-response relationships are used in risk assessment and the type of information that can be obtained from the dose-response curve. Risk assessment takes advantage of the ability of the dose-response curve to quantitate the susceptibility of individuals in an exposed population to a substance of concern. Dose-response assessment determines the relationship between the extent (magnitude) of exposure and the probability of occurrence of health effects. For pharmaceuticals, safety ratios such as the therapeutic index and margin of safety are derived. "Safe levels" of exposure such as reference

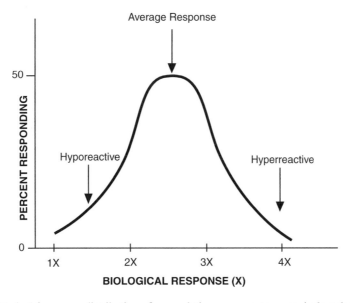

FIGURE 24.11 Typical frequency distribution of a population response to an equivalent dose of biologically active agent. This type of response represents the variability that occurs within biological systems and is the basis for the concept of dose response in pharmacology and toxicology. This figure demonstrates that within any population, both hyporeactive and hyperreactive individuals can be expected to exist and must be addressed in a risk assessment.

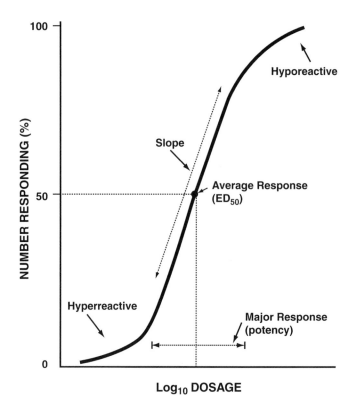

FIGURE 24.12 Typical sigmoid cumulative dose-response curve for a toxic effect which is symmetrical about the average (50% response) point. Note dosage is presented on a log scale. The major response (potency) occurs around the average response. The midpoint of the curve is referred to as the median effective dose for the effect being considered (ED_{50}). If mortality is the endpoint, this point is referred to as the median lethal dose (LD_{50}). The 95% confidence limits are the narrowest at the midpoint (see Figure 24.14) which makes this the point most useful for comparison of toxicity between chemicals. The slope of the curve is determined by the increase in response as a function of incremental increases in dosage. A steep slope indicates a majority of a population will respond within a narrow dose range, while a flatter curve indicates that a much wider dose range is required to affect a majority of the exposed population (see Figure 24.15). Hyperreactive and hyporeactive individuals are at the extreme left and rights sides of the curve, respectively. (From Ballantyne, *Hazardous Materials Toxicology: Clinical Principles of Environmental Health*, 1992.[16] With permission.)

dose (RfD), acceptable daily intake (ADI), and permissible exposure limits (PEL) for pollutants, food additives, and industrial chemicals, respectively, are estimated from dose-response.

The above values are determined for substances demonstrated to have a threshold below which an effect of concern is not expected to occur. Where thresholds are assumed not to exist, such as for carcinogens, virtually safe doses (VSD) or exposures are determined by extrapolation of the dose-response curve to levels of risk deemed acceptable by society. The reliability of this approach is compromised by the uncertainty associated with modeling the low-dose region of the dose-response curve.

The quality of a dose-response assessment is only as good as the data with which the dose-response curve was generated. Dose-response assessment, coupled with exposure assessment, allows the risk of exposure to a chemical to be characterized, which ultimately is the purpose of the risk assessment process. The more accurate the dose-response and exposure assessment, the more realistic the risk characterization will be.

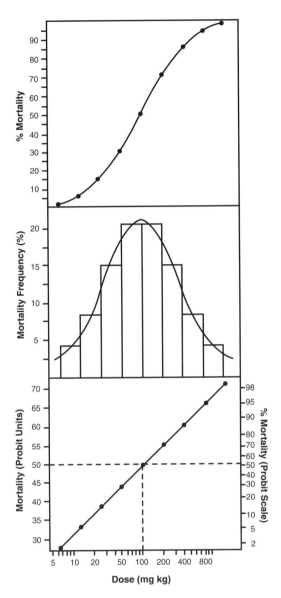

FIGURE 24.13 Various ways of presenting dose-response data. The abscissa is a log dosage of the chemical. The ordinate of the top panel is percent mortality producing a sigmoidal curve (see Figure 24.12); a bell-shaped curve is produced when the ordinate is mortality frequency (middle panel); the response is linearized when the ordinate is in probit units (bottom panel). (From Klaassen and Eaton, *Casarett and Doull's Toxicology: The Basic Science of Poisons*, 4th ed., 1991.[17] With permission of McGraw-Hill.)

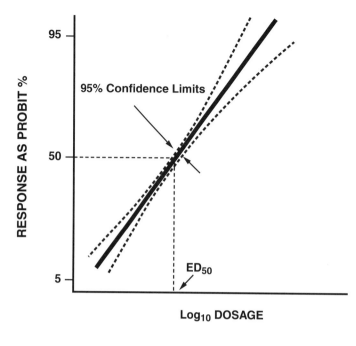

FIGURE 24.14 Dosage-mortality curve showing 95% confidence limits. These limits show the uncertainty associated with the dose-response curve resulting from the use of small numbers of animals. The confidence limits are narrowest at the ED_{50} (or LD_{50}). (From Ballantyne, *Hazardous Materials Toxicology: Clinical Principles of Environmental Health*, 1992.[16] With permission.)

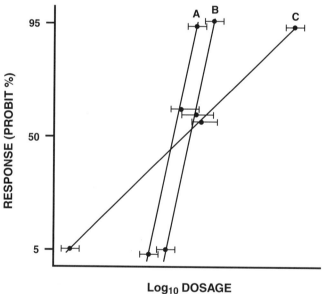

FIGURE 24.15 Influence of slopes of dosage-mortality data on the interpretation of LD_{50} data. All three materials (A, B, and C) have overlapping 95% confidence limits at the 50% response level and are therefore of comparable LD_{50}. Materials A and B have parallel dose-response lines and overlapping confidence limits at 5% and 95%; therefore, these two materials are of comparable lethal toxicity over a wide range of doses. Material C with a shallower slope has significantly different LD_5 and LD_{95} values, and therefore over a wide range of doses has a differing lethal toxicity to materials A and B. With materials A and B, due to the steep slope of the dose-response line, a much larger proportion of the population will be affected by small incremental increases in dosage. With material C, there may be a greater hazard for the hyperreactive groups, because the LD_5 lies at a much lower dosage than for A and B. (From Ballantyne, *Hazardous Materials Toxicology: Clinical Principles of Environmental Health*, 1992.[16] With permission.)

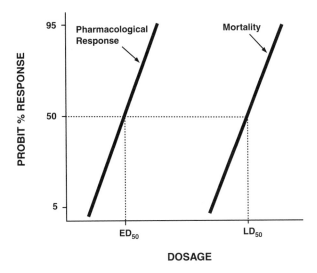

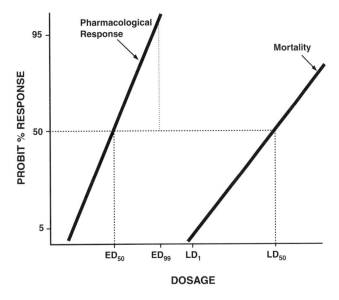

FIGURE 24.16 A simplistic method for assessing "safety ratios" for drugs is by comparing the ratio of the therapeutically effective dose (ED_{50}) and lethal dose (LD_{50}); this ratio of LD_{50}/ED_{50} is referred to as the therapeutic index (TI_{50}). For parallel pharmacological effect and lethality dose-response lines, the therapeutic index will be similar over a wide range of doses (upper figure). The therapeutic index may be misleading if the dose-response lines for pharmacological and lethal effects are not parallel (lower figure). As shown in this figure, the margin based on LD_{50} and ED_{50} may be reasonable. However, due to the shallow slope of the mortality dose-response line, the therapeutic index will be significantly lower at the 1% and 5% level, thus the hyperreactive group may be at greater risk. In such a case, a better index of safety will be the ratio of the LD_1/ED_{99} which is referred to as the margin of safety. (From Ballatyne, *Hazardous Materials Toxicology: Clinical Principles of Environmental Health,* 1992.[16] With permission.)

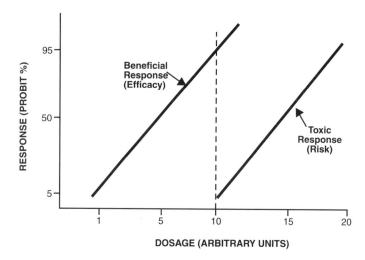

FIGURE 24.17 In situations where the beneficial (desired) dose-response curve of a pharmaceutical overlaps the toxic (side effect) dose-response curve of the drug, risk benefit determinations are made to assess the safety of the drug for its intended use. In making such decisions, many factors must be considered including the necessity for the drug, its intended use, and the type and severity of the side effect associated with the drug. For example, if the drug has some life-saving effect but produces nausea, the maximum dosage might be greater than 10 units to insure efficacious treatment. Some patients would have to tolerate the nausea. An example of such a drug would be a chemotherapeutic agent. Conversely, nausea would not be tolerated if associated with a decongestant. For such a drug, the maximum dose would be kept below 10 units. (Adapted from Lowrance, 1976.[15])

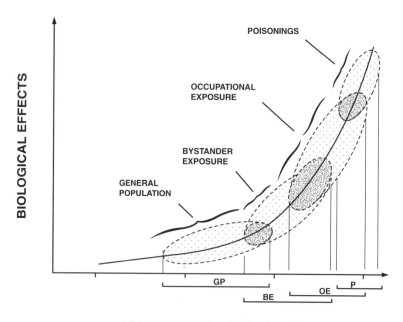

FIGURE 24.18 A theoretical dose-response relationship indicating the range of dosage (mg/kg of body weight) of a toxicant to which representative human populations might be exposed. Poisonings (P) tend to occur over a relatively narrow range, whereas in occupational exposures (OE) the range would be somewhat broader. Overlapping with occupational exposure, the dosage range to which bystanders would be exposed (BE) would be broader still, whereas the general population (GP) would encounter a dosage range of possibly one to three orders of magnitude. (From Ecobichon, *The Basis of Toxicity Testing,* 1992.[6] With permission.)

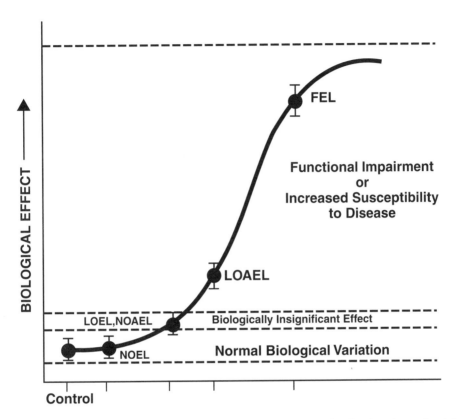

FIGURE 24.19 A dose-response curve from a typical toxicological study showing dose-related indices commonly used in risk assessment. A well-designed study should include dose levels which produce a Frank Effect (FEL), a Lowest Observable Adverse Effect (LOAEL), and either a Lowest Observable Effect (LOEL), a No Observable Adverse Effect (NOAEL), or a No Observable Effect (NOEL). A FEL is a dose or exposure level that produces unmistakable *adverse* health effects that cause functional impairment or increased susceptability to disease; a LOAEL is the lowest dose or exposure level that produces an *adverse* health effect; a LOEL is the lowest dose or exposure level that produces an observable effect, but not to a degree which would be expected to have a significant impact on the health of the animal (the LOEL is sometimes confused with a LOAEL); a NOAEL is the highest dose or exposure level at which no *adverse* health effects are observed which are capable of functional impairment or increase susceptability to disease (the NOAEL can be equivalent to the LOEL); a NOEL is the highest dose or exposure level at which no effects are observed outside of the range of normal biological variation for the species and strain under study. The effect, if any, observed at the NOEL should not be statistically significant when compared with the control group. (Adapted from Ecobichon, 1992.[18])

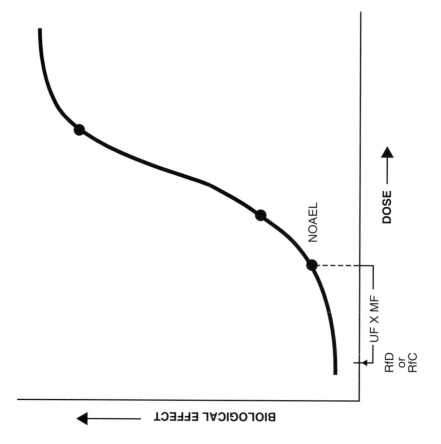

FIGURE 24.20 A dose-response curve from a typical toxicology study showing the relationship of the Reference Dose (RfD) and Reference Concentration (RfC) to the No Observable Adverse Effect Level (NOAEL). The RfD and RfC are determined from data developed from a subchronic or chronic animal study and represents an estimate of the level of exposure to which the human population (including sensitive subpopulations) can be exposed during a lifetime without deleterious effects. The RfD and RfC are used by EPA for noncarcinogenic effects having a threshold. The RfD and RfC are derived by dividing the NOAEL by the product of several uncertainty factors (UF) and a modifying factor (MF) (*see* Table 24.55 for a description of commonly used UF and MF). Depending on the degree of uncertainty associated with the data, the RfD and RfC can span several orders of magnitude from the NOAEL. The reference values (RfD and RfC) are similar in concept to FDA's Acceptable Daily Intake (ADI) and OSHA's Permissible Exposure Limit (PEL).

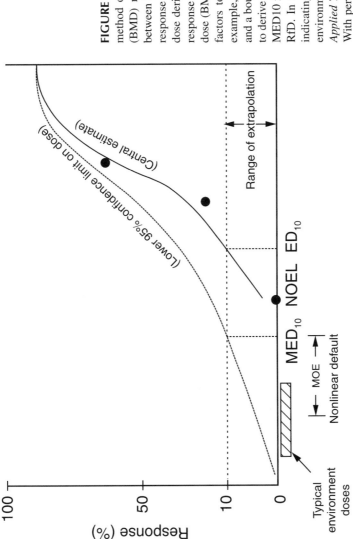

FIGURE 24.21 An alternative approach to the NOAEL method of deriving reference doses is the benchmark dose (BMD) method. In this approach, an effect level (usually between 1 and 10% response rate) is identified from the dose-response curve (solid line) and a bounding estimate on that dose derived (dotted line). A bound on the dose evoking the response of interest is identified and this value, the benchmark dose (BMD) is once again divided by appropriate uncertainty factors to derive a reference dose or concentration. In this example, the dose causing a 10% response is chosen (ED10) and a bounding estimate (dotted line) on this response is used to derive the BMD or minimum effective dose (MED10). The MED10 is then divided by an uncertainty factor to derive the RfD. In this case, the margin of exposure (MOE) is shown indicating where the MED10 is found in relation to the typical environmental exposure. (From Gargas et al., *General and Applied Toxicology,* 1999,[78] Grove's Dictionaries, New York. With permission.)

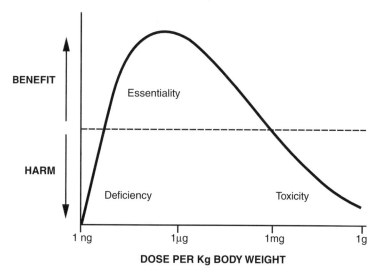

FIGURE 24.22 Harmful effects associated with a substance (deficiency and toxicity) can be produced at both low and high doses. Examples of such materials include metals that act as cofactors for essential biochemical processes. Note the wide range in the dosage scale. Because of the large uncertainty factors associated with risk assessment, the estimated safe exposure levels of such substances may fall at or near the levels which result in deficiency. This emphasizes the sometimes ultraconservative approaches used in the risk assessment process. (Modified from Crone, 1986.[19])

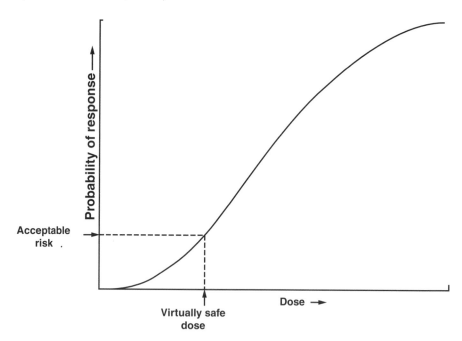

FIGURE 24.23 The determination of a Virtually Safe Dose (VSD). Applied by regulatory agencies for carcinogens which are assumed not to have a threshold, the VSD is defined as the exposure level which is not expected to produce an excess of cancers beyond that which is deemed acceptable to society (acceptable risk). Acceptable risk is generally considered to be 1×10^{-6} (one in one million) but can range between 10^{-4} and 10^{-7} depending on the chemical of concern and the circumstances of the exposure. (Reprinted from Munro, I.C. and Krewski, D.R., *FD. Chem. Toxicol.*, 19, 549, 1981,[20] with kind permission from Elsevier Science, The Boulevard, Langford Lane, Kidlington OX5168B UK.)

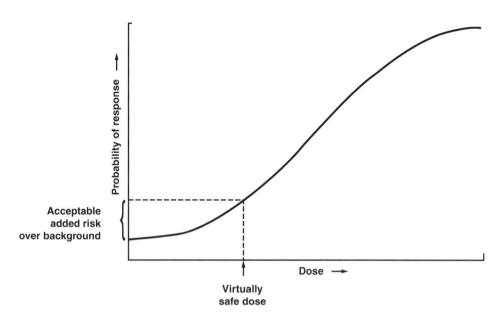

FIGURE 24.24 The determination of a Virtually Safe Dose (VSD) in the presence of background. (Reprinted from Munro, I.C. and Krewski, D.R., *FD. Chem. Toxicol..* 19, 549, 1981,[20] with kind permission from Elsevier Science, The Boulevard, Langford Lane, Kidlington OX5168B UK.)

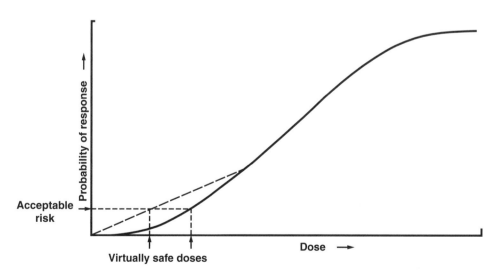

FIGURE 24.25 The effect of linear extrapolation of a sublinear dose-response curve on the determination of a virtually safe dose (VSD). (Reprinted from Munro, I.C. and Krewski, D.R., *FD. Chem. Toxicol.,* 19, 549, 1981,[20] with kind permission from Elsevier Science, The Boulevard, Langford Lane, Kidlington OX5168B UK.)

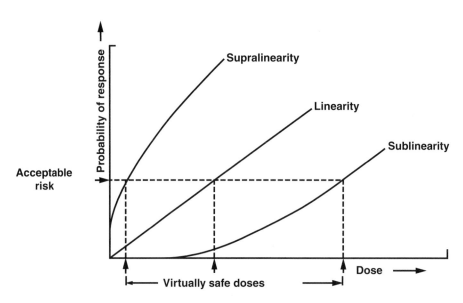

FIGURE 24.26 The effect of the shape of the dose-response curve on the determination of a virtually safe dose (VSD). (Reprinted from Munro, I.C. and Krewski, D.R., *FD. Chem. Toxicol.*, 19, 549,1981,[20] with kind permission from Elsevier Science, The Boulevard, Langford Lane, Kidlington OX5168B UK.)

TABLE 24.8
Mathematical Models Used in the Determination of Low-Dose Response Relationships for Potentially Carcinogenic Agents

Model	Description	Probability of a Test Animal Responding at Dose Level "d"	Shape of Parameter	Low-Dose Response
One-hit	Based on the concept that a response will occur after the target has been "hit" by a single biologically effective unit of dose	$1 - \exp^{-\beta d}$	$\beta > 0$	Linear at low doses
Multihit	Based on an extension of the one-hit model assuming that more than one hit is required to induce a response	$\int_{o}^{\beta d} (u^{k-1}e^{-u} / r(k))du$	$k > 0$ $\beta > 0$	Linear at low doses only when the shape parameters are equal to unity
Weibull		$1 - \exp^{-\beta d^m}$	$m > 0$ $\beta > 0$	When shape parameters are curves approaching zero at slower than linear or sublinear rate
Multistage	Based on the assumption that the induction of irreversible self-replicating toxic effects is the result of a number of random biological events, the time of each being in strict linear proportion to the dose rate.	$1 - \exp - \sum_{i=L}^{k} \alpha_i d^i$	k, an integer $\alpha_i > 0$ $i = 1 \rightarrow k$	Linear at low doses only when the linear coefficient B_i is positive; the relationship is sublinear otherwise

Data from Van Ryzin, 1980,[21] Van Ryzin and Rai, 1980,[22] and Munro and Krewski, 1981.[20] From Ecobichon, *The Basis of Toxicity Testing*, 1992.[18] With permission.

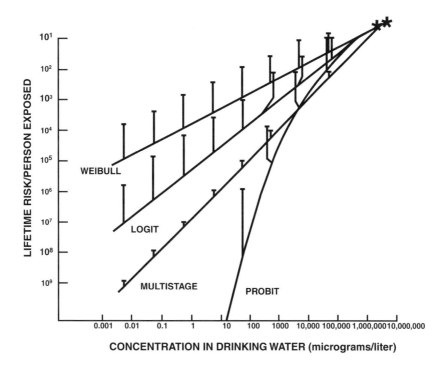

FIGURE 24.27 Dose-response curves extrapolated with data from a chronic bioassay (represented by the starred points in the upper right-hand corner of the figure) using the Weibull, Logit, Multistage, and Probit models. The curves are drawn from the point estimates with the vertical bars indicating the upper 95% confidence limit. The lower 95% confidence limit is the horizontal axis. This figure demonstrates the degree of variability (as much as several orders of magnitude) which can occur between the curves generated by the various models. (Modified from U.S. Environmental Protection Agency, 1984.[12])

SECTION 4. EPIDEMIOLOGY

Epidemiology, the study of the distribution and determinants of disease in human populations, is one of the tools used in the hazard identification step of the risk assessment process (see Figure 24.1). Despite the many problems inherent to epidemiological studies including various biases, confounding factors, and inadequate quantitation of exposures, these studies offer a major advantage over those conducted with animals: the direct observation of effects in humans.

Much of the uncertainty associated with risk assessment results from the extrapolation of animal data to humans. Quality epidemiology studies can significantly reduce or eliminate such uncertainty. For this reason, human data are preferred over animal data for risk assessment (see Table 24.1). Usually, however, the availability of quality epidemiological studies is limited, and human, animal and *in vitro* data are used together in a "weight-of-evidence" approach to the risk assessment process.

Most toxicologists will encounter epidemiological data at some point in their careers. Epidemiology has its own unique methodology, measurement indices, and terminology. Much of the information from these studies is reported as relative risks, rates, ratios, and proportions. This section provides the toxicologist with an overview of epidemiological study designs, their uses and limitations, and the type of information they provide. In addition, general information on incidence and causation is provided for human cancer and reproductive and developmental effects; endpoints are frequently the focus of epidemiological studies. Knowledge of such information is useful for evaluating the design and interpreting the results of human studies.

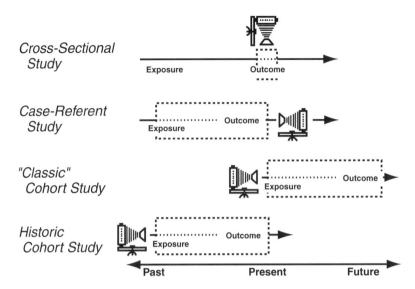

FIGURE 24.28 Common epidemiological study designs. The cross-sectional study takes a snapshot of both exposure and outcome at a particular point in time. In the case-referent study, the investigator identifies the outcome and looks back at the exposure. The cohort study can be done from two perspectives. Both approaches identify exposure groups and follow them to observe outcomes; however, one is done historically on past events, and the other identifies current exposures and follows the study members forward. (From Selevan, *Occupational and Environmental Reproductive Hazards: A Guide for Clinicians,* 1993.[23] With permission.)

TABLE 24.9
Human Data Commonly Used in Risk Assessment

Study Type	Alternative Terms	Comments on Use
Cross-sectional	Prevalence, survey	Sampling of a population at a given point in time to assess prevalence of a disease. Most useful for studying chronic diseases of high frequency. Cannot measure incidence. Although associations may be drawn with prevalent cases, the temporal and causal order of such associations cannot be determined.
Case-control	Retrospective, dose or case-referent, case history	Compares previous exposure in subjects with disease with one or more groups of subjects without disease. Selection of cases and noncases can be controlled. Exposures cannot be controlled. If exposure data available, a NOEL may be identified. Exposure history may be difficult to reconstruct outside of an occupational setting. Recall and other biases are possible due to retrospective evaluation. Allows estimation of relative odds of exposure in cases and controls but not absolute risk.
Cohort	Longitudinal, prospective, incidence	Population or sample of subjects at risk of disease observed through time for outcome of interest. May fail to detect rare outcome. Many factors can be controlled for reduced bias (prospective design). Dose-response curves may be constructed if dose or exposure data available. Allows estimation of absolute and relative risk.
Clinical trials		Type of cohort study in which investigator controls treatment (exposure). Generally not applicable to environmental issues. Intervention trials in which an exposure is removed or changed (e.g., medication, smoking, diet) are useful for evaluating causality.
Experimental studies		Controlled human exposures generally of low dose and limited exposure time. Used for hazard identification, dose-response, and risk characterization.
Case reports		Suggests nature of acute endpoints. Cannot be used to support absence of hazard.

Modified from Piantadosi, 1992,[24] U.S. Environmental Protection Agency, 1989.[25]

TABLE 24.10
Epidemiological Terms

Annual crude death rate $= \dfrac{\text{Total number of deaths during a given year}}{\text{total population at midyear}} \times 1000$

Annual specific death rate $= \dfrac{\text{total number of deaths in a specific group during a given year}}{\text{total population in the specific group at mid year}} \times 100$

Proportional mortality rate $= \dfrac{\text{total number of deaths in a specific group}}{\text{Total number of deaths}} \times 100$

Infant mortality rate (IMR) $= \dfrac{\text{Infant deaths}}{\text{Total lives births}}$

Standard mortality rate (SMR) $= \dfrac{\text{Observed deaths}}{\text{Expected deaths}}$

Cause-of-death ratio $= \dfrac{\text{Deaths from a specific cause over a period of time}}{\text{Total deaths due to all causes in the same time period}} \times 100$

Incidence rate $= \dfrac{\text{Number of new cases over a period of time}}{\text{Population at risk over the same time period}}$

Prevalence rate $= \dfrac{\text{Number of existing cases at a point in time}}{\text{total population}}$

Relative risk (risk ratio) $= \dfrac{\text{Incidence among the exposed}}{\text{Incidence among the nonexposed}}$

Attributal risk (risk difference) $=$ Incidence among the exposed $-$ Incidence among the nonexposed

Relative odds ratio $= \dfrac{\text{Number of exposed individuals with disease}}{\text{Number of exposed individuals without disease}}$
$\times \dfrac{\text{Number of nonexposed individuals without disease}}{\text{Number of nonexposed individuals with disease}}$

Source: Selevan, 1993,[23] Hallenbeck and Cunningham, 1986,[4] Gamble and Battigelli, 1978.[26]

TABLE 24.11
Steps in the Investigation of a Cancer Cluster

1. Each case of cancer must be identified and confirmed. Histopathology and medical records should be reviewed for accuracy of diagnosis.
2. The time of occurrence of the cancer case should be identified. Employees working for the company during this time should be evaluated. This step of the investigation can be affected by a changing workforce.
3. The observed number of cases should be compared with the expected number of cases. The expected number of cases may be obtained from cancer registries. This comparison should be age standardized, because the majority of cancer occurs in older individuals. Comparison of the observed number of cases with the expected number allows for the calculation of a standard mortality ratio (SMR). An SMR greater than one may indicate an excess of cancer.
4. After the types of cancer are identified, determination should be made of whether a particular cell type or target organ is overrepresented in the population being studied.
5. The latency period must be evaluated. Latency is the time from the onset of exposure to a certain chemical or environment to appearance of clinical disease. The latency period for solid tumors is 15–20 years, and for hernatological tumors, 5–10 years. If an individual is noted to have cancer after a recent exposure, then the latency period is too short to implicate the chemical or the environment as the cause.
6. Confounding and contributing factors must be evaluated. These include smoking, substance and drug abuse, a family history of cancer, multiple exposures to other chemicals or potential carcinogens, or employment in an industry that has been associated with carcinogenesis.

TABLE 24.11 *(Continued)*
Steps in the Investigation of a Cancer Cluster

7. There may be a particular job or site in an area of industry that is overrepresented in cases of cancer. The standard mortality ratio may not show an elevation of cancer cases in the industry overall, but specific jobs or sites may show an excess of deaths if separate SMRs are calculated for these sites and job descriptions.
8. If an excess of similar cases exists, then the issue of causation must be addressed. A chemical may be responsible, and further investigation is warranted. If there is a mixture of cancer types, then this is unlikely to be a true cancer cluster. If there is overrepresentation by a particular job, environment, or chemical exposure than a cluster may indeed be occurring. If there is no pattern of common exposures or job site locations, then the chances of a cluster are diminished.
9. An environmental assessment and industrial hygiene review is warranted to determine whether exposures to potential carcinogens are occurring. Previous environment surveys should be reviewed and appropriate environmental monitoring conducted as needed.
10. The investigation should conclude that:
    a. cluster is not present
    b. a cluster may be present but is inconsistent with an occupational or environmental exposure cause
    c. a cluster is present and could be related to a chemical or environmental exposure; or
    d. the cluster is definitely related to the exposure.
    If an exposure or occupational setting is implicated, then aggressive corrective action must be undertaken.

From Piantadosi and Sullivan, *Hazardous Materials Toxicology: Clinical Principals of Environmental Health,* 1992.[27] With permission.

TABLE 24.12
Overall Evaluation of Human and Animal Evidence about the Carcinogenicity of 597 Agents[a]

	Humans				
Animals	**Sufficient**	**Limited**	**Inadequate**	**No Adequate Data**	**Total**
Sufficient	21 (3.5)	12 (2.0)	47 (7.9)	123 (20.6)	203 (34.0)
Limited	8 (1.3)	1 (0.2)	28 (4.7)	124 (20.8)	161 (27.0)
Inadequate	6 (1.0)	1 (0.2)	33 (5.5)	164 (27.5)	204 (34.2)
No adequate data	1 (0.2)	0	1 (0.2)	24 (4.0)	26 (4.4)
Lack of carcinogenicity	0	0	1 (0.2)	2 (0.3)	3 (0.5)
Total	36 (6.0)	14 (2.3)	110 (18.4)	437 (73.2)	597 (100.0)

[a] Classified are 597 agents from the 1987 IARC database. As can be seen for 36 agents (6%), sufficient evidence of carcinogenicity in humans exists. Of the 36 human carcinogens, 15 (41.7%) did not show sufficient evidence of carcinogenicity in animals. For one of these agents, no adequate animal data existed. In contrast, for 203 agents (34%), sufficient evidence of carcinogenicity in experimental animals is available. Only 21 of these 203 agents (10.3%) also proved to be a human carcinogen. This is partly due to the fact that for 123 agents, no adequate human data existed. Nevertheless, for 59 of the 203 agents (29%), the existing human evidence resulted in an evaluation that differed from the categorization based on animal evidence. The majority of agents that seemed to be carcinogenic in animals did not seem to produce clear and positive results in humans. For agents with sufficient evidence based on human epidemiology, the correspondence with animal experimental data is weak.

Data from IARC, 1987,[28] from Meijers et al., 1992.[29] With permission.

TABLE 24.13
Estimates on Causes of Cancer

Factor	USA, 1981		Birmingham England, 1979 Estimate (%)		USA, 1977 Estimate (%)	
	Estimate (%)	Range (%)	Male	Female	Male	Female
Tobacco	30	25–40	30	7	28	8
Alcohol	3	2–4	5	3	4	1
Tobacco/alcohol						
Diet	35	10–70	30	63	40	57
Life style						
Food additives	<1	–5–2				
Reproduction and sexual behavior	7	1–13				
Occupation	4	2–8	6	2	4	2
Industrial products	<1	<1–2				
Pollution	2	<1–5				
Sunlight			10	10		
Ionizing radiation					8	8
Geophysical factors	3	2–4	1	1		
Iatrogenic (drugs and medical procedures)	1	0.5–3	1	1		
Infection	10?	1–?				
Exogenous hormones					—	4
Congenital			2	2	16	20
Unknown			15	11		

Data from Doll and Peto, 1981,[30] Higginson and Muir, 1979,[31] Wynder and Gori, 1977,[32] from Weisburger, *Dangerous Properties of Industrial Materials*, 1984.[33] With permission.

TABLE 24.14
Top 12 Most Frequently Observed Site-Specific Cancers in Humans in the United States for the 2-Year Period 1986–1987[a] with Estimated Ranking for Year 2000

	Males and Females		Males		Females	
	Site	Rate	Site	Rate	Site	Rate
A. Cancer Incidence Rates						
1.	Breast	61.3	(1)[b] Prostate gland	94.2	(1)[b] Breast	112.1
2.	Lung and bronchus	56.6	(2) Lung and bronchus	82.0	(3) Colon/rectum	41.7
3.	Colon/rectum	49.8	(3) Colon/rectum	61.2	(2) Lung and bronchus	38.1
4.	Prostate gland	38.2	(4) Urinary bladder	32.4	(4) Cervix uteri, corpus and uterus	30.0
5.	Urinary bladder	18.1	(5) Non-Hodgkin's lymphoma	17.1	(6) Ovary	13.9
6.	Cervix uteri, corpus and uterus	16.3	(7) Oral and pharynx	16.4	(5) Non-Hodgkin's lymphoma	11.0
7.	Non-Hodgkin's lymphoma	13.8	(9) Leukemia	13.0	(7) Melanoma of skin	10.0
8.	Melanoma of skin	11.2	(6) Melanoma of skin	12.9	(9) Pancreas	7.6
9.	Oral and pharynx	10.9	(8) Kidney	11.7	(8) Urinary bladder	7.6
10.	Leukemia	9.7	(11) Stomach	10.6	(10) Leukemia	7.4
11.	Pancreas	8.8	(10) Pancreas	10.6	(11) Thyroid gland	6.1
12.	Kidney	8.4	(12) Larynx	8.2	(12) Brain and nervous system	5.8
B. Cancer Mortality Rates						
1.	Lung and bronchus	47.4	(1) Lung and bronchus	74.5	(1)[b] Lung and bronchus	27.6
2.	Colon/rectum	20.2	(3) Colon/rectum	24.5	(2) Breast	27.2
3.	Prostate gland	15.3	(2) Prostate gland	24.4	(3) Colon/rectum	16.8
4.	Pancreas	9.2	(4) Pancreas	10.0	(5) Ovary	7.7
5.	Pancreas	8.4	(6) Leukemia	8.3	(4) Pancreas	7.2
6.	Leukemia	6.3	(10) Stomach	7.2	(8) Cervix uteri, corpus and uterus	6.7
7.	Non-Hodgkin's lymphoma	5.8	(5) Non-Hodgkin's lymphoma	7.1	(7) Leukemia	4.9
8.	Stomach	4.9	(7) Esophagus	5.8	(6) Non-Hodgkin's lymphoma	4.8
9.	Ovary	4.3	(4) Urinary bladder	5.7	(9) Brain and nervous system	3.3
10.	Brain and nervous system	4.1	(12) Brain and nervous system	4.9	(10)[c] Stomach	3.2
11.	Kidney	3.4	(11) Kidney	4.8	(10)[c] Multiple myeloma	2.4
12.	Urinary bladder	3.3	(8) Liver	3.7	(11) Kidney	2.3

[a] Age adjusted rates per 100,000 population

[b] Values in brackets are relative ranking based on year 2000 estimates.

[c] Predicted rate for stomach and multiple myeloma is the same for year 2000.

Data from Ries et al., 1990[34] and American Cancer Society, 2000.[36] Original table from Huff et al., 1991.[35]

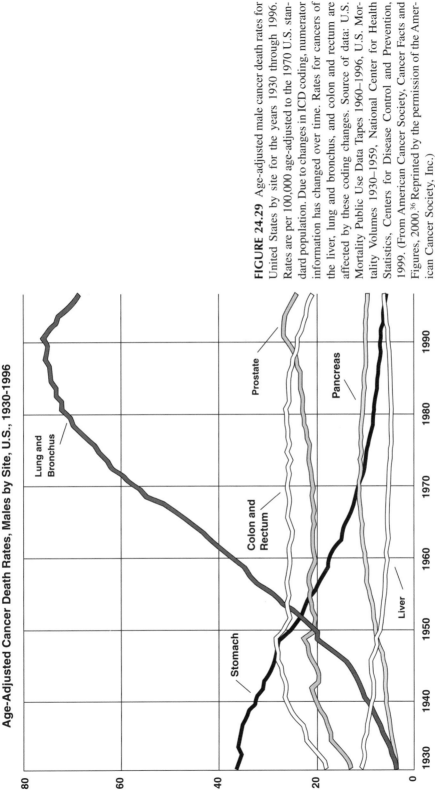

FIGURE 24.29 Age-adjusted male cancer death rates for United States by site for the years 1930 through 1996. Rates are per 100,000 age-adjusted to the 1970 U.S. standard population. Due to changes in ICD coding, numerator information has changed over time. Rates for cancers of the liver, lung and bronchus, and colon and rectum are affected by these coding changes. Source of data: U.S. Mortality Public Use Data Tapes 1960–1996, U.S. Mortality Volumes 1930–1959, National Center for Health Statistics, Centers for Disease Control and Prevention, 1999. (From American Cancer Society, Cancer Facts and Figures, 2000.[36] Reprinted by the permission of the American Cancer Society, Inc.)

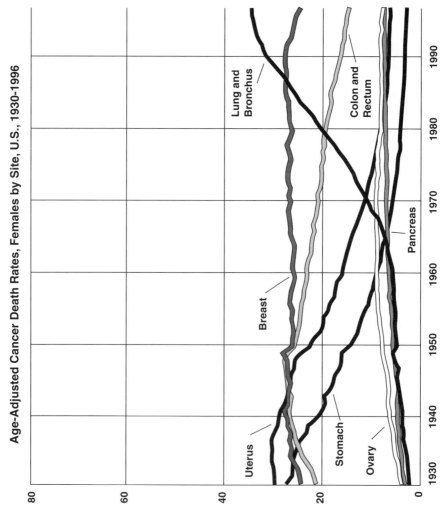

Age-Adjusted Cancer Death Rates, Females by Site, U.S., 1930–1996

FIGURE 24.30 Age-adjusted female cancer death rates for United States by site for the years 1930 through 1996. Rates are per 100,000 age-adjusted to the 1970 U.S. standard population. Uterus cancer death rates are for uterine cervix and uterine corpus combined. Due to changes in ICD coding, numerator information has changed over time. Rates for cancers of the uterus, ovary, lung and bronchus, and colon and rectum are affected by these coding changes. Source of data: U.S. Mortality Public Use Data Tapes 1960–1996, U.S. Mortality Volumes 1930–1959, National Center for Health Statistics, Centers for Disease Control and Prevention, 1999. (From American Cancer Society, Cancer Facts and Figures, 2000.[36] Reprinted by the permission of the American Cancer Society, Inc.)

TABLE 24.15
Cancer Mortality Rates per 100,000 for Women by Indicated Age Group for the Years 1962 to 1987

Year	25–29	30–34	35–39	40–44	45–49	50–54	55–59	60–64	65–69	70–74	75–79	80–84	85+	ACMR[a]
1962	12.8	26.3	49.7	87.8	145.0	220.0	283.9	389.3	513.1	628.7	798.5	1031	1279	136.1
1963	13.6	24.9	50.5	87.0	146.9	214.3	294.6	383.7	509.2	632.3	795.3	1014	1301	136.6
1964	13.0	26.9	49.6	88.1	144.3	220.9	292.3	378.2	509.2	620.7	778.4	999.3	1260	136.2
1965	12.9	27.3	47.8	88.6	144.7	219.3	296.3	381.4	511.1	638.4	793.8	985.2	1276	137.9
1966	12.6	25.7	48.3	87.3	146.1	217.4	296.7	378.1	515.6	640.0	783.9	987.1	1296	138.8
1967	12.0	24.0	47.6	86.9	145.3	217.8	298.0	385.6	515.6	654.6	779.6	974.3	1270	140.2
1968	11.3	24.2	48.7	86.3	146.0	221.3	298.4	391.4	510.0	653.4	795.4	944.2	1273	141.6
1969	11.1	23.7	46.5	87.6	143.7	215.4	302.1	389.0	513.7	645.7	781.9	971.5	1276	142.0
1970	11.9	22.3	46.6	83.2	146.0	220.1	307.3	384.0	499.3	630.1	828.8	993.8	1096	144.3
1971	11.6	22.7	43.0	85.2	143.1	217.1	302.0	398.9	511.2	659.6	805.1	953.4	1260	145.0
1972	11.4	22.0	43.3	82.7	144.6	214.3	309.2	388.4	507.1	654.3	820.7	965.5	1174	147.2
1973	10.8	21.5	43.7	78.0	143.9	213.3	314.9	399.6	502.3	643.8	838.1	958.2	1143	148.4
1974	11.1	20.8	42.8	79.1	141.9	212.6	314.6	412.8	494.8	661.3	840.7	990.3	1134	151.0
1975	10.3	20.1	39.5	77.7	139.5	212.7	309.4	411.8	485.9	667.6	847.8	1000	1128	152.1
1976	10.5	20.7	39.5	74.1	135.3	216.2	311.5	425.6	505.1	672.1	862.9	1008	1159	156.0
1977	9.8	20.2	37.6	74.3	136.4	215.6	312.8	433.2	517.1	666.8	875.3	1028	1144	158.6
1978	9.9	19.3	35.5	75.0	135.3	216.8	310.3	439.3	520.9	676.7	891.8	1055	1139	161.4
1979	9.3	18.9	36.9	71.2	129.1	215.3	309.7	432.8	530.8	664.3	893.0	1057	1124	162.1
1980	9.6	18.8	37.6	71.6	128.5	212.4	307.5	423.0	542.8	686.4	820.5	1030	1255	163.6
1981	9.0	18.1	36.4	69.1	125.5	211.2	309.7	419.1	551.0	673.9	827.7	1025	1244	164.7
1982	8.7	18.5	35.7	68.7	125.6	208.7	310.6	428.0	564.9	683.7	840.9	1017	1256	167.8
1983	8.7	17.5	35.8	67.1	122.7	206.8	312.4	434.2	558.9	712.7	839.1	1041	1253	170.1
1984	8.9	17.8	36.8	69.6	122.8	207.3	313.5	440.0	573.7	714.8	860.7	1073	1271	173.5
1985	8.5	18.0	35.0	66.8	124.2	206.0	311.7	447.5	571.1	731.9	868.1	1072	1263	175.1
1986	8.7	17.2	35.0	68.8	121.3	203.4	303.8	444.0	579.9	750.8	874.6	1077	1277	176.8
1987	8.4	17.2	35.0	63.1	120.4	203.8	304.6	444.4	577.2	743.8	892.9	1081	1283	178.0

Age (Years)

[a] Annual crude mortality rates (ACMR).

From Riggs, 1992.[37] With permission.

TABLE 24.16
Cancer Mortality Rates per 100,000 for Men by Indicated Age Group for the Years 1962 to 1987

Year	| Age (Years)													ACMR[a]
	25–29	30–34	35–39	40–44	45–49	50–54	55–59	60–64	65–69	70–74	75–79	80–84	85+	
1962	14.1	21.1	34.7	63.9	123.0	228.1	371.3	574.2	832.1	1036	1272	1565	1850	164.2
1963	14.2	22.0	35.5	64.2	124.8	228.2	381.2	573.2	858.1	1067	1295	1545	1884	166.5
1964	15.2	22.4	36.3	67.9	123.5	230.6	382.5	586.5	853.3	1076	1313	1525	1803	167.0
1965	14.8	21.1	37.0	67.4	124.9	230.7	393.2	591.2	868.5	1113	1325	1567	1842	169.7
1966	14.1	21.5	36.8	69.1	126.2	238.3	391.8	598.1	871.3	1137	1357	1572	1812	172.0
1967	13.8	21.2	36.4	67.3	126.9	236.1	398.1	608.7	874.1	1181	1394	1572	1833	174.9
1968	14.1	21.0	37.2	69.2	130.4	239.5	400.4	628.7	882.7	1220	1406	1585	1816	178.0
1969	14.5	19.9	36.9	70.7	128.5	237.1	406.5	626.7	881.0	1209	1436	1594	1829	178.8
1970	13.4	19.6	34.8	69.9	132.2	239.7	412.3	629.6	890.4	1164	1494	1755	1722	182.1
1971	14.0	20.9	34.9	68.1	128.8	236.1	405.5	635.3	903.5	1232	1548	1668	1812	182.1
1972	12.8	18.5	34.5	67.7	132.5	231.7	420.6	627.5	899.3	1229	1570	1792	1917	185.7
1973	13.1	18.4	35.5	65.7	135.5	232.1	408.7	633.0	901.1	1223	1580	1807	2018	187.1
1974	11.9	17.6	33.1	64.8	138.1	242.7	410.1	649.1	904.0	1249	1633	1849	1985	191.1
1975	12.4	18.2	31.3	64.3	133.6	240.9	400.2	642.7	902.3	1271	1624	1899	1987	192.3
1976	11.9	16. 6	30.6	63.5	133.5	241.5	405.2	656.1	912.6	1276	1686	1938	2042	196.6
1977	12.5	16.6	31.3	63.3	130.4	245.3	404.4	660.5	911.9	1292	1710	1969	2102	200.0
1978	11.4	17.1	30.2	62.2	130.8	251.8	403.1	666.4	920.7	1298	1721	2065	2137	203.5
1979	11.6	15.9	29.0	61.5	129.0	248.1	405.3	660.4	930.2	1291	1744	2073	2130	205.6
1980	11.3	15.8	29.3	61.6	128.1	246.7	414.8	645.1	947.5	1292	1656	2034	2368	205.3
1981	10.5	14.9	28.5	60.4	127.6	244.7	413.9	637.1	939.4	1284	1625	2006	2351	204.5
1982	10.0	16.2	28.8	58.4	124.6	244.0	412.7	644.2	954.2	1277	1671	2027	2410	207.6
1983	10.3	15.6	28.2	56.7	123.6	236.4	418.5	639.7	929.9	1300	1689	2070	2386	209.6
1984	9.9	16.1	28.0	58.8	119.0	238.0	424.4	644.3	929.5	1298	1674	2110	2427	211.0
1985	10.3	16.0	28.7	59.5	119.8	233.3	416.4	651.7	925.5	1297	1686	2127	2414	212.5
1986	10.7	16.3	27.8	57.9	117.4	230.2	406.7	647.7	925.0	1304	1679	2155	2460	213.5
1987	9.4	14.8	26.9	54.0	115.2	230.6	408.6	653.6	922.8	1302	1684	2156	2475	214.8

[a] Annual crude mortality rates (ACMR).

From Riggs, 1992.[37] With permission.

TABLE 24.17
Probability (%) of Developing Invasive Cancers Over Selected Age Intervals, by Sex, United States, 1994–1996[a]

		Birth to 39	40–59	60–79	Birth to Death
All Sites[b]	Male	1.61 (1 in 62)	8.17 (1 in 12)	33.65 (1 in 3)	43.56 (1 in 2)
	Female	1.94 (1 in 52)	9.23 (1 in 11)	22.27 (1 in 4)	38.11 (1 in 3)
Breast	Female	0.43 (1 in 235)	4.06 (1 in 25)	6.88 (1 in 15)	12.56 (1 in 8)
Colon and Rectum	Male	0.06 (1 in 1,579)	0.85 (1 in 124)	3.97 (1 in 29)	5.64 (1 in 18)
	Female	0.05 (1 in 1,947)	0.67 (1 in 149)	3.06 (1 in 33)	5.55 (1 in 18)
Lung and Bronchus	Male	0.04 (1 in 2,592)	1.29 (1 in 78)	6.35 (1 in 16)	8.11 (1 in 12)
	Female	0.03 (1 in 2,894)	0.94 (1 in 106)	3.98 (1 in 25)	5.69 (1 in 18)
Prostate	Male	<1 in 10,000	1.90 (1 in 53)	13.69 (1 in 7)	15.91 (1 in 6)

[a] Of those free of cancer at beginning of age interval. Based on cancer cases diagnosed during 1994–1996. The "1 in" statistic and the inverse of the percentage may not be equivalent due to rounding.

[b] Excludes basal and squamous cell skin cancers and *in situ* carcinomas except urinary bladder.

Data source: DEVCAN Software, Version 4.0, Surveillance, Epidemiology and End Results Program, 1973–1996, Division of Cancer Control and Population Sciences, National Cancer Institute.

Table from American Cancer Society *Cancer Facts and Figures 2000*,[36] with permission.

TABLE 24.18
Cancer Death Rates Per 100,000 Population for Selected Countries: Males

	All Sites	Oral	Colon and Rectum	Prostate	Lung and Bronchus	Stomach	Leukemia
United States (a)	156.0	3.2	15.2	15.9	52.3	4.4	6.3
Canada (b)	156.2	3.8	16.1	16.4	50.0	6.2	5.5
Mexico (b)	85.0	1.9	3.6	12.8	16.2	9.7	3.9
Chile (d)	142.5	2.1	7.0	16.0	20.5	32.2	4.2
Columbia (d)	97.7	2.1	4.8	12.6	14.3	21.4	4.3
Venezuela (d)	104.3	2.5	5.9	20.3	19.4	16.8	4.1
United Kingdom (a)	164.2	2.9	18.0	16.6	46.6	9.5	4.7
France (b)	188.2	11.3	16.6	15.8	46.5	7.2	5.6
Germany (a)	169.5	6.5	20.8	16.6	45.4	12.0	5.5
Netherlands (b)	182.3	2.8	17.7	19.4	62.0	10.3	5.7
Russian Federation (b)	237.1	9.1	18.2	7.2	70.5	36.9	5.1
Poland (c)	204.9	6.3	16.4	11.1	71.3	18.9	5.6
Australia (b)	156.7	4.1	20.2	19.0	38.8	6.6	6.1
China (d, e)	149.9	2.6	7.9	—	37.3	26.9	3.7
Japan (g)	155.2	3.1	17.1	5.1	31.7	30.2	4.1

Note: Rates are age-adjusted to the World Health Organization world standard population. a = 1994–1997, b = 1994–1995, c = 1994–1996, d = 1994 only, e = oral cancer mortality rate includes nasopharynx only, f = 1995–1996, g = 1995–1997.

Data source: Mortality Database 1994–1997, World Health Organization, 1999.

Table adapted from American Cancer Society, *Cancer Facts and Figures, 2000.*[36]

TABLE 24.19
Cancer Death Rates Per 100,000 Population for Selected Countries: Females

	All Sites	Oral	Colon and Rectum	Breast	Lung and Bronchus	Uterus (Cervix)	Stomach	Leukemia
United States (a)	108.3	1.1	10.4	20.0	26.6	2.4	2.0	3.7
Canada (b)	106.6	1.2	10.3	21.5	23.0	1.9	3.0	3.2
Mexico (b)	78.9	0.7	3.3	9.3	6.0	14.0	7.1	3.1
Chile (d)	105.3	0.6	6.7	12.1	6.4	10.6	11.7	2.7
Columbia (d)	89.1	1.2	5.1	9.1	6.8	9.9	13.1	3.7
Venezuela (d)	90.0	1.2	6.2	11.8	9.3	10.8	9.7	3.1
United Kingdom (a)	116.5	1.1	11.6	24.5	20.5	3.0	3.9	3.0
France (b)	84.8	1.3	9.6	19.6	6.1	1.6	2.8	3.3
Germany (a)	103.3	1.2	14.0	21.7	9.4	2.8	6.3	3.5
Netherlands (b)	108.0	1.0	12.7	26.0	13.6	1.7	4.2	3.1
Russian Federation (b)	107.6	1.1	12.6	16.1	7.0	5.0	15.3	3.5
Poland (c)	107.6	1.1	11.0	16.1	11.1	7.3	6.8	3.5
Australia (b)	98.2	1.2	13.3	19.9	13.6	2.6	2.7	3.6
China (d, e)	83.5	1.1	6.4	5.0	15.8	3.0	12.7	3.0
Japan (g)	75.7	0.8	9.9	7.7	8.5	1.9	12.3	2.5

Note: Rates are age-adjusted to the World Health Organization world standard population. a = 1994–1997, b = 1994–1995, c = 1994–1996, d = 1994 only, e = oral cancer mortality rate includes nasopharynx only, f = 1995–1996, g = 1995–1997.

Data source: Mortality Database 1994–1997, World Health Organization, 1999.

Table adapted from American Cancer Society, *Cancer Facts and Figures, 2000.*[36]

TABLE 24.20
Known[a] and Suspect[b] Human Carcinogens

Agents, Substances, Mixtures or Exposure Circumstances Known To Be Human Carcinogens

Aflatoxins
Alcoholic Beverage Consumption
4-Aminobiphenyl (4-Aminodiphenyl)
Analgesic Mixtures Containing Phenacetin
Arsenic and Certain Arsenic Compounds
Asbestos
Azathioprine
Benzene
Benzidine
bis(Chloromethyl) Ether and Technical-Grade Chloromethyl Methyl Ether
1,3-Butadiene
1,4-Butanediol Dimethylsufonate
Cadmium and Cadmium Compounds
Chlorambucil

1-(2-Chloroethyl)-3-(4-methylcyclohexyl)-1-nitrosourea (MeCCNU)
Chromium Hexavalent Compounds
Coke Oven Emissions
Conjugated Estrogens
Cyclophosphamide
Cyclosporin A
Diethylstilbestrol

TABLE 24.20 *(Continued)*
Known[a] and Suspect[b] Human Carcinogens

Dyes that Metabolize to Benizidine
- Direct Black 38
- Direct Blue 6

Environmental Tobacco Smoke
Erionite
Ethylene Oxide
Melphalan
Methoxsalen with Ultraviolet A Therapy (PUVA)
Mustard Gas
2-Naphthylamine
Radon
Silica, Crystalline (Respirable Size)
- Quartz
- Cristobalite
- Tridymite

Smokeless Tobacco
Solar Radiation and Exposure to Sunlamps or Sunbeds
Soots
Strong Inorganic Acid Mists Containing Sulfuric Acid
Tamoxifen
Tars and Mineral Oils
Thiotepa
Thorium Dioxide
Tobacco Smoking
Vinyl Chloride

Agents, Substances, Mixtures or Exposure Circumstances Reasonably Anticipated to be Human Carcinogens
Acetaldehyde
2-Acetylaminofluorene
Acrylamide
Acrylonitrile
Adriamycin®
2-Aminoanthraquinone
o-Aminoazotoluene
1-Amino-2-methylanthraquinone
Amitrole
o-Anisidine Hydrochloride
Azacitidine
Benzotrichloride
Beryllium and Certain Beryllium Compounds
bis(Chloroethyl) nitrosourea
Bromodichloromethane
Butylated Hydroxyanisole
Carbon Tetrachloride
Ceramic Fibers (Respirable Size)
Chlorendic Acid
Chlorinated Paraffins (C_{12}-60% Chlorine)
1-(2-Chloroethyl)-3-cyclohexyl-l-nitrosourea
Chloroform
3-Chloro-2-methylpropene

TABLE 24.20 *(Continued)*
Known[a] and Suspect[b] Human Carcinogens

4-Chloro-*o*-phenylenediamine

Chloroprene

p-Chloro-*o*-toluidine and *p*-Chloro-*o*-toluidine Hydrochloride

Chlorozotocin

C.I. Basic Red 9 Monohydrochloride

Cisplatin

p-Cresidine

Cupferron

Dacarbazine

Danthron

DDT (Dichlorodiphenyltrichloroethane)

2,4-Diaminoanisole Sulfate

2,4-Diaminotoluene

1,2-Dibromo-3-chloropropane

1,2-Dibromoethane (Ethylene Dibromide)

1,4-Dichlorobenzene

3,3′-Dichlorobenzidine and 3,3′-Dichlorobenzidine Dihydrochloride

1,2-Dichloroethane

Dichloromethane

1,3-Dichloropropene (Technical Grade)

Diepoxybutane

Diesel Exhaust Particulates

Di(2-ethylhexyl) Phthalate

Diethyl Sulfate

Diglycidyl Resorcinol Ether

3,3′-Dimethoxybenzidine and 3,3′-Dimethoxybenzidine Dihydrochloride

4-Dimethylaminoazobenzene

3,3′-Dimethylbenzidine

Dimethylcarbamoyl Chloride

1,1-Dimethylhydrazine

Dimethyl Sulfate

Dimethylvinyl Chloride

1,4-Dioxane

Disperse Blue 1

Epichlorohydrin

Estrogens (Not Conjugated): Estradiol-17β

Estrogens (Not Conjugated): Estrone

Estrogens (Not Conjugated): Ethinylestradiol

Estrogens (Not Conjugated): Mestranol

Ethylene Thiourea

Ethyl Methanesulfonate

Formaldehyde (Gas)

Furan

Glasswool (Respirable Size)

Glycidol

Hexachlorobenzene

Hexachloroethane

Hexamethylphosphoramide

Hydrazine and Hydrazine Sulfate

Hydrazobenzene

Iron Dextran Complex

TABLE 24.20 *(Continued)*
Known[a] **and Suspect**[b] **Human Carcinogens**

Isoprene

Kepone®

Lead Acetate and Lead Phosphate

Lindane and Other Hexachlorocyclohexane Isomers

2-Methylaziridine (Propylenimine)

4,4′-Methylenebis(2-chloroaniline) (MBOCA)

4-4′-Methylenebis(*N,N*-dimethylbenzenamine)

4.4′-Methylenedianiline and Its Dihydrochloride

Methyl Methanesulfonate

N-Methyl-*N*′-nitro-*N*-nitrosoguanidine

Metronidazole

Michler's Ketone

Mirex

Nickel and Certain Nickel Compounds

Nitrilotriacetic Acid

o-Nitroanisole

Nitroarenes

- 1,6-Dinitropyrene
- 1,8-Dinitropyrene
- 6-Nitrochrysene
- 1-Nitropyrene
- 4-Nitropyrene

Nitrofen

Nitrogen Mustard Hydrochloride

2-Nitropropane

N-Nitrosodi-*n*-butylamine

N-Nitrosodiethanolamine

N-Nitrosodiethylamine

N-Nitrosodimethylamine

N-Nitrosodi-*n*-propylamine

N-Nitroso-*N*-ethylurea

4-(*N*-Nitrosomethylamino)-1-(3-pyridyl)-l-butanone (NNK)

N-Nitroso-*N*-methylurea

N-Nitrosomethylvinylamine

N-Nitrosomorpholine

N-Nitrosonornicotine

N-Nitrosopiperidine

N-Nitrosopyrrolidine

N-Nitrososarcosine

Norethisterone

Ochratoxin A

4.4′-Oxydianiline

Oxymetholone

Phenacetin

Phenazopyridine Hydrochloride

Phenolphthalein

Phenoxybenzamine Hydrochloride

Phenytoin

Polybrominated Biphenyls

Polychlorinated Biphenyls

Polycyclic Aromatic Hydrocarbons, 15 Listings

TABLE 24.20 *(Continued)*
Known[a] and Suspect[b] Human Carcinogens

- Benz[*a*]anthracene
- Benzo[*b*]fluoranthene
- Benzo[*j*]fluoranthene
- Benzo[*k*]fluoranthene
- Benzo[*a*]pyrene
- Dibenz[*a, h*] acridine
- Dibenz[*a, j*]acridine
- Dibenz[*a,h*]anthracene
- 7*H*-Dibenzo[*c,g*]carbazole
- Dibenzo[*a,e*]pyrene
- Dibenzo[*a,h*]pyrene
- Dibenzo[*a,i*]pyrene
- Dibenzo[*a,l*]pyrene
- Indeno[1,2,3-*cd*]pyrene
- 5-Methylchrysene

Procarbazine Hydrochloride
Progesterone
1,3-Propane Sultone
β-Propiolactone
Propylene Oxide
Propylthiouracil
Reserpine
Safrole
Selenium Sulfide
Streptozotocin
Sulfallate
*2,3,7,8-Tetrachlorodibenzo-*p*-dioxin (TCDD)
Tetrachloroethylene
Tetrafluoroethylene
Tetranitromethane
Thioacetamide
Thiourea
Toluene Diisocyanate
o-Toluidine and *o*-Toluidine Hydrochloride
Toxaphene
Trichloroethylene
2,4,6-Trichlorophenol
1,2,3-Trichloropropane
Tris(2,3-dibromopropyl) Phosphate
Urethane
4-Vinyl-l-cyclohexene Diepoxide

[a] Known carcinogens are defined as those substances for which evidence from human studies indicates that there is a causal relationship between exposure to the substance and human cancer.

[b] Suspect carcinogens (substances which may reasonably be anticipated to be human carcinogens) are defined as those substances for which there is limited evidence of carcinogenicity in humans or sufficient evidence of carcinogenicity in experimental animals.

* This substance has been proposed for upgrade to the Known Human Carcinogen category.

From U.S Department of Health and Human Services, Public Health Service, National Toxicology Program *The 9th Report on Carcinogens, 2000.*[38]

TABLE 24.21
Reproductive Endpoints to Indicate Reproductive Dysfunction

Sexual dysfunction: decreased libido; impotence.

Sperm abnormalities: decreased number; decreased motility; abnormal morphology.

Subfecundity: abnormal gonads, ducts of external genitalia; abnormal pubertal development; infertility of male or female origin; amenorrhea; anovulatory cycles; delay in conception.

Illness during pregnancy and parturition; toxemia; hemorrhage.

Early fetal loss (to 28 weeks).

Late fetal loss (after 28 weeks) and stillbirth.

Intrapartum death.

Death in first week.

$\left.\begin{array}{c} \\ \\ \\ \\ \end{array}\right\}$ Perinatal death

Decreased birth weight.

Change in gestational age at delivery: prematurity; postmaturity.

Altered sex ratio.

Multiple births.

Birth defects, major and minor.

Chromosome abnormalities, in fetal deaths, at amniocentesis, in perinatal deaths, in livebirths.

Infant death.

Childhood morbidity.

Childhood malignancies.

Age at menopause.

From Warburton, 1981.[39] With permission.

TABLE 24.22
Possible Environmental Risk Factors for Spontaneous Abortion

Factor(s)	Comment
Parental age	Advanced maternal age associated with increase in trisomic and chromosomally normal abortions
Socioeconomic status	Increased risk of chromosomally normal abortion among socially disadvantaged populations; results may be confounded by differences in ethnicity, patterns of medical care utilization, environmental exposures, etc.
Previous abortion	Conflicting evidence regarding role of multiple, prior, induced abortions; may depend on method of termination; prior spontaneous losses increase risk of recurrence; repeat losses to the same woman tend to be chromosomally normal
Immunological factors	Increased risk of chromosomally normal losses; important etiological factor in recurrent abortion
Hormonal factors	Luteal phase defects implicated in recurrent abortion; in utero diethylstilbestrol (DES) exposure associated with increased risk of spontaneous loss; no increased loss rate among users of oral contraceptives
Chronic diseases	Risk in diabetics relates to degree of glucose control; some studies show increased loss rates among untreated epileptics, others do not; systemic lupus erythematosus associated with increased risk; role of thyroid diseases remains unclear
Anatomic abnormalities	Uterine anomalies associated with increased risk of chromosomally normal loss; cervical incompetence increases risk of mid trimester abortion; risk factors include prior cervical surgery (dilatation and curettage, amputation, conization), DES exposure, parity
Maternal fever	Increased risk of chromosomally normal abortion; difficult to separate role of fever from infection itself
Cigarette smoking	Modest dose-related effect on risk for chromosomally normal abortion; in one study, increased risk found only in socially disadvantaged women
Alcohol	Dose-related increase in risk of chromosomally normal loss; in one study, effect noted only in socially disadvantaged women
Irradiation	Possible association with aneuploid abortion (triploidy, possibly trisomy)

Modified from Kline, et al., 1989.[40] from Shepard et al., *Occupational and Environmental Reproductive Hazards: A Guide to Clinicians,* 1993.[41] With permission.

TABLE 24.23
Probabilities of Spontaneous Abortion

Time from Ovulation	Probability of Fetal Death in Gestation Interval (%)
1–6 days	54.6
7–13 days	24.7
14–20 days	8.2
3–5 wk	7.6
6–9 wk	6.5
10–13 wk	4.4
14–17 wk	1.3
18–21 wk	0.8
22–25 wk	0.3
26–29 wk	0.3
30–33 wk	0.3
34–37 wk	0.3
38+ wk	0.7

Modified from Kline and Stein, 1985,[47] from McGuigan, *Hazardous Materials Toxicology: Clinical Principles of Environmental Health*, 1992.[10] With permission.

TABLE 24.24
Factors Known to Cause Fetal Growth Retardation in Humans

Maternal
  Genetic
  Stature
  Maternal diseases (e.g., chronic pulmonary disease, sickle cell anemia)
  Malnutrition
  Hypoxia (high altitude)
  Immunological factors
  Metabolic diseases
  Uterine anomalies
  After induced abortion
  Maternal addiction (e.g., heroin)
  Smoking (nicotine?)
  Alcoholism
  Socioeconomic influences
Fetal
  Genetic and chromosomal (e.g., trisomies 13, 15, and 21 and Turner's syndrome)
  Congenital malformations (e.g., anencephaly and cardiac malformations) Rh Hemolytic disease
  Twin-to-twin transfusion
  Endocrine disorders
  Hydroamnios
  Multiple gestation (twins)
  Infections (e.g., rubella, cytomegalovirus, syphilis, toxoplasmosis, malaria)
  Nonionizing radiation
  Certain drugs (e.g., aminopterin, busulfan)

TABLE 24.24 *(Continued)*
Factors Known to Cause Fetal Growth Retardation in Humans

Placental

Metabolic disturbances

"Placental insufficiency," postmature "aged" placenta, reduced uteroplacental circulation

Abnormal implantation (e.g., *placenta previa*)

Single umbilical artery

Velamentous insertion of umbilical cord

Circumvallate placenta

Abruptio placentae

Infarctions

Avascularity of chorionic villi

Hemangioma

Fibrinous exudation

Modified from Persaud, 1979,[42] from Rousseaux and Blakley, *Handbook of Toxicologic Pathology*, 1991.[43] With permission.

TABLE 24.25
Frequency of Selected Adverse Pregnancy Outcomes in Humans

Event	Frequency per 100	Unit
Spontaneous abortion, 8–28 wk	10–20	Pregnancies or women
Chromosomal anomalies in spontaneous abortions, 8–28 wk	30–40	Spontaneous abortions
Chromosomal anomalies from amniocentesis	2	Amniocentesis specimens
Stillbirths	2–4	Stillbirths and livebirths
Low birthweight <2500 g	7	Livebirths
Major malformations	2–3	Livebirths
Chromosomal anomalies	0.2	Livebirths
Severe mental retardation	0.4	Children to 15 yr of age

Modified from National Foundation/March of Dimes, 1981,[44] from Manson and Wise, Casarett and Doull's Toxicology: *The Basic Science of Poisons,* 4th ed., 1991.[45] With permission of McGraw-Hill.

TABLE 24.26
Criteria for Recognizing a New Teratogen in the Human

1. An abrupt increase in the frequency of a particular defect or association of defects (syndrome)
2. Coincidence of this increase with a known environmental change, such as widespread use of a new drug
3. Known exposure to the environmental change at a particular stage of gestation yielding a characteristically defective syndrome
4. Absence of other factors common to all pregnancies yielding infants with the characteristic defect

Data from Wilson, 1977,[48] from Ecobichon, *The Basis of Toxicity Testing*, 1992.[49] With permission.

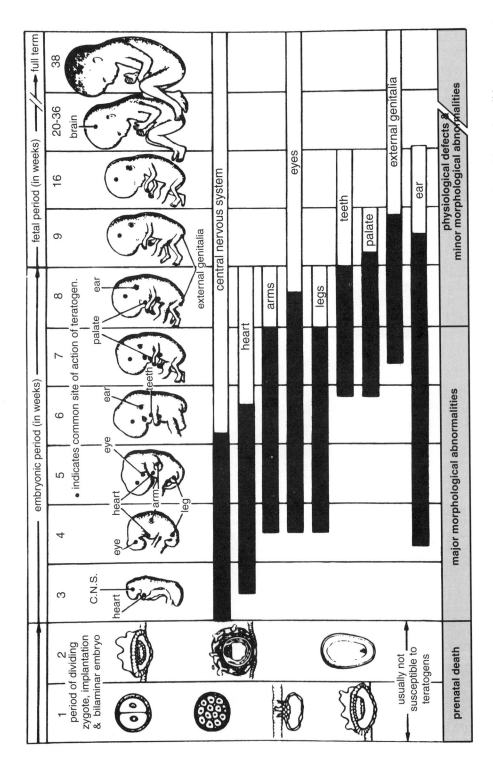

FIGURE 24.31 Schematic diagram of critical periods of human development. For organs and structures indicated within horizontal bars, the solid area represents periods of high sensitivity to teratogens; clear areas represent less sensitive periods. (From Moore, *The Developing Human: Clinically Oriented Embryology*, 5th ed., 1993.[46] With permission.)

TABLE 24.27
Causes of Malformation in Humans

Unknown	65–70%
Genetic defects	20%
Drugs/environmental chemicals	4–6%
Chromosomal abnormalities	3–5%
Maternal infections	2–3%
Maternal metabolic imbalances	1–2%
Maternal reactions	<1%
Potentiative interactions	?

Modified from Wilson, 1977,[48] from McGuigan, *Hazardous Materials Toxicology: Clinical Principles of Environmental Health*, 1992.[10] With permission.

TABLE 24.28
Incidence of Human Birth Defects per 1000

Defect	Spontaneous Abortuses	Elective Termination	Stillborn and Premature	Newborns
Neural tube defects	14	2.4	4.4	0.9
Spina bifida and cephaly	—[c]	—	—	0.9
Hydrocephalus	—	—	—	0.4
Heart malformations	—	—	—	3.0
Cleft palate	1.3	1.1	4.0	2.7
Cleft palate and cleft lip	6.9	3.2	8.0	0.4
Hypospadias[a]	—	—	—	5.1
Clubfoot	—	—	—	2.6
Cyclopia	2.7	2.1	—	0
Polydactyly	2.7	2.8	—	1.4
Sirenomelia[b] and caudal regression	4.2	—	—	0
Defects of intestines and/or trachea	—	—	—	0.5
Kidney inadequacy	—	—	—	0.1
Down's syndrome	—	—	—	0.8
Turner's syndrome	90	—	—	0.05
Total anomalies	200	—	90–140	20–30

[a] Displacement of opening of urinary tract from top of penis and genital organs in varying degrees of underdevelopment.

[b] Union of the legs with partial or complete fusion of the feet.

[c] No data found.

Data from Shepard et al., 1989,[50] Fantel and Shepard, 1987,[51] MMWR, 1982.[52] Modified from Shepard et al., 1993,[41] Crone, 1986.[53]

TABLE 24.29
Known Human Teratogens

Radiation	Drugs chemicals
Therapeutic	Androgenic hormones
Radioiodine	Aminopterin
Atomic weapons	Cyclophosphamide
Infections	Busulfan
Rubella virus	Thalidomide
Cytomegalovirus	Mercury, organic
Herpes simplex virus	Chlorobiphenyls
Toxoplasmosis	Diethylstilbestrol
Venezuelan equine encephalitis virus	Diphenylhydantoin
Syphilis	Trimethadione
Maternal metabolic imbalances	Coumarin anticoagulants
Cretinism	Valproic acid
Diabetes	Antithyroid drugs
Phenylketonuria	Tetracyclines
Virilizing tumors, metabolic conditions	13-cis-retinoic acid
Alcoholism	Lithium
Hyperthermia	Methimazole
Rheumatic disease and congenital heart block	

From *Manson and Wise, Casarett and Doull's Toxicology: The Basic Science of Poisons,* 4th ed., 1991.[45] With permission of McGraw-Hill. From *Manson and Wise, Casarett and Doull's Toxicology: The Basic Science of Poisons,* 4th ed., 1991.[45] With permission of McGraw-Hill.

TABLE 24.30
Etiologic Agents for Congenital Malformations in Humans and Domestic Animals[a]

Agent	Effect
Alcohol	Pre- and postnatal growth retardation, MR, unusual facial features, congenital heart defects, urogenital defects, skeletal defects
Amantadine hydrochloride (±)	Congenital heart defect, pulmonary atresia
Aminopterin	Hydrocephaly, CP, meningocele, meningomyelocele, reduced derivatives of first bronchial arch
Anogyrine (Lupins)	Crooked calf disease, scoliosis, arthrogyropsis, CP
Anesthetics	Increased spontaneous abortions, CNS defects, musculoskeletal defects
Benztropine mesylate (±)	Left colon syndrome
Boric acid (±)	Increased risk for major malformation, especially cataracts
Bromide (±)	Short stature, small cranium, congenital heart disease
Busulfan (±)	CP, eye defects, generalized cytomegaly
Calcium carbonate	CNS defects
Carbon monoxide	CNS defects
Wild black cherry	Syrinomyelia, rudimentary external genitalia, anal atresia, blindly ending colon (pigs)
Chlorambucil (±)	Renal agenesis
Chloroquine (±)	Congenital deafness, chorioretinitis, hemihypertrophy
Cigarette smoking	Increased spontaneous abortion, prematurity, IUGR
Clomiphene (±)	Anencepaly, microcephaly
Coniine (Conium maculatum)	Arthrogryposis, scoliosis

TABLE 24.30 *(Continued)*
Etiologic Agents for Congenital Malformations in Humans and Domestic Animals[a]

Agent	Effect
Copper deficiency	"Swayback," enzootic ataxia (sheep)
Coumarin derivatives	Nasal hypoplasia, calcific stippling of dicumarol, warfarin secondary epiphyses, hydrocephaly
Cyclopamine (*Veratum californicum*)	Cyclopia, CP, cerebral defects
Cyclophosphamide (±)	Ectrodactyly, brachydactyly, flattened nasal bridge
Dextroamphetamine	Atrial and ventricular septal defect, biliary sulfate (±) atresia, facial clefts
Diabetes	Caudal regression syndrome, CP, defects of branchial arches
Diazepam	Facial clefts, CP
Diethylstilbestrol	Hypospadias, male and female pseudohermaphroditism, vaginal adenocarcinoma
Diphenylhydantoin	CL/CP, congenital heart disease, microcephaly, hypoplasia of nails and distal phalanges
Enovid-R (oral progestin) (±)	Female pseudohermaphroditism
17-α-Ethinyltestosterone	Female pseudohermaphroditism
Ethionamide (±)	Congenital heart defects, spina bifida, gastrointestinal atresia
Fasting, starvation	Hydrocephaly, meningomyelocoele
Fluorine	Mottled tooth enamel
5-Fluorouracil (±)	Radial aplasia, imperforate anus, esophageal aplasia, hypoplasia of duodenum, lung, and aorta
Folic acid deficiency	Neural tube defects
Griseofulvin	CP (cats)
17-Hydroxyprogesterone (±)	Female pseudohermaphroditism
Hypertension	IUGR, microcephaly, patent ductus arteriosus, hypotonia of skeletal and gut musculature
Hyperthermia	Microcephaly, microphthalmia, anencephaly, spina bifida
Hypervitaminosis A	Ectopic ureter, CP, craniofacial defects, skeletal malformations
Hypoxia (±)	Decreased birth weight, patent ductus arteriosus (may be a postnatal effect)
Imipramine (±)	Limb reduction deformities
Indomethacin (±)	Pulmonary artery changes
Insulin (±)	Fetal deaths, multiple congenital anomalies
Iodine deficiency	Endemic cretinism, hyperthyroidism
Iodine excess	Congenital goiter, hypothyroidism
Isoniazid (±)	Increased risk for malformations
Isotretinoin	Hydrocephaly, micrognathia, low-set ears, microcephaly, microphthalmia, malformed skull, ventricular septal defect
Lathyrism (Lathyrus)	Poorly developed muscles and connective tissue, dissecting aneurysms of aorta, spinal malformations, CP (domestic animals)
Lead	Increased stillbirth and spontaneous abortion, MR
Lithium carbonate	Epstein's anomaly
Locoweed (*Astragolus, Oxytropis*)	Arthrogryposis
Lysergic acid (±)	Increased spontaneous abortions
Marijuana (±)	IUGR, developmental delays
Medroxyprogesterone (±)	Female pseudohermophroditism, hypospadias
Meprobonate (±)	Congenital heart defect, increased malformation rate with no specific pattern
Mercury	Cerebral palsy, microcephaly, MR
Methallibure	Contractures of distal extremities, distorted mandible and cranial bones, dysplasia of renal cortex (pigs)
Methimazole (±)	Midline defect of scalp
Methotrexate	Absence of frontal bone, premature craniosynostosis, rib defects, ectrodactyly
Methyltestosterone	Female pseudohermaphroditism

TABLE 24.30 *(Continued)*
Etiologic Agents for Congenital Malformations in Humans and Domestic Animals[a]

Agent	Effect
Myasthenia gravis	Congenital contractures
Neguvon	Congenital tremors with hypoplasia of cerebellum (pigs)
Oral contraceptives (±)	Congenital heart defects, limb reduction deformities
Oxytetracycline	Stains deciduous tooth enamel
O-Penicillamine	Lax skin, inguinal hernia, flexion contractures of knee and hip
Phenothiazine (±)	Increased malformation rate
Phenylalanine excess (maternal PKU)	Microcephaly, IUGR, congenital heart defects, dislocation of hips, strabismus
Phenylpropanolamine	Eye and ear defects, hypospadias
Phenobarbital (±)	Fetal hydontoin-like syndrome
Polychlorinated biphenyls	Cola-colored babies, IUGR, exophthalmus, staining of skin and gums
Pregnancy test tablets (±)	Neural tube defects, congenital heart defects
Primidone (±)	Low nasal bridge, ocular hypertelorism, pulmonic stenosis
Progesterone (±)	Hypospadias
Propylthiouracil	Congenital goiter
Quinine (±)	Congenital deafness, hydrocephaly, limb, facial, gastrointestinal and urogenital defects
Reserpine (±)	Congenital lung cysts
Rheumatic disease of mother (especially systemic lupus erythematosus)	Congenital heart block
Organic solvents (±)	Neural tube defects, hydrocephaly, congenital heart defects, talipes
Streptomycin (±)	Congenital deafness
Testosterone	Female pseudohermaphroditism
Tetracycline	Staining of enamel of deciduous or permanent teeth
Thalidomide	Limb reduction anomalies, polydactyly, ear defects, facial hemangioma, esophageal or duodenal atresia, tetralogy of Fallot, renal agenesis
Tobacco stalk	Arthrogryposis (pigs)
Trimethadione	Cp, cardiac defects, V-shaped eyebrows, developmental delays, low-set ears, irregular teeth
Valproic acid	Microcephaly, facial dysmorphology, congenital heart defect, neural tube defect
Virilizing tumor	Female pseudohermaproditism
Vitamin D excess (±)	Supravalvular aortic stenosis, elfin faces, MR
X-irradiation	Microcephaly, MR, hydrocephaly, CP, hypospadias, hypoplastic genitalia, IUGR, microphthalmia, cataracts, strabismus, retinal degeneration and pigment changes, skeletal defects
Zinc deficiency	Anencephaly, achondrogenesis

[a] MR, mental retardation; CNS, central nervous system; CL/CP, cleft lip/cleft palate; lUGR, intrauterine growth retardation; (±), questionable association.

From Rousseaux and Blakley *Handbook of Toxicologic Pathology*, 1991.[43] With permission.

SECTION 5. RELATIVE RISK TABLES

As an aid for making risk comparisons, this section contains reference risk values for death from various types of cancer and for factors believed to cause cancer. In addition, risk values for various occupations, lifestyles, and activities are also presented. For Tables 24.31–24.34, refer to the cited source for information on how these values were determined and the uncertainty associated with them.

In the risk assessment process, risk is expressed in quantitative terms that form the basis for risk management decisions. Generally, carcinogens are regulated to "safe" exposure levels based on risk levels considered "acceptable" to society. Regulatory agencies such as the U.S. Environmental Protection Agency consider a risk of 1×10^{-6} or one in one million to be acceptable. However, this number can vary from 10^{-4} to 10^{-7} depending on the substance of concern and the circumstances of the exposure.

Quantitative risk is a difficult concept for the general public to comprehend. It is often necessary to put risk in perspective to convey the magnitude of an unfamiliar risk. A risk of one in one million is easier to relate to when it is compared to a familiar reference point, e.g., the risk of death from driving an automobile.

Risk comparisons are useful in two other ways: to compare the risks of alternative options and to gauge the importance of different causes of the same hazard.[54] In the former case, an example would be a risk comparison between a new and existing chemical to show the value of introducing the new product. An example of the latter type of comparison would be the ranking of the risk associated with various environmental factors suspected of causing of lung cancer to determine where remediation efforts would have the greatest impact.

Risk comparisons should not be used to attempt to trivialize or make a risk more acceptable. The acceptability of risk is a matter of perception based on numerous subjective qualitative factors related to a hazard's perceived "dreadfulness" and how well it is understood (see Figure 24.10). Risks that are similar quantitatively, but differ qualitatively, will not be perceived as equally acceptable. Risks perceived as voluntary are considered more acceptable than risks perceived as involuntary. For example, the risk of developing cancer from smoking may be viewed as more acceptable than the risk of developing lung cancer from an air pollutant, even though the risk from smoking may be several orders of magnitude greater.

Where possible, risks of similar qualitative characteristics should be compared. Avoid "apples and oranges" comparisons such as comparing the uncontrollable to the controllable, technological to natural, involuntary to voluntary, etc. The reader is referred to the National Research Council's publication entitled *Improving Risk Communication*[54] for a detailed discussion of the uses, misuses, and pitfalls associated with risk comparisons.

TABLE 24.31
Lifetime Risk and Annual Average Risk of Death from Cancer in the United States[a]

Type	Lifetime Risk	Average Annual Risk
All cancers	0.20	2.8×10^{-3}
Buccal cavity, pharynx, respiratory	0.050	7.2×10^{-4}
Digestive organs and peritoneum	0.053	7.5×10^{-4}
Bone, connective tissue, skin, breast	0.022	3.1×10^{-4}
Genital organs	0.022	3.2×10^{-4}
Urinary tract	0.008	1.2×10^{-4}
Leukemia, other blood and lymph	0.018	2.6×10^{-4}
Other	0.019	2.7×10^{-4}

[a] The uncertainty in all these values is about 20%.

From Crouch and Wilson, *Assessment and Management of Chemical Risks*, 1984.[55] With permission.

TABLE 24.32
Cancer Risks from Radiation Exposures

Type	Average Annual Risk
Natural background (average U.S., sea level)	2×10^{-5}
U.S. average medical diagnostic X-ray	2×10^{-5}
Excess due to living in masonry building rather than wood	5×10^{-6}
Cosmic rays	
Airline pilot (50 h/mo at 12-km altitude)	4×10^{-5}
One transcontinental round trip by air per year	1×10^{-6}
Frequent airline passenger (4 h/wk)	1×10^{-5}
Living in Colorado compared with New York	8×10^{-6}
Camping at 15,000 ft for 4 mo/yr	2×10^{-6}

From Crouch and Wilson, *Assessment and Management of Chemical Risks*, 1984.[55] With permission.

TABLE 24.33
Everyday Cancer Risks from Common Carcinogens

Action	Average Annual Risk	Uncertainty
One 12.5-oz diet soda daily (saccharin)	1×10^{-5}	Factor of ~10
Average personal saccharin consumption	2×10^{-6}	Factor of ~10
4 tbsp peanut butter per day (aflatoxins)	8×10^{-6}	Factor of ~10
One pint of milk per day (aflatoxins)	2×10^{-6}	Factor of ~10
Miami/New Orleans drinking water	1×10^{-6}	Factor of ~10
1/2-lb charcoal broiled steak/week (cancer only; heart attack etc., extra)	3×10^{-7}	Factor of ~10
Average smoker (cancer only)	1.2×10^{-3}	Factor of 3 (human data)
(all effects)	3×10^{-3}	Factor of 3 (human data)
Person sharing room with smoker	1×10^{-5}	Factor of ~10
Air pollution (polycyclic organics)	1.5×10^{-5}	Factor of ~10

From Crouch and Wilson, *Assessment and Management of Chemical Risks*, 1984.[55] With permission.

TABLE 24.34
Risk of Death in the United States

	Annual Risk of Death
Industry Group	
Trade	5.3×10^{-5}
Manufacturing	8.2×10^{-5}
Service and government	1.0×10^{-4}
Transport and public utilities	3.7×10^{-4}
Agriculture	6.0×10^{-4}
Construction	6.1×10^{-4}
Mining and Quarrying	9.5×10^{-4}
More Finely Divided Grouping	
Farming	3.6×10^{-4}
Stone quarries and mills	5.9×10^{-4}
Police officers (in line of duty)	2.2×10^{-4}
Railroad employee	2.4×10^{-4}
Steelworker-(accident only)	2.8×10^{-4}
Firefighter	8.0×10^{-4}
Accident	
Motor vehicle	2.4×10^{-4}
All home accidents	1.1×10^{-4}
Fall	6.2×10^{-5}
Drowning	3.6×10^{-5}
Fire	2.8×10^{-5}
Inhalation/ingestion of objects	1.5×10^{-5}
Accidental poisoning	1.4×10^{-5}
Firearms (accidents)	1.0×10^{-5}
Electrocution	5.3×10^{-6}
Tornado	6×10^{-7}
Flood	6×10^{-7}
Lightning	5×10^{-7}
Tropical cyclone/hurricane	3×10^{-7}
Bite/sting	2×10^{-7}
Sport	
Professional stunting	$<1 \times 10^{-2}$
Air show/air racing and acrobatics	5×10^{-3}
Flying amateur/home built aircraft	3×10^{-3}
Sport parachuting	2×10^{-3}
Professional aerial acrobatics	$<2 \times 10^{-4}$
Hang gliding	8×10^{-4}
Mountaineering	6×10^{-4}
Glider flying	4×10^{-4}
Scuba diving	4×10^{-4}
Spelunking	$<1 \times 10^{-4}$
Boating	5×10^{-5}
College football	3×10^{-5}
Hunting	3×10^{-5}
Swimming	3×10^{-5}
Ski racing	2×10^{-5}

Modified from Crouch and Wilson, *Assessment and Management of Chemical Risks*, 1984.[55] With permission.

SECTION 6. STANDARD RISK ASSESSMENT
REFERENCE VALUES*

The risk assessment process involves extrapolation of dose-response data from animals to humans and quantitative estimates of human exposure. For this to be accomplished, a detailed understanding of interspecies differences, population diversity, and environmental factors is critical. Comparative quantitative morphological, physiological, and biochemical information is required for different species. The heterogeneity of exposed populations with respect to such factors as age, lifestyle, and activity patterns must be characterized. Measurements of environmental factors affecting the distribution and fate of the substance from source to exposed human must be obtained (see Figure 24.7).

Accurate data for the type of information described above are not always available. Although exposure determinations are best made at the site where people live and work, problems of sampling, unequal distribution of exposure, fluctuations in environmental conditions, and many other confounding factors make accurate representative measurements difficult to obtain. Characterizing the diversity and lifestyles of a population becomes more difficult as both the size of the population and the area of the exposure increases. The accuracy and relevance of limited data developed for diverse populations spread out over vast areas is questionable. The cost of characterizing such a population becomes prohibitive. For this reason, estimates, rather than actual measurements, are most often used in risk assessment. However, the use of standard values of this sort introduces a source of uncertainty regarding the relevance of the values to the exposed population.

Risk assessment usually relies on a combination of measured and estimated values. The more accurate and representative the measured values, the more realistic will be the risk assessment because the quality of the conclusions will only be as good as the information on which the assessment is based.

This section presents standard comparative reference values useful for extrapolating animal exposures to humans. Also provided are standard values related to human lifestyles and activity patterns needed for making exposure estimates. Reference values for environmental factors affecting fate and distribution are beyond the scope of this book.

The reference values presented may differ from values available from other sources and should not be considered to be more valid than those which can be obtained elsewhere. The reference values presented in this section, however, reasonably represent the available data. The reader is cautioned that these values may not be reliable for all situations. To the extent possible, the use of standard values in risk assessment should be avoided where accurate and reliable measurements can be made from the real world.

---

* See Chapter 33, Section 2 for additional information.

TABLE 24.35
The Duration of Studies in Experimental
Animals and Time Equivalents in the Human

Species	\multicolumn{5}{c}{Duration of Study In Months}				
	1	3	6	12	24
\multicolumn{6}{c}{*Percent of life span*}					
Rat	4.1	12	25	49	99
Rabbit	1.5	4.5	9	18	36
Dog	0.82	2.5	4.9	9.8	20
Pig	0.82	2.5	4.9	9.8	20
Monkey	0.55	1.6	3.3	6.6	13
\multicolumn{6}{c}{*Human equivalents (in months)*}					
Rat	34	101	202	404	808
Rabbit	12	36	72	145	289
Dog	6.5	20	40	81	162
Pig	6.5	20	40	81	162
Monkey	4.5	13	27	61	107

Modified from Paget, 1970.[56] From Ecobichon, *The Basis of Toxicity Testing*, 1992.[57] With permission.

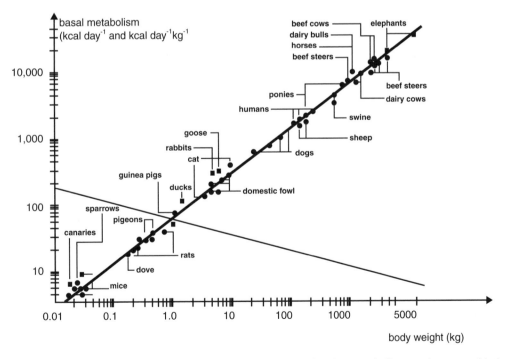

FIGURE 24.32 Interspecies extrapolation of metabolic rate showing that metabolic rates increase with the three-fourths power of body weight ($BW^{0.75}$) for species covering a broad size range. (From Kleiber, M., *Physiol. Rev.*, 27:511, 1947, The American Physiological Society, with permission.)

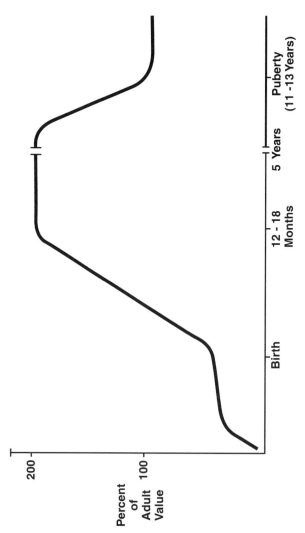

FIGURE 24.33 Schematic representation of development changes in hepatic metabolism and renal elimination. Prenatally and at birth, function is less than 50% of adult values. During infancy and early childhood, function increases beyond adult values. During puberty, values decline toward typical adult levels. These changes are important to consider in a risk assessment because they can have significant impact on the risk of exposure to substances that undergo biotransformation and/or renal elimination. (From Mortensen, *Similarities and Differences Between Children and Adults: Implications for Risk Assessment*, © 1992 International Lifesciences Institute. Used with permission. All rights reserved.)

TABLE 12.36
Summary of Drug Absorption in Neonates, Infants, and Children

	Neonate	Infants	Children
Physiological Alteration			
Gastric Emptying Time	Irregular	Increased	Slightly increased
Gastric pH	>5	4 to 2	Normal (2–3)
Intestinal Motility	Reduced	Increased	Slightly increased
Intestinal Surface Area	Reduced	Near adult	Adult pattern
Microbial Colonization	Reduced	Near adult	Adult pattern
Biliary Function	Immature	Near adult	Adult pattern
Muscular Blood Flow	Reduced	Increased	Adult pattern
Skin Permeability	Increased	Increased	Near adult pattern
Possible Pharmacokinetic Consequences			
Oral Absorption	Erratic — reduced	$\uparrow$ rate	Near adult pattern
I.M. Absorption	Variable	Increased	Adult pattern
Percutaneous Absorption	Increased	Increased	Near adult pattern
Rectal Absorption	Very efficient	Efficient	Near adult pattern
Pre-systemic Clearance	< adult	> adult	> adult ($\uparrow$ rate)

Note: Direction of alteration given relative to expected normal adult pattern. Data contained in the above table reflect developmental differences that might be expected in healthy pediatric patients. Certain conditions/disease states might modify the function and/or structure of the absorptive surface area, GI motility, and/or systemic blood flow impacting on the rate or extent of absorption. Generally, neonate ≤ 1 month of age, infants = 1–24 months of age, children = 2–12 years of age. As the age limits defining these developmental stages are somewhat arbitrary, some overlap in the functional capacity between these stages should be expected. Because physiological development is a dynamic process, it should be kept in mind that functional changes occur incrementally over time and do not abruptly change from one age group to another.

From, with permission, Table 24-1 "Summary of Drug Absorption in Neonates, Infants and Children" of the *Handbook of Basic Pharmacokinetics,* 5th Edition,[80] p 307. © 1999 by the American Pharmaceutical Association. Originally adapted from Morselli, P.L., 1983.[79]

TABLE 24.37
Plasma Protein Binding and Drug Distribution in Neonates, Infants, and Children

	Neonate	Infants	Children
Physiological Alteration			
Plasma Albumin	Reduced	Near normal	Near adult pattern
Fetal Albumin	Present	Absent	Absent
Total Proteins	Reduced	Decreased	Near adult pattern
Total Globulins	Reduced	Decreased	Near adult pattern
Serum Bilirubin	Increased	Normal	Normal adult pattern
Serum Free Fatty Acids	Increased	Normal	Normal adult pattern
Blood pH	7.1–7.3	7.4 (normal)	7.4 (normal)
Adipose Tissue	Scarce ($\uparrow$CNS)	Reduced	Generally reduced
Total Body Water	Increased	Increased	Near adult pattern
Extracellular Water	Increased	Increased	Near adult pattern
Endogenous Maternal Substances (Ligands)	Present	Absent	Absent

TABLE 24.37 *(Continued)*
Plasma Protein Binding and Drug Distribution in Neonates, Infants, and Children

	Neonate	Infants	Children
Possible Pharmacokinetic Consequences			
Free Fraction	Increased	Increased	Slightly increased
Apparent Volume of Distribution			
Hydrophilic drugs	Increased	Increased	Slightly increased
Hydrophobic drugs	Reduced	Reduced	Slightly decreased
Tissue/Plasma Ratio	Increased	Increased	Slightly increased

Note: Direction of alteration given relative to expected normal adult pattern. Generally, neonate ≤ 1 month of age, infants = 1–24 months of age, children = 2–12 years of age. As the age limits defining these developmental stages are somewhat arbitrary, some overlap in the functional capacity between these stages should be expected. Because physiological development is a dynamic process, it should be kept in mind that functional changes occur incrementally over time and do not abruptly change from one age group to another.

From, with permission, Table 24-2 "Plasma Protein Binding and Drug Distribution" of the *Handbook of Basic Pharmacokinetics,* 5th Edition,[80] p. 309. © 1999 by the American Pharmaceutical Association. Originally adapted from Morselli, P.L., 1983.[79]

TABLE 24.38
Renal Function in the Neonate, Infant, and Child

	Neonate	Infants	Children
Physiological Alteration			
Kidney/Body Weight Ratio	Increased	Increased	Near adult values
Glomerular Filtration Rate	Reduced	Normal (by 12 mo)	Normal adult values
Active Tubular Secretion	Reduced	Near normal	Normal adult values[a]
Active Tubular Reabsorption	Reduced	Near normal	Normal adult values
Proteins present in urine	Present (30%)	Low to absent	Normally absent
Urinary Acidification Capacity	Low	Normal (by 1 mo.)	Normal adult activity
Urine Output (ml/hr/kg)	3 to 6	2 to 4	1 to 3
Urine Concentrating Capacity	Reduced	Near normal	Normal adult values
Possible Pharmacokinetic Consequences			
Active Drug Excretion	Reduced	Near normal	Normal adult pattern
Passive Drug Excretion	Reduced to Increased	Increased	Normal adult pattern
Excretion of Basic Drugs	Increased	Increased	Near normal

Note: Direction of alteration given relative to expected normal adult patterns. Generally, neonate ≤ 1 month of age, infants = 1–24 months of age, children = 2–12 years of age. As the age limits defining these developmental stages are somewhat arbitrary, some overlap in the functional capacity between these stages should be expected. Because physiological development is a dynamic process, it should be kept in mind that functional changes occur incrementally over time and do not abruptly change from one age group to another.

[a] Denotes slight increase in excretion rate for basic compounds.

From, with permission, Table 24-6 "Renal Function in the Neonate, Infant and Child" of the *Handbook of Basic Pharmacokinetics,* 5th Edition,[80] p. 315. © 1999 by the American Pharmaceutical Association. Originally adapted from Morselli, P.L., 1983.[79]

TABLE 24.39
Drug Metabolism in the Neonate, Infant, and Child

	Neonate	Infants	Children
Physiological Alteration			
Liver/Body Weight Ratio	Increased	Increased	Slightly increased
Cylochromes P450 Activity	Reduced	Increased	Slightly increased
Blood Esterase Activity	Reduced	Normal (by 12 mo)	Adult pattern
Hepatic Blow Flow	Reduced	Increased	Near adult pattern
Phase 11 Enzyme Activity	Reduced	Increased	Near adult pattern
Possible Pharmacokinetic Consequences			
Metabolic Rates	Reduced	Increased	Near adult pattern[a]
Pre-systemic Clearance	Reduced	Increased	Near adult pattern
Total Body Clearance	Reduced	Increased	Near adult pattern[a]
Inducibility of Enzymes	More evident	Slightly increased	Near adult pattern[a]

Note: Direction of alteration given relative to expected normal adult patterns. Generally, neonate ≤ 1 month of age, infants = 1–24 months of age, children = 2–12 years of age. As the age limits defining these developmental stages are somewhat arbitrary, some overlap in the functional capacity between these stages should be expected. Because physiological development is a dynamic process, it should be kept in mind that functional changes occur incrementally over time and do not abruptly change from one age group to another.

[a] Denotes assumption of adult pattern of activity after the conclusion of puberty. The activity of all drug metabolizing enzymes is generally higher before vs. after puberty.

From, with permission, Table 24-5 "Drug Metabolism in the Neonate, Infant and Child" of the *Handbook of Basic Pharmacokinetics,* 5th Edition,[80] p. 314. © 1999 by the American Pharmaceutical Association. Originally adapted from Morselli, P.L., 1983.[79]

TABLE 24.40
Developmental Patterns for the Ontogeny of Important Drug Metabolizing Enzymes in Man

Enzyme(s)	Known Developmental Pattern
Phase I Enzymes	
CYP2D6	Low to absent in fetal liver but present at 1 week of age. Poor activity (i.e., 20% of adult) by 1 month. Adult competence by 3 to 5 years of age.
CYP2C19, CYP2C9	Apparently absent in fetal liver. Low activity in first 2 to 4 weeks of life with adult activity reached by approximately 6 months. Activity may exceed adult levels during childhood and declines to adult levels after conclusion of puberty.
CYP1A2	Not present in appreciable levels in human fetal liver. Adult levels reached by approximately 4 months and exceeded in children at 1 to 2 years of age. Adult activity reached after puberty.
CYP3A7	Fetal form of CYP3A which is functionally active (and inducible) during gestation. Virtually disappears by 1 to 4 weeks of postnatal when CYP3A4 activity predominates but remains present in approximately 5% of individuals.
CYP3A4	Extremely low activity at birth reaching approximately 30 to 40% of adult activity by 1 month and full adult activity by 6 months. May exceed adult activity between 1 to 4 years of age, decreasing to adult levels after puberty.
Phase II Enzymes	
NAT2	Some fetal activity by 16 weeks gestation. Poor activity between birth and 2 months of age. Adult phenotype distribution reached by 4 to 6 months with adult activity reached by 1 to 3 years.
TPMT	Fetal levels approximately 30% of adult values. In newborns, activity is approximately 50% higher than adults with phenotype distribution which approximates adults. Exception is Korean children where adult activity is seen by 7 to 9 years of age.
UGT	Ontogeny is isoform specific. In general, adult activity is reached by 6 to 24 months of age.
ST	Ontogeny is isoform specific and appears more rapid than that for UGT. Activity for some isoforms may exceed adult levels during infancy and early childhood.

Abbreviations include: CYP, cytochrome P450; NAT2, N-acetyltransferase-2; TPMT, thiopurine methyltransferase; UGT, glucuronosyltransferase and ST, sulfotransferase.

From, with permission, Table 24-4 "Developmental Patterns for the Ontogeny of Important Drug Metabolizing Enzymes in Man" of the *Handbook of Basic Pharmacokinetics,* 5th Edition,[80] p. 3122. © 1999 by the American Pharmaceutical Association. Originally adapted from Leeder, J.S., and Kearns, G.L., 1997.[81]

TABLE 24.41
Comparative Mammalian Reference Values for Relative Dose Calculations

Species	Average Life Span (yrs)	Body Weight (kg)	Food Consumption (g/day)	Food Consumption Factor[a]	Water Consumption (ml/day)	Inhalation Rate (m³/day)
Human	70	70	2000	0.028	1400	20
Mouse	1.5–2	0.03	4	0.13	6	0.052
Rat	2	0.35	18	0.05	50	0.29
Hamster	2.4	0.14	12	0.083	27	0.13
Guinea pig	4.5	0.84	34	0.040	200	0.40
Rabbit	7.8	3.8	186	0.049	410	2
Cat	17	3	90	0.030	220	1.2
Dog	12	12.7	318	0.025	610	4.3
Monkey (Rhesus)	18	8	320	0.040	530	5.4

[a] Fraction of body weight consumed per day as food

Modified from U.S. Environmental Protection Agency, 1985.[60]

TABLE 24.42
Reference Comparative Physiological Values[a,b]

Parameter	Mouse	Rat	Human
Tissue Perfusion (% of Cardiac Output)			
Brain	7.5 (2.0–13.0)	1.2	14.0 (13.0–15.0)
Heart	4.4 (2.8–6.0)	2.9	3.3 (2.6–4.0)
Kidney	24.8 (14.6–35.0)	17.8	22.0
Liver (total)	21.0	18.6 (17.0–26.0)	26.5 (26.0–27.0)
Liver (arterial only)	8.4	6.7	—[c]
Viscera	30.3	26.3	30.0
Adipose tissue	—[c]	4.5 (4.0–5.0)	4.7 (4.5–5.0)
Tissue Volume (% of Body Weight)			
Heart	0.4	0.5	0.6
Kidney	1.5	0.9 (0.9–1.0)	1.1 (0.4–1.5)
Liver	5.0 (4.0–5.9)	4.0 (3.7–4.2)	3.0 (2.4–4.0)
GI tract	6.8	4.3 (3.0–5.5)	3.8 (3.0–4.5)
Fat	7.6 (4.0–9.8)	8.4 (7.0–9.0)	15.5 (9.0–23.1)
Blood	7.6	7.2 (4.9–9.0)	7.2
Muscle	59.0 (45.0–73.0)	59.0 (50.0–73.0)	52.4 (43.4-73.0)
Skin	14.5	16.0	4.3
Marrow	2.7	—[c]	2.5 (2.1–2.8)
Skeletal tissue	9.0	—[c]	—[c]
Cardiac Output			
Absolute (liters/min)	0.0129	0.1066	5.59
	(0.110–0.160)	(0.0730–0.1340)	(4.60–6.49)
Relative (liters/min · kg)	0.535	0.327	0.080
	(0.440–0.711)	(0.248–0.646)	—[c]
Alveolar Ventilation (liters/min)			
	0.026	0.080	4.6
	(0.012–0.039)	(0.075–0.085)	(4.0–5.8)
Minute Volume			
Absolute (liters/min)	0.038	0.169	7.4
	(0.024–0.052)	(0.057–0.336)	(6.0–9.0)
Relative (liters/min · kg)	1.533	0.780	0.089
	(1.239–1.925)	(0.142–2.054)	(0.014-0.127)
Respiratory Frequency (breaths/min)			
	171	117	14
	(100–213)	(60–153)	(10–16)

[a] Mean of reported values. Brackets contain range of reported values from which mean was calculated. Absence of range indicates value was from a single report.

[b] Values presented are for unanesthetized animals.

[c] No data found.

Data derived from U.S. Environmental Protection Agency, 1988.[61]

TABLE 24.43
Body Fluid Volumes for Men and Women

Parameter	Adult Male[a] Volume (liters)	Adult Male[a] % of Bodyweight	Adult Female[b] Volume (liters)	Adult Female[b] % of Bodyweight
Total body water	45.0	60	33.0	55
Extracellular water	11.25	15	9.0	15
Intracellular water	33.75	45	24.0	40
Total blood volume	5.4	7.2	4.3	7.2
Plasma volume	3.0	—	2.6	—
Erythrocyte volume	2.4	—	1.7	—

[a] Volumes calculated for an adult male with a bodyweight of 75 kg and a hematocrit of 45%.

[b] Volumes calculated for an adult female with a bodyweight of 60 kg and a hematocrit of 40%.

Adapted from Plowchalk et al., 1993.[62]

TABLE 24.44
Comparative Mammalian Organ Weights (g/100 g Body Weight)

Species	Brain	Heart	Adrenals	Kidneys	Lungs	Liver	Spleen	Testes
Human	1.96	0.42	0.02	0.41	0.73	2.30	0.25	0.04
Mouse	1.35	0.68	0.02	2.60	0.66	5.29	0.32	0.62
Rat	0.46	0.32	0.01	0.70	0.40	3.10	0.20	0.92
Monkey (Rhesus)	2.78	0.38	0.02	0.54	1.89	2.09	0.14	0.03
Dog	0.59	0.85	0.01	0.30	0.94	2.94	0.45	0.15
Rabbit	0.40	0.35	0.02	0.70	0.53	3.19	0.04	0.13
Hamster	0.88	0.47	0.02	0.53	0.46	5.16	—	—
Guinea pig	1.33	0.53	0.07	1.17	1.18	5.14	0.21	0.65
Cat	0.77	0.45	0.02	1.07	1.04	2.59	0.29	0.07

TABLE 24.45
Typical Human Exposure Values Used in Risk Assessments

Body weight

Young child (1–2 yr)	13 kg
Older child (5 yr)	20 kg
Typical adult	70 kg
male	78 kg
female	60 kg

(see Table 24.46 for more specific children's weight relative to age)

Lifespan   75 yr

Inhalation rate

Typical adult

male	15.2 m³/day
female	11.3 m³/day
Child (<1 yr)	4.5 m³/day
Child (1–12 yr)	8.7 m³/day

TABLE 24.45 *(Continued)*
Typical Human Exposure Values Used in Risk Assessments

Industrial worker (8-hr work shift)	10 m³/day
Industrial worker (24 hr total)	20 m³/day
Reasonable worst case	30 m³/day
(see Table 24.52 for inhalation rates relative to age and degree of activity)	

Drinking water ingestion rate
Adult (average)	1.4 liters/day (21 mL/kg-day)
Adult (90th percentile)	2.0 liters/day (34 mL/kg-day)
Infant (<10 kg)	1.0 liter/day

Food consumption rate
Total average meat intake	2.1 g/kg-day
Total average vegetable intake	4.3 g/kg-day
Total average fruit intake	3.4 g/kg-day
Total average dairy intake	8.0 g/kg-day
Total grain intake	4.1 g/kg-day
Total average fish intake	20.1 g/day
Adult total food intake	2000 g/day

Breast milk intake rate
Average	742 mL/day
Upper percentile	1,033 mL/day

Exposed skin surface
Typical adult	0.20 m²
Reasonable worst case	0.53 m²
Swimming or bathing (average)	
male	1.94 m²
female	1.69 m²
(see Tables 24.48–24.50 for more specific information relative to age and body parts)	

Soil ingestion rate
Children	
average	100 mg/day
upper percentile	400 mg/day
pica child	10 grams/day
Adult (average)	50 mg/day

Activities (also Table 24.51)
a. Showering (typically one event/day)	
Average	10 min/day
95th percentile	35 min/day
(a 5 min shower is estimated to use 40 gallons of water)	
b. Bathing (typically one event/day)	
Median	20 min/event
90th percentile	45 min/event
c. Time indoors	
children (ages 3–11)	19 hr/day
adults	21 hr/day
average residence volume	369 m³
d. Time outdoors	
children (ages 3–11)	5 hr/day
adults	1.5 hr/day

Source: U.S. Environmental Protection Agency, 1989,[63] 1997.[82]

TABLE 24.46
Mean Body Weight (kg) of Children by Age

Age (years)	Boys	Girls	Both
Less than 3	11.9	11.2	11.6
3–5	17.6	17.1	17.4
6–8	25.3	24.6	25.0
9–11	35.7	36.2	36.0
12–14	50.5	50.7	50.6
15–17	64.9	57.4	61.2

Modified from U.S. Environmental Protection Agency, 1989.[63]

TABLE 24.47
Constants for Estimating Surface Area of Mammals[a]

Species	Constant (K)
Rat	9.6
Mouse	9.0
Rabbit	10.0
Guinea pig	9.0
Monkey	11.8
Dog	11.0
Cat	8.7

[a] $A = KW^{2/3}$ where A = surface area (cm^2); K = constant; W = body weight (g).

Data derived from Spector, 1956.[64]

TABLE 24.48
Median Total Body Surface Area (m^2) for Humans by Age

Age (years)	Males	Females
3–5	0.728	0.711
6–8	0.931	0.919
9–11	1.16	1.16
12–14	1.49	1.48
15–17	1.75	1.60
Adult	1.94	1.69

Modified from U.S. Environmental Protection Agency, 1989.[63]

TABLE 24.49
Total Body Surface Area (m²) For Humans by Height and Weight

Body Weight (kg)	Height (cm) 20	30	40	50	60	70	80	90	100	110	120	130	140	150	160	170	180	190	200	210	220	230	240	250	260
5	.18	.20	.23	.26	.29	.33	.37	.42	.48	.55	.62														
10		.35	.36	.38	.41	.44	.48	.52	.57	.64	.69	.76													
15					.54	.57	.60	.63	.67	.72	.77	.83	.89												
20							.68	.72	.76	.80	.85	.91	.97												
25								.80	.84	.88	.93	.98	1.03	1.03	1.15										
30									.92	.96	1.01	1.05	1.10	1.09	1.22	1.28									
35										1.04	1.08	1.12	1.17	1.16	1.29	1.35									
40										1.11	1.15	1.20	1.25	1.23	1.36	1.42	1.42	1.55							
45											1.23	1.27	1.32	1.30	1.43	1.48	1.48	1.61							
50											1.30	1.34	1.39	1.37	1.49	1.54	1.54	1.67	1.74						
55											1.37	1.42	1.46	1.44	1.55	1.61	1.60	1.73	1.80						
60											1.44	1.48	1.52	1.50	1.62	1.67	1.67	1.79	1.85	1.92					
65												1.54	1.58	1.57	1.68	1.73	1.73	1.85	1.91	1.97					
70												1.61	1.65	1.63	1.75	1.80	1.79	1.91	1.96	2.02	2.08				
75												1.68	1.72	1.70	1.81	1.86	1.85	1.96	2.02	2.07	2.13				
80												1.74	1.78	1.76	1.86	1.91	1.91	2.02	2.07	2.13	2.18	2.25			
85												1.81	1.84	1.82	1.92	1.97	1.96	2.07	2.13	2.18	2.24	2.31			
90												1.87	1.90	1.88	1.98	2.03	2.02	2.13	2.18	2.24	2.30	2.36			
95													1.97	1.94	2.05	2.09	2.08	2.18	2.24	2.30	2.36	2.42	2.48		
100													2.03	2.01	2.12	2.16	2.14	2.24	2.30	2.35	2.41	2.47	2.54		
105													2.10	2.07	2.18	2.22	2.20	2.31	2.35	2.41	2.47	2.53	2.60		
110													2.17	2.14	2.24	2.28	2.26	2.36	2.41	2.47	2.53	2.58	2.65		
115													2.23	2.21	2.30	2.33	2.32	2.42	2.47	2.53	2.58	2.64	2.71	2.73	
120														2.27	2.36	2.39	2.38	2.48	2.53	2.58	2.63	2.70	2.77	2.78	
125														2.33	2.42	2.45	2.43	2.53	2.58	2.63	2.69	2.76	2.83	2.84	2.93
130														2.39	2.47	2.51	2.49	2.59	2.63	2.68	2.75	2.82	2.88	2.90	2.97
135														2.44	2.53	2.56	2.54	2.64	2.69	2.74	2.81	2.87	2.93	2.95	3.02
140														2.50	2.58	2.62	2.60	2.70	2.74	2.80	2.87	2.93	2.98	3.00	3.08
145														2.55	2.63	2.67	2.66	2.75	2.80	2.86	2.92	2.98	3.04	3.06	
150														2.61	2.69	2.73	2.71	2.81	2.86	2.92	2.97	3.03	3.09		
155														2.66	2.74	2.78	2.77	2.87	2.92	2.97	3.03	3.08			
160														2.72	2.80	2.83	2.83	2.92	2.97	3.02	3.08				
165														2.77	2.86	2.89	2.88	2.97	3.02	3.07					
170															2.91	2.94	2.93	3.03	3.07						
175															2.96	2.99	2.98	3.08							
180															3.01	3.04	3.03								
185															3.06	3.09	3.08								

From Spector: *Handbook of Biological Data*, 1956.[64] With permission.

TABLE 24.50
Percentage of Total Body Surface Area by Part

Age (years)	Head	Trunk	Arms	Hands	Legs	Feet
<1	18.2	35.7	13.7	5.3	20.6	6.54
1 < 2	16.5	35.5	13.0	5.68	23.1	6.27
2 < 3	14.2	38.5	11.8	5.30	23.2	7.07
3 < 4	13.6	31.9	14.4	6.07	26.8	7.21
4 < 5	13.8	31.5	14.0	5.70	27.8	7.29
5 < 6	—[a]	—	—	—	—	—
6 < 7	13.1	35.1	13.1	4.71	27.1	6.90
7 < 8	—	—	—	—	—	—
8 < 9	—	—	—	—	—	—
9 < 10	12.0	34.2	12.3	5.30	28.7	7.58
10 < 11	—	—	—	—	—	—
11 < 12	—	—	—	—	—	—
12 < 13	8.74	34.7	13.7	5.39	30.5	7.03
13 < 14	9.97	32.7	12.1	5.11	32.0	8.02
14 < 15	—	—	—	—	—	—
15 < 16	—	—	—	—	—	—
16 < 17	7.96	32.7	13.1	5.68	33.6	6.93
17 < 18	7.58	31.7	17.5	5.13	30.8	7.28
Adult (male)	7.8	35.9	14.1	5.2	31.2	7.0
Adult (female)	7.1	34.8	14.0	5.1	32.4	6.5

[a] No data found.

Modified from U.S. Environmental Protection Agency, 1989.[63]

TABLE 24.51
**Activity Pattern Data Aggregated for Three
Microenvironments by Activity Level**

Microenvironment	Activity Level	Average Hours in Each Microenvironment at Each Activity Level
Indoors	Resting	9.82
	Light	9.82
	Moderate	0.71
	Heavy	0.098
	Total	20.4
Outdoors	Resting	0.505
	Light	0.505
	Moderate	0.65
	Heavy	0.12
	Total	1.77
In transportation vehicle	Resting	0.86
	Light	0.86
	Moderate	0.05
	Heavy	0.0012
	Total	1.77

From U.S. Environmental Protection Agency, 1989.[63]

TABLE 24.52
Summary of Human Inhalation Rates for Men,
Women, and Children by Activity Level (m³/hour)[a]

	Resting[b]	Light[c]	Moderate[d]	Heavy[e]
Adult male	0.7	0.8	2.5	4.8
Adult female	0.3	0.5	1.6	2.9
Average adult[f]	0.5	0.6	2.1	3.9
Child, age 6	0.4	0.8	2.0	2.4
Child, age 10	0.4	1.0	3.2	4.2

[a] Values of inhalation rates for males, females, and children presented in this table represent the mean of values reported for each activity level in USEPA (1985).[60]

[b] Includes watching television, reading, and sleeping.

[c] Includes most domestic work, attending to personal needs and care, hobbies, and conducting minor indoor repairs and home improvements.

[d] Includes heavy indoor cleanup, performance of major indoor repairs and alterations, and climbing stairs.

[e] Includes vigorous physical exercise and climbing stairs carrying a load.

[f] Derived by taking the mean of the adult male and adult female values for each activity level.

From U.S. Environmental Protection Agency, 1989.[63]

SECTION 7. PHYSIOLOGICALLY BASED PHARMACOKINETIC MODELING

This section provides standard values for rodent and human physiological and biochemical parameters used in physiologically based pharmacokinetic (PBPK) modeling. With more emphasis being placed on internal (tissue) dose for quantitating exposure between species, PBPK modeling is finding increasing use in the risk assessment process.

Figure 24.34 shows a typical PBPK model consisting of a series of compartments representing organ and tissue groups with realistic blood flows. Each tissue group is described mathematically by a series of differential equations which express the rate of change of a chemical of concern in each compartment. The rate of exchange between compartments is based on species-specific physiological parameters. Unlike data-based pharmacokinetic models, PBPK models are limited within the constraints placed on the model by the unique physiological values for each species modeled. Because PBPK models use species-specific values, interspecies extrapolations can be performed whereas data-based pharmacokinetic models are limited to intraspecies extrapolation. Herein lies the value of PBPK models in risk assessment.

No one PBPK model can represent the kinetics of all chemicals. The number of compartments and their interrelationships will vary depending on the nature of the chemical being modeled. More specific physiological values than those presented in this section can be used to adjust for variations in strain, sex, age, body weight, etc. of the species being modeled.

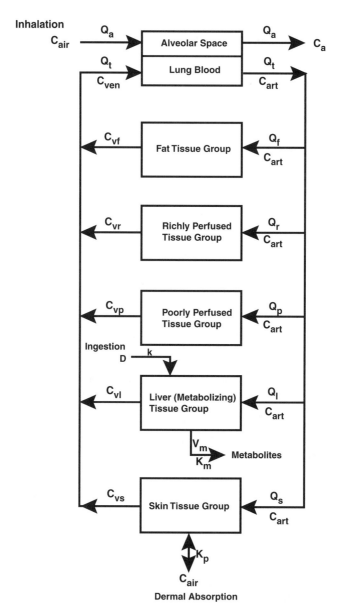

FIGURE 24.34 Diagram of typical physiologically based pharmacokinetic model (PBPK). Cart = concentration in arterial blood (mg/liter); Cven = concentration in venous blood (mg/liter); Cvf, Cvr, Cvp, Cvl, Cvs = venous concentrations in tissue groups corresponding, respectively, to fat, richly perfused, poorly perfused, liver, and skin tissue groups; Cair = concentration in inhaled air (mg/liter); Ca = concentration in alveolar air (mg/liter); D = gavage dose (mg); k = gut absorption time constant (min⁻¹). Other abbreviations with reference values can be found in Table 24.53. (From Chen and Hoang, *Health Risk Assessment: Dermal and Inhalation Exposure and Absorption of Toxicants*, 1993.[65] With permission.)

TABLE 24.53
Reference Physiological and Biochemical Values Used in PBPK Models

Parameter	Abbreviation	Rats	Mice		Human
			Male	Females	
Body weight (kg)		0.35	0.035	0.025	70
Alveolar ventillation rate (liters/min)	Qa	0.083	0.035	0.028	7.5
Blood flow rate (liters/min)					
Cardiac output	Qt	0.104	0.023	0.019	6.2
To fat tissue group	Qf	0.0092	0.002	0.0017	0.31
To richly perfused tissue group	Qr	0.0434	0.0012	0.0097	2.76
To poorly perfused tissue group	Qp	0.0074	0.0035	0.00195	1.26
To liver tissue group	Ql	0.0389	0.0058	0.0048	1.55
To skin tissue group	Qs	0.0052	0.00115	0.00095	0.31
Tissue volume (liters)					
Of fat tissue group	Vf	0.0315	0.0038	0.0027	14
Of richly perfused tissue group	Vr	0.015	0.0021	0.0015	3.5
Of poorly perfused tissue group	Vp	0.220	0.0273	0.0195	36.4
Of liver tissue group	Vl	0.0140	0.0017	0.0012	1.72
Of skin tissue group	Vs	0.035	0.00035	0.00025	7
Partition coefficient					
Blood/air	N	18.9	16.9		10.3
Skin/air	Ps/a	—	—		505.4
Fat tissue/blood	Pf	108.994	121.893		108.994
Richly perfused tissue/blood	Pr	3.179	4.159		3.719
Poorly perfused tissue/blood	Pp	1.058	1.183		3.72
Liver/blood	Pl	3.719	4.159		3.72
Skin/blood	Ps	—	—		505.4
Metabolic constants					
Maximum velocity of metabolism (mg/min)	Vm	0.00586	0.0039	0.003	0.703
Michaelis constant (mg/liter)	Km	2.9378	1.472	1.472	32.043
Absorption coefficients					
Skin Permeability (cm/hr)	Kp	0.668	—	—	0.17

Modified from Chen and Hoang, *Health Risk Assessment; Dermal and Inhalation Exposure and Absorption of Toxicants*, 1993.[65] With permission.

TABLE 24.54

EPA Recommended Reference Physiological Values for Use in PBPK Modeling

Parameter	Mouse	Rat	Human
Body weight (Kg)	0.025	0.25	70.0
Tissue volumes (liters)			
Liver	0.0014	0.01	1.82
	(0.055)[a]	(0.04)	(0.026)
Fat	0.0025	0.0175	13.3
	(0.10)	(0.07)	(0.19)
VRG[b]	0.0013	0.0125	3.5
	(0.05)	(0.05)	(0.05)
MG[c]	0.0175	0.1875	43.4
	(0.70)	(0.75)	(0.62)
Cardiac output (liters/min)	0.017	0.083	6.2
Tissue perfusion (liters/min)			
Liver	0.0043	0.0208	1.61
	(0.25)[d]	(0.25)	(0.26)
Fat	0.0015	0.0075	0.31
	(0.09)	(0.09)	(0.05)
VRG	0.0087	0.0423	2.73
	(0.51)	(0.51)	(0.44)
MG	0.0026	0.0125	1.55
	(0.15)	(0.15)	(0.25)
Minute volume (liters/min)	0.037	0.174	7.5
Alveolar ventilation (liters/min)	0.025	0.117	5.0

[a] Values in parentheses are tissue volumes as fractions of body weight.
[b] Vessel-rich group (brain, heart, kidney, viscera).
[c] Muscle group (muscle and skin).
[d] Values in parentheses are tissue perfusion as fractions of cardiac output.

Modified from U.S. Environmental Protection Agency, 1988.[61]

SECTION 8. RISK ASSESSMENT CALCULATIONS

Contained in this section are equations for calculations commonly performed in risk assessments. Equations (1) through (4) are for various dose/exposure conversions. Lifetime average daily dose (LADD) for a variety of exposure scenarios can be calculated using Equations (6) through (11). These equations can also be used to calculate maximum daily dose (MDD), sometimes referred to as average daily dose (ADD), by eliminating the lifetime factor (LT) from the denominator and adjusting the numerator for a single day of exposure by removing the exposure duration (ED) factor.

The numerator in Equations (6) through (11) contains absorption (bioavailability) factors to adjust for the fraction of substance actually absorbed (internal dose). Absorption factors may not be found in similar equations from other sources because in the absence of specific data, the value for absorption defaults to one. Additional exposure-modifying factors are used occasionally in the numerator. For example, a meteorological factor for adjusting the exposure for the number of days of precipitation could be used where such an event would limit exposure to dust from contaminated soil. The more data of this type available to express actual exposure, the more accurate will be the calculated estimate of exposure and the more realistic the risk assessment based on this information.

TABLE 24.55
Risk Assessment Calculations

1. Human Equivalent Dose (HED)

$$HED = (\text{Animal dose}) \times \left(\frac{\text{Human body weight}}{\text{Animal body weight}} \right)^{1/3}$$

2. ppm – mg/m³ Conversion

$$PPM = \frac{(mg/m^3) \times (R)}{(MW)}$$

where   ppm = exposure concentration as ppm; mg/m³ = exposure concentration as mg/m³; R universal gas constant (24.5 at 25°C and 760 mm Hg); MW = molecular weight.
* (See below)

3. Airborne Concentration to Equivalent Oral Dose*

$$EOD = \frac{(C) \times (EL) \times (MV) \times (AF) \times (10^{-6})}{(BW)}$$

where   EOD = equivalent oral dose (mg/kg); C = concentration of substance in air (mg/m³); EL = exposure length (min); MV = minute volume, species specific (ml/min); AF = absorption factor (fraction of inhaled substance absorbed), default = 1; 10^{-6} = conversion factor m³ ↔ ml; BW = body weight (kg).
* "See below"

4. Oral Dose to Equivalent Airborne Concentration*

$$EAC = \frac{(OD) \times (BW)}{(MV) \times (AF) \times (EL) \times (10^{-6})}$$

where   EAC = equivalent airborne concentration (mg/m³); OD = oral dose (mg/kg); BW = body weight (kg); MV = minute volume, species specific (ml/min); AF = absorption factor, fraction of inhaled substance absorbed; (default = 1) EL = exposure length (min); 10^{-6} = Conversion factor m³ ↔ ml.

* Caution should be exercised when using Equations 3 and 4. These give crude approximations in that the time period will be set and protracted for inhalation and may be either bolus for gavage studies or averaged over the entire day for feeding and drinking water studies. They assume that there will be no chemical reactivity associated with oral administration, no portal entry effects and that the target organ effects will be the same regardless of the route of administration.

5. Lifetime Exposure (h)

Lifetime = (hours exposed) × (days exposed) × (weeks exposed) × (years exposed)
exposure   per day   per week   per year

6. Exposure from Ingestion of Contaminated Water

$$LADD = \frac{(C) \times (CR) \times (ED) \times (AF)}{(BW) \times (TL)}$$

where   LADD = lifetime average daily dose (mg/kg/day); C = concentration of contaminant in water (mg/liter); CR = water consumption rate (liters/day); ED = exposure duration (days); AF = absorption factor (fraction of ingested contaminant absorbed) default = 1 (dimensionless); BW = body weight (kg); TL = typical lifetime (days).

7. Exposure from Dermal Contact with Contaminated Water

$$LADD = \frac{(C) \times (SA) \times (EL) \times (AR) \times (ED) \times (SV) \times (10^{-9})}{(BW) \times (TL)}$$

TABLE 24.55 *(Continued)*
Risk Assessment Calculations

where   LADD = lifetime average daily dose (mg/kg/day); C = concentration of contaminant in water (mg/liter); SA = surface area of exposed skin (cm^2); EL = exposure length (min/day); AR = absorption rate (μg/cm^2/min); SV = specific volume of water (1 liter/kg); ED = exposure duration (days); 10^{-9} = conversion factor (kg → μg); BW = body weight (kg); TL = typical lifetime (days).

8. Exposure from Ingestion of Contamination Soil

$$LADD = \frac{(C) \times (CR) \times (ED) \times (AF) \times (FC) \times (10^{-6})}{(BW) \times (TL)}$$

where   LADD = lifetime average daily dose (mg/kg/day); C = concentration of contaminant in soil (mg/kg); CR = Soil consumption rate (mg/day); ED = exposure duration (days); AF = absorption factor (fraction of ingested contaminant absorbed) default 10 = (dimensionless); FC = fraction of total soil from contaminated source; 10^{-6} = conversion factor kg ↔ mg; BW = body weight (kg); TL = typical lifetime (days).

9. Exposure from Dermal Contact with Contaminated Soil

$$LADD = \frac{(C) \times (SA) \times (BF) \times (FC) \times (SDF) \times (ED) \times (10^{-6})}{(BW) \times (TL)}$$

where   LADD = lifetime average daily dose (mg/kg/day); C = concentration of contaminant in soil (mg/kg); SA = surface area of exposed skin (cm^2); BF = bioavailability factor (percent absorbed/day); FC = fraction of total soil from contaminated source; SDF = soil deposition factor; amount deposited per unit area of skin (mg/cm^2/day); ED = exposure duration (days); BW = body weight (kg); TL = typical lifetime (days).

10. Exposure from Inhalation of Contaminated Particles in Air

$$LADD = \frac{(C) \times (PC) \times (IR) \times (RF) \times (EL) \times (AF) \times (ED) \times (10^{-6})}{(BW) \times (TL)}$$

where   LADD = lifetime average daily dose (mg/kg/day); C = concentration of contaminant on particulate (mg/kg); PC = particulate concentration in air (mg/m^3); IR = inhalation rate (m^3/hr); RF = respirable fraction of particulates; EL = exposure length (hr/day); AF = absorption factor (fraction of inhaled contaminant absorbed) default = 1; ED = exposure duration (days); 10^{-6} = conversion factor kg ↔ mg; BW = body weight (kg); TL = typical lifetime (days).

11. Exposure from Inhalation of Vapors

$$LADD = \frac{(C) \times (IR) \times (EL) \times (AF) \times (ED)}{(BW) \times (TL)}$$

where   LADD = lifetime average daily dose (mg/kg/day); C = concentration of contaminant in air (mg/m^3); IR = inhalation rate (m^3/hr); EL = exposure length (hr/day); AF = absorption factor (fraction of inhaled contaminant absorbed) default = 1; ED = exposure duration (days); BW = body weight (kg); TL = typical lifetime (days).

12. Calculation of an RfD

$$RfD = \frac{(NOAEL)}{(UFs) \times (MF)}$$

where   RfD = reference dose (mg/kg/day); UFs = uncertainty factors — Generally multiples of 10 (although 3 or 1 are occasionally used depending on the strength and quality of the data). The following uncertainty factors are usually used:

UF

10 Accounts for variation in the general population. Intended to protect sensitive subpopulations (an additional factor of 10 has been proposed to account for an increased sensitivity of children over adults).

10 Used when extrapolating from animals to humans. Intended to account for interspecies variability between humans and animals.

TABLE 24.55 *(Continued)*
Risk Assessment Calculations

10 Used when a NOAEL is derived from a subchronic rather than a chronic study in calculating a chronic RfD.
10 Applied when a LOAEL is used instead of a NOAEL. Intended to account for the uncertainty in extrapolating from LOAELs to NOAELs.
MF = modifying factor; multiple of 1 to 10; intended to reflect a professional qualitative assessment of the uncertainty in the critical study from which the NOAEL is derived as well as the overall quality of the database. Accounts for the uncertainty not addressed by the UFs.

13. Estimating an LD_{50} of a Mixture

$$\frac{1}{\text{Predicted LD}_{50}} = \frac{Pa}{\text{LD}_{50}\text{ of Component a}} = \frac{Pb}{\text{LD}_{50}\text{ of Component b}} + \cdots \frac{Pn}{\text{LD}_{50}\text{ of Component n}}$$

where   P = fraction of components in the mixture.

14. Estimation of Maximal Attainable Air Concentration of a Chemical

$$\text{MAAC} = \frac{(vp) \times (mw) \times (10^6)}{(760) \times (R)}$$

where   MAAC = maximal attainable air concentration (mg/m³); vp = vapor pressure of the chemical (mm Hg) at 25°C; mw = molecular weight in grams; 760 = atmospheric pressure at 25°C; R = 24.5 (universal gas constant at 25°C and 760 mm Hg).

Note: In the absence of analytical measurements, this equation can give a worst case estimate of the theoretically achievable air concentration of a volatile chemical at equilibrium in any size room with no ventilation and an infinite source of chemical. Actual air concentrations could be lower depending on physical properties of the chemical, the amount of chemical being used, room ventilation, and other handling practices but not exceed the MAAC.

15. Haber's Rule

$$C \times t = k$$

where   C = exposure concentration, t = time, and k = a constant
Note: Haber's rule has been historically used to relate exposure concentration and duration to a toxic effect. Basically, this concept states that exposure concentration and exposure duration may be reciprocally adjusted to maintain a cumulative exposure constant (k) and that this cumulative exposure constant will always reflect a specific toxic response. In general terms, it states that the shorter the time of exposure, the higher the concentration that will be needed to achieve the same toxic effect as occurs with a longer period of exposure at lower concentrations. The inverse relationship of concentration and time may be valid when the toxic response to a chemical is equally dependent upon the concentration and the exposure duration. However, work by ten Berge et al. (1986) with acutely toxic chemicals revealed chemical-specific relationships between exposure concentration and exposure time that were often exponential rather than linear. This relationship can be expressed by the Equation $C^n \times t = k$, where n represents a chemical specific, and even toxic endpoint specific, exponent. The relationship described by this equation is basically the form of a linear regression analysis of the log-log transformation of a plot of C vs t. ten Berge et al. examined the airborne concentration (C) and short term exposure time (t) relationship relative to lethal responses for approximately 20 chemicals and found that the empirically derived value of n ranged from 0.8 to 3.5 among this group of chemicals. Hence, these workers showed that the value of the exponent (n) in the equation $C^n \times t = k$ quantitatively defines the relationship between exposure concentration and exposure duration for a given chemical and for a specific toxic or health effect endpoint. Haber's Rule is the special case where n = 1. As the value of n increases, the plot of concentration vs time yields a progressive decrease in the slope of the curve. In short, the best expression for extrapolation over several time points is $C^n \times t = k$, where the value for n is derived from existing data.

TABLE 24.55 *(Continued)*
Risk Assessment Calculations

As this edition went to press, the approach to time scaling in acute studies was being reviewed in the Standing Operating Procedures of the National Advisory Committee on Acute Exposure Guideline Levels for Hazardous Substances with a planned publication by the National Academy of Science in 2001.
References

DRAFT Standing Operating Procedures of the National Advisory Committee on Acute Exposure Guideline Levels for Hazardous Substances. October 1, 1998.

Haber, F. Zur Geschichte des Gaskrieges, in, *Funf Vortrage aus den Jahren*, 1920–1923. Springer-Verlag, Berlin, 76–92, 1924.

Rinehart, W.E. and Hatch, T., *Ind. Hyg. J.*, 25: 545–553, 1964.

ten Berge, W.F. Zwart, A., and Applemen, L.M., *J. Hazard. Materials*, 13: 301–309, 1986.

Witschi, H.P., *Toxicol. Sci.*, 50: 164–168, 1999.

16. Time-Weighted Average (TWA) for an 8-Hr Workday

$$\text{TWA} = \frac{C_1 T_1 + C_2 T_2 + \dots C_n T_n}{8}$$

where C_n = concentration measured during a period of time (<8 h); T_n = duration of the period of exposure in hours at concentration C_n ($\Sigma T = 8$).

17. Risk for Noncarcinogens (Hazard Index)

$$\text{Risk} = \frac{\text{MDD}}{\text{ADI}}$$

If: Risk > 1, A potential risk exists which may be significant.
    Risk < 1, Risk is insignificant.
where   MDD = maximum daily dose; ADI = acceptable daily intake.

18. Lifetime Risk for Carcinogens

$$\text{Risk} = (\text{LADD}) \times (\text{SF})$$

If: Risk = 10^{-6}, risk is insignificant; 10^{-6} – 10^{-4} , possible risk; 10^{-4}, risk may be significant.
where   LADD = lifetime average daily dose (mg/kg/day); SF = slope factor or cancer potency factor $(\text{mg/kg/day})^{-1}$ (chemical and route specific)

19. Total Risk from a Single Contaminant via Multiple Exposure Pathways

$$\text{Total} = \Sigma \text{ risks from all exposure pathways}$$

Example: Total risk (from a contaminant in water) = (risk from ingestion) + (risk from showering) + (risk from swimming)

20. Total Risk from Multiple Contaminants via a Single Exposure Pathway

$$\text{Total risk} = \Sigma \text{ risks from all contaminants in the media}$$

Example:
Total risk from contaminants A, B, and C in water = Total risk from contaminant A + Total risk from contaminant B + Total risk from contaminant C

Note: For calculations 19 and 20: total risk < 1 is insignificant; total risk > 1 may be significant. Both of these methods are extremely conservative and can greatly overestimate risk.

Source: Paustenbach and Leung, 1993,[67] Environ Corporation, 1990,[69] U.S. Environmental Protection Agency, 1989,[63] U.S. Environmental Agency, 1989,[66] Lynch, 1979.[68]

SECTION 9. TOXICITY CLASSIFICATIONS

This section presents some common classification schemes based on acute lethality and carcinogenicity. Classifications can be based on other toxic effects such as skin irritancy, contact sensitization potential, teratogenicity, etc. The reader is referred to other sections of the handbook or the referenced literature for other classification schemes.

Although classification schemes based on lethality are useful for ranking chemicals, caution should be exercised when using such classifications to communicate risk information or to make risk management decisions. The median lethal dose is not the only determinant of toxicity. Consideration must also be given to the slope of the dose-response curve. Two substances having identical LD_{50} values could vary significantly in the slope of their dose-response curves and pose much different risks to hyperreactive individuals (see Figure 24.15). Moreover, classifications of this type can relay a false sense of security because other determinants of toxicity are not addressed in a classification based on lethality. For example, a teratogenic substance could be classified as "slightly toxic" based solely on its LD_{50}. Classification schemes should only be used with a clear understanding of their inherent limitations.

TABLE 24.56
Combined Tabulation of Toxicity Classes

		Various Routes of Administration			
Toxicity Rating	Commonly Used Term	LD_{50} Single Oral Dose Rats	Inhalation 4-hr Vapor Exposure Mortality 2/6–4/6 Rats	LD_{50} Skin Rabbits	Probable Lethal Dose for Man
1	Extremely toxic	≤1 mg/kg	<10 ppm	≤5 mg/kg	A taste, 1 grain
2	Highly toxic	1–50 mg	10–100 ppm	5–43 mg/kg	1 teaspoon, 4 cc
3	Moderately toxic	50–500 mg	100–1000 ppm	44–340 mg/kg	1 ounce, 30 gm
4	Slightly toxic	0.5–5 g	1000–10,000 ppm	0.35–2.81 g/kg	1 cup, 250 gm
5	Practically nontoxic	5–15 g	10,000–100,000 ppm	2.82–22.59 g/kg	1 quart, 1000 gm
6	Relatively harmless	>15 g	>100,000 ppm	>22.6 g/kg	>1 quart

From Hodge and Sterner, *Am. Ind. Hygiene Assoc. Q.*, 1949.[70] With permission.

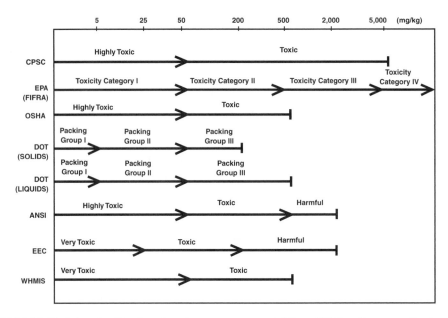

FIGURE 24.35 Toxicity classifications based on rat acute oral LD$_{50}$. CPSC = Consumer Product Safety Commission; EPA = U.S. Environmental Protection Agency (FIFRA = Federal Insecticide, Fungicide and Rodenticide Act); OSHA = U.S. Occupational Safety and Health Administration; DOT = U.S. Department of Transportation; ANSI = American National Standards Institute; EEC = European Economic Community; WHMIS = Workplace Hazardous Materials Information System (Canada). Use the following example of the DOT (solids) classification as an aid for interpreting the values of this figure: Packing Group I (≤5 mg/kg); Packing Group II (>5 mg/kg to ≤ 50mg/kg); Packing Group III (>50 mg/kg to ≤200 mg/kg). (Modified from Schurger and McConnell, Eastern Chemicals, 1989.[71])

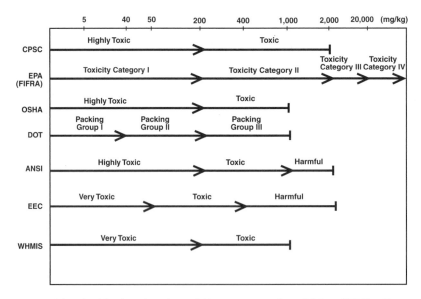

FIGURE 24.36 Toxicity classifications based on rabbit or rat acute dermal LD$_{50}$. CPSC = Consumer Product Safety Commission; EPA = U.S. Environmental Protection Agency; FIFRA = Federal Insecticide, Fungicide and Rodenticide Act; OSHA = U.S. Occupational Safety and Health Administration; DOT = U.S. Department of Transportation; ANSI = American National Standards Institute; EEC = European Economic Community; WHMIS = Workplace Hazardous Materials Information System (Canada). Refer to the legend for Figure 24.35 for an aid to interpreting the values of this figure. (Modified from Schurger and McConnell, Eastman Chemicals, 1989.[71])

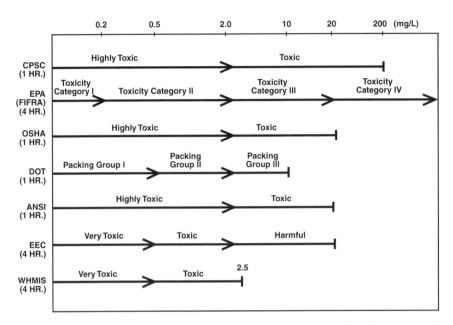

FIGURE 24.37 Toxicity classifications based on rat acute inhalation LC_{50}. CPSC = Consumer Product Safety Commission; EPA = U.S. Environmental Protection Agency; FIFRA = Federal Insecticide, Fungicide and Rodenticide Act; OSHA = U.S. Occupational Safety and Health Administration; DOT = U.S. Department of Transportation; ANSI = American National Standards Institute; EEC = European Economic Community; WHMIS = Workplace Hazardous Materials Information System (Canada). Refer to the legend for Figure 24.35 for an aid to interpreting the values of this figure. (Modified from Schurger and McConnell, Eastman Chemicals, 1989.[71])

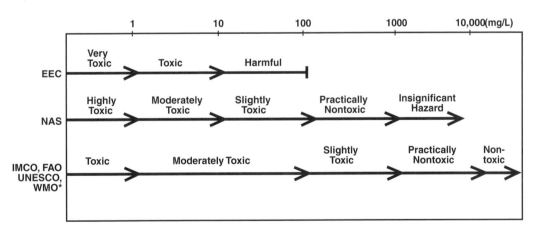

*Values are for Acute Threshold Limits, Not LC_{50}

FIGURE 24.38 Aquatic toxicity classifications based on fish LC_{50}. EEC = European Economic Community; NAS = U.S. National Academy of Sciences; IMCO = Inter-Government Maritime Consultive Organization; FAO = Food and Agriculture Organization; UNESCO = United Nations Educational, Scientific and Cultural Organization; WMO = World Meterological Organization. Refer to the legend of Figure 24.35 for an aid to interpreting the values of this figure.

TABLE 24.57
EPA, IARC, and EEC Classification Systems for Carcinogens

Agency	Category	Classification	Description
United States Environmental Protection Agency (EPA)*	A	Carcinogenic to humans	Sufficient evidence from epidemiology studies to support a casual association
	B1	Probably carcinogenic to humans	Limited evidence in humans from epidemiology studies
	B2	Probably carcinogenic to humans	Sufficient evidence from animal studies but inadequate or no data in humans
	C	Possibly carcinogenic to humans	Limited or equivocal evidence from animal studies but inadequate or no data in humans
	D	Not classifiable as to human carcinogenicity	Inadequate or no data from animals and inadequate or no data in humans
	E	Evidence of noncarcinogenicity for humans	No evidence of carcinogenicity in a least two animal species and no evidence in humans
International Agency for Research on Cancer (IARC)	1	Carcinogenic to humans	Sufficient epidemilogical evidence for carcinogenicity in humans or sufficient evidence of carcinogenicity from animal studies with strong evidence for a carcinogenic mechanism relevant to humans.
	2A	Probably carcinogenic to humans	Sufficient evidence from animal studies and limited evidence in humans
	2B	Possibly carcinogenic to humans	Sufficient evidence from animal studies but inadequate evidence in humans or limited evidence in humans and less than sufficient evidence in animals
	3	Not classifiable as to human carcinogenicity	Inadequate data to classify
	4	Not carcinogenic	Sufficient evidence of noncarcinogenicity in humans and/or animals
European Economic Community (EEC)	1	Known to be carcinogenic to humans	Sufficient evidence to establish a casual association between human exposure and cancer
	2	Regarded as if carcinogenic to humans	Sufficient evidence to provide a strong presumption that human exposure may result in cancer. Based on long-term animal studies and/or other relevant information
	3	Causes concern due to possible carcinogenic effects	Inadequate information to make a satisfactory assessment. Some evidence from animal studies but insufficient to place in category 2.

Adapted from Ecobichon, 1992,[12] European Economic Community, 1993.[72]

Note: As this edition went to print, the EPA was proposing a revision of its carcinogen classification scheme[83]. The proposal was for a classification using three categories of descriptors for human carcinogenic potential: "known/likely," "cannot be determined," and "not likely." Each category would have associated subdesciptors to further define the conclusion. The descriptors and subdescriptors would be standardized for consistent use from case to case. Proposed descriptors and subdescriptors are:

Known/likely: For chemicals that are:

- known to cause cancer in humans *from epidemiology and/or experimental evidence demonstrating causality.*

- to be treated as if known to cause cancer in humans *based on plausible causality and strong experimental evidence.*

- likely to cause cancer in humans due to tumors *resulting from modes of action that are relevant to human* carcinogenicity.

- likely to cause cancer in humans based on data that are at the *high end of the weights of evidence* typical of this group

- likely to cause cancer in humans based on data that are at the *low end of the weights of evidence typical of this group*

Cannot be determined: For chemicals whose:

- carcinogenic potential cannot be determined but for which there is *suggestive* evidence that raises concern for carcinogenicity

- carcinogenic potential cannot be determined *due to conflicting data*

- carcinogenic potential cannot be determined *due to inadequate data*

- carcinogenic potential cannot be determined *due to no data* exisiting

Not likely: For chemicals that are:

- not likely to be carcinogenic to humans *based on animal studies*

- not likely to be carcinogenic to humans, having only *effects not relevant to humans* (e.g. alpha$_{2u}$ -globulin accumulation)

- not likely to be carcinogenic to humans *based on dose and/or route of exposure*

- not likely to be carcinogenic to humans *based on extensive human experience*

TABLE 24.58
Criteria for Determining the Human Relevance of Animal Bioassay Results

Supportive	Not Supportive
Same exposure route as for humans	Different exposure route than for humans
Tumors with several types of exposure	Tumors with only one type of exposure (not relevant to humans)
Tumors in several species	Tumors in only one species
Tumor site correspondence	No site correspondence across species
Tumors at multiple sites	Tumors at only one site
Tumors at sites of low spontaneous occurrence	Tumors at sites with high background incidence
Tumors in tissues analogous to human tissues	Tumors in animal tissues not relevant to humans
No evidence of cellular toxicity at the target site	Tumors only in organs displaying cellular toxicity
Tumors appear early in life	Tumors detectable only late in life
Tumors progress rapidly (benign to malignant)	Benign tumors only
Tumors usually fatal	Tumors not fatal
Similar metabolism (biotransformation) in animals and humans	Metabolic pathways differ in humans and animals
Genotoxic	Nongenotoxic
DNA-reactive	No reaction with DNA
Mechanism of tumorogenesis relevant to humans	Mechanism of tumorogenesis does not occur in humans
Structural similarity to known human carcinogens	Little structural similarity to known human carcinogens
No evidence for disruption of homeostasis	Homeostasis disrupted

Modified from Ashby et al., 1990.[73] With permission.

SECTION 10. GLOSSARY: RISK ASSESSMENT TERMS, ABBREVIATIONS, AND ACRONYMS[69,74-76]

Absorbed dose The amount of a substance penetrating across the exchange boundaries of an organism and into body fluids and tissues after exposure.

Absorption To take in a substance through a body surface such as the lungs, gastrointestinal tract, or skin and ultimately into body fluids and tissues.

Acceptable daily intake (ADI) A value used for noncarcinogenic effects which represents a daily dose that is very likely to be safe over an extended period of time. An ADI is similar to an RfD (defined below) but less strictly defined.

Acceptable risk A risk level that is deemed by society to be acceptable.

ACGIH American Conference of Governmental Industrial Hygienists.

Acute exposure One or a series of short-term exposures generally lasting less than 24 h.

Administered dose The amount of a substance given to a human or test animal in determining dose-response relationships, especially through ingestion or inhalation (see Applied Dose). Administered dose is actually a measure of exposure, because even though the substance in "inside" the organism once ingested or inhaled, administered dose does not account for absorption (*see* Absorbed Dose).

Adverse effect A biochemical change, functional impairment, or pathological lesion that either singly or in combination adversely affects the performance of the whole organism, or reduces an organism's ability to respond to an additional environmental challenge.

Adenoma A benign tumor originating in the covering tissue (epithelium) of a gland.

Additivity An interaction in which the combined effect of two or more chemicals is approximately equal to the sum of the effect of each chemical alone.

Aerosol A suspension of liquid or solid particles in a gaseous medium.

Aggregate risk The sum of individual increased risks of an adverse health effect in an exposed population.

Allergen An antigenic substance capable of eliciting an allergic response.

Ambient Encompassing or surrounding area.

Anaphylaxis An exaggerated reaction to an antigen to which an organism has been sensitized previously.

Anergy Diminished reactivity to specific antigens.

Annual Incidence The number of new cases of disease occurring or predicted to occur in a population over a year.

ANPR Advanced Notice of Proposed Rulemaking.

Antagonism An interaction in which the combined effect of two chemicals is less than the sum of the effect of each chemical alone; the chemicals either interfere with each other's actions, or one interferes with the action of the other.

Antigen A substance that induces the formation of antibodies and interacts with its specific antibody. Antigens may be introduced into the body or may be formed within the body.

Applied dose The amount of a substance given to a human or test animal in determining dose-response relationships, especially through dermal contact. Applied dose is actually a measure of exposure, because it does not take absorption into account (see Absorbed Dose).

Atrophy Reduction in the size of a structure or organ resulting from lack of nourishment or functional activity, death and reabsorption of cells, diminished cellular proliferation, pressure, ischemia, or hormone changes.

ATSDR Agency for Toxic Substance and Disease Registry.

AWQC Ambient Water Quality Criteria.

BEL Biological Exposure Index.

Benign A condition of a neoplasm (tumor) in which the morphological and behavioral characteristics of the tumor differ minimally from the tissue from which it originates. A benign neoplasm (as distinct from malignant) may expand, but remains encapsulated, and has limited potential to invade local structure and proliferate.

Bioaccumulation Progressive increase in amount of a chemical in an organism or part of an organism that occurs because the rate of intake exceeds the organism's ability to remove the substance from the body.

Bioavailability A measure of the degree to which a dose of a substance becomes physiologically available to the body tissues depending on absorption, distribution, metabolism, and excretion rates.

Bioconcentration Same as bioaccumulation; refers to the increase in concentration of a chemical in an organism.

Biological endpoint The biological processes, responses, or effects assessed.

Biological half-life The time required for the concentration of a chemical present in the body or in a particular body compartment to decrease by one-half through biological processes such as metabolism and excretion.

Biological markers/monitoring Measuring chemicals or their metabolites in biological materials (e.g., blood, urine, breath) to estimate exposure, or to detect biochemical changes in the exposed subject before or during the onset of adverse health effects. Sometimes refers to a specific indicator for a particular disease/functional disturbance.

Biological significant effect A response in an organism or other biological system that is considered to have a substantial or noteworthy effect (positive or negative) on the well-being of the biological system. Used to distinguish statistically significant effects or changes, which may or may not be meaningful to the general state of health of the system.

Biotransformation An enzymatic chemical alteration of a substance within the body that generally leads to a more excretable metabolite, sometimes producing a more toxic form of the substance.

Block group/enumeration district (BG/ED) The smallest geographic areas used by the Bureau of Census in conducting the population census. Block groups are designated for urban areas, whereas enumeration districts are designated for rural areas. BG/EDs data are frequently incorporated into exposure models to estimate population exposure to environmental pollutants.

CAA Clean Air Act.

CAG Carcinogen Assessment Group — EPA.

Cancer A malignant new growth. Cancers are divided into two broad categories: carcinoma and sarcoma.

Cancer potency factor (CPF) The statistical 95% upper confidence limit on the slope of the dose-response relationship at low doses for a carcinogen. Values are in units of lifetime risk per unit dose (mg/kg/day). A plausible upper bound on risk is derived by multiplying the extended lifetime average daily dose (LADD) by the CPF.

Carcinogen A substance that is able to produce malignant tumor growth.

Carcinogenic Able to produce malignant tumor growth. Operationally benign tumors are often included.

Carcinogenic process A series of stages at the cellular level after which cancer can develop in an organism. It is hypothesized that there are at least three stages: initiation, promotion, and progression.

Carcinoma A malignant tumor of epithelial cell origin (e.g., skin, lung, breast), tending to infiltrate the surrounding tissue and give rise to metastases.

Case-control study A retrospective epidemiological study in which individuals with the disease under study (cases) are compared with individuals without the disease (controls) to contrast the extent of exposure in the diseased group with the extent of exposure in the controls.

CBI Confidential Business Information.

CDC Center for Disease Control.

CEC Chemical Evaluation Committee — NTP.

Ceiling limit A concentration limit in the work place that should not be exceeded, even for a short time, to protect workers against frank health effects.

CERCLA Comprehensive Environmental Response, Compensation, and Liability Act of 1980.

CFR Code of Federal Regulations.

Chemical mixture Any combination of two or more substances.

Chronic exposure Long-term exposure usually lasting 6 months to a lifetime.

Clearance The disappearance of a compound from a specific organ or body compartment or the whole body.

CNS Central Nervous System.

Cohort study A study of a group of persons sharing a common experience (e.g., exposure to a substance) within a defined time period; the experiment is used to determine whether an increased risk of a health effect (disease) is associated with that exposure.

Complete carcinogen Chemicals that are capable of inducing tumors in animals or humans without supplemental exposure to other agents. Complete refers to the three stages of carcinogenesis (initiation, promotion, and progression), which are hypothesized to be needed to induce cancer.

Confidence limit The confidence interval is a range of values that has a specified probability (e.g., 95 percent) of containing a given parameter or characteristic. The confidence limit often refers to the upper value of the range (e.g., upper confidence limit).

Control group A group of subjects observed in the absence of the exposure agent for comparison with exposed groups.

CPSA Consumer Product Safety Act.

CPSC Consumer Product Safety Commission.

Critical endpoint A chemical may elicit more than one toxic effect (endpoint), even in one test animal, in tests of the same or different duration (acute, subchronic, and chronic exposure studies). The doses that cause these effects may differ. The critical endpoint used in the dose-response assessment is the one that occurs at the lowest dose. In the event that data from multiple species are available, it is often the most sensitive species that determines the critical endpoint. This term is applied in the derivation of risk reference doses.

Cross-sectional study An epidemiological study assessing the prevalence of a disease in a population. These studies are most useful for conditions or diseases that are not expected to have a long latent period and do not cause death or withdrawal from the study population. Potential bias in case ascertainment and exposure duration must be addressed when considering cross-sectional studies.

CSWG Chemical Selection Working Group — NTP.

CWA Clean Water Act.

Cytochrome P-448 and P-450 Enzymes that are important in the detoxification by biotransformation of many chemical substances. Cytochrome P-448 and P-450 enzymes, integral in the metabolic activation and detoxification of many compounds, are found primarily in the liver and, to a lesser extent, in the lung and other tissues.

Cytotoxicity Producing a specific toxic action on cells.

De minimus risk From the legal maxim *"de minimus non curat lex"* or "the law is not concerned with trifles." As related to risk assessment of carcinogens, it is commonly interpreted to mean that a lifetime risk of 1×10^{-6} is a *de mininius* level of cancer risk (i.e., insignificant and therefore acceptable) and is of no public health consequence.

DNA adduct A lesion in the DNA formed by covalent binding of an exogenous chemical to one of the nucleotide bases. DNA adducts are frequently the precursors to changes in the sequence of nucleotides (mutations).

DNA cross-link A lesion in the DNA formed by the covalent binding of an exogenous chemical to two nucleotide bases, one each on opposing strands of the DNA. DNA cross-links usually prevent DNA replication and are lethal to cells attempting to divide.

Deposition Specific to air toxics, the adsorption on the respiratory tract surface of inhaled, gaseous, or particulate pollutants. Also, adsorption of a gaseous or particulate air pollutant at the surface of the ground, vegetation, or water.

Dermal Related to the skin.

Dermatitis Inflammation of the skin.

Detoxification Reduction of a chemical's toxic properties by means of biotransformation processes, to form a more readily excreted, or a less toxic chemical than the parent compound.

Developmental toxicity Adverse effects on the developing organism. Adverse developmental effects may be detected at any point in the life span of the organism. Major manifestations of developmental toxicity include: death of the developing organism, induction of structural abnormalities (teratogenicity), altered growth, and functional deficiency.

Dispersion model A mathematical model or computer simulation used to predict the movement of airborne or waterborne contaminants. Models take into account a variety of mixing mechanisms that dilute effluents and transport them away from the point of emission.

Disposition The movement and fate of chemicals in the body, including absorption, distribution, biotransformation, and excretion.

Dose The amount of substance administered to an animal or human generally expressed as the weight or volume of the substance per unit of body weight (e.g., mg/kg, ml/kg).

Dose-response relationship A relationship between (1) the dose, often actually based on "administered dose" (i.e., exposure) rather than absorbed dose and (2) the extent of toxic injury produced by that chemical. Response can be expressed either as the severity of injury or proportion of exposed subjects affected. A dose-response assessment is one of the steps in a risk assessment.

Dosimetry In general, the measurement or modeling of the amount, rate, and distribution of a drug or toxicant especially as it pertains to producing a particular biological effect.

Duration of exposure Generally referred to in toxicology as acute (one-time), subacute (repeated over several weeks), subchronic (repeated for a fraction of a lifetime), and chronic (repeated for nearly a lifetime).

DWEL Drinking Water Equivalent Level.

ECAD Existing Chemical Assessment Division.

EEC European Economic Community.

Embryo In mammals, the stage in the developing organism at which organs and organ systems are developing. For humans, this involves the stage of development between the second through eighth weeks (inclusive) postconception.

Embryotoxicity Any toxic effect on the conceptus as a result of exposure during the embryonic stages of development. These effects may include malformations and variations, altered growth, *in utero* death, and altered postnatal function.

Endemic Present in a community or among a group of people; said of a disease prevailing continually in a region.

Endpoint An observable or measurable biological or chemical event used as an index of the effect of a chemical on a cell, tissue, organ, organism, etc.

Environmental fate The destiny of a chemical or biological pollutant after release into the environment. Environmental fate involves temporal and spatial considerations of transport, transfer, storage, and transformation.

EPA Environmental Protection Agency.

Epidemiology The study of the occurrence and distribution of a disease or physiological condition in human populations and of the factors that influence this distribution.

Epigenetic Alterations in the expression of genes by mechanisms other than changes in the nucleotide sequence of DNA.

ETS Emergency Temporary Standard.

Excess risk An increased risk of disease above the normal background rate.

Excretion Elimination or discharge of chemicals from the body. Chemicals may be excreted through feces, urine, exhaled breath, etc.

Exposure Contact of an organism with a chemical, physical, or biological agent. Exposure is quantified as the amount of the agent available at the exchange boundaries of the organism (e.g., skin, lungs, digestive tract) and available for absorption.

Exposure, direct Exposure of an organism to a chemical via the medium in which it was initially released into the environment.

Exposure, indirect Exposure of an organism to a chemical involving multimedia transport from the source to the exposed organism (e.g., chemicals deposited onto soil or consumption of fruits and vegetable containing pesticide residues).

Exposure assessment Measurement or estimation of the magnitude, frequency, duration, and route of exposure of subjects to substances in the environment. The exposure assessment also describes the nature of exposure and the size and nature of the exposed populations, and is one of the steps in risk assessment.

Exposure frequency The number of times an exposure occurs in a given period. The exposure(s) may be continuous, discontinuous but regular (e.g., once daily), or intermittent.

Exposure rate The rate at which external exposure is delivered.

Extrapolation An estimate of response or quantity at a point outside the range of the experimental data. Also refers to the estimation of a measured response in a different species or by a different route than that used in the experimental study of interest (i.e., species-to-species, route-to-route, acute-to-chronic, high-to-low).

FDA Food and Drug Administration.

FD&CA Food Drug and Cosmetic Act.

Fence line concentration Modeled or measured concentrations of pollutants found at the boundaries of a property on which a pollution source is located. Usually assumed to be the nearest location at which an exposure of the general population could occur.

Fertility The ability to achieve conception and to produce offspring. For litter-bearing species, the number of offspring per litter is also used as a measure of fertility. Reduced fertility is sometimes referred to as subfertility.

Fetus The postembryonic stage of the developing young. In humans, from the end of the second month of pregnancy up to birth.

FHSA Federal Hazardous Substance Act.

FIFRA Federal Insecticide, Fungicide and Rodentcide Act.

First pass effect Reduction in a substance's systemic availability resulting from metabolism or excretion by the first major organ of contact with such capability after the absorption process. This phenomenon is often associated with the lung or liver.

Frank effect level (FEL) Related to biological responses to chemical exposures (compare with NOAEL and LOEL); the exposure level that produces an unmistakable adverse health effect (such as inflammation, severe convulsions, or death).

Functional developmental toxicity Alterations or delays in functional competence of an organism or organ system after exposure to an agent during critical periods of development pre- and/or postnatally.

Gamma multihit model A dose-response model that can be derived under the assumption that the response is induced if the target site has undergone some number of independent biological events (hits).

Gavage Experimental exposure regimen in which a substance is administered to an animal into the stomach via a tube.

Gene The simplest complete functional unit in a DNA molecule. A linear sequence of nucleotides in DNA that is needed to synthesize a protein and/or regulate cell function. A mutation in one or more of the nucleotides in a gene may lead to abnormalities in the structure of the gene product or in the amount of gene product synthesized.

Genome A term used to refer to all the genetic material carried by a cell.

Genotoxic A broad term that usually refers to a chemical which has the ability to damage DNA or the chromosomes. This can be determined directly by measuring mutations or chromosome abnormalities or indirectly by measuring DNA repair, sister-chromatid exchange, etc.

Germ cell A cell capable of developing into a gamete [ovum (egg) or sperm].

GI Gastrointestinal.

GRAS Generally Recognized as Safe.

HA Health Advisory.

Hazard The inherent ability of a substance to cause an adverse effect under defined conditions of exposure.

Hazard identification The process of determining whether exposure to a substance is causally related to the incidence and/or severity of an adverse health effect (e.g., cancer, birth defects, organ-specific toxicity etc.). Hazard identification involves gathering and evaluating data on the types of health injury or disease that may be produced by a chemical and on the conditions of exposure under which injury or disease is produced. Hazard identification is the first step in the risk assessment process.

Hazard index The ratio of the maximum daily dose (MDD) to the acceptable daily intake (ADI) used to evaluate the risk to noncarcinogens. A value of less than 1 indicates the risk from the exposure is likely insignificant; a value greater than 1 indicates a potentially significant risk.

HBROEL Health-Based Recommended Occupational Exposure Limits (Europe).

HEAST Health Effects Assessment Summary Tables.

Hemangiosarcoma A malignant neoplasm characterized by rapidly proliferating, extensively infiltrating, anaplastic cells derived from blood vessels and lining of blood-filled spaces.

Homeostasis Maintenance of normal, internal stability in an organism by coordinated responses of the organ systems.

HSL Hazardous Substances List.

Human equivalent dose The human dose of an agent expected to induce the same type of severity of toxic effect that an animal dose has induced.

Hyperplasia The abnormal multiplication or increase in the number of normal cells in normal arrangement in a tissue.

Hypersensitivity Exaggerated response by the immune system to an allergen sometimes used incorrectly in a nonimmune sense to indicate increased susceptibility to the effects of a pollutant.

IARC International Agency for Research on Cancer.

Immediately dangerous to life and health (IDLH) A concentration representing the maximum level of a pollutant from which an individual could escape within 30 minutes without escape-impairing symptoms or irreversible health effects.

Incidence The number of new cases of a disease within a specified time period. It is frequently presented as the number of new cases per 1,000, 10,000 or 100,000. The incidence rate is a direct estimate of the probability or risk of developing a disease during a specified time period.

Individual risk The increased risk for a person exposed to a specific concentration of a toxicant.

Indoor/outdoor ratio The ratio of the indoor concentration of an air pollutant to the outdoor concentration of that pollutant.

Inflammation A protective tissue response to injury that serves to destroy, dilute, or wall-off both the injurious agent and the injured tissue. It is characterized by symptoms such as pain, heat, redness, swelling, and loss of function.

Ingestion Intake of a substance through the mouth.

Inhalation Intake of a substance through the lungs.

Initiator An agent capable of starting but not necessarily completing the process of producing an abnormal, uncontrolled growth of tissue usually by altering a cell's genetic material. Initiated cells may or may not be transformed into tumors.

Interspecies Between different species.

Interspecies scaling factors Numerical values used in the determination of equivalent doses between species (e.g., frequently a known animal dose is scaled to estimate an equivalent human dose). The U.S. EPA's cancer risk assessment guidelines (50 FR 33992) note that commonly used dosage scales include milligram per kilogram body weight per day, parts per million in soil or water or air, milligram per square meter body surface area per day, and milligrain per kilogram body weight per lifetime. The guidelines for carcinogen assessment generally recommend using the surface area approach unless there is evidence to the contrary. The dose as mg/kg of body weight/day is generally used to scale between species for noncancer effects of chemicals after dermal, oral, or parenteral exposure.

Intramuscular Within the muscle; refers to injection.

Intraperitoneal Within the membrane surrounding the organs of the abdominal cavity; refers to injection.

Intraspecies Within a particular species.

Intravascular Within the blood vessels; refers to injection, usually into the veins (intravenous or IV).

In vitro Tests conducted outside the whole body in an artificially maintained environment, as in a test tube, culture dish, or bottle.

In vivo Tests conducted within the whole living body.

Involuntary risk A risk that impinges on an individual without their awareness or consent.

Latency The period of time between exposure to an injurious agent and the manifestation of a response.

Lesion A pathological or traumatic discontinuity of tissue or loss of function.

LC_{LO} (lethal concentration low) The lowest concentration of a chemical required to cause death in some of the population after exposure for a specified period of time and observed for a specified period of time after exposure. Refers to inhalation time exposure in the context of air toxics (may refer to water concentration for tests of aquatic organisms or systems).

LC_{50} (median lethal concentration) The concentration of a chemical required to cause death in 50% of the exposed population when exposed for a specified time period and observed for a specified period of time after exposure. Refers to inhalation exposure concentration in the context of air toxics (may refer to water concentration for tests of aquatic organisms or systems).

LD_{LO} (lethal dose low) The lowest dose of a chemical required to cause death in some of the population after noninhalation exposure (e.g., injection, ingestion), for a specified observation period after exposure.

LD_{50} (median lethal dose) The dose of a chemical required to cause death in 50% of the exposed population after noninhalation exposure (e.g., injection, ingestion), for a specified observation period after exposure.

Lifetime average daily dose (LADD) The total dose received over a lifetime multiplied by the fraction of a lifetime during which exposure occurs, expressed in mg/kg body weight/day.

Lifetime risk A risk that results from lifetime exposure.

Limited evidence According to the U.S. EPA carcinogen risk assessment guidelines, limited evidence is a collection of facts and accepted scientific inferences that suggests the agent may be causing an effect but the suggestion is not strong enough to be an established fact.

Local effect A biological response occurring at the site of first contact between the toxic substance and the organism.

Logit model A dose-response model that can be derived under the assumption that the individual tolerance level is a random variable following the logit distribution.

Lower respiratory tract That part of the respiratory tract below the larynx.

Lowest observed adverse effect level (LOAEL) The lowest dose or exposure level of a chemical in a study at which there is a statistically or biologically significant increase in the frequency or severity of an *adverse* effect in the exposed population compared with an appropriate, unexposed control group.

Lowest observed effect level (LOEL) In a study, the lowest dose or exposure level of a chemical at which a statistically or biologically significant effect is observed in the exposed population compared with an appropriate unexposed control group. The effect is generally considered not to have an adverse effect on the health and survival of the animal. This term is occasionally misused in place of a LOAEL.

Lymphoma Any abnormal growth (neoplasm) of the lymphoid tissues. Lymphoma usually refers to a malignant growth and thus is a cancer.

Male reproductive toxicity The occurrence of adverse effects on the male reproductive system, which may result from exposure to substances. The toxicity may be expressed as alterations to the male reproductive organs and/or the related endocrine system. The manifestation of such toxicity may include alteration in sexual behavior, fertility, pregnancy outcomes, or modifications in other functions that are dependent on the integrity of the male reproductive system.

Malformation A permanent structural change in a developing organism that may adversely affect survival, development, or function. Compare with variation.

Malignant A condition of a neoplasm (tumor) in which it has escaped normal growth regulation and has demonstrated the ability to invade local or distant structures, thereby disrupting the normal architecture or functional relationships of the tissue system.

Margin of exposure (MOE) The ratio of the no-observed-adverse-effect level (NOAEL) to the estimated human exposure. The MOE formerly was referred to as the margin of safety (MOS).

Mass median aerodynamic diameter (MMAD) Median of the distribution of mass with respect to the aerodynamic diameter of a particle.

Maximum contaminant level (MCL) The maximum level of a contaminant permissible in water as defined by regulations promulgated under the Safe Drinking Water Act.

Maximum daily dose (MDD) Maximum dose received on any given day during a period of exposure generally expressed in mg/kg body weight/day.

Maximum individual risk (MIR) The increased risk for a person exposed to the highest measured or predicted concentration of a toxicant.

Maximum likelihood estimate (MLE) A statistical best estimate of the value of a parameter from a given data set.

Maximum tolerated dose (MTD) The highest dose of a toxicant that causes toxic effects without causing death during a chronic exposure and that does not decrease the body weight by more than 10%.

Media The air, water, soil, and biota (plants or animals that transport chemicals on or in their tissues) that make up the physical pathway between the source of a chemical and an exposed individual.

Metaplasia The abnormal transformation of an adult, fully differentiated tissue of one kind into a differentiated tissue of another kind.

Metastasis The transfer of a disease, or its local manifestations, from one part of the body to another. In cancer, this relates to the appearance of neoplasms in parts of the body remote from the site of the primary tumor. This is a characteristic of malignancy.

Microenvironment The immediate local environment or an organism.

MLE *See* Maximum likelihood estimate.

Model A mathematical representation of a natural system intended to mimic the behavior of the real system, allowing description of empirical data, and predictions about untested states of the system.

Modifying factor (MF) A factor that is greater than zero and less than or equal to 10; used in the operational derivation of a reference dose. Its magnitude depends on an assessment of the scientific uncertainties of the toxicological database not explicitly treated with standard uncertainty factor (e.g., number of animals tested). The default value for the MF is 1.

Morbidity The number of sick individuals or cases of disease in a population.

Morphology Study of the form or structure of cells, tissues, organs, or organisms.

Morphometry Quantitative measure of morphology.

Mortality The number of individual deaths in a population.

Multistage model A mathematical function used to extrapolate the probability of incidence of disease from a bioassay in animals using high doses, to that expected to be observed at the low doses that are likely to be found in chronic human exposure. This model is commonly used in quantitative carcinogenic risk assessments where the chemical agent is assumed to be a complete carcinogen and the risk is assumed to be proportional to the dose in the low region.

Mutagenic Ability to cause a permanent change in the structure of DNA. More specific than, but often used interchangeably with, genotoxic.

Mutation Changes in the composition of DNA, generally divided according to size into "gene mutations" (changes with a single gene) and "chromosome mutations" (affecting larger portion of the chromosome, or the loss or addition of an entire chromosome). A "heritable mutation" is a mutation that is passed from parent to offspring and therefore was present in the germ cell of one of the parents. Somatic cell mutations may result in cancer.

NAAQS National Ambient Air Quality Standards.

Necrosis Death of areas of tissue or bone, usually as individual cells, as groups of cells, or in localized areas. Necrosis can be caused by cessation of blood supply, physical agents such as radiation, or chemical agents.

Neonatal Newly born; in humans, up to 6 weeks of age.

Neoplasia The pathological process that results in the formation and growth of a tumor, i.e., a neoplasm.

Neoplasm A new and abnormal growth of tissue, such as a tumor.

NESHAPS National Emission Standards for Hazardous Air Pollutants.

Neurotoxicity Ability to damage nervous tissue.

Noncarcinogen A substance that has been demonstrated not to increase the incidence of cancer.

Nonthreshold toxicant An agent considered to produce a toxic effect from any dose; any level of exposure is deemed to involve some risk. Usually used only in regard to carcinogenesis.

No-observed-adverse-effect level (NOAEL) The highest experimental dose at which there is not statistically or biologically significant increases in frequency or severity of *adverse* health effects, as seen in the exposed population compared with an appropriate, unexposed population. Effects may be produced at this level, but they are not considered to be adverse.

No-observed-effect level (NOEL) The highest experimental dose at which there are no statistically or biologically significant increases in frequency or severity of toxic effects seen in the exposed compared with an appropriate unexposed population.

NOS Not Otherwise Specified.

NPDWR National Primary Drinking Water Regulation.

NPL National Priorities List.

NTP National Toxicology Program.

Occupational exposure limit (OEL) A generic term denoting a variety of values and standards, generally time-weighted average concentrations of airborne substances to which a worker can be exposed during defined work periods.

OERR Office of Emergency and Remedial Response.

OMB Office of Management and Budget.

Oncogene A naturally occurring gene that specifies the synthesis of a protein that is involved in normal cellular processes. Alterations in the structure or function of oncogenes are associated with the development of some cancers.

Oncogenesis The origin and growth of a neoplasm.

One-hit model A mathematical model that assumes a single biological event can initiate a response.

Organogenesis The development of specific body structures or organs from undifferentiated tissue. In humans, this relates primarily to weeks 2 through 8 (inclusive) postconception.

OSHA Occupational Safety and Health Administration.

OSWER Office of Solid Waste and Emergency Response.

OTS Office of Toxic Substances.

PAH Polycyclic Aromatic Hydrocarbon.

Permissible exposure limit (PEL) Limits developed to indicate the maximum airborne concentration of a contaminant to which an employee may be exposed for a specific duration.

Pharmacokinetics The field of study concerned with defining, through measurement or modeling, the absorption, distribution, metabolism, and excretion of drugs or chemicals in a biological system as a function of time.

PHS Public Health Service.

Physiologically based pharmacokinetics Pharmacokinetics (see above) based on measured physiological variables such as blood flows through organs, etc.

Population at risk A group of subjects with the opportunity for exposure to a chemical.

Population variability The concept of differences in susceptibility of individuals within a population to toxicants due to variations such as genetic differences in metabolism and response of biological tissue to chemicals.

Portal of entry effects Biological response at the site of entry (e.g., the lungs, stomach) of a toxicant into the body.

Potency A comparative expression of chemical or drug activity measured in terms of the relationship between the incidence or intensity of a particular effect and the associated dose of a chemical to a given or implied standard of reference. Can be used for ranking the toxicity of chemicals.

Potential The inherent toxicological properties of a chemical, i.e., the possibility that toxicity can occur with no concern for its likelihood or severity.

ppb Parts per billion.

ppm Parts per million.

Prevalence The percentage of a population that is affected with a particular disease at a given time.

Prop. 65 California Safe Drinking Water and Toxic Enforcement Act of 1986.

Probit model A dose-response model that can be derived assuming that individual tolerance is a random variable following log normal distribution.

Promotion The second hypothesized stage in a multistage process of cancer development. The conversion of initiated cells into tumorigenic cells.

q_1^* The symbol used to denote the 95% upper bound estimate of the linearized slope of the dose-response curve in the low-dose region as determined by the multistage model.

RCRA Resource Conservation and Recovery Act of 1976.

Reactivity Tendency of a substance to undergo chemical change.

Reference dose (RfD) An estimate (with uncertainty spanning perhaps an order of magnitude or more) of the daily exposure to the human population (including sensitive-subpopulations) that is likely to be without deleterious effects during a lifetime. The RfD is reported in units of mg of substance/kg body weight/day for oral exposures, or mg of substance/m^3 of air breathed for inhalation exposures (RfC).

Reproductive toxicity Harmful effects on fertility, gestation, or offspring, caused by exposure of either parent to a substance.

Respiratory rate The frequency of a complete cycle of a breath (inhalation and exhalation).

Retention The state of being held in a specific location. Used to refer to the amount of an inhaled material that remains in the lung (pulmonary retention) or to the amount of a toxicant dose that remains in the body or body compartment for a specified period of time.

RfD *See* Reference dose.

RI Remedial investigation.

RI/FS Remedial investigation and feasibility study.

Risk The probability that an adverse effect will occur under a particular condition of exposure.

Risk assessment The scientific activity of evaluating the toxic properties of a chemical and the conditions of human exposure to it to ascertain both the likelihood that exposed humans will be adversely affected and to characterize the nature of the effects they may experience. May contain some or all of the following four steps.

    Hazard identification The determination of whether a particular chemical is or is not causally linked to particular health effects(s).

    Dose-response assessment The determination of the relation between the magnitude of exposure and the probability of occurrence of the health effects in question.

    Exposure assessment The determination of the extent of human exposure.

Risk characterization The description of the nature and often the magnitude of human risk, including attendant uncertainty.

Risk characterization The final step of a risk assessment, which is a description of the nature and often the magnitude of human risk, including attendant uncertainty.

Risk management The decision-making process that uses the results of risk assessment to produce a decision about environmental action. Risk management includes consideration of technical, scientific, social, economic, and political information.

Risk-specific dose The dose corresponding to a specified level of risk.

RMCL Recommended Maximum Contaminant Level.

Route of exposure The means by which toxic agents gain access to an organism (e.g., ingestion, inhalation, dermal exposure, intravenous, subcutaneous, intramuscular, intraperitoneal administration).

RTECS Registry of Toxic Effects of Chemical Substances.

SARA Superfund Amendments and Reauthorization Act of 1986.

Sarcoma A malignant tumor arising in connective tissue and composed primarily of anaplastic cells resembling supportive tissue.

SDWA Safe Drinking Water Act.

Sensitization An allergic condition that usually affects the skin or lungs. Once exposure to a substance has caused a reaction, the individual may be sensitized to that substance and further exposure even at low levels may elicit an adverse reaction.

Short-term exposure limit (STEL) A time-weighted average OEL that the American Conference of Government and Industrial Hygienists (ACGIH) indicates should not be exceeded any time during the work day. Exposures at the STEL should not be longer than 15 minutes and should not be repeated more than four times per day. There should be at least 60 minutes between successive exposure at the STEL.

Slope factor *See* Cancer potency factor.

SNUR Significant New Use Rule.

Somatic cells All cells other than germ cells or gametes.

Squamous cell carcinoma A malignant neoplasm derived from squamous epithelium.

Standardized mortality ratio The number of deaths, either total or cause-specific, in a given group expressed as a percentage of the number of deaths that could have been expected if the group has the same age- and sex-specific rates as the general population. Used in epidemiological studies to adjust mortality rates to a common standard so that comparisons can be made among groups.

Statistically significant effect In statistical analysis of data, a health effect that exhibits differences between a study population and a control group that are unlikely to have arisen by chance alone.

STEL *See* Short-term exposure limit.

Structure-activity relationship Relationships of biological activity or toxicity of a chemical to its chemical structure or substructure.

Subchronic exposure Exposure to a substance spanning approximately 10% of the lifetime of an organism.

Subcutaneous A method of exposure in which the substance is injected beneath the skin.

Surface area scaling factor The intra- and interspecies scaling factor most often used for cancer risk assessment by the U.S. EPA to convert an animal dose to a human equivalent dose: milligrams per square meter surface area per day. Body surface area is proportional to basal metabolic rate; the ratio of surface area to metabolic rate tends to be constant from one species to another. Because body surface area is approximately proportional to an animal's body weight to the 2/3 power, the scaling factor can be reduced to milligrams per body weight$^{2/3}$.

Synergism Interaction in which the combined effect of two or more chemicals is greater than the sum of the effect of each chemical alone.

Systemic Pertaining to or affecting the body as a whole or acting in a portion of the body other than the site of entry.

Target organ/system An organ or functional system (e.g., respiratory, immune, excretory, reproductive systems) that demonstrates toxicity to a specific chemical; not necessarily the organ/system with the highest accumulation of the chemical, but rather that which elicits a toxic response(s) of concern.

TBREL Toxicology-Based Recommended Exposure Limits (Dutch).

TC$_{LO}$ (toxic concentration low) The lowest concentration of a substance in air required to cause a toxic effect in some of the exposed population.

TD$_{LO}$ (toxic dose low) The lowest dose of a substance required to cause a toxic effect in some of the exposed population.

Teratogenicity The property of a chemical to cause structural or functional defects during the development of an organism.

Threshold limit value (TLV) The concentration of a substance below which no adverse health effects are expected to occur for workers assuming exposure for 8 hours per day, 40 hours per week. TLVs are published by the American Conference of Governmental Industrial Hygienists (ACGIH).

Threshold toxicant A substance showing an apparent level of effect that is a minimally effective dose, above which a response occurs; below that dose, no response is expected.

Time-weighted average (TWA) An approach to calculating the average exposure during a specified time period.

Total dose The sum of doses received from multiple routes of exposure.

Toxicant Any synthetic or natural chemical with an ability to produce adverse health effects.

Toxic effect Any change in an organism that results in impairment of functional capacity of the organism (as determined by anatomical, physiological, biochemical, or behavioral parameters); causes decrements in the organism's ability to maintain its normal function; or enchances the susceptibility of the organism to the deleterious effects of other environmental influences.

Toxicology The multidisciplinary study of toxicants, their harmful effects on biological systems, and the conditions under which these harmful effects occur. The mechanisms of action, detection, and treatment of the conditions produced by toxicants are studied.

TSCA Toxic Substances Control Act.

Tumor An abnormal growth of tissue, a neoplasm.

Uncertainty In the conduct of risk assessment (hazard identification, dose-response assessment, exposure assessment, risk characterization) the need to make assumptions or best judgments in the absence of precise scientific data creates uncertainties. These uncertainties, expressed qualitatively and sometimes quantitatively, attempt to define the usefulness of a particular evaluation in making a decision based on the available data.

Uncertainty factor (UF) One of several, generally 10-fold factors, applied to a NOAEL or a LOAEL to derive a reference dose (RfD) from experimental data. UFs are intended to account for (a) the variation in the sensitivity among the members of the human population, (b) the uncertainty in extrapolating animal data to human, (c) the uncertainty in extrapolating from data obtained in a less-than-lifetime exposure study to chronic exposure, and (d) the uncertainty in using a LOAEL rather than a NOAEL for estimating the threshold region.

Unit cancer risk A measure of the probability of an individual developing cancer as a result of exposure to a specified unit ambient concentration. For example, an inhalation unit cancer risk of 3.0×10^{-4} near a point source implies that if 10,000 people breathe a given concentration of a carcinogenic agent (e.g., 1 μg/m^3) for 70 years, three of the 10,000 will develop cancer as a result of this exposure. In water, the exposure unit is usually 1 μg/L, whereas in air it is 1 μg/m^3.

Upper bound cancer risk assessment A qualifying statement indicating that the cancer risk estimate is not a true value in that the dose-response modeling used provides a value that is not likely to be an underestimate of the true value. The true value may be lower than the upper bound cancer risk estimate and it may even be close to zero. This results from the use of a statistical upper confidence limit and from the use of conservative assumptions in deriving the cancer risk estimate.

Upper 95% confidence limit Assuming random and normal distribution, this is the range of values below which a value will fall 95% of the time.

USP United States Pharmacopeia.

Variation A divergence in the developing organism beyond the usual range of structural constitution that may not adversely affect survival or health. A specific category in the evaluation of developmental effects.

Voluntary risk Risk that an individual has consciously decided to accept.

Water quality criteria Nonregulatory guidance values used to identify a safe concentration of a pollutant or contaminant in ambient waters.

Weight of evidence The extent to which the available biomedical data support the hypothesis that a substance causes an effect in humans. For example, the following factors increase the weight of evidence that a chemical poses a hazard to humans: an increase in the number of tissue sites affected by the agent; an increase in the number of animal species, strains, sexes, and number of experiments and doses showing a response; the occurrence of a clear-cut dose-response relationship as well as a high level of statistical significance in the occurrence of the adverse effect in treated subjects compared with untreated controls; a dose-related shortening of the time of occurrence of the adverse effect; etc.

WHO World Health Organization.

WQC Water quality criteria.

Xenobiotic A substance not normally present in the environment, such as a pesticide or pollutant.

REFERENCES

1. U.S. Environmental Protection Agency, *General Quantitative Risk Assessment Guidance for Non-Cancer Health Effects,* ECAP-CIN-538M, 1989, cited in Hooper et al.[3]
2. National Research Council, *Risk Assessment in the Federal Government,* National Academy Press, Washington, D.C., 1983.
3. Hooper, L. D., Oehme, F. W., and Krieger, G. R., Risk assessment for toxic hazards, in *Hazardous Materials Toxicology: Clinical Principles of Environmental Health,* Sullivan, J. B. and Krieger, G. R., Eds., Williams and Wilkins, Baltimore, 1992, chap. 7.
4. Hallenbeck, W. H. and Cunningham K. M., Qualitative evaluation of human and animal studies, in *Quantitative Risk Assessment for Environmental and Occupational Health,* Lewis Publishers, Chelsea, MI, 1986, chap. 3.
5. Zbinden, G., *Progress in Toxicology,* vol. 1, Springer-Verlag, New York, 1973.
6. Ecobichon, D. J., *The Basis of Toxicity Testing,* CRC Press, Boca Raton, FL, 1992, chap. 2.
7. Ballantyne, B. and Sullivan, J. B., Basic principles of toxicology, in *Hazardous Materials Toxicology: Clinical Principles of Environmental Health,* Sullivan, J. B. and Krieger, G. R., Eds., Williams and Wilkins, Baltimore, 1992, chap. 2.
8. Paul, M., Clinical evaluation and management, in *Occupational and Environmental Reproductive Hazards: A Guide for Clinicians,* Williams and Wilkins, Baltimore, 1993, chap. 10.
9. Chow, A. W. and Jewesson, P. J., Pharmacokinetics and safety of antimicrobial agents during pregnancy, *Rev. Infect. Dis.,* 7, 288, 1985.

10. McGuigan, M. A., Teratogenesis and reproductive toxicology, in *Hazardous Materials Toxicology: Clinical Principles of Environmental Health,* Sullivan, J. B. and Krieger, G. R., Eds., Williams and Wilkins, Baltimore, 1993, chap. 16.

11. Lowe, J. A. et al., in *Health Effects of Municipal Waste Incineration,* CRC Press, Boca Raton, FL, 1990.

12. U.S. Environmental Protection Agency, *Techniques for the Assessment of the Carcinogenic Risk to the U.S. Population Due to Exposure from Selected Volatile Organic Compounds from Drinking Water via the Ingestion, Inhalation and Dermal Routes,* Cothern, C. R., Coniglio, W. A., and Marcus, W. L., Eds., Office of Drinking Water, NTIS, PB 84-213941, 1984.

13. U.S. Environmental Protection Agency, Reported in *Pesticide and Toxic Chemical News,* Oct. 19, 34, 1988.

14. Morgan, M. G., Risk analysis and management, *Scientific American,* 269, 32, 1993.

15. Lowrance, W. M., *Of Acceptable Risk: Science and the Determination of Safety,* William Kaufmann, Los Altos, 1976, chap. 3.

16. Ballantyne, B., Exposure-dose-response relationships, in *Hazardous Materials Toxicology: Clinical Principles of Environmental Health,* Sullivan, J. B. and Krieger, G. R., Eds., Williams and Wilkins, Baltimore, 1993, chap. 3.

17. Klaassen, C. D. and Eaton, D. L., Principles of toxicology, in *Casarett and Doull's Toxicology: The Basic Science of Poisons,* 4th ed., Doull, J., Klaassen, C. D., and Anders, M. O., Eds., Pergamon Press, New York, 1991, chap. 2.

18. Ecobichon, D. J., *The Basis of Toxicity Testing,* CRC Press, Boca Raton, FL, 1992, chap. 7.

19. Crone, H. D., *Chemicals and Society: A Guide to the New Chemical Age,* Cambridge University Press, Cambridge, 1986, chap. 4.

20. Munro, I. C. and Krewski, D. R., Risk assessment and regulatory decision making, *Food Cosmet. Toxicol.,* 19, 549, 1981.

21. Van Ryzin, J., Quantitative risk assessment, *J. Occup. Med.,* 22, 321, 1980.

22. Van Ryzin, J. and Rai, K., The use of quantal response data to make predictions, in *The Scientific Basis of Toxicity Assessment,* Witschi, H. R., Ed., Elsevier/North-Holland, New York, 1980, 273.

23. Selevan, S. G., Epidemiology, in *Occupational and Environmental Reproductive Hazards: A Guide for Clinicians,* Paul, M., Ed., Williams and Wilkins, Baltimore, 1993, chap. 9.

24. Piantadose, S., Epidemiology and principles of surveillance regarding toxic hazards in the environment, in *Hazardous Materials Toxicology: Clinical Principles of Environmental Health,* Sullivan, J. B. and Krieger, G. R., Eds., Williams and Wilkins, Baltimore, 1992, chap. 6.

25. U. S. Environmental Protection Agency, *Interim Methods for the Development of Inhalation Reference Doses,* Blackburn, K., Dourson, M., Erdreich, L., Jarabek, A. M., and Overton, J., Jr., Environmental Criteria and Assessment Offices, EPA1600/8-88/066F, 1989.

26. Gamble, J. F. and Battigelli, M. C., Epidemiology, in *Patty's Industrial Hygiene and Toxicology,* 3rd rev. ed. vol. I., Clayton, G. D. and Clayton, F. E., Eds., John Wiley & Sons, New York, 1978, chap. 5.

27. Piantadosi, S. and Sullivan, J. B., Chemical and environmental carcinogenesis, in *Hazardous Materials Toxicology: Clinical Principles of Environmental Health,* Sullivan, J. B. and Krieger, G. R., Eds., Williams and Wilkins, Baltimore, 1992, chap. 8.

28. IARC Working Group on the Evaluation of Carcinogenic Risk, Overall evaluations of carcinogenicity: An updating of IARC monographs, in *IARC Monographs on the Evaluation of Carcinogenic Risks to Humans,* Vols. 1 to 42, Suppl. 7, Lyon, France, 1987.

29. Meijers, J. M. M., Swaen, G. M. H., Schreiber, G. H., and Sturmans, F., Occupational epidemiological studies in risk assessment and their relation to animal experimental data, *Regul. Toxicol. Pharmacol.,* 16, 215, 1992.

30. Doll, B. and Peto, R., The causes of cancer: quantitative estimates of avoidable risks of cancer in the United States today, *J. Natl. Cancer Inst.,* 68, 1191, 1981.

31. Higginson, J. and Muir, C. S., Environmental carcinogenesis: misconceptions and limitations to cancer control, *J. Natl. Cancer Inst.,* 63, 1291, 1979.

32. Wynder, E. L. and Gori, G. B., Contribution of the environment to cancer incidence: an epidemiologic exercise, *J. Natl. Cancer Inst.,* 58, 825, 1977.

33. Weisburger, E. K., Industrial and environmental cancer risks, in *Dangerous Properties of Industrial Materials,* 6th ed., Sax, N. I., Ed., Van Nostrand Reinhold, New York, 1984, section 3.

34. Ries, L. A. G., Hankey, B. F., and Edwards, B. K., Eds., *Cancer Statistics Review, 1973–1987,* National Cancer Institute, Bethesda, MD, 1990.

35. Huff, J., Cirvello, J., Haseman, J., and Bucher, J., Chemicals associated with site-specific neoplasia in 1394 long term carcinogenesis experiments in laboratory rodents, *Environ. Health Perspect.*, 93, 247, 1991.

36. American Cancer Society, *Cancer Facts and Figures*, 2000.

37. Riggs, J. E., Rising cancer mortality in the United States, 1962–1987: evidence against environmental causation, *Regul. Toxicol. Pharmacol.*, 16, 81, 1992.

38. U.S. Department of Health and Human Services, Public Health Service, National Toxicology Program, *Ninth Annual Report on Carcinogens*, 2000.

39. Warburton, I., Measurement of reproductive effects in human populations: selected outcomes for study, in *Symposium on Criteria for Assessment of Health Effects at Chemical Disposal Sites*, Rockefeller University, New York, 1981.

40. Kline, J., Stein, Z., and Susser, M., *Conception to Birth: Epidemiology of Prenatal Development*, Oxford University Press, New York, NY, 1989.

41. Shepard, T. H., Fantel, A. G., and Mirkes, P. E., Developmental toxicology: prenatal period, in *Occupational and Environmental Reproductive Hazards: A Guide to Clinicians*, Paul, M., Ed., Williams and Wilkins, Baltimore, 1993, chap. 4.

42. Persaud, T. V. N., Teratogenic mechanisms, in *Advances in the Study of Birth Defects*, vol. 1, University Park Press, Baltimore, 1979.

43. Rousseaux, C. G. and Blakley, P. M., Fetus, in *Handbook of Toxicologic Pathology*, Haschek, W. M., and Rousseaux, C. G., Eds., Academic Press, San Diego, 1991, chap. 25.

44. National Foundation/March of Dimes: Report of Panel II. Guidelines for reproductive studies in exposed human populations, In: *Guidelines for Studies of Human Populations Exposed to Mutagenic and Reproductive Hazards*, Bloom, A. D., Ed., The Foundation, New York, 1981, 37.

45. Manson, J. M. and Wise, L. D., Teratogens, in *Cassarett and Doull's Toxicology: The Basic Science of Poisons*, 4th ed., Amdur, M. O., Doull, J., and Klaassen, C. D., Eds., Pergamon Press, New York, 1991, chap. 7.

46. Moore, K. L., *The Developing Human: Clinically Oriented Embryology*, 5th ed., Saunders, Philadelphia, 1993.

47. Kline, J. and Stein, Z., Very early pregnancy, in *Reproduction Toxicology*, Dixon, R. L., Ed., Raven Press, New York, 1985, 259.

48. Wilson, J. G., Teratogenic effects of environmental chemicals, *Fed. Proc.*, 36, 1698, 1977.

49. Ecobichon, D. J., *The Basis of Toxicity Testing*, CRC Press, Boca Raton, FL, 1992, chap. 5.

50. Shepard, T. H., Fantel, A. G., and Fitzsimmon, J., Congenital defect rates among spontaneous abortuses: twenty years of monitoring, *Teratology*, 39, 325, 1989.

51. Fantel, A. G. and Shepard, T. H., Morphological analysis of spontaneous abortuses, in *Spontaneous and Recurrent Abortion*, Bennett, M. J. and Edmons, D. K., Eds., Blackwell Publications, Oxford, 1987, 8.

52. MMWR, *Annual Summary 1981*, Morbidity and Mortality Weekly Report, 30, No. 54, 108, 1981.

53. Crone, H. D., *Chemicals and Society: A Guide to the New Chemical Age*, Cambridge University Press, Cambridge, 1986, chap. 7.

54. National Research Council, *Improving Risk Communication*, Committee on Risk Perception and Communication, Commission on Behavioral and Social Sciences and Education, Commission on Physical Sciences, Mathematics and Resources, National Academy Press, Washington, D.C., 1989.

55. Crouch, E. A. C. and Wilson, R., Inter-risk comparisons, in *Assessment and Management of Chemical Risks*, Rodricks, J. V. and Tardiff, R. G., Eds., American Chemical Society, Washington, D.C., 1984, chap. 7.

56. Paget, G. E., Ed., *Methods in Toxicology*, Blackwell Scientific Publishers, Oxford, 1970, 49.

57. Ecobichon, D. J., *The Basis of Toxicity Testing*, CRC Press, Boca Raton, FL, 1992, chap. 4.

58. Kleiber, M., *The Fire of Life: An Introduction to Animal Energetics*, John Wiley & Sons, New York, 1961.

59. Mortensen, M. E., Mercury toxicity in children, in *Similarities and Differences Between Children and Adults: Implications for Risk Assessment*, Guzelian, P. S., Henry, C. J., and Olin S. S., Eds., ISLI Press, Washington, D.C., 1992, 204.

60. U.S. Environmental Protection Agency, *Development of Statistical Distributions or Ranges of Standard Factors Used in Exposure Assessments*, Office of Health and Environmental Assessments, EPA No. 600/8-85/010, NTIS, PB85-242667, 1985.

61. U.S. Environmental Protection Agency, *Reference Physiological Parameters in Pharmacokinetic Modeling,* Arms, A. D. and Travis, C. C., Office of Risk Analysis, EPA No., 600/6-88/004, 1988.

62. Plowchalk, D., Meadows, M. J., and Martinson, D. R., Comparative approach to toxicokinetics, In: *Occupational and Environmental Reproductive Hazards, A Guide for Clinicians,* Paul, M., Ed., Williams and Wilkins, Baltimore, 1993, chap. 3.

63. U.S. Environmental Protection Agency, *Exposure Factors Handbook,* Konz, J. J., Lisi, K., Friebele, E., and Dixon, D. A., Office of Health and Environmental Assessments, EPA No. 600/8-89/043, 1989.

64. Spector, W. S., Ed., *Handbook of Biological Data,* W.B. Saunders, Philadelphia, 1956, 175.

65. Chen, C. W. and Hoang, K-C., Incorporating biological information into the assessment of cancer risk to humans under various exposure conditions and issues related to high background tumor incidence rates, in *Health Risk Assessment: Dermal and Inhalation Exposure and Absorption of Toxicants,* Wang, R. G. M., Knaak, J. B., and Maibach, H. I., Eds., CRC Press, Boca Raton, FL, 1993, chap. 21.

66. U.S. Environmental Protection Agency, *Risk Assessment Guidance for Superfund, Vol. 1: Human Health Evaluation Manual,* Office of Emergency and Remedial Response, EPA No. 540/1-89/002, 1989.

67. Paustenbach, D. J. and Leung, H-W., Techniques for assessing the health risks of dermal contact with chemicals in the environment, in *Health Risk Assessment: Dermal and Inhalation Exposure and Absorption of Toxicants,* Wang, R. G. M., Knaak, J. B, and Maibach, H. I., Eds., CRC Press, Boca Raton, FL, 1993, chap. 23.

68. Lynch, J. R., Measurement of worker exposure, in *Patty's Industrial Hygiene and Toxicology, Vol. III. Theory and Rationale of Industrial Hygiene Practice,* Cralley, L. V. and Cralley, L. J., Eds., John Wiley & Sons, New York, 1979, chap. 6.

69. Environ Corporation, *Risk Assessment Guidance Manual,* Allied Signal Inc., Morristown, NJ, 1990.

70. Hodge, H. C. and Sterner, J. H., *Am. Ind. Hyg. Assoc. Q.,* 10, 4, 1949.

71. Schurger, M. G. and McConnell, F., Eastman Chemicals, Kingsport, TN, 1989.

72. European Economic Community (EEC), l8th Adaptation to technical progress, Directive 93/21/EEC, *Off. J. Europ. Econ. Commun.,* 36, No. L110A/61, May 5, 1993.

73. Ashby, J., Doerrer, N. G., Flamm, F. G., Harris, J. E., Hughes, D. H., Johannsen, F. R., Lewis, S. C., Krivanek N, D., McCarthy, J. F., Moolenaar, R. J., Raabe, G. K., Reynolds, R. C., Smith, J. M., Stevens, J. T., Teta, M. J., and Wilson, J. D., A scheme for classifying carcinogens, *Regul. Toxicol. Pharmacol.,* 12, 270, 1990.

74. U.S. Environmental Protection Agency, *Glossary of Terms Related to Health, Exposure and Risk Assessment,* Air Risk Information Support Center, EPA No. 450/3-88/016, 1989.

75. Balls, M., Blaauboer, B., Brusick, D., Frazier, J., Lamb, D., Pemberton, M., Reinhardt, C., Roberfroid, M., Rosenkrantz, H., Schmid, B., Spielmann, H., Stammati, A-L., and Walum, E., Report and recommendations of the CAAT/ERGATT Workshop on the Validation of Toxicity Test Procedures, *ALTA,* 18, 313, 1990.

76. Hallenbeck, W. H. and Cunningham, K. M., Eds., *Quantitative Risk Assessment for Environmental and Occupational Health,* Lewis Publishers, Chelsea, MI, 1986, Appendix 2.

77. *Low-Dose Extrapolation of Cancer Risks: Issues and Perspectives,* International Life Sciences Institute, Washington, D.C., 1995, p 188.

78. Gargas, M. L., Finley, B. L., Pustenbach, D. J., and Long, T. F., Environmental health risk assessment: theory and practice, in *General and Appied Toxicology,* Ballantyne, B., Marrs, T. C., and Syversen, T., Eds., Grove's Dictionary, New York, 1999, chap. 82.

79. Morselli, P. L., Clinical pharmacology of the prenatal period and early infancy, *Clin. Pharmacokinetics,* 17 (Suppl. 1), 13, 1989.

80. Ritschel, W. A. and Kearns, G. L., *Handbook of Basic Pharmacokinetics,* 5th ed., American Pharmaceutical Association, Washington, D.C., 1999.

81. Leeder, J. S. and Kearns, G. L., Pharmacogenetics in pediatrics: implications for practice, *Pediatr. Clin. North Am.,* 44, 55, 1997.

82. U. S. Environmental Protection Agency, *Exposure Factors Handbook,* Wood, P., Phillips, L., Adenuga, A., Koontz, M., Rector, H., Wilkes, C., and Wilson, M., National Center for Environmental Assessment, EPA/ 600/p-95/002Fa, 1997.

83. U. S. Environmental Protection Agency, *Proposed Guidelines for Carcinogen Risk Assessment,* Office of Research and Development, EPA/600/p-92/003C, 1996.

25 Regulatory Toxicology in the United States: An Overview

Michael J. Derelanko, Ph.D., D.A.B.T., F.A.T.S.

CONTENTS

SECTION 1. INTRODUCTION

The following tables present an overview of U.S. federal agencies and major legislation regulating toxic substances.[1-3] More detailed information is presented elsewhere in the handbook or can be obtained from the references cited. Other legislation regulating toxic substances exists at the federal, state, and local levels, but a discussion of such legislation is beyond the scope of this book.

TABLE 25.1
Principal U.S. Regulatory Agencies Having Involvement with Toxicology

Agency	Agency Description	General Coverage
Food and Drug Administration (FDA)	A unit of the Department of Health and Human Services	• Drugs and foods • Food additives and cosmetics • Medical devices • Biologicals
Environmental Protection Agency (EPA)	Independent agency, not a part of a cabinet department	• Pesticides and Sterilants • Industrial chemicals • Air pollutants • Industrial waste
Occupational Safety and Health Administration (OSHA)	Unit of the Department of Labor	• Occupational exposure

TABLE 25.1 *(Continued)*
Principal U.S. Regulatory Agencies Having Involvement with Toxicology

Agency	Agency Description	General Coverage
Consumer Product Safety Commission (CPSC)	Independent commission	• Consumer products
Department of Agriculture (USDA)	Cabinet Department	• Veterinary biologicals • Administers the Animal Welfare Act covering the well being and humane treatment of warm-blooded lab animals. Currently, birds, rats, and mice are excluded. But efforts are underway that may result in their inclusion in the future.

TABLE 25.2
Major U.S. Federal Legislation Involving Toxic Substances

Statute	Code of Federal Regulations (CFR) Citation	Description
Clean Air Act (CAA)	40 CFR 50–80	Administered by EPA. Deals with control of hazardous air pollutants. Sets national standards for air quality, sources that produce air pollution, emission of noxious air pollutants, and motor vehicles.
Clean Water Act (CWA)	40 CFR 100–140, 400–470	Administered by EPA. Limits water pollution from industrial and municipal sources; provides funding for municipal sewage treatment construction; allows recovery of costs in mitigation of hazardous substance spills; emphasizes the importance of controlling toxic pollutants and encourages waste-treatment experimentation.
Comprehensive Environmental Response, Compensation and Liability Act (CERCLA)	40 CFR 300	Administered by EPA. Known as "Superfund." Requires cleanup of hazardous substances released into air, water, and land; covers both new releases and old dumpsites; establishes reportable quantities (RQs) for certain hazardous substances.
Consumer Product Safety Act (CPSA)	16 CFR 1015–1402	Administered by CPSC. Regulates products that pose unreasonable risk of injury or illness to consumers; establishes safety standards; promotes research into causes and prevention of product-related deaths, illness, and injuries.
Federal Food, Drug, and Cosmetic Act (FFDCA)	21 CFR 1–1300	Administered by FDA. Forbids the marketing of any food containing additives or nonadditives that render it injurious to health; requires the safety of food additives to be demonstrated; requires premarket approval of all new drugs based on demonstration of safety and efficacy; regulates the testing, marketing, and use of medical devices; regulates the distribution of cosmetics which pose a risk of more than transitory harm if used as intended; and mandates safety testing of color additives.

TABLE 25.2 *(Continued)*
Major U.S. Federal Legislation Involving Toxic Substances

Statute	Code of Federal Regulations (CFR) Citation	Description
Federal Hazardous Substances Act (FHSA)	16 CFR 1500–1512	Adminsitered by CPSC. Regulates, primarily through labeling requirements, hazardous substances used by consumers that are toxic, corrosive, combustible, radioactive, or generate pressure. Contains detailed criteria for determining toxicity.
Federal Insecticide, Fungicide, and Rodenticide Act (FIFRA)	40 CFR 162–180	Administered by EPA. Regulates all pesticides marketed in the United States through registration requirements. Safety and efficacy must be demonstrated such that no unreasonable risk to man and the environment is indicated.
Food Quality Protection Act (FQPA)	—	Administered by EPA. Amends FIFRA and FFDCA. Intended to update and resolve inconsistencies in the two major pesticide statutes; regulates pesticides to a reasonable-certainty-of-no-harm safety standard; mandates a single, health-based standard for all pesticides in all foods; provides special protection of infants and children; expedites approval of safer pesticides; creates incentives for the development effective crop protection tools; requires periodic re-evaluation of pesticide registrations and tolerances; addresses screening for endocrine active substances.
Hazardous Materials Transportation Act (HMTA)	49 CFR 106–107, 171–179	Administered by the Department of Transportation (DOT). Regulates hazardous materials shipped by road, air, or rail; specifies packaging, labeling, and shipping requirements.
Occupational Safety and Health Act (OSHA)	29 CFR 1910, 1915, 1918, 1926	Administered by the Occupational Safety and Health Administration (OSHA). Requires employers to provide safe working conditions; prescribes mandatory occupational safety and health standards including exposure limits for toxic chemicals; requires assessment of chemical hazards and notification of workers of such hazards (requires material safety data sheets). Established the National Institutes of Occupational Safety and Health (NIOSH).
Poison Prevention Packaging Act (PPPA)	16 CFR 1700–1704	Administered by CPSC. Sets standards for packaging of hazardous household products.
Resource Conservation and Recovery Act (RCRA)	40 CFR 240–271	Administered by EPA. Regulates the activities of generators, transporters, and those who treat, store, or dispose of hazardous wastes; establishes a list of waste substances considered hazardous; establishes a manifest system to track the generation, transportation, and disposal of hazardous wastes. Under RCRA, methods for treating, storing, and disposing of wastes are prescribed; location design and construction of treatment facilities are governed; qualifications for ownership, training, and financial responsibility of treatment facilities are established.
Safe Drinking Water Act (SDWA)	40 CFR 140–149	Administered by EPA. Sets standards for drinking water to protect public health. Maximum contaminant levels (MCLs) are prescribed. Includes provisions specifically designed to protect underground sources of drinking water. As of August, 1996, amended to address screening of endocrine active substances.

TABLE 25.2 *(Continued)*
Major U.S. Federal Legislation Involving Toxic Substances

Statute	Code of Federal Regulations (CFR) Citation	Description
Toxic Substances Control Act (TSCA)	40 CFR 700–799	Administered by EPA. Regulates the production, processing, importation, and use of chemical substances that present an unreasonable risk to health or the environment; requires notification of production of a new chemical or significant new use of an existing chemical; testing may be required for hazard assessment for high volume/high exposure chemicals; requires record keeping and reporting requirements of significant health effects.

TABLE 25.3
Federal Regulatory Programs Involved with Toxicological Testing

Agency	Authority	Statute	Program
CPSC	Consumer product exposures	Federal Hazardous Substances Act; Consumer Product Safety Act; Poison Prevention Packaging Act	Hazard Assessment and Reduction Program and Regulated Products Program
DOI[a]	Drug and management chemical for fisheries	Fish and Wildlife Coordination Act; Federal Insecticide, Fungicide and Rodenticide Act (FIFRA); Federal Food, Drug and Cosmetic Act (FFDCA)	Chemical-Drug Registration Program, National Biological Survey
	Non-Toxic Shot Program	Migratory Bird Treaty Act	Office of Migratory Bird Management, Fish and Wildlife Service
DOT[b]	Exposure to hazardous materials in transport	Federal Hazardous Materials Transportation Law	Research and Special Programs Administration
EPA	Pesticides	FIFRA	Office of Pesticide Programs
	Industrial chemicals	Toxic Substances Control Act	Office of Pollution Prevention and Toxics
FDA	Biologicals	FFDCA; Public Health Service Act	Center for Biologics Evaluation and Research
	Medical devices Radioactive materials	FFDCA	Center for Devices and Radiological Health
	Pharmaceuticals	FFDCA	Center for Drug Evaluation and Research
	Food and color additives, cosmetics	FFDCA	Center for Food Safety and Applied Nutrition
	Veterinary drugs	FFDCA	Center for Veterinary Medicine
OSHA	Worker exposures	OSHA	Directorate of Health Standards Programs

TABLE 25.3 *(Continued)*
Federal Regulatory Programs Involved with Toxicological Testing

Agency	Authority	Statute	Program
USDA	Genetically engineered plants, microbes, and arthropods	Plant Pest Act	APHIS[c]
	Veterinary biologicals and diagnostics	Virus, Serum, Toxin Act	APHIS[c]
	Non-food compounds on foods	Federal Meat Inspection Act; Poultry Products Inspection Act	Food Safety Inspection Service

[a] Department of the Interior
[b] Department of Transportation
[c] Animal and Plant Health Inspection Service. Program has authority, but no routine toxicity testing requirements.

Source: ICCVAM (ntp-server.niehs.nih.gov/htdocs/iccvam/REGUL.html).

REFERENCES

1. United States Environmental Protection Agency, Draft Report: Principles of Neurotoxicity Risk Assessment, *Federal Register,* Vol. 58, no. 148, 41556–41549, 1993.
2. Wexler, P., *Information Resources in Toxicology,* 2nd ed., Elsevier, New York, 1988, chap. 10, pp. 245–249.
3. Merrill, R. A., Regulatory toxicology, in *Casarett and Doull's Toxicology: The Basic Science of Poisons,* 4th ed., Amdur, M.D., Doull, J., and Klaassen, C.D., Eds., Pergamon Press, New York, 1991, chap. 30, pp. 970–984.

26 Regulatory Toxicology: U.S. EPA/Chemicals (TSCA)

Henry C. Fogle, M.S

CONTENTS

0-8493-0370-2/02/$0.00+$1.50
© 2002 by CRC Press LLC

SECTION 1. INTRODUCTION

This chapter outlines parts of the Toxic Substances Control Act (TSCA) which relate to toxicology and will be of particular interest to toxicologists. Brief descriptions are provided indicating the role that the U.S. Environmental Protection Agency (EPA) has in the implementation of this law and the handling and use of toxicological information. Descriptions of health and environmental data associated with the different sections of TSCA are also provided. References from which the data presented in this chapter were gathered and sources for additional information are included.

SECTION 2. EPA AND THE TOXIC SUBSTANCES CONTROL ACT (TSCA)

The U.S. EPA was created in 1970. It is the federal agency responsible for the administration of environmental protection laws in the United States including the Toxic Substances Control Act, U.S. Public Law 94-469. TSCA was created by the U.S. Congress in 1976 to "protect human health and the environment by requiring testing and necessary use restrictions on certain chemical substances and for other purposes."[1] This law became effective in the United States on January 1, 1977 and is codified in Title 40 of the U.S. Code of Federal Regulations.

The EPA's Office of Prevention, Pesticides, and Toxic Substances (OPPTS) works directly with TSCA implementation. This office "… is responsible for the development of national strategies for the control of toxic substances; criteria for assessing chemical substances; standards for test protocols for chemicals; rules and procedures for industry reporting and regulations for the control of substances deemed to be hazardous to man or the environment; enforcement of standards; and evaluating and assessing the impact of new chemicals and chemicals with new uses to determine the potential risk to health and/or the environment and, if needed, develop appropriate restrictions. The EPA coordinates activities on the assessment and control of toxic substances. Additional activities include control and regulation of pesticides and reduction in their use to assure human safety and protection of environmental quality; establishment of tolerance levels for pesticides which occur in or on food; monitoring of pesticide residue levels in food, humans, and nontarget fish, wildlife and their environments; investigation of pesticide accidents; and coordination of the Agency pollution prevention program."[1]

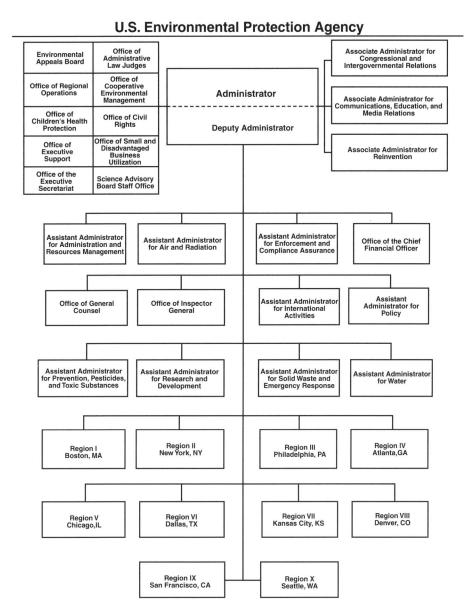

FIGURE 26.1 The EPA headquarters is in Washington, D.C. The Office of the EPA Administrator provides overall supervision to the EPA. This figure was provided by the EPA,[2] 1999.

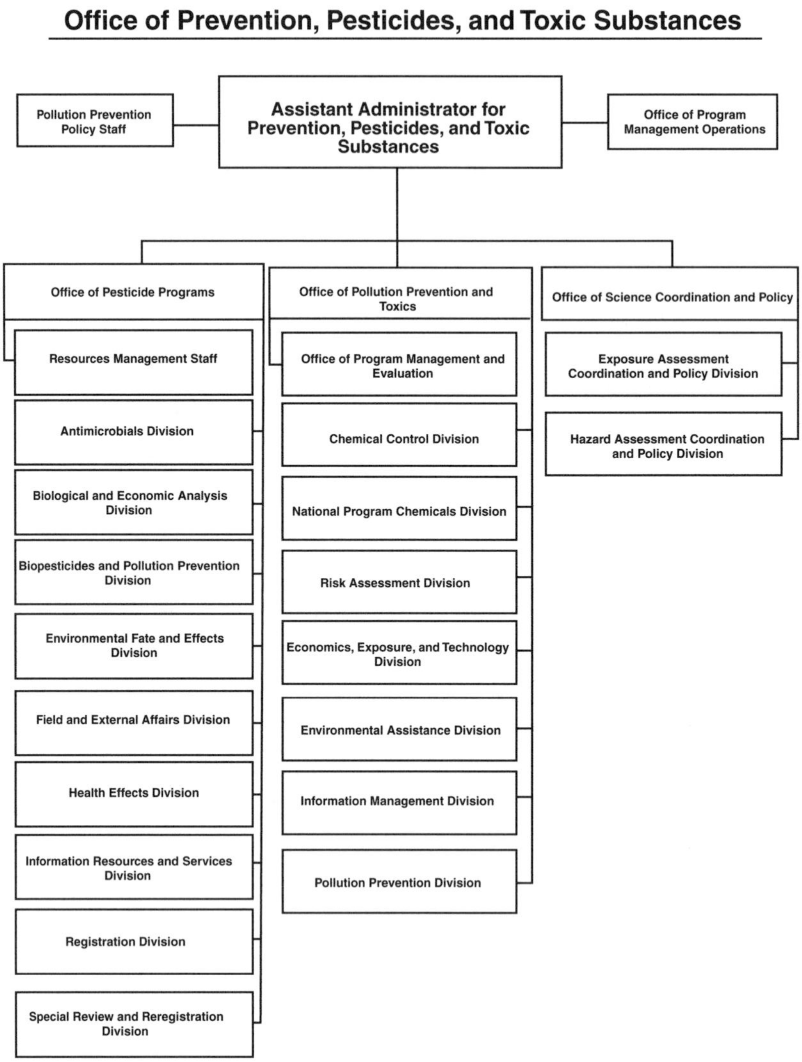

Office of Prevention, Pesticides, and Toxic Substances

FIGURE 26.2 The Assistant Administrator for Prevention, Pesticides, and Toxic Substances administers TSCA. This figure was provided by the EPA,[2] 1999.

TABLE 26.1
Location of EPA Regional Offices and their Homepages

Region	Regional Office	Information Telephone Number	Homepage
I	Boston, MA	(888) 372-7341	www.epa.gov/region01
II	New York, NY	(212) 637-3000	www.epa.gov/region02
III	Philadelphia, PA	(800) 438-2474	www.epa.gov/region03
IV	Atlanta, GA	(404) 562-9900	www.epa.gov/region04
V	Chicago, IL	(312) 353-2000	www.epa.gov/region05
VI	Dallas, TX	(214) 665-6444	www.epa.gov/region06
VII	Kansas City, KS	(913) 551-7000	www.epa.gov/region07
VIII	Denver, CO	(303) 312-6312	www.epa.gov/region08
IX	San Francisco, CA	(415) 744-1702	www.epa.gov/region09
X	Seattle, WA	(206) 553-1200	www.epa.gov/region10

EPA Regional Offices and State Breakdown

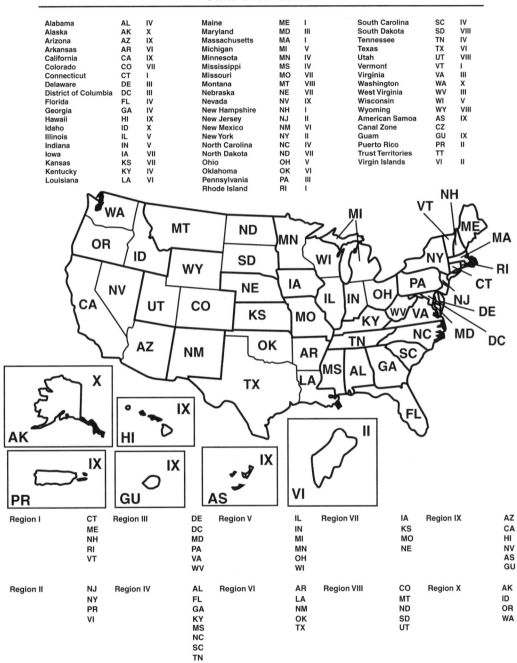

State	Abbr	Region
Alabama	AL	IV
Alaska	AK	X
Arizona	AZ	IX
Arkansas	AR	VI
California	CA	IX
Colorado	CO	VII
Connecticut	CT	I
Delaware	DE	III
District of Columbia	DC	III
Florida	FL	IV
Georgia	GA	IV
Hawaii	HI	IX
Idaho	ID	X
Illinois	IL	V
Indiana	IN	V
Iowa	IA	VII
Kansas	KS	VII
Kentucky	KY	IV
Louisiana	LA	VI
Maine	ME	I
Maryland	MD	III
Massachusetts	MA	I
Michigan	MI	V
Minnesota	MN	IV
Mississippi	MS	IV
Missouri	MO	VII
Montana	MT	VIII
Nebraska	NE	VII
Nevada	NV	IX
New Hampshire	NH	I
New Jersey	NJ	II
New Mexico	NM	VI
New York	NY	II
North Carolina	NC	IV
North Dakota	ND	VII
Ohio	OH	V
Oklahoma	OK	VI
Pennsylvania	PA	III
Rhode Island	RI	I
South Carolina	SC	IV
South Dakota	SD	VIII
Tennessee	TN	IV
Texas	TX	VI
Utah	UT	VIII
Vermont	VT	I
Virginia	VA	III
Washington	WA	X
West Virginia	WV	III
Wisconsin	WI	V
Wyoming	WY	VIII
American Samoa	AS	IX
Canal Zone	CZ	
Guam	GU	IX
Puerto Rico	PR	II
Trust Territories	TT	
Virgin Islands	VI	II

Region I		Region III		Region V		Region VII		Region IX	
	CT		DE		IL		IA		AZ
	ME		DC		IN		KS		CA
	NH		MD		MI		MO		HI
	RI		PA		MN		NE		NV
	VT		VA		OH				AS
			WV		WI				GU

Region II		Region IV		Region VI		Region VIII		Region X	
	NJ		AL		AR		CO		AK
	NY		FL		LA		MT		ID
	PR		GA		NM		ND		OR
	VI		KY		OK		SD		WA
			MS		TX		UT		
			NC						
			SC						
			TN						

FIGURE 26.3 EPA Regional Offices and State Breakdown. This figure was provided by the EPA,[2] 1999.

SECTION 3. *TSCA SECTION 4:* TESTING OF EXISTING CHEMICAL SUBSTANCES

A. BACKGROUND

TSCA Section 4 relates to testing of "existing chemicals." Existing chemicals are chemical substances that are listed on the *Toxic Substances Control Act Chemical Substances Inventory* (often referred to as "The TSCA or EPA Inventory"). Section 4 gives the EPA authority to require toxicological testing of selected substances, or mixtures containing one or more of those substances, to clarify or substantiate potential health or environmental hazards and risks. Testing may be required if the EPA believes that a substance may present an unreasonable risk of injury to health or the environment or if there may be significant exposure because of potential for use and/or the quantity produced or released into the environment. (See 56 FR 32294, July 15, 1991[3] for details.)

Although several federal agencies and EPA program offices can request the EPA to consider Section 4 test rules for chemical substances, the main source of such a request or recommendation is the Interagency Testing Committee (ITC). The ITC is an advisory committee directed by TSCA to establish testing priorities for TSCA-regulatable chemical substances and mixtures. It also recommends the kinds of tests that should be performed under TSCA Section 4. In making a recommendation, the ITC considers all available data on and potential for carcinogenic, mutagenic, teratogenic, and chronic toxic effects, as well as a substance's ability to bioaccumulate or cause adverse environmental effects. The ITC maintains a "TSCA Section 4(e) Priority Testing List" and transmits revisions of the list in the form of a "report" to the EPA administrator every 6 months for EPA action and publication in the Federal Register.

The EPA can issue a Section 4 Test Rule, arrange for testing by way of a consent agreement with industry manufacturers, or determine that additional testing isn't necessary. The types of testing generally associated with Section 4 Test Rules fall into the following three categories:

1. Health Effects Testing: Includes general toxicity, exposure assessment, specific organ/tissue toxicity, neurotoxicity, and/or metabolism.
2. Environmental Effects Testing: Includes aquatic and terrestrial toxicity testing.
3. Chemical Fate Testing: Includes the determination of selected physical and chemical properties, transport processes as well as testing to determine transformation processes.

Test data may be developed according to the following standard guidelines:

1. Standard EPA Testing guidelines: 40 CFR 795, 796, 797, and 798.[4] (On Aug. 15, 1997 the EPA OPPT issued revised TSCA test guidelines (62 FR 438201)
2. Organization for Economic Cooperation and Development (OECD) testing guidelines available from the OECD Publication and Information Center, 1750 Pennsylvania Ave., N.W., Washington, D.C. 20006; Telephone (202) 785-6323.
3. EPA's pesticide assessment guidelines as published by the National Technical Information Service (NTIS), 5285 Port Royal Road, Springfield, VA 22161; Telephone (703) 487-4650.

All studies conducted by industry under TSCA Section 4 must be performed in accordance with established test methods ("guidelines") and must adhere strictly to EPA's Good Laboratory Practice Standards regulations (see 40 CFR Part 792).

TABLE 26.2
Substances Currently Related to Section 4 Activity
(see note at end of Table 26.3)

Chemical Group	CAS Numbers		
Acetonitrile	75-05-8		
Acrylamide	79-06-1		
Acrylic acid	79-10-7		
Alkyl epoxides	558-30-5	1464-53-5	2404-44-6
	2855-19-8	3234-28-4	3266-23-7
	7320-37-8	7390-81-0	18633-25-5
	22092-38-2	67860-04-2	
Alkyl phthalates	84-66-2	84-74-2	85-68-7
	85-69-8	117-81-7	131-11-3
	3648-20-2	27554-26-3	68515-42-4
	68515-47-9	68515-48-0	68515-49-1
	68515-50-4	68515-51-5	
Alkyl tin compounds	77-58-7	1185-81-5	25168-21-2
	25168-24-5	25852-70-4	26636-01-1
	54849-38-6		
Anilines	62-53-3	88-74-4	89-63-4
	95-51-2	95-76-1	95-82-9
	97-02-9	99-09-2	99-30-9
	100-01-6	106-47-8	108-42-9
	121-87-9	554-00-7	608-27-5
	634-93-5	635-22-3	827-94-1
	1817-73-8	6283-25-6	
Anthraquinone,9,10	84-65-1		
Antimony compounds	1309-64-4	1345-04-6	7440-36-0
Aryl phosphates	78-33-1	115-86-6	1241-94-7
	1330-78-5	2528-36-1	25155-23-1
	26967-76-0	28108-99-8	28109-00-4
	29761-21-5	34364-42-6	56803-37-3
	64532-97-4	65652-41-7	
Benzidine dyes	72-57-1	91-92-9	91-96-3
	573-58-0	992-59-6	1937-37-7
	2150-54-1	2429-71-2	2429-73-4
	2429-74-5	2429-79-0	2429-81-4
	2429-82-5	2429-83-6	2429-84-7
	2586-57-4	2586-58-5	2586-60-9
	2602-46-2	2610-05-1	2893-80-3
	3476-90-2	3530-19-6	3567-65-5
	3626-28-6	4335-09-5	5422-17-3
	6358-29-8	6360-54-9	6426-67-1
	6449-35-0	6507-81-9	6637-88-3
	6656-03-7	6739-62-4	7082-31-7
	8014-91-3	10401-50-0	16071-86-6
	16143-79-6	20282-70-6	

TABLE 26.2 *(Continued)*
Substances Currently Related to Section 4 Activity
(see note at end of Table 26.3)

Chemical Group	CAS Numbers		
Biphenyl	92-52-4		
Bis(2-ethylhexyl) terephthalate	6422-86-2		
Bisphenol A	80-05-7		
Brominated flame retardants I	1163-19-5	3194-55-6	32534-81-9
	32536-52-0	37853-59-1	
Butyl glycolyl butyl phthalate	85-70-1		
Butylene oxide, 1,2	106-88-7		
C.I. disperse blues	3618-72-2	3618-73-3	3956-55-6
	21429-43-6		
C9 Aromatic hydrocarbons	70693-06-0		
Carbofuran intermediates	13414-54-5	13414-55-6	68298-46-4
Chlorendic acid	115-28-6		
Chlorinated benzenes	87-61-6	95-50-1	95-94-3
	106-46-7	108-90-7	120-82-1
	608-93-5	634-66-2	634-90-2
Chlorinated naphthalenes	90-13-1	1321-64-8	1321-65-9
	1335-87-1	1335-88-2	2234-13-1
	28699-88-9		
Chlorinated paraffins	2-00-6	2-01-7	2-02-8
	2-03-9		
Chloro-1,3-butadiene,2-	126-99-8		
Chlorobenzotrifluoride,4-	98-56-6		
Chloromethane	74-87-3		
Chlorotoluene,2-	95-49-8		
Commercial hexane	1-00-3	96-37-7	
Cresols	95-48-7	106-44-5	108-39-4
	1319-77-3		
Crotonaldehyde	4170-30-3		
Cumene	98-82-8		
Cyclohexane	110-82-7		
Cyclohexanone	108-94-1		
Developmental/ reproductive toxicity	57-10-3	74-97-5	75-15-0
	79-31-2	95-80-7	100-21-0
	104-76-7	107-13-1	111-11-5
	120-80-9	123-30-8	27193-86-8
Di-*tert*-butylphenol,2,6-	128-39-2		

TABLE 26.2 *(Continued)*
Substances Currently Related to Section 4 Activity
(see note at end of Table 26.3)

Chemical Group	CAS Numbers		
Dibromo(dibromoethyl) cyclohexane	3322-93-8		
Dichlorobenzotrifluoride,3,4	328-84-7		
Dichloroethylene,1,1-	75-35-4		
Dichloromethane	75-09-2		
Dichloropropane,1,2-	78-87-5		
Diethylene glycol butyleth/ac	112-34-5	124-17-4	
Diethylenetriamine	111-40-0		
Diisodecyl phenyl phosphite	25550-98-5		
Dioxolane,1,3-	646-06-0		
Ethylene oxide	75-21-8		
Ethylenebis (oxyethylene) diacetate	111-21-7		
Ethylhexanoic acid,2	149-57-5		
Ethylhexanol,2	104-76-7		
Fluoroalkenes	75-02-5	75-38-7	116-14-3
	116-15-4	359-11-5	677-21-4
Formamide	75-12-7		
Glycidols	101-90-6	106-90-1	106-91-2
	106-92-3	122-60-1	126-80-7
	556-52-5	930-37-0	1675-54-3
	2210-79-9	2224-15-9	2238-07-5
	2425-01-6	2425-79-8	2426-08-6
	2461-15-6	2461-18-9	2530-83-8
	2897-60-1	3072-84-2	3101-60-8
	3188-83-8	3568-29-4	4016-11-9
	4016-14-2	5026-74-4	5255-75-4
	5493-45-8	6178-32-1	7195-45-1
	7328-97-4	7422-52-8	7665-72-7
	13236-02-7	13561-08-5	14228-73-0
	15965-99-8	16245-97-9	17557-23-2
	17963-04-1	20217-01-0	22421-59-6
	26447-14-3	26761-45-5	32568-89-1
	35243-89-1	38304-52-8	38954-75-5
	54208-63-8	60501-41-9	61578-04-9
	67786-03-2	68081-84-5	68134-06-5
	68134-07-6	68517-02-2	68609-96-1
	68609-97-2	68959-23-9	68987-80-4
	69155-42-6	71033-08-4	71808-64-5
	72319-24-5	74398-71-3	75150-13-9
Halogenated alkyl epoxides	106-89-8	694-17-7	3083-23-6
	3083-25-8	3132-64-7	3583-47-9

TABLE 26.2 *(Continued)*
**Substances Currently Related to Section 4 Activity
(see note at end of Table 26.3)**

Chemical Group	CAS Numbers		
Hexachlorobutadiene	87-68-3		
Hexachlorocyclopentadiene	77-47-4		
Hexachloroethane	67-72-1		
Hexachloronorbomadiene	3389-71-7		
Hexafluoropropylene oxide	428-59-1		
Hexamethylene diisocyanate	822-06-0		
Hydroquinone	123-31-9		
Isophorone	78-59-1		
Isopropanol	67-63-0		
Isopropyl biphenyl/DPBP	25640-78-2	69009-90-1	
Mercaptobenzothiazole,2-	149-30-4		
Mesityl oxide	141-79-7		
Methyl ethyl ketoxime	96-29-7		
Methyl isobutyl ketone/MEK	78-93-3	108-10-1	
Methyl *tert*-butyl ether	1634-04-4		
Methylenedianiline,4,4-	101-77-9		
Methylpyrrolidone,*N*-	872-50-4		
Naphthenate salts	61789-36-4	61789-51-3	61790-14-5
Chemicals recommended due to specific neuro toxicity concerns	60-29-7	64-17-5	67-64-1
	71-36-3	78-83-1	78-93-3
	108-10-1	108-88-3	109-99-9
	110-80-5	123-86-4	141-78-6
	628-63-7	1330-20-7	
Nitrobenzene	98-95-3		
Nonylphenol,4-branched	84852-15-3		
Octamethylcyclotetrasiloxane	556-67-2		
Chemicals recommended for testing by the Office of Drinking Water	75-00-3	75-34-3	79-34-5
	103-65-1	108-67-8	
Chemicals recommended for testing by the Office of Solid Waste	54-11-5	62-44-2	72-20-8
	72-57-1	70-30-4	74-93-1
	74-95-3	74-87-3	75-34-3
	75-44-5	75-25-2	75-87-6
	75-70-7	79-19-6	79-22-1
	76-01-7	84-74-2	85-44-9
	81-07-2	94-75-7	95-50-1
	94-58-6	96-23-1	97-63-2

TABLE 26.2 *(Continued)*
Substances Currently Related to Section 4 Activity
(see note at end of Table 26.3)

Chemical Group	CAS Numbers		
	95-94-3	98-87-3	100-01-6
	98-86-2	101-55-3	103-85-5
	100-02-7	106-51-4	107-10-8
	106-46-7	108-31-6	108-60-1
	107-12-0	109-77-3	110-75-8
	109-06-8	111-91-1	120-58-1
	111-54-6	123-33-1	123-63-7
	122-09-8	131-11-3	131-89-5
	126-98-7	353-50-4	494-03-1
	134-32-7	541-73-1	542-76-7
	506-68-3	598-31-2	606-20-2
	591-08-2	616-23-9	636-21-5
	608-93-5	757-58-4	765-34-4
	640-19-7	2136-89-2	3288-58-2
	1464-53-5	5216-25-1	5344-82-1
	3689-24-5	16532-79-9	20830-81-3
	7803-55-6		
Oleylamine	112-90-3		
Pentabromoethylbenzene	85-22-3		
Phenoxyethanol,2-	122-99-6		
Phenylenediamines	95-54-5	95-70-5	95-80-7
	95-83-0	99-56-9	106-50-3
	108-45-2	108-71-4	137-09-7
	496-72-0	541-69-5	541-70-8
	614-94-8	615-05-4	615-28-1
	615-45-2	615-46-3	624-18-0
	823-40-5	1197-37-1	2687-25-4
	3663-23-8	5042-55-7	5131-58-8
	5131-60-2	5307-02-8	5307-14-2
	6219-71-2	6219-77-8	6369-59-1
	15872-73-8	16245-77-5	18266-52-9
	20103-09-7	25376-45-8	39156-41-7
	42389-30-0	62654-17-5	65879-44-9
	66422-95-5	67801-06-3	68015-98-5
	68239-80-5	68239-82-7	68239-83-8
	68459-98-3	68966-84-7	
Polychlorinated terphenyls	61788-33-8		
Polyhalogenated dibenzodioxins	1-06-9	1-07-0	79-94-7
	79-95-8	82-68-8	85-22-3
	87-10-5	87-61-6	87-65-0
	87-84-3	89-61-2	89-64-5
	89-69-0	92-04-6	94-74-6
	94-75-7	94-81-5	94-82-6
	95-50-1	95-56-7	95-57-8

TABLE 26.2 *(Continued)*
Substances Currently Related to Section 4 Activity
(see note at end of Table 26.3)

Chemical Group	CAS Numbers		
	95-77-2	95-88-5	95-94-3
	95-95-4	97-50-7	99-28-5
	99-30-9	99-54-7	106-37-6
	106-46-7	108-70-3	108-86-1
	108-90-7	117-18-0	118-75-2
	118-79-6	120-36-5	120-82-1
	120-83-2	320-72-9	348-51-6
	350-30-1	488-47-1	576-24-9
	583-78-8	608-71-9	615-58-7
	615-67-8	626-39-1	827-94-1
	933-75-5	1163-19-5	1940-42-7
	2577-72-2	3772-94-9	4162-45-2
	21850-44-2	25327-89-3	32534-81-9
	32536-52-0	37853-59-1	37853-61-5
	55205-38-4		
Propylene oxide	75-56-9		
Pyridine	110-86-1		
Quinone	106-51-4		
Sodium *N*-methyl-*N*-oleoyltaurine	137-20-2		
Sodium cyanide	143-33-9		
Tetrabromobisphenol A	79-94-7		
Tetramethylbutylphenol	140-66-9		
Toluene	108-88-3		
Tributyl phosphate	126-73-8		
Trichloroethane,1,1,1 -	71-55-6		
Triethylene glycolethers	112-35-6	112-50-5	143-22-6
Tris(2-chloroethyl) phosphite	140-08-9		
Tris(2-ethylhexyl) trimellitate	3319-31-1		
UF Resins	9011-05-6		
Vinylcyclohexene,4-	100-40-3		
Xylenes	95-47-6	106-42-3	108-38-3
	1330-20-7		

TABLE 26.3
Summaries of Test Data are Available for the Following Substances which Have Been Tested under TSCA Section 4 (see note at end of this table)

Chemical Summary No.	Chemical Substance or Group	Federal Register Date Announcing Receipt of Section 4 Test Data				
G001	Acetonitrile	11/02/84				
G002	Acrylamide	07/27/83	02/06/85	05/01/86	10/31/86	
G003	Alkyl epoxides					
G004	Alkyl phthalates	12/01/82	03/23/83	07/27/83	11/25/83	02/10/84
		05/02/84	07/26/84	11/02/84	05/03/85	11/12/85
		02/06/85	02/24/86	05/01/86	08/01/86	10/31/86
		01/20/87	12/14/89	04/13/90	04/26/90	12/04/90
		08/28/91				
G005	Alkyl tin compounds					
G006	Anilines	11/09/88	06/13/89	08/04/89	08/16/89	08/31/89
		09/28/89	10/13/89	10/25/89		
G007	9,10-Anthraquinone	11/09/88	01/18/89	04/13/89	09/18/89	
G008	Antimony metal, trioxide, and sulfide	02/24/86	08/01/86	01/20/87		
G009	Aryl phosphate base stocks	11/12/85	02/24/86			
G010	Benzidine-, *o*-Toluidine-, *o*-Dianisidine-based dyes					
G011	Biphenyl	10/22/87	05/18/88	06/22/88	08/01/88	10/26/88
		01/12/89	03/29/89			
G012	Bis(2-ethylhexyl)terephthalate (DOTP)	02/06/85	05/03/85	11/12/85	02/24/86	08/01/86
		01/20/87				
G013	Bisphenol A (BPA)	11/12/85	04/22/88			
G014	Butyl glycolyl butyl phthalate (BGBP)					
G015	1,2-Butylene oxide	05/02/84				
G016	C.I. Disperse blues	12/04/90	01/22/91	03/22/91	05/29/91	
G017	C$_9$ Aromatic hydrocarbon fraction	03/01/88	06/22/88	07/21/88	08/31/89	
G018	Carbofuran intermediates (Cls)					
G019	Chlorendic acid (CA)					
G020	Chlorinated benzenes	05/02/84	01/20/87	01/14/88	08/31/88	10/26/88
		12/06/88	05/17/89			
G021	Chlorinated naphthalenes					
G022	Chlorinated paraffins	08/24/82	12/01/82	03/23/83	05/04/83	07/27/83
		11/25/83	02/10/84	07/26/84	11/02/84	05/03/85
G023	4-Chlorobenzotrifluoride (4-CBTF)	05/04/83	11/25/83	05/02/84	02/06/85	
G024	2-Chloro-,3-butadiene (Chloroprene)					
G025	Chloromethane	07/26/84				
G026	2-Chlorotoluene (2-CT)	08/24/82	12/01/82	03/23/83	05/04/83	07/27/83
		11/25/83	02/10/84	05/02/84	02/06/85	08/07/85
		02/24/86	08/01/86	10/31/86		

TABLE 26.3 *(Continued)*
Summaries of Test Data are Available for the Following Substances which Have Been Tested under TSCA Section 4 (see note at end of this table)

Chemical Summary No.	Chemical Substance or Group	Federal Register Date Announcing Receipt of Section 4 Test Data				
G027	Commercial hexane	08/04/89 09/30/92	12/21/89	07/02/90	03/14/90	05/16/91
G028	Cresols	07/21/88 07/20/89	09/27/88 12/21/89	12/20/88	02/16/89	04/13/89
G029	Crotonaldehyde	12/04/90				
G030	Cumene	07/21/87	09/28/89	01/04/90	03/27/90	
G031	Cyclohexane					
G032	Cyclohexanone	11/02/84	08/01/86	01/20/87		
G033	1,2-Dibromo-4-(1,2-dibromoethyl) cyclohexane (TBEC)					
G034	2,6-Di-*tert*-butylphenol (DTBT)					
G035	3,4-Dichlorobenzotrifluoride (DCBTF)	08/01/88	10/26/88	12/20/88		
G036	1,1 –Dichloroethylene					
G037	Dichloromethane	05/03/85				
G038	1,2-Dichloropropane (DCP)	12/06/88	03/17/89	05/17/89	06/13/89	07/02/90
G039	Diethylene glycol butyl ether/acetate (DGBE/DGBA)	10/22/87	08/04/89	10/13/89		
G040	Diethylenetriamine (DETA)	01/20/87	10/02/87	05/27/88	07/01/88	04/22/91
G041	Diisodecyl phenyl phosphite (PDDP)	06/05/90				
G042	1,3-Dioxolane	08/07/85	02/24/86			
G043	Ethylenebis (oxyethylene) diacetate (TGD)					
G044	Ethylene oxide					
G045	2-Ethylhexanoic acid (EHA)	07/21/87	01/14/88	07/08/88		
G046	2-Ethylhexanol (EH)	07/21/87	02/14/92	03/10/92		
G047	Fluoroalkenes	05/01/86 09/27/88 03/29/89	08/01/86 10/26/88 01/22/91	05/27/88 11/09/88 04/22/91	06/06/88 12/06/88 08/19/92	08/31/88 03/02/89
G048	Formamide	02/10/84	08/07/85			
G049	Glycidol and derivatives					
G050	Halogenated alkyl epoxides (HAE)					
G051	Hexachloro-1,3-butadiene (HCBD)					
G052	Hexachlorocyclopentadiene (HCCP)					
G053	Hexachloroethane (HCE)					
G054	1,2,3,4,7,7-Hexachloronorbornadiene (HEX-BCH)					

TABLE 26.3 *(Continued)*
Summaries of Test Data are Available for the Following Substances which Have Been Tested under TSCA Section 4 (see note at end of this table)

Chemical Summary No.	Chemical Substance or Group	Federal Register Date Announcing Receipt of Section 4 Test Data				
G055	Hexafluoropropylene oxide (HFPO)					
G056	1,6-Hexamethylene diisocyanate (HDI)					
G057	Hydroquinone	02/24/86	05/01/86	08/01/88	11/28/88	01/04/90
G058	Isophorone	02/10/84	02/06/85	05/03/85		
G059	Isopropanol	06/21/90	12/29/90	03/22/91	05/02/91	06/02/92
G060	Isopropyl biphenyl/Diisopropyl biphenyl (IPBP/DPBP)					
G061	2-Mercaptobenzothiazole (MBT)	10/31/86 01/25/91	01/20/87	04/22/87	11/08/89	05/11/90
G062	Mesityl oxide (MO)	07/01/92	11/13/92			
G063	Methyl *tert*-butyl ether	08/04/89 10/13/89	05/17/89 07/19/90	06/13/89 12/14/92	08/04/89	08/16/89
G064	Methyl ethyl ketoxime (MEKO)	01/25/91	05/16/91	07/24/91	04/28/92	
G065	4,4′-Methylenedianiline (4,4′-MDA)					
G066	Methyl isobutyl ketone/Methyl ethylketone (MIBK/MEK)	11/25/83	02/10/84	02/06/85		
G067	*N*-Methylpyrrolidone (NMP)					
G068	Naphthenate salts	07/26/84	04/22/87			
G069	Nitrobenzene					
G070	4-Nonylphenol, branched (4-NP)	09/11/90 05/21/92	12/28/90	03/22/91	06/18/91	01/28/92
G071	Octamethylcyclotetrasiloxane (OMCTS)	12/14/89 05/02/91	02/01/90 08/15/92	05/11/90	06/05/90	02/12/91
G072	Office of Drinking Water (ODW) Chemicals					
G073	Office of Solid Waste (OSW) Chemicals	02/16/89 01/04/90	03/17/89 04/13/90	07/20/89	08/16/89	11/21/89
G074	Oleylamine	08/07/85	11/12/85	10/25/89	12/21/89	
G075	Pentabromoethylbenzene (PEB)					
G076	2-Phenoxyethanol (2-PE)	07/26/84	08/07/85	01/20/87	07/21/87	10/22/87
G077	Phenylenediamines (PDAs)	02/24/86 07/28/92	12/04/90 02/09/93	12/28/90 02/19/93	02/12/91	05/16/91
G078	Polychlorinated terphenyls (PCT)					
G079	Polyhalogenated dibenzodioxins/furans (HDDs/HDFs)	12/21/89 12/14/92	02/01/90	05/30/90	06/23/92	11/13/92
G080	Propylene oxide	11/12/85	02/24/86	10/22/87	01/14/88	

TABLE 26.3 *(Continued)*
Summaries of Test Data are Available for the Following Substances which Have Been Tested under TSCA Section 4 (see note at end of this table)

Chemical Summary No.	Chemical Substance or Group	Federal Register Date Announcing Receipt of Section 4 Test Data				
G081	Pyridine					
G082	Quinone					
G083	Sodium *N*-methyl-*N*-oleoyltaurine (SMOT)					
G084	Tetrabromobisphenol A (TBBPA)	12/06/88	03/02/89	04/13/89	07/10/89	09/18/89
G085	4-(1,1,3,3-Tetramethylbutyl)-phenol (TMBP)	02/06/85	01/20/87			
G086	Toluene					
G087	Tributyl phosphate (TBP)	04/13/90 02/09/93	07/19/90	12/04/90	04/22/91	01/28/92
G088	1,1,1-Trichloroethane (TCEA)	08/01/86 06/25/91	07/15/87	12/04/90	02/12/91	05/29/91
G089	Triethylene glycol ethers	04/13/90	04/26/90	12/04/90	04/06/92	
G090	Tris(2-chloroethyl) phosphite (TCEP)					
G091	Tris(2-ethylhexyl)trimellitate (TOTM)	02/06/85 08/01/86	08/07/85	11/12/85	02/24/86	05/01/86
G092	UF Resins					
G093	Xylenes					
G094	Multi-substance rule: Developmental/ Reproductive toxicity					
G095	Multi-substance rule: Neurotoxicity					
G096	Brominated Flame Retardants I					
G097	4-Vinylcyclohexene (VCH)	08/19/92	11/13/92			
G098	Sodium cyanide					
G099	Acrylic acid					

Note: The information provided in Tables 26.2 and 26.3 changes from year to year due to addition of chemical substances to be tested under TSCA Section 4 and receipt of new test data. By year 2000 the EPA received over 600 studies for approximately 150 chemicals. **For the most recent information, access the EPA's OPPT Chemical Testing and Information gathering home page at [www.epa.gov/opptintr/chemtest] or consult the latest available edition of 40 CFR Part 799.**

B. The Master Testing List (MTL)

Currently there are 79,745 chemical substances listed on the TSCA Inventory and all are referred to as being "existing chemicals." They can be produced, imported, and used for commercial purposes in the United States without prior notification to the EPA. An EPA program, "The Existing Chemicals Program," focuses on potential health and environmental risks related to about 1400 of the existing chemicals, all of which are produced in quantities > 10,000 pounds per year. Polymers are not emphasized because they are generally considered to be of relatively little concern, mainly due to limited bioavailability.

The EPA's Existing Chemicals Risk Management Program consists of two phases. The first phase, "Risk Management One (RM1)," involves consideration of a substance's hazards and exposure potential by an interdisciplinary EPA committee called the RM1 Committee. Health and environmental effects and exposure data are usually provided to the EPA by The Interagency Testing Committee (ITC) as well as other EPA offices and state agencies. Substances believed to pose the highest potential risk of injury to health or the environment are identified by the RM1 Committee and lists are developed for possible follow-up activity (exposure reduction, toxicity testing, or regulatory action) by industry and/or the EPA. Such substances are prioritized according to potential risk with those of the highest priority being placed on a "Master Testing List (MTL)." The MTL has been used by the EPA since 1990 to set the testing agenda under Section 4 of TSCA. The MTL is not an EPA "rule" and is not published in the *Federal Register*, although a notice of its availability is published in the *Federal Register*.

Since the initial MTL in 1990, the EPA has placed over 500 specific chemical substances and 10 categories of substances on the MTL.

The second phase of the EPA's Existing Chemicals Risk Management Program is referred to as the "Risk Management Two (RM2)" phase. Substances are selected from a "risk reduction list" prepared by the RM1 committee based on potential or known toxicity, potential or known exposure, and the extent to which pollution prevention may be achieved. Strategies to reduce or eliminate risk through pollution prevention are developed and recommendations are provided by the EPA to industry for voluntary adoption. RM2 assessments can also lead to required testing by industry via Section 4, "findings" under Sections 4(F) and 9(A) of TSCA, and enforcement action.

TABLE 26.4
Codes for Testing Recommended for Selected Substances on the 1992 MTL[a]

Health Effects		Environmental Effects		Environmental Fate	
ACUTE	Acute toxicity	ACUTE EE	Acute toxicity	BIOC	Bioconcentration
CARC	Carcinogenicity	CHR EE	Chronic toxicity	DEGR	Biodegradation
CHR	Chronic toxicity	SIDS EE	Screening data	MONIT	Monitoring
DEVEL	Developmental toxicity	OTHR EE	Other	PCHM	Physical chemical property
DNEURO	Developmental neurotoxicity			TSPT	Transport/Transformation
EPID	Epidemiology			SIDS EF	Screening data
IMUN	Immunotoxicity			OTHR EF	Other
MUTA	Mutagenicity				
NEURO	Neurotoxicity				
PK	Pharmacokinetics				
PCHR	Prechronic toxicity/14–28 day				
REPRO	Reproductive toxicity				
SCHR	Subchronic toxicity/90 day				
SIDS	Screening data				
OTHR	Other				

[a] These codes are used in Table 26.5.

TABLE 26.5
EPA 1992 Master Testing List[a] (see note at end of Table 26.7)

CAS No.	Chemical Name	Health or Environmental Effects and Environmental Fate Testing Needs (See Table 26.4 for Codes)
None	Commercial hexane	CARC, DEVEL, MUTA, NEURO, PK, REPRO, SCHR
None	Dioxins, polyhalogenated dibenzo-*p*-	
None	Furans, polyhalogenated dibenzo-	
50-00-0	Formaldehyde	Characterization of emissions/exposures (Health)
50-81-7	*L*-Ascorbic acid	
57-10-3	Hexadecanoic acid	DEVEL
57-13-6	Urea	
59-67-6	Pyridinecarboxylic acid, 3-	
60-29-7	Diethyl ether	NEURO
67-63-0	Isopropanol	CARC, MUTA, SCHR, PK, DEVEL, REPRO, NEURO
67-64-1	Acetone	REPRO, NEURO
70-55-3	Benzenesulfonamide, 4-methyl-	
71-36-3	Butanol, 1-	REPRO, NEURO
71-55-6	Trichloroethane, 1,1,1-	DNEURO, NEURO, MUTA
74-85-1	Ethylene	
74-87-3	Chloromethane	PCHR, SCHR
74-97-5	Bromochloromethane	REPRO
75-00-3	Chloroethane	PCHR, SCHR
75-02-5	Vinyl fluoride	CARC, MUTA
75-15-0	Carbon disulfide	REPRO
75-34-3	Dichloroethane, 1,1-	PCHR, SCHR
75-35-4	1,1-Dichloroethylene	CARC, PK
75-38-7	Vinylidene fluoride	CARC, MUTA, REPRO
75-54-7	Silane, dichloromethyl-	
75-69-4	Fluorotrichloromethane	PCHR, SCHR
75-77-4	Silane, chlorotrimethyl-	
75-78-5	Silane, dichlorodimethyl-	
75-79-6	Silane, trichloromethyl-	
75-86-5	Acetone cyanhydrin	
75-91-2	Hydroperoxide, 1,1-dimethylethyl-	
75-98-9	2,2-Dimethylpropanoic acid	
76-03-9	Trichloroacetic acid	
77-99-6	Propanediol, 2-ethyl-2-(hydroxymethyl)-1,3	
78-33-1	Phosphate, tris(*tert*-butylphenyl)	DEVEL, NEURO, REPRO, CHR EE, DEGR
78-40-0	Triethyl phosphate	
78-83-1	Isobutyl alcohol	CARC, DEVEL, PK, REPRO, NEURO
78-84-2	Propanal, 2-methyl-	
78-93-3	Methyl ethyl ketone	
78-97-7	Propanenitrile, 2-hydroxy-	
79-00-5	1,1,2-Trichloroethane	PCHR, SCHR
79-10-7	Acrylic acid	DEVEL, PK, REPRO
79-11-8	Chloroacetic acid	
79-31-2	Methylpropanoic acid, 2-	DEVEL
79-34-5	Tetrachloroethane, 1,1,2,2-	PCHR, SCHR
79-92-5	Camphene	
79-94-7	Tetrabromobisphenol A	OTHR EF

TABLE 26.5 *(Continued)*
EPA 1992 Master Testing List[a] (see note at end of Table 26.7)

CAS No.	Chemical Name	Health or Environmental Effects and Environmental Fate Testing Needs (See Table 26.4 for Codes)
80-05-7	Bisphenol A	
80-43-3	Dicumyl peroxide	
81-11-8	Benzenesulfonic acid, 2,2′-(1,2-) ethenedi-	
82-45-1	1-Aminoanthraquinone	
87-10-5	Tribromosalicylanilide, 3,4′,5-	OTHR EF
88-72-2	Nitrotoluene, 2	
89-61-2	Benzene, 1,4-dichloro-2-nitro	
92-70-6	2-Hydroxy-3-naphthoic acid	
95-48-7	*o*-Cresol	
95-54-5	Phenylenediamine, *ortho*	NEURO, ACUTE EE, CHR EE, TSPT
95-73-8	2,4-Dichlorotoluene	
95-80-7	Diaminotoluene, 2,4-	DEVEL, REPRO
96-29-7	Methyl ethyl ketoxime	CARC, NEURO, DEVEL, REPRO, MUTA
97-65-4	Butanedioic acid, methylene-	
98-56-6	Benzene, -chloro-4-(trifluoromethyl)-	
98-86-2	Acetophenone	DEVEL, MUTA, NEURO, PK, REPRO, SCHR
99-09-2	Nitroaniline, 3-	
100-21-0	Terephthalic acid	REPRO
100-40-3	Vinylcyclohexene, 4-	MUTA, PK, SCHR, TSPT
100-52-7	Benzaldehyde	
101-54-2	1,4,-Benzenediamine, N-pheny-	
101-68-8	Methylenediphenyl diisocyanate, 4,4′-	
101-72-4	Benzenediamine, *N*-(1-methylethyl)-*N*′-phenyl-, 1,4	
101-90-6	Resorcinol diglycidyl ether	
102-01-2	Acetoacetanilide	
102-71-6	Triethanolamine	
103-23-1	Di(2-ethylhexyl) adipate	DEVEL, NEURO, REPRO, CHR EE, DEGR, PCHM
103-65-1	Propylbenzene, *n*-	PCHR, SCHR
104-76-7	Ethylhexanol, 2-	DEVEL
104-90-5	2-Picoline, 5-ethyl-	
104-94-9	Aniline, 4-methoxy-	
105-05-5	Benzene, 1,4-diethyl-	
105-76-0	Maleic acid, dibutyl ester	
105-99-7	Di-butyl adipate	
106-42-3	*p*-Xylene	
106-50-3	Phenylenediamine, *para*-	NEURO, ACUTE EE, CHR EE, TSPT
106-90-1	Glycidyl acrylate	CARC, MUTA, SCHR
106-91-2	Glycidyl methacrylate	DEVEL, MUTA, SCHR
106-92-3	Allyl glycidyl ether	DEVEL, MUTA, NEURO, REPRO, SCHR
106-98-9	Butene, 1-	
107-01-7	Butene, 2-	
107-13-1	Acrylonitrile	DEVEL
107-21-1	Ethylene glycol	
107-22-2	Glyoxal	
107-64-2	1-Octadecanaminium, *N,N*-dimethyl-*N*-octad	
107-66-4	Phosphoric acid, dibutyl ester	

TABLE 26.5 *(Continued)*
EPA 1992 Master Testing List[a] (see note at end of Table 26.7)

CAS No.	Chemical Name	Health or Environmental Effects and Environmental Fate Testing Needs (See Table 26.4 for Codes)
108-01-0	Dimethylaminoethanol	
108-10-1	Methyl isobutyl ketone	NEURO
108-24-7	Acetic anhydride	
108-44-1	*m*-Toluidine	
108-45-2	Phenylenediamine, meta-	NEURO, MUTA, ACUTE EE, CHR EE, TSPT
108-67-8	Trimethylbenzene, 1,3,5-	PCHR, SCHR
108-78-1	Melamine	
108-83-8	Heptanone, 2,6-dimethyl-,4	
108-89-4	Pyridine, 4-methyl-	
108-94-1	Cyclohexanone	
108-95-2	Phenol	NEURO, PK, REPRO, SCHR
108-98-5	Thiophenol	CARC, DEVEL, MUTA, NEURO, PK, REPRO, ACUTE EE, CHR EE, DEGR, TSPT, PCHM
108-99-6	Pyridine, 3-methyl-	
109-06-8	Pyridine, 2-methyl-	
109-55-7	1-Amino-3-dimethylamino propane	
109-69-3	Chlorobutane, 1-	
109-99-9	Tetrahydrofuran	NEURO
110-27-0	Isopropyl myristate	
110-30-5	Octadecanamide, *N,N'*-1,2-ethanediylbis-	
110-80-5	Ethoxyethanol, 2-	NEURO
110-82-7	Cyclohexane	ACUTE, CARC, DEVEL, MUTA, NEURO, PK, REPRO, SCHR
110-91-8	Morpholine	
111-11-5	Octanoic acid, methyl ester	DEVEL
111-40-0	Diethylenetriamine	
111-42-2	Diethanolamine	
111-46-6	Diethylene glycol	
111-66-0	1-Octane	
111-69-3	1,4-Dicyanobutane	
112-18-5	*N,N*-Dimethyidodecylamine	
112-24-3	Triethylene tetramine	
112-35-6	Ethanol, 2-[2-(2-methoxyethoxy)ethoxy]-	
112-41-4	1–Dodecene	
112-50-5	Triethylene glycol, monoethyl ether	
112-53-8	Dodecanol, 1-	
112-72-1	1-Tetradecanol	
112-90-3	9-Octadecen-1-amine, (Z)-	
112-92-5	Octadecanol, 1-	
115-11-7	2-Methylpropene	
115-18-4	3-Buten-2-ol,2-methyl	
115-19-5	3-Butyn-2-ol,2-methyl-	
115-86-6	Triphenyl phosphate	DEVEL, NEURO, REPRO, CHR EE, DEGR
115-96-8	Tris(2-chloroethyl)phosphate	SIDS
116-15-4	Hexafluoropropene	
118-69-4	2,6-Dichlorotoluene	
118-75-2	Chloranil	OTHR EF
118-79-6	2,4,6-Tribromophenol	OTHR EF

TABLE 26.5 *(Continued)*
EPA 1992 Master Testing List[a] (see note at end of Table 26.7)

CAS No.	Chemical Name	Health or Environmental Effects and Environmental Fate Testing Needs (See Table 26.4 for Codes)
120-61-6	Dimethyl terephthalate	DEVEL, NEURO, REPRO, ACUTE EE, CHR EE, DEGR
120-78-5	Benzthiazole disulfide	
120-80-9	Hydroxyphenol, *o*-	DEVEL
120-82-1	Trichlorobenzene, 1,2,4-	CARC
121-14-2	Benzene, 1-methyl-2,4-dinitro-	
121-33-5	Vanillin	
121-69-7	Dimethylaniline, *N,N*-	DEVEL, MUTA, NEURO, PK, REPRO, SCHR, ACUTE EE, CHR EE, DEGR
122-60-1	Phenyl glycidyl ether	NEURO, REPRO
123-01-3	Dodecylbenzene	
123-30-8	Aminophenol, *p*-	DEVEL
123-31-9	Hydroquinone	
123-38-6	Propanal	
123-72-8	Butyraldehyde	
123-77-3	Diazenedicarboxamide	
123-86-4	Butyl acetate, *n*-	NEURO
124-09-4	1,6-Hexanediamine	
124-18-5	*n*-Decane	
126-30-7	Propanediol,2,2-dimethyl-,1,3,-	
126-58-9	1,3-Propanediol,2,2′-[oxybis-(methylene)]	
126-73-8	Tributyl phosphate	CARC, DEVEL, MUTA, NEURO, OTHR, PK, REPRO, ACUTE EE, CHR EE, PCHM, TSPT
126-80-7	1,3-Bis[3-(2,3-epoxypropoxy)-propyl] tetramethyldisiloxane	
126-99-8	Chloroprene	
127-19-5	Dimethylacetamide	
128-39-2	Di-*tert*-butylphenol	ACUTE EE, CHR EE, DEGR, TSPT
135-19-3	2-Napththol	
140-66-9	Phenol,4-(1,1,3,3-tetramethylbutyl)-	
141-78-6	Ethyl acetate	DEVEL, MUTA, NEURO, REPRO, CARC
141-79-7	Mesityl oxide	SIDS
143-33-9	Sodium cyanide	ACUTE EE, CHR EE, TSPT
147-14-8	C.I. Pigment Blue 15	
149-57-5	Ethyl hexanoic acid, 2-	
151-21-3	Sodium lauryl sulfate	
156-43-4	Benzenamine, 4-ethoxy-	
294-62-2	Cyclododecane	
482-89-3	3H-Indol-3-one, 2-(1,3-dihydro-3-oxo-) 2H-	
504-60-9	Pentadiene,1,3-	
512-56-1	Phosphoric acid, trimethyl ester	
527-60-6	Phenol,2,4,6-trimethyl-	
536-90-3	Benzenamine, 3-methoxy-	
556-52-5	Glycidol	MUTA, NEURO, REPRO
556-67-2	Octamethylcyclotetrasiloxane	
576-26-1	Dimethylphenol 2,6-	DEVEL, MUTA, NEURO, REPRO, ACUTE EE, CHR EE, DEGR, TSPT
584-03-2	Butanediol, 1,2-	

TABLE 26.5 *(Continued)*
EPA 1992 Master Testing List[a] (see note at end of Table 26.7)

CAS No.	Chemical Name	Health or Environmental Effects and Environmental Fate Testing Needs (See Table 26.4 for Codes)
590-86-3	Butanal, 3-methyl-	
592-41-6	1-Hexene	
611-06-3	Benzene, 2,4-dichloro-1-nitro-	
623-91-6	2-Butenedioic: acid (E)-, diethyl ester	
628-63-7	Amyl acetate, *n*-	NEURO
629-11-8	Hexamethylene glycol	
629-59-4	Tetradecane	
693-23-2	Dodecanedioic acid	
793-24-8	1,4-Benzenediamine, *N*-(1,3-) dimethylbutyl	
822-06-0	Hexamethylene diisocyanate, 1,6-	CARC, DEVEL, MUTA, NEURO, PK, REPRO, PCHM
836-30-6	Benzenamine, 4-nitro-*N*-phenyl-	
872-05-9	Decene, *n*-	
872-50-4	Methylpyrrolidone, *N*-	CARC, NEURO, PK, SCHR, MUTA, DEVEL, REPRO
930-37-0	Methyl glycidyl ether	
1000-82-4	Methylol urea	
1120-36-1	1-Tetradecene	
1163-19-5	Decabromodiphenyl ether	ACUTE EE, CHR EE, OTHR, BIOC, DEGR, MONIT, PCHM, TSPT, CHR, DEVEL, MUTA, NEURO, REPRO, OTHR EF
1241-94-7	Ethylhexyl diphenyl phosphate, 2-	DEVEL, NEURO, REPRO, CHR EE, DEGR
1309-64-4	Antimony trioxide	EPID
1330-78-5	Tricresyl phosphate	DEVEL, NEURO, REPRO, CHR EE, DEGR
1634-04-4	Methyl *tert*-butyl ether	CARC, MUTA, NEURO, DEVEL, REPRO
1675-54-3	Bisphenol A diglycidyl ether	CARC, DEVEL, MUTA, NEURO, REPRO, SCHR
1758-73-2	Methanesulfinic acid, aminoimino-	
1854-26-8	2-Imidazolidinone, 4,5-dihydroxy-1,3-bis	
1879-09-0	6-*tert*-Butyl-2,4-xylenol	
1912-24-9	Atrazine	
2210-79-9	Cresyl glycidyl ether, *O*-	DEVEL, MUTA, NEURO, SCHR
2224-15-9	Ethylene glycol diglycidyl ether	
2238-07-5	Diglycidyl ether	
2402-79-1	Tetrachloropyridine, 2,3,5,6-	
2425-01-6	Hydroquinone diglycidyl ether	
2425-79-8	Butanediol diglycidyl ether, 1,4-	MUTA, NEURO, SCHR
2426-08-6	Butyl glycidyl ether, *n*-	CARC, DEVEL, MUTA, NEURO, REPRO, SCHR
2431-50-7	Butene,2,3,4-trichloro, 1-	
2461-15-6	Ethylhexyl glycidyl ether, 2-	CARC, MUTA, SCHR
2461-18-9	Lauryl glycidyl ether	
2524-03-0	Dimethyl chlorothiophosphate	
2524-04-1	Diethyl chlorothiophosphate	
2528-36-1	Di(*n*-butyl)phenyl phosphate	DEVEL, NEURO, REPRO, CHR EE, DEGR
2530-83-8	Glycidoxypropyltrimethyoxysilane, γ-	CARC, DEVEL, MUTA, NEURO, REPRO, SCHR
2581-34-2	Phenol,3-methyl-4-nitro	

TABLE 26.5 *(Continued)*
EPA 1992 Master Testing List[a] (see note at end of Table 26.7)

CAS No.	Chemical Name	Health or Environmental Effects and Environmental Fate Testing Needs (See Table 26.4 for Codes)
2897-60-1	3-(Methyidiethoxysilyl)propyl glycidyl ether	
3039-83-6	Ethenesulfonic acid, sodium salt	
3072-84-2	Tetrabromobisphenol A diglycidyl ether, 2,2′,6,6′-	
3101-60-8	Butylphenyl glycidyl ether, *p-tert-*	
3188-83-8	2-Methylol-4,4′-isopropylidene diphenol diglycidyl ether	
3194-55-6	Hexabromocyclododecane	CARC, CHR, DEVEL, MUTA, NEURO, REPRO, ACUTE EE, CHR EE, OTHR EE, BIOC, DEGR, PCHM, TSPT
3209-22-1	Benzene, 1,2-dichloro-3-nitro	
3568-29-4	Glycerol 1,3-diglycidyl ether	
3926-62-3	Acetic acid, chloro-, sodium salt	
4016-11-9	Ethyl glycidyl ether	
4016-14-2	Isopropyl glycidyl ether	
4162-45-2	Tetrabromobisphenol-A-bis(ethoxyla)	OTHR EF
4170-30-3	Crotonaldehyde	CHR EE
4259-15-8	Phosphorodithioic acid, *O,O*-bis(2-ethyln-)	
4461-52-3	Methoxymethanol	
4979-32-2	*N,N*-Dicyclohexyl-2-benzothiazolesulfenam	
5026-74-4	4-(Diglycidylamino)phenyl, glycidyl ether	MUTA
5255-75-4	Nitrophenyl glycidyl ether, *p*-	
5281-04-9	D and C Red No. 7	
5392-40-5	Citral	
5493-45-8	Diglycidyl ester of hexahydrophthalic acid	CARC, MUTA, SCHR
6178-32-1	*p*-Nonylphenyl glycidyl ether	
6386-38-5	Benzenepropanoic acid, 3,5-bis(1,1-dimethylethyl)-	
6419-19-8	Phosphonic acid, [nitrilotris(methylene)]tris-	
6742-54-7	Benzene, undecyl-	
6846-50-0	2,2,4-Trimethyl-1,3-pentanediol ester	
7195-45-1	Diglycidyl ester of phthalic acid	
7328-97-4	1,1,2,2-Tetra(*p*-hydroxyphenyl)ethane tetraglycidyl ether	
7422-52-8	3-[Bis(trimethylsiloxy)methyl]-propyl glycidyl ether	
7665-72-7	Butyl glycidyl ether, *tert-*	SCHR
9011-05-6	Urea-formaldehyde resins/formaldehyde	
11631-19-5	Decabromodiphenyloxide	
13236-02-7	Glycerol triglycidyl ether	
13561-08-5	Diglycidylphenyl glycidyl ether, 2,6-	
13674-84-5	2-Propanol, 1-chloro-, phosphate (3:1)	
14228-73-0	Bis(glycidyloxymethyl)cyclohexane, 1,4-	
15965-99-8	Hexadecyl glycidyl ether	
16245-97-9	Octadecyl glycidyl ether, *n*-	
17557-23-2	Neopentyl glycol diglycidyl ether	CARC, SCHR
17963-04-1	3-(Dimethylethoxysilyl) glycidyl ether	
20217-01-0	Dibromophenyl glycidyl ether, 2,4-	
22421-59-6	Dibromo-4-methylphenyl glycidyl ether, 2,6	
24800-44-0	Tripropylene glycol	
25155-23-1	Phosphate, trixylyl	DEVEL, NEURO, REPRO, CHR EE, DEGR

TABLE 26.5 *(Continued)*
EPA 1992 Master Testing List[a] **(see note at end of Table 26.7)**

CAS No.	Chemical Name	Health or Environmental Effects and Environmental Fate Testing Needs (See Table 26.4 for Codes)
25265-77-4	Propanoic acid, 2-methyl-, monoester	
25327-89-3	Tetrabromobisphenol-A, allyl ether	OTHR EF
26444-49-5	Phosphoric acid, methylphenyldiphenyle	
26447-14-3	Cresyl glycidyl ether (mixed isomers)	
26761-45-5	Glycidyl ester of neodecanoic acid	DEVEL,MUTA,NEURO,SCHR
26967-76-0	Phosphate, tris(isopropylphenyl)	DEVEL,NEURO,REPRO,CHR EE,DEGR
27193-86-8	Dodecylphenol	DEVEL
28108-99-8	Isopropylphenyl diphenyl phosphate	DEVEL, NEURO, REPRO, CHR EE, DEGR
28629-66-5	Phosphorodithioic acid, *O,O*-diisooctyl	
29171-20-8	6-Octen-1-yn-3-ol, 3,7-dimethyl-	
29590-42-9	Iso-octyl acrylatc	
29761-21-5	Isodecyl diphenyl phosphate	DEVEL, NEURO, REPRO, CHR EE, DEGR
32534-81-9	Pentabromodiphenyl ether	CARC, CHR, DEVEL, MUTA, NEURO, REPRO, ACUTE EE, CHR EE, OTHR EE, BIOC, DEGR, MONIT, PCHM, TSPT, OTHER EF
32536-52-0	Octabromodiphenyl ether	CARC, CHR, DEVEL, MUTA, NEURO, REPRO, ACUTE EE, CHR EE, OTHR EE, BIOC, DEGR, MONIT, PCHM, TSPT, OTHR EF
32568-89-1	3-(2-Glycidyloxypropyl)-l-glycidol-5,5-dimethyl-hydantoin	
35243-89-1	Dibromopropyl glycidyl ether, 1,2-	
37853-59-1	Ethane, 1,2-bis(2,4,6-tribromophenoxy)-	CARC, CHR, DEVEL, MUTA, NEURO, REPRO, ACUTE EE,CHR EE, OTHR EE, BIOC, DEGR, MONIT, PCHR, OTHR EF, TSPT
37971-36-1	Butanetricarboxylic acid, 1,2,4-	
38304-52-8	1,3-Bis(5,5-dimethyl-l-glycidyl-hydantoin-3-yl)-2-glycidyl	
38954-75-5	Tetradecyl glycidyl ether	
54208-63-8	Bisphenol F diglycidyl ether	
56803-37-3	Phosphate, *tert*-butylphenyl diphenyl	DEVEL, NEURO, REPRO, CHR EE, DEGR
60501-41-9	Oleyl glycidyl ether	
61578-04-9	Cumylphenyl glycidyl ether, *p*-	
65652-41-7	Phosphate, bis(*tert*-butylphenyl)phenyl	DEVEL, NEURO, REPRO, CHR EE, DEGR
67786-03-2	[Bis(*r*-glycidyloxyphenyl)]-(2-glycidyl oxyphenyl)methane	
68081-84-5	Alkyl (C10–CI6)glycidyl ether	SCHR
68134-06-5	Dimethylbutyl glycidyl ether, 1,3-	
68134-07-6	Methylheptyl glycidyl ether, 6-	
68517-02-2	Tris(4-hydroxyphenyl)propane-triglycidyl ether	
68609-96-1	Alkyl (C8–C10) glycidyl ether	REPRO, SCHR
68609-97-2	Alkyl (C12–C14) glycidyl ether	DEVEL, MUTA, NEURO, SCHR
68611-64-3	Urea-formaldehyde resin	
68937-41-7	Phenol isopropylated phosphate	DEVEL, NEURO, REPRO, CHR EE, DEGR
68959-23-9	Hexanetriol triglycidyl ether, 1,2,6-	
68987-80-4	Alkyl (C6–C12) glycidyl ether	
69155-42-6	1,1,1,3,5,7,7,7-Octamethyl-3,5,-bis(6,7-epoxy-4-oxaheptyl)-	

TABLE 26.5 *(Continued)*
EPA 1992 Master Testing List[a] (see note at end of Table 26.7)

CAS No.	Chemical Name	Health or Environmental Effects and Environmental Fate Testing Needs (See Table 26.4 for Codes)
71033-08-4	2,2-Bis[(*p*-2-glycidyloxy-3-butoxypropyloxy)-phenyl]propane	
71808-64-5	Dimethoxysilane, (3-glycidoxy-propyl) (3-chloropropyl)-	
72319-24-5	2,2′-[(1-Methylethylidene)bis[4,1-phenyleneoxy-3,1-propanediyloxy-4,1-phenylene(1-methyl-ethylidene)-4,1-phenyleneoxymethylene]bis-	
74398-71-3	1,2,3-Propanetriyl ester of 12-(oxiranylmethoxy)-9-octadecanoic acid	
75150-13-9	2,4-Dibromo-6-methylphenyl glycidyl ether	DEVEL, MUTA, NEURO, SCHR
84852-15-3	Nonylphenol, 4-branched	CHR EE, ACUTE EE, PCHM, BIOC
97380-66-3	Urea-formaldehyde resin	
142844-00-6	Refractory ceramic fibers	Characterization of emissions/exposures (Health)

[a] The lack of a code does not indicate that no testing is needed. Where no code is indicated, the testing needs may be obtained from the proposed EPA Section 4 test rule or the relevant report to EPA from ITC, OPPT, OECD, CPSC, or OW. (See EPA's December 1992 MTL Document.) ITC = The Interagency Testing Committee; OPPT = EPA's Office of Pollution Prevention and Toxics; OECD = The Organization for Economic Cooperation and Development; CPSC = The Consumer Product Safety Commission; OW = EPA's Office of Water.

Source: U.S. Environmental Protection Agency, 1992.[5]

TABLE 26.6
Deletions from the MTL Since 1990[a] (see note at end of Table 26.7)

Chemical Name	CAS Registry No.
Propylene oxide	75-56-9
Isophorone	78-59-1
1,2-Dichloropropane	78-87-5
Methyl ethyl ketone	78-93-3
Biphenyl	92-52-4
o-Cresol	95-48-7
Cumene	98-82-8
p-Cresol	106-44-5
1,4-Dichlorobenzene	106-46-7
Methyl isobutyl ketone	108-10-1
m-Cresol	108-39-4
Cyclohexanone	108-94-1
Diethylenetriamine	111-40-0
Diethylene glycol butyl ether	112-34-5
Triethylene glycol monomethyl ether	112-35-6
Oleylamine	112-90-3
Tetrafluoroethene	116-14-3
Hexafluoropropene	116-15-4
2,4-Dinitrotoluene	121-14-2
2-Phenoxyethanol	122-99-6
Hydroquinone	123-31-9
Diethyleneglycol butyl ether acetate	124-17-4
2-Mercaptobenzothiazole	149-30-4

TABLE 26.6 *(Continued)*
Deletions from the MTL Since 1990ᵃ (see note at end of Table 26.7)

Chemical Name	CAS Registry No.
2-Ethylhexanoic acid	149-57-5
2,6-Dinitrotoluene	606-20-2
1,3-Dioxolane	646-06-0
Antimony sulfide	1345-04-6
Disperse blue 79	3618-72-2
2-Phenoxyethanol acetate	6192-44-5
Antimony	7440-36-0
Diisodecylphenyl phosphite	25550-98-98-5
C-9 Aromatic Mixture	NONE
Chlorinated Paraffins (9 materials of various levels of chlorination and chain lengths)	NONE

In addition, the Interagency Testing Committee (ITC) removed the following quaternary ammonium compounds from the MTL:

Imidazolium quaternary ammonium	68142-86-1
Ethoxylated quaternary ammonium	68410-69-5
Ethoxylated quaternary ammonium	68413-04-7
Imidazolium quaternary ammonium	72643-82-6

ᵃ TSCA Section 4 test results and the rationale for removing substances from the MTL stored in the "adminstrative record" at the EPA in Washington, D.C. (For more information, see section 3(c) of this chapter)

TABLE 26.7
Categories of Substances on the 1992 Master Testing List[5] (see note at end of table)

1. Air toxics	Need additional data to determine risk posed by Hazardous Air Pollutants listed under section 112 of the Clean Air Act Amendments.
2. Carpet	Need to characterize Total Volatile Organic Compound (TVOC) emissions to indoor air from carpets, carpet cushions (pads), and carpet adhesives. (See 56 FR 67317, December 30, 1991 for Carpet Policy Dialogue results.)
3. Interior architectural coatings	Need to characterize specific chemical emissions and TVOC emissions from indoor air sources such as paints, varnishes, and other coatings.
4. "Categories of Concern" in EPA's New Chemicals Program	EPA has identified 40 chemical categories that are of particular concern relative to potential health or environmental effects. The EPA is gathering additional test and exposure data to improve their understanding of the risks presented when reviewing PMN substances within these categories.
5. Persistent bioaccumulates	EPA needs data to confirm persistence/bioaccumulation potential and environmental effects predicted by SAR analysis.
6. Polychlorinated dioxins/furans (D/F) in wood and paper pulp sludge	The EPA is contemplating a testing program to include the determination of D/F concentrations in pulp and paper mill sludge and an evaluation of the environmental fate and ecological effects of D/F in sludge produced by pulp and paper mill wastewater treatment plants.
7. Respirable fibers	EPA intends to investigate potential inhalation health hazards and better characterize the potential for human exposure to synthetic and naturally occurring respirable fibers.
8. SARA Section 104	EPA intends to require toxicological testing under TSCA Section 4 when data needs are identified through the development of Toxicological Profiles.
9. Chemicals on the Toxics Release Inventory (TRI)	EPA intends to develop screening level test data for chemicals in the TRI which relate to high production volumes and high environmental releases.

Note: The most current information relating to the MTL and Tables 26.5, 26.6, and 26.7 can be obtained electronically by accessing the OPPT home page [http://www.epa.gov/opptintr/chemtest/mtlintro.htm].

C. Sources for Additional Information on Section 4 and the MTL

Information regarding the MTL can be obtained from the Director of the Environmental Assistance Division (TS-799), Office of Pollution Prevention and Toxics, U.S. Environmental Protection Agency, 401 M Street SW, Washington, D.C. 20460, (202) 554-1404 (TSCA Hotline) or (202) 554-0557. TSCA Section 4 test results and the results of the EPA's review of the test data are available to the public through summaries that are added to TSCATS which is a publicly accessible computerized database.

Information as to the basis for RM1 and RM2 decisions for each substance reviewed is available in a central collection point called the "administrative record." Such information includes:

- Exposure and hazard information
- Recommendations from EPA work groups as to information needs and associated decision rationale
- Summaries of major toxicological or exposure studies considered
- Summaries of Risk Management (RM) meetings
- "Letters of concern" sent by EPA to industry and the industry responses
- Relevant comments or correspondence from other parties outside of the EPA

Information from the administrative record can be obtained in person by going to room G-004 of the Northeast Mall, EPA Headquarters, 401 M Street, SW, Washington, D.C. from 12:00 noon to 4:00 pm Monday through Friday (photocopy facilities are available) or upon request by calling (202) 260-7099. Information from the administrative record may also be obtained by writing to:

> The TSCA Public Docket (TS-793)
> Attention: RMI Process
> Office of Pollution Prevention and Toxics
> U.S. Environmental Protection Agency
> 401 M Street SW
> Washington, D.C. 20460

SECTION 4. *TSCA SECTION 5:* PREMANUFACTURING NOTIFICATION

TSCA Section 5 requires that a manufacturer (or importer) submit a Premanufacturing Notification (PMN) or one of several possible exemption applications to the EPA before a substance is manufactured or imported for commercial purposes in the United States (if the substances is not on the *Toxic Substances Control Act Chemical Substance Inventory* also referred to as "The TSCA or EPA Inventory"). There are exemptions to this requirement which allow a manufacturer or importer to handle, process, conduct research and development, test market, and even produce in low volume for commercial purposes (see CFR, Title 40, Part 720, Sections 30, 36, and 38; and Part 723, Sections 50, 175, and 250).[1] Some exemptions require prior EPA notification and approval while others do not. In all cases, detailed recordkeeping is required to comply with TSCA Section 5.

Section 5 of TSCA does not require that toxicological testing be performed before a PMN submittal (unless the PMN substance is subject to a Section 4 test rule). However, if the manufacturer or importer has toxicological data, it must be included with the PMN submittal. If the PMN substance is subject to a TSCA Section 4 Test Rule, the submitter must submit the test data specified in the rule as part of the PMN. The EPA reports that only about 50% of the PMNs filed are accompanied by toxicological test data.

The EPA has 90 days to review the PMN to determine whether or not manufacture and use of the PMN substance is likely to present an unreasonable risk of injury to health or the environment. On completion of the review, the EPA may allow the substance to be manufactured or imported, it may prohibit manufacture or importation, or it may impose restrictions or conditions to which the manufacturer or importer must adhere. The EPA can also discontinue or extend the 90-day review period if there is insufficient toxicological or exposure information available for the EPA scientists to make a risk assessment. In this case, a submitter may obtain the needed additional information so that the EPA can continue the review, the submitter can perform toxicological testing under a Section 5(e) consent order while manufacturing with restrictions, or the submitter may elect not to perform the testing requested by the EPA and simply withdraw the PMN which will end the PMN review process and the substance cannot be placed into commerce.

The EPA will consider any toxicological and exposure data that are submitted with the PMN along with other information already in their possession from other sources to make their health and environmental risk assessments. The EPA uses exposure models, structure-activity relationships, health, safety, and environmental information obtained through other sections of TSCA (e.g., Sections 8(e), 8(d), and Section 4), and the experience of different health, safety, and environmental disciplines during their review of each PMN substance.

There is a specific form used for PMN submittals (EPA form 7710-25 revised 5/95). Although there is not a specific page or section for toxicological data, the PMN must include any test and exposure data that the submitter has on file which relates to the potential health and environmental effects of the PMN substance or mixture(s) containing the substance. The submitter should include all exposure and hazard information in his possession which relates to the manufacture, processing, use, distribution, and disposal of the PMN substance. With regard to toxicological data, any scientifically valid test protocol is acceptable to the EPA as long as it is reliable and is conducted in accordance with Good Laboratory Practice (GLP) Standards. (See 40 CFR 792.[4]) The submitter will need to verify to the EPA that the test protocol is valid and that GLPs were followed.

Status of the EPA review of TSCA Section 5 notifications (PMNs, exemption applications, etc.) that have been submitted to the EPA, may be determined by the public by accessing [www.epa.gov/opptintr/chemtest/index.htm].

Based on years of reviewing hazards and risks associated with chemical substances, "Categories of Chemicals" were developed by the EPA to facilitate the review of new substances for which PMNs are submitted under Section 5 of TSCA. These categories may serve as a guide for PMN submitters indicating possible concerns for the different types of substances and the types of test data that might be useful in addressing those concerns. In general, the message to PMN submitters, toxicologists, and risk assessors is that, as done by the EPA *after* receipt of a PMN, the health and environmental hazards and risks associated with the production, use, and ultimate disposal of the PMN substance should be addressed and new data should be acquired, if needed, before the new substance is placed into commerce, preferably before the PMN is submitted.

In addition to the toxicological testing guidelines published in the U.S. Code of Federal Regulations, Title 40,[4] specific information on test protocols, conditions, testing options, and schemes for testing new chemical substances can be obtained from the EPA's New Chemicals Branch at (202) 260-3725.

The information provided in Tables 26.7 through 26.9 was extracted from an EPA document entitled "TSCA New Chemicals Program (NCP) Chemical Categories"[6] (paper or electronic). This document can be obtained from the EPA by calling the TSCA Assistance Office at (800) 424-9065 (toll-free), or (202) 554-1404 or by e-mail [tsca-hotline@epamail.epa.gov]. It describes potential health and/or environmental concerns for each of 52 categories and the basis for those concerns along with suggestions of possible testing strategy, testing triggers, conditions under which the substances may present the different levels of concern, and related literature references. Table 26.8 provides a brief summary of possible toxicological concerns, and details relative to those concerns.

TABLE 26.8
Chemical Categories with Health or Environmental Concerns and a Brief Description of Those Concerns

Category	Concern
Acid Chlorides (includes carbonyl and sulfochlorides) R-C[=O]Cl and (S[=O]Cl) where R is aliphatic or aromatic	Toxic to aquatic organisms. Concern is greater if the log octanol/water partition coefficient (log K_{ow}) > 8 or if molecular weight (mol. wt) < 1000.
Dyes *Acid* (anionic or negatively charged) and *Amphoteric* (positive and negative charges on the same molecule	Many of these dyes are toxic to fish and aquatic organisms particularly if the substance is water-soluble and mol. wt. is around 1000 or less.
Dyes Cationic (any dye with one or more net positive charges)	Water-soluble cationic dyes are toxic to fish, daphnids, and algae, whereas poorly soluble dyes tend to be toxic only to algae.
Acrylamides	The acrylamides of greatest concern are those with a labile substituent, e.g., methylol acrylamides, that may release acrylamide *per se* under metabolic conditions. Members of this class are considered potential carcinogens, heritable mutagens, developmental or reproductive toxicants, potential neurotoxins, and are toxic to aquatic organisms.
R_1 = H (acrylamides) 　　**= CH$_3$ (methacrylamides)** **R_2 = can be anything**	Structures with an acrylamide equivalent wt. ≤ 5000 are presumed not to pose a hazard under any condition. Inhalation concerns are generally confined to acrylamides with mol. wt. < 1000. Species with mol. wt. < 500 are of concern when there is potential for dermal exposure.
Acylates and Methacrylates Any molecular structure containing one or more of the following reactive groups: **acrylate, CH$_2$=CH–C(=O–)–O** **methacrylate, CH$_2$=C(=C–)–O**	There is potential concern for irritation and sensitization; toxicity is also a concern, particularly if the log of the oct/water partition coefficient (Log P) < 5. Environmental toxicity concerns are typically confirmed to species with mol. wt. < 1000.
Aldehydes **R–C (=O)–H**	Aldehydes are ionizable in water and can exhibit excess aquate toxicity in addition to narcosis. Aldehydes with mol. wt. > 1000 are of less concern than those with mol. wt. < 1000.
Aliphatic Amines (regardless of types of substitution) Amine oxides and polyamines (e.g., di, tri, tetra, penta, etc.) are included in this category.	Can be highly toxic to all groups of freshwater organisms (i.e., fish, aquatic invertebrates, and green algae). Generally, members of this category will have mol. wt. < 1000, and may present environmental toxicity. The "typical" substance of concern is a polymer with a substantial fraction of species with mol. wt. < 1000 and pendant trimethoxy or triethoxysilane groups. There is concern for irreversible lung toxicity if such substances are inhaled. Alkoxysilane structures are presumed not to pose a hazard under any conditions if the siloxy equivalent weight is ≥ 1000 and the alkyl substituents are larger than ethyl groups. The degree of concern depends on the relative abundance of lower molecular weight species in the polymer.
Aluminum Compounds	There is concern for aquatic toxicity. This concern relates to water-soluble forms of aluminum (i.e., salts and hydroxides) particularly if the water solubility is >1 ppb.

TABLE 26.8 *(Continued)*
Chemical Categories with Health or Environmental Concerns and a Brief Description of Those Concerns

Category	Concern
Dyes: Aminobenzothiazole AZO (category also includes their phenyl ring-substituted derivatives)	There are oncogenicity and mutagenicity concerns. There is also potential for liver, thyroid toxicity, and neurotoxicity. Exotoxity concerns generally relate to chronic toxicity.
Carboxylic Acid Anhydrides (includes any substance which contains one or more carboxylic acid anhydride groups)	Concern for health effects are confined to species with mol. wt. < 1000. Potential for pulmonary sensitization; also developmental or reproductive toxicity (if mol. wt. < 500) Structures with a carboxylic acid anhydride equivalent weight of ≥ 5000 are presumed not to pose a hazard under any conditions.
Anilines (includes monoanilines and polyanilines)	Aquatic toxicity depending on K_{ow}, mol. wt. and substitutions. Acute toxicity is expected if log K_{ow} < 7.38 and mol. wt. is < 1000. Certain anilines are subject to rapid direct and indirect photolysis under environmental conditions.
Azides	There is concern for environmental toxicity if mol. wts. < 1000.
Dianilines Must have at least two phenyl rings with a bridging carbon, oxygen, nitrogen, or sulfur. Each terminal phenyl ring must have a primary amino group (or a group that can be readily metabolized to a primary amino group) either meta- or para- to the bridging atom. Compounds with one or more additional phenyl ring(s), with or without ring substituents and one or more bridging atoms are also included in this category.	Potential carcinogens and mutagens. Also potential retinotoxic agents. Also potential reproductive and systemic toxicants.
Benzothriazoles	Because it is expected that these compounds need to be absorbed to be toxic, only compounds with mol. wt. < 1000 are expected to manifest environmental toxicity. Acute toxicity is expected if log K_{ow} ≤ 5.0 and mol. wt. < 1000. Although this is especially true for liquids, solids will vary in toxicity depending on the melting point. Only chronic toxicity is expected when log K_{ow} > 5.0 and < 8.0, and mol. wt. < 1000. Aerobic biodegradation is expected to be the dominant route of transformation in the environment.
Benzotriazole — hindered phenols	Health effects (systemic, dermal sensitization, and reproductive toxicity) may vary depending on the nature of the ring substitutes. See "phenol" for environmental concerns.
Boron Compounds (includes borates, organoborates, borate esters, boron hydrides, boranes, and boroxines)	All boron hydrides are highly toxic for mammals (more toxic than borates). The major environmental hazard concerns for this category are for chronic toxicity toward fish and toxicity toward green algae. Boron compounds that have water solubilities ≥ 1.0 ppb and mol. wt. near or below 1000 are likely to present environmental hazards.
Cobalt	There are major environmental concerns (daphnids and algae) related to cobalt compounds with water solubilities > 1.0 pp and mol. wts. near or below 1000.

TABLE 26.8 *(Continued)*
Chemical Categories with Health or Environmental Concerns and a Brief Description of Those Concerns

Category	Concern
Surfactants Cationic (quaternary ammonium)	Cationic surfactants are biocidal to a wide array of species in the environment. Toxicity increases with increasing chain length up to 16 carbons and then decreases as the chain length increases further. Little ecotoxicity is expected when the carbon chain length exceeds 22 carbons.
Surfactants: Nonionic (any nonionizable structure having a surfactant activity is considered a member of this category, i.e., alkyl ethoxylates)	Acute aquatic toxicity increases with the hydrophobic chain length up to 16–18 carbons. Aquatic toxicity is decreased with increasing number of ethoxylate or propoxylate groups. Toxic to a wide variety of aquatic organisms.
Surfactants: Anionic (any molecular structure with a net negative charge and having surfactant activity)	Toxic to a wide variety of aquatic organisms.
Diazoniums (aromatic only) Aliphatic diazoniums are not included and are very explosive	Diazoniums need to be absorbed to be toxic. Those with mol. wt. < 1000 are of particular concern. The concern is acute and chronic ecotoxicity. Diazoniums are expected to be subject to rapid direct and indirect photolysis under environmental conditions and are also expected to slowly hydrolyze to phenols.
Dithiocarbamates (and their metal salts)	The concern is ecotoxicity. Many members of this category are commercial insecticides, fungicides, disinfectants, rodenticides, antioxidants, slimicides, algalicides, bactericides, and heavy metal chelators. Their mode of toxic action apparently results from interference with metalloenzymes in living cells.
Expoxides (includes any structure with one or more epoxy groups)	Health concerns for epoxides are for cancer and reproductive effects. There is greater concern for primary epoxides than for epoxides with substitutions on both of the epoxy carbons. Structures with epoxy equivalent weights ≥ 1000 are presumed not to pose a hazard under any conditions. Concerns are confined to those epoxides with mol. wt. < 500 if the exposure is limited to the dermal route.
Esters (includes all esters, vinyl esters, propargylic esters, aliphatic and aromatic esters, carboxylic acid esters, and sulfonate esters)	These compounds need to be absorbed to be toxic, therefore, compounds with mol. weights > 1000 are not of concern. The concern is aquatic toxicity. The toxicity for vinyl, allylic, and propargylic esters is expected to be greater than for simple esters. The toxicity seems to decrease with increasing K_{ow}. Esters are subject to both abiotic and biotic hydrolysis and aerobic biodegradation. Aerobic biodegradation is expected to be the dominant route to transformation in the environment.
Ethylene Glycol Ethers $R-(OCH_2\ CH_2)n-OR^1$ Where n = 1, 2, or 3 R = alkyl C_7 or less or phenyl or alkyl substituted phenyl. R^1 = H or alkyl C_7 or less or any group that can be chemically or metabolically removed to yield a glycol ether.	Short-cjaom ethylene glycol ethers are absorbed by all routes of exposures and have caused irritation of skin, eyes, and mucous membranes; hemolysis, bone-marrow damage, and leukopenia of both lymphocytes and granulocytes; direct and indirect kidney damage; liver damage, immunotoxicity, and central nervous system depression. Some are also developmental and reproductive toxicants.

TABLE 26.8 *(Continued)*
Chemical Categories with Health or Environmental Concerns and a Brief Description of Those Concerns

Category	Concern
Hydrazines and related compounds (includes any structure, which contains any of the following functional groups: hydrazine, hydrazone; hydrazide, or semicarbazide.)	There are concerns for carcinogenicity and chronic effects to liver, kidney, and blood. There are also ecotoxicity concerns. There is particular concern if the mol. wt. < 500. There is greater concern for substances with few substitutions on the functional group than for those with multiple substitutions.
Hindered Amines	The concern with substances in this category is that they may be toxic to the immune system, liver, blood, the male reproductive system, and the gastrointestinal tract. The primary health concern relates to the potential for inhalation exposure.
Imides (includes all imides and maleimides; substitutions may be aliphatic, aromatic, and/or halogens)	Halogenated imides are used as fungicides, bactericides, slimicides, and algicides. It is assumed that these compounds need to be absorbed to be toxic, therefore, compounds with mol. wt. < 1000 are of greater concern. The primary toxicity concern is for aquatic organisms.
Diisocyanates (includes any substances containing two or more isocyanate groups) $R-(N=C=O)_{\geq 2}$	Diisocyanates are of concern because of potential dermal and pulmonary sensitization and other lung effects. Aromatic isocyanates may be potential carcinogens. Structures with an isocyanate equivalent weight of ≥ 5000 are presumed not to pose a hazard under any conditions. The primary concern is for substances with mol. wt. < 1000. There is particular concern if there is potential for inhalation exposure.
Beta-Napthylamines (monosulfonated) Azo dyes are also included in category	Potential carcinogens and mutagens (genotoxic). Concern is restricted to those compounds where the sulfonate or sulfatoethylsulfone group is on the ring distal to the beta-amino group. The EPA has data indicating that compounds where the sulfonate group is on the proximal ring are unlikely to be carcinogenic.
Neutral Organics (includes nonreactive nonionizable organic substances such as alcohols, ketones, ethers, alkyl halides, and aromatic hydrocarbons; also nonionic or neutral dyes)	"Neutral organics" are believed to be environmentally toxic because of their ability to produce simple narcosis in aquatic species. Therefore, the concern is ecotoxicity. The molecular weights of neutral organics of concern are generally < 1000 and the octanol/water partition coefficients (log P) are < 8.
Nickel Compounds (includes all organic and inorganic soluble complexes of nickel) Nickel-complexed dyes and strong ion pairs between nickel and anionic surfactants are not included	Nickel produces acute and chronic toxicity to aquatic organisms over a wide range of concentrations. As water hardness (as $CaCo_3$) decreases, toxicity increases; and as salinity decreases, toxicity increases. Nickel compounds, e.g. nickel refinery dust and its major component nickel subsulfide, have been shown to be carcinogenic in humans.
Lanthanides or Rare Earth Metals	The only toxicity data for this category are for La [7439-91-0]. Soluble salts of La are known to exhibit chronic toxicity toward fish and algae.

TABLE 26.8 *(Continued)*
Chemical Categories with Health or Environmental Concerns and a Brief Description of Those Concerns

Category	Concern
Organotins	Known to affect carbonate metabolism and other metabolic processes. Compounds which have a mol. wt. < 1000 and transform to organotin compounds with mol. wts. < 1000 are of greatest concern. Some of these compounds can be irritating and/or corrosive to the skin and eyes. Acute oral and dermal exposures can result in systemic effects, primarily neurotoxicity. There are also concerns for immunotoxicity and aquatic toxicity.
Peroxides Any molecular structure containing one or more of the following functional groups is in this category: dialkyl peroxide, alkyl hydroperoxide, peroxy ester, diacyl peroxide, peroxy acid.	Members of this category may be carcinogenic. There are also ecotoxicity and environmental fate concerns.
Phenols (includes monophenols, polyhydroxy phenols, and polyphenols)	It is assumed that these compounds need to be absorbed to be toxic, so the compounds of greater concern have mol. wt. < 1000. The primary concern is for acute and chronic toxicity to aquatic organisms. Phenols are subject to indirect photolysis under environmental conditions.
Pigments (Dichlorobenzidine based)	There are oncogenicity/mutagenicity concerns based on potential for release of 3,3[1]–dichlorobenzidine and the presence of residual dicholorobenzidine (DCB). DCB is a known animal carcinogen, a suspect human carcinogen, and is known to bioconcentrate in the tissues of aquatic organisms. Concern for the "intact" pigment is restricted to uses at temperatures exceeding 200°C.
Pigments/Dyes (Triarylmethane) with solubilizing groups	Oncogenicity, developmental and reproductive toxicity concerns. Pigments that have negligible water solubility with little or no bioavailability do not exhibit these concerns.
Phenolphthaleins	There is a health concern (carcinogenicity) for phenolphthanlein and derivities of phenolphthalein (based on oral studies).
Phosphinate Esters	Metabolically active and exhibit excess aquatic toxicity (fish and aquatic invertebrates and green algae) in addition to narcosis. Phosphinate esters with mol. wt. < 1000 are of more concern than those with mol. wt. > 1000.
Polyanionic Polymers (and Monomers) There are two subcategories that are of concern: 1. Polyaromatic sulfates 2. Polyacrylates with free carboxyl groups (includes monomers with two or more acid groups and which act like organic acid chelators)	Compounds must be water-soluble or water self-dispersing to be in this category. Molecular weights are generally >1000. The concern is toxicity to aquatic organisms (ecotoxicity).
Polycationic Polymers (includes any polymer that exists in the environment with multiple positive charges, i.e., polyamines, polyquaternary ammonium, polysulfonium, and polyphosphonium compounds)	The concern is ecotoxicity (fish, invertebrates, and algae). It is presumed that these compounds act on the surface of organisms and need not be absorbed. The polymers must be water soluble or water dispersible and the molecular weights are generally > 300.

TABLE 26.8 *(Continued)*
Chemical Categories with Health or Environmental Concerns and a Brief Description of Those Concerns

Category	Concern
Polynitroaromatics (includes all di-and tri-nitroaromactics)	It is believed that these compounds need to be water soluble to be toxic, therefore the concern is for compounds with mol. wt. < 1000. There is a concern for toxicity toward the aquatic environment. Polynitroaromatics are expected to be subject to rapid direct and indirect photolysis under environmental conditions.
Rosin (includes rosin, abietinic acid, sylvic acid, their salts, and polymeric forms whose mol. wt. < 1000.	It is believed that these compounds need to be water soluble to be toxic. There is a concern for toxicity toward the aquatic environment.
Stilbene, derivatives of 4,4-bis (triazin-2-ylamino)	There are developmental/reproductive toxicity concerns for this category based on analogy to water-soluble sulfonated derivatives of 4,4-bis(triazin-2-ylamino) stilbene. Ecotoxicity concerns are low.
Substituted Triazines (includes aromatic and unsaturated compounds; members of this category typically have mol. wts. < 1000)	The concern is for ecotoxicity. Many members of this category are herbicides, which are used to control both aquatic and terrestrial plants. Their mode of toxic action is generally considered to be inhibition of photosynthesis.
Thiols (or mercaptans)	Compounds with mol. wt. < 1000 present environmental concerns.
Vinyl Esters (a carboxylic acid ester with at least one vinyl group, $CH_2=CH-$, attached to an organic acid radical; structure must include a vinyl group and an acid group)	An example of this category is vinyl acetate. Primary concerns are oncogenicity (mutagenicity data supports a cancer concern), neurotoxicity, reproductive toxicity, and environmental toxicity. (See "Esters" category.)
Vinyl Sulfones (includes compounds that can generate a vinyl sulfone given the right conditions)	An example of this group is a "fiber-reactive dye" bearing one or more vinyl sulfone precursors, or vinyl sulfones. For persons who inhale or ingest a vinyl sulfone, there is concern for carcinogenicity based on the potent mutagenicity of vinyl sulfone and methylvinyl sulfone. EPA's experience has been mainly with water-soluble, fiber-reactive dyes with mol. wt. < 1000.
Soluble Complexes of Zinc (zinc-complexed acid dyes and strong ion pairs between zinc and anionic surfactants are not included in this category)	Zinc can produce acute and chronic toxicity to freshwater organisms over a range of concentrations. Zinc has been shown to reduce the growth of various aquatic plants, (algae appear to be the most sensitive group). Acute toxicity is affected by water hardness while chronic toxicity is not. The aquatic concerns are based on the toxicity of the following Zn salts: sulfate, chloride, phosphate, and nitrate.
Zironium Compounds (includes inorganic salts of zirconium (Zr), complexes between Zr and organic salts, and organo-zirconium compounds; dues complexed with Zr are not included)	Soluble salts Zr are known to be moderately toxic to algae and fish. Zirconium is more toxic in soft water than in hard water. The toxicity of Zr salts and Zr complexes with organic acids are expected to be related to their water solubility, mol. wt., and their octanol/water partition coefficient. Compounds with mol. wt. < 1000 are not expected to be absorbed by aquatic organisms even if they are water soluble. Only water-soluble Zr compounds with mol. wt. < 1000 are expected to be toxic.

Source: U.S. Environmental Protection Agency Document entitled "TSCA New Chemicals Program (NCP) Chemical Categories" (June, 1998 Revision).

TABLE 26.9
Health-Related Toxicological Testing and Chemical or Environmental Fate Testing Associated with "Chemical Categories" [6]

Test	Test Guidelines[6]
Dermal sensitization	40 CFR 798, 4100
Pulmonary sensitization by method of Karol (or equivalent)	*Toxicol. Appl. Pharmacol.*, 68, 229–241, 1983
90-day dermal subchronic toxicity	40 CFR 798.2250
90-day oral subchronic toxicity	40 CFR 798.2650
90-day inhalation subchronic toxicity	40 CFR 798.2450
Functional observational battery	40 CFR 798.6050
Neuropathology	40 CFR 798.6400
Oral or dermal developmental toxicity study	40 CFR 798.4900
Inhalation developmental toxicity study	40 CFR 798.4350
Two-year carcinogenicity test	40 CFR 798.3300
Two-year cancer bioassay	40 CFR 798.3260
Rodent dominant lethal assay	40 CFR 798.5450
Rodent heritable translocation test	40 CFR 798.5460
In vitro mouse micronucleus assay in bone marrow by IP route	40 CFR 798.5395
Mouse lymphoma test	40 CFR 798.5300
Ames test	40 CFR 798.5265
Ames test with prival modification	*Mutat. Res.* 138, 33–47, 1984
Unscheduled DNA synthesis test in rat hepatocytes	40 CFR 798.5550
The cat acute oral retinopathy screening study	Protocol to be approved by EPA
Combined repeated dose toxicity (with reproduction/developmental toxicity screen test)	OECD Guideline, 422
Prenatal development toxicity	40 CFR 799.9370
2 — Generation reproduction test	40 CFR 799.9380
Immunotoxicity	OPPTS 870.7800 (EPA)

Chemical or Environmental Fate Testing

Water solubility	40 CFR 796.1840/40 CFR 796-1860
K_{ow}	40 CFR 796.1570/40 CFR 796.1550/ 40 CFR 796.1720
Vapor pressure	40 CFR 796.1950
Melting point and range	40 CFR 796.1300/OECD 102
Boiling point and range	40 CFR 796.1220/OPPTS 830.7220 (EPA)
Physical state	OPPTS 830.6303 (EPA)

TABLE 26.10
Ecosystem-Related Toxicological Testing Associated with "Chemical Categories" [6]

Test	Test Guidelines[6]
Hydrolysis rate as a function of pH and temperature	40 CFR 796.3500
Acute fish toxicity test	40 CFR 797.1400
Acute Daphnid toxicity test	40 CFR 797.1300
Acute green algae toxicity test (static)	40 CFR 797.1050
Acute fish toxicity test with humic acid	40 CFR 797.1400
Fish — toxicity — migration test	OPPTS 850.1085
Testing using natural sediments and organisms known to ingest sediment (benthic organisms)	Protocol available from the EPA
Chronic fish early life stage toxicity test	40 CFR 797.1600
Chronic daphnid partial life cycle toxicity test	40 CFR 797.1330 or 40 CFR 797.1350
Chronic algal toxicity test	40 CFR 797.1050
Early seedling growth test	40 CFR 797.2800
Earthworm acute toxicity test	40 CFR 795.150
Soil microbial community bioassay	40 CFR 797.3700
Plant whole life cycle test	40 CFR 797.2830
Plant uptake test	40 CFR 797.2850
Avian acute oral toxicity test	40 CFR 797.2175
Avian reproductive toxicity test	40 CFR 797.2130 or 40 CFR 797.2150
Direct and indirect photolysis screening test	40 CFR 796.3765 or 40 CFR 796.3700
Aerobic aquatic biodegradation	40 CFR 796.3100
Modified sturm test	40 CFR 796.3260
Closed bottle test	40 CFR 796.3200
Modified OECD screening test	40 CFR 796.3240
Modified MITI test (I)	40 CFR 796.3220
Modified AFNOR test	40 CFR 796.3180
Fate test for inherent biodegradability in soil	40 CFR 796.3400
Jar test to determine the settling rate and extent of removal of suspended solids from solution	Protocol available from the EPA
Simulation test — aerobic sewage treatment: coupled units test (Env.Fate)	40 CFR 796.3300
Activated sludge adsorption isotherm test	Protocol available from EPA
Soil and sediment adsorption isotherm test	40 CFR 796.2750

SECTION 5. *TSCA SECTION 8(c):* ALLEGATIONS OF SIGNIFICANT ADVERSE REACTIONS

TSCA Section 8(c) requires that manufacturers, processors, and distributors of chemical substances and mixtures maintain records as to allegations that chemical substances might cause significant adverse reactions to health or the environment. It is primarily a recordkeeping rule, whereas TSCA Sections 8(e) and 8(d) are reporting rules. Employee health-related allegations arising from any employment-related exposure must be retained for 30 years. Any other record of alleged significant adverse reactions must be retained for 5 years. Examples of "other" records include allegations of human health effects listed in Table 26.11 suffered by nonemployees, or environmental effects alleged by employees or nonemployees such as those listed in Table 26.11. The Section 8(c) rule exempts "known" human effects as described in the scientific literature, Material Safety Data Sheets, or on a product label. However, an effect is not a "known human effect" if:

1. It is a significantly *more severe* effect than described previously.
2. It is a manifestation of a toxic effect following a significantly shorter exposure period or lower exposure level than described.
3. It is a manifestation of a toxic effect by an exposure route different from that described in public information.

For additional information about TSCA Section 8(c), see latest edition of 40 CFR part 717.

TABLE 26.11
Examples of Adverse Reactions,[a] Subject to TSCA 8(c)

Health Effects	Environmental Effects
• Long-lasting or irreversible damage, e.g., cancer or birth defects.	• Gradual or sudden changes in the composition of animal or plant life in an area (including fungal or microbial organisms).
• Partial or complete impairment of bodily functions, e.g., reproductive disorders, neurological disorders, or blood disorders.	• Abnormal number of deaths of organisms (e.g., fish kills).
• An impairment of *normal activities* experienced by all or most of the persons exposed at one time.	• Reduction of the reproductive success or the vigor of a species.
• An impairment of normal activities which is experienced *each time* an individual is exposed.	• Reduction in agricultural productivity, whether crops or livestock.
	• Alterations in the behavior or distribution of a species.
	• Long-lasting or irreversible contamination of components of the physical environment, especially in the case of ground water, surface water, and soil resources that have limited self-cleansing capability.

[a] Significant adverse reactions are reactions that *may* indicate a substantial impairment of normal activities, or long-lasting or irreversible damage to health or the environment.

SECTION 6. *TSCA SECTION 8(d):* REPORTING OF HEALTH AND SAFETY STUDIES

Section 8(d) of TSCA requires that manufacturers (includes importers) of specified chemical substances (or mixtures containing those substances) submit unpublished health or environmentally related studies in their possession to the EPA. Such submittals may include epidemiological data, occupational/environmental exposure data, or health/environmental toxicology studies. The TSCA Section 8(d) regulations with specific reporting requirements are defined in the Code of Federal Regulations, Title 40, Part 716.[4] TSCA defines a health and safety study as being any study of any effect of a chemical substance on health or the environment. The specific substances as well as certain categories of substances that are or have been subject to TSCA Section 8(d) in the past can be found in the Code of Federal Regulations, Title 40, Part 716, Section 120. [4] The Final Rule providing details of the TSCA Section 8(d) reporting requirements was published in the 9-15-86 *Federal Register*, Volume 51, page 32720.[7]

A manufacturer or processor who intends to conduct a new study relating to a chemical substance on the 8(d) list must submit a notice of initiation to the EPA when the study is started and the final report must be submitted to the EPA upon completion of the study. However, findings that constitute "substantial risk" information under Section 8(e) must be reported to the EPA within 15 working days of its receipt. This means that it might be necessary to report *some* observations to EPA even as the test is in progress.

TABLE 26.12
Examples of Information Typically Reported under TSCA Section 8(d)

- Mutagenicity, carcinogenicity, or teratogenicity data.
- Studies indicating potential for neurotoxicity or behavioral disorders.
- Studies of sensitization, pharmacological effects, mammalian absorption/distribution/metabolism/excretion, cumulative/additive/synergistic effects, and acute/subchronic/chronic health or environmental effects.
- Test data relating to ecological/environmental effects on invertebrates, fish, or other aquatic animals/plants.
- Assessments of human or environmental exposure including workplace exposure data where the data are analyzed with respect to potential health or environmental effects.
- Monitoring data when analyzed to determine the degree of exposure of a listed 8(d) substance to humans or the environment and related effects.

TABLE 26.13
Examples of Information Not Reportable under TSCA 8(d)

- Studies that have been published in the scientific literature (TSCA is looking for "unpublished" data).
- Data previously submitted to the EPA under Sections 8(e), 4 or 5 or for EPA's information (FYI submissions).
- Data relating to substances which are *not* listed on EPA's Section 8(d) list (See 40 CFR 716.120).
- Monitoring data (workplace or environmental) that were collected and analyzed more than 5 years before the substance was placed on the 8(d) list.
- Data previously submitted to the EPA under TSCA Section 8(d) by trade associations on behalf of member companies.

SECTION 7. *TSCA SECTION 8(e):* SUBSTANTIAL RISK NOTIFICATION

Section 8(e) of TSCA requires that any person who manufactures, imports, processes, or distributes in commerce a chemical substance or mixture of substances and who obtains information which "reasonably" supports the conclusion that the substance or mixture presents a substantial risk of injury to health or the environment must inform the EPA Administrator of such information (unless it is known that the EPA Administrator already has knowledge of the information).

The TSCA 8(e) reporting requirements became effective on January 1, 1977 and the EPA issued a proposed policy statement on September 9, 1977 (42 FR 45362).[8] A "Statement of Interpretation and Enforcement Policy; Notification of Substantial Risk" describing the types of information subject to TSCA 8(e) reporting and the procedures for doing so, was published in the *Federal Register* on March 16, 1978 (43 FR 11110).[9]

- Section 8(e) of TSCA is an information-gathering tool directed at new-found serious chemical hazards and/or exposures.
- Information that meets the reporting criteria *need not* establish *conclusively* that a sub-stantial risk actually exists. Key criteria to be considered when determining whether new-found information is reportable or not are the seriousness of the adverse effect, the potential for human or environmental exposure to the substance or mixture, and whether the information is already known by the EPA Administrator or not.
- Substances *not* subject to TSCA 8(e) reporting requirements (exempt by definition) are:
  1. Pesticides that are in commerce solely for use as pesticides. A chemical substance which is in the process of research and development (R & D) as a pesticide *is* subject to TSCA 8(e) reporting *until* an application for an "Experimental Use Permit" (EUP) is submitted to the EPA or the substance/mixture is registered under FIFRA.
  2. Tobacco or tobacco products.
  3. Source materials, special nuclear materials and byproducts (as defined in the 1954 Atomic Energy Act and relevant regulations).
  4. Foods, food additives, drugs, cosmetics, and devices (as defined in the Federal Food, Drug, and Cosmetic Act) when manufactured, imported, processed, or distributed in U.S. commerce as a food, food additive, drug, cosmetic, or device.
- All chemical substances (except those exempted by definition) including but not limited to R & D chemical substances, laboratory reagents, polymers, intermediates (whether isolated or not!), catalysts byproducts, impurities, and TSCA-covered microorganisms and products therefrom are subject to the TSCA 8(e) reporting requirements.

On February 1, 1991, the EPA announced a "one time" voluntary TSCA Section 8(e) "Compliance Audit Program (CAP)" in 51 FR 4128.[10] Modifications to this program were later published in the *Federal Register* on April 26, 1991 (56 FR 19514)[11] and on June 20, 1991 (56 FR Part IV). In June 1991, the EPA published a "TSCA Section 8(e) Reporting Guide"[13] which includes complete copies of the EPA's Federal Register announcements of the Section 8(e) CAP and its modifications as well as the original 1978 FR notice. Much of the "Reporting Guide" is presented in basic question and answer format addressing the most common questions asked about TSCA Section 8(e). This Reporting Guide may be obtained by calling the TSCA Hotline at (202) 554-1404, by telefax (202) 554-5603, or by letter addressed to:

The TSCA Assistance Information Service
Environmental Assistance Division
Office of Toxic Substances (TS-799)
U.S. Environmental Protection Agency
401 M Street, SW
Washington, D.C. 20460

Between January 1, 1977 and September 30, 1990 more than 2,600 TSCA 8(e) submissions (including supplemental and follow-up submissions) providing a broad range of toxicity and exposure data for a wide variety of chemical substances were received and reviewed by the EPA.

Summaries of these submissions are provided in Table 26.14 and Figure 26.4. The basis for these summaries is seven bound volumes (compendiums) of "status reports" published by the EPA containing evaluations of all TSCA 8(e) submissions between January 1, 1977 and September 30, 1990. They are identified as follows: NTIS PB No. 80-22/609[14] covering January 1, 1977 to June 30, 1979; NTIS PB No. 81-145732[15] covering July 1, 1979 to January 31, 1980; NTIS PB No. 83-187815[16] covering February 1, 1980 to December 31, 1982; NTIS PB No. 87-129409[17] covering January 1, 1983 to December 31, 1984; NTIS PB No. 87-176004[18] covering January 1, 1985 to December 31, 1986; NTIS PB No. 89-182687[19] covering January 1, 1987 to December 31, 1988; NTIS PB No. 91-233643[20] covering January 1, 1989 to September 30, 1990. Copies of these compendiums may be purchased from the National Technical Information Service (NTIS) by calling (703)487-4600 or writing to:

> The National Technical Information Service
> U.S. Department of Commerce
> 5285 Port Royal Road
> Springfield, VA 22161

Starting with October 1, 1990, the EPA began preparing "summaries" rather than "status reports" for TSCA Section 8(e) submissions. They contain a detailed accounting of toxicological and exposure information that was presented in the 8(e) submission, and copies can be obtained through the TSCA Hotline (202)554-1404. Also available through the TSCA Hotline is a *TSCA Section 8(e) database* that contains a ranking system used by the EPA's Office of Pollution Prevention and Toxics to prioritize Section 8(e) submissions *by toxicity concern*.

From October 1, 1991 to August 27, 1993, more than 7,900 TSCA 8(e) notices were submitted to EPA's Office of Pollution Prevention and Toxics. Most of these were submitted by 123 companies that voluntarily participated in the EPA's CAP program. These are sometimes referred to as being "CAP submissions." These submissions are currently under review by EPA but, based on a preliminary analysis, it appears that 35 to 40% will be categorized as providing information indicating a high degree of hazard associated with the chemical substance involved.

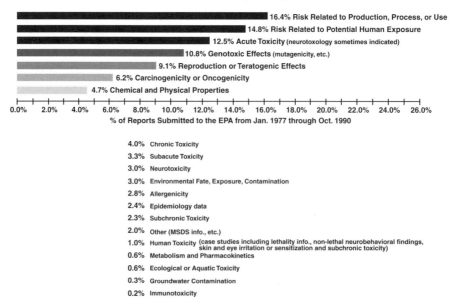

GENERAL NATURE OF TSCA 8(e) REPORTS

16.4% Risk Related to Production, Process, or Use
14.8% Risk Related to Potential Human Exposure
12.5% Acute Toxicity (neurotoxology sometimes indicated)
10.8% Genotoxic Effects (mutagenicity, etc.)
9.1% Reproduction or Teratogenic Effects
6.2% Carcinogenicity or Oncogenicity
4.7% Chemical and Physical Properties

0.0% 2.0% 4.0% 6.0% 8.0% 10.0% 12.0% 14.0% 16.0% 18.0% 20.0% 22.0% 24.0% 26.0%
% of Reports Submitted to the EPA from Jan. 1977 through Oct. 1990

4.0% Chronic Toxicity
3.3% Subacute Toxicity
3.0% Neurotoxicity
3.0% Environmental Fate, Exposure, Contamination
2.8% Allergenicity
2.4% Epidemiology data
2.3% Subchronic Toxicity
2.0% Other (MSDS info., etc.)
1.0% Human Toxicity (case studies including lethality info., non-lethal neurobehavioral findings, skin and eye irritation or sensitization and subchronic toxicity)
0.6% Metabolism and Pharmacokinetics
0.6% Ecological or Aquatic Toxicity
0.3% Groundwater Contamination
0.2% Immunotoxicity

FIGURE 26.4 This information was derived from Compendiums of TSCA 8(e) Status Reports (7) Volumes.[14–20]

TABLE 26.14
TSCA Section 8(e) Submittals (includes Supplemental and Follow-up Submittals)

Information Type	1-1-77 to 6-30-79	7-1-79 to 1-31-80	2-1-80 to 12-31-82	1-1-83 to 12-31-84	1-1-85 to 12-31-86	1-1-87 to 12-31-88	1-1-89 to 9-30-90	Total
Acute toxicity (animal and human)	97	5	44	34	38	42	72	332
Subacute toxicity (animal data)	0	0	12	11	17	15	32	87
Subchronic toxicity (animal data)	12	0	5	6	10	11	17	61
Chronic toxicity (animal and human)	3	0	4	17	23	29	30	106
Human toxicity (case studies)	25	3	0	0	0	0	0	28
Allergenicity (animal and human)	12	0	8	8	11	18	17	74
Immunotoxicity (animal and human)	0	0	0	0	2	1	2	5
Epidemiology data	4	0	9	3	17	11	20	64
Human exposure	0	3	42	37	63	67	181	393
(Accidental)	(0)	(0)	(7)	(2)	(2)	(2)	(7)	
(Monitoring data)	(0)	(0)	(12)	(6)	(12)	(8)	(17)	
(Product composition/contamination)	(0)	(3)	(23)	(29)	(49)	(57)	(157)	
Metabolism and pharmacokinetics	0	0	2	2	9	2	1	16
Carcinogenicity and oncogenicity	38	12	26	19	21	27	22	165
Mutagenicity, clastogenicity, cell transformation, DNA effects/repair	36	6	47	69	50	35	46	289
Neurotoxicity	8	0	7	5	8	10	41	79
Reproduction, developmental, or teratogenic effects	24	2	22	8	16	32	138	242
Chemical and physical properties	4	3	4	24	36	32	22	125
Eco/aquatic toxicity	0	0	1	3	1	3	8	16
Environmental fate, exposure, contamination	25	8	15	4	7	8	13	80
Groundwater contamination	0	0	3	0	0	2	2	7
Risk related to production process or use	0	0	0	43	82	94	217	436
Other	17	0	0	3	4	6	24	54

Source: U.S. Environmental Status Reports.[14-20]

SECTION 8. ADDITIONAL SOURCES OF TSCA-RELATED
INFORMATION

1. **The Toxic Substances Control Act Test Submissions on-line database** (TSCATS), sponsored by the EPA's Office of Prevention, Pesticides, and Toxic Substances, Office of Pollution Prevention and Toxics. The EPA number for information about TSCATS is (202) 382-3524. Also, TSCATS can be accessed through any PC with a communications package or standard modem/terminal/phone setup. Direct dial or telecommunications systems can access CIS (The TSCATS online vendor).

   A. TSCATS contains unpublished, nonconfidential business information data used to monitor health, ecological, and safety effects of the toxic chemicals used within industries.

   B. TSCATS contains citations and abstracts of studies relating to chemicals regulated under TSCA Sections 4, 8(d), and 8(e). Specifically, information such as purpose of study, methodology, health effect, and route of administration is included. TSCATS also contains information about case reports and episodic incidents, such as spills. Also included is information submitted by industries for EPA information purposes (FYI submittals). These submittals contain information on human exposure, toxicity test results, environmental fate, epidemiology, and other information that may be helpful for risk assessment.

   C. The TSCATS database is updated quarterly and offers search with on-line and off-line print capabilities.

   D. A TSCATS User Guide and file description is available from vendors. Fees for on-line access and for tape and microfiche versions are established by the vendors. (National Library of Medicine TOXLINE (301) 496-6193; Chemical Information Systems TSCATS (800) CIS-USER; Dialog Information Services File 156 (800) 3-DIALOG; STN International TOXLIST (614) 421-3600. All of these services charge for accessing their files).

   E. TSCATS fact sheet is available through [http://www.epa.gov/opptintr/cie/tscats.htm]

2. **The Toxic Substances Control Act Assistance Information Service:** telephone (202) 554-1404, fax number (202) 554-5603 (for document requests only). Publications such as *Federal Register* notices and other documents that provide information on TSCA regulatory activities are available.

3. **Toxic Substances Dockets** maintained by the EPA at 401 M Street, SW, Washington, D.C.: telephone (202) 260-7099. The EPA's Office of Pollution Prevention and Toxics (OPPT) Public Information Section houses the official copies of all OPPT administrative records supporting regulatory decisions promulgated under TSCA. Dockets generally contain the following types of supporting documentation: *Federal Register* notices; various health, environmental, and exposure assessment documents; published references; communications; records/transcripts of public and informal meetings; records of informal hearings; public comments, and test data. The EPA maintains and operates a public reading room which is equipped with a photocopier, fiche-to-fiche copier, and fiche reader/printer.

   1. Health and Environmental Assessment Reports are maintained by the EPA's Office of Research and Development and Office of Health and Environmental Assessment (OHEA) in Washington, D.C.: telephone number (202) 260-7345. The OHEA is EPA's focal point for the scientific assessment of the degree of risks imposed by environmental pollutants in varying exposure situations related to human health and ecological systems. The OHEA prepares a variety of health, risk, and exposure assessments and publishes guidelines and methods documents, journal articles, and symposia proceedings. Such documents include but are not limited to the following:

- Air Quality Criteria Documents: Evaluations of the available scientific literature on the health effects of criteria pollutants. (For more information about "criteria pollutants," see 40 CFR, Part 50.)
- Drinking Water Criteria Documents Evaluations of health effects of data on pharmacokinetics, human exposure, acute and chronic toxicity to animals and humans, epidemiology and mechanisms of toxicity, with specific emphasis on data providing dose-response information.
- Exposure Assessments: Assessments of the magnitude, frequency, duration, and route of human exposures occurring at a specific site as a result of an industrial operation or the dumping of hazardous materials.
- Guidelines and Methodologies: Inclusion of the range of assumptions, models, and data to provide the scientific basis for evaluating risk and assuring credibility, consistency, and uniformity in assessments used to support regulatory decisions.
- Health Assessment Documents: Evaluations of the known health data, including carcinogenicity, mutagenicity, and developmental and reproductive effects, from exposure to particular chemicals and compounds.
- Health Effects Assessments: Brief, quantitatively oriented, preliminary assessments of relevant health effects data.
- Health and Environmental Effects Documents: Summaries of the literature concerning health hazards associated with environmental exposure to particular chemicals or chemical compounds.
- Risk Assessments: Carcinogenicity, mutagenicity, developmental toxicity, and reproductive effects. These are analyses of varying length and scope of scientific data on chemical substances as these data relate to human health.
- Ambient Water Quality Criteria Documents: Assessments of the potential risk of adverse effects of a pollutant on aquatic life and on human health.

Specific reports may be ordered from: (1) the EPA's Center for Environmental Research Information, 26 West Martin Luther King Drive, Cincinnati, OH 45268 (telephone number (513) 569-7502) or (2) The National Technical Information Service, 5285 Port Royal Road, Springfield, VA, 22161 (telephone number (703) 487-4650).

5. **EPA Scientific Computer Models:** A sampling of models developed by the EPA is as follows:
   - Assessment Tools for the Evaluation of Risk
   - Biodegradation of Environmental Chemicals Modeled with Aquatic, Relative-Rate Coefficients
   - Exposure Analysis Modeling System II
   - Food and Gill Exchange of Toxic Substances
   - Littoral Ecosystem Risk Assessment Model
   - Multimedia Exposure Assessment Model

The EPA Model Clearinghouse can provide information on EPA scientific models; telephone number (919) 541-5683.

6. Specific Questions
   A. For answers to policy questions, e.g., what kind of regulatory action might be taken under a particular section of TSCA given certain information about toxicity and potential exposure (questions of regulation), call:
   - The EPA's Health and Environmental Review Division (HERD) (202) 260-1241.
   - If the question is environmentally related, call the Environmental Effects Branch (EEB) of HERD, (202) 260-1237.
   - If the question is related to human health, call the Health Effects Branch (HEB) of HERD, (202)260-1513.

B. For answers to questions about Quantitative Structure Activity Relationships (QSAR), call the Environmental Effects Branch (EEB) of HERD, (202)260-1237. (Current use of QSARs by the EPA is limited to the estimation of physical chemical properties, acute aquatic toxicity, and bioconcentration factors.)

C. Questions relating to regulations of new or existing chemical substances (Section 4 and Section 5 regulations) should be directed to the EPA's Chemical Control Division, (202)260-3749.

D. Questions as to EPA's thoughts regarding what testing would be most appropriate to answer particular questions or what protocols should be used should be directed to the Health Effects Branch (202)260-1513 or the Environmental Effects Branch (202)260-1237 of HERD. Information can also be found in the Code of Federal Regulations Title 40.

E. Questions related to existing publicly available toxicological data that have been submitted to the EPA under Sections 8(d) and 8(e) should be directed to the Information Management Division, (202)260-3938, and/or the TSCA Information Management Branch, (202)260-0425.

F. Questions as to whether particular data need to be submitted to the EPA under Sections 8(e) or 8(d) should be directed to the Chemical Screening and Risk Assessment Division of the Office of Pollution Prevention and Toxics, (202)260-3442.

G. Environmental or health-related questions pertaining to pesticides should be directed to one of the two following EPA offices: The Environmental Fate and Effects Division, (202)305-7695; or The Health Effects Division, (202)305-7351. (Pesticides are regulated under the Federal Insecticide, Fungicide, and Rodenticide Act (FIFRA), as amended. Substances regulated under FIFRA are not subject to the TSCA regulations insofar as they are actually manufactured, processed, or distributed in commerce for use as a pesticide. If a pesticide has multiple uses only some of which are regulated under FIFRA, it *will* be subject to the TSCA regulations.)[21]

H. **To determine the phone number or location of a particular EPA office, contact the "EPA locator" at (202) 260-2090.**

TABLE 26.15
EPA Web Addresses Relating to TSCA[22]

Web Addresses

Subject	Website
Office of Pollution Prevention & Toxics Home Page	www.epa.gov/opptintr
Aqueous & Semi-aqueous Solvent Chemicals	www.epa.gov/opptintr/solvents
Asbestos Program	www.epa.gov/opptintr/asbestos
OPPT Chemical Fact Sheets	www.epa.gov/opptintr/chemfact
Chemical Right-to-Know Program High Production Volume (HPV) Challenge Program	www.epa.gov/chemrtk
Chemical Registry System	www.epa.gov/crs
Children's Health Test Rule	www.epa.gov/opptintr /shemrtk/childhlt.htm
Community-Based Environmental Protection	www.epa.gov/opptintr/cbep
HPV Chemical List	www.epa.gov/opptintr /chemrtk/hpvchmlt.htm
Chemical Spill Information	www.chemicalispill.org
Chemicals on Reporting Rules List	www.epa.gov/opptintr/CORR
40 CFR Sections 700–799	www.epa.gov/docs/epacfr40/chapt-I.info/subch-R
Design for the Environment Program	www.epa.gov/opptintr/dfe

TABLE 26.15 *(Continued)*
EPA Web Addresses Relating to TSCA[22]

Web Addresses

Subject	Website
Electronic Products Recovery	www.epr2@nsc.org
Environment Reporting Requirements	www.pwbrc.org
Endocrine Disruptors Screening and Testing Program	www.epa.gov/opptintr/opptendo
Envirofacts	www.epa.gov/enviro/indexjava.html
Environmental Accounting Project	www.epa.gov/opptintr/acctg
Environmental Monitoring for Public Access and Community Tracking	www.epa.gov/empact
Environmentally Preferable Purchasing	www.epa.gov/opptintr /epp
EPP Pilot Projects-Internet Tools	www.epa.gov/opptintr/cleaners/select
Exposure Assessment Tools and Models	www.epa.gov/opptintr/exposure
Great Lakes Binational Toxics Strategy	www.epa.gov/bns
Green Chemistry Program	www.epa.gov/greenchemistry
Harmonized Test Guidelines	www.epa.gov/opptsfrs/home/guidelin.htm
Integrated Risk Information System	www.epa.gov/ORD/dbases/iris
Interagency Testing Committee	www.epa.gov/opptintr /itc
Inventory Update Rule Amendments 1998 IUR Electronic Reporting	www.epa.gov/opptintr/iur98
Lead Programs	www.epa.gov/opptintr/lead
National Lead Information Center	www.nsc.org/lead/nlic.htm
National Service Center for Environmental Publications	www.epa.gov/ncepilhom
New Chemicals Program	www.epa.gov/opptintr/newchms
New Chemicals Program Chemical Categories Report	www.epa.gov/opptintr/newchms/chemcat
New Chemicals Chemistry Assistance Manual for PMN Submitters	www.epa.gov/opptintr/chem-pmn
New Chemicals Program Weekly Postings	www.epa.gov/opptintr/newchms/dropstat.htm
The New Chemicals Pollution Prevention Recognition Program	www.epa.gov/opptintr/newchms/p2.htm
Online Library System (OLS)	www.epa.gov/natlibra/ols.htm
Persistent, Bioaccumulative and Toxics (PBT) Initiative	www.epa.gov/pbt
PCB Regulations	www.epa.gov/opptintr/pcb
Pollution Prevention	www.epa.gov/opptintr/p2home
Pollution Prevention Information Clearinghouse	www.epa.gov/opptintr/library/ppicdist.htm
Pollution Prevention Resource Exchange (P2RX)	www.epa.gov/p2/p2rxfact.htm
P2 Integration in Regional Program Management — Private Sector Partnerships — Region 5	www.deq.state.mi.us
Prevention Tools — Region 5	www.epa.gov/reg5cra/wptdiv/p2pages/toolbox.htm
Recognition and Award Programs	www.epa.gov/region07/specinit/p2/98awards.htm
Risk Screening Environmental Indicators Model	*www.epa.gov/opptintr/env_ind/index.html*
Small Business Assistance Program	www.epa.gov/ttn/sbap
OPPT Tribal Program	www.epa.gov/opptintr/tribal
Toxic Release Inventory	www.epa.gov/opptintr/tri
TSCA Biotechnology	www.epa.gov/opptintr/biotech
TSCA Chemical Testing Program Master Testing List	www.epa.gov/opptintr/chemtest
TSCA Federal Registers	www.epa.gov/fedrgstr/EPA-TOX
TSCA-related pre-1994 Federal Registers	www.epa.gov/opptsfrs/home/histox.htm
TSCA 8(e) Triage	www.epa.gov/opptintr/8etriag
Vermont Environmental Assistance Partnership	www.veap.org
Voluntary Initiative for Source Reduction	www.nrdc.org/nrdcpro/msri/msriinx.html

REFERENCES

1. U.S. Environmental Protection Agency, *Access EPA*, EPA 220B-92-014, 1992.
2. U.S. EPA, *Headquarters Telephone Directory*, EPA 208-B-99-001, 1999.
3. *Federal Register,* FR 32294, July 15, 1991.
4. *Code of Federal Regulations*, CFR Title 40.
5. EPA Dec. 1, 1992 MTL Document.
6. U.S. EPA, *TSCA New Chemicals Program (NCP) Chemical Categories*; Revised June 1998.
7. *Federal Register,* vol 51, September 15, 1986.
8. *Federal Register*, vol 42 FR 45362, September 9, 1977.
9. *Federal Register,* vol 43 FR 11110, March 16, 1978.
10. *Federal Register,* vol. 51 FR 4128, February 1, 1991.
11. *Federal Register,* vol. 56 FR 19514, April 26, 1991.
12. *Federal Register,* vol. 56 FR Part IV, June 20, 1991.
13. U.S. EPA, *TSCA Section 8(e) Reporting Guide*, June 1991.
14. EPA Status Report, PB No. 80-22/609.
15. EPA Status Report, PB No. 81-145732.
16. EPA Status Report, PB No. 83-187815.
17. EPA Status Report, PB No. 87-129409.
18. EPA Status Report, PB No. 87-176004.
19. EPA Status Report, PB No. 89-182687.
20. EPA Status Report, PB No. 91-233643.
21. *Federal Register,* vol. 42, FR 64585, December 23, 1977.
22. EPA Review of OPPT Program Activities (1998–1999) EPA 745-K-99-003; Dec 1999.

27 Regulatory Toxicology: U.S. EPA/Pesticides (FIFRA)

Jane E. Harris, Ph.D.

CONTENTS

SECTION 1. INTRODUCTION

Pesticides are used to control unwanted insects, fungi, weeds, microbes, and rodents. They are intended to protect human health from diseases or toxins, to increase the yield of crops, and to improve the natural beauty of the environment. For example, insecticides can be used to control the following: insects that transmit bacterial or viral diseases or allergens to humans or plants; insects that directly eat crops or parts of plants, shrubs, or trees; termites, carpenter and fire ants, and cockroaches; or grubs and worms that feed on the roots of turf and field crops. Fungicides are used to prevent the destruction of plants, trees, or grasses and to keep crops untainted by mycotoxins. Herbicides act by selectively killing weeds that compete with crops for nutrients in soil and water, and thereby can indirectly increase crops yields. Herbicides are also used on turf to improve the aesthetics of lawns around the home and golf courses and for total vegetation control to eliminate unwanted vegetation around railroad tracks, rights of way, fences, etc. Algicides are also used aquatically to improve water flow, which in turn may prevent flooding. Antimicrobial agents are used to kill bacteria and viruses, and thereby limit the spread of infectious agents in the home, hospitals, restaurants, and food-processing establishments. Finally, rodenticides are intended to kill rodents that spread diseases and excrement in food-storage areas or in urban areas where garbage is concentrated.

Fundamentally, pesticides are medicines developed to treat diseases and to prevent both the spread of disease and predator destruction of trees, shrubs, grasses, and crops. As a result, pesticides prevent the vector-borne spread of diseases to humans and plants, and increase crop yields, which help provide an inexpensive source of fruits and vegetables necessary for maintaining optimum human health. Further, antifungal agents prevent fungal contamination of agricultural crops with mycotoxins that can be extremely toxic and, in some cases, carcinogenic to humans.

SECTION 2. FIFRA

The original legislation, entitled the Federal Insecticide, Fungicide, and Rodenticide Act (FIFRA), was passed in 1947 and assigned labeling authority of pesticides to the Department of Agriculture. The most significant amendment to FIFRA occurred in 1972; the amendment transferred most regulatory authority of pesticides to the newly formed (1970) Environmental Protection Agency (EPA). Under this amendment, pesticides would be registered as either general-use or restricted-use pesticides, the latter requiring handling by a *certified* pesticide handler only, who would be certified by the states. This amendment also required that pesticides not only be registered with the EPA, but also be reregistered with the EPA, assuring that reevaluation of the safety of a pesticide would be performed periodically using up-to-date safety standards. Additional federal actions since 1972, with the most recent entitled "The Food Quality Protection Act" (FQPA, 1996), are all intended to expand the requirements and standards for registering and reregistering pesticides to protect humans, especially children, and the environment by minimizing the level of risk in the use of pesticides, i.e., by providing a standard of "reasonable certainty of no harm."

A. OFFICE OF PESTICIDE PROGRAMS

The Office of Pesticide Programs (OPP), which regulates the pesticide industry under FIFRA, is within the Office of Prevention, Pesticides, and Toxic Substances (OPPTS) (Table 27.1). The Health Effects Division requires that mammalian toxicology testing be performed to evaluate the risk to humans from pesticide use. The Environmental Fate and Effects Division requires ecological toxicology testing and environmental fate analyses to determine potential risks to birds, fish, wildlife, invertebrates, and nontarget plants in both terrestrial and aquatic environments.

TABLE 27.1
Office of Pesticide Programs Contact Information[a]

Office of Pesticide Programs Divisions

- Antimicrobials
- Biological and Economic Analyses
- Biopesticides and Pollution Prevention
- Environmental Fate and Effects
- Field and External Affairs

- Health Effects Division
- Information Resources and Services
- Registration
- Special Review and Reregistration

Mailing Address:
U.S. Environmental Protection Agency
Office of Pesticide Programs (Division Mail Code)
Ariel Rios Building
1200 Pennsylvania Ave. NW
Washington, D.C. 20460

Location:
Office of Pesticide Programs
Crystal Mall #2,
1921 Jefferson Davis Highway
Arlington, VA
(18th St. and Clark Place, diagonally across from the Crystal City Metro Stop)
Nearest Stop on the Washington Metro Line: Crystal City on the Yellow or Blue Line

Environmental Fate and Effects Division
Mail Code: 7507C
Fax: 703-305-6309

EFED is responsible for evaluating and validating environmental data submitted on pesticide properties and effects (includes ecotoxicology).

TABLE 27.1 *(Continued)*
Office of Pesticide Programs Contact Information[a]

Health Effects Division
Mail Code: 7509C
Fax: 703-305-5147

HED is responsible for reviewing and validating data on properties and effects of pesticides, as well as characterizing and assessing exposure and risks to humans and domestic animals (mammalian toxiocolgy).

[a] See www.epa/pesticides/contacts.htm for detailed contact information.

B. TESTING REQUIREMENTS

For pesticides, whose general-use patterns include terrestrial, aquatic, and greenhouse uses for both food crops and nonfood, as well as forestry, domestic outdoor and indoor uses for nonfood, a broad selection of toxicology studies is used to screen each chemical for the purposes of dietary, worker, and nonworker risk assessments. These requirements for testing were proposed in the *Federal Register* (October 24, 1984) and are now listed in 40 CFR 158.340. For the studies listed in Table 27.2, the EPA 870 Series Data Requirements/Test Guidelines are available (Table 27.3).

Although acute and short-term studies may be conducted by various routes of exposure, e.g., dermal, inhalation, oral intubation (gavage), longer-term studies are generally performed by administering the pesticide in the diet, which is consistent with general long-term exposure of humans to pesticide residues in the food. However, these pesticides are tested to a maximum tolerated dose or a limit dose of 1000 mg/kg body weight/day [approximately 20,000 ppm in the rat (S-D) and 7000 ppm in the mouse (CD-1)], whereas most foods have no detectable pesticide residues and, when present, are often found only in ppb ranges.

For certain classes of chemicals, such as pesticides (usually insecticides) with neurotoxic activity, the Office of Pesticide Programs (Health Effects Division) at the EPA now requires for new registrations or reregistration, both acute and subchronic (90-day) neurotoxicity studies in rats and, for organophosphate cholinesterase inhibitors, acute and 28-day delayed neurotoxicity studies in hens, including measurements of neuropathy target esterase. Other conditionally required studies, which may be requested depending on results (triggers) from the above studies or on specific-use patterns, include the following studies in rats: subchronic (90-day) dermal or inhalation studies (particularly for indoor residential exposures), chronic neurotoxicity studies, dermal penetration studies, and immunotoxicity studies. Following the passage of the 1996 FQPA, which requires evaluation of potential increased sensitivity of infants and children, the EPA requested that the developmental neurotoxicity study in rats be performed for pesticides showing neurotoxic activity and more recently, subtle disruption of the endocrine system.

Some of the above studies may be waived depending on the use pattern of the pesticide. For example, a pesticide used only on golf courses may have the chronic/oncogenicity studies and reproduction studies waived and a 90-day dermal toxicity study substituted for the subchronic feeding study in rats. It should also be noted that the acute battery of six studies and occasionally the 21/28-day dermal toxicity studies are required for registration, not only of the active ingredient but also of all end-use formulations, unless waivers for these studies are granted by the EPA.

Finally, there is a new class of pesticides, referred to as biopesticides and microbial pest control agents (MPCA). These include pheromones and other naturally occurring compounds, bacteria, algae, fungi, viruses, protozoa, and plant pesticides, as defined in 40 CRF 152.20. Biological and biologically derived pesticides are generally naturally occurring or strain improved, either by natural selection or by deliberate genetic manipulation.

Because biopesticides are specific to the target species and typically have a unique or nontoxic mode of action, the EPA published in 1983, and amended in 1989, testing guidelines classified as subdivison M of the Pesticide Assessment Guidelines. The testing requirements are a tiered system; the first tier consists of a battery of short-term tests designed to evaluate potential toxicity, infectivity, and pathogenicity of the biopesticide (OPPTS Series 885, Group C). Both the design and extent of testing are determined on a case-by-case basis by the EPA to minimize unnecessary testing but to assure that sufficient testing is performed to make scientifically sound regulatory decisions. Ecological and nontarget organism, and environmental expression testing (OPPTS Series 885, Groups D and E) also have been grouped in tiers.

TABLE 27.2
Typical Toxicology Studies Required for Pesticides[a]

- Six acute studies — rat oral, dermal, inhalation, and primary eye (rabbit) and skin (rat) irritation, and dermal sensitization (guinea pig)
- 21/28-day dermal toxicity study
- Subchronic (90-day) feeding studies in rodents and nonrodents (e.g., dogs)
- Chronic feeding studies in rodents and nonrodents
- Oncogenicity studies in two species of rodents (rat and mice preferred)
- Prenatal developmental toxicity studies in rodents and nonrodents (rats and rabbits preferred)
- Two-generation reproduction study in rodents
- General metabolism/pharmacokinetic study in rodents (usually rats)
- Genotoxicity studies — *in vitro* gene mutation (bacterial and mammalian cells), structural chromosomal aberration (e.g., rodent, *in vivo*), and other genotoxic effects

[a] Additional studies may be required or some of the above studies waived on a case-by-case basis (see text).

TABLE 27.3
Series 870 — Health Effects Test Guidelines

OPPTS No.	Name	Existing Numbers			EPA Pub. No. 712–C–
		OPPT	OPP	OECD	
Group A — Acute Toxicity Test Guidelines					
870.1000	Acute toxicity testing — background	None	None	None	98–189
870.1100	Acute oral toxicity	798.1175	81–1	401	98–190
870.1200	Acute dermal toxicity	798.1100	81–2	402	98–192
870.1300	Acute inhalation toxicity	798.1150	81–3	403	98–193
870.2400	Acute eye irritation	798.4500	81–4	405	98–195
870.2500	Acute dermal irritation	798.4470	81–5	404	98–196
870.2600	Skin sensitization	798.4100	81–6	406	98–197
Group B — Subchronic Toxicity Test Guidelines					
870.3050	Repeated dose 28-day oral toxicity study in rodents	None	None	407	00–366
870.3100	90-day oral toxicity in rodents	798.2650	82–1	408	98–199
870.3150	90-day oral toxicity in nonrodents	None	82–1	409	98–200
870.3200	21/28-day dermal toxicity	None	82–2	410	98–201
870.3250	90-day dermal toxicity	798.2250	82–3	411	98–202
870.3465	90-day inhalation toxicity	798.2450	82–4	413	98–204
870.3550	Reproduction/development toxicity screening test	None	None	421	00–367
870.3650	Combined repeated dose toxicity with the reproduction/development toxicity screening test	None	None	422	00–368

TABLE 27.3 *(Continued)*
Series 870 — Health Effects Test Guidelines

OPPTS No.	Name	Existing Numbers			EPA Pub. No. 712–C–
		OPPT	OPP	OECD	
870.3700	Prenatal developmental toxicity study	798.4900	83–3	414	98–207
870.3800	Reproduction and fertility effects	798.4700	83–4	416	98–208
	Group C — Chronic Toxicity Test Guidelines				
870.4100	Chronic toxicity	798.3260	83–1	452	98–210
870.4200	Carcinogenicity	798.3300	83–2	451	98–211
870.4300	Combined chronic toxicity/carcinogenicity	798.3320	83–5	453	98–212
	Group D — Genetic Toxicity Test Guidelines				
870.5100	Bacterial reverse mutation test	798.5100, .5265	84–2	471	98–247
870.5140	Gene mutation in *Aspergillus nidulans*	798.5140	84–2	None	98–215
870.5195	Mouse biochemical specific locus test	798.5195	84–2	None	98–216
870.5200	Mouse visible specific locus test	798.5200	84–2	None	98–217
870.5250	Gene mutation in *Neurospora crassa*	798.5250	84–2	None	98–218
870.5275	Sex-linked recessive lethal test in *Drosophila melanogaster*	798.5275	84–2	477	98–220
870.5300	*In vitro* mammalian cell gene mutation test	798.5300	84–2	476	98–221
870.5375	*In vitro* mammalian chromosome aberration test	798.5375	84–2	473	98–223
870.5380	Mammalian spermatogonial chromosomal aberration test	798.5380	84–2	483	98–224
870.5385	Mammalian bone marrow chromosomal aberration test	798.5385	84–2	475	98–225
870.5395	Mammalian erythrocyte micronucleus test	798.5395	84–2	474	98–226
870.5450	Rodent dominant lethal assay	798.5450	84–2	478	98–227
870.5460	Rodent heritable translocation assays	798.5460	84–2	485	98–228
870.5500	Bacterial DNA damage or repair tests	798.5500	84–2	None	98–229
870.5550	Unscheduled DNA synthesis in mammalian cells in culture	798.5550	84–2	482	98–230
870.5575	Mitotic gene conversion in *Saccharomyces cerevisiae*	798.5575	84–2	481	98–232
870.5900	*In vitro* sister chromatid exchange assay	798.5900	84–2	479	98–234
870.5915	*In vivo* sister chromatid exchange assay	798.5915	84–2	None	98–235
	Group E — Neurotoxicity Test Guidelines				
870.6100	Acute and 28-day delayed neurotoxicity of organophosphorus substances	798.6450, .6540, .6560	81–7, 82–5, 82–6	418, 419	98–237
870.6200	Neurotoxicity screening battery	798.6050, .6200, .6400	81–8, 82–7, 83–1	424	98–238
870.6300	Developmental neurotoxicity study	None	83–6	None	98–239
870.6500	Schedule-controlled operant behavior	798.6500	85–5	None	98–240
870.6850	Peripheral nerve function	798.6850	85–6	None	98–241
870.6855	Neurophysiology: Sensory evoked potentials	798.6855	None	None	98–242
	Group F — Special Studies Test Guidelines				
870.7200	Companion animal safety	None	None	None	98–349
870.7485	Metabolism and pharmacokinetics	798.7485	85–1	417	95–244
870.7600	Dermal penetration	None	85–3	None	98–350
870.7800	Immunotoxicity	None	85–7	None	98–351

Source: http://www.epa.gov/docs/OPPTS_Harmonized/870_Health_Effects_Test_Guidelines/Master/harmon.pdf.

SECTION 3. RISK ASSESSMENTS

Acute studies, including toxicity, irritation, and sensitization studies, especially on end-use formulations, are intended to provide hazard evaluations to label these formulations with proper handling procedures and to indicate personal protective equipment needed to prevent dermal and inhalation exposure by operators and workers. Short-term, repeat-dose studies are more aptly used for risk assessments performed for operators during mixing, loading, and applying pesticides and during reentry onto sprayed fields especially when harvesting crops. These shorter-term studies also support risk assessments when exposure to homeowners may potentially occur from pesticides applied to turf, shrubs, or trees around the house or inside the home for pest control. Finally, longer-term studies, including the two-generation reproduction study, are generally used for chronic dietary risk assessments for infants, children, and adults from potential residues in foods. More recently, the EPA has included in its evaluations acute dietary risk assessments. These are based on acute and/or short-term toxicity studies, such as acute neurotoxicity or developmental toxicity, which evaluate toxicological end points after a single dose or short-term exposure.

In general, the hazard assessment for acute and chronic dietary exposure from residues in food and water is performed by the EPA by identifying the lowest "no observable adverse effect level" (NOAEL) for the most sensitive parameter and species. The NOAEL is generally divided by 100 to adjust for interspecies (tenfold) and intraspecies (tenfold) sensitivities, i.e., between the experimental animal and human and within the human population, respectively. If uncertainties exist in the database or if adverse effects are evaluated as more problematic, additional safety factors, i.e., 2, 3, or 10, may be applied. Moreover, with the passage of the FQPA, an extra tenfold safety factor (i.e., a total uncertainty factor of 1000) to account for the uncertain potential for children and infants to show an increased sensitivity (e.g., special susceptibility to neurological effects) may be applied in addition to the tenfold factor already used for intraspecies sensitivities within the human population. Pediatric toxicology not only has become a major issue at the EPA, but also has become a focus for testing at the FDA to predict pediatric pharmacology/toxicity prior to clinical trials in children. Further, quantitative risk assessments, which entail multistage modeling, upper 95% confidence limits, and linear extrapolation, are applied for some pesticides identified with oncogenic activity in mice and/or rats. For these latter calculations, cancer risks for the general population above 1 in 1 million are typically considered limiting for registration purposes.

Worker and nonworker (e.g., residential) nondietary exposures from both dermal and inhalation sources are compared with the most sensitive NOAELs from available toxicity studies. Dividing these NOAELs by estimated exposures provide margins of exposure (MOEs), which again are expected to reach at least 100-fold. Passage of the FQPA has also required the EPA to consider both aggregate exposure of a single pesticide if exposure may be anticipated from different sources, i.e., food, water and residential environments, and multiple daily exposures from a group of pesticides with a common mechanism of action, e.g., cholinesterase inhibitors. The EPA is attempting to develop new methodologies for pesticide risk assessments to evaluate these very complex issues.

Finally, ecotoxicological assessments must be performed on pesticides that are applied to the environment to assess the following: acute and life-cycle (or reproductive) effects on fish (freshwater and marine), birds, aquatic invertebrates (e.g., daphnia and mysid shrimp), earthworms, honeybees, plants (terrestrial and aquatic), and wild mammals. A very thorough review of requirements for toxicity testing for pesticides in the United States and the European Union can be found in Sumner et al.[1]

REFERENCE

1. Sumner, D.D., Luempert, L.G., and Stevens, J.T., Agricultural chemicals: the Federal Insecticide, Fungicide and Rodenticide Act and a review of the European Community regulatory process, in *Regulatory Toxicology*, Chengelis, C.P., Holson, J.F., and Gad, S.C., Eds., Raven Press, New York, 1995, 133–163.

28 Regulatory Toxicology: U.S. FDA/Pharmaceuticals

William J. Powers, Jr., Ph.D., D.A.B.T.

CONTENTS

0-8493-0370-2/02/$0.00+$1.50
© 2002 by CRC Press LLC

SECTION 1. INTRODUCTION

The following information is designed as an introductory guide to regulatory toxicology for a toxicologist in the pharmaceutical industry. The section on FDA organization will be helpful when trying to determine the particular part of FDA with which to interact. Some of the more commonly required topics are also addressed, e.g., NDA Format, User Fees, Pregnancy Categories, Guidelines for Animal Toxicity Testing, and GRAS Substances.

SECTION 2. ORGANIZATIONAL STRUCTURE OF THE FOOD AND DRUG ADMINISTRATION (FDA)[1]

The FDA is part of the U.S. Government Department of Health and Human Services — Public Health Service. The name "Food and Drug Administration" was first provided by the Agriculture Appropriation Act of 1931, although similar law enforcement functions had been in existence under different organizational titles of the Food and Drug Act of 1906.

The FDA's activities are directed toward protecting the health of the nation against impure and unsafe foods, drugs and cosmetics, and other potential hazards. Figure 28.1 shows an overview of the organization of the Food and Drug Administration. The organization and functions of some of the key groups or centers are shown in Figures 28.2 through 28.8. The FDA website is www. FDA. gov.

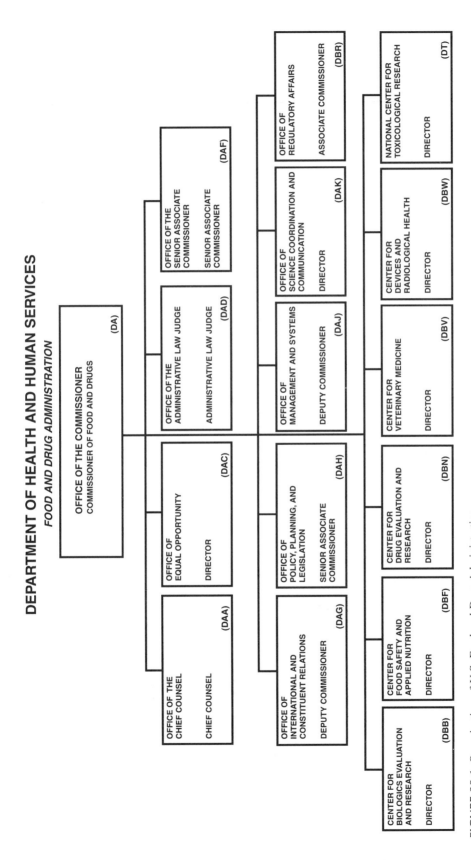

DEPARTMENT OF HEALTH AND HUMAN SERVICES

FOOD AND DRUG ADMINISTRATION

FIGURE 28.1 Organization of U.S. Food and Drug Administration

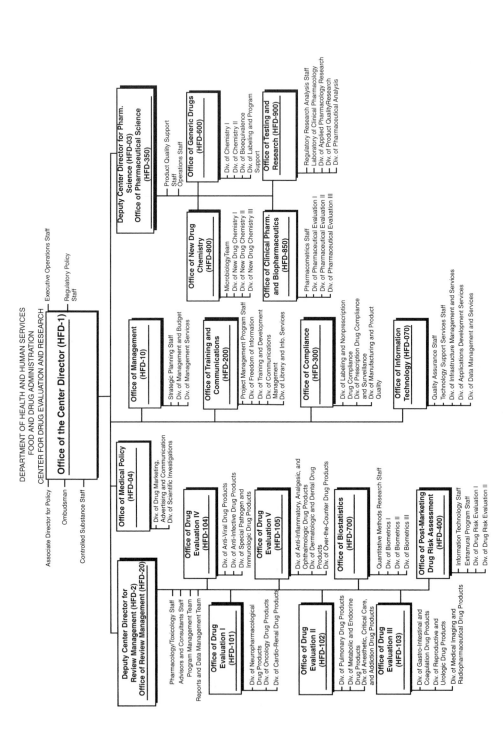

FIGURE 28.2 The Center for Drug Evaluation and Research develops policy with regard to the safety, effectiveness, and labeling of all drug products for human use and reviews and evaluates new drug applications (NDAs) and investigational new drug applications (INDs). It develops and implements standards for the safety and effectiveness of all over-the-counter drugs and monitors the quality of marketed drug products through product testing, surveillance, and compliance programs.

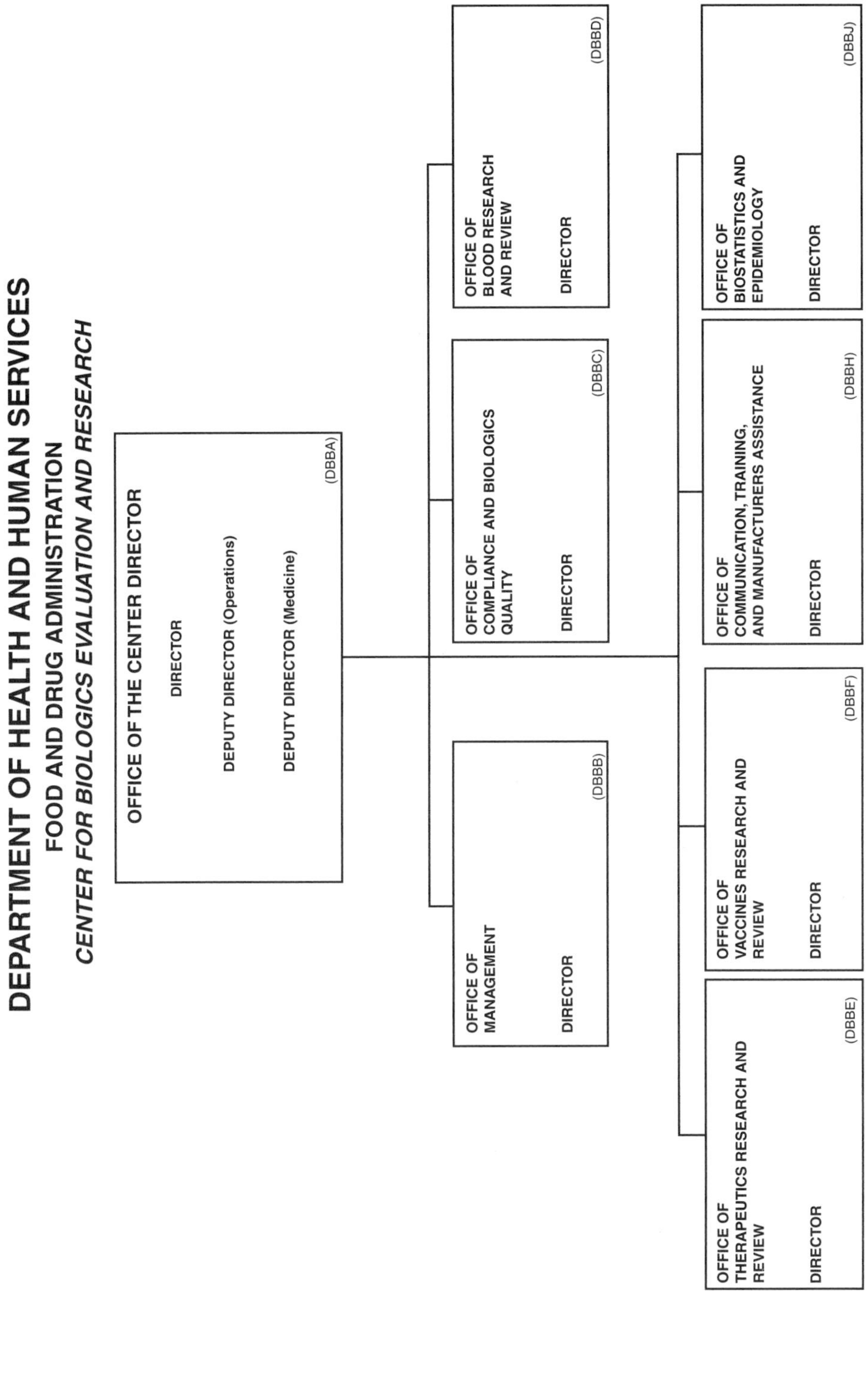

FIGURE 28.3 The Center for Biologics Evaluation and Research administers regulation of biological products under the biological product control provisions of the Public Health Service Act and applicable provisions of the Federal Food, Drug and Cosmetic Act. It provides primary scientific focus for coordination of the AIDS program (including vaccine and diagnostic tests development). It inspects manufacturers' facilities for compliance with standards, tests products submitted for release, establishes written and physical standards, and approves licensing of manufacturers to produce biological products (PLAs).

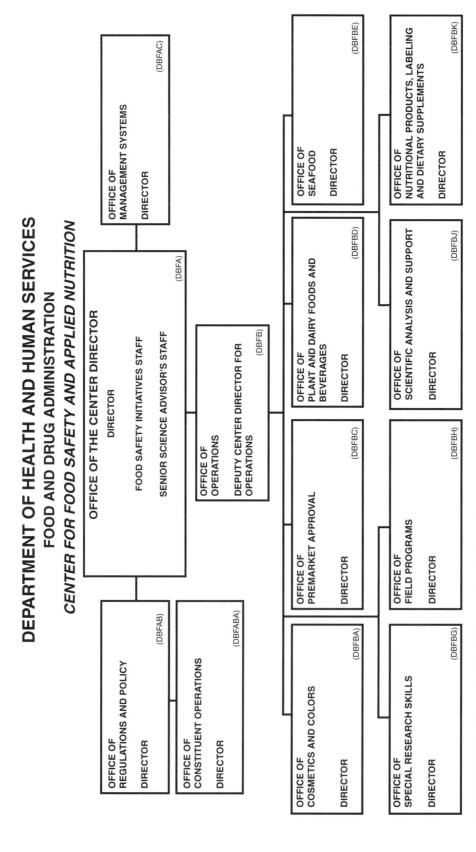

FIGURE 28.4 The Center for Food Safety and Applied Nutrition conducts research and develops standards on the composition, quality, nutrition, and safety of food and food additives, colors, and cosmetics. It conducts research designed to improve the detection, prevention, and control of contamination that may be responsible for illness or injury conveyed by foods, colors, and cosmetics and coordinates and evaluates the FDA's surveillance and compliance programs related to foods, colors, and cosmetics. This Center also regulates the safe use of food and color additives.

DEPARTMENT OF HEALTH AND HUMAN SERVICES
FOOD AND DRUG ADMINISTRATION
CENTER FOR VETERINARY MEDICINE

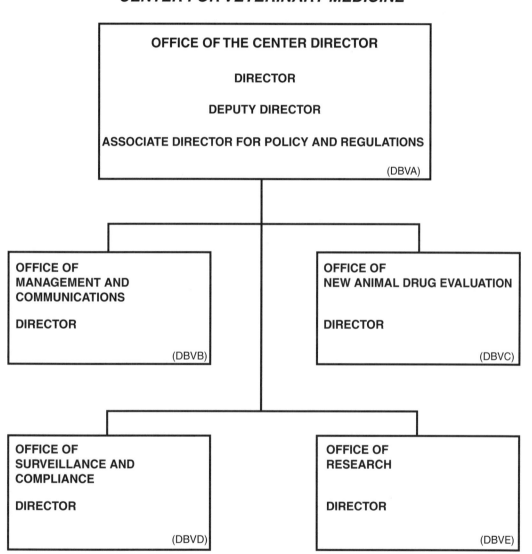

OFFICE OF THE CENTER DIRECTOR

DIRECTOR

DEPUTY DIRECTOR

ASSOCIATE DIRECTOR FOR POLICY AND REGULATIONS

(DBVA)

OFFICE OF MANAGEMENT AND COMMUNICATIONS

DIRECTOR

(DBVB)

OFFICE OF NEW ANIMAL DRUG EVALUATION

DIRECTOR

(DBVC)

OFFICE OF SURVEILLANCE AND COMPLIANCE

DIRECTOR

(DBVD)

OFFICE OF RESEARCH

DIRECTOR

(DBVE)

FIGURE 28.5 The Center for Veterinary Medicine develops and conducts programs with respect to the safety and efficacy of veterinary preparations and devices.

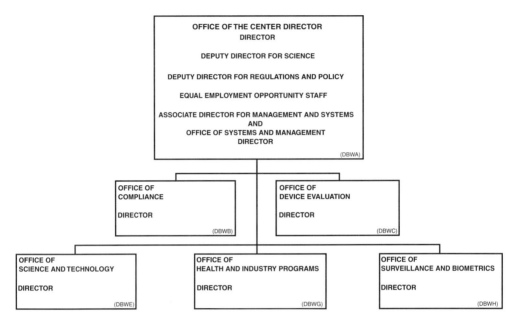

FIGURE 28.6 The Center for Devices and Radiological Health develops and implements a national program designed to control unnecessary exposure of humans to and ensure the safe and efficacious use of potentially hazardous ionizing and non-ionizing radiation.

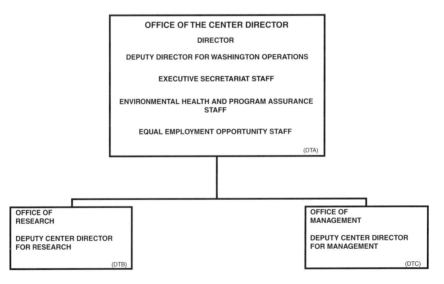

FIGURE 28.7 The National Center for Toxicological Research conducts research programs to study the biological effects of potentially toxic chemical substances found in the environment, emphasizing the determination of the health effects resulting from long-term, low-level exposure to chemical toxicants.

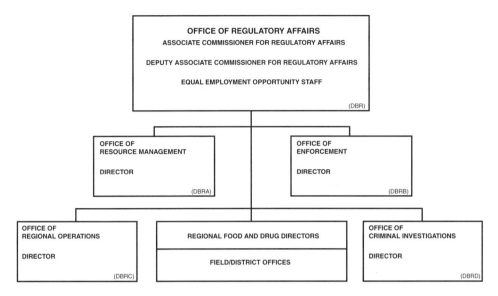

FIGURE 28.8 The Office of Regulatory Affairs advises and assists the commissioner and other key officials on compliance-related matters.

SECTION 3. GUIDELINE FOR THE FORMAT AND CONTENT OF NONCLINICAL PHARMACOLOGY/TOXICOLOGY SECTION OF A NEW DRUG APPLICATION[2]

The FDA has published a guideline that describes an acceptable format for organizing and presenting the pharmacology and toxicology data required in the nonclinical section of the application. These guidelines pertain only to organization of existing data, not specific study requirements.

A. Drug Identification

All drugs used in studies should be prominently identified by appropriate code numbers. Chemical names and structures should also be provided. Where appropriate, batch or lot numbers should be included.

B. Animals

When more than one species is used, these data should be reported in the following relative order, males preceding females: mouse, rat, hamster, other rodent(s), rabbit, dog, monkey, other nonrodent mammal(s), nonmammals. Data for "normal" adult animals should precede that for infant, geriatric, or disease-model animals.

C. Route and Mode of Administration

Discussions of studies for each species should first represent the intended clinical route followed by data for other routes in the following relative order: oral, intravenous, intramuscular, interperitoneal, subcutaneous, inhalation, topical, other *in vivo*, *in vitro*.

D. Doses

Multidose data should be displayed from the lowest to the highest dose. In multigroup studies, results should be presented in order of increasing dosage: untreated control, vehicle control, low dose, middle dose(s), high dose, positive or comparative control(s).

E. Order of Presentation of Studies

Rather than using a chronological sequence for presentation of studies, the following order is recommended by FDA:

Pharmacology Studies
Acute Toxicity Studies
Multidose Toxicity Studies (Subchronic/Chronic, Carcinogenicity)
Special Toxicity Studies (Irritation, Sensitization, Antigenicity, etc.)
Reproduction Studies
Mutagenicity Studies
Absorption, Distribution, Metabolism, Excretion (ADME) Studies

FDA's regulations describe certain conditions under which the agency may refuse to file (RTF) an application (21 CFR 314.101). A portion of this provision states "The application is incomplete because it does not on its face contain information required under section 505(b), section 505(j), or section 507 of the act and §314.50 or §314.94." As part of its program to improve efficiency of the new drug review process, CDER has further clarified its practices regarding RFTs.[3] In the past, decisions to refuse to file an application by CDER were based on extreme deficiencies, e.g., the total omission of a needed section or the absence of any study that was considered an adequate well-controlled study.

It is now CDER's position that the past practice of submitting an incomplete or inadequate application and then "repairing" it in the course of an extended review period is extremely inefficient and a waste of limited FDA resources. It is similarly wasteful of industry resources. CDER has therefore applied §314.101(d)(3) to refuse to file applications that at the time of submission are not reviewable and at least potentially approvable as submitted. Accepting an application that is obviously in need of extensive repair is unfair to those sponsors who have fulfilled their scientific and legal obligations by submitting a complete quality application. The incomplete application, submitted prematurely, may delay review of the latter more complete application from another industry sponsor.

An application that has required major repair during review will also usually prove to be one with a prolonged review time. FDA has committed, in response to User Fee legislation (Prescription Drug User Fee Act of 1992), to providing a comprehensive action letter to sponsors within 6 to 12 months of submission. (*Note:* Refusal to file an application should not be confused with refusal to approve the application after full review by the agency.) Good FDA-industry interactions and use of pre-NDA meetings will improve submissions and help to identify applications whose submissions would be premature.

There are three circumstances under which FDA has generally exercised its RTF authority:

1. Omission of a section of the NDA required under 21 CFR 314.50, or presentation of a section in so haphazard a manner as to render it incomplete on its face.
2. Clear failure to include evidence of effectiveness compatible with the statute and regulations.
3. Omission of critical data, information or analyses needed to evaluate effectiveness and safety or provide adequate directions for use.

In 1992, CDER shared with industry a 45-Day Worksheet used by the division to facilitate initial 45-day review of NDAs for the RTF process.[4] The NDA sections reviewed for filability are: Biopharmaceutical, Clinical, Manufacturing and Controls, Microbiology, Pharmacology, and Project Management.

The specific items listed under Pharmacology (Toxicology is included in this section) are:

1. On its face, is the pharmacology section of the NDA organized in a manner to allow substantive review to begin?
2. Is the pharmacology section of the NDA indexed and paginated in a manner to allow substantive review to begin?
3. On its face, is the pharmacology section of the NDA legible so that substantive review can begin?
4. Are all required(*) and requested IND studies completed and submitted in this NDA (carcinogenicity, mutagenicity, teratogenicity,* effects on fertility,* juvenile studies, acute adult studies,* chronic adult studies,* maximum tolerated dosage determination, dermal irritancy, ocular irritancy, photocarcinogenicity, animal pharmacokinetic studies, etc.).
5. If the formulation to be marketed is different from the formulation used in the toxicology studies, has the sponsor made an appropriate effort to either repeat the studies using the marketed product or to explain why such repetition should not be required?
6. Are the proposed labeling sections relative to pharmacology appropriate (including human dose multiples expressed in either mg/m^2 or comparative serum/plasma levels) and in accordance with 201.57?
7. Has the sponsor submitted all special studies/data requested by the division during presubmission discussions with the sponsor?
8. On its face, does the route of administration used in the animal studies appear to be the same as the intended human exposure route? If not, has the sponsor submitted a rationale to justify the alternative route?
9. Has the sponsor submitted a statement(s) that all of the pivotal pharmacology/toxicology studies have been performed in accordance with the GLP regulations (21 CFR 58) or an explanation for any significant deviations?
10. Has the sponsor submitted a statement(s) that the pharmacology/toxicology studies have been performed using acceptable, state-of-the-art protocols which also reflect agency animal welfare concerns?

SECTION 4. FDA USER FEE PROGRAM

The passage of the Prescription Drug User Fee Act of 1992 had a significant impact on the drug development process in the pharmaceutical industry and has resulted in a shortening of the average review time. The intent of the program was to provide additional resources to FDA with the aim of expediting the review of submissions, e.g., NDAs, PLAs, etc.

Benefits to the consumer include the availability of new drugs more quickly while benefits to the pharmaceutical industry include faster and more predictable reviews, well-defined expectations, and conservation of resources. The program was expected to be re-evaluated after several years and adjusted as appropriate.

Based on projected resource needs at FDA for the period 1993–1997, three types of user fees (application fees, establishment fees, and product fees) were established along with an escalating fee schedule for each type of user fee.

Application fees for new NDAs and PLAs/ELAs increased from $100,000 to $233,000 from 1993 to 1997, with the fee for supplements/amendments increasing from $50,000 to $116,000. At the time of the filing, 50% of the application fee is paid; the remaining 50% is paid when the FDA issues an action letter (i.e., a list of actions necessary to place the application in condition for approval). If there is a refusal-to-file action, 50% of the initial payment is refunded.

The user fees can be waived or reduced under certain conditions, e.g., if necessary to protect the public health or if the fee presents a significant barrier to innovation (orphan drugs), ANDAs. The increased resources generated by this program are focused on three key areas at FDA: 1) increase in headcount; 2) information systems (CANDAs); and 3) project management.

Performance goals and standards were also established by FDA to ensure that the additional resources produced measurable results. FDA's 5-year goals were to reach action (i.e., issue an "action letter" as described above) on priority NDAs and PLAs within 6 months, standard NDAs and PLAs within 12 months, and priority supplements within 6 months. The action letter was expected to completely delineate any additional work or information needed to secure approval. Moreover, the resubmitted "complete" application was to be acted on by FDA within 6 months.

The user fee program and associated performance goals by FDA have resulted in the following changes.

A. PRESUBMISSION

- Applications must be *complete* and *organized:* increased emphasis on the quality of the initial filing to avoid additional user fees and to benefit from increased opportunities for expedited review.
- Issues must be identified *prior* to the submission and discussed with reviewers so that these issues are handled appropriately in the submission.
- Increased emphasis on "reviewability."
- Inappropriate "bundling" of products in one application are no longer accepted.

As part of this initiative, there has been increased emphasis on end-of-Phase II meetings and pre- NDA meetings as FDA seeks to increase its partnership with industry in the clinical development process. Likewise, advisory committee meetings/input are expected to occur not only after Phase III but at the end of Phase II as part of the planning process for Phase III programs.

B. POSTSUBMISSION

The most significant change postsubmission was FDA's elimination of the large number of industry-initiated amendments (not including required items such as the 4-month safety update). There are now strict limitations on any amendments containing substantive new information requiring additional FDA review and evaluation. Sponsors have also been pushed to reduce the time for responses to FDA questions and to advise reviewers of the projected time frames for submitting these responses.

From an industry perspective, the changes have been beneficial because they link both FDA and the industry to a *predictable* time frame for action. Moreover, if the application is not approvable in its initial form, sponsors will receive a complete list of actions required for it to be approvable and can expect a 6-month review of the resubmitted application.

SECTION 5. FDA PREGNANCY CATEGORIES

FDA has assigned "Pregnancy Categories" to approved drugs based on potential to produce reproductive toxicity. These categories can be omitted from drug labeling only if the drug is not absorbed systematically and the drug is known not to have a potential for indirect harm to the fetus. These categories are used in drug product labeling and are:

A. Pregnancy Category A

If adequate and well-controlled studies in pregnant women have failed to demonstrate a risk to the fetus in the first trimester of pregnancy (and there is no evidence of a risk in later trimesters), the labeling shall state:

Pregnancy Category A. Studies in pregnant women have not shown that (name of drug) increases the risk of fetal abnormalities if administered during the first (second, third, or all) trimester(s) of pregnancy. If this drug is used during pregnancy, the possibility of fetal harm appears remote. Because studies cannot rule out the possibility of harm, however, (name of drug) should be used during pregnancy only if clearly needed.

The labeling shall also contain a description of the human studies. If animal reproduction studies are available and they fail to demonstrate a risk to the fetus, the labeling shall also state: "Reproduction studies have been performed [kinds of animal(s)] at doses up to (×) times the human dose and have revealed no evidence of impaired fertility or harm to the fetus due to (name of drug)." The labeling shall also contain a description of available data on the effect of the drug on the later growth, development, and functional maturation of the child.

B. Pregnancy Category B

If animal reproduction studies have failed to demonstrate a risk to the fetus and there are no adequate and well-controlled studies in pregnant women, the labeling shall state:

Pregnancy Category B. Reproduction studies have been performed in [kind(s) of animal(s)] at doses up to (×) times the human dose and have revealed no evidence of impaired fertility or harm to the fetus due to (name of drug). There are, however, no adequate and well-controlled studies in pregnant women. Because animal reproduction studies are not always predictive of human response, this drug should be used during pregnancy only if clearly needed.

If animal reproduction studies have shown an adverse effect (other than decrease in fertility), but adequate and well-controlled studies in pregnant women have failed to demonstrate a risk to the fetus during the first trimester of pregnancy (and there is no evidence of a risk in later trimesters), the labeling shall state:

Pregnancy Category B. Reproduction studies in [kind(s) of animals(s)] have shown (describe findings) at (×) times the human dose. Studies in pregnant women, however, have not shown that (name of drug) increases the risk of abnormalities when administered during the first (second, third, or all) trimester(s) of pregnancy. Despite the animal findings, it would appear that the possibility of fetal harm is remote, if the drug is used during pregnancy. Nevertheless, because the studies in humans cannot rule out the possibility of harm, (name of drug) should be used during pregnancy only if clearly needed.

The labeling shall also contain a description of the human studies and a description of available data on the effect of the drug on the later growth, development, and functional maturation of the child.

C. PREGNANCY CATEGORY C

If animal reproduction studies have shown an adverse effect on the fetus, if there are no adequate and well-controlled studies in humans, and if the benefits from the use of the drug in pregnant women may be acceptable despite its potential risks, the labeling shall state:

Pregnancy Category C. (Name of drug) has been shown to be teratogenic (or to have an embryocidal effect or other adverse effect) in [name(s) of species] when given in doses (×) times the human dose. There are no adequate and well-controlled studies in pregnant women. (Name of drug) should be used during pregnancy only if the potential benefit justifies the potential risk to the fetus.

The labeling shall contain a description of the animal studies. If there are no animal reproduction studies and no adequate and well-controlled studies in humans, the labeling shall state:

Pregnancy Category C. Animal reproduction studies have not been conducted with (name of drug). It is also not known whether (name of drug) can cause fetal harm when administered to a pregnant woman or can affect reproduction capacity. (Name of drug) should be given to a pregnant woman only if clearly needed.

The labeling shall contain a description of any available data on the effect of the drug on the later growth, development, and functional maturation of the child.

D. PREGNANCY CATEGORY D

If there is positive evidence of human fetal risk based on adverse reaction data from investigational or marketing experience or studies in humans, but the potential benefits from the use of the drug in pregnant women may be acceptable despite its potential risks (for example, if the drug is needed in a life-threatening situation or serious disease for which safer drugs cannot be used or are ineffective), the labeling shall state:

"Pregnancy Category D. See 'Warnings' section." Under the "Warnings" section, the labeling states: (Name of drug) can cause fetal harm when administered to a pregnant woman. (Describe the human data and any pertinent animal data.) If this drug is used during pregnancy, or if the patient becomes pregnant while taking this drug, the patient should be apprised of the potential hazard to the fetus.

E. PREGNANCY CATEGORY X

If studies in animals or humans have demonstrated fetal abnormalities or if there is positive evidence of fetal risk based on adverse reaction reports from investigational or marketing experience, or both, and the risk of the use of the drug in a pregnant woman clearly outweighs any possible benefit (for example, safer drugs or other forms of therapy are available), the labeling shall state:

"Pregnancy Category X. See 'Contraindications' section." Under "Contraindications," the labeling shall state: (Name of drug) may (can) cause fetal harm when administered to a pregnant woman. (Describe the human data and any pertinent animal data.) (Name of drug) is contraindicated in women who are or may become pregnant. If this drug is used during pregnancy, or if the patient becomes pregnant while taking this drug, the patient should be apprised of the potential hazard to the fetus.

F. NONTERATOGENIC EFFECTS

Under this heading the labeling shall contain other information on the drug's effects on reproduction and the drug's use during pregnancy that is not required specifically by one of the pregnancy categories, if the information is relevant to the safe and effective use of the drug. Information required under this heading shall include nonteratogenic effects in the fetus or newborn infant (for example, withdrawal symptoms or hypoglycemia) that may occur because of a pregnant woman's chronic use of the drug for a preexisting condition or disease.

SECTION 6. SYNOPSIS OF GENERAL FDA GUIDELINES FOR ANIMAL TOXICITY TESTING STUDIES

Acceptance of the IND submission by FDA allows a sponsor to initiate clinical studies divided into three phases. Phase I clinical studies are usually conducted in a small number normal subjects (20–80). Women of childbearing potential are normally excluded because preclinical reproductive toxicity studies have not been conducted at this stage of drug development. This practice is now a topic of debate both within the industry and the Agency. The purpose of Phase I studies is to determine safety in humans, define the ADME characteristics of drug, to approximate the clinical dose, and to define the preferred route of administration. To conduct Phase I studies, acute, subchronic, and possibly specialty preclinical studies are required. Favorable results in Phase I clinical studies warrants conducting additional preclinical studies, e.g., chronic, carcinogenicity, and teratology.

Phase II clinical studies are conducted in patients with disease (approximately 200–300) and are carefully controlled. Additional pharmacology, safety, efficacy, and dosing information is gathered.

Phase III clinical studies are large clinical trials whose objective is to prove statistical efficacy, safety, and the most desirable dosage regimen. Phase III studies are designed to support product approval.

A variety of preclinical safety (toxicity) studies are conducted during the course of the Phase I, II, and III clinical trials which can occur over a period of 3 to 7 years. The purpose of animal safety studies is not so much to directly extrapolate animal data to human, as to use animal models to characterize potentially adverse physiological changes that might be expected to occur in a biological system in response to the administration of a particular drug. The basic type of toxicity studies are:

Acute: 2 species* (few days duration)
Subchronic: 2 species* (2 weeks to 6 months)

Chronic: 2 species* (12 to 18 months)
* The two species are usually one rodent (typically rat) and one nonrodent (dog or primate)
Carcinogenicity: 2 rodents (18 months to 2 + years)
Reproductive Toxicity
    Segment I: rats
    Segment II: rats, rabbits
    Segment III: rats
Specialty studies (mutagenicity, antigenicity, dermal/ocular irritation, mucosal irritation, etc.,
    depending on drug type and clinical usage)

The duration of animal studies depends on the duration of clinical usage (Table 28.1).

TABLE 28.1
Duration of Animal Studies Based on Duration of Clinical Use

Duration of Clinical Usage	Animal Studies
Several days	2 weeks; 2 species
1 month	3 months; 2 species
3 months	6 months; 2 species
> 3 months	6 months; rodent
	12 months; nonrodent
	Rat and mouse 24-month carcinogenicity

The following is a brief summary of the Segment reproductive toxicology studies. Refer to Chapters 11 and 12 for additional information.

1. **Segment I: Reproductive and Fertility Studies in Rats**

    • All reproductive parameters from exposure of gametes to F_2 generation
    • Dosing: males and females before mating; females through end of lactation

2. **Segment II: Teratology**

    • Pregnant females dosed during period of organogenesis
    • Rats: Gestational days 6–15 of 21
    • Rabbits: Gestational days 6–18 of 31
    • Evaluate the teratogenic effects on soft tissue and skeletal tissues of fetus

3. **Segment III: Peri-Postnatal**

    • Pregnant females dosed on gestational days 15 through postpartum day 21
    • Examines late gestational, parturition, and lactation effects

SECTION 7. SUBSTANCES GENERALLY RECOGNIZED AS SAFE

TABLE 28.2
Substances Generally Recognized as Safe (GRAS)[6]

Multiple Purpose GRAS Food Substances	Dietary Supplements (Con't)	Chemical Preservatives (Con't)
Citric acid	Magnesium oxide	Potassium bisulfite
Glutamic acid	Magnesium phosphate	Potassium metabisulfite
Glutamic acid hydrochloride	Magnesium sulfate	Potassium sorbate
Hydrochloric acid	Magnesium chloride	Sodium ascorbate
Phosphoric acid	Manganese citrate	Sodium bisulfite
Sodium acid pyrophosphate	Manganese gluconate	Sodium metabisulfite
Aluminum sulfate	Manganese glycerophosphate	Sodium sorbate
Aluminum ammonium sulfate		Sodium sulfite
Aluminum potassium sulfate	**Sequestrants**	Sulfur dioxide
Aluminum sodium sulfate	Citric acid	Tocopherols
Caffeine	Sodium acid phosphate	
Calcium citrate	Calcium citrate	**Dietary Supplements**
Calcium phosphate	Calcium diacetate	Manganese sulfate
Caramel	Calcium hexametaphosphate	Manganous oxide
Glycerin	Monobasic calcium phosphate	Niacin
Methylcellulose	Dipotassium phosphate	Niacinamide
Monoammonium glutamate	Disodium phosphate	D-Pantothenyl alcohol
Monopotassium glutamate	Isopropyl citrate	Potassium chloride
Potassium citrate	Monoisopropy citrate	Potassium glycerophosphate
Silica aerogel	Potassium citrate	Pyridoxine hydrochloride
Sodium carboxymethylcellulose	Sodium citrate	Riboflavin
Sodium caseinate	Sodium gluconate	Riboflavin-5-phosphate
Sodium citrate	Sodium hexametaphosphate	Sodium pantothenate
Sodium phosphate	Sodium metaphosphate	Sodium phosphate
Sodium aluminum phosphate	Sodium phosphate	Thiamine hydrochloride
Sodium tripolyphosphate	Sodium pyrophosphate	Thiamine mononitrate
High fructose corn syrup	Tetra sodium pyrophosphate	Tocopherols
Triethyl citrate	Sodium tripolyphosphate	α–Tocopherol acetate
	Stearyl citrate	Vitamin A
Dietary Supplements		Vitamin A acetate
Ascorbic acid	**Stabilizers**	Vitamin A, palmitate
Linoleic acid	Chondrus extract	Vitamin B_{12}
Biotin		Vitamin D_2
Calcium carbonate	**Anticaking Agents**	Vitamin D_3
Calcium citrate	Aluminum calcium silicate	Zinc chloride
Calcium glycerophosphate	Calcium silicate	Zinc gluconate
Calcium oxide	Magnesium silicate	Zinc oxide
Calcium pantothenate	Sodium aluminosilicate	Zinc stearate
Calcium phosphate	Sodium calcium aluminosilicate	Zinc sulfate
Calcium pyrophosphate	hydrated	
Carotene	Tricalcium silicate	**Nutrients**
Choline bitartrate		Ascorbic acid
Choline chloride	**Chemical Preservatives**	Biotin
Copper gluconate	Ascorbic acid	Calcium citrate
Ferric phosphate	Erythorbic acid	Calcium phosphate
Ferric pyrophosphate	Sorbic acid	Calcium pyrophosphate
Ferric sodium pyrophosphate	Thiodipropionic acid	Choline bitartrate
Ferrous gluconate	Ascorbyl palmitate	Choline chloride
Ferrous lactate	Butylated hydroxyanisole	Manganese hypophosphite
Ferrous sulfate	Butylated hydroxytoluene	Sodium phosphate
Inositol	Calcium ascorbate	Tocopherols
Iron reduced	Calcium sorbate	α-Tocopherol acetate
	Dilauryl thiodipropionate	Zinc chloride

Source: Section 21, CFR PART 182.

SECTION 8. GLOSSARY

ADME Absorption, Distribution, Metabolism and Excretion

ANDA Abbreviated New Drug Company

CANDA Computer-Assisted New Drug Application

CBER FDA's Center for Biologics Evalution and Research: division charged regulating biological products

CDER FDA's Center for Drug Evaluation and Research: division charged with developing and enforcing policy with regard to the safety, effectiveness, and labeling of all drug products for human use

ELA Establishment License Application for a biologic

FDA Food and Drug Administration: federal agency charged with issuing regulations on safety of foods, drugs, and cosmetics in United States

IND Investigational New Drug Application: a request to initiate clinical study of a new drug product

NDA New Drug Application: a request for approval to market new drugs

PLA Product License Application for a biologic

REFERENCES

1. U.S. Government Manual, 1992/1993 Office of the Federal Register, National Archive and Records Administration.
2. Food and Drug Administration, *Guideline for the Format and Content of the Nonclinical Pharmacology/Toxicology Section of an Application,* Center for Drugs and Biologics, Department of Health and Human Services.
3. Food and Drug Administration, *New Drug Evaluation Guidance Document,* refusal to file, July 12, 1993.
4. Lumpkin, M. M., 45-day worksheets, participants at the commissioner's industry exchange meeting, Philadelphia, PA, May 28, 1992.
5. 21 CFR Ch. 1 (4-1-87 Edition) 201.57.
6. 21 CFR Part 182, Substance Generally Recognized as Safe, Ch. 1 (4-1-92 Edition) 181.33.

29 Regulatory Toxicology: Medical Devices

Steven J. Hermansky, Pharm.D., Ph.D., D.A.B.T.

CONTENTS

0-8493-0370-2/02/$0.00+$1.50
© 2002 by CRC Press LLC

SECTION 1. INTRODUCTION

Although the use of medical devices has a long history, modern medical use of devices only became realistic as an effective therapeutic intervention as the use of aseptic techniques expanded in the late 1800s. The first devices were, of course, fashioned from materials found in nature. Often, materials were obtained from domesticated animals. For example, leather was sculptured to form replacements for lost ears and noses and goose trachea was used as tubing in the measurement of arterial pressure. In all cases, key to the search for successful device materials was identifying materials with appropriate mechanical properties while minimizing the potential for adverse biological reactions.

Although tissues obtained from domestic animals continue to be used for medical devices, material science has continued to develop and now includes many forms of metal, ceramic, plastics, and other synthetic polymers. The role of toxicology in medical device development is to ensure that the materials selected for use in devices are safe for their intended use. As in all disciplines of toxicology, the safety tests used to evaluate a device material must be appropriate to the route and duration of exposure. This chapter provides information, related to both testing and regulatory strategies, intended to be beneficial to the medical device researcher.

Even though the difference between a medical device and a drug may seem obvious, the clarity of the distinction is becoming blurred as therapeutic interventions become more complex and disease specific. The difference between a drug and a device can generally be summarized by the simple observation that a drug is independent of its physical form as long as the physical form allows for systemic absorption of the active drug. However, a medical device is generally dependent upon its physical form to exert its therapeutic (biologic) effect. There are multiple examples of therapeutic medicaments that are not easily classified as either a drug or a device based upon their mechanism of action and intended therapeutic effect. The specific issues associated with the categorization of a treatment modality as either a device or drug is beyond the scope of this chapter.

This chapter is divided into six sections including this introduction. The second section presents a historical perspective to medical device testing. The history of medical device toxicology continues to be important to the researcher since regulatory guidelines are continuing to evolve in this rapidly developing field. Furthermore, the "history" of this area of toxicology is recent memory to many researchers, and historical terminology is important in many current discussions. The third section focuses on the varied and often confusing regulatory arena for medical devices. The development of the European Community and publication of the International Standards Organisation (ISO) guideline documents have had significant impact on the medical device manufacturer. The regulatory arena continues to evolve and the information in this chapter presents a snapshot of the landscape. The fourth section attempts to provide the researcher with some basic references necessary to understand the rationale behind the selection of toxicity tests for any given material or medical device. The fifth section provides some basic information relevant to the nuances of testing solid materials and devices using models originally designed to evaluate the potential toxicity of soluble or semisoluble chemicals and drugs. The standard models have, therefore, been modified to provide information useful to the process of assessing the potential risk associated with materials/medical devices, and this section attempts to provide some information associated with the nature of the modifications. The sixth and final section provides some basic definitions for terms frequently used in the evaluation of the safety of medical devices.

SECTION 2. HISTORICAL PERSPECTIVE

Because of the difficulties encountered when attempting to evaluate the safety of a solid test article, a historical description of the development of medical devices is considered useful to anyone evaluating medical devices for safety. The inherent safety of "natural" materials was often assumed. This, of course, was not always supported under use conditions.

Synthetic materials originally selected for medical use were chosen primarily for their physical attributes. These were materials first created for military, commercial, or industrial purposes. Since these materials were essentially considered to be inert and stable in the biological environment, the safety of medical device materials initially focused on sterility. However, as the developing device industry evolved and the devices were intended to treat increasingly complex conditions, materials were increasingly scrutinized for appropriateness for use in the biological environment.

As researchers examined the biological effects of medical device materials, whether synthetic or natural, under use conditions, adverse events were increasingly noted.[1] Therefore, a need for methods to determine the safety of materials was recognized by both the medical device industry and regulatory agencies, and the focus of medical device material identification shifted from purely performance to a combination of performance and safety. To that end, the industry became aware that a procedure was necessary for predicting which materials could be used safely.[2]

Since plastics were already a common material used in many varied devices, a set of tests designed by the U.S. Pharmacopoeia (USP) for classifying plastics using a series of biological tests was selected as a guidance.[3] In this classification system, the proposed end use of the plastic, including the nature and extent of expected biological interaction, as well as possible solutions (e.g., drug vehicles) that may contact the plastic, is used as a guide to determine for which class the plastic should be qualified. Then, to determine whether the plastic is suitable for that class, a series of biological reactivity tests must be conducted. Representative samples of the plastic are used for the biological reactivity testing using specific methods prescribed by the USP. If the results of the tests are acceptable, as defined by the USP, for all the tests in the selected class, the plastic is considered to have met the requirements for that class (Table 29.1 presents a summary of the tests to be successfully conducted for each class). It is important to note that the class into which a plastic is placed is not related to its physical form or chemistry but is defined by the tests conducted and successfully completed.

Although the classification of plastics by the USP methods are not generally considered to address adequately the safety of medical devices, a knowledge of the classes is important for the material researcher since some plastic raw materials may be identified using a plastic classification. This classification may therefore provide the researcher with a baseline indication of the appropriateness of the raw material for possible use in a device. It is important to note that the plastic class does not indicate safety of the plastic raw material in the final device and it is the responsibility of the device manufacturer to substantiate safety of the final device utilizing appropriate test methods. To that end, in 1976, the U.S. Congress passed the Medical Device Amendments to the Food, Drug, and Cosmetic Act. Critical wording of this Act necessitated an emphasis on the nature of the end use of a medical device in the assessment of safety parameters. Furthermore, the focus of safety testing was the final device, as intended for use, rather than individual raw materials to be used in the device.

In part to address the requirements of this Act, the U.S. Food and Drug Administration (FDA), in collaboration with Canada and Great Britain, drafted a guidance document in 1987 for medical devices, known as the Tripartite Agreement. This agreement utilized a matrix approach of intimacy and duration of tissue contact to categorize a medical device based upon its intended use. This assumed that more critical medical devices (that is, those implanted into the body, life supporting, and/or life sustaining) would, by definition, have a greater intimacy of tissue contact and a longer duration of that contact.[4] Based upon the category determined by the parameters of the Tripartite matrix, the necessary safety evaluations that had to be successfully completed before the device could be marketed were identified.

The intended use of a device, specifically, the intimacy of tissue contact combined with the duration of this contact, as initially defined by the Tripartite Agreement would dominate the selection of safety tests for a specific device both then and now. However, other criteria for categorization of medical devices have been recognized, including whether the device has direct or indirect contact with biological tissues (see below), and today considerations for medical device testing may include

TABLE 29.1
Classification of Plastics[a]

Class I
- *Saline extract* of sample evaluated using the systemic injection and intracutaneous reactivity tests

Class II
- *Saline extract* of sample evaluated using the systemic injection and intracutaneous reactivity tests
- *Ethyl alcohol in saline (5% v/v) extract* evaluated using the systemic injection and intracutaneous reactivity tests

Class III
- *Saline extract* of sample evaluated using the systemic injection and intracutaneous reactivity tests
- *Ethyl alcohol in saline (5% v/v) extract* evaluated using the systemic injection and intracutaneous reactivity tests
- *PEG 400 extract of sample* evaluated using the systemic injection test (ip)
- *Vegetable oil extract of sample* evaluated using the systemic injection test (ip)

Class IV
- *Saline extract* of sample evaluated using the systemic injection and intracutaneous reactivity tests
- *Ethyl alcohol in saline (5% v/v) extract* evaluated using the systemic injection and intracutaneous reactivity tests
- *Vegetable oil extract of sample* evaluated using the systemic injection (ip) and intracutaneous reactivity tests
- *Sample (not extract)* implanted into the muscle of an animal and evaluated for macroscopically visible signs of inflammation

Class V
- *Saline extract* of sample evaluated using the systemic injection and intracutaneous reactivity tests
- *Ethyl alcohol in saline (5% v/v) extract* evaluated using the systemic injection and intracutaneous reactivity tests
- *PEG 400 extract of sample* evaluated using the systemic injection (ip) and intracutaneous reactivity tests
- *Vegetable oil extract of sample* evaluated using the systemic injection (ip) and intracutaneous reactivity tests

Class VI
- *Saline extract* of sample evaluated using the systemic injection and intracutaneous reactivity tests
- *Ethyl alcohol in saline (5% v/v) extract* evaluated using the systemic injection and intracutaneous reactivity tests
- *PEG 400 extract of sample* evaluated using the systemic injection (ip) and intracutaneous reactivity tests
- *Vegetable oil extract of sample* evaluated using the systemic injection (ip) and intracutaneous reactivity tests
- *Sample (not extract)* implanted into the muscle of an animal and evaluated for macroscopically visible signs of inflammation

[a] If a plastic raw material is considered to meet the requirements of one of these classes, testing of a representative sample of that plastic would have met the acceptable standards for all of the very specific, biological reactivity tests listed below that class. See the USP, 1994, for the specific testing parameters and criteria for meeting the individual test procedures.

Notes: All systemic tests are dosed by the intravenous route of administration unless noted in the table as being dosed by the intraperitoneal (ip) route of administration. PEG 400 = polyethylene glycol 400, which may be diluted with saline prior to conducting the biological assay.

Source: USP.[8]

inductive and inflammatory responses, general toxicity, specific organ toxicity, immunotoxicity, reproductive toxicity, genetic toxicity, and carcinogenicity.

The Tripartite Agreement has recently been replaced by a more international series of guidance documents that continue to be prepared and refined. The ISO has led the current efforts to establish a series of international medical device guidelines. The ISO guidance documents maintained the matrix approach of the Tripartite Agreement and proposed a guidance document in 1992. The focal point of the guidance was ISO 10993-1: Biological Evaluation of Medical Devices — Part 1: Guidance on Selection of Tests. Additional supporting documents have been and continue to be developed. The title of other parts of the ISO 10993 guidance are shown in Table 29.2 although not all guidance documents are finalized. The ISO 10993 guidance documents have become the standard for manufacturers desiring to market medical devices in Europe, Japan, and the United States. The ISO 10993 series of documents were formally adopted by the FDA, with modification,

TABLE 29.2
ISO 10993 — Biological Evaluation of Medical Devices

Part	Title
1	Guidance on selection of tests
2	Animal welfare requirements
3	Tests for genotoxiciity, carcinogenicity, and reproductive toxicity
4	Selection of tests for interaction with blood
5	Tests for cytotoxicity: *in vitro* methods
6	Tests for local effects after implantation
7	Ethylene oxide sterilization residuals
8	Clinical investigation
9	Degradation of materials related to biological testing
10	Tests for irritation and sensitization
11	Tests for systemic toxicity
12	Sample preparation and reference materials
13	Identification and quantification of degredation products from polymers
14	Identification and quantification of degredation products from ceramics
15	Identification and quantification of degredation products from metals and alloys
16	General guidance on toxicokinetic study design for degradation products and leachables
17	Establishment of allowable limits for leachable substance
18	Chemical characterization of materials
ISO/DIS 14155	Clinical investigation of medical devices
ISO/DIS 12891	Implants for surgery — retrieval and analysis of surgical implants

in 1995. Therefore, the ISO guidance documents will be the focus of information presented in this chapter. However, the ISO 10993 guidance documents are dynamic and the reader is encouraged to ensure that the most up-to-date information is available before initiating any testing.

SECTION 3. REGULATION OF MEDICAL DEVICES

A. UNITED STATES

There are several methods of classification of devices in the United States. The method used will depend upon the specific use for the device and, importantly, by whom and how the device is intended to be used. The FDA has established specific classifications for nearly 2000 different generic classes of devices. These different types of devices are further grouped into 16 "panels" based upon medical specialties. The 16 panels and some representative classes of devices are presented in Table 29.3. The panels and generic class description (name) of the device helps the manufacturer to identify whether its proposed device has already been assessed and placed into a generic classification by the FDA. The FDA has further assigned each of these generic classes of devices to one of three regulatory classes. The assignment of a regulatory class is based upon the level of control the FDA considers to be necessary to ensure the safety and effectiveness of the device when manufactured and marketed as intended. The three FDA regulatory classes and requirements that apply to each, along with some examples, are shown in Table 29.4.

To market a device in the United States, the manufacturer must determine whether a regulatory submission is necessary. Generally, a submission to FDA will be necessary to market a medical device in the United States unless the FDA has published a notice indicating that this generic class of device is exempt from the premarket notification procedure. Devices exempted by FDA for submission are generally Class I devices for which the FDA considers general manufacturing controls to be sufficient to ensure the safety and efficacy of the device for the patient and/or user.

When it has been determined that a submission to FDA is necessary prior to marketing a device in the United States, the manufacturer must then determine the type of submission. In the United States, the two forms of submission are the premarket notification, or 510(k), and the premarket approval, or PMA. Most devices on the market in the United States are Class II and, therefore, most devices are cleared for commercial distribution in the United States by the 510(k) process. Most class I devices are exempt from the need for a regulatory submission and most class III devices require a premarket approval application (see below) prior to marketing in the United States. Although it is beyond the scope of this chapter to describe the specific issues associated with these submissions, a brief description of each is provided.

Areas that generally must be addressed in a regulatory submission required for either the 510(k) or PMA are shown in Table 29.5. Preferred organization of the data for a regulatory submission in the United States is shown in Table 29.6.

The 510(k) is a submission to the FDA demonstrating that the proposed noncritical and non-exempt device (generally Class II) is as safe and as effective (that is, substantially equivalent) to a legally marketed device that was or is currently on the U.S. market. Therefore, an important aspect of the 510(k) process is identification of the previously marketed, substantially equivalent device for use in comparison with the proposed device. Substantial equivalence of the marketed and proposed device is established based upon a number of factors, but the two devices do not have to be identical. The need for toxicological/safety testing will be, at least partially, based on the similarity of the two devices including materials and manufacturing practices. Clearly, the manufacturer must provide, at the least, adequate safety information on any new materials in the new device.

The PMA process is used by the FDA to evaluate the safety and effectiveness of noncritical and nonexempt devices (usually Class II) for which a currently marketed, substantially equivalent device cannot be identified as well as most critical devices (Class III). Because of the level of risk associated with the use of critical devices, the FDA determines that these devices require a rigorous regulatory submission prior to marketing. To substantiate safety and efficacy, the PMA process requires more information than is presented during a comparison to a preexisting device. Therefore, each critical device marketed in the United States must be individually shown to be safe and effective.

TABLE 29.3
FDA Panels of Devices with Example Devices

Clinical chemistry and clinical toxicology devices
  Urinary pH (nonquantitative) test system
  Blood specimen collection device
  High-pressure liquid chromatography system for clinical use
  Pipetting and diluting system for clinical use
  Breath alcohol test system
  Codeine test system
Hematology and pathology devices
  Cytocentrifuge
  Occult blood test
  Prothrombin time test
  Automated slide stainer
Immunology and microbiology device
  Automated colon counter
  Enriched culture medium
Anesthesiology devices
  Pressure regulator
  Emergency airway needle
  Oxygen mask
  Ventilator tubing
Cardiovascular devices
  Blood pressure alarm
  Blood pressure cuff
  Stethoscope
  Ear oximeter
  Pacemaker lead adapter
  Vascular clamp
  Defibrillator (including paddles)
Dental devices
  Caries detection device
  Resin applicator
  Preformed plastic denture tooth
  Root canal post
  Dental injecting needle
  Dental floss
  Manual toothbrush
Ear, nose, and throat devices
  Hearing aid
  Ossicular replacement device
  Tympanostomy tube
  Otoscope
  External nasal splint

Gastroenterology–urology devices
  Stomach pH electrode
  Hemorrhoidal ligator
  Ostomy pouch and accessories
General and plastic surgery devices
  Chin prosthesis
  Occlusive wound dressing
  Surgeon's glove
  Skin marker
  Sutures
General hospital and personal use device
  Patient scale
  Elastic bandage
  Suction snakebite kit
  Tongue depressor
Neurological devices
  Cutaneous electrode
  Neurosurgical headrest
  Aneurysm clip
  Implanted neuromuscular stimulator
Obstetrical and gynecological devices
  Endometrial brush
  Fetal blood sampler
  Obstetric forceps
  Condom
  Menstrual tampon
Ophthalmic devices
  Visual acuity chart
  Ophthalmoscope
  Artificial eye
  Contact lens and solutions
Orthopedic devices
  Joint prosthesis (many)
  Cast components
Physical medicine devices
  Cane
  Mechanical chair
  Arm sling
  Hot or cold disposable pack
Radiology devices
  Bone densitometer
  Ultrasonic pulsed doppler imaging system

TABLE 29.4
Three Regulatory Classes

Class I. General Controls (with or without exemptions)
    Least perceived risk to device user and/or patient
        Stethoscope
        Canes and crutches
Class II. General Controls and Performance Standards (with or without exemptions)
        Mercury thermometer
        Condom
        Blood pressure cuff
Class III. General Controls and Premarket Approval
    Most perceived risk to device user and/or patient
        Pacemaker
        Implanted neuromuscular stimulator
        Replacement heart valve

TABLE 29.5
Areas to be Addressed in a Regulatory Submission to the FDA

Intended use
Indications for use
Target population
Design
Materials
Performance
Sterility
Biocompatibility
Mechanical safety
Chemical safety
Anatomical sites
Human factors
Energy used and/or delivered
Compatibility with the environment and other devices
Where used
Standards met
Electrical safety
Thermal safety
Radiation safety

For 510(k): To market a noncritical and nonexempt device (generally Class II)

Selection of predicate device that is as safe and as effective (that is, substantially equivalent) to a legally marketed device that was or is currently on the U.S. market

TABLE 29.6
Presentation of Data for Regulatory Submission to the FDA

To facilitate FDA review of the data, analysis, and conclusions in the application, the manufacturer and contract laboratory, if used, should check the following:

- Logical presentation of the biocompatibility data
- Scientific soundness of the test method and data analysis
- Relevance of the test program to the device and the intended use
- Completeness of the summary report of the tests or studies

The summary of test results should be presented in a table format in each report whenever possible. Each study or test attachment report should contain sufficient and well-organized information in reasonable detail so that the FDA reviewer can determine:

- What exact material or device was tested
- What tests were performed
- How the tests were performed
- What the test results were

A description of the tests and the results obtained are essential; and reasonable and sufficient details of all test procedures and results should be submitted to the FDA. For biocompatibility studies, manufacturers should use a standard scoring system for each test method, if a standard scoring system exists. Each test report should include the following:

- Name and address of the manufacturer of the item tested
- Name and technical description of the item tested
- Name and address of the laboratory where the tests were conducted
- Test methods including the scoring method
- Number of samples and replicates tested
- Any control data needed to establish the validity of the test
- The date when the tests were conducted
- Summary report(s) of results obtained
- Analysis, interpretation of results, and conclusions

B. EUROPE

In Europe, the 15 original member states (along with several more recently added member states) of the European Community have authored, reviewed, and accepted a common method by which manufacturers must evaluate and qualify their proposed devices prior to marketing. The Active Implantable Medical Device Directive and the Medical Device Directive define the legal framework accepted by the member states through which medical devices are regulated (see Table 29.7 for the components of this basic framework). Through the directives and system of Notified and Competent Bodies, many devices must meet essential requirements prior to being marketed. As in the United States, devices must be evaluated for safety and efficacy to ensure that they do not harm the patient, clinician, or any third party. Also similar to the United States, there is a system of classification determined by the Medical Device Directives as shown, with examples, in Table 29.8.

For most medical devices, the independent Notified Body often signifies that the device may be marketed in the European Community by granting the manufacturer the right to label the product or its packaging with a "CE marking," which signifies that the manufacturer has adequately proved the safety and efficacy of the proposed device. In theory, a CE marking obtained through a Notified Body appointed by the government agency of one of the member states gives the manufacturer the right to market the subject device in any one of the member states. However, any of the individual member states may, at any time, implement a safeguard clause and require additional testing to evaluate the device further to ensure that the CE marking was not incorrectly granted.

TABLE 29.7
Hierarchy of European Regulation of Medical Devices

European Commission
  Multicountry body consisting of weighted membership from member countries
CEN/CENELEC
  Committees for European Standards
  (CEN: European Committee for Standardization)
  (CENELEC: European Committee for Electrotechnical Standardization)
Competent Authorities
  Government agency that approves and monitors Notified Bodies
  Coordinates complaint management and device noncompliance issues
  Qualified to issue the final assessment certificate once an adequate technical file has been submitted and reviewed
Accreditation Bodies
  Agency/group that works with Notified Bodies to provide assurance ("accreditation") to further ensure testing standards
    have been met
  Review quality systems
Notified Bodies
  Address quality systems and may perform some testing; must be "notified" for each product line for which they are
    responsible
  The Notified Bodies must remain a legally separate entity from manufacturers
Manufacturer

TABLE 29.8
European Classifications as Defined by the Active Implantable Medical Device Directive and the Medical Device Directive (MDD)

- Placement of a device into a class is based upon risk and duration of use
- The intended use determines the class placement
- For combination devices and devices with accessories, each part of the device must be placed into a class and the highest
  class placement applies to the entire device
- There is no connection between the MDD classifications and FDA classifications

Class I
  Most basic classification for medical devices
  Wheelchairs
  Surgical instruments
Class IIa
  Short-term surgically invasive devices
  Some active, noninvasive devices
Class IIb
  Energy/substance delivering
  Utilizes or emits ionizing radiation
  Long-term surgically invasive devices
Class III
  Most cardiovascular and CNS devices

SECTION 4. DETERMINING TOXICOLOGY TESTING NEEDS

Once toxicology testing has been determined to be necessary, the specific tests to be performed must be identified by the manufacturer. The FDA and European Community both generally use the ISO 10993 Biological Evaluation of Medical Devices in the evaluation of manufacturers' biological safety testing program for medical devices regardless of the specific regulatory submission made — 510(k), PMA, or for a CE marking. As noted above, the testing recommended by the ISO guidelines utilize a categorization of the device based on the specific nature of the interaction of the device and component parts with the body.

The ISO standard 10993-1 as modified by the FDA (Table 29.9) summarizes the initial toxicology tests necessary for a proposed device based on the "Nature of Body Contact": noncontact, surface-contacting (skin, mucosal membranes, and breached or compromised surfaces), external communicating (blood path, indirect; tissue/bone/dentris communicating and circulating blood), or implant devices and by the duration of contact: limited exposure (≤24 h), prolonged exposure (> 24 h to 30 days), or permanent contact (>30 days). Testing requirements increase as intimacy and duration of contact of the device increase.

Using the expected intimacy of contact and duration of contact for the proposed device, the intimacy and duration categories can be determined and, therefore, the required tests for biological evaluation identified. Effects on reproduction (including developmental effects) and biodegradation may be considered for specific materials/devices depending upon the intended end use. Additional tests for specific target organ toxicity such as immunotoxicity or neurotoxicity may be necessary, depending on the characteristics of the intended use of the device including the intimacy and duration of contact. Table 29.10 provides examples of some medical devices and the corresponding body contact categories.

The intended use of the device as well as the experience with and knowledge of the materials used in its manufacture must be considered during the determination of which tests to conduct. To that end, the ISO 10993 standard is intended to be used as a guide, and, therefore, the final decision on which tests to be conducted must be made by individuals qualified in material biology and/or toxicology. The establishment of the safety assessment plan for a device should be made by the appropriate professionals, qualified by training and experience using interpretation and judgment, when considering the factors relevant to the device or its materials, the intended use, and current knowledge of the device and its materials provided by scientific literature and previous clinical experience.[5]

There are several specific situations for which ISO 10993 is *not* applicable and should not be used. Even though many of the materials used in these applications are the same, it is important that the researcher be familiar with these cases to ensure that the ISO guidance documents are not inappropriately applied to these situations. For example, packaging materials for drugs and biologics are not considered medical devices. Furthermore, several special standards for specific categories of devices are available for guidance. The researcher must ensure that the proposed device would not be included in one of these specific guidance documents before proceeding with the selection of testing methods.

For all toxicological end points, a stepwise approach to selection of tests is recommended. The researcher should first conduct a comprehensive literature review to ensure that animal studies are not inappropriately conducted. The literature search should be followed, as appropriate, by relevant *in vitro* assays and, finally, *in vivo* assays in animals if the end point has not been resolved. To aid the manufacturer, the FDA has assembled a biocompatability flowchart for the selection of toxicity tests for 510(k)s (Figure 29.1).

TABLE 29.9
The ISO Standard 10993-1 Guidance for Selection of Biocompatibility Tests as Modified by the FDA

Device Categories		Contact Duration[b]	Cytotoxicity	Sensitization	Irritation or Intractuaneous	Systemic Toxicity (Acute)	Subchronic Toxicity	Genotoxicity	Implantation	Hemocompatability	Chronic Toxicity	Carcinogenicity
Body Contact[a]												
Surface devices	Skin	A	x	x	x							
		B	x	x	x							
		C	x	x	x							
	Mucosal membrane	A	x	x	x							
		B	x	x	x	o	o		o			
		C	x	x	x	o	x	x	o		o	
	Breached or compromised surfaces	A	x	x	x	o						
		B	x	x	x	o	o		o			
		C	x	x	x	o	x	x	o		o	
External communicating devices	Blood path, indirect	A	x	x	x	x				x		
		B	x	x	x	x	o			x		
		C	x	x	o	x	x	x	o	x	x	x
	Tissue/bone/dentin communicating+	A	x	x	x	o						
		B	x	x	o	o	o	x	x			
		C	x	x	o	o	o	x	x		o	x
	Circulating blood	A	x	x	x	x		o^		x		
		B	x	x	x	x	o	x	o	x		
		C	x	x	x	x	x	x	o	x	x	x
Implant devices	Tissue/bone	A	x	x	x	o						
		B	x	x	o	o	o	x	x			
		C	x	x	o	o	o	x	x		x	x
	Blood	A	x	x	x	x			x	x		
		B	x	x	x	x	o	x	x	x		
		C	x	x	x	x	x	x	x	x	x	x

[a] See text.

[b] A = limited (24 h); B = prolonged (24 h to 30 days); C = permanent (>30 days). See text.

[c] x = ISO Evaluation Tests for Consideration; o = additional tests that may be applicable.

Note: + Tissue includes tissue fluids and subcutanous spaces; ^ for all devices used in extracorporial circuits.

Source: Adapted from FDA General Program Memorandum G95-1, Tables 1 and 2.

TABLE 29.10
Examples of Body Contact Categories as Determined by the ISO 10993-1 Guidance Matrix

	Body Contact Category	Examples
Surface Devices	Skin	Stethoscope head Electrodes Compression bandages Surgical gowns
	Mucosal membrane	Examination gloves Inhalers Endotracheal tubes Urinary catheters External feeding tubes
	Breached or compromised surface	Bandages, dressings Wound patches Occlusive tapes
External communicating devices	Tissue/bone/dentin communicating	Surgical gloves Laparoscopes Endoscopes
	Blood path indirect	Hypodermic needles Extension sets Transfer sets Blood transfusion sets
	Circulating blood	IV catheters Dialysis tubing Hemodialyzers Oxygenator
Implant devices	Tissue/bone	Bone/dental cements Cerebrospinal drains Implanted drug delivery port Orthopedic joints, pins, plates, screws Pacemakers
	Blood	Blood monitors Heart valves Vascular grafts Internal drug delivery catheter Permanent pacemaker electrodes

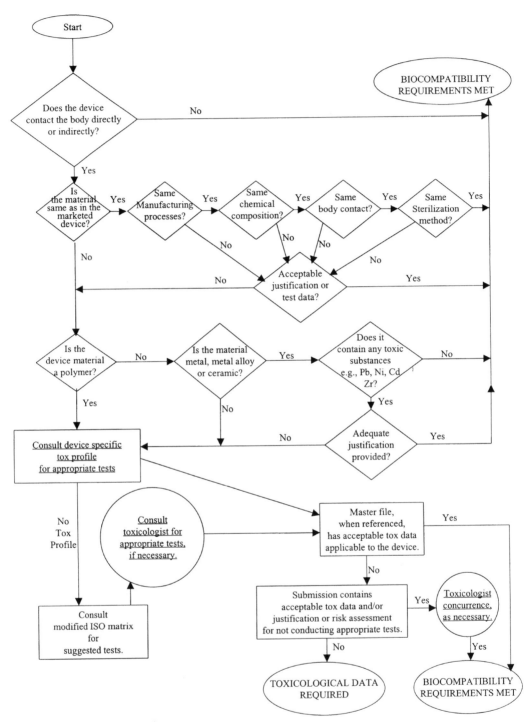

FIGURE 29.1 Biocompatibility flowchart for the selection of toxicity tests for 510(k)s. (Adapted from FDA General Program Memorandum G95-1, Attachment C.)

SECTION 5. TESTING METHODS

A. Use of Extracts

Devices, unlike drugs and chemicals, cannot be easily administered to animals in carefully measured, exact doses in varying amounts so that a dose–response relationship can be established. Device materials can include metal, fabric, silicone, and ceramics — none of which is easily administered in its final form to biological systems. Furthermore, these materials are not generally considered to be bioavailable under conditions of normal use in that they do not typically fully break down in a biological environment or they break down at a such a slow rate that biologically significant changes may not be detected for many years.[4] However, the potential for the effects of any biological components of the material as well as other chemicals that may be more bioavailable must be evaluated prior to final use of the material in a device. Chemicals other than the primary constituent of the material that may be bioavailable may include contaminants, processing aids, unreacted monomer, etc.

The task presented to the manufacturer/material scientist is to prepare the material and any other chemicals in a way that introduces the relevant chemicals to the biological system such that any potential biological effects can be observed and measured. It can be argued that total dissolution of the material using an aggressive solvent and/or physical pulverization would not generally be relevant for a material that is not intended to dissolve under normal use as a medical device component. Thus, an approach to safety evaluation that is both relevant and sufficiently challenging to the biological system must be designed.

To be available to cause a systemic effect, a chemical must migrate away from the site of tissue contact. The biological environment is a complex mixture of hydrophobic (nonpolar) and hydrophilic (polar) microenvironments. Therefore, the incubation of a material/device in a hydrophobic solution (e.g., vegetable oil) and a hydrophilic solution (e.g., saline) should dissolve or "leach" the potentially bioavailable chemicals out of the material. The potentially bioavailable chemicals should remain in the solutions after incubation and the administration of the resulting incubation solutions to a biological system would expose that system to the chemicals that may cause systemic effects. These chemicals, which may diffuse away from the device when in contact with a biological environment, are often called "leachables." Examples of extraction solutions are provided in Table 29.11.

To ensure that the leachables are present in the saline or oil incubation solutions at relevant concentrations, the incubation conditions must be considered. The ratio of material to incubation solution should be sufficient to ensure that the amount of leachables is likely to expose the biological test system to the chemical adequately so that an effect, if it occurs, will be detected. Of course, the appropriate ratio for each material under every exposure condition is impossible to calculate since the specific leachable chemicals are generally unknown. However, as a general rule, the ratio of material to solution should greatly exceed the anticipated ratio to be encountered under final-use conditions. The relevance of the safety testing program could well be challenged if, during regulatory review, it is discovered that the ratio of material to solution is less than the anticipated exposure under final-use conditions. The device industry and regulatory agencies have designed a specific set of ratios that are considered to be appropriate for most materials under most conditions. Examples of these standard ratios are provided in Table 29.12.

In addition to the ratio of material to solution, the length of time that the material is exposed to the biological system must also be considered. It can be assumed that the laws of physics apply to biological systems in that the longer the material is in contact with the biological system, an increasing percentage of the leachable chemical will diffuse away from the material and become biologically available. Unfortunately, it is not practical for the development of products nor the advancement of science to incubate materials and/or devices in saline and oil for 20 years before a material can be used in a device intended for chronic use in a patient. Therefore, the device industry and regulatory agencies have applied another law of physics in which the diffusion rate of a chemical toward equilibrium is increased at higher temperaturers. As with ratios of material to solution extraction, a specific set of temperatures to be used during extraction have been designed. The standard extraction conditions are presented in Table 29.13. In general, extraction temperatures approximating the normal human body temperature (37°C) should only be used when the body contact duration for the device is anticipated to be brief or when the integrity of the material may be compromised by using higher temperatures.

The selection of the specific conditions to be used during extraction for any material or device is dependent upon many factors, including the potential for the material to degrade physically at the selected incubation temperature, the proposed end use of the material in the device, the anticipated time of exposure under routine-use conditions of the device, and several others. The material scientist is encouraged to select these conditions carefully.

TABLE 29.11
Extraction Solutions — Common Examples

Polar (hydrophilic) liquid
    Saline
    Culture media (without sera)
    Distilled water
Nonpolar (hydrophobic) liquid
    Cottonseed oil
    Sesame oil
Other extraction liquids (may be used for specific issues and "Class" testing)
    Polyethylene glycol 400 (diluted to physiological osmotic pressure)
    Ethanol/saline (5% v/v)

TABLE 29.12
Extraction Ratios — Common Examples

Thickness (mm)	Extraction Ratio (± 10%)	Examples of Materials
≤ 0.5	6 cm²/ml	Metal; synthetic polymer; ceramic; film, sheet, and tubing wall
> 0.5	3 cm²/ml	Metal; synthetic polymer; ceramic; tubing wall; slab; molded items
≤ 1.0	3 cm²/ml	Elastomer
> 1.0	1.25 cm²/ml	Elastomer
Irregular	0.1–0.2 g/ml; 6 cm²/ml	Pellets, molded parts

TABLE 29.13
Temperature and Time Conditions — Common Examples

$37 \pm 1°C$ for 24 ± 2 h
$37 \pm 1°C$ for 72 ± 2 h
$50 \pm 2°C$ for 72 ± 2 h
$70 \pm 2°C$ for 24 ± 2 h
$121 \pm 2°C$ for 1.0 ± 0.2 h

B. BIOCOMPATIBILITY TESTS

The potential toxicity associated with the use of the device/material is often evaluated by dosing the incubation solutions (extracts), now rich with leachable compounds, to appropriate biological systems. The methods used to detect possible toxicity associated with the solutions are generally standard toxicological methods slightly modified for the use of extracts. Most important of these modifications is the obvious need to conduct two tests for each toxicology end point since two extracts exist for each device/material (hydrophobic and hydrophilic). Therefore, each test must be run in duplicate to evaluate both extracts for each end point.

A second modification to standard toxicology tests is necessary because of the dilute nature of the extracts. In spite of attempts to use high material-to-solution ratios and increased temperatures of incubation, the concentration of leachable chemicals within the solution will likely be quite low. Therefore, the dose volume of solution administered to the test system must be as high as feasible to ensure detection of any potential effects.

A third modification of standard tests is the need to adapt the study to the physical nature of the extract. Thus, both the hydrophilic and hydrophobic extracts from a device that will be in contact with the blood should be evaluated for the potential to cause systemic toxicity. However, the hydrophobic (a vegetable oil) extract cannot be injected directly into the bloodstream at a sufficiently high dose without immediately killing the animals via lipid emboli. Therefore, this extract is administered to the animals by an alternative route. Obviously, the oral or dermal routes of exposure would be inappropriate because of significant differences in absorption and metabolism potential and, therefore, the intraperitoneal route of exposure is used as the most relevant alternative. Similarly, a saline extract cannot be added directly to many *in vitro* systems because of toxicity, and the extract medium must be altered to ensure successful dosing.

The risk assessment process must also be modified to adapt to these differences between standard toxicology tests and the methods used to evaluate the extracts of medical devices. It is important to recognize that the level of uncertainty is increased when extracts are used since the actual test article (the material/device) is one more level removed from the human exposure condition. Because of this added level of uncertainty accompanying the use of extracts, physical pieces or, better yet, miniature devices can be prepared and evaluated in toxicology tests individually designed to evaluate the material/device. However, the time and cost associated with the preparation of miniature devices may be prohibitive even though the miniature "device" need not be an exact duplicate, nor does it have to be functional to be used for evaluation of toxicology. The miniature device only needs to maintain the same basic ratios of materials to be used in the device and to be of appropriate size to provide a sufficient "dose" of the materials to the test animals. If a miniature device can be devised and produced in a timely and cost-effective manner, the difficulty of adapting toxicology tests to evaluate a physical piece or pieces of plastic, fabric, or other solid material may eliminate the possibility of conducting the study. In spite of these complexities, which necessitate the use of extracts for most toxicology evaluations of medical devices, the researcher is encouraged to consider the use of solid materials since this approach eliminates the uncertainty introduced into the risk assessment process by the use of extracts.

As a final note to the preparation of materials for evaluation of materials/devices, the researcher must recognize that the procedures used to sterilize devices are generally accepted to have the potential to change the physical characteristics of the component materials. These physical changes also have the potential to affect the biocompatibility of the material/device.[6] Therefore, materials to be used in toxicology testing, whether they are extracted, used to create miniature devices, or sectioned into implantable aliquots, should be sterilized using the procedures to be used to sterilize the final device prior to use in humans. Therefore, a final modification to standard toxicology testing procedures is the possible need to evaluate a material/device in a multiple series of tests to ensure that all forms of sterilization considered to be acceptable for the device do not negatively impact the biocompatability of the device or component parts. A guidance document regarding sterilization procedures has been prepared (ISO 10993-12).

In determining testing requirements for medical devices, as for other test articles to be evaluated for toxicity, it is important to consider previously conducted study results or published literature before initiating a study using animals.[7] To that end, the Animal Welfare Act has defined a responsibility for the individual researcher and, therefore, the manufacturer to consider all information before initiating animal testing.

Studies often conducted during the safety evaluation of medical devices are presented in Table 29.14.

TABLE 29.14
Studies Often Conducted during the Safety Evaluation of Medical Devices

Cytotoxicity
- *In vitro* test that utilizes cell culture techniques
- Used primarily to evaluate the potential for local toxic effects
- Often used as an initial biological screen for new materials or changes to existing formulations (for example, existing materials sterilized by a new method)

Sensitization
- Methods used most frequently utilize guinea pigs as the test organism
- Study duration of guinea pig assays is approximately 6 weeks
- Evaluates the sensitization component of the immunological response of the biological system to foreign materials
- Delayed hypersensitivity (Type IV) allergic reaction is the specific biological reaction evaluated in this study
- Both natural and synthetic materials can produce sensitization reactions and the potential morbidity that may be caused by sensitization of an individual to a device is significant
- All materials considered for use in medical devices should be evaluated for the potential to cause sensitization
- The local lymph node assay (LLNA) utilizing mice is becoming more widely accepted as a method (study duration is approximately 1 week)
- Using human volunteers to evaluate sensitization should be considered for some applications
- Study duration of human studies is approximately 6 weeks

Skin Irritation (Topical)
- Generally uses albino rabbits as the test model because of high potential for observable skin reaction in this model
- Most obviously used to evaluate potential for a topical product to produce skin irritation at the site of application
- Evaluation of treatment sites uses standardized scoring criteria to allow for a calculation of a "Primary Irritation Index" (combined severity of erythema and edema scores)
- For materials/devices intended to be in contact with abraded skin and/or open wounds, testing for skin irritation needs to be expanded to include animals in which the epidermis has been abraded using appropriate methods
- Study duration is approximately 3 days

Skin Irritation (Intracutaneous Reactivity)
- Uses albino rabbits as the test model because of high potential for observable skin reaction in this model
- Extracts injected into the surface layers of the skin (approximately between the epidermis and dermis)
- Evaluation of injection sites uses standardized scoring criteria similar to topical testing
- Has become a standard test to help evaluate the potential for many materials/devices, regardless of their intended final use, to produce a local reaction at the site of tissue contact
- Study duration is approximately 3 days

Acute Systemic Toxicity
- Utilizes mice injected with extracts by either the intravenous or intraperitoneal route
- Designed to evaluate the potential for harmful effect(s) to occur distant from the site of tissue contact
- Evaluation for toxic effects generally follows standard toxicological methods including death, weight loss, and clinical signs
- Study duration is approximately 3 days

Implantation
- Used as a direct measure of the local irritation potential of materials/devices in direct contact with living tissue

TABLE 29.14 *(Continued)*
Studies Often Conducted during the Safety Evaluation of Medical Devices

- Implanted test article may be a small piece of a device component, a specific part of a final device, or an entire device
- Design often includes implantation of a standard control material into same animals (at distant sites) as the test article to serve as an irritant control
- Site of implantation is generally a large muscle of a laboratory animal (often an albino rabbit) due to ease of placement and subsequent gross and histopathological scoring of any tissue changes
- Care must be taken during test article preparation to avoid the inadvertent presence of any sharp edges/corners on the test article that may bias the results of the test by causing inflammation due to the shape of the test article
- Basic muscle implantation techniques do not absolutely require microscopic evaluation of the implantation site, but histology should be used as frequently as possible to maximize the potential to detect biologically significant reactions to the test article
- Attempts should be made to evaluate the tissue response macroscopically and microscopically without disturbing the test article location in the tissue since removal of the test article may also remove some inflammatory tissue from the site
- Specialized studies using implantation into the intended site of use of the device should be considered
- Method of inserting (implanting) the test article into the tissue has the potential to impact the results of the study
- Study duration can be 5 days to several months depending on proposed end use of the device

Hemocompatibility
- Evaluates the potential for a material/device to effect the formed cellular elements of the blood (cells/platelets) as well as to activate the coagulation and/or complement systems of the circulation
- Frequently conducted using *in vitro* assays in which the end point is red blood cell lysis, coagulation, etc.
- Assays generally use the blood from laboratory animals although this has been challenged due to possible differences in cell friability and, therefore, use of donated human blood may be considered
- Potential biological significance of hematological changes caused by materials/devices in contact with the blood suggests that *in vivo* testing should be considered when standard *in vitro* studies are inconclusive
- Study duration is generally very brief (less than 1 day)

Genotoxicity
- Assays evaluate the potential for test article to induce genetic changes including mutations and/or altered chromosomal structure
- *In vitro* studies including the Ames assay and chromosomal aberration are frequently used
- *In vivo* studies such as the mouse micronucleas assay may also be utilized
- Study duration varies with the specific assay

Subchronic/Chronic Systemic Toxicity
- These assays should only be conducted for devices used repeatedly (same device frequently on the same patient or different devices used frequently on the same patient)
- Studies are typically individually designed for specific devices
- Test system may be virtually any laboratory animal model and should be selected based upon the desired end point of the study
- Evaluation for toxic effects generally follows standard toxicological methods including death, weight loss, clinical signs, clinical pathology, hematology, and histopathology (of local tissue effects as well as possible target organs)
- These assays may be conducted by evaluating implanted materials (obviously, test and control articles must be placed into different animals for these assays) or by repeatedly dosing animals with freshly prepared extracts
- Study duration may be as short as 2 weeks or as long as several years depending upon the desired end point of the study

Carcinogencity
- Rarely required for device materials
- Test system is generally mice or rats
- Evaluation for carcinogenicity end point follows standard toxicological methods and is dependent upon hematology and histopathology
- These assays may be conducted by evaluating implanted materials (obviously, test and control articles must be placed into different animals for these assays) or by repeatedly dosing animals with freshly prepared extracts
- Study duration (including significant time to complete histopathological evaluation) is at least 2 years and is often close to 3 years

SECTION 6. GLOSSARY

Agar Diffusion Cytotoxicity Assay A cytotoxicity assay (also called the agar overlay method) using cultured mammalian cells in which the material/device is placed in contact with a layer of agar which, in turn, is in direct contact with the cells, and, after a prescribed period of incubation, the cells are examined for signs of toxicity resulting from exposure to the test article.

Annex Quality conformity assessment as defined by the European Medical Device Directives. Annex I through VII are defined.

Biocompatibility The science of determining the suitability of a material for a proposed contact with biological tissues. It is important to note that a material determined to be "biocompatible" for one application (e.g., for a device intended to be in contact only with the intact surface of the skin) may not be biocompatible for another application in which it will be implanted into a body cavity. Therefore, the term *biocompatibility* is dependent upon the suitability of the safety evaluation as it relates to the intended use of the material.

Biomaterial A material that has direct or indirect patient contact. A biomaterial (also termed a *biomedical material*) may be composed of any synthetic or natural rubber or fiber, polymeric or elastomeric formulation, alloy, ceramic, bonding agent, ink, or other nonviable substance, including tissue rendered nonviable, used as a device or any part thereof.

Biomedical material Synonymous with biomaterial.

CE marking A "passport" that can allow a manufacturer to circulate its products freely within the European marketplace. The marking applies only to products regulated by European health, safety, and environmental protection legislation (product directives). This is estimated to include more than 50% of the goods currently exported from the United States to Europe including medical devices. CE is short for a French phrase, *Confomite Europeene.*

Class testing The testing of plastics for biological reactivity according to predetermined testing requirements defined by the USP.

Combination product A product containing both a drug and device component that are physically, chemically, or otherwise combined to result in a medical product that is used therapeutically as a single entity. In the case of a combination product, the medical device component of the product must be evaluated for safety according to device requirements (as addressed in this chapter) while the drug component must be fully evaluated as necessary for drugs. The final, combined finished product will also need to be evaluated for safety.

Design dossier Documentation similar to a Technical File that is submitted to a Notified Body. Defined in Annex II, Section 4 of the Medical Device Directives.

Direct contact When the materials of a device are in direct (that is, intimate) contact with the surface or tissues of the body (adhesive bandages, pacemaker leads, as well as dialysis chambers are examples).

Direct Contact Cytotoxicity Assay A cytotoxicity assay using cultured mammalian cells in which the material/device is placed in direct contact with the cells and, after a prescribed period of incubation, the cells are examined for signs of toxicity resulting from exposure to the test article.

Elution Cytotoxicity Assay A cytotoxicity assay using cultured mammalian cells in which the material/device is extracted in culture media before the media is used to culture the cells. The cells are then incubated in the extracted media for a prescribed period and the cells examined for signs of toxicity resulting from exposure to the test article.

Essential requirements The basic documentation requirements for a manufacturer to obtain a CE marking. Many devices require additional documentation to obtain a CE marking.

Requirements are based upon perceived risk. Defined in Annex I of the Medical Device Directives.

Extract A solution produced by the incubation of a material/medical device in an appropriate vehicle. After incubation, the vehicle contains the soluble chemicals (or leachables) that have dissolved out of or off of the material/medical device and this combination of soluble chemicals in the vehicle is considered to be an extract.

Indirect contact When the materials of a device do not contact the surface or tissues of the body but the materials of the device may influence the body. That is, a solution or material contacts the device, may become contaminated with leachables from the device, and then contacts the body. An example is an intravenous (iv) bag.

ISO International Standards Organisation.

Leachable A chemical that may, under anticipated-use conditions, dissolve away from a material or device when in contact with a biological system and, therefore, has the potential to produce a biological effect that may be distant from the site of tissue contact.

Medical device Any instrument, apparatus, appliance, material, or other article, including software, whether used alone or in combination, intended by the manufacturer for use by human beings solely or principally for the purpose of diagnosis, prevention, monitoring, or treatment; alleviation of disease, injury, or handicap; investigation, replacement, or modification of the anatomy or of a physiological process; control of conception; and that which does not achieve its principal intended action of the human body by pharmaceutical, immunological, or metabolic means, but may be assisted in its function by such means (ISO 10993-1).

Predicate device A previously marketed device that is substantially equivalent to a proposed device. The predicate device is used as a comparison to the proposed device to establish safety and efficacy.

Processing aid A material that contacts the product during the manufacturing process and, therefore, has a potential for affecting product quality and/or may elicit a biological response following the use of a medical device. Solvents, cleaning products, lubricants, and mold-release agents are examples of processing aids.

Technical documentation All documents supporting a European CE Marking.

Technical file European documentation for a medical device including the essential requirements data, product specifications, and manufacturing data.

Type examination Testing of a device by a European Notified Body. Defined in Annex II, Section 3 of the Medical Device Directives.

USP Negative Control Plastic RS A standardized plastic produced by the USP for use as a control material in some biocompatibility assays.

REFERENCES

1. Rubin, J.P. and Yaremchuk, M.J., Complications and toxicities of implantable biomaterials used in facial reconstructive and aesthetic surgery: a comprehensive review of the literature, *Plast. Reconstr. Surg.*, 100, 1336, 1997.
2. Gotman, I., Characteristics of metals used in implants, *J. Endourol.*, 11, 383, 1997
3. Northup, S.J., Strategies for biological testing of biomaterials, *J. Biomater. Appl.*, 2, 132, 1987.
4. Pinchuk, L., A review of the biostability and carcinogenicity of polyurethanes in medicine and the new generation of "biostable" polyurethanes, *J. Biomater. Sci. Polym. Ed.*, 6, 225, 1994.
5. ANSI/AAMI, 10993-1: Biological evaluation of medical devices — Part 1, Guidance on selection of tests, 1997.
6. Nair, P.D., Currently practiced sterilization methods — some inadvertent consequences, *J. Biomater. Appl.*, 10, 121, 1995.

7. Schwindaman, D., Federal regulation of experimental animal use in the United States of America, *Rev. Sci. Tech.*, 13, 247, 1994.

8. *U.S. Pharmacopoeia 23/National Formulary 18, 1995 edition*, United States Pharmacopeial Convention, Inc., Rockville, MD, 1994, chap. 88.

30 Regulatory Toxicology: Consumer Products

Dennis J. Naas, B.S.

CONTENTS

0-8493-0370-2/02/$0.00+$1.50
© 2002 by CRC Press LLC

SECTION 1. OVERVIEW

When a chapter on consumer products was first contemplated, its scope seemed quite straightforward and limited. The interest was to develop a chapter or section that related to the Consumer Product Safety Commission (CPSC), its makeup and authority, and the requirements and guidelines for toxicity safety testing of consumer products to aid the practicing industrial toxicologist. The chapter was intended to provide general information on typical testing programs a consumer products company might follow in developing health and toxicity safety information on such consumer products as household and personal hygiene products.

However, when one fully considers the term *consumer product* in a broad sense, the scope of this subject rapidly expands. For example, certainly, in the traditional sense and use of the term, standard household cleaning products are consumer products that are regulated under the Consumer Product Safety Act (CPSA) via the CPSC. However, a household cleaning product that contains an antimicrobial agent and is labeled as a disinfectant is regulated under the Federal Insecticide, Fungicide, and Rhodenticide Act (FIFRA), as administered by the Environmental Protection Agency (EPA), because it contains a pesticide. Also consider the area of personal hygiene products, i.e., "cosmetics." This general category includes such diverse products as shaving creams, shampoos, antibacterial liquid soaps, sunscreens, and athlete's foot treatments, certainly all available directly to the consumer, i.e., consumer products. However, the first two types of products are regulated under the Food, Drug and Cosmetic Act (FDCA) as cosmetics, while the last three, because they contain an "active" ingredient, are regulated via the Over-the-Counter (OTC) Drug Monograph. And although both the FDCA and the OTC are administered by the Food and Drug Administration (FDA), the requirements for marketing these two types of products are quite different. And the above product classes are not included in the special regulatory environments that exist for two other types of consumer products, art materials and dietary supplements.

At least ten major U.S. federal regulations exist under which consumer products may be regulated (Table 30.1). As illustrated above, consumer products represent an extremely broad and diverse collection of substances, materials, and products, even if considered only within the context of the U.S. market and regulatory environment, as will be the case in this chapter. For the purposes of this discussion, a consumer product is considered to be any product customarily produced or distributed for sale to or for consumption by the individual customer. Exceptions to this definition are foods and food additives, which are specially regulated by the FDCA/FDA, fuels, which are regulated primarily based on physiochemical hazard rather than toxicity, FIFRA/EPA-regulated pesticides available directly to the consumer, and prescription drugs, which are subjected by the FDA to the most comprehensive safety assessments in existence.

General consumer product classes and the corresponding federal regulations and administering agencies are presented in Table 30.2. Consumer product class definitions are presented in Table 30.3. The primary focus of this chapter is on safety/toxicity testing of consumer products that are regulated under CPSA/CPSC, i.e., household products and art supplies (as defined herein). The CPSA/CPSC also regulates consumer products on the basis of physiochemical properties such as explosive potential, flammability, corrosivity, etc., as well as common household items (beds, clothing, toys, etc.) primarily on the basis of physical safety. These aspects of CPSA/CPSC regulation will not be addressed. While a comprehensive discussion of all intricacies related to consumer product testing, safety, labeling, and other regulatory considerations is beyond the scope of this chapter, some limited discussion of these other considerations is provided, as well as references on resources from which further information can be obtained. Aside from recognizing OTC drug products as a type of consumer product and briefly describing the responsible regulatory acts and agencies, the topic of OTC drug product safety evaluation, registration, and regulation will not be further discussed in this chapter.

TABLE 30.1
Federal Regulations and Regulatory Agencies for Consumer Products in the United States

Regulation	Acronym	Year Promulgated	Administrating Agency
Federal Trade Commission Act	FTCA	1914	FTC
Food, Drug, and Cosmetic Act	FDCA	1938	FDA
The Investigational New Drug/New Drug Application Process	IND/NDA	1938	FDA
Federal Insecticide, Fungicide, and Rodenticide Act	FIFRA	1947	EPA
Federal Hazardous Substances Act	FSHA	1960	CPSC
Color Additives Amendments to the FDCA	CAA	1960, 1962	FDA
Fair Packaging and Labeling Act	FPLA	1966	FDA
Poison Prevention and Packaging Act	PPPA	1970	CPSC
Over-the-Counter Drug Monograph Process	OTC	1972	FDA
Labeling of Hazardous Art Materials Act	LHAMA	1988	CPSC
Dietary Supplement Health and Education Act	DSHEA	1994	FDA

Note: FTC = Federal Trade Commission.

TABLE 30.2
General Consumer Product Classes and Corresponding Regulations/Regulatory Agencies

Product Class	Regulation/Agency	Product Class Examples
Household products	FHSA/CPSC PPPA/CPSC	Window cleaner, silicone caulk, floor wax, antifreeze
Art supplies	LHAMA/CPSC PPPA/CPSC	Children's coloring books, crayons, glues
Cosmetics	FDCA/FDA CAA/FDA FPLA/FDA FTCA/FTC	Shaving cream, shampoo, deodorants
Disinfectant household products	FIFRA/EPA PPPA/CPSC	Lysol® products,[a] Tilex®,[b]
Dietary supplements	DSHEA/FDA FTCA/FTC	Ephedrine, ginkoba, ginseng
OTC drug products	OTC/FDA IND-NDA/FDA	Treatments for athlete's foot, antibacterial soap, sunscreen

[a] Registered trademark of Reckitt & Coleman, Inc., Montvale, NJ.
[b] Registered trademark of the Clorox Company, Oakland, CA.

TABLE 30.3
General Consumer Product Class Definitions

Class	Definition
Household product	This may be viewed generally as a default category of products customarily manufactured or distributed for sale for consumption or use, or customarily stored by, individuals in or about the household that do not fall into other classes. Items such as toys, bunk beds, matches, charcoal briquettes, lighters, electrical appliances, etc. are household products regulated under CPSA/CPSC; however, their regulation is based primarily on physical safety of the consumer and not on chemical toxicity hazard. For the purposes of this discussion, household products may be considered as chemicals or chemical mixtures to which consumers are exposed that do not fall into any of the other classes listed below.
Art material	"Any raw or processed material, or manufactured product, marketed or represented by the producer or repackager as intended for and suitable for [use by] artists or crafts people of any age who create, or recreate in a limited number, largely by hand, works which may or may not have a practical use, but in which aesthetic considerations are paramount" (16 CFR 1500.14).
Cosmetic	"A product which enhances appearance, aids in personal hygiene and does not affect the structure or function of the skin."[1]
Disinfectant household product	Household products containing an active ingredient present to produce a specific biocidal (usually antimicrobial) effect that are marketed directly to the consumer. These materials are not intended for direct human application/exposure.
Dietary supplement	Any product that is not a food or either a direct or indirect food additive, that is intended for ingestion as a supplement to the diet.
OTC drug product	Nonprescription drug or cosmetic-like products marketed directly to the consumer, deliberately ingested or applied, containing an active ingredient present to produce a specific desired (usually biological) effect.

SECTION 2. CONSUMER PRODUCT SAFETY COMMISSION

The CPSC was formed as an independent commission (agency) on May 14, 1973 under the provisions of the Consumer Product Safety Act (CPSA). The complete text pertaining to the CPSC is located in the Code of Federal Regulation, CFR 16 Parts 1000 through 1750. The stated purposes of the commission are (16 CFR 1000.1):

- To protect the public against unreasonable risks of injury associated with consumer products;
- To assist consumers in evaluating the comparative safety of consumer products;
- To develop uniform safety standards for consumer products and to minimize conflicting state and local regulation; and
- To promote research and investigation into the causes and prevention of product-related deaths, illnesses, and injury.

In addition to administering the CPSA, the CPSC administers three legislative acts pertinent to consumer product safety as defined herein, the Federal Hazardous Substances Act (FHSA, 16 CFR 1500.1 through 1500.13), the Labeling of Hazardous Art Materials Act [LHAMA, CFR 1500.14(b)(8)], and the Poison Prevention Packaging Act (PPPA, 16 CFR 1700 through 1750), passed initially in 1960, 1988, and 1970, respectively.

Products regulated under CPSC do not have to be "registered" prior to marketing, unlike chemicals and products regulated by other agencies, i.e., the EPA under both the Toxic Substances Control Act (TSCA) and FIFRA, and drugs and food additives regulated by the FDA. Thus, responsibility for appropriate safety stewardship of CPSC-regulated products falls almost exclusively to the producers and manufacturers.

The CPSC is empowered to develop uniform safety standards for consumer products. In the event that a standard to "protect the public from the unreasonable risk of injury" adequately cannot be developed, the CPSC is further empowered to ban the product or impose specific labeling or packaging requirements. However, some previous attempts to ban products containing specific materials or to require special labeling have been successfully challenged in the courts.

SECTION 3. WHEN TO PERFORM ANIMAL SAFETY TESTING

Perhaps the most confounding question facing the industrial toxicologist today is when to perform animal safety testing on a consumer product. No clear-cut formula exists to help make this determination. The testing considered, required, or recommended to satisfy one regulatory body may impact many other aspects of product commercialization (Material Safety Data Sheet contents, product labeling, U.S. Department of Transportation packaging classification, EPA TSCA Section 8e Significant Risk Notification, etc.). Increasing pressures to conserve laboratory animal resources must be balanced against the obligation to bring products to market responsibly. International regulatory considerations, in an increasingly global commercial environment, further confound the issue.

The CPSC has well-defined labeling requirements and warning phrases based on the results of specific acute toxicity testing in animals. Undesirable warning phrases on package labels, i.e., "over-warning," can clearly represent a competitive disadvantage. However, "under-warning" can be equally or more disadvantageous in this highly litigious society.

The actual engagement of safety testing in animals can be a labor- and capital-intensive endeavor and should not be undertaken lightly. The toxicologist and company must be prepared to potentially accept and subsequently deal with an unexpected result. Internal testing resources have greatly diminished in recent years. Therefore, the use of external contract research organizations has become increasingly common. Considerations on laboratory selection and study design, conduct, and monitoring are presented in a subsequent section of this chapter.

The following guidelines are offered to the industrial toxicologist evaluating the need for animal safety testing on a "new" consumer product:

- Determine as precisely as possible, by ingredient material and their quantities, the chemical composition of the product. Most are mixtures.
- Determine if, in the mixing of the ingredient materials combined to make the product, any reactions have or may have occurred to create a substance not originally present. The identification of a reaction product at this point could have several outcomes, depending upon the material that was formed. Inadvertent synthesis of a highly toxic reaction product would almost certainly halt further commercialization efforts, although this can sometimes be resolved via process refinement. Formation of a previously unknown substance or new chemical entity (NCE) could trigger testing, halt commercialization, cause process refinement, or require the toxicologist to perform a structure–activity relationship type of assessment on the new chemical. A reaction to form a known substance would simply result in this material being considered as one of the components in the final product, assessed in the same manner as one of the original ingredient materials. In a reactive process, the relative quantities of the original components would change; such changes should also be taken into account when assessing the toxicity hazard potential of the final product. CPSC addresses the assessment/testing of potentially hazardous mixtures as follows: "It may not be possible to reach a fully satisfactory decision concerning the toxic, irritant, corrosive, flammable, sensitizing, or

pressure-generating properties of a substance [mixture] from what is known about its components or ingredients. The mixture itself should be tested."(16 CFR 1500.5).

- Determine the relevant route or routes of human exposure. For example, a liquid household cleaner will or may come into contact with the skin, eyes, and possibly be ingested, and therefore data by these routes of exposure should be available. However, virtually no opportunity exists for inhalation exposure; therefore, data by this route would not necessarily be required. A spray oven cleaner does pose an inhalation exposure risk, as well as potential for exposure by the other routes. Therefore, information regarding the toxicity hazard by the inhalation route should be available for such a product. In general, data need to be available or testing needs to be performed only by relevant exposure routes. A new application for an existing product, e.g., a liquid cleaner made available in spray form, could trigger testing by a route of exposure not previously evaluated.

- The total potential exposure to the product should be assessed, in terms of both the frequency of exposure and the dose received at each exposure. This information may be used to determine the adequacy of existing toxicity data and/or in the design of any studies that may be performed. Single-exposure, short-term (acute) data or studies are the minimum needed to classify a substance and in most cases will satisfy CPSC requirements with respect to hazard identification and labeling.

- Evaluate the toxicity information available for the chemical or substances that comprise the product. Physiochemical factors such as pH, volatility, physical form, viscosity, etc., should be taken into account. The data should be reviewed for consistency, completeness, currency, and general quality. The reliability of the source of the information or data must be carefully considered; some resources are generally more reliable than others. A peer-reviewed publication of a study conducted under Good Laboratory Practice standards (GLPs) should be given much greater credence than a single sentence or two from a Material Safety Data Sheet (MSDS) obtained from a second party. Full study reports, when available, are preferable to abstracts. More recent studies tend to be of higher quality and thus more reliable than older ones because of the now-routine conduct of toxicity/safety studies under GLPs.

A multitude of resources exists from which to obtain toxicity data as well as other physiochemical and hazard information on chemicals of commercial interest. A listing of examples of such resources is provided at the end of this chapter (see Table 30.12).

Thus, the ultimate question that the industrial toxicologist must answer is "Does sufficient toxicity data of adequate type and quality exist to responsibly, safely, and efficiently bring this product to market without an unreasonable risk of injury to the consumer?" If the answer to this question is no, appropriate studies to address the data inadequacies must be performed.

SECTION 4. DESIGN, CONDUCT, AND MONITORING OF SAFETY/TOXICITY STUDIES IN ANIMALS

A. GOOD LABORATORY PRACTICES

Animal toxicity/safety studies conducted in support of consumer product marketing and/or registration should be conducted under GLPs. Several such federal standards exist; the EPA has promulgated two sets of GLPs, one for TSCA (40 CFR Part 792) and one for FIFRA (40 CFR Part 160). In addition, the FDA has issued Good Laboratory Practice for Nonclinical Laboratory Studies (21 CFR Part 58). For practical intents and purposes, these standards are essentially identical. Studies to support products regulated exclusively by CPSA/CPSC may be conducted under any of these sets of GLPs. Studies intended to support product registration under the jurisdiction of other regulatory agencies should follow the appropriate respective set of GLPs.

An important note to manufacturers/producers who may sponsor or conduct GLP studies concerns test substance/article characterization. All the above GLP standards require test substance/article characterization prior to starting the test. Although it is not explicitly stated that this characterization be carried out under GLPs, the presence of this passage within the standards certainly implies this to be the case.

B. ANIMAL WELFARE

It is strongly recommended that the test facility be accredited by the Association for Assessment and Accreditation of Laboratory Care International (AAALAC International). Participation in this accreditation program is voluntary. Accreditation is based on thorough triannual inspection by a team of animal welfare experts of all facilities, equipment, procedures, and practices relating to the laboratory's care, maintenance, and management of its animal resources, in accordance with federal animal welfare laws. AAALAC International accreditation helps provide assurance of the welfare and humane treatment of the animals used for testing.

C. STUDY PROTOCOL

The study protocol is the controlling document with respect to study conduct. In accordance with the applicable GLPs, it should contain all information necessary to execute the project according to the stated study objective.

D. LABORATORY SELECTION

With respect to externally contracted studies, all major regulatory agencies hold the study sponsor legally responsible for its conduct and results, not the testing facility. From this aspect, some level of monitoring external studies, including on-site inspections, is both prudent and common practice. Literally dozens of testing facilities able to conduct the studies to support consumer product marketing/registration are in operation. Unfortunately, no objective mechanism exists for evaluating their capabilities, competence, or quality. Laboratory selection factors may include personal knowledge, the laboratory's reputation, professional references, prestudy site inspections, proximity, personnel, governmental agency inspections, study fees, and other factors. In the absence of knowledge in this area, utilization of the services of an independent professional consultant familiar with the contract research organization industry may be highly valuable.

E. STUDY DESIGN CONSIDERATIONS

Animal toxicity/safety studies are not often conducted solely to support marketing of a consumer product in the United States under CPCA/CPCS/FHSA. The potential for product penetration into other, especially international, markets may require more rigorous testing than that described in FHSA.

Some types of studies performed in accordance with other federal and/or international testing guidelines, while providing more information than required by the FHSA test methods, could yield results perfectly acceptable for arriving at an FHSA classification. For example, an acute oral toxicity study done to comply with either the EPA Office of Prevention, Pesticides and Toxic Substances (OPPTS) Guideline No. 870.1100 or the Organisation for Economic Cooperation and Development (OECD) Test Guideline No. 401 should produce an LD_{50} value that can be used to assign an FHSA classification. The same can be said for determination of acute dermal toxicity (EPA OPPTS Guideline No. 870.1200 or OECD Test Guideline No. 402). However, this is not always the case. Other major regulatory bodies usually require determination of the acute inhalation LC_{50} based on a 4-h exposure duration, while the FHSA is based on a 1-h exposure. Whereas extrapolation is possible, a 4-h exposure to the same concentration is obviously more likely to cause acute toxicity than a 1-h exposure. Similarly, primary dermal irritation is assessed under EPA

OPPTS and OECD test guidelines following a 4-h rather than a 24-h exposure. So while a study of a substance that caused severe irritation or corrosion in an OPPTS or OECD design could certainly be used to classify under FHSA, a minimally to moderately irritating result in such a study would not be useful for FHSA classification. Similar logic can be applied to primary eye irritation testing, with the difference being the OPPTS and OECD designs utilize only three rabbits whereas the FHSA design requires at least six.

With proper planning and foresight, studies can be designed to meet or exceed the requirements of multiple regulatory agencies, thereby responsibly utilizing laboratory animal resources, maximizing the information obtained from the studies and its subsequent use, while minimizing product development time and costs without compromising consumer safety.

Ultimately, the design of animal toxicity/safety studies must be such that previously identified data inadequacies are addressed, future data needs are anticipated and addressed to greatest extent reasonably possible, and the studies are acceptable to the regulatory body (or bodies) of interest.

SECTION 5. SAFETY ASSESSMENT OF CONSUMER PRODUCTS

A. HOUSEHOLD PRODUCTS

Toxicity/safety test methods, evaluation methods, classification criteria, and definitions for household products are presented and described in Tables 30.4 through 30.10.

TABLE 30.4
Federal Hazardous Substances Act Methods for Assessing Dermal and Eye Toxicity

	Acute Dermal Toxicity[a]	Primary Dermal Irritancy[b]	Eye Irritation[c]
Test species	Albino rabbits	Albino rabbits	Albino rabbits
n	10 (per dose level)[d]	6	6
Dose levels	Sufficient to enable the calculation of an LD_{50}	0.5 ml/site (liquids) 0.5 g/site (solids; semisolids)[e]	0.1 ml (liquids) 100 mg (solids; pastes)[f]
Chemical exposure duration	24 h	24 h	24–72 h[g]
Observation period (following exposure)	14 days	24 and 72 h	24, 48, and 72 h
Comments	Fully occlusive, impervious wraps are used[h] The skin of the test site is abraded Result: The LD_{50} is the median dose at which 50% mortality is observed.	Fully occlusive, impervious wraps are used[h] At least one intact and one abraded site are employed per animal Scoring: see Table 30.5	One eye is treated; contalateral eye serves as control Eyes are not washed for at least 24 h after exposure Scoring: see Table 30.7
Classification	See Table 30.10	See Tables 30.6 and 30.10	See Tables 30.8 and 30.10

[a] 16 CFR 1500.40.

[b] 16 CFR 1500.41.

[c] 16 CFR 1500.42.

[d] Normally five animals/sex/dose level are employed.

[e] Solids should be dissolved in an appropriate solvent and the solution applied as directed for liquids.

[f] For powders, flakes, granular materials, or other particulate, 0.1 ml of compacted material shall be used whenever this volume weighs <100 mg.

[g] Use of a multiple animal holder for restraint during exposure is indicated in the FHSA test method. However, current animal welfare considerations may preclude such complete immobilization.

[g] A single does is instilled; exposure may theoretically continue until study termination at 72 hours.

TABLE 30.5
Federal Hazardous Substances Act Primary Dermal Irritation Scoring Method[a]

Skin Reaction	Value[b]
Erythema and eschar	
No erythema	0
Very slight erythema (barely perceptible)	1
Well-defined erythema	2
Moderate to severe erythema	3
Severe erythema (beet red) to slight eschar formation (injury in depth)	4
Edema	
No edema	0
Very slight edema (barely perceptible)	1
Slight edema (area edges well defined by definite raising)	2
Moderate edema (raised approximately 1 mm)	3
Severe edema (raised >1 mm and extending beyond the area of exposure)	4

[a] Taken from 16 CFR 1500.41.

[b] The "value" recorded is the average value for six or more animals subjected to the test.

TABLE 30.6
Example Calculation of a Primary Dermal Irritation Score According to the Method Described in the Federal Hazardous Substances Act[a]

Skin Reaction	Exposure Time, h	Value[b]
Erythema and eschar		
Intact Skin	24	3
	72	2
Abraded Skin	24	4
	72	3
Subtotal		*12*
Edema		
Intact Skin	24	0
	72	1
Abraded Skin	24	1
	72	2
Subtotal		*4*
Total Score		**16**

Primary Irritation Score[c]: $16 \div 4 = 4$ Classification[d]: Not an irritant

[a] Taken from 16 CFR 1500.42.

[b] The "value" recorded is the average value for six or more animals subjected to the test.

[c] To calculate the primary irritation score, intact and abraded sites are evaluated, at 24 and 72 h after exposure, according to the scoring method presented in Table 30.5. The four values for erythema and eschar are added together for a subtotal (12 in this example). The four values for edema are added together for a second subtotal (4 in this example). The two subtotals are added together to give an overall total score (16 in this example). This total score is then divided by 4 to give the primary irritation score. The material can then be classified.

[d] Substances/products whose Primary Irritation Score is ≥ 5 are classified as "irritants" under FHSA.

TABLE 30.7
Recommended Scoring System for Primary Eye Irritation[a,b]

Ocular Reaction	Score[c]
Cornea	
Opacity — Degree of density (area most dense taken for reading)	
No ulceration or opacity	0
Scattered or diffuse areas of opacity (other than slight dulling of luster), details of iris still clearly visible	1*
Easily discernible translucent area, details of iris slightly obscured	2*
Nacreous area, no details or iris visible, size of pupil barely discernible	3*
Opaque cornea, iris not discernible through opacity	4*
Iris	
Normal	0
Markedly deepened rugae, congestion, swelling, moderate circumcorneal hyperemia, or injection (any of these or combination of any thereof), iris still reacting to light (sluggish reaction is positive)	1*
No reaction to light, hemorrhage, gross destruction (any or all of these)	2*
Conjunctivae	
Redness (refers to palpebral and bulbar conjunctivae, excluding cornea and iris)	
Blood vessels normal	0
Some blood vessels definitely hyperemic	1
Diffuse crimson color with individual vessels not discernible	2*
Diffuse, beefy red	3*
Chemosis (refers to lids and/or nictitating membranes)	
No swelling	0
Any swelling above normal (includes nictitating membranes)	1
Obvious swelling with partial eversion of lids	2*
Swelling with lids about half closed	3*
Swelling with lids more than half closed	4*

[a] Grading scale for scoring ocular lesions, as published in EPA-OPPTS Health Effects Test Guideline 870.2400 (1998).

[b] Reading of reactions is facilitated by the use of a binocular loupe, handheld slit lamp, or other means. After recording the scores at 24 h, the eyes may be further examined through the use of sodium fluoride solution and ultraviolet light to aid in the detection of corneal damage.

[c] Starred (*) scores indicate a positive response. If any animal receives one or more scores that are starred, the animal is considered to exhibit a positive response for eye irritation.

TABLE 30.8
Federal Hazardous Substances Act Criteria for Classification as an Eye Irritant[a]

Ocular Reactions for Individual Animals	Test Result
Corneal ulceration (other than stippling)	Positive
Corneal opacity (other than slight dulling of luster)	Positive
Inflammation of the iris (other than deepening of the folds or a slight circumcorneal injection of the blood vessels)	Positive
Conjunctival swelling with partial eversion of the eyelids or a diffuse crimson-red coloration with individual vessels not discernible	Positive

Group Result ($n = 6$)	FHSA Classification
4–6 animals in the test group exhibit a positive reaction	Eye irritant
2–3 animals in the test group exhibit a positive reaction	Inconclusive[b]
0–1 animals in the test group exhibit a positive reaction	Nonirritant

[a] 16 CFR 1500.42.

[b] If two to three animals exhibit a positive response, the test is repeated using new test animals. If three or more animals in the second test exhibit positive reactions, the material is classified as an eye irritant under FHSA. If one to two animals in the second test exhibit a positive response, a third test is conducted using new test animals. If one or more animals in the third test exhibit a positive response, the material is classified as an eye irritant under FHSA.

TABLE 30.9
Recommended Methods for Assessing Oral and Inhalation Toxicity[a]

	Acute Oral Toxicity	Acute Inhalation Toxicity (Gases and Vapors)	Acute Inhalation Toxicity (Dusts and Mists)
Test species	Albino rats (200–300 g)	Albino rats (200–300 g)	Albino rats (200–300 g)
n (per dose level)	10[b]	10[b]	10[b]
Dose levels	5000, 500, and 50 mg/kg[c]	200,000, 20,000, or 200 ppm[c,d]	2 mg/l[e]
Chemical exposure duration	Single oral gavage	Single 1-h exposure	Single 1-h exposure
Observation period (following exposure)	14 days	14 days	14 days
Comments	Rats should be fasted approximately 18 h before dosing	Either whole-body or nose-only exposure methods may be used	Either whole-body or nose-only exposure methods may be used
Classification	See Table 30.10	See Table 30.10	See Table 30.10

[a] Adapted from 16 CFR 1500.3. LD_{50}/LC_{50} data from previously conducted acceptable studies may be used to assign a classification; however, some end points routinely included in studies for other regulatory agencies (clinical observation, gross necropsy, etc.) need not necessarily be included in an LD_{50}/LC_{50} study done solely for FHSA classification purposes. LD_{50}/LC_{50} studies can be designed to satisfy multiple regulatory agencies; refer to EPA OPPTS Series 870 — Health Effects Test Guidelines (870.1100 for oral and 870.1300 for inhalation) or OECD Guidelines for Testing of Chemicals, No. 401 (oral) and No. 403 (inhalation).

[b] Normally five animals/sex/dose level are employed.

[c] Testing is initiated using the highest dose level only. If less than 50% mortality occurs at this (or any subsequent) level, no further testing is done and the LD_{50}/LC_{50} is estimated accordingly. If mortality is ≥ 50%, the next lower level is tested until the appropriate LD_{50}/LC_{50} estimation can be made.

[d] The highest exposure level may be limited to the saturated vapor concentration.

[e] 16 CFR 1500.3 discusses testing results up to 200 mg/l in the labeling classification of dusts and mists based on acute inhalation toxicity. Dusts or mists with an estimated or calculated 1-h LC_{50} ≤ 2 mg/l are classified under FHSA as highly toxic. Dusts or mists with an estimated or calculated LC_{50} > 2 mg/l and ≤ 200 mg/l are classified as toxic. It is presumed that dusts and mists having an LC_{50} > 200 mg/l are considered nontoxic, but this is not explicitly stated. All major federal and international testing guidelines specify maximum limit test exposure levels of 2 to 5 mg/l (for 4 h). Exposure duration aside, the toxicological relevance of a 200 mg/l exposure concentration is highly questionable. Achieving relevant airborne concentrations 40 times below this level is technically challenging. Further, physical laws for aerosol particle behavior limit minimum (respirable) particle size, even in experimental test atmospheres.[2] Based on these considerations, and in the absence of a clear benefit in doing so, inhalation testing of dusts and mists above 2 mg/l is not recommended.

TABLE 30.10
Hazard Classification under the Federal Hazardous Substances Act[a]

Term	Definition
Hazardous substance	"Any substance or mixture of substances which is toxic, corrosive, an irritant, a strong sensitizer, flammable or combustible, or generates pressure through decomposition, heat or other means, if such substance or mixture of substances may cause substantial personal injury or substantial illness during or as a proximate result of any customary or reasonably foreseeable handling or use, including reasonably foreseeable ingestion by children." *Definition includes*: • Any substance that, by regulation, the CPSC finds meets the requirements noted in the definition above; • Radioactive substances, with respect to the way these substances are used in a particular class of article or as packaged, that the CPSC deems sufficiently hazardous to require labeling in accordance to the FHSA to protect public health; • Toys or articles intended for use by children that, by regulation the CPSC finds, in accordance with section 3(e) of the FHSA, presents an electrical, mechanical, or thermal hazard;. • Any article which is not itself a pesticide within the meaning of FIFRA, but which is a hazardous substance within the meaning of FHSA by reason of bearing or containing such a pesticide. *Definition excludes*: • Pesticides subject to regulation under FIFRA; • Foods, drugs, cosmetics subject to the FDCA; • Substances intended as fuels when stored in containers and used in the heating, cooking, or refrigeration system of a house; • Source materials, special nuclear material, or by-product material as defined by the Atomic Energy Act of 1954, as amended, and regulations issued pursuant thereto by the Atomic Energy Commission.
Toxic	Any substance that has the capacity to produce personal injury or illness through ingestion, inhalation, or absorption through body surfaces. The definition is expanded to include the specifics listed below. This classification also applies to any substance that is "toxic" (but not "highly toxic") on the basis of human experience.
Acute toxicity	Unless specified, the studies listed below require a sufficient number of rats to give a statistically significant result and are to be in conformity with good scientific practices. In the acute studies, rats are exposed once and are observed for 14 days. *Acute Oral Toxicity* $LD_{50} > 50$ mg/kg and < 5000 mg/kg Substances with an $LD_{50} > 500$ mg/kg and < 5000 mg/kg, may be considered for some labeling exemptions if it can be shown that the labeling is not needed because of the physical form of the material, the size or closure of the container, human experience with the article, or other relevant factors. *Acute Inhalation Toxicity* 1-h LC_{50} in rats is > 200 ppm and ≤ 20,000 ppm (gas or vapor), *or* 1-h LC_{50} in rats is > 2 mg/l and ≤ 200 mg/l (dust or mist), if such concentration is likely to be encountered by humans when the substance is used in any reasonably foreseeable manner *Acute Dermal Toxicity*[b] $LD_{50} > 200$ mg/kg and ≤ 2000 mg/kg
Chronic toxicity[c]	A substance is toxic because it presents a chronic hazard if it falls into one of the following categories: *Carcinogen* — Substance is or contains a known or probable human carcinogen *Neurotoxicant* — Substance is or contains a known or probable human neurotoxicant *Developmental or reproductive toxicant* — Substance is or contains a known or probable human developmental or reproductive toxicant

TABLE 30.10 *(Continued)*
Hazard Classification under the Federal Hazardous Substances Act[a]

Term	Definition
Highly toxic	Any substance that falls into any one of the categories listed below. If the CPSC finds that available data on human experience with any substance indicate results different from those obtained on animals in the dosages and concentrations specified below, the human data take precedence. These studies involve a single exposure of 10 rats (oral, inhalation) or 10 rabbits (dermal) to the test substance followed by a 14-day observation period. *Acute Oral Toxicity* $LD_{50} \leq 50$ mg/kg *Acute Inhalation Toxicity* 1-h $LC_{50} \leq 200$ ppm (gas or vapor), *or* 1-h $LC_{50} \leq 2$ mg/l (dust or mist), provided such concentration is likely to be encountered by man when the substance is used in any reasonably foreseeable manner. *Acute Dermal Toxicity*[b] $LD_{50} \leq 200$ mg/kg
Corrosive	Any substance that in contact with living tissue will cause visible destruction or irreversible alterations in the tissue by chemical action at the site of exposure. This does not include the effect of chemical action on inanimate surface (e.g., corrosive to aluminum or steel). A substance would be considered corrosive if tested as described in 16 CFR 1500.41 and visible destruction or irreversible alteration of the tissue at the site of contact was observed.
Irritant	Any substance not corrosive within the meaning above, which on immediate, prolonged, or repeated contact with normal living tissue will induce a local inflammatory response. This includes substances classified as primary skin irritants and eye irritants according to 16 CFR 1500.41 and 16 CFR 1500.42, or where there are human data to indicate the material is an irritant to the skin or eyes.
Strong sensitizer	A substance that will cause, on normal living tissue through an allergic or photodynamic process, a hypersensitivity that becomes evident on reapplication of the same substance and that is designated as such by the CPSC. Before designating the substance as a strong sensitizer, the CPSC will consider the frequency of occurrence and the severity of reaction, and from these data will conclude that the substance has a significant potential to produce hypersensitivity.
Sensitizer	A substance that will induce an immunologically-mediated (allergic) response, including photosensitivity, that becomes evident upon re-exposure to the same substance. Occasionally it may induce a response on first exposure by virtue of active sensitization.
Normal living tissue	The allergic response occurs in normal living tissues, including skin and other organs such as the respiratory system or gastrointestinal tract, either singularly or in combination, following sensitization by contact, ingestion, or inhalation.
Strong	The CPSC shall consider the available data for a number of factors, including quantitative or qualitative risk assessment, frequency of occurrence and range of severity of reactions in healthy or susceptible populations, experimental animal and human data (considering dose–response relationships) with human data taking precedence, potency or bioavailability data, cross-reactivity, threshold of human sensitivity, epidemiological studies, case histories, occupational studies, and other appropriate *in vivo* or *in vitro* studies.
Severity	The minimal severity reaction required for classification as a "strong" sensitizer is a clinically important allergic reaction. This may include: substantial illness, physical discomfort, distress, hardship, and functional or structural impairment. These reactions may require medical treatment or may produce loss of functional activities.
Significant potential	A relative determination that must be made separately for each substance. It may be based on the chemical or functional properties of the substance, documented medical evidence of allergic reactions obtained from epidemiological studies or individual case reports, controlled *in vitro* or *in vivo* experiments, or susceptibility profiles in normal or allergic subjects.

[a] 16 CFR 1500.3.

[b] Method according to 16 CFR 1500.40.

[c] Detailed criteria for assigning a chronic toxicity classification to a material are located in 16 CFR 1500.135.

B. Art Materials

The Labeling of Hazardous Art Materials Act (LHAMA), promulgated in 1988, set standards for the evaluation and labeling of art materials (as defined earlier) for chronic toxic hazard potential. A key component of this act is that the producer or repackager of art materials is required to have the product formulation reviewed by a certified physician or toxicologist for potential chronic toxicity hazards.

The reviewer would normally perform a component-based assessment on the product, which is then used to arrive at appropriate precautionary labeling. The Act indicates that the reviewer shall make the labeling recommendation(s). The requirements for labeling are set forth in the standard of the American Society for Testing and Materials identified as ASTM D-4236, the provisions of which are contained in 16 CFR 1500.2.

In order for a thorough review to be performed, it is essential that a complete and accurate description of the product formula be available. The regulations specify that (with certain exceptions) this be held in confidence by the reviewer; however, unless the reviewer is an employee of the manufacturer or repackager, additional contractual assurances of confidentiality should be considered.

As for many consumer products, art materials are usually mixtures of many chemicals and toxicity test results on the final formulation or product are rarely available. Therefore, not only the individual components, but also the amount (percentage, usually by weight) of each component must be known to perform a full evaluation. The physical form of the final product, use exposure scenarios, potential for chemical reaction in the mixture during processing and sensitive populations, especially children, must all be taken into account when assessing the product.

On occasion, component information or final product formulation information is not available or is extremely difficult to obtain. In such cases, it may be appropriate to perform an empirical determination of the product composition analytically.

It is important to recognize that the LHAMA labeling requirements do not diminish the effect of required acute toxicity hazard warnings. The focus of LHAMA is on requiring precautionary warnings for chronic adverse health effects, defined as "a persistent toxic effect that develops over time from a single, prolonged or repeated exposure to a substance" (16 CFR 1500.14). Under this definition, such obvious hazards as carcinogenicity, developmental or reproductive toxicity, and neurotoxicity are considered chronic adverse effects. In addition, such less obvious toxicities as permanent skin scarring, irreversible ocular damage (especially to the cornea), sensitization or a permanent adverse effect to any other organ system meet the LHAMA definition of a chronic adverse effect. Further, the Act specifically cites a concern for harm to a nursing infant; therefore, the potential for any of the substances present to be expressed in human milk must also be assessed.

C. Cosmetics

In 21 CFR 720.4, the FDA describes 13 categories of cosmetics that contain at total of 66 different product types. In addition, each category contains provision for "other" products that do not specifically fit one of the preassigned product types. A listing of these categories and product types is presented in Table 30.11.

Premarket approval of cosmetics (as previously defined) is not required, and, in fact, there is no regulatory statute that requires any product safety testing for cosmetics. The manufacturer is responsible for assuring the safety of its cosmetic products and no product can be marketed if it contains "a poisonous or deleterious substance which may render it injurious to health" (FDCA, Section 601). [Note: The safety of color additives must be demonstrated with reasonable certainty according to the 1960 Color Additives Amendment to the FDCA.]

The industrial toxicologist is responsible for determining the level of testing necessary and appropriate for the safe introduction of cosmetic products into commerce. For many decades, this consisted of a fairly standard battery of acute tests for oral toxicity in rats, dermal toxicity in rabbits, primary dermal and ocular irritancy in rabbits, and dermal sensitization testing in guinea pigs. If appropriate, based on the intended-use pattern, acute inhalation testing in rats, or longer-term studies by the appropriate route of exposure may also have been conducted. While the merits of such animal testing and use shall likely forever remain in debate, this historical testing has provided an enormous body of safety and toxicity data for cosmetic ingredients and final products against which current ingredients, products, and reformulations can be compared. Since relatively few new chemicals or substances are entering the cosmetic product chain, the need for new safety studies in animals has continued to diminish. Cosmetic producers now rely more on historical safety data, structure–activity assessments, component assessments, and certain validated *in vitro* testing to document and demonstrate the safety of their products. If testing is needed, standard toxicity testing protocols appropriate for the route of administration and potential exposure are used.

Aside from the standard resources that can provide toxicity information on chemicals, several excellent resources targeted to the cosmetic industry are available. The *International Journal of Toxicology* (Taylor & Francis, publishers), the official journal of the American College of Toxicology, periodically dedicates an entire issue to the in-depth evaluation of a few to several cosmetic ingredients. These reports are issued by the Cosmetic Ingredient Review (CIR) Expert Panel as supported by the Cosmetic, Toiletry, and Fragrance Association, Inc. The CIR also publishes reports independently. The *International Journal of Toxicology* also periodically dedicates an entire issue to the publication of acute toxicity data. To date, data on approximately 500 Chemical Abstract Services-registered chemicals have been published.

In vitro alternatives to animal testing continue to hold promise and to be developed for use in the safety assessment of cosmetics, cosmetic ingredients, and other materials and products. However, to date, only one *in vitro* test system has gained wide and formal acceptance in the U.S. regulatory community. The Corrositex® (InVitro International, Irvine, CA) has been accepted by the FDA, EPA, and CPSC as a suitable substitute for dermal corrosion data developed in animals, *provided* a positive result is obtained.

Cosmetic manufacturers routinely file their cosmetic product ingredient composition (21 CFR 720) and register their production/manufacturing sites (21 CFR 710) with the FDA. Purported adverse reactions to cosmetics are reported to the FDA by the manufacturer (21 CFR 730). These are technically considered to be voluntary programs, but participation within the cosmetic industry is essentially complete.

TABLE 30.11
Cosmetic Product Categories[a]

Category	Product Types
Baby products	Shampoos
	Lotions
	Oils
	Powders
	Creams
	Other baby products
Bath preparations	Bath oils, tablets, salts
	Bubble baths
	Bath capsules
	Other bath preparations
Eye makeup preparations	Eyebrow pencil
	Eyeliner
	Eye shadow
	Eye lotion
	Eye makeup remover
	Mascara
	Other eye makeup preparations

TABLE 30.11 *(Continued)*
Cosmetic Product Categories[a]

Category	Product Types
Fragrance preparations	Colognes and toilet waters
	Perfumes
	Powders (dusting and talcum; excluding aftershave talc)
	Sachets
	Other fragrance preparations
Hair preparations (noncoloring)	Hair conditioners
	Hair sprays (aerosol fixatives)
	Hair straighteners
	Permanent waves
	Rinses (noncoloring)
	Shampoos (noncoloring)
	Tonics, dressings, and other hair grooming aids
	Wave sets
	Other hair preparations
Hair coloring preparations	Hair dyes and colors (all types requiring caution statement and patch test)
	Hair tints
	Hair rinses (coloring)
	Hair shampoos (coloring)
	Hair color sprays (aerosol)
	Hair lighteners with color
	Hair bleaches
	Other hair coloring preparations
Makeup preparations (not eye)	Blushers (all types)
	Face powders
	Foundations
	Leg and body paints
	Lipstick
	Makeup bases
	Rouges
	Makeup fixatives
	Other makeup preparations
Manicuring preparations	Basecoats and undercoats
	Cuticle softeners
	Nail creams and lotions
	Nail extenders
	Nail polish and enamel
	Nail polish and enamel removers
	Other manicuring preparations
Oral hygiene products	Dentifrices (aerosol, liquid, pastes, and powders)
	Mouthwashes and breath fresheners (liquids and sprays)
	Other oral hygiene products
Personal cleanliness	Bath soaps and detergents
	Deodorants (underarm)
	Douches
	Feminine hygiene deodorants
	Other personal cleanliness products

TABLE 30.11 *(Continued)*
Cosmetic Product Categories[a]

Category	Product Types
Shaving preparations	Aftershave lotions
	Beard softeners
	Men's talcum
	Preshave lotions (all types)
	Shaving cream (aerosol, brushless, and lather)
	Shaving soap (cakes, sticks, etc.)
	Other shaving preparations
Skin care preparations (creams, lotions, powders, and sprays)	Cleansing (cold creams, cleansing lotions, liquids, and pads)
	Depilatories
	Face and neck (excluding shaving preparations)
	Body and hand (excluding shaving preparations)
	Foot powders and sprays
	Moisturizing
	Night
	Paste masks (mud packs)
	Skin fresheners
	Other skin preparations
Suntan preparations	Suntan gels, creams, and liquids
	Indoor tanning preparations
	Other suntan preparations

[a] Taken from 21 CFR 720.4.

D. DISINFECTANT HOUSEHOLD PRODUCTS

Because they contain a pesticide, usually an antimicrobial agent, disinfectant household products bearing a label claim for antimicrobial activity are subject to regulation and registration via the EPA FIFRA. Data development and registration for approval to market as a disinfectant must be sought following the standard EPA FIFRA process described elsewhere in this book.

Data required for submission may include, but are not necessarily limited to (as appropriate for the intended use), product chemistry, residue chemistry, environmental fate, toxicology, reentry protection, aerial drift evaluation, toxicity to wildlife and aquatic organisms, protection of plant and nontarget insects.

Assessments of the pure and technical grades of the active substance may need to be performed, as well as information on intentionally added inert ingredients, metabolites of active or inert ingredients, the end-use product, the end-use product plus recommended vehicles or adjuvants, or any additional substance that could act as a synergist to the product for which registration is sought (40 CFR 158.75).

Previously developed data may be used provided they were done under GLPs, meet the purposes of the regulation, and permit sound scientific judgments to be made. The Pesticide Assessments Guidelines contain the standards for conducting acceptable tests (although results from studies conducted using other appropriate protocols are acceptable), guidance on evaluation and reporting of data, definitions of terms, further guidance on when data are required, and examples of acceptable protocols. These guidelines are available through the National Technical Information Service, 5285 Port Royal Road, Springfield, VA 22161 (703-487-4650).

E. DIETARY SUPPLEMENTS

The regulatory environment for dietary supplements is relatively new and evolving. The Dietary Supplement Health and Education Act (DSHEA) was enacted in 1994, primarily under the jurisdiction of the FDA. For dietary supplements, the FDA oversees safety, manufacturing, and product information, including claims, while the FTC regulates advertising.

DSHEA applies only to "new" dietary supplements, i.e., those containing an ingredient not marketed in the United States before 1994. Manufacturers desiring to market such a product have two choices. One is to submit to FDA information that supports the conclusion that the new ingredient can reasonably be expected to be safe, i.e., that it does not present a significant or unreasonable risk of illness or injury under the recommended conditions of use. This information must be submitted at least 75 days before the product is expected to go on the market and is made available to the public 90 days after the FDA receives it. The second option for manufacturers is to ask the FDA to establish conditions under which the new ingredient would reasonably be expected to be safe. As of January 1999, no such petitions had been received.

Contrast the above with food additives, which, if not generally recognized as safe (GRAS), are subject to the FDA approval process for new food ingredients *before* marketing. The food additive manufacturers must conduct extensive, often expensive, and long-term safety studies to meet this regulatory burden of proof of safety.

This is further contrasted against the regulatory and approval requirements for drugs. Dietary supplements, which often make curative-, preventative-, or treatment-like claims, are not required to undergo clinical studies for effectiveness, safety, interactions with other substances, or determination of appropriate dosages.

Issues concerning the safety assessment of dietary supplements via epidemiological types of studies are numerous. In the absence of controlled studies, an uncertain history of use must be relied upon. Many dietary supplements are derived from plants. Plant types, identification, and nomenclature vary regionally as well as internationally. The source, or origin, of the material used to prepare or manufacture the dietary supplement can be a source of variability and contamination. Biomarkers for exposure have not generally been established and therefore estimates of exposure are difficult to obtain. The potential effects of mixtures of dietary supplements and possible interactive effects must also be considered.

Existing dietary supplements may or may not be manufactured under Good Manufacturing Practices (GMPs). DSHEA authorizes the FDA to establish GMPs for dietary supplements. The FDA has sought public comment on establishing GMPs for dietary supplements if conventional food GMPs are inadequate.

Certain dietary supplement manufacturers trade associations are striving toward self-regulation. For example, industry-specific GMPs have been devised by the Council for Responsible Nutrition, which are voluntarily followed by some manufacturers. Limited safety testing of dietary supplements, using studies similar to the "upper limit protocols" for vitamins and minerals proposed by the National Academy of Sciences, has some support in the industry.

SECTION 6. RESOURCES FOR REGULATORY AND TOXICTY INFORMATION

TABLE 30.12
Resources for Regulatory and Toxicity Information

Name	Source of Availability
American College of Government Industrial Hygienists (ACGIH)	http://www.acgih.org
Cosmetic Ingredient Review (CIR)	cirinfo@cir-safety.org
Code of Federal Regulations (CFR)	http://www.access.gpo.gov/nara/cfr/
Consumer Product Safety Commission (CPSC)	http://www.cpsc.gov
Environmental Protection Agency (EPA)	http://www.epa.gov
EPA Integrated Risk Information System (IRIS)	http://www.epa.gov/iris/
EPA Office of Pesticide Programs (OPP)	http://www.epa.gov/pesticides/
EPA Technical Documents	http://www.epa.gov/epahome/techdoc.htm
Food and Drug Administration (FDA)	http://www.fda.gov
Grateful Med V2.6.2	http://igm.nlm.nih.gov
International Agency for Research on Cancer (IARC)	http://www.iarc.fr/index.html
International Journal of Toxicology	Taylor & Francis, Philadelphia, PA (publisher)
Medline	http://igm.nlm.nih.gov
Medscape	http://www.medscape.com/
MSDSs	http://www.ilpi.com/msds/index.chtml
Organisation for Economic Cooperation and Development (OECD)	http://www.oecd.org
Office of Prevention, Pesticides, and Toxic Substances (OPPTS)	http://www.epa.gov/internet/oppts/
Patty's Industrial Hygiene and Toxicology	Available in book form or on CD-ROM from John Wiley & Sons, New York (publisher)
Toxline®	Available via Grateful Med V2.6.2
Toxic Substances Control Act Test Submissions (TSCATS), via The Right to Know Network	http://www.rtk.net/tscatsinputstandard.html

REFERENCES

1. Jackson, E.M., Consumer products: cosmetics and topical over-the-counter drug products, in *Regulatory Toxicology*, Chengelis, C., Holson, J.F., and Gad, S.C., Eds., Raven Press, New York, 1995, chap. 5.
2. Anonymous, Commentary — recommendations for the conduct of acute inhalation limit tests (prepared by Technical Committee of the Inhalation Specialty Section, Society of Toxicology), *Fundam. Appl. Toxicol.*, 18, 321–327, 1992.

31 Regulatory Toxicology: Notification of New Substances in the European Union

Michael J. Derelanko, Ph.D., D.A.B.T., F.A.T.S.

CONTENTS

SECTION 1. INTRODUCTION

Requirements for notification of new substances in the European Union are established under Council Directive 92/32/EEC of April 30, 1992 amending for the seventh time Directive 67/548/EEC on the approximation of the laws, regulations, and administrative provisions relating to the classification, packaging, and labeling of dangerous substances.[1] The purposes of the 7th Amendment are to approximate laws, regulations, and administrative provisions of the Member States on: a) the notification of substances; b) the exchange of information on notified substances; c) the assessment of the potential risk to humans and the environment of notified substances; d) classification, packaging, and labeling of dangerous substances.

Testing requirements are linked to quantities of substances marketed with yearly production and cumulative thresholds triggering the type of tests. There are reduced notification requirements for substances placed on the market in quantities of less than 1 tonne per year per manufacturer. Production at greater than 1 tonne per year or 5 tonnes cummulative requires base set testing.

Once a notification has been made at more than 1 tonne, any quantity of substance may be supplied. However, the competent authority must be informed when the 10, 100, or 1,000 tonnes per year thresholds have been exceeded or the 50, 500, or 5,000 tonnes cumulative thresholds have been reached.

All tests (including physiochemical) must be conducted to GLP and European Community (EC) test guidelines. The adequacy of existing test data which were generated by methods other than stated in the EC guidelines will be decided on a case-by-case basis.

In the absence of any indication from the Competent Authority to the contrary, substances notified at less than 1 tonne per year may be placed on the market no sooner than 30 days after receipt by the Authority of a dossier in conformity with the Directive. In the absence of any indications from the Competent Authority to the contrary, substances notified at greater than 1 tonne per year may be placed on the market no sooner than 60 days after receipt by the Authority of a dossier in conformity with the Directive.

The following information is intended as a brief overview of the requirements for notification of new substances in the European Union. Readers are referred to the referenced legislation for a detailed description of the requirements. Those unfamiliar with the notification procedure are advised to contact consultants specializing in notifications. Several European contract laboratories offer such services including advice on legislation, conduct of studies, preparation and submission of the notification in the relevant language, conduct of discussions and negotiations with competent authorities, and advice on and negotiation of higher level testing programs.

TABLE 31.1
Exemptions from Notification

- Medicinal products[a]
- Veterinary products
- Cosmetic products
- Waste
- Foodstuffs
- Animal feedstuffs
- Pesticides
- Radioactive substances
- Other substances or preparations covered by equivalent European Community (EC) notification or approval procedures

[a] Active ingredients only, chemical intermediates are not exempt.

Source: Brooker.[2]

TABLE 31.2
Notification of a New Substance: Who Makes the Notification and to What Country

a. Substances manufactured in the European Community
  - Notification is made by the manufacturer to the Competent Authority in the country of manufacture.
  - A change of manufacturer or a change of country of manufacture will require a new notification.
b. Substances manufactured outside of the European Community
  - A single notification is made to the Competent Authority of the country in which they are resident by a person designated by the manufacturer as its 'sole' representative. This person must be established within the community, need not be the importer, but must list all importations and quantities introduced onto the European market.
or
  - A separate notification is made by each importer.

Source: Brooker.[2]

TABLE 31.3
Notification of a New Substance: Information and
Test Data Required

Annual Total	Cumulative Total	Data Requirements (Refer to Table 31.5)
< 10 kg		Exempt
10–100 kg		Annex VII C
100–1,000 kg	500 kg	Annex VII B
> 1,000 kg (1 tonne)	5,000 kg	Annex VII A
> 10 tonnes	50 tonnes	Level 1 (may be required[a])
> 100 tonnes	500 tonnes	Level 1
> 1,000 tonnes	5,000 tonnes	Level 2

[a] Testing at 10/50 tonnage thresholds will depend on the nature of the chemical, its uses, and the results of existing tests.

Source: Brooker.[2]

TABLE 31.4
Information Common to All Notifications

Identity
- Identity of manufacturer and notifier
- Location of production site
- Identity of addresses of importers
- Name(s) of substance
- Molecular and structural formula
- Composition of substance
- Methods of detection and determination
- Physical state of the substance at 20°C and 101.3 kPa

Substance information
- Production — sufficient information to allow an approximate but realistic estimation of human and environmental exposure. Precise details (e.g., those of a commercially sensitive nature) are not required.
- Technological process
- Exposure estimates
- Proposed uses
- Quantities
- Methods and precautions for handling, storage, and transport
- Emergency measures
- Packaging
- Ways of rendering the substance harmless
- Classification and proposed labeling

Source: Brooker.[2]

TABLE 31.5
Data Requirements for Notification

Annex VII C
(Supply at 10–100 kg/yr)

Flash point/flammability
Acute toxicity (oral or inhalation)

Annex VII B
(Supply at 100–1,000 kg/yr or 500 kg cumulative)

Melting point/boiling point	Eye irritation
Water solubility	Skin sensitization
Partition coefficient (*n*-octanol/water)	Ames
Flashpoint/flammability	
Vapor pressure (may be required)	Biodegradation
	Daphnia acute toxicity test (may be required)
Acute toxicity (oral or inhalation)	
Skin irritation	

Annex VII A
"The Base Set"
(Supply at > 1,000 kg/yr or 5,000 kg cumulative)

Melting point/boiling point	Flash point flammability
Relative density	Explosive properties
Vapor pressure	Self-Ignition temperature
Surface tension	Oxidizing properties
Water solubility	Granulometry
Partition/coefficient (*n*-octanol/water)	
	Ames test
Acute toxicity (2 routes)	*In vitro* cytogenetics
Skin irritation	Reproductive toxicity screen
Eye irritation	Toxicokinetic assessment (derived from base set data)
Skin sensitization	
28-day repeat dose toxicity	
	Biodegradation
Acute toxicity for fish	Hydrolysis as a function of pH
Acute toxicity for *Daphnia*	Soil adsorption/desorption screen
Algal growth inhibition	
Bacterial inhibition	

Level 1 Studies[a] Annex VIII
(Supply at > 10[b] or 100 tonnes/yr or 50[b] tonnes cumulative)

Analytical method development	21-day *Daphnia* toxicity
Physiochemical properties of thermal decomposition products	Further fish toxicity studies
	Bioaccumulation study
	Test on higher plants
Fertility study (one generation)	Earthworm toxicity
Teratology study	Inherent biodegradation
Subchronic/chronic toxicity study	Further adsorption/desorption
Additional mutagenicity studies	
Basic toxicokinetics	

Level 2 Studies[c] Annex VIII
(Supply at > 1,000 tonnes/yr or 5,000 tonnes cumulative)

Chronic toxicity study	Additional test for accumulation, degradation,
Carcinogenicity study	and mobility

TABLE 31.5 *(Continued)*
Data Requirements for Notification

(Level 2 continued)

Fertility study (2-generation)	Additional test for adsorption/desorption
Developmental toxicity (peri- and postnatal)	Further fish toxicity studies
Teratology study (different species from level 1)	Bird toxicity studies
	Toxicity studies with other organisms

Biotransformation
Pharmacokinetics
Additional test to investigate organ or system toxicity

[a] Studies required at level 1 are on a negotiated basis. Negotiations begin once a trigger tonnage has been exceeded. Studies chosen will be based on 1) the quantity supplied, 2) the results of the Base-Set Tests, and 3) the degree of exposure to humans and the environment.

[b] Testing at the 10/50 tonnage thresholds will depend on the nature of the chemical, its uses, and the results of earlier tests.

[c] Studies required at level 2 are on a negotiated basis. Negotiations begin once a trigger tonnage has been exceeded. Studies chosen will be based on: 1) the quantity supplied, 2) the results of earlier tests, and 3) the degree of exposure to humans and the environment.

Source: Brooker.[2]

TABLE 31.6
Comparison of the Notification Requirements of the EU and Selected Countries

Study	OECD[a]	EC[b]	Switzerland[c]	Austria[d]	Canada[e]	Australia[f]
Spectra	√	√	√	√	√	√
Melting point	√[g]	√	√	√	√	√[g]
Boiling point	√[g]	√	√	√	√	√[g]
Relative density	√	√	√	√	√	√
Vapour pressure	√	√	√	√	√	√
Surface tension		√	√	√		
Water solubility	√	√	√	√	√	√
Partition coefficient	√	√	√	√	√	√
Fat solubility	√		√[h]	√	√	
Dissociation constant	√		√		√	√
Granulometry	√	√	—[i]		√	√
Henry's Law constant			—[i]			
Volatility from water			—[i]			
Complex formation constants			—[i]			
Stability			—[i]			
Viscosity			—[i]			
Permeability			—[i]			
Flash point (liquids)		√		√		√
Flammability tests		√		√		√
Explosivity		√		√		√
Oxidizing properties		√		√		√
Autoflammability		√		√		√
Acute oral toxicity	√	√	—[o]	√	√	√
Acute dermal toxicity	√	√[k]	—[o]	√[k]	√[k]	√[k]
Acute inhalation toxicity	√	√[k]	—[o]	√[k]	√[k]	√[k]
Skin irritation	√	√	—[o]	√	√	√
Eye irritation	√	√	—[o]	√		√
Skin sensitization	√	√	—[o]	√	√	√

TABLE 31.6 *(Continued)*
Comparison of the Notification Requirements of the EU and Selected Countries

Study	OECD[a]	EC[b]	Switzerland[c]	Austria[d]	Canada[e]	Australia[f]
Subacute toxicity	✓	✓	—[j]	✓	✓	✓
Ames test	—[l]	✓	✓	✓	✓	✓
In vitro chromosome aberration test	—[l]	✓	✓	✓[m]	✓	✓
Mouse micronucleus test	—[l]	—[n]	—[j]	—[m]	✓[o]	✓[p]
Mouse lymphoma, assay	—[l]	—[q]	—[j]			
Acute fish toxicity	✓	✓	✓	✓	✓	✓
Acute *Daphnia* toxicity		✓	✓	✓	✓	✓
Algal growth inhibition	✓	✓	—[i]			✓
Daphnia reproduction study	✓		✓			✓
Fish bioaccumulation			—[i]			—[r]
Earthworm toxicity				✓		
Ready biodegradability	✓	✓	✓	✓	✓	✓
Activated sludge respiration inhibition		✓[s]				
Abiotic degradation by hydrolysis	✓	✓[t]	✓	✓	✓	✓
Soil adsorption/desorption screening test	✓	✓[u]	—[i]		✓	✓
Anaerobic biodegradation			—[i]			
Soil biodegradation			—[i]			
Photolysis			—[i]			

[a] The MPD is recommended by the OECD for adequate hazard assessment of new chemical substances. (MPD = minimum premarketing data set).

[b] Full notification for supply in the EC at 1 tonne per annum (or 5 tonnes cumulative) under the "Seventh Amendment" Council Directive 92/32/EEC. Note that a screening test for toxicity to reproduction will also be required as part of the Base Set when a suitable method has been developed.

[c] These are the minimum data requirements for notification under the Swiss Ordinance on Environmentally Hazardous Substances.

[d] Full notification for supply in Austria at 1 tonne per annum under the Austrian Chemicals Law.

[e] These are the data of Schedule III of the Imminent Canadian New Substances Notification Regulations to permit supply at above 10 tonnes per annum (or over 50 tonnes cumulative).

[f] Full notification for supply in Australia at 1 tonne per annum under the National Industrial Chemicals Notification and Assessment Scheme (NICNAS).

[g] It is adequate to determine either the melting point or boiling point, whichever is most appropriate.

[h] Solubility in an organic solvent is adequate as an alternative to fat solubility.

[i] These additional studies may be required if the minimum data are inadequate for full environmental assessment.

[j] Available toxicity studies are evaluated for notification under the Swiss Ordinance on Environmentally Hazardous Substances and also under the Order relating to Toxic Substances.

[k] The choice of exposure route for the second acute toxicity study depends on the respirability of the substance evaluated from the granulometry test and the likely human exposure route.

[l] The OECD MPD specifies that mutagenicity should be evaluated.

[m] The second mutagenicity test for notification in Austria can be either the *in vitro* chromosome aberration test or an *in vivo* study such as the mouse micronucleus test, although the former may be preferred from an animal welfare viewpoint and be consistent with other notification schemes.

[n] The mouse micronucleus test or an *in vivo* chromosome aberration test will normally be required immediately after notification in the EC if any of the *in vitro* Base Set mutagenicity tests are positive.

[o] The third mutagenicity study required for notification in Canada can be either the mouse micronucleus test or the *in vivo* chromosome aberration test.

[p] The mouse micronucleus test has been agreed with the Australian regulatory authorities as an alternative to the dominant lethal assay suggested in the official guidelines.

[q] The mouse lymphoma assay or HPRT locus test is required as part of the EC Base Set if the Ames test is positive.

[r] A fish bioaccumulation study may be needed if the substance is not "readily biodegradable" and has a high partition coefficient.

[s] The activated sludge respiration inhibition test is conducted on nonbiodegradable substances to establish whether the lack of biodegradation is caused by toxicity to microorganisms, and also to predict if adverse effects on sewage treatment plants could occur.

[t] Required for substances which are not "readily biodegradable."

[u] A soil adsorption/desorption screening test is part of the Base Set, but notifications will be accepted without this until the proposed reverse-phase high-performance liquid chromatography method is finalized, as an alternative to the OECD screening test.

Source: Knight.[3]

TABLE 31.7
Selected OECD Guidelines for Testing of Chemicals

Mammalian:

#401	acute oral toxicity, LD_{50}
#402	acute dermal toxicity
#403	acute inhalation toxicity
#404	acute dermal irritation/corrosion
#405	acute eye irritation
#406	contact sensitization
#407	repeated dose 28-day oral toxicity (rodent)
#408	repeated dose 90-day oral toxicity (rodent)
#409	repeated dose 90-day oral toxicity (non-rodent)
#410	repeated dose 28-day dermal toxicity
#411	repeated dose 90-day dermal toxicity
#412	repeated dose 28-day inhalation toxicity
#413	repeated dose 90-day inhalation toxicity
#414	developmental toxicity study
#415	one generation reproduction
#416	two generation reproduction
#417	metabolism and pharmacokinetics
#418	acute exposure delayed neurotoxicity of organophosphorus substances
#419	repeated exposure delayed neurotoxicity of organophosphorus substances
#420	acute oral toxicity, fixed dose procedure
#421	reproductive/developmental toxicity screen
#422	combined repeated dose 28-day oral toxicity/ developmental toxicity screen
#423	acute oral toxicity, acute toxic class
#424	neurotoxicity screening battery
#425	acute oral toxicity, up and down method
#451	carcinogenicity
#452	chronic toxicity
#453	combined chronic toxicity/carcinogenicity

Genetox:

#471	reverse mutation assay/*Salmonella* (Ames test)
#472	reverse mutation assay/*E. coli*
#473	*In vitro* mammalian chromosome aberration test
#474	micronucleus test
#475	*In vivo* bone marrow mammalian chromosome aberration test
#476	*In vitro* mammalian cell gene mutation test (mouse lymphoma)
#477	sex-linked recessive lethal test (*Drosophila*)
#478	rodent dominant lethal test (mouse)
#479	*in vitro* sister chromatid exchange (SCE) assay
#480	gene mutation assay/*Saccharomyces*
#481	mitotic recombination assay/*Saccharomyces*
#482	*In vivo* unscheduled DNA synthesis (UDS)
#483	mammalian spermatogonial chromosome aberration assay
#484	mouse spot test
#485	mouse heritable translocation assay
#486	mitotic recombination assay/*Saccharomyces*

Ecotox/Aquatic:

#106	absorption/desorption
#201	algal growth inhibition
#202	acute toxicology/*Daphnia*

TABLE 31.7 *(Continued)*
Selected OECD Guidelines for Testing of Chemicals

#203	acute toxicity/fish
#204	14-day prolonged toxicity/fish
#205	avian dietary toxicity
#206	avian reproduction
#207	acute toxicity/earthworm
#208	terrestrial plant growth test
#209	activated sludge respiration inhibition
#210	fish early life-stage toxicity
#211	21-day *Daphnia* reproduction
#301	ready biodegradability
#302	inherent biodegradability
#305	bioaccumulation/fish

TABLE 31.8
Risk (R) Phrases Used in the European Community (EU)

R1:	Explosive when dry
R2:	Risk of explosion by shock, friction, fire or other sources of ignition
R3:	Extreme risk of explosion by shock, friction, fire or other sources of ignition
R4:	Forms very sensitive explosive metallic compounds
R5:	Heating may cause an explosion
R6:	Explosive with or without contact with air
R7:	May cause fire
R8:	Contact with combustible material may cause fire
R9:	Explosive when mixed with combustible material
R10:	Flammable
R11:	Highly flammable
R12:	Extremely flammable
R14:	Reacts violently with water
R15:	Contact with water liberates extremely flammable gases
R16:	Explosive when mixed with oxidizing substances
R17:	Spontaneously flammable in air
R18:	In use may form flammable/explosive vapor-air mixture
R19:	May form explosive peroxides
R20:	Harmful by inhalation
R21:	Harmful in contact with skin
R22:	Harmful if swallowed
R23:	Toxic by inhalation
R24:	Toxic in contact with skin
R25:	Toxic if swallowed
R26:	Very toxic by inhalation
R27.	Very toxic in contact with skin
R28:	Very toxic if swallowed
R29:	Contact with water liberates toxic gas
R30:	Can become highly flammable in use
R31:	Contact with acids liberates toxic gas
R32:	Contact with acids liberates very toxic gas
R33:	Danger of cumulative effects
R34:	Causes burns
R35:	Causes severe burns

TABLE 31.8 *(Continued)*
Risk (R) Phrases Used in the European Community (EU)

R36:	Irritating to the eyes
R37:	Irritating to the respiratory system
R38:	Irritating to the skin
R39:	Danger of very serious irreversible effects
R40:	Possible risk of irreversible effects*

* (As this book went to press, it seemed likely that the R40 phrase would be changed to "Limited evidence of a carcinogenic effect." The current phrase above would be allocated to R68.)

R41:	Risk of serious damage to the eyes
R42:	May cause sensitisation by inhalation
R43:	May cause sensitisation by skin contact
R44:	Risk explosion if heated under confinement
R45:	May cause cancer
R46:	May cause heritable genetic damage
R48:	Danger of serious damage to health by prolonged exposure
R49:	May cause cancer by inhalation
R50:	Very toxic to aquatic organisms
R51:	Toxic to aquatic organisms
R52:	Harmful to aquatic organisms
R53:	May cause long term adverse effects in the aquatic environment
R54:	Toxic to flora
R55:	Toxic to fauna
R56:	Toxic to soil organisms
R57:	Toxic to bees
R58:	May cause long term adverse effects to the environment
R59:	Dangerous for the ozone layer
R60:	May impair fertility
R61:	May cause harm to the unborn child
R62:	Possible risk of impaired fertility
R63:	Possible risk of harm to the unborn child
R64:	May cause harm to breastfed babies
R68:	Possible risk of irreversible effects*

* (As this book went to press, it seemed likely that the R40 phrase above would be allocated under R68.)

Combination of Particular Risks

R14/15:	Reacts violently with water, liberating extremely flammable gases
R15/29:	Contact with water liberates toxic, extremely flammable gas
R20/21:	Harmful by inhalation and in contact with skin
R20/21/22:	Harmful by inhalation, in contact with skin and if swallowed
R20/22:	Harmful by inhalation and if swallowed
R21/22:	Harmful in contact with skin and if swallowed
R23/24:	Toxic by inhalation and in contact with skin
R23/24/25:	Toxic by inhalation, in contact with skin, and if swallowed
R23/25:	Toxic by inhalation and if swallowed
R24/25:	Toxic in contact with skin and if swallowed
R26/27:	Very toxic by inhalation and in contact with skin
R26/27/28:	Very toxic by inhalation, in contact with skin and if swallowed
R26/28:	Very toxic by inhalation and if swallowed
R27/28:	Very toxic in contact with skin and if swallowed
R36/37:	Irritating to eyes, respiratory system

TABLE 31.8 *(Continued)*
Risk (R) Phrases Used in the European Community (EU)

R36/37/38:	Irritating to eyes, respiratory system and skin
R36/38:	Irritating to eyes and skin
R37/38:	Irritating to respiratory system and skin
R39/23:	Toxic: danger of very serious irreversible effects through inhalation
R39/23/24:	Toxic: danger of very serious irreversible effects through inhalation and in contact with skin
R39/23/24/25:	Toxic: danger of very serious irreversible effects through inhalation, in contact with skin and if swallowed
R39/23/25:	Toxic: danger of very serious irreversible effects through inhalation and if swallowed
R39/24:	Toxic: danger of very serious irreversible effects in contact with skin
R39/24/25:	Toxic: danger of very serious irreversible effects in contact with skin and if swallowed
R39/25:	Toxic: danger of very serious irreversible effects if swallowed
R39/26:	Very Toxic: danger of very serious irreversible effects through inhalation
R39/26/27:	Very Toxic: danger of very serious irreversible effects through inhalation and in contact with skin
R39/26/27/28:	Very Toxic: danger of very serious irreversible effects through inhalation, in contact with skin and if swallowed
R39/26/28:	Very Toxic: danger of very serious irreversible effects through inhalation and if swallowed
R39/27:	Very Toxic: danger of very serious irreversible effects in contact with skin
R39/27/28:	Very Toxic: danger of very serious irreversible effects in contact with skin and if swallowed
R39/28:	Very Toxic: danger of very serious irreversible effects if swallowed
R40*/20:	Harmful: possible risk of irreversible effects through inhalation
R40*/20/21:	Harmful: possible risk of irreversible effects through inhalation and in contact with skin
R40*/20/21/22:	Harmful: possible risk of irreversible effects through inhalation, in contact with skin and if swallowed
R40*/20/22:	Harmful: possible risk of irreversible effects through inhalation and if swallowed
R40*/22:	Harmful: possible risk of irreversible effects if swallowed
R40*/21:	Harmful: possible risk of irreversible effects in contact with skin
R40*/21/22:	Harmful: possible risk of irreversible effects in contact with skin and if swallowed

* (See potential phrase change for R40.)

R42/43:	May cause sensitisation by inhalation and skin contact
R48/20:	Harmful: danger of serious damage to health by prolonged exposure through inhalation
R48/20/21:	Harmful: danger of serious damage to health by prolonged exposure through inhalation and in contact with skin
R48/20/21/22:	Harmful: danger of serious damage to health by prolonged exposure through inhalation, in contact with skin and if swallowed
R48/20/22:	Harmful: danger of serious damage to health by prolonged exposure through inhalation and if swallowed
R48/21:	Harmful: danger of serious damage to health by prolonged exposure in contact with skin
R48/21/22:	Harmful: danger of serious damage to health by prolonged exposure in contact with skin and if swallowed
R48/22:	Harmful: danger of serious damage to health by prolonged exposure if swallowed
R48/23:	Toxic: danger of serious damage to health by prolonged exposure through inhalation
R48/23/24:	Toxic: danger of serious damage to health by prolonged exposure through inhalation and in contact with skin
R48/23/24/25:	Toxic: danger of serious damage to health by prolonged exposure through inhalation, in contact with skin and if swallowed
R48/23/25:	Toxic: danger of serious damage to health by prolonged exposure through inhalation and if swallowed
R48/24:	Toxic: danger of serious damage to health by prolonged exposure in contact with skin
R48/24/25:	Toxic: danger of serious damage to health by prolonged exposure in contact with skin and if swallowed
R48/25:	Toxic: danger of serious damage to health by prolonged exposure if swallowed
R50/53:	Very toxic to aquatic organisms, may cause long-term adverse effects in the aquatic environment
R51/53:	Toxic to aquatic organisms, may cause long-term adverse effects in the aquatic environment
R52/53:	Harmful to aquatic organisms, may cause long-term adverse effects in the aquatic environment

SECTION 2. GLOSSARY[1]

(As relates to the 7th Directive for Notification of New Substances in the European Community.)

A. General

EINECS European Inventory of Existing Commercial Substances. This inventory contains the definitive list of all substances deemed to be on the Community market on 18 September 1981. It is a closed list searchable by CAS number and chemical name.

ELINCS European List of New Chemical Substances. The list contains the EEC number, notification number, trade name, classification, and in some cases the IUPAC name.

Notification Document, with the requisite information, presented to the competent authority of a Member State.

Placing on the market The making available of a substance to third parties. Incorporation into the community customs territory shall be deemed to be placing on the market.

Polymer A substance consisting of molecules characterized by the sequence of one or more types of monomer units and comprising a simple weight majority of molecules containing at least three monomer units which are covalently bound to at least one other monomer unit or other reactant and consists of less than a simple weight majority of molecules of the same molecular weight. Such molecules must be distributed over a range of molecular weights wherein differences in the molecular weight are primarily attributable to differences in the number of monomer units. In the context of this definition a "monomer unit" means the reacted form of a monomer in a polymer.

Preparations Mixtures or solutions composed of two or more substances.

Process-oriented research and development The further development of a substance in the course of which pilot plant of production trials are used to test the fields of application of the substance.

Scientific research and development Scientific experimentation, analysis or chemical research carried out under controlled conditions; it includes the determination of intrinsic properties, performance, and efficacy, as well as scientific investigation related to product development.

Substances Chemical elements and their compounds in the natural state or obtained by any production process, including any additive necessary to preserve the stability of the products and any impurity deriving from the process used, but excluding any solvent which may be separated without affecting the stability of the substance or changing its compositions.

B. Toxicological

Carcinogenic substances Substances or preparations which, if they are inhaled or ingested or if they penetrate the skin, may induce cancer or increase its incidence.

Corrosive substances Substances or preparations which may, on contact with living tissues, destroy them.

Environmental toxic substances Substances and preparations which are dangerous for the environment: substances and preparations which, were they to enter the environment, would or may present an immediate or delayed danger for one or more components of the environment.

Harmful substances Substances and preparations that may cause death or acute or chronic damage to health when inhaled, swallowed, or absorbed via the skin.

Irritant substances Noncorrosive substances and preparations which, through immediate, prolonged, or repeated contact with the skin or mucus membrane, may cause inflammation.

Mutagenic substances Substances and preparations which, if they are inhaled or ingested or if they penetrate the skin, may induce heritable genetic defects or increase their incidence.

Reprotoxic substances Substances and preparations which, if they are inhaled or ingested or if they penetrate the skin, may produce, or increase the incidence of, nonheritable adverse effects in the progeny and/or an impairment of male or female reproductive functions or capacity.

Sensitizing substances Substances and preparations which, if they are inhaled or if they penetrate the skin, are capable of eliciting a reaction of hypersensitization such that on further exposure to the substance or preparation, characteristic adverse effects are produced.

Toxic substances Substances and preparations which in low quantities cause death or acute or chronic damage to health when inhaled, swallowed, or absorbed via the skin.

Very toxic substances Substances and preparations which in very low quantities cause death or acute or chronic damage to health when inhaled, swallowed, or absorbed via the skin.

REFERENCES

1. Council Directive 92/32/EEC, April 30, 1993, amending for the seventh time Directive 67/548/EEC on the approximation of the laws, regulations and administrative provisions relating to the classification, packaging and labeling of dangerous substances, *Official Journal of the European Community,* 35, No. L-154, pp. 1–29, 1992.
2. Brooker, P.C., personal communication, Huntingdon Research Centre, Huntingdon, U.K., 1993.
3. Knight, D.J., personal communication, Safepharm Laboratories, Derby, U.K., 1993.

ADDITIONAL RELATED INFORMATION

TABLE 31.9
OECD Screening Information Data Set (SIDS) Studies

- Physical Chemistry
  - ➢ Melting point
  - ➢ Boiling point
  - ➢ Vapor pressure
  - ➢ Octanol/water partition coefficient
- Environmental fate
  - ➢ Photodegradation (estimation)
  - ➢ Hydrolysis-stability in water (estimation)
  - ➢ Transport/distribution (fugacity model)
  - ➢ Inherent biodegradation
- Ecotoxicology
  - ➢ Acute toxicity to fish
  - ➢ Acute toxicity to *Daphnia*
  - ➢ Algal growth inhibition
- Genetic Toxicology
  - ➢ Bacterial mutation assay (Ames)
  - ➢ *In vitro* chromosomal aberration
  - or
  - ➢ *In vivo* chromosomal aberration
- Mammalian toxicology
  - ➢ Acute oral toxicity
  - ➢ Acute dermal toxicity
  - ➢ 28-day oral toxicity
  - ➢ Reproduction/developmental toxicity screening
  - or
  - Combined repeat dose toxicity/reproduction

Note: For more information on SIDS program visit www.oecd.org/ehs/sidsman.htm.

---

32 Regulatory Toxicology: Notification of New Substances in Canada, Korea, Australia, and China

Henry C. Fogle, B.S., M.S.

CONTENTS

SECTION 1: CANADA

The importation or manufacture of chemical substances in Canada is controlled by New Substance Notification Regulations, which implement requirements outlined in Section 26 of the Canadian Environmental Protection Act (CEPA). The information that must be included in the notification and timing are explained in the New Substance Notification Regulations, Part I (Chemicals), Part II (Polymers), and Part III (Administrative and Testing Requirements). The amount of information required and the government review periods are dependent on the type of substance, the quantity to be imported or manufactured, specific use, etc. Parts I, II, and III of these regulations were published in the *Canada Gazette,* Part II on April 6, 1994 and have been in effect since July 1, 1994. A modification to these regulations was published in Part II of the *Canada Gazette* on December 28, 1994. Copies of CEPA and the notification regulations with guidelines and related notification forms may be obtained from Environment Canada at:

New Substances Division
Commercial Chemicals Evaluation Branch
Environment Canada
14th Floor
Place Vincent Massey
Ottawa, Ontario, Canada KIA OH3
Telephone: (800) 567-1999 (toll-free within Canada)
           (819) 953-7156 (outside Canada)

0-8493-0370-2/02/$0.00+$1.50
© 2002 by CRC Press LLC

Most of the definitions, classifications, and procedures used in the United States under the Toxic Substances Control Act (TSCA) have been adopted by Canada. However, unlike TSCA in the United States, Canada has a "menu" of required toxicological test data similar to the European Union (see Chapter 31, Table 31.6). A "new substance" is one that is not on the Canadian Domestic Substances List (DSL). There are *quantity triggers* for the amount of information that must be included in a new substance notification (NSN), starting from the basic Schedule I (720 kg/calendar year), through Schedule II (71,000 kg/calendar year), to Schedule III (710,000 kg/calendar year). The amount of toxicological and physicochemical data required is directly related to the quantity to be commercialized in Canada.

There are a number of categories where "reduced information packages" are allowed. Details regarding toxicological and physicochemical test data required for different categories and different volume levels (there are three different schedules based on quantity and ten other schedules based on use and nature of the substance) are described in *Guidelines for Notification and Testing of New Substances: Chemical and Polymers.* These guidelines, as well as copies of CEPA and the DSL, may be obtained from Environment Canada at 1-800-567-1999 or, if calling from outside of Canada, 819-953-7156.

The test conditions and procedures used to generate the required test data must be consistent with the Organisation for Economic Cooperation and Development (OECD) Guidelines for Testing of Chemicals. The laboratory practices used to develop test data included in new substance notifications must be consistent with the Principles of Good Laboratory Practice (GLP) set out by the OECD. Some deviations from these GLPs and published OECD testing guidelines might be acceptable but they should be discussed with Environment Canada before inclusion in the NSN.

SECTION 2: KOREA

Chemical control in Korea is covered by legislation and regulations under the administration and control of two ministries: the Ministry of the Environment (MOE) and the Ministry of Labor (MOL). The Toxic Chemicals Control Law (TCCL) is administered by the MOE and the Industrial Safety and Health Law (ISHL) is administered by the MOL. In Korea, there are three types of notifications requiring differing amounts of data:

1. A "Full Notification"
2. A "Simplified or Reduced Notification" for chemical substances listed on the inventories of at least two other countries (before 1991) and certain polymers (requires acute toxicity and an Ames test)
3. A "Polymer Notification" for substances meeting the definition of a polymer by the OECD, the European Union, or the United States (TSCA).

The Korean Chemical Control Law (the TCCL) requires that a notification be approved prior to the importation or manufacture of a new chemical substance for commercial purposes in Korea. A "new" substance is defined as a chemical substance that does not appear on the Korean Existing Core Inventory (KECI) which was published in 1992. (In 1996, about 5000 substances on the MOL inventory were added to KECI.) If a product is composed of a mixture of two or more substances, each component must either be exempt from notification or notified prior to import/manufacture and commercialization in Korea.

Although MOE must evaluate and approve notifications related to substances to be produced or shipped into Korea for the first time, "existing chemicals" that are on KECI must be "certified" before entry through customs will be permitted (certification is provided by the Korean Toxic Chemicals Management Association, KTCMA, on behalf of MOE). A notification must also be approved by MOL, but efforts are being made to integrate the two systems. Notification is accomplished through the use of a specific "Notification of Manufacture/Import of Chemical Substances" form. Test data regarding the toxicity of the notified substance must be included in the notification for evaluation by MOE. Such data must include acute toxicity (e.g., oral, dermal, and inhalation toxicity as tested on mammalia, i.e., rats or mice). Inhalation toxicity data are required for volatile liquids or gases. Data on mutagenicity must include a reverse-mutation assay, a chromosomal aberration assay, and, if either of these tests are positive, *in vivo* nonbacteriological tests (e.g., micronucleus assays in mouse bone marrow) must be performed. Data on biological degradability may also be required. Additional details can be obtained from the MOE, the Toxic Substance Division, 1-JoongAng-dong, KwaChun-shi, Kyungki-do, Korea 427-760; telephone (02) 504-9288; fax (02) 504-9280.

Information relating to the MOL can be obtained from the Work Environment Division, 1-JoongAng-dong, Kwa-Chun-shi, Kyungki-do, Korea 427-760; telephone (02) 500-5635; fax (02) 503-4545.

The address for the Korean Toxic Chemicals Management Association (KTCMA) is 5th Floor, Jungwon Bldg., 1556-8, Seocho-dong, Secho-ku, Seoul, Korea; telephone (02) 587-698217; fax (02) 587-6988.

SECTION 3. AUSTRALIA

The Australian Industrial Chemicals (Notification and Assessment) Act 1989 provides for a national scheme for the notification and assessment of industrial chemicals to protect people and the environment from potential and harmful effects prior to import, manufacture, or use of a chemical substance for commercial purposes. The scheme, known as the National Industrial Chemicals Notification and Assessment Scheme (NICNAS), began operating in July 1990 and is administered by the National Occupational Health and Safety Commission (Worksafe Australia), which also performs the primary toxicological assessment and the occupational health and safety assessments. The Department of Arts, Sport, the Environment, Tourism and Territories undertakes the environmental hazard assessment, while the Department of Community Services and Health carries out the public health assessment. Under this Australian law, a new chemical substance is one that is not listed on the Australian Inventory of Chemical Substances (AICS). If a chemical substance is listed on AICS, a notification and assessment is not required. Five years after a new substance is issued an assessment certificate by the Director of NICNAS, the identity of that substance will be listed on AICS.

The information required for a full notification essentially corresponds to the OECD minimum premarketing set of data (MPD), and is detailed in Parts A, B, and C of the schedule to the Act. OECD toxicological testing guidelines are recommended, but equivalent methods are accepted. Tests must be performed in compliance with GLP, and Australian Codes of Practice on GLP are to be in harmony with OECD GLP principles.

The Australian notification scheme has varying data requirements for different classes of notifiable industrial chemicals. In general, more data are required if the quantity is greater, the chemical is not site-limited, and the class of the chemical is more likely to be hazardous. The exact requirements for data also vary depending on exposure potential, potential uses, and the characteristics of the chemical.

A full package of data, similar to the premarketing data set of the OECD, is required for a standard notification, which includes information on mammalian toxicity, ecotoxicity and biodegradability/bioaccumulation (see Chapter 31, Table 31.6).

A chemical substance cannot be introduced into Australia until it has been assessed and a certificate issued. There is a statutory period of 90 days allowed for government assessment of new chemical notifications. A secondary notification is required if any one of a number of circumstances change after the initial assessment. These include a significant new use or change of use that is likely to increase the risk of adverse effects to health or the environment, a significant increase in production, and new information on the hazardous properties of the chemical. Special conditions for secondary notification can also be set at the time of the initial assessment.

Sources of information on NICNAS are as follows:

- AICS, Vols. 1 and 2, 1992
- *Chemical Gazette,* Commonwealth of Australia Gazette, published monthly
- Annual Reports, The Operation of the Industrial Chemicals (Notification and Assessment) Act of 1989
- Handbook for Notifiers, National Industrial Chemicals Notification and Assessment Scheme (NICNAS), Worksafe Australia, GPO Box 58, Sydney, NSW 2001. It contains AICS on microfiche and the legislation, as well as detailed guidance regarding NICNAS

SECTION 4. PEOPLES REPUBLIC OF CHINA

The Peoples Republic of China (PRC) has regulations governing the importation (registration) of chemical "products" (as opposed to chemical substances). Such products to be registered can be a single chemical substance or a mixture of several chemical substances. It is the "product" that must be registered, not the chemical substance (unless the product happens to be a single specific chemical substance). The product must be registered under the product name that appears on the container label and the Material Safety Data Sheet (MSDS). If a number of products are very similar in characteristics and content, that number of products can be registered as a "group" or category of products.

The regulations relating to this registration requirement is entitled "Regulations for Environmental Management of the First Import of Chemical and the Import and Export of Toxic Chemicals," May 1994. (The PRC is currently in the process of modifying these regulations and in the future, plans to implement a new law to be called the New Chemical Environmental Pollution Control Law.) Currently, any "product" that is a chemical substance or that contains a chemical substance must be registered with the State Environmental Protection Administration (SEPA) prior to shipment into the PRC for commercial purposes. There are exemptions to this registration requirement, which may apply (similar to notification exemptions in other countries). Upon approval of the "product" registration application, SEPA provides the importer with a "Registration Certificate." There are registration fees associated with different types of chemical products that have different degrees of toxicity. Currently, the product registration does not require new toxicological testing. Typically, a good MSDS explaining the hazards related to the products and proper handling and disposal is acceptable along with the completed form.

Currently, the PRC is also receiving nominations for an inventory of "chemical substances" that have been or are currently being shipped into the PRC. At this time, placement of such chemical substances on this inventory is voluntary and is not a regulatory requirement. This opportunity to place a chemical substance on the PRC inventory may change in 2001 or 2002. This inventory is not currently linked to the "product" regulation process (but may be when the law is modified).

Copies of forms and instructions needed to register chemical products to be shipped into the PRC can be obtained from:

Director
The Chemical Registration Center of the State Environmental Production Administration (CRC-SEPA)
Beiyuan, Beijin 100012, P.R. China
Tel: +86-10-8491-5286
Fax: +86-10-8491-3897
http://www.crc-sepa.org.cn (contains English versions of forms)

SECTION 5: WORLDWIDE INTERNET ADDRESSES RELATING TO CHEMICAL PRODUCTS

TABLE 32.1
Worldwide Internet Addresses Relating to Chemical Products

Country	Description	Address
Australia	WorkSafe Australia: WorkSafe Online	http://www.allette.com.au/worksafe/home.htm
		http://www.worksafe.gov.au
	Chemicals in Australia	http://jimi.vianet.net.au/~acted/reg_home.htm
	National Industrial Chemicals Notifications and Assessment Scheme	http://www.nicnas.gov.au
Peoples Republic of China (PRC)	China — Laws and Regulations of the PRC	http://www.qis.net/chinalaw/
	China Environmental Protection Agency	http://www.ihei.com/
	The Chemical Registration Center	http://www.crc-sepa.org.cn./home.english.htm
Hong Kong	Environmental Protection Department	http://www.info.gov.hk/epd
Indonesia	BAPEDAL Environment Ministry	http://www.bapedal.go.id
Japan	Ministry of Labor	http://www.mol.go.jp/english/index.htm
		http://www.mx.eic.or.jp.eanet/
	Environmental Agency	http://www.yahoo.com/Regional/Countries/Japan
Korea	Ministry of the Environment	http://www.moenv.go.kr/english/index.htm
	Ministry of Labor	http://www.molab.go.kr/English/English.html
	Ministry of Environment	http://www.moenv.go.kr/english/index.html
		http://www.me.go.kr/english/
Malaysia	Malaysian Ministries	http://www.smpke.jpm.my/
	Ministry for Science and Technology	http://mastic.gov.my/
New Zealand	Department of Labor	http://www.dol.govt.nz/
	Ministry of the Environment	http://www.mfe.govt.nz/
Philippines	Environmental Management Bureau	http://www.psdn.org.ph/emb
Singapore	Ministry of the Environment	http://www.gov.sg.env/
	Ministry of Labor	http://www.gov.sg.mol/
Taiwan	Environmental Protection Administration	http://www.epa.gov.tw/english/
Thailand	Ministry of Industry	http://www.tisi.go.th/moi/index.html
	MOSTE Ministry for Science	http://www.nectec.or.th/bureaux/moste/moste.html/
The European Union	European Governments on the WWW	http://www..lrz-muenchen.de/~a2c0133/222/govt.eur
	The European Directory	http://www.ukshops.co.uk:8000/thedoor.html
	Full text of the last 20 days' publication of the EU Official Journal	http://europa.eu.int/eur-lex/en/oj/index.html
Canada	CEPA Publications	http://www.doe.ca/tandi/cepa/etitles.html
	Environment Canada–Commercial Chemicals Web site	http://www.ec.gc.ca/ccebl/eng/psap/html
	Health Canada	http://www.hwc.ca/links/english.html
	Chemical Sustances on Canada's Domestic Substances List and Nondomestic Substances List	http://www.2.ec.gc.ca/ccebl/cas_e.html
	DSL Catagorization and Screening Program	http://www.ec.gc.ca/cceb1/ese/eng/dslprog.htm
		http://www.ec.gc.ca/cceb1/ese/fre/dslprog.htm
	Canada Gazette Web site	www.canada.gc.ca/gazette/hompar/_e.html

33 Miscellaneous Information of Toxicological Significance

Mannfred A. Hollinger, Ph.D. and
Michael J. Derelanko, Ph.D., D.A.B.T, F.A.T.S.

CONTENTS

0-8493-0370-2/02/$0.00+$1.50
© 2002 by CRC Press LLC

SECTION 1. LD$_{50}$ VALUES

TABLE 33.1
LD$_{50}$ Values of Common Xenobiotics (mg/kg unless stated otherwise)

	Dermal	IV	IP	IM	SC	PO
Acetaldehyde						
Rabbit		300			1,200	
Rat					640	1,900
Acetaminophen						
Rat			500			338
Acetanilide						
Mouse			820			
Rat			800			800
Acetone cyanohydrin						
Rabbit	17					
Acetylsalicylic acid						
Mouse			495			1,100
Rat			500			1,500
Guinea pig						1,200
Rabbit						1,800
Dog						3,000
Acetylcholine						
Mouse		20	>125		170	3,000
Rat		22			250	2,500
Rabbit		0.3				
Cat					10	
Aconitine						
Mouse		6.9				20
Albuterol sulfate						
Mouse						>2,000
Rat						>2,000
Alfentanil HCl						
Mouse		73				
Rat		45				
Guinea pig		75				
Dog		75				
Allobarbital						
Rat					110	50
Alloxan						
Mouse		200	350			
Allopurinol						
Rat						4,500
Allylamine						
Mouse						57
Rat						106
Allyl chloride						
Rat						700
α-Prodine						
Mouse		54	73		98	
Rat			22		23	90
Guinea pig		18				

TABLE 33.1 *(Continued)*
LD$_{50}$ Values of Common Xenobiotics (mg/kg unless stated otherwise)

	Dermal	IV	IP	IM	SC	PO
Rabbit		18.5				
Alprazolam						
Rat						331–2,171
Altretamine						
Mouse						437
Rat						1,050
Amidephrine						
Mouse					1,990	>6,000
Amiloride (base)						
Mouse						56
Rat						36–85
Aminocaproic						
Mouse		3 g/kg				12 g/kg
Rat		3.2 g/kg				16.4 g/kg
Aminoglutethimide						
Rat		156				1,800
Dog		>100				>100
Aminohippurate sodium						
Mouse, female		7.22 g/kg				
Aminophenazone						
Mouse		184			350	1,850
Rat		110				1,380
Rabbit						160
Dog						150
Aminophylline						
Mouse						540
Rabbit		150				
Aminopyrine						
Mouse		184			350	1,850
Rat			248			1,700
Amitriptyline						
Mouse		27	76		328	289
Rat		10	72		1,290	530
Rabbit		9.9				446
Dog		10	72			200
Ammonium fluorosilicate						
Guinea pig						150
Amobarbital						
Rat		128	115			160
Rabbit		75				575
Dog		75				125
Amphetamine						
Mouse		25	120			22
Rat			125		160	60.5
Rabbit						85
Aniline						
Rat						440

TABLE 33.1 *(Continued)*
LD$_{50}$ Values of Common Xenobiotics (mg/kg unless stated otherwise)

	Dermal	IV	IP	IM	SC	PO
Anileridine (base)						
Mouse		25	53		100	128
Rat			45		163	175
o-Anisidine						
Mouse						1,300
Rat						1,400
Rabbit						2,900
p-Anisidine						
Mouse						1,400
Rat						2,000
Rabbit						870
Antazoline						
Rat					1.1 mmol/kg	
Antipyrine						
Mouse					1,000	1,800
Rat						1,800
Apomorphine						
Dog		80				
Aprobarbital						
Rat					100	
Arsenic pentoxide						
Mouse						50–100
Rat						8
Arsenic trioxide						
Mouse						30–60
Rat						13–30
Asparaginase						
Mouse		500K I.U./kg				
Rabbit		22K I.U./kg				
Atracurium besylate						
Mouse, male		1.9				
Mouse, female		2				
Rat, male		1.3			283	
Atrazine						
Rat						1.2 g/kg
Atropine						
Mouse		90	250		900	400
Rat			280			750
Guinea pig			400			1,100
Auranofin						
Mouse						310
Rat						265
Azacyclonol						
Mouse		177	220		350	650
Azapetine						
Mouse		27	210	600	725	460
Rabbit		28				
Dog		50				
Azathioprine						
Mouse						2,500

TABLE 33.1 *(Continued)*
LD$_{50}$ Values of Common Xenobiotics (mg/kg unless stated otherwise)

	Dermal	IV	IP	IM	SC	PO
Rat						400
Aziridine						
Rat						15
Guinea pig	14					
Barbital						
Mouse			760			600
Barium chloride						
Mouse			500			
Rat					178	
Beclomethasone dipropionate						
Mouse						>1 g/kg
Rat						>1 g/kg
Bemegride						
Mouse		20	45		43	100
Rat		16.3	23.5		30.5	
Guinea pig		26.5				
Rabbit		25				
Benactyzine						
Mouse			100–130		250	350
Rat			100–130			
Benztropine						
Mouse		25			103	94
Rat					353	
Betaxolol						
Mouse						350–920
Rat						860–1,050
Bethanechol chloride						
Mouse						1,510
Bethanidine						
Mouse		12	150		260	520
Biperiden						
Mouse		56				545
Rat						750
Dog						340
Bisacodyl						
Mouse						17,500
Rat						4,320
bis(2-chloroethyl)-ether						
Rat						75–150
Bitolterol mesylate						
Mouse						6,575
Rat						5,650
Bretylium						
Mouse		20	49		72	400
Bromoacetic acid						
Mouse						100

TABLE 33.1 *(Continued)*
LD$_{50}$ Values of Common Xenobiotics (mg/kg unless stated otherwise)

	Dermal	IV	IP	IM	SC	PO
Bromomethane						
Rat						214
1-Bromopropane						
Rat						4,000
Buformin						
Mouse						380
Rat						320
Bulbocapnine						
Mouse					195	
Bupivacaine HCl						
Mouse			6–8		38–54	
Bupropion HCl						
Mouse, male						544
Mouse, female						636
Rat, male						607
Rat, female						482
Buspirone						
Mouse						655
Rat						196
Dog						586
Monkey						356
Busulfan						
Mouse						120
1,4-Butynediol						
Rat						104
Guinea pig						130
Butyronitrile						
Mouse		50				
Rat						140–220
Cadmium chloride						
Rat						88
Cadmium cycanide						
Rat						16
Cadmium fluoride						
Guinea pig						150
Cadmium nitrate						
Mouse						100
Cadmium oxide						
Rat						72–296
Caffeine						
Mouse		100				1,200
Rat		105	245		250	200
Dog		175				
Calcium chloride						
Rat			500			4,000
Capreomycin sulfate						
Mouse					514	
Captan						
Rat						9,000–1,500

TABLE 33.1 *(Continued)*
LD$_{50}$ Values of Common Xenobiotics (mg/kg unless stated otherwise)

	Dermal	IV	IP	IM	SC	PO
Carbachol						
Mouse		0.3			3	15
Rat		0.1			4	40
Carbamazepine						
Mouse			350			1,100–3,570
Rat						3,850–4,025
Rabbit						1,500–2,680
Guinea pig						920
Carbenicillin						
Mouse						3,600
Rat						2,000
Dog						>500
Rat		450				1,320
Rabbit		124				
Carbromal						
Rabbit						500–700
Dog						450
Cefoxitin sodium						
Mouse, female		8 g/kg				
Rat			>10 g/kg			
Rabbit		>1 g/kg				
Ceftazidime						
Rabbit		>2 g/kg				
Cefuroxime sodium						
Mouse						>10 g/kg
Centchroman						
Mouse			400			
Chloral hydrate						
Mouse			890			
Rat					620	500
Chloralose						
Mouse			200			
Chlorambucil						
Mouse						123
Chlordiazepoxide						
Mouse		95	268		530	720
Rat		165			800	2,000
Rabbit		36				590
Dog						1,000
Chlorisondamine						
Mouse		24			401	
Rat		28				
Chloroacetic acid						
Mouse						165
Rat						76
Chloroacetonitrile						
Mouse						139
Rat						220
p-Chloroaniline						
Rat						310

TABLE 33.1 *(Continued)*
LD$_{50}$ Values of Common Xenobiotics (mg/kg unless stated otherwise)

	Dermal	IV	IP	IM	SC	PO
1-Chloro-2,4-dinitro-benzene						
Rat						1,070
2-Chloroethanol						
Rat						58–95
Chloromethyl methyl ether						
Rat						817
p-Chloronitrobenzene						
Rat						810
Chloroprocaine HCl						
Mouse		97			950	
Chlorothiazide						
Mouse		1,120				8,510
Rat			1,386			10,000
Dog		1,000				>1,000
Chlorpheniramine						
Mouse						162
Chlorpromazine						
Mouse		26	92		300	319
Rat		29	74		542	493
Rabbit		235				
Dog		228				
Chlorprothixene (2%)						
Mouse						350
Chlorprothixene (5% suspension)						
Mouse						220
Chlorprothixene (injectable)						
Mouse			>125			
Cimetidine						
Mouse		140				2–5,000
Rat		110				6,000
Clemastine						
Mouse						730
Rat						3,550
Dog						175
Clomethiazole						
Mouse		220				800
Clomipamine						
Mouse						630
Rat						1,450
Clonazepam						
Mouse						>2,000
Rat						>2,000
Clonidine HCl						
Mouse						206
Rat						465

TABLE 33.1 *(Continued)*
LD$_{50}$ Values of Common Xenobiotics (mg/kg unless stated otherwise)

	Dermal	IV	IP	IM	SC	PO
Clotrimazole						
Mouse						700–1,000
Rat						700–1,000
Rabbit						700–1,000
Cocaethylene						
Mouse			60			
Cocaine						
Mouse		75–100	95			
Rat		17.5	70		250	
Rabbit		17				
Dog		22				
Codeine						
Mouse		68	130		183	395
Rat		55	102		332	542
Rabbit		60			32	
Colchicine						
Mouse		1.75	3.5		3.1	
Rat		1.7			4	
Cat		0.25				
Coniine						
Rabbit						56
Guinea pig						150
Cortisone acetate						
Mouse female			1,405			
m-Cresol						
Rat						2,020
o-Cresol						
Rat						1,350
p-Cresol						
Rat						1,800
Crotonaldehyde						
Mouse						240
Cyanamide						
Rat						125
Cyclobarbital						
Rat						205
Rabbit						450
Dog						250
Cyclobenzaphine HCl						
Mouse						338
Rat						425
Cycloserine						
Mouse						5,290
Cyclosporine						
Mouse		148				2,329
Rat		104				1,480
Rabbit		46				>1,000
Cyproheptadine						
Mouse		23	55		107	125
Rat			52			295

TABLE 33.1 *(Continued)*
LD$_{50}$ Values of Common Xenobiotics (mg/kg unless stated otherwise)

	Dermal	IV	IP	IM	SC	PO
Dactinomycin						
Rat		0.46				
Decamethonium						
Mouse		0.75				
Rabbit		0.2				
Desipramine						
Mouse, male						290
Rat, female						320
Desmetryn						
Rat						1,390
Dexamethasone						
Mouse, female						6.5 g/kg
Dexamethasone						
sodium phosphate						
Mouse, female		794				
Dextroamphetamine						
Mouse		14.3	72.2		84	37
Rat					200	80
Dextromoramide						
Mouse						220
o-Dianisidine						
Rat						1,920
2,4-Diaminophenol						
Rat						240
Diazepam						
Mouse			220			970
Rat						1,200
Rabbit		8.8				
Dog						1,000
N-(2-Chloroethyl)-						
dibenzylamine						
Mouse			800			
Dibozane						
Mouse			260			
Rabbit		43				
3,4-Dichloroaniline						
Mouse						740
Rat						648
Dichloroisoproterenol						
Mouse		48	132			
2,2'-dichloro-4,4'-						
methylenedianiline						
Mouse						880
1,1-Dichloro-1-nitro-						
ethane						
Rat						410
Dichlorphenamide						
Mouse						1,710
Rat						2,600

TABLE 33.1 *(Continued)*
LD$_{50}$ Values of Common Xenobiotics (mg/kg unless stated otherwise)

	Dermal	IV	IP	IM	SC	PO
Dicyclomine HCl						
Mouse						625
Dicumarol						
Mouse		64	350			233
Rat		52				542
Guinea pig		59				
N,N-Diethylaniline						
Rat						782
Diethylcarbamazine						
Mouse						550
Rat						395
Diethylene glycol						
diacrylate						
Rat						770
Rabbit	180					
Diethylpropion HCl						
Mouse						600
Rat						250
Dog						225
Diflunisal						
Mouse, female						500
Rat, female						826
Digitoxin						
Mouse					22.2	32.7
Rat					16.4	23.8
Guinea pig						>100
Digoxin						
Guinea pig		0.355				
Dihydroergotamine						
Mouse		118				
Rat		110				
Rabbit		25				
Cat					68	
Diisopropyl fluoro-						6
phosphate						
Mouse					3.7	36.8
Rat				1.8	3	6
Rabbit	0.34				1	9.8
Cat	1.6					
Dog	3.4				3	
Monkey	0.25					
Diltiazem HCl						
Mouse		60				415–740
Rat		38				560–810
Dog						>50
Dimethindene						
Rat		26.8				618.2
Guinea pig						888
Dog		45				

TABLE 33.1 *(Continued)*
LD$_{50}$ Values of Common Xenobiotics (mg/kg unless stated otherwise)

	Dermal	IV	IP	IM	SC	PO
N,N-Dimethylaniline						
Rat						1,410
Dimethylnitrosamine						
Rat						26
Dimethyl phenyl-piperazinium						
Mouse			40	27.5		365
Rat						2,000
Dimethyl sulfate						
Rat						440
Dimethyl sulfoxide						
Mouse			14,700			
Dog						>10,000
2,4-Dinitrophenol						
Rat					25	30
Rabbit						200
Dog		30		20	22	25
2,4-Dinitrotoluene						
Rat						268
Diphenhydramine						
Mouse		31	84		127	164
Rat		42	82		475	500
Guinea pig			75			
Rabbit		10				
Dog		24				
Disopyramide phos-phate						
Mouse						700
Rat						580
Dyclonine						
Mouse						90
Rat			31			176
Diphenylamine						
Rat						3,300
Doxapram HCl						
Mouse		75				
Rat		75				
Cat		40–80				
Dog		40–80				
Doxazosin						
Mouse						>1,000
Rat						>1,000
Doxepine						
Mouse		20				165
Rat		16				400
Doxycycline						
Mouse		175				1,600
Dropempine						
Mouse						420
Rat			125			370

TABLE 33.1 *(Continued)*
LD$_{50}$ Values of Common Xenobiotics (mg/kg unless stated otherwise)

	Dermal	IV	IP	IM	SC	PO
Econazole						
Mouse						462
Rat						668
Guinea pig						272
Dog						>160
Edrophonium						
Mouse		9	37		130	600
Rabbit		28.5				
Dog		15				
Enalaprilat						
Mouse, female		3,740–5,890				2,000
Rat						2,000
Ephedrine						
Mouse						1,550
Rat					650	
Epinephrine						
Mouse		0.5	4		1.47	50
Rat		0.98		3.5	5	
2,3-Epoxy-1-propanol						
Mouse						431
Rat						420
Rabbit	1980					
2,3-Epoxypropyl acrylate						
Rat						214
Rabbit	400					
Ergometrine						
Mouse		144				
Ergotamine						
Mouse		52				
Rat		62				
Rabbit		3.55				
Cat					11	
Ethacrynic acid						
Mouse						627
Ethacrynate sodium						
Mouse		175				
Ethanol						
Mouse		1,953	7,260		8,285	9,488
Rat			5,000			13,600
Guinea pig			5,560			
Rabbit						9,500
Ethinamate						
Rat						331
Dog						314
Ethosuximide						
Mouse						1,530
Rat						1,820
N-Ethylaniline						
Mouse						500

TABLE 33.1 *(Continued)*
LD$_{50}$ Values of Common Xenobiotics (mg/kg unless stated otherwise)

	Dermal	IV	IP	IM	SC	PO
Rat						290
Rabbit	4,700					
Ethyl biscoumacetate						
Mouse						880
Rat						880
Rabbit						1,100
Ethyl chloroacetate						
Rabbit	230					
Ethyl chloroformate						
Mouse						15
Rat						270
Rabbit	7,120					
Ethylene dibromide						
Rat	300					
Rabbit	300					
Ethylene oxide						
Mouse						365
Rat						330
Ethyl methacrylate						
Rat						16g/kg
Ethylmorphine						
Mouse					200	
Ethylnorepinephrine						
Mouse		117				
Etilefrine						
Mouse						1,600
Etrentinate						
Rat			>4,000			>4,000
Mouse			>4,000			>4,000
Fentenyl citrate						
Rat		3				
Mouse		11.2				
Cat		1				
Dog		14				
Monkey		0.03				
Floxuridine						
Mouse		880				
Rat		670				
Rabbit		94				
Dog		157				
Fluoroacetic acid						
Mouse			10		16	8
Rat			0.4	5	2.5	2.5
Guinea pig			0.35			
Rabbit		0.25				
Cat		0.2				
Dog		0.06				
Monkey		4				
Fluorouracil						
Mouse		340				

TABLE 33.1 *(Continued)*

LD$_{50}$ Values of Common Xenobiotics (mg/kg unless stated otherwise)

	Dermal	IV	IP	IM	SC	PO
Rat		165				
Rabbit		27				
Dog		32				
Flurazepam						
Mouse						870
Rat						1,230
Flurbiprofen						
Mouse			200			750
Rat			400			160
Fominoben						
Mouse		100				2,000
Rat		100				2,000
Fosinopril						
Rat						2,600
2-Furaldehyde						
Rat						127
Furosemide						
Rat						4,600
Rabbit						800
Dog						2,000
Gadopentetate dimeglumine						
Mouse		5–12.5mmol/kg				
Rat		10–15 mmol/kg				
Gallamine						
Mouse		4.3	9.6		17.4	425
Rat		5.5			25	
Rabbit		0.65		2.5	3	100
Dog		0.8				
Glucagon						
Mouse		300				
Glutethimide						
Mouse			350			
Guanethidine						
Mouse		22				
Rat		23			1,000	
Haloperidol						
Mouse		13			54	144
Rat		19				
Harmaline						
Mouse		120				
HC Blue No. 2						
Rat						1,250–5,000
Hemicholinium						
Mouse			0.064			
Rat			0.45			
Heparin						
Mouse		1,780				
Hexachlorophene						
Rat		7.5	30			70

TABLE 33.1 *(Continued)*
LD$_{50}$ Values of Common Xenobiotics (mg/kg unless stated otherwise)

	Dermal	IV	IP	IM	SC	PO
Hexamethonium						
Mouse		21	42		484	
Hexobarbital						
Mouse			340			468
Rat			280			468
Rabbit		80				
Hexocyclium						
Mouse		10.5	55		360	600
Histamine						
Guinea pig		0.18				
Homatropine						
Mouse			60		650	1,400
Rat			82		800	1,200
Guinea pig			120			1,000
Hydralazine						
Mouse			83			
Rat						180
Hydrazine						
Rat						60
Hydrochlorothiazide						
Mouse	884		578		1,470	3,080
Rat			234		1,270	6,190
Rabbit	461					
Dog	250					
Hydrocordone						
Mouse					9	
Hydrocortisone						
Mouse, female			1,740			
Hydromorphone						
Mouse		88			84	
Hydroquinone						
Rat						700
Hydroxyzine						
Rat		45				1,000
Hyoscyamine-sulfate						
Rat						375
Ibuprofen						
Mouse			320			800
Rat					1,300	1,600
Imipramine						
Mouse		35	115		189	400
Rat		22	79		250	625
Rabbit		18				
Iodoacetic acid						
Mouse						83
Rat						60
Iodomethane						
Rat						76
Iohexol						
Mouse		24.2 g iodine/kg				

TABLE 33.1 *(Continued)*
LD$_{50}$ Values of Common Xenobiotics (mg/kg unless stated otherwise)

	Dermal	IV	IP	IM	SC	PO
Rat		15 g iodine/kg				
Ipratropium bromide						
Mouse						1,001–2,010
Rat						1,667–4,000
Dog						400–1,300
Iproniazid						
Mouse		725	690	683	750	968
Rat						383
Rabbit		150				150
Isocarboxazid						
Mouse			110			173
Rat			199			280
Isoflurophate						
Mouse						37
Isoniazid						
Mouse		153	132	140	160	142
Rat		398			533	650
Rabbit		94			151	
Dog		50				
Isoprenaline						
Mouse						2,221
Isoproterenol						
Mouse		128	300			450
Guinea pig					0.32	270
Dog		50				
Isosorbide dinitrate						
Rat						1,100
Ketamine						
Mouse		65	360.6			680
Rat		62				490
Labetalol						
Mouse		50–60				600
Rat		50–60				>2 g/kg
Lactulose						
Mouse						48.8 ml/kg
Rat						>30 ml/kg
Lauremine oxide (0.3%)						
Rat						>20g/kg
Levallorphan						
Mouse			184			949
Rat			185			949
Levocarnitine						
Mouse						19.2 g/kg
Levorphanol						
Mouse		41.5	73		187	285
Rat					110	150
Rabbit		20				

TABLE 33.1 *(Continued)*
LD$_{50}$ Values of Common Xenobiotics (mg/kg unless stated otherwise)

	Dermal	IV	IP	IM	SC	PO
Lidocaine HCl						
Mouse		31.5			400	457
Rat						459
Lignocaine						
Mouse		35	122			520
Lisinopril						
Mouse						>20 g/kg
Rat						>20 g/kg
Loperamide						
Rat		5.92				
Lysergide						
Mouse		54				46
Rat						16
Rabbit		3				
Malononitrile						
Mouse						18.6
Mebendazole						
Mouse						1,280
Rat						1,280
Guinea pig						1,280
Rabbit						1,280
Dog						>640
Cat						>640
Mebutamate						
Mouse			460			550
Rat			410			1,160
Mecamylamine						
(base)						
Mouse		21	39		93	92
Rat			54		145	171
Guinea pig			52		127	144
Mechlorethamine						
HCl						
Mouse		2				
Rat		1.6				
Meclofenoxate						
Mouse		330				1,750
Meclozine						
Mouse						1,600
Menadiol sodium						
diphosphate						
Mouse		500				6,172
Rat		400				5,250
Mepenzolate						
Mouse		9.8				900
Rat		21.8				1,100
Meperidine						
Mouse		50	150		195	178
Rat		34	93		200	170
Rabbit		30				500

TABLE 33.1 *(Continued)*
LD$_{50}$ Values of Common Xenobiotics (mg/kg unless stated otherwise)

	Dermal	IV	IP	IM	SC	PO
Mephenesin						
Mouse		186	471			990
Rat						625
Rabbit		125				
Mephenoxalone						
Mouse						3,820
Mephentermine						
Mouse			110			
Mephenytoin						
Mouse						560
Guinea pig			215			
Rabbit						430
Cat						190
Mepivacaine						
Mouse		23–35			280	
Meprobamate						
Mouse			710			980
Rat		350				1,600
Rabbit		260				
Mercaptopurine						
Mouse			250			
Mercury (II) bromide						
Mouse						35
Rat	100					1
Mercury (II) chloride						
Rat						1
Mercury (II) cyanide						
Mouse						33
Rat						26
Mercury (II) nitrate						
Rat						26
Mercury (II) oxide						
Mouse						22
Rat	315					18
Mescaline						
Mouse			500			
Rat			370			
Metaraminol						
Mouse						99
Rat						240
Methacholine-Cl						
Mouse						1,100
Rat						750
Methacrylonitrile						
Rat						0.25 ml/kg
Methadone						
Mouse		17	38		33	93.7
Rat		10	23		12	95
Guinea pig					54	
Monkey					15	

TABLE 33.1 *(Continued)*
LD$_{50}$ Values of Common Xenobiotics (mg/kg unless stated otherwise)

	Dermal	IV	IP	IM	SC	PO
Methamphetamine						
Mouse		10	15			232
Methaqualone						
Rat		100				300
Metharbital						
Mouse		500				500
Methotrexate						
Mouse			4.5			
Methoxamine						
Mouse			92			
N-Methylaniline						
Rabbit						280
Methylatropine						
Mouse		7	250			
2-Methylazindine						
Rat						19
Methyl chloroformate						
Mouse	1,750					
Rabbit	7,120					
Rat						60
Methyldopa						
Mouse		1,900	406			5,300
Rat			647			7,490
Rabbit						713
Methyldopate HCl						
Mouse		321				
Methylergonovine						
Mouse		85				187
Rat		23				93
Rabbit		2.6				4.5
Methyl isocyanate						
Mouse						120
Rat						69
Rabbit	0.22 ml/kg					90
1-Methyl-3-nitro-l-nitrosoguanidine						
Rat						90
Methyloxirane						
Rat						520–1,140
Methylpentynol						
Mouse						525
Rat						300–900
Guinea pig						534
Methylphenidate						
Mouse			450		470	680
Rat		48				367
Metyrapone						
Rat						521
Miconazole nitrate						
Mouse						578

TABLE 33.1 *(Continued)*
LD$_{50}$ Values of Common Xenobiotics (mg/kg unless stated otherwise)

	Dermal	IV	IP	IM	SC	PO
Rat						>640
Guinea pig						276
Dog						>160
Minoxidil						
Mouse		51	1,000–1,300			2,500
Rat		49				1,300–2,000
Morphine						
Mouse		275	500		500–700	745
Rat		237	500		266–572	905
Guinea pig					391	
Rabbit			500		600	
Muscarine						
Mouse		0.23				
Nalorphine						
Mouse		190	590	0.4	670	
Naloxone						
Mouse		150				565
Rat		109				
Naltrexone						
Mouse						1,100
Rat						1,450
Guinea pig						1,490
Naphazoline						
Mouse		170				
Rat				385		
Rabbit		0.8				
Naproxen						
Mouse						1,234
Rat						543
Hamster						4,110
Dog						>1,000
Neostigmine						
Mouse		0.36	0.62	0.31	0.8	14.4
Rat		0.16		0.42	0.37	
Rabbit				0.31		
Nialamide						
Mouse			742			1,000
Rat						1,700
Nicotine						
Mouse		7.1				3.3
Rat					33.5	>24
Rabbit		9.4				
Dog		5				
Nicotinic acid						
Rat						7,000
Nifedipine						
Mouse		16				490
Rat		4				1,020
Nikethamide						
Mouse			174			

TABLE 33.1 *(Continued)*
LD$_{50}$ Values of Common Xenobiotics (mg/kg unless stated otherwise)

	Dermal	IV	IP	IM	SC	PO
Rat		191	300		470	
Rabbit			225			
Nitrazepam						
Mouse						1,800
Rat						2,000
m-Nitroaniline						
Rat						535
ø-Nitroaniline						
Rat						1,600
p-Nitroaniline						
Rat						750
Nitrofurazone						
Mouse						747
Rat					30	590
2-Nitro-*p*-anisidine						
Rat						14,100
2-Nitronaphthalene						
Rat						4,400
2-Nitropropane						
Rat						720
o-Nitrotoluene						
Rat						891
p-Nitrotoluene						
Mouse						1,231
Rat						2,144
5-Nitro-*o*-toluidine						
Rat						574
Nitroprusside						
Mouse		8.4				
Rat		11.2				
Rabbit		2.8				
Dog		5				
Nizatidine						
Mouse		232				
Rat		301				
Norephedrine						
Rabbit		75				
Norepinephrine						
Rat					29	132
Noscapine						
Rat						800
Obidoxime						
Mouse		100	200			2,240
Rat		100	200			
Rabbit		100	200			
Octreotide acetate						
Mouse		72				
Rat		18				
Orciprenaline						
Mouse						4,800

TABLE 33.1 *(Continued)*
LD$_{50}$ Values of Common Xenobiotics (mg/kg unless stated otherwise)

	Dermal	IV	IP	IM	SC	PO
Osmium tetroxide						
Mouse						162
Ouabain						
Mouse			20			
Rat					97	
Guinea pig				0.26		
Cat		0.11				
Oxazepam						
Mouse			>1,500			7,500
Oxilorphan						
Mouse		32			315	
Oxotremorine						
Mouse			5			
Papaverine						
Mouse		33.1	750			2,500
Rat			63		420	745
Paracetamol						
Rat						3,700
Paraldehyde						
Mouse						1,650
Guinea pig			1,230			
Rabbit		450				
Cat		450				
Dog		500				3,500
Paraquat (mmol/kg)						
Mouse			0.12			0.66
Rat			0.12			0.57–0.94
Guinea pig			0.018			0.19
Cat						0.22
Pargyline						
Mouse			370			680
Rat			142			300
Cat			200			
Dog						175
Monkey			150			
Pentachlorophenol						
Rat	96					
Pentazocine-HCl						
Mouse						3,570
Pentobarbital						
Mouse		80	130	124	107	280
Rat			75			118
Guinea pig			50	70		
Rabbit		45				275
Cat						100
Pentolinium						
Mouse		29	36			512
Pentylenetetrazol						
Mouse		51	92		101	162

TABLE 33.1 *(Continued)*
LD$_{50}$ Values of Common Xenobiotics (mg/kg unless stated otherwise)

	Dermal	IV	IP	IM	SC	PO
Rat			70		100	
Perphenazine						
Mouse			70			
Phalloidine						
Mouse			1.9			
Phenacetin						
Mouse						1,030–2,000
Rat						1,650
Phenazone						
Rat						1,800
Phenelzine						
Mouse		157			150	156
p-Phenetidine						
Mouse						530
Rat						580
Pheniprazine						
Mouse		60.6	122		95	73
Rat		44.5			45.3	34.1
Phenobarbital						
Mouse			340		230	325
Rat			190		200	660
Rabbit		185				
Cat						175
Phenoxybenzamine						
Mouse						1,535
Rat						2,500
Guinea pig						500
Phentolamine						
Mouse						1,000
Rat		75			275	1,250
Phentolamine						
mesylate						
Mouse						1,000
Rat						1,250
Phenylbutazone						
Mouse		123	336			417.5
Rat		150	215			650–1,000
Rabbit						146
m-Phenylenediamine						
Rat						650
p-Phenylenediamine						
Rat						98
Phenylephedrine						
Mouse		21	1,000		70	120
Rat					92	350–1,120
Phenylhydrazine						
Mouse						175
Rat						188
Rabbit						80
Guinea pig						80

TABLE 33.1 *(Continued)*
LD$_{50}$ Values of Common Xenobiotics (mg/kg unless stated otherwise)

	Dermal	IV	IP	IM	SC	PO
Phenyl oxirane						
Rat						4,290
Rabbit	930–1,060					
Phenytoin						
Mouse			200			490
Rat			280			
Rabbit		125				
Phloroglucinol						
Rat			3,180		4,850	5,200
Physostigmine						
Mouse			1		0.54	3
Phytonadione (1%)						
Mouse		52 ml/kg				
Phytonadione						
Mouse			>25 g/kg			>25 g/kg
4-Picoline						
Rat						1,290
Rabbit	270					14.8
Picrotoxin						
Mouse			7.2		7	14.8
Rat		3	6.5			
Pilocarpine						
Mouse			500			
Pimozide						
Mouse						>5, 100
Rat						>5,100
Dog						40
Pipradrol						
Mouse			94		240	365
Rat		30			240	180
Rabbit		15				
Potassium bromate						
Rat			50–200			200–400
Potassium cyanide						
Mouse					6	16
Potassium fluoro-silicate						
Guinea pig						500
Pralidoxime						
Mouse		90	155	180		4,100
Rat		96		150		
Guinea pig				168		
Rabbit		95				
Praziquantel						
Mouse						2,500
Rat						2,500
Prednisolone phosphate disodium						
Mouse, female			1,190			

TABLE 33.1 *(Continued)*
LD$_{50}$ Values of Common Xenobiotics (mg/kg unless stated otherwise)

	Dermal	IV	IP	IM	SC	PO
Prenylamine						
Mouse						200
Rat						1,000
Primidone						
Mouse						600–800
Rat						1,500–2,000
Proadifen						
Mouse		60	117.5			538
Rat			163			2,140
Probenecid						
Mouse		458	230		1,156	1,666
Rat			394		611	1,604
Rabbit		304				
Dog		270				
Probucol						
Mouse						>5 g/kg
Rat						>5 g/kg
Procaine						
Mouse		45	230	630	800	500
Rat		50	250	1,600	2,100	
Guinea pig		51				
Rabbit		57				
Dog		62.4				
Prochlorperazine						
Mouse		92	125		350	750
Rat						1,800
Prodilidine						
Mouse		91			194	318
Rat		74			188	253
Promazine						
Mouse		38		113		216–485
Rat		17–29		233		343–650
Rabbit		21				125
Promethazine						
Mouse		28–75	150	216	750	375–575
Rat		20–45		250	225	480
Guinea pig		42.5				
Rabbit		19				
Prontalol						
Mouse		50	124			900
Rat		50				900
Propanidid						
Mouse		90				
Rat		80				
Dog		80				
Rabbit		75				
Propantheline						
Rat					298	370
Propargyl alcohol						
Mouse						50

TABLE 33.1 *(Continued)*
LD$_{50}$ Values of Common Xenobiotics (mg/kg unless stated otherwise)

	Dermal	IV	IP	IM	SC	PO
Rat						55
Guinea pig						60
Propiverine						
Mouse		113				490
Rat		29				2,100
Rabbit		13				620
Propofol						
Mouse		53				
Propoxyphene HCl						
Mouse					204	282
Rat					131	230
Propoxyphene napsylate						
Mouse						915
Rat						647
Rabbit						>183
Dog						>183
Propranolol						
Mouse		27	114			380
Rat						533
Propyl chloroformate						
Mouse						650
Protoveratrine						
Mouse		0.05	0.4			
Rat					0.6	5
Rabbit		0.05			0.11	
Cat					0.5	
Protriptyline						
Mouse		37			192	269
Pseudoephedrine						
Mouse						726
Rat			202			2,206
Rabbit						1,177
Psilocin						
Mouse		74				
Rat		75				
Psilocybine						
Mouse		285				
Rat		280				
Pyrethrin						
Rat						1,500
Pyrilamine						
Mouse		30	102		150	235
Rat					150	
Guinea pig		24.4			70	
Quinidine						
Mouse		69	190	200		594
Rat		23.1				1,000
Cat		21.6				

TABLE 33.1 *(Continued)*
LD$_{50}$ Values of Common Xenobiotics (mg/kg unless stated otherwise)

	Dermal	IV	IP	IM	SC	PO
Ramipril						
Mouse						10–11 g/kg
Rat						10–11 g/kg
Ranitidine HCl						
Mouse		77				
Rat		83				
Reserpine						
Mouse			70			390–500
Rat		18				
Resorcinol						
Rat						370
Guinea pig						370
Rifampin						
Mouse						885
Rat						1,720
Rabbit						2,120
Ritodrine						
Mouse						540
Rabbit		64				
Rotenone						
Rat						100–300
Salicylamide						
Mouse		313				1,400
Rat						1,200
Rabbit			600			3,000
Scopolamine						
Mouse			153.5		590	
Secobarbital						
Cat						50
Selenium						
Rat						6,700
Selenium disulfide						
Rat						138
Selenium monosulfide						
Mouse						370
Selenium tetrachloride						
Guinea pig					19	
Semicarbazide						
Mouse		125.6	23.3		125.5	176
Serotonin						
Mouse		160	868	750		
Rat		30	117			
Sodium bromide						
Mouse					5,020	7,000
Rat						3,500
Sodium fluoride						
Rat						200
Sodium tetradecyl sulfate						
Mouse		90				

TABLE 33.1 *(Continued)*
LD$_{50}$ Values of Common Xenobiotics (mg/kg unless stated otherwise)

	Dermal	IV	IP	IM	SC	PO
Rat		72–128				
Solanine						
Rat			75			590
Rabbit			20–23			
Sheep						225
Sotalol						
Mouse			670			2,600
Rat			680			3,450
Rabbit						1,000
Dog			330			
g-Strophanthine						
Guinea pig				0.26		
Stearyl Heptanoate						
Rat						>5g/kg
Strychnine						
Mouse			0.98		0.85	
Rat			0.09–1.4		1.2	16.2
Succinylcholine						
Mouse		0.75	4			125
Rabbit		1				
Sulfacetamide						
Mouse						16.5 g/kg
Sulfadimethoxine						
Rat						>4,000
Rabbit						>2,000
Sulfafurazole						
Rat						>10,000
Rabbit						>2,000
Sulfaguanidine						
Mouse						15,000
Sulfamethoxazole						
Mouse						3,200
Sufentanil citrate						
Mouse		17				
Rat		10.5				
Guinea pig		12.5				
Dog		10.1–19.5				
Sulfamethoxazole						
Mouse						2,300
Rat						3,000
Rabbit						>2,000
Sulfanilamide						
Mouse						3,700–4,300
Rat						3,900–10,000
Dog						2,000
Sulfasalazine						
Mouse						>12 g/kg
Sulfisoxazole						
Mouse						5,700
Rat						>10,000

TABLE 33.1 *(Continued)*
LD$_{50}$ Values of Common Xenobiotics (mg/kg unless stated otherwise)

	Dermal	IV	IP	IM	SC	PO
Rabbit						>2,000
Syrosingopine						
Rat		50				
Talinolol						
Mouse						600–1,450
Rat						1,180–2,580
Terbutaline						
Mouse						3,000
Rat						18,000
Terconazole						
Rat, male						1,741
Rat, female						849
Dog, male						1,280
Dog, female						640
Terfenadine						
Mouse						>5,000
Rat						>5,000
Rat newborn						438
Tetrabenazine						
Mouse		150			400	
Tetracaine						
Mouse		6.6				
Guinea pig		15.6				
Dog		4.3				
1,1,2,2-Tetrabromo-ethane						
Mouse						269
Rat	5,250					1,100
Rabbit						400
Guinea pig						400
1,1,2,2-Tetrachloro-ethane						
Rat						800
2,3,4,5-Tetrachloro-phenol						
Mouse						400
Rat						140
Guinea pig						250
2,3,4,6-Tetrachloro-phenol						
Mouse						109
Rabbit	250					
Tetraethylammonium						
Mouse		29	56			655
Rat		63	115			
Rabbit		72				
Dog		55				
Tetrahydrocannabinol						
Mouse			510			

TABLE 33.1 *(Continued)*
LD$_{50}$ Values of Common Xenobiotics (mg/kg unless stated otherwise)

	Dermal	IV	IP	IM	SC	PO
Tetryzoline						
Mouse		39				
Thebaine						
Rat						13.9
Theophylline						
Mouse						350
Thioglycolic acid						
Rat						114
Rabbit	848					
Thioguanine						
Rat, male						823
Rat, female						740
Thiram						
Rat						865
Rabbit						210
Thiopental						
Mouse		112	200			350
Rat		67.5	120			
Guinea pig		55	57.5			
Rabbit		40				600
Dog		55				150
Timolol maleate						
Mouse, female						1,190
Rat, female						900
Tocinide HCl						
Mouse						800
Rat						1,000
Guinea pig						230
Tolazoline						
Mouse			500			
o-Tolidine						
Rat						404
Toluene-2,4-diiso-cyanate						
Rat						5,800
o-Toluidine						
Rat						670
Rabbit	3,250					
P-Toluidine						
Mouse						794
Rat						656
Rabbit	890					
Toxaphene						
Rat						40–120
Tranylcypromine						
Mouse		37				38
Trazodone						
Mouse		96				610
Rat						486

TABLE 33.1 *(Continued)*
LD$_{50}$ Values of Common Xenobiotics (mg/kg unless stated otherwise)

	Dermal	IV	IP	IM	SC	PO
Rabbit						560
Triamterene						
Mouse						300–380
Triazolam						
Mouse						>1,000
Rat						>5,000
Trichloroacetonitrile						
Rat						250
Rabbit	900					
Trichloronitromethane						
Rat						250
Trichlorotrinitroben-						
zene						
Rat						30 g/kg
Trichothecene						
Rat		0.75				
Guinea pig		1.3				
Trifluperidol						
Mouse						988
Rat						113
Trifluoperazine						
Mouse		36				442
Rat						740
Dog		60				
Trimethadione						
Mouse		2,000	1,800			2,200
Rat					2,200	
Rabbit			1,500	1,500		
Trimipramine						
Mouse						250
Tripelennamine						
Mouse		17	70		75	210
Rat		13			225	570
Guinea pig					30.2	155
Triphenyltin acetate						
Rat						140
Rabbit						30
Triphenyltin						
hydroxide						
Mouse						245
Rat						46
Tubocurarine						
Mouse			0.14			
Rat			0.25			
Rabbit		0.35				

TABLE 33.1 *(Continued)*
LD$_{50}$ Values of Common Xenobiotics (mg/kg unless stated otherwise)

	Dermal	IV	IP	IM	SC	PO
Ursodiol						
Mouse						>7,500
Rat						>5,000
Vancomycine HCl						
Mouse		400				
Rat		319				
Veratradine						
Mouse		0.42	1.35			
Rat		3.5				
Vidarabine						
Mouse						>5,020
Rat						>5,020
Vinyl chloride						
Rat						500
Vinyl cyclohexene diepoxide						
Rat						2,130
Rabbit	620					
Warfarin						
Mouse		165				374
Rat		186				323
Guinea pig						182
Rabbit		150				800
Dog		250				250
2,4-Xylenol						
Mouse	1,040					
Rat						3,200
2,5-Xylenol						
Mouse						383
2,6-Xylenol						
Mouse	920					980
Rat						296
Zinc phosphide						
Mouse						40
Rat						2.7–40.5
Rabbit	2,000–5,000					40
Cat						250
Zoxazolamine						
Mouse			376			825
Rat			102			376
Dog		117				

Data taken from *Drug Dosage in Laboratory Animals: A Handbook,* R.E. Borchard, C.D. Barnas, and L.G. Eltherington, Eds., CRC Press, Boca Raton, FL, 1992; *Chemical Safety Data Sheets,* Vols. 4a and 4b, Royal Society of Chemistry, Indispensable Publications Ltd., Bugbrooke, Northamptonshire, U.K., 1991; *Physician Desk Reference,* 47 ed., Medical Economics Data, Montvale, NJ, 1993; *Toxicological Analysis,* R. Klaus Müller, Ed., Ullstein Mosby GmbH & Co., KG, Berlin, 1992.

TABLE 33.2
Radiation LD$_{50}$ Values for Different Species

Species	LD$_{50}$ (Midline Absorbed Dose, Rads)
Sheep	155
Burro	155
Swine	195
Goat	230
Dog	265
Man	270(?)
	243(?)
	255(?)
Rabbit	840
Mouse	900
Rat	900
Hamster	900
Gerbil	1,059
Wild mice	1,100–1,200
Desert mice	
Praomys formusus	1,300
Praomys longimembris	1,520
Guinea pig	255(?)
Monkey	398
Marmoset	200

From *CRC Handbook of Radiobiology*, Kedar N. Prasad, 1984. With permission.

SECTION 2. TABLES OF COMPARATIVE ANATOMICAL, PHYSIOLOGICAL, AND BIOCHEMICAL DATA

TABLE 33.3
Comparison of Physiological Parameters for Different Body Organs

Organ	Weight (kg)	Percent of Body Volume	Percent Water	Blood Flow (ml/min)	Plasma Flow (ml/min)	Blood Flow (ml/kg)	Blood Flow Fraction
Adrenal glands		0.03		25	15		
Blood	5.4	7	83	5,000			
Bone	10	16	22	250	150		
Brain	1.5	2	75	700	420	780	
Fat	10	10	10	200	120		0.05
Heart	0.3	0.5	79	200	120	250	
Kidneys	0.3	0.4	83	1,100	660	1,200	
Liver	1.5	2.3	68	1,350	810	1,500	0.25
Portal				1,050	630		
Arterial				300	180		
Lungs	1.0	0.7	79	5,000	3,000		
Muscle	30	42	76	750	450	900	0.19
Skin	5	18	72	300	180	250	
Thyroid gland	0.03	0.03		50	30		
Total body		100	60	5,000	3,000		

Source: Modified from Illing, *Xenobiotic Metabolism and Disposition: The Design of Studies on Novel Compounds*, CRC Press, Boca Raton, FL, 1989. Data are for hypothetical 70-kg human.

TABLE 33.4
Comparison of the Blood Flow/Perfusion and Oxygen Consumption of Liver, Lung, Intestine, and Kidney of the Rat *In Vivo* and in Organ Perfusion[a]

Parameter (unit)	Liver	Lung	Intestine	Kidney
In vivo				
Blood flow (ml min^{-1})	13–20	55–70	5–8	4–6
Blood pressure S/D (torr)	150/100	25/10	150/100	150/100
pO$_2$-arterial (torr)	95	40	95	95
pO$_2$-venous (torr)	40	100	50	70
O$_2$-consumption (µl min^{-1})	500–800	From air	40–160	100–200
In perfusion				
Perfusion flow (ml min^{-1})	30–50	50	6	20–35
Perfusion pressure (torr)	100–120	10–20	100–120	100–120
pO$_2$-arterial (torr)	600	600	400	600
pO$_2$-venous (torr)	200	?	180	400
max. O$_2$-supply[b] (µl min^{-1})	380–630	?	120[c]	120–220

[a] These values are indications of the most common values measured for the various organs in a rat of 250 to 300 g. The figures provided for the kidney apply to a single kidney. The values measured in organ perfusions may differ greatly, depending on the set-up, method of gassing, etc. S = systolic; D = diastolic.

[b] Calculated from pO$_2$ arterial, pO$_2$-venous, and perfusion flow.

[c] With 20% FC-43 emulsion in KRB; other figures apply to KRB buffer without erythrocytes or oxygen carrier. (KRB = Krebs-Ringer buffer.)

From *Toxicology: Principles and Applications*, CRC Press, Boca Raton, FL, 1996. With permission.

TABLE 33.5
Comparison of Respiratory Volume and Alveolar Ventilation in Relation to Animal Weight

Species	Weight (g)	Respiratory Volume per Minute (cm^3)	Respiratory Volume per Minute (cm^3) ÷ Weight (g)	Alveolar Ventilation (l/hr) ÷ Weight (g)
Mouse	19.8	24.5	1.24	0.067
Cotton rat	76.8	39.6	0.52	
Hamster	91.6	60.9	0.67	
White rat	112.8	72.9	0.65	0.070
Guinea pig	466.0	155.6	0.33	
Rabbit	2,069.0	800.0	0.39	
Monkey	2,682.0	863.5	0.32	
Human	68,500.0	8,732.0	0.13	0.005

Source: Modified from Calabrese, *Principles of Animal Extrapolation*, Lewis Publishers, Chelsea, MI, 1991.

TABLE 33.6
Comparison of Dosage by Weight and Surface Area

Species	Weight (g)	Dosage (mg/kg)	Dose (mg/animal)	Surface Area (cm²)	Dosage (mg/cm²)
Mouse	20	100	2	46	0.043
Rat	200	100	20	325	0.061
Guinea pig	400	100	40	565	0.071
Rabbit	1,500	100	150	1,270	0.118
Cat	2,000	100	200	1,380	0.145
Monkey	4,000	100	400	2,980	0.134
Dog	12,000	100	1,200	5,770	0.207
Human	70,000	100	7,000	18,000	0.388

Source: Casarett and Doull's *Toxicology,* 4th ed., M. O. Amdur, J. Doull, and C. D. Klassen, Eds., Pergamon Press, New York, 1991. With permission.

TABLE 33.7
Relationship Between Body Weight and Body Surface Area in a Number of Vertebrates

Species	Weight (g)	Surface Area (cm²)
Mouse	20	46
Rat	200	325
Guinea pig	400	565
Rabbit	1,500	1,270
Cat	2,000	1,380
Monkey	4,000	2,980
Dog	12,000	5,770
Man	70,000	18,000

From Toxicology: Principles and Applications, CRC Press, Boca Raton, FL, 1996. With permission.

TABLE 33.8
Comparison of Bile Flow and Hepatic Blood Flow Rates in Various Species

Species	Liver Weight as Percentage of Total Body Weight	Hepatic Blood Flow Rate (ml Blood per 100 g Liver/min)	Bile Flow Rate (ml Bile per kg Body Weight/Day)
Rat	3.36	79	28.6–47.1
Guinea pig	3.86	—	228
Rabbit	3.2	74	118
Cat	3.59	35–48	14
Dog	2.94	82	12
Hen	1.53	—	14
Sheep	2.97	—	12
Monkey	2.09	—	28

From Calabrese, *Principles of Animal Extrapolation,* Lewis Publisher, Chelsea, MI, 1991. With permission.

TABLE 33.9
Comparison of the pH Value of Contents of Different Parts of the Alimentary Tract in Various Species

Species (No. Examined)	Stomach[a]		Small Intestine Portion				Cecum	Colon	Feces[a]
	A	P	1	3	5	7			
Monkey (3)	4.8	2.8	5.6	5.8	6.0	6.0	5.0	5.1	5.5
Dog (3)	5.5	3.4	6.2	6.2	6.6	7.5	6.4	6.5	6.2
Cat (6)	5.0	4.2	6.2	6.7	7.0	7.6	6.0	6.2	7.0
Ox (3)	6.0	2.4	6.7	7.0	7.3	7.9	7.0	7.4	7.5
Sheep (3)	6.4	3.0	5.7	6.6	7.7	8.0	7.3	7.8	8.0
Horse (3)	5.4	3.3	6.7	7.0	7.3	7.9	7.0	7.4	7.5
Pig (20)	4.3	2.2	6.0	6.2	6.9	7.5	6.3	6.8	7.1
Rabbit (11)	1.9	1.9	6.0	6.8	7.5	8.0	6.6	7.2	7.2
Guinea Pig (6)	4.5	4.1	7.6	7.7	8.1	8.2	7.0	6.7	6.7
Rat (7)	5.0	3.8	6.5	6.7	6.8	7.1	6.8	6.6	6.9
Mouse (3)	4.5	3.1	—	—	—	—	—	—	—
Hamster (3)	6.9	2.9	6.1	6.6	6.8	7.1	7.1	—	—
Gerbil (3)	5.5	3.8	6.7	7.0	7.8	8.2	7.0	7.4	7.5
Fowl (6)	4.9	4.2	5.8	6.2	7.0	7.8	7.0	—	7.6
Duck (3)	5.0	4.5	6.1	6.5	7.4	8.0	—	—	7.3

[a] A = Anterior portion of stomach; P = posterior portion; feces = contents of posterior rectum.

From Calabrese, *Principles of Animal Extrapolation,* Lewis Publisher, Chelsea, MI, 1991. With permission.

TABLE 33.10
Comparison of Enzyme Activity in the Small Intestine of Several Species

Species	Enzymatic Activity in the Small Intestine as a Percentage of That in the Liver					
	Ethylmorphine N-Demethylase	Biphenyl Hydroxylase	Aniline Hydroxylase	AHH	Cytochrome c Reductase	Cytochrome P-450
Rabbit	18.6	14.1	20.4	30.0	75.7	34.6
Guinea pig	23.3	16.4	19.8	37.4	78.7	12.4
Cat	ND[a]	9.3	ND	4.6	42.0	ND
Mouse	ND	9.0	ND	6.0	79.6	4.0
Hamster	ND	6.8	ND	5.7	60.7	13.0

[a] ND = not detectable.

From *Toxicology: Principles and Applications,* CRC Press, Boca Raton, FL, 1996. With permission.

TABLE 33.11
Comparison of pH Values in Some
Human Body Compartments

Blood	7.35–7.45
Oral cavity	6.2–7.2
Stomach (at rest)	1.0–3.0
Duodenum	4.8–8.2
Jejunum	6.3–7.3
Ileum	7.6
Colon	7.8–8.0
Rectum	7.8
Cerebral fluid	7.3–7.4
Vagina	3.4–4.2
Urine	4.8–7.5
Sweat	4.0–6.8
Milk	6.6–7.0

From *Toxicology: Principles and Applications,* CRC
Press, Boca Raton, FL, 1996. With permission.

TABLE 33.12
Comparison of the Size of the Absorptive Surface
of the Various Parts of the Gastrointestinal Tract

Oral cavity	0.02
Stomach	0.1–0.2
Small intestine	100
Large intestine	0.5–1.0
Rectum	0.04–0.07

From *Toxicology: Principles and Applications,* CRC Press, Boca
Raton, FL, 1996. With permission.

TABLE 33.13
Comparison of Physiological Characteristics of Experimental Animals and Humans

| Species | Body Wt. (kg) | Surface Area (cm²) | Energy Metabolism[a] | | Cardiac Function | | | | | Arterial Blood Pressure (mm Hg) | |
			cal/kg/day	cal/m²/day	Heart Wt. (g/100g)	Heart Rate (beats/min)	Stroke Vol (ml/beat)	Cardiac Output (l/min)	Cardiac Index (l/m²/m)	Systolic	Diastolic
Rat	0.1–0.5	0.03–0.06	120–140 (B)	760–905 (B)	0.24–0.58	250–400	1.3–2.0	0.015–0.079	1.6	88–184	58–145
Rabbit	1–4	0.23	47 (B)	810	0.19–0.36	123–330	1.3–3.8	0.25–0.75	1.7	95–130	60–90
Monkey	2–4	0.31	49 (B)	675	0.34–0.39	165–240	8.8	1.06	—	137–188	112–152
Dog	5–31	0.39–0.78	34–39 (B)	770–800 (B)	0.65–0.96	72–130	14–22	0.65–1.57	2.9	95–136	43–66
Man	54–94	1.65–1.83	23–26 (B)	790–910 (B)	0.45–0.65	41–108	62.8	5.6	3.3	92–150	53–90
Pig	100–250	2.9–3.2	14–17 (B)	1,100–1,360 (B)	0.25–0.40	55–86	39–43	5.4	4.8	144–185	98–120
Ox	500–800	4.2–8.0	15 (B)	1635 (B)	0.31–0.53	40–58	244	146	—	121–166	80–120
Horse	650–800	5.8–8.0	25 (R)	2,710–2,770 (R)	0.39–0.94	23–70	852	188	4.4	86–104	43–86

[a] B = basal; R = resting.

Source: Mitruka, B.M. and Rawnsley, H.M., *Clinical Biochemical and Hematological Reference Values in Normal Experimental Animals*, Masson Publishing, New York, 1977. With permission.

TABLE 33.14

Comparison of Certain Physiological Values of Experimental Animals and Humans

Species	Body Temperature (°C)	Whole Blood Volume (ml/ kg body wt)	Plasma Volume (ml/kg body wt)	Plasma pH	Plasma CO_2 content (mM/l)	CO_2 Pressure (mm Hg)
Mouse	36.5 ± 0.70	74.5 ± 17.0	48.8 ± 17.0	7.40 ± 0.06	22.5 ± 4.50	40.0 ± 5.40
Rat	37.3 ± 1.40	58.0 ± 14.0	31.3 ± 12.0	7.35 ± 0.09	24.0 ± 4.70	42.0 ± 5.70
Hamster	36.0 ± 0.50	72.0 ± 15.0	45.5 ± 7.50	7.39 ± 0.08	37.3 ± 2.50	59.0 ± 5.00
Guinea pig	37.9 ± 0.95	74.0 ± 7.00	38.8 ± 4.50	7.35 ± 0.09	22.0 ± 6.60	40.0 ± 9.80
Rabbit	38.8 ± 0.65	69.4 ± 12.0	43.5 ± 9.10	7.32 ± 0.03	22.8 ± 8.60	40.0 ± 11.5
Chicken	41.4 ± 0.25	95.5 ± 24.0	65.6 ± 12.5	7.52 ± 0.04	23.0 ± 2.50	26.0 ± 4.50
Cat	38.6 ± 0.70	84.6 ± 14.5	47.7 ± 12.0	7.43 ± 0.03	20.4 ± 3.50	36.0 ± 4.60
Dog	38.9 ± 0.65	92.6 ± 29.5	53.8 ± 20.1	7.42 ± 0.04	21.4 ± 3.90	38.0 ± 5.50
Monkey	38.8 ± 0.80	75.0 ± 14.0	44.7 ± 13.0	7.46 ± 0.06	29.3 ± 3.8	44.0 ± 4.8
Pig	39.3 ± 0.30	69.4 ± 11.5	41.9 ± 8.90	7.40 ± 0.08	30.2 ± 2.5	43.0 ± 5.60
Goat	39.5 ± 0.60	71.0 ± 14.0	55.5 ± 13.0	7.41 ± 0.09	25.2 ± 2.8	50.0 ± 9.40
Sheep	38.8 ± 0.80	58.0 ± 8.50	41.9 ± 12.0	7.48 ± 0.06	26.2 ± 5.00	38.0 ± 8.50
Cattle	38.6 ± 0.30	57.4 ± 5.00	38.8 ± 2.50	7.38 ± 0.05	31.0 ± 3.0	48.0 ± 4.80
Horse	37.8 ± 0.25	72.0 ± 15.0	51.5 ± 12.0	7.42 ± 0.03	28.0 ± 4.00	47.0 ± 8.50
Man	36.9 ± 0.35	77.8 ± 15.0	47.9 ± 8.70	7.39 ± 0.06	27.0 ± 2.00	42.0 ± 5.00

Source: Mitruka, B. M. and Rawnsley, H. M., *Clinical Biochemical and Hematological Reference Values in Normal Experimental Animals,* Masson Publishing, New York, 1977. With permission.

TABLE 33.15

Comparison of Biochemical Components in Urines of Normal Experimental Animals and Humans

Component (mg/kg body wt/day) or Property	Rat	Rabbit	Cat	Dog	Goat	Sheep
Volume (ml/kg body wt/day)	150–350	20.0–350	10.0–30.0	20.0–167	7.0–40.0	10.0–40.0
Specific gravity	1.040–1.076	1.003–1.036	1.020–1.045	1.015–1.050	1.015–1.062	1.015–1.045
pH	7.30–8.50	7.60–8.80	6.00–7.00	6.00–7.00	7.5–8.80	7.50–8.80
Calcium	3.00–9.00	12.1–19.0	0.20–0.45	1.00–3.00	1.00–3.40	1.00–3.00
Chloride	50.0–75.0	190–300	89.0–130	5.00–15.0	186–376	—
Creatinine	24.0–40.0	20.0–80.0	12.0–30.0	15.0–80.0	10.0–22.0	5.80–14.5
Magnesium	0.20–1.90	0.65–4.20	1.50–3.20	1.70–3.00	0.15–1.80	0.10–1.50
Phosphorous, inorganic	20.0–40.0	10.0–60.0	39.0–62.0	20.0–50.0	0.5–1.6	0.10–0.50
Potassium	50.0–60.0	40.0–55.0	55.0–120	40.0–100	250–360	300–420
Protein, total	1.20–6.20	0.74–1.86	3.10–6.82	1.55–4.96	0.74–2.48	0.74–2.17
Sodium	90.4–110.	50.0–70.0	—	2.00–189.	140.–347.	0.80–2.00
Urea nitrogen (g/kg/day)	1.00–1.60	1.20–1.50	0.80–4.00	0.30–0.50	0.14–0.47	0.11–0.17
Uric acid	8.00–12.0	4.00–6.00	0.20–13.0	3.1–6.0	2.00–5.00	2.00–4.00

	Swine	Cattle	Horse	Monkey	Man
Volume (ml/kg body wt/day)	5.00–30.0	17.0–45.0	3.0–18.0	70.0–80.0	8.60–28.6
Specific gravity	1.010–1.050	1.025–1.045	1.020–1.050	1.015–1.065	1.002–1.040

	Swine	Cattle	Horse	Monkey	Man
pH	6.25–7.55	7.60–8.40	7.80–8.30	5.50–7.40	4.80–7.80

TABLE 33.15 *(Continued)*
Comparison of Biochemical Components in Urines of Normal Experimental Animals and Humans

Calcium	—	0.10–3.60	—	10.0–20.0	0.60–8.30
Chloride	—	10.0–140.	81.0–120	80.0–120.	40.0–180.
Creatinine	20.0–90.0	15.0–30.0	—	20.0–60.0	15.0–30.0
Magnesium	—	2.00–7.00	—	3.20–7.10	0.42–2.40
Phosphorous, inorganic	—	0.01–6.20	0.05–2.00	9.00–20.6	10.0–15.0
Potassium	—	240–320.	—	160–245.	16.0–56.0
Protein, total	0.33–1.49	0.25–2.99	0.62–0.99	0.87–2.48	0.81–1.86
Sodium	—	2.00–40.0	—	—	25.0–94.0
Urea nitrogen (g/kg/day)	0.28–0.58	0.05–0.06	0.20–0.80	0.20–0.70	0.20–0.50
Uric acid	1.00–2.00	1.00–4.00	1.00–2.00	1.00–2.00	0.80–3.00

Source: Mitruka, B. M. and Rawnsley, H. M., *Clinical Biochemical and Hematological Reference Values in Normal Experimental Animals*, Masson Publishing, New York, 1977. With permission.

TABLE 33.16
Comparison of Some Biochemical/Physiological/Morphological Differences of Potential Toxicological Significance Between Rats and Humans

	Rat	Human
A. Skin characteristics		
1. Stratum corneum		Much thicker than rat
2. Dermal vasculature		Much thicker than rat
3. Sweat glands	Missing from general body surface; eccrine sweat glands located in foot pads to moisten frictional surface	Numerous coiled tubular sweat glands (100–600/m²)
4. Hair follicles	Densely haired with up to 4000 hairs/cm²	Much fewer hairs, with 40–70 hairs/cm² on skin of the trunk and limbs
5. Dermal absorption based on the above characteristics	Considerably more efficient absorber than humans for a wide variety of organic compounds	
B. Respiratory parameters		
1. Histamine content (µg/g)	15.8	27.7
2. Exogenous histamine catabolism (%)	44.2	29.2
3. Histamine release (%) µg/g		
Compound 48/80	17.1	43.2
Cotton dust	0.0	16.1
4. Lung morphometry		
a. Branching angles	Decreases with increasing depth in the lung	Increases with increasing depth in the lung
b. Symmetry	Less than humans	
c. Diameter ratio of daughter branches at bifurcation	Greater than humans	
d. Number of diversions of tracheobronchial tree	More variable than humans	
5. Mucus flow patterns	13.5 mm/min	15 mm/min
6. Bronchial glands	Absence	Numerous
7. Position of lung to ground	Horizontal	Vertical

TABLE 33.16 *(Continued)*

Comparison of Some Biochemical/Physiological/Morphological Differences of Potential Toxicological Significance Between Rats and Humans

	Rat	Human
8. Breathing	Obligate nose breathers	
C. Gut flora location	Numerous flora in stomach and proximal small intestine	Little or no flora in stomach and proximal small intestine
	Numerous flora in distal small intestine, large intestine, rectum, and feces	Similar to rat
D. Estimated β-glucuronidase activity		
Proximal small intestine	Very high (304.0 units)	0.02 units
Distal small intestine	Very high (1,341.0 units)	0.09 units
E. Plasma protein binding	Generally not as extensive a binder as the human; a number of leading researchers feel that it is not possible to adequately predict the extent of human binding with the rat model	
F. Biliary excretion	The rat is perhaps the most efficient biliary excreter, whereas limited evidence suggests that the human is not an efficient excreter of intermediately weighted compounds.	
G. Metabolism		
1. Conjugations		
Sulfate	Less active than human	
Glucuronidation	More active than human	
Acetylation	Effective	Humans display both effective and slow acetylator phenotypes
Deacetylation	Displays a relatively low ability	Human data inadequate to assess 100% conjugation with glycine
Amino acid with carboxylic acid substrates		
Benzoic acid	80–100% conjugation with glycine	Strongly favors glutamine conjugation
Phenylacetic acid	Strongly favors glycine conjugation	
2. Rodanese activity (liver)	Considerably more active than humans	
3. Epoxide hydrase	Less active in humans	
4. Red blood cell enzymes that prevent oxidant stress (in values relative to humans, which are given as 1)		
Glutathione peroxidase	10.2	1
Glutathione reductase	0.2	1
Catalase	0.2	1
Glucose-6-phosphate dehydrogenase	2.4	1
Superoxide dismutase	1.7	1
Methemoglobin reductase	2.4	1
5. Comparison of rat versus human for 23 substances according to qualitative and quantitative similarity of metabolic pathway	Good predictor 4 of 23; Invalid predictor 8 of 23	

TABLE 33.16 *(Continued)*
Comparison of Some Biochemical/Physiological/Morphological Differences of Potential Toxicological Significance Between Rats and Humans

	Rat	Human
6. Concentration of urine	Typical laboratory rat has the ability to concentrate its urine approximately 2 times as much as that of humans, as indicated by urine/plasma ratios; the desert rat will concentrate its urine 4–5 times more than humans	
H. Dermatotoxicity 　1. Ocular 　2. Skin	Practical reasons preclude its widespread use as a predictive model (e.g., not sufficiently docile); the rabbit is the model of choice for historical reasons and practical considerations: docility, large skin surface, large nonpigmented eyes	
3. Allergic hypersensitivity	The rat is *not* a good model, because it does not produce anaphylactic antibodies in response to the diversity of allergens, which humans do; the guinea pig model is favored in such studies for qualitative predictions.	
I. DNA repair	In absolute terms, less efficient than humans in excision repair; when adjusted for the influence of life span, little difference between these species is found; more efficient than humans in postreplicative repair.	
J. Teratogenicity	Prolonged dependence of the rat (up to the 20–25th somite) on the inverted yolk sac placenta during organogenesis as compared with higher mammals, especially humans (5th somite), thereby making the rodent generally much more susceptible to teratogens than humans.	
K. High-risk animal models 　1. Respiratory 　　a. Asthma	Rats are not considered appropriate; with the exception of humans, dogs are the only animal that develop a defined hypersensitivity disease related to aeroallergens.	
b. Bronchitis	Rats are not considered an appropriate model, because of its version of chronic respiratory disease that involves bronchitis displays, excessive inflammation, and involvement of the pulmonary parenchyma.	

TABLE 33.16 *(Continued)*
Comparison of Some Biochemical/Physiological/Morphological Differences of Potential Toxicological Significance Between Rats and Humans

	Rat	Human
2. Cardiovascular		
a. Atherosclerosis	The rat is generally not considered a very effective model, because it is very resistant to developing this disease.	
b. Hypertension	Numerous predictive rat strains exist; the rat is the animal of choice.	

From *Principles of Animal Extrapolation*, Calabrese, E. J., Ed., Lewis Publishers, Chelsea, MI, 1991. With permission.

TABLE 33.17
Permittivity and Conductivity of Biological Tissues

ϵ: Relative permittivity
σ: Conductivity in S/m (siemens per meter)
All values refer to 37°C.
Frequencies are those commonly used for therapy.

Material	Wt % Water	13.56 MHz ϵ	13.56 MHz σ	27.12 MHz ϵ	27.12 MHz σ	433 MHz ϵ	433 MHz σ	915 MHz ϵ	915 MHz σ	2450 MHz ϵ	2450 MHz σ
Artery	—	—	—	—	—	—	—	—		43	1.85
Blood	—	155	1.16	110	1.19	66	1.27	62	1.41	60	2.04
Bone											
With marrow	44–55	11	0.03	9	0.04	5.2	0.11	4.9	0.15	4.8	0.21
In Hank's solution		28	0.021	24	0.024	—	—	—	—	—	—
Bowell (plus contents)	60–82	73	—	49	—	—	—	—	—	—	—
Brain											
White matter	68–73	182	0.27	123	0.33	48	0.63	41	0.77	35.5	1.04
Grey matter	82–85	310	0.40	186	0.45	57	0.83	50	1.0	43	1.43
Fat	5–20	38	0.21	22	0.21	15	0.26	15	0.35	12	0.82
Kidney	78–79	402	0.72	229	0.83	60	1.22	55	1.41	50	2.63
Liver	73–77	288	0.49	182	0.58	47	0.89	46	1.06	44	1.79
Lung	80–83										
Inflated		42	0.11	29	0.13	—	—	—		—	—
Deflated		94	0.29	57	0.32	35	0.71	33	0.78	—	—
Muscle	73–78	152	0.74	112	0.76	57	1.12	55.4	1.45	49.6	2.56
Ocular tissues											
Choroid	78	240	0.97	144	1.0	60	1.32	55	1.40	52	2.30
Cornea	75	132	1.55	100	1.57	55	1.73	51.5	1.90	49	2.50
Iris	77	240	0.90	150	0.95	59	1.18	55	1.18	52	2.10
Lens cortex	65	175	0.53	107	0.58	55	0.80	52	0.97	48	1.75
Lens nucleus	—	50.5	0.13	48.5	0.15	31.5	0.29	30.8	0.50	26	1.40
Retina	89	464	0.90	250	1.0	61	1.50	57	1.55	56	2.50
Skin	60–76	120	0.25	98	0.40	47	0.84	45	0.97	44	1.85
Spleen	76–81	269	0.86	170	0.93	—	—	—	—	—	—
Tumor tissues											
Hemangiopericytoma		136	1.10	106	1.14	57	1.37	55.4	1.61	50	2.86

TABLE 33.17 *(Continued)*
Permittivity and Conductivity of Biological Tissues

ε: Relative permittivity
σ: Conductivity in S/m (siemens per meter)
All values refer to 37°C.
Frequencies are those commonly used for therapy.

Material	Wt % Water	13.56 MHz ε	σ	27.12 MHz ε	σ	433 MHz ε	σ	915 MHz ε	σ	2450 MHz ε	σ
Intestinal leiomysarcoma	309	0.83	183	0.91	62	1.23	60	1.49	54	2.63
Splenic hematoma	297	0.64	243	0.74	54	0.93	52	1.06	49	1.89
Rat hepatoma D23	305	0.74	178	0.87	—	—	—	—	—	—
Canine fibrosarcoma	48	0.18	29	0.19	(Before hyperthermia)					
	30	0.65	19	0.66	(After 43°C hyperthermia)					
Mouse KHT tumor	—	—	135	—	61	1.12	60	1.61	54	2.56

Note: The dielectric properties of the same tissue types from different animals have been found to be similar. The data given in this table should be considered as representing average values, and the likely spread of the electrical properties for each tissue type can be estimated from the range of tissue water contents.

These data have been derived from Pethig, R., *IEEE Trans. Elec. Insul. El-19,* 453, 1984, from which full references may be obtained. The electrical properties of other biological materials at other frequencies have been tabulated by Geddes, L. A. and Baker, L. E., *Med. Biol. Eng.,* 5, 271, 1967 and by Stuchly, M. A. and Stuchly, S. S., *J. Microwave Power* 15, 19, 1980. From *Handbook of Chemistry and Physics,* Lide, D. R., Ed., CRC Press, Boca Raton, FL, 1990. With permission.

SECTION 3. MATHEMATICS, SYMBOLS, PHYSICAL CONSTANTS, CONVERSIONS, AND STATISTICS

A. SYMBOLS

TABLE 33.18
Greek Alphabet

Greek Letter		Greek Name	English Equivalent	Greek Letter		Greek Name	English Equivalent
A	α	Alpha	a	N	ν	Nu	n
B	β	Beta	b	Ξ	ξ	Xi	x
Γ	γ	Gamma	g	O	o	Omicron	o
Δ	δ	Delta	d	Π	π	Pi	p
E	ε	Epsilon	ĕ	P	ρ	Rho	r
Z	ζ	Zeta	z	Σ	σ	ē Sigma	s
H	η	Eta	ē	T	τ	Tau	t
Θ	θ	Theta	th	Y	υ	Upsilon	u
I	ι	Iota	i	Φ	φ	φ Phi	ph
K	κ	Kappa	k	X	χ	Chi	ch
Λ	λ	Lambda	l	Ψ	ψ	Psi	ps
M	μ	Mu	m	Ω	ω	Omega	ō

See end of section for source.

B. CONVERSIONS

The Système international d'unités (International System of Units) or SI is a modernized version
of the metric system. The primary goal of the conversion to SI units is to revise the present confused
measurement system and to improve test-result communications. The SI has 7 basic units from
which other units are derived:

TABLE 33.19
Base Units of SI

Physical Quantity	Base Unit	SI Symbol
Length	meter	m
Mass	kilogram	kg
Time	second	s
Amount of substance	mole	mol
Thermodynamic temperature	kelvin	K
Electric current	ampere	A
Luminous intensity	candela	cd

See end of section for source.

Combinations of these base units can express any property, although for simplicity, special
names are given to some of these derived units.

TABLE 33.20
Representative Derived Units

Derived Unit	Name and Symbol	Derivation from Base Units
Area	square meter	m^2
Volume	cubic meter	m^3
Force	newton (N)	$kg \cdot m \cdot s^{-2}$
Pressure	pascal (Pa)	$kg \cdot m^1 \cdot s^{-2}$ (N/m^2)
Work, energy	joule (J)	$kg \cdot m^2 \cdot s^{-2}$ ($N \cdot m$)
Mass density	kilogram per cubic meter	kg/m^3
Frequency	hertz (Hz)	s^{-1}
Temperature	degree Celsius (°C)	°C = °K − 273.15
Concentration		
Mass	kilogram/liter	kg/l
Substance	mole/liter	mol/l
Molality	mole/kilogram	mol/kg
Density	kilogram/liter	kg/l

See end of section for source.

Prefixes to the base unit are used in this system to form decimal multiples and submultiples.
The preferred multiples and submultiples listed below change the quantity by increments of 10^3 or
10^{-3}. The exceptions to these recommended factors are indicated by the asterisk.

TABLE 33.21
Prefixes and Symbols for Decimal
Multiples and Submultiples

Factor	Prefix	Symbol
10^{18}	exa	E
10^{15}	beta	P
10^{12}	tera	T
10^{9}	giga	G
10^{6}	mega	M
10^{3}	kilo	k
10^{2}*	hecto	h
10^{1}*	deka	da
10^{-1}*	deci	d
10^{-2}*	centi	c
10^{-3}	milli	m
10^{-6}	micro	μ
10^{-9}	nano	n
10^{-12}	pico	p
10^{-15}	femto	f
10^{-18}	atto	a

See end of section for source.

To convert xenobiotic concentrations to or from SI units: Conversion factor (CF) = 1000/mol. wt.; conversion *to* SI units: μg/ml $\times$CF = μmol/l; conversion *from* SI units: μmol/l $\div$ CF = μg/ml.

TABLE 33.22
Conversion of Human Hematological Values from Traditional Units into SI Units

Constituent	Traditional Units	Multiplication Factor	SI Units
Clotting time	Minutes	0.06	ks
Prothrombin time	Seconds	1.0	arb. unit
Hematocrit (erythrocytes, volume fraction)	%	0.01	1
Hemoglobin	g/100 ml	0.6205	mmol/l
Leukocyte count (leukocytes, number concentration)	per mm^3	10^6	10^9/l
Erythrocyte count (erythrocytes, number concentration)	million per mm^3	10^6	10^{12}/l
Mean corpuscular volume (MCV)	μ^3	1.0	fl
Mean corpuscular hemoglobin (MCH) (Erc-Hemoglobin, amount of substance)	pg	0.06205	fmol
Mean corpuscular hemoglobin concentration (MCHC) (Erc-Hemoglobin, substance concentration)	%	0.6205	mmol/l
Erythrocyte sedimentation rate	mm/hour	1.0	arb.unit
Platelet count (Blood platelets, number concentration)	mm^3	10^6	10^9/l
Reticulocyte count (Erc-Reticulocytes, number fraction)	% red cells	0.01	1

Source: Young, D. S., *N. Engl. J. Med.,* 292, 795, 1975. With permission.

TABLE 33.23
Conversion of Laboratory Values from Traditional Units into SI Units

Constituent	Traditional Units	Multiplication Factor	SI Units
Amylase	Units/l	1.0	arb · unit
Bilirubin (direct)	mg/100 ml	43.06	µmol/l
conjugated	mg/100 ml	17.10	µmol/l
total	mg/100 ml	17.10	µmol/l
Calcium	mg/100 ml	0.2495	mmol/l
Carbon dioxide	mEq/1	1.0	mmol/l
Chloride	mEq/1	1.0	mmol/l
Creatine phosphokinase (CPK)	mU/ml	0.01667	µmol S^{-1}/l
Creatinine	mg/100 ml	88.40	µmol/l
Glucose	mg/100 ml	0.05551	mmol/l
Lactic dehydrogenase	mU/ml	0.01667	µmol S^{-1}/l
Cholesterol	mg/100 ml	0.02586	mmol/l
Magnesium	mEq/l	0.50	mmol/l
P_{CO_2}	mm Hg	0.1333	kPa
pH		1.0	1
P_{O_2}	mm Hg	0.133	kPa
Phosphatase, acid	Sigma	278.4	nmol S^{-1}/l
Phosphatase, alkaline	Bodansky	0.08967	nmol S^{-1}/l
Phosphorus, inorganic	mg/100 ml	0.3229	nmol/l
Protein, total	g/100 ml	10	g/l
Protein, electrophoreses			
Albumin	% total	0.01	1
Globulin, α_1	% total	0.01	1
α_2	% total	0.01	1
β	% total	0.01	1
γ	% total	0.01	1
Potassium	m Eq/l	1.0	mmol/l
Sodium	m Eq/l	1.0	mmol/l
Transaminase (SGOT) (aminotransferase)	Karmen	0.008051	µmol S^{-1}/1
Urea nitrogen	mg/100 ml	0.3569	mmol/l
Uric acid	mg/100 ml	0.65948	mmol/l

Source: Young, D. S., *N. Engl. J. Med.*, 292, 795, 1975. With permission.

TABLE 33.24
Calculation of Milliequivalent Weight, Creatinine Clearance, and Surface Area of Children

To calculate milliequivalent weight: $\text{mEq} = \dfrac{\text{Gram molecular weight / valence}}{1000}$

$\text{mEq} = \dfrac{\text{mg}}{\text{eq wt}}$

Equivalent weight or eq wt $= \dfrac{\text{Gram molecular weight}}{\text{Valence}}$

Commonly Used mEq Weights

Chloride	35.5 mg = 1 mEq	Magnesium	12 mg = 1 mEq
Sodium	23 mg = 1 mEq	Potassium	39 mg = 1 mEq
Calcium	20 mg = 1 mEq		

TABLE 33.24 *(Continued)*
Calculation of Milliequivalent Weight, Creatinine Clearance, and Surface Area of Children

To calculate creatinine clearance (Ccr) from serum creatinine:

$$\text{Male: Ccr} = \frac{\text{Weight (kg)} \times (140 - \text{age})}{72 \times \text{serum creatinine (mg / dl)}} \quad \text{Female: Ccr} = 0.85 \times \text{calculation for males}$$

To calculate ideal body weight (kg):

Male = 50 kg + 2.3 kg (each inch > 5ft) Female = 45.5 kg + 2.3 kg (each inch > 5ft)

To approximate surface area (ml) of children from weight (kg):

Weight Range (kg)	≈ Surface Area (m²)
1–5	$(0.05 \times \text{kg}) + 0.05$
6–10	$(0.04 \times \text{kg}) + 0.10$
11–20	$(0.03 \times \text{kg}) + 0.20$
21–40	$(0.02 \times \text{kg}) + 0.40$

To calculate body surface area (BSA) in adults and children:
1) Dubois method:

$$\text{SA (cm}^2\text{) wt (kg)}^{0.425} \times \text{ht (cm)}^{0.725} \times 71.84$$

$$\text{SA (m}^2\text{)} = K \times \sqrt[3]{\text{wt}^2} \text{ (kg)} \quad \text{(common } K \text{ value 0.1 for toddlers, 0.103 for neonates)}$$

2) Simplified method:

$$\text{BSA(m}^2) = \sqrt{\frac{\text{ht(cm)} \times \text{wt(kg)}}{3,600}}$$

TABLE 33.25
Table for Predicting Human Half-Life of Xenobiotics from Rat Half-Life

Rat Half-life (Hours)	Lower			Human Half-Life Estimate (Hours)	Upper		
	95%	90%	80%		80%	90%	95%
0.01	0.019	0.025	0.034	0.106	0.327	0.451	0.598
0.02	0.034	0.045	0.062	0.189	0.574	0.790	1.045
0.03	0.048	0.064	0.087	0.264	0.799	1.098	1.450
0.04	0.062	0.081	0.111	0.335	1.011	1.387	1.830
0.05	0.074	0.098	0.134	0.404	1.213	1.664	2.193
0.06	0.087	0.114	0.156	0.469	1.408	1.930	2.543
0.07	0.099	0.130	0.178	0.533	1.598	2.189	2.882
0.08	0.110	0.146	0.199	0.596	1.782	2.441	3.213
0.09	0.122	0.161	0.220	0.657	1.963	2.687	3.536
0.1	0.13	0.18	0.24	0.72	2.14	2.93	3.85
0.2	0.24	0.31	0.43	1.27	3.78	5.17	6.79
0.3	0.34	0.44	0.60	1.78	5.28	7.21	9.47
0.4	0.43	0.56	0.77	2.26	6.70	9.14	12.00
0.5	0.51	0.68	0.92	2.72	8.05	10.99	14.42
0.6	0.60	0.79	1.07	3.17	9.36	12.77	16.76
0.7	0.68	0.89	1.22	3.60	10.63	14.51	19.04

TABLE 33.25 *(Continued)*
Table for Predicting Human Half-Life of Xenobiotics from Rat Half-Life

Rat Half-life (Hours)	Lower			Human Half-Life Estimate (Hours)	Upper		
	95%	90%	80%		80%	90%	95%
0.8	0.76	1.00	1.36	4.02	11.88	16.20	21.26
0.9	0.84	1.10	1.50	4.44	13.09	17.86	23.44
1	0.92	1.20	1.64	4.84	14.29	19.49	25.57
2	1.63	2.13	2.91	8.60	25.40	34.66	45.47
3	2.27	2.98	4.07	12.04	35.59	48.58	63.76
4	2.88	3.78	5.16	15.28	45.24	61.76	81.09
5	3.46	4.54	6.20	18.39	54.49	74.42	97.74
6	4.02	5.28	7.21	21.39	63.46	86.69	113.88
7	4.56	5.99	8.19	24.31	72.18	98.64	129.61
8	5.08	6.68	9.14	27.15	80.71	110.32	144.99
9	5.60	7.36	10.06	29.94	89.07	121.77	160.08
10	6.1	8.0	11.0	32.7	97.3	133.0	174.9
20	10.7	14.1	19.4	58.1	174.0	238.3	313.9
30	14.9	19.7	27.0	81.3	244.6	335.6	442.4
40	18.8	24.9	34.1	103.2	311.6	427.9	564.7
50	22.6	29.8	41.0	124.1	376.1	516.9	682.7
60	26.2	34.6	47.5	144.4	438.6	603.3	797.2
70	29.6	39.2	53.9	164.1	499.5	687.5	909.1
80	33.0	43.6	60.1	183.3	559.2	770.0	1018.7
90	36.3	48.0	66.1	202.1	617.7	851.1	1126.4
100	39.5	52.3	72.0	220.6	675.2	930.8	1232.4
200	68.9	91.4	126.5	391.9	1214.2	1679.5	2230.5
300	95.2	126.7	175.7	548.6	1712.7	2374.3	3159.3
400	119.8	159.7	221.7	696.4	2186.8	3036.7	4046.6
500	143.2	191.0	265.6	837.9	2643.8	3676.1	4904.4
600	165.5	221.1	307.7	974.7	3087.5	4297.9	5739.6
700	187.1	250.1	348.5	1107.6	3520.5	4905.5	6556.7
800	208.1	278.3	388.1	1237.3	3944.6	5501.3	7358.6
900	228.5	305.8	426.8	1364.3	4361.2	6086.9	8147.4
1000	248.4	332.7	464.6	1488.9	4771.1	6663.7	8925.0
1100	267.9	359.0	501.7	1611.3	5175.1	7232.7	9692.5

Note: The following examples indicate how this table is used. For a xenobiotic with a rat half-life of 0.8 h, the prediction or best guess of the human half-life is 4.02 h. The table indicates that the actual half-life would fall between 1.0 and 16.2 h with a confidence of 90%. Values falling between those indicated in the table can be linearly interpolated, for example, a rat half-life of 2.7 h gives a human half-life of 11.01 h.

From Bachmann, K. M., Pardoe, D., and White, D., Scaling basic toxicokinetic parameters from rat to man, *Environ. Health Perspect.*, 104, 400–407, 1996. With permission.

TABLE 33.26
Table for Predicting Human Volume of Distribution from Rat Volume of Distribution

Rat volume	Lower			Human Volume	Upper		
(l/kg)	95%	90%	80%	Estimate (l/kg)	80%	90%	95%
0.01	0.002	0.003	0.004	0.011	0.031	0.041	0.054
0.02	0.004	0.005	0.007	0.020	0.057	0.076	0.099
0.03	0.006	0.008	0.011	0.029	0.082	0.109	0.141
0.04	0.008	0.010	0.014	0.038	0.105	0.141	0.182
0.05	0.010	0.013	0.017	0.046	0.128	0.172	0.222
0.06	0.012	0.015	0.020	0.055	0.151	0.202	0.261
0.07	0.013	0.017	0.023	0.063	0.174	0.232	0.299
0.08	0.015	0.019	0.026	0.071	0.196	0.261	0.337
0.09	0.017	0.022	0.029	0.079	0.217	0.290	0.374
0.1	0.019	0.024	0.032	0.087	0.239	0.319	0.411
0.2	0.035	0.045	0.060	0.164	0.445	0.593	0.762
0.3	0.051	0.065	0.087	0.236	0.641	0.853	1.096
0.4	0.066	0.085	0.113	0.307	0.831	1.105	1.419
0.5	0.081	0.104	0.139	0.376	1.016	1.352	1.735
0.6	0.096	0.123	0.164	0.443	1.198	1.593	2.045
0.7	0.111	0.142	0.189	0.510	1.377	1.832	2.350
0.8	0.125	0.160	0.213	0.575	1.554	2.067	2.652
0.9	0.139	0.178	0.237	0.640	1.729	2.299	2.950
1	0.15	0.20	0.26	0.70	1.90	2.53	3.25
2	0.29	0.37	0.49	1.32	3.57	4.75	6.09
3	0.41	0.53	0.70	1.91	5.16	6.87	8.82
4	0.53	0.69	0.91	2.48	6.71	8.93	11.47
5	0.65	0.84	1.18	3.03	8.23	10.96	14.08
6	0.77	0.99	1.32	3.58	9.72	12.95	16.64
7	0.88	1.14	1.51	4.11	11.19	14.92	19.17
8	0.99	1.28	1.71	4.64	12.65	16.86	21.68
9	1.11	1.42	1.90	5.17	14.09	18.79	24.17
10	1.21	1.56	2.08	5.69	15.52	20.70	26.63
20	2.25	2.90	3.88	10.66	29.32	39.20	50.54
30	3.22	4.16	5.57	15.40	42.60	57.04	73.63
40	4.15	5.37	7.20	19.99	55.54	74.46	96.23
50	5.06	6.54	8.78	24.48	68.24	91.59	118.48
60	5.94	7.69	10.33	28.88	80.77	108.50	140.45
70	6.80	8.81	11.84	33.22	93.14	125.22	162.21
80	7.65	9.91	13.34	37.49	105.39	141.79	183.79
90	8.48	11.00	14.81	41.72	117.54	158.23	205.22

Note: See note of previous table for examples of how this table is used.

From Bachmann, K. M., Pardoe, D., and White, D., Scaling basic toxicokinetic parameters from rat to man, *Environ. Health Perspect.*, 104, 400–407, 1996. With permission.

TABLE 33.27
Approximate Metric and Apothecary Weight Equivalents

Metric	Apothecary	Metric	Apothecary
1 gram (g)	= 15 grains	0.05g (50 mg)	= 3/4 grain
0.6 g (600 mg)	= 10 grains	0.03 g (30 mg)	= 1/2 grain
0.5 g (500 mg)	= 7½ grains	0.015 g (15 mg)	= 1/4 grain
0.3 g (300 mg)	= 5 grains	0.001 g (1 mg)	= 1/80 grain
0.2 g (200 mg)	= 3 grains	0.6 mg	= 1/100 grain
0. 1 g (100 mg)	= 1½ grains	0.5 mg	= 1/120 grain
0.06 g (60 mg)	= 1 grain	0.4 mg	= 1/150 grain

Approximate household, apothecary, and metric volume equivalents

Household	Apothecary	Metric
1 teaspoon (t or tsp)	= 1 fluidram (f_3)	= 4 or 5 ml[a]
1 tablespoon (T or tbs)	= ½ fluidounce (f_3)	= 15 ml
2 tablespoons	= 1 fluidounce	= 30 ml
1 measuring cupful	= 8 fluidounces	= 240 ml
1 pint (pt)	= 16 fluidounces	= 473 ml
1 quart (qt)	= 32 fluidounces	= 946 ml
1 gallon (gal)	= 128 fluidounces	= 3,785 ml

[a] 1 ml = 1 cubic centimeter (cc); however, ml is the preferred measurement term today.

See end of section for source.

TABLE 33.28
Conversion Factors — Metric to English

To Obtain	Multiply	By
Inches	Centimeters	0.3937007874
Feet	Meters	3.280839895
Yards	Meters	1.093613298
Miles	Kilometers	0.6213711922
Ounces	Grams	$3.527396195 \times 10^{-2}$
Pounds	Kilograms	2.204622622
Gallons (U.S. Liquid)	Liters	0.2641720524
Fluid ounces	Milliliters (cc)	$3.381402270 \times 10^{-2}$
Square inches	Square centimeters	0.1550003100
Square feet	Square meters	10.76391042
Square yards	Square meters	1.195990046
Cubic inches	Milliliters (cc)	$6.102374409 \times 10^{-2}$
Cubic feet	Cubic meters	35.31466672
Cubic yards	Cubic meters	1.307950619

See end of section for source.

TABLE 33.29
Conversion Factors — English to Metric[a]

To Obtain	Multiply	By
Microns	Mils	**25.4**
Centimeters	Inches	**2.54**
Meters	Feet	**0.3048**
Meters	Yards	**0.9144**
Kilometers	Miles	**1.609344**
Grains	Ounces	28.34952313
Kilograms	Pounds	**0.45359237**
Liters	Gallons (U.S. Liquid)	**3.785411784**
Millimeters (cc)	Fluid ounces	29.57352956
Square centimeters	Square inches	**6.4516**
Square meters	Square feet	**0.09290304**
Square meters	Square yards	**0.83612736**
Milliliters (cc)	Cubic inches	**16.387064**
Cubic meters	Cubic feet	$2.831684659 \times 10^{-2}$
Cubic meters	Cubic yards	0.764554858

[a] Boldface numbers are exact; others are given to ten significant figures where so indicated by the multiplier factor. See end of section for source.

TABLE 33.30
Conversion Factors — General[a]

To Obtain	Multiply	By
Atmospheres	Feet of water @ 4°C	2.950×10^{-2}
Atmospheres	Inches of mercury @ 0°C	3.342×10^{-2}
Atmospheres	Pounds per square inch	6.804×10^{-2}
Pascal	Millibar	1×10^{2}
Pascal	Millimeter mercury 0°C	1.33×10^{2}
Pascal	Pound per square inch	6.894×10^{3}
BTU	Foot-pounds	1.285×10^{-3}
BTU	Joules	9.480×10^{-4}
Cubic feet	Cords	**128**
Degree (angle)	Radians	57.2958
Ergs	Foot-pounds	1.356×10^{7}
Feet	Miles	5,280
Feet of water @ 40°C	Atmospheres	33.90
Foot-pounds	Horsepower-hours	1.98×10^{6}
Foot-pounds	Kilowatt-hours	2.655×10^{6}
Foot-pounds per min	Horsepower	3.3×10^{4}
Horsepower	Foot-pounds per sec	1.818×10^{-3}
Inches of mercury @ 0°C	Pounds per square inch	2.036
Joules	BTU	1.054.8
Joules	Foot-pounds	1.35582
Kilowatts	BTU per min	1.758×10^{-2}
Kilowatts	Foot-pounds per min	2.26×10^{-5}

TABLE 33.30 *(Continued)*
Conversion Factors — General[a]

To Obtain	Multiply	By
Kilowatts	Horsepower	0.745712
Knots	Miles per hour	0.86897624
Miles	Feet	1.894×10^{-4}
Nautical miles	Miles	0.86897624
Radians	Degrees	1.745×10^{-2}
Square feet	Acres	**43,560**
Watts	BTU per min	17.5796

[a] Boldface numbers are exact; others are given to ten significant figures where so indicated by the multiplier factor. See end of section for source.

See www.onlineconversion.com for other conversions.

TABLE 33.31
Temperature Factors[a]

$$F = 9/5 \, (°C) + 32$$
Fahrenheit temperature = 1.8 (temperature in kelvins) − 459.67
$$°C = 5/9 \, [(°F) - 32)]$$
Celsius temperature = temperature in kelvins − 273.15
Fahrenheit temperature = 1.8 (Celsius temperature) + 32

Conversion of Temperatures		
From	**To**	
°Celsius	°Fahrenheit	$t_F = (t_c \times 1.8) + 32$
	Kelvin	$T_K = t_c + 273.15$
	°Rankine	$T_R = (t_c + 273.15) \times 18$
°Fahrenheit	°Celsius	$T_Y = \dfrac{t_F - 32}{1.8}$
	Kelvin	$T_k = \dfrac{t_F - 32}{1.8} + 273.15$
	°Rankine	$T_R = t_f + 459.67$
Kelvin	°Celsius	$t_c = T_K - 273.15$
	°Rankine	$T_R = T_K \times 1.8$
°Rankine	°Farenheit	$t_F = T_R - 459.67$
	Kelvin	$T_K = \dfrac{t_R}{1.8}$

[a] Boldface numbers are exact; others are given to ten significant figures where so indicated by the multiplier factor. See end of section for source.

TABLE 33.32
Temperature Conversions

°F	°C	°F	°C	°F	°C	°F	°C	°F	°C
−10	−23.3	35	+1.6	85	29.4	135	57.2	185	85.0
−5	−20.5	40	4.4	90	32.2	140	60.0	190	87.8
0	−17.8	45	7.2	95	35.0	145	62.8	195	90.5
+5	−15.0	50	10.0	100	37.8	150	65.5	200	93.3
10	−12.2	55	12.8	105	40.5	155	68.3	205	96.1
15	−9.4	60	15.5	110	43.3	160	71.1	210	98.9
20	−6.6	65	18.3	115	46.1	165	73.9	212	100
25	−3.9	70	21.1	120	48.9	170	76.6		
30	−1.1	75	23.9	125	51.6	175	79.4		
32	0	80	26.6	130	54.4	180	82.2		

TABLE 33.33
Table of Equivalents

Kg	= 1,000 g, 1 million mg, 2.2 lbs
g	= 1,000 mg, 1 million µg, approx. 0.035 oz
mg	= 1,000 µg, 1 million ng
µg	= 1,000 ng
1	= approx. 1 quart, approx. 33 oz
lb	= 16 oz, 454.5 g, 0.45 kg
oz	= 28.4 g
acre	= 4,047 m^2
hectare	= 2.5 acres

When referring to the concentration of a chemical in food or other medium:

mg/kg	= ppm, µg/g
mg/l	= ppm = 0.0001%
µg/kg	= ppb, ng/g
ng/kg	= ppt
ppm	= mg/kg, µg/g
ppb	= µg/kg, ng/g
ppt	= ng/kg

See end of section for source.

HOW MANY MOLECULES?

To calculate the number of molecules in any quantity of a chemical, one needs to know the weight of a mole of the chemical and the number of molecules in a mole. A mole of any chemical is its molecular weight expressed in grams. Avogadro's number, 6×10^{23}, is the number of molecules in a mole.

The number of molecules in 10 µg of benzpyrene is calculated as follows: the molecular weight of benzpyrene is 252; therefore, a mole would weigh 252 g. 252 g is equal to 2.52×10^8 µg. The number of molecules in a µg is obtained by dividing the number of molecules in a mole by the number of µg in a mole. For benzpyrene, 6×10^{23} divided by 2.52×10^8 equals 2.4×10^{15}. The number of molecules in 10 µg benzpyrene would be 10 times as much, or 2.4×10^{16}.

TABLE 33.34
Overview of Units Used to Express the Concentration of a Substance

Compartment	Units	Abbreviation	Conversion[a]
Air (gases)	$\mu g\ m^{-3}$		1 $\mu g\ m^{-3}$ is V/A $\mu l\ m^{-3}$
	$\mu mol\ m^{-3}$		1 $\mu mol\ m^{-3}$ is V $\mu l\ m^{-3}$
	$\mu l\ m^{-3}$	ppbv	
	μl^{-1}	ppmv	
Water	$\mu g\ l^{-1}$	ppb	
	$mg\ l^{-1}$	ppm	
	$\mu mol\ l^{-1}$	μM	1 $\mu mol\ l^{-1}$ is A $\mu g\ l^{-1}$
Soil	$\mu g\ kg^{-1}$	ppb	
	$mg\ kg^{-1}$	ppm	
	$\mu g\ g^{-1}$	ppm	
	$\mu mol\ g^{-1}$		1 $\mu mol\ g^{-1}$ is A $\mu g\ g^{-1}$

[a] A = molecular weight of the substance; V = molar volume at current pressure and temperature.

See end of section for source.

TABLE 33.35
Conversions of Nucleic Acids and Proteins

I. Weight conversions
  1 mg = 10^{-6} g
  1 ng = 10^{-9} g
  1 pg = 10^{-12} g
  1 fg = 10^{-15} g

II. Spectrophotometric conversions
  1A_{260} unit of double-stranded DNA = 50 $\mu g/ml$
  1A_{260} unit of single-stranded DNA = 33 $\mu g/ml$
  1A_{260} unit of single-stranded RNA = 40 $\mu g/ml$

III. DNA molar conversions
  1 μg of 1,000 bp DNA = 1.52 pmol (3.03 pmol of ends)
  1 μg of pBR322 DNA = 0.36 pmol DNA
  1 pmol of 1,000 bp DNA = 0.66 μg
  1 pmol of pBR322 DNA = 2.8 μg

IV. Protein molar conversions
  100 pmol of 100,000 MW protein = 10 μg
  100 pmol of 50,000 MW protein = 5 μg
  100 pmol of 10,000 MW protein = 1 μg

V. Protein/DNA conversions
  1 kb of DNA = 333 amino acids of coding capacity = 3.7×10^4 MW
  10,000 MW protein = 270 bp DNA
  30,000 MW protein = 810 bp DNA
  50,000 MW protein = 1.35 kb DNA
  100,000 MW protein = 2.7 kb DNA

TABLE 33.36
Conversion of Radioactivity Units from mCi and μCi to MBq

mCi	MBq	mCl	MBq	μCi	MBq	μCi	MBq
200	7,400	10	370	1,000	37.0	80	2.96
150	5,550	9	333	900	33.3	70	2.59
100	3,700	8	296	800	29.6	60	2.22
90	3,330	7	259	700	25.9	50	1.85
80	2,960	6	222	600	22.2	40	1.48
70	2,590	5	185	500	18.5	30	1.11
60	2,220	4	148	400	14.8	20	0.74
50	1,850	3	111	300	11.1	10	0.37
40	1,480	2	74.0	200	7.4	5	0.185
30	1,110	1	37.0	100	3.7	2	0.074
20	740			90	3.33	1	0.037

See end of section for source.

TABLE 33.37
Conversion Formula for Concentration of Solutions

A = Weight per cent of solute   G = Molality
B = Molecular weight of solvent   M = Molarity
E = Molecular weight of solute   N = Mole fraction
F = Grams of solute per liter of solution   R = Density of solution grams per cc

Concentration of Solute SOUGHT	Concentration of Solute — GIVEN				
	A	N	G	M	F
A	—	$\dfrac{100N \times E}{N \times E + (1-N)B}$	$\dfrac{100G \times E}{1,000 + G \times E}$	$\dfrac{M \times E}{10R}$	$\dfrac{F}{10R}$
N	$\dfrac{\dfrac{A}{E}}{\dfrac{A}{E} + \dfrac{100-A}{B}}$	—	$\dfrac{B \times G}{B \times G + 1,000}$	$\dfrac{B \times M}{M(B-E) + 1,000R}$	$\dfrac{B \times F}{F(B-E) + 1,000R \times E}$
G	$\dfrac{1,000A}{E(100-A)}$	$\dfrac{1,000N}{B - N \times B}$	—	$\dfrac{1,000M}{1,000R - (M \times E)}$	$\dfrac{1,000F}{E(1,000R - F)}$
M	$\dfrac{10R \times A}{E}$	$\dfrac{1,000R \times N}{N \times E + (1-N)B}$	$\dfrac{1,000R \times G}{1,000 + E \times G}$	—	$\dfrac{F}{E}$
F	10AR	$\dfrac{1,000R \times N \times E}{N \times E + (1-N)B}$	$\dfrac{1,000R \times G \times E}{1,000 + G \times ES}$	$M \times E$	—

Source: Handbook of Chemistry and Physics, Lide, D. R., Ed., CRC Press, Boca Raton, FL, 1990. With permission.

C. PHYSICAL CONSTANTS

TABLE 33.38
General Physical Constants

Equatorial radius of the earth = 6378.388 km = 3963.34 miles (statute).

Polar radius of the earth = 6356.912 km = 3949.99 miles (statute).

1 degree of latitude at 40° = 69 miles.

1 international nautical mile = 1.15078 miles (statute) = 1852 m = 6076.115 ft.

Mean density of the earth = 5.522 g/cm^3 = 344.7 lb/ft^3

Constant of gravitation (6.673 ± 0.003) × 10^{-8} cm^3 gm^{-1}s^{-2}.

Acceleration due to gravity at sea level, latitude 45° = 980.6194 cm/s^2 = 32.1726 ft/s^2.

Length of seconds pendulum at sea level, latitude 45° = 99.3575 cm = 39.1171 in.

1 knot (international) = 101.269 ft/min = 1.6878 ft/s = 1.1508 miles (statute)/h.

1 micron = 10^{-4} cm.

1 ångstrom = 10^{-5} cm.

Mass of hydrogen atom = (1.67339 ± 0.0031) × 10^{-24} g.

Density of mercury at 0°C = 13.5955 g/ml.

Density of water at 3.98°C = 1.000000 g/ml.

Density, maximum, of water, at 3.98°C = 0.999973 g/cm^3.

Density of dry air at 0°C. 760 mm = 1.2929 g/l.

Velocity of sound in dry air at 0°C = 331.36 m/s – 1087.1 ft/s.

Velocity of light in vacuum = (2.997925 ± 0.000002) × 10^{10} cm/s.

Heat of fusion of water 0°C = 79.71 cal/g.

Heat of vaporization of water 100°C = 539.55 cal/g.

Electrochemical equivalent of silver = 0.001118 g/s international amp.

Absolute wavelength of red cadmium light in air at 15°C. 760 mm pressure = 6438.4696 Å.

Wavelength of orange-red line of krypton 86 = 6057.802 Å.

Source: Handbook of Electrical Engineering, Dorf, R. C., Ed., CRC Press, Boca Raton, FL, 1993. With permission.

TABLE 33.39
Summary of the 1986 Recommended Values of the Fundamental Physical Constants

Quantity	Symbol	Value	Units	Relative Uncertainty (ppm)
Speed of light in vacuum	c	299,792,458	ms^{-1}	(exact)
Permeability of vacuum	μ_o	4π × 10^{-7}	N A^{-2}	
		= 12.566 370614...	10^{-7} N A^{-2}	(exact)
Permittivity of vacuum	ε_o	1/ $\mu_o c^2$		
		= 8.854 187 817...	10^{-12} F m^{-1}	(exact)
Newtonian constant of gravitation	G	6.672 59(85)	10^{-11} m^{-3} kg^{-1} s^{-2}	128
Planck constant	h	6.626 0755(40)	10^{-3} J s	0.60
$h/2\pi$	h	1.054 572 66(63)	10^{-3}J s	0.60
Elementary charge	e	1.602 177 33(49)	10^{-19} C	0.30
Magnetic flux quantum. $h/2e$	Φ_o	2.067 834 61(61)	10^{-15} Wb	0.30
Electron mass	m_e	9.109 3897(54)	10^{-31} kg	0.59
Proton mass	m_p	1.672 6231(10)	10^{-27} kg	0.59
Proton-electron mass ratio	m_p/m_e	1836.152701(37)		0.020
Fine-structure constant, $\mu_0 c e^2/2h$	α	7.297 353 08(33)	10^{-3}	0.045

TABLE 33.39 *(Continued)*
Summary of the 1986 Recommended Values of the Fundamental Physical Constants

Quantity	Symbol	Value	Units	Relative Uncertainty (ppm)
Inverse fine-structure constant	α^{-1}	137 035 9895(61)		0.045
Rydberg constant, $m_e c \alpha^2 / 2h$	R_x	10 973 731.534(13)	m^{-1}	0.0012
Avogadro constant	$N_A L$	6.022 1367(36)	$10^{23} mol^{-1}$	0.59
Faraday constant, $N_A e$	F	96 485.309(29)	$C\ mol^{-1}$	0.30
Molar gas constant	R	8.314 510(70)	$J\ mol^{-1}\ K^{-1}$	8.4
Boltzmann constant, R/N_A	k	1.380 658(12)	$10^{-23}\ J\ K^{-1}$	8.5
Stefan-Boltzmann constant, $(\pi r^9/60)k^9/h^7 c^7$	σ	5.670 51(19)	$10^{-8}\ W\ m^{-2}\ K^{-4}$	34
Non-SI units used with SI				
Electronvolt. $(e/C)J = (e)J$	eV	1.602 17733(40)	$10^{-19}\ J$	0.30
(Unified) atomic mass unit.	u	1.660 5402(10)	$10^{-27}\ kg$	0.59
$1\ u = m_u = 1/12m(^{12}C)$				

Note: An abbreviated list of the fundamental constants of physics and chemistry based on a least-squares adjustment with 17 degrees of freedom. The digits in parentheses are the one-standard-deviation uncertainty in the last digits of the given value. Since the uncertainties of many entries are correlated, the full covariance matrix must be used in evaluating the uncertainties of quantities computed from them.

Source: Handbook of Electrical Engineering, Dorf, R. C., Ed., CRC Press, Boca Raton, FL, 1993. With permission.

TABLE 33.40
Standard Atomic Weights (1987)

(Scaled to A_r (^{12}C) = 12)

The atomic weights of many elements are not invariant but depend on the origin and treatment of the material. The footnotes to this table elaborate the types of variation to be expected for individual elements. The values of A_r (E) and uncertainty U_r (E) given here apply to elements as they exist naturally on earth.

Name	Symbol	No.	Atomic Weight		Footnotes	
Actinium*	Ac	89				A
Aluminium	Al	13	26.981539(5)			
Americium*	Am	95				A
Antimony (Stibium)	Sb	51	121.75(3)			
Argon	Ar	18	39.948(1)	g	r	
Arsenic	As	33	74.92159(2)			
Astatine*	At	85				A
Barium	Ba	56	137.327(7)			
Berkelium*	Bk	97				A
Beryllium	Be	4	9.012182(3)			
Bismuth	Bi	83	208.98037(3)			
Boron	B	5	10.811(5)	g	m	r
Bromine	Br	35	79.904(1)			
Cadmium	Cd	48	112.411(8)	g		
Caesium	Cs	55	132.90543(5)			
Calcium	Ca	20	40.078(4)	g		

TABLE 33.40 *(Continued)*
Standard Atomic Weights (1987)

(Scaled to A_r (^{12}C) = 12)

The atomic weights of many elements are not invariant but depend on the origin and treatment of the material. The footnotes to this table elaborate the types of variation to be expected for individual elements. The values of A_r (E) and uncertainty U_r (E) given here apply to elements as they exist naturally on earth.

Name	Symbol	No.	Atomic Weight	Footnotes		
Californium*	Cf	98				A
Carbon	C	6	12.011(1)		r	
Cerium	Ce	58	140.115 (4)	g		
Chlorine	Cl	17	35.4527(9)			
Chromium	Cr	24	51.9961(6)			
Cobalt	Co	27	58.93320(1)			
Copper	Cu	29	63.546(3)		r	
Curium*	Cm	96				A
Dysprosium	Dy	66	162.50(3)	g		
Einsteinium*	Es	99				A
Erbium	Er	68	167.26(3)	g		
Europium	Eu	63	151.965(9)	g		
Fermium*	Fm	100				A
Fluorine	F	9	18.9984032(9)			
Francium*	Fr	87				A
Gadolinium	Gd	64	157.25(3)	g		
Gallium	Ga	31	69.723(1)			
Germanium	Ge	32	72.61(2)			
Gold	Au	79	196.96654(3)			
Hafnium	Hf	72	178.49(2)			
Helium	He	2	4.002602(2)	g	r	
Holmium	Ho	67	164.93032(3)			
Hydrogen	H	1	1.00794(7)	g	m	r
Indium	In	49	114.82(1)			
Iodine	I	53	126.90447(3)			
Iridium	Ir	77	192.22(3)			
Iron	Fe	26	55.847(3)			
Krypton	Kr	36	83.80(1)	g	m	
Lanthanum	La	57	138.9055(2)	g		
Lawrencium*	Lr	103				A
Lead	Pb	82	207.2(1)	g	r	
Lithium	Li	3	6.941(2)	g	m	r
Lutetium	Lu	71	174.967(1)	g		
Magnesium	Mg	12	24.3050(6)			
Manganese	Mn	25	54.93805(1)			
Mendelevium*	Md	101				A
Mercury	Hg	80	200.59(3)			
Molybdenum	Mo	42	95.94(1)			
Neodymium	Nd	60	144.24(3)	g		
Neon	Ne	10	20.1797(6)	g	m	
Neptunium*	Np	93				A
Nickel	Ni	28	58.69(1)			
Niobium	Nb	41	92.90638(2)			

TABLE 33.40 *(Continued)*
Standard Atomic Weights (1987)

(Scaled to A_r (^{12}C) = 12)

The atomic weights of many elements are not invariant but depend on the origin and treatment of the material. The footnotes to this table elaborate the types of variation to be expected for individual elements. The values of A_r (E) and uncertainty U_r (E) given here apply to elements as they exist naturally on earth.

Name	Symbol	No.	Atomic Weight	Footnotes		
Nitrogen	N	7	14.00674(7)	g	r	
Nobelium*	No	102				A
Osmium	Os	76	190.2(1)	g		
Oxygen	O	8	15.9994(3)	g	r	
Palladium	Pd	46	105.42(1)	g		
Phosphorus	P	15	30.973762(4)			
Platinum	Pt	78	195.08(3)			
Plutonium*	Pu	94				A
Polonium*	Po	84				A
Potassium (Kalium)	K	19	39.0983(1)			
Praseodymium	Pr	59	140.90765(3)			
Promethium*	Pm	61				A
Protactinium*	Pa	91				A
Radium*	Ra	88				A
Radon*	Rn	86				A
Rhenium	Re	75	186.207(1)			
Rhodium	Rh	45	102.90550(3)			
Rubidium	Rb	37	85.4678(3)	g		
Ruthenium	Ru	44	101.07(2)	g		
Samarium	Sm	62	150.36(3)	g		
Scandium	Sc	21	44.955910(9)			
Selenium	Se	34	78.96(3)			
Silicon	Si	14	28.0855(3)		r	
Silver	Ag	47	107.8682(2)	g		
Sodium (Natrium)	Na	11	22.989768(6)			
Strontium	Sr	38	87.62(1)	g	r	
Sulfur	S	16	32.066(6)		r	
Tantalum	Ta	73	180.9479(1)			
Technetium*	Tc	43				A
Tellurium	Te	52	127.60(3)	g		
Terbium	Tb	65	158.92534(3)			
Thallium	Tl	81	204.3833(2)			
Thorium*	Th	90	232.0381(1)	g		Z
Thulium	Tm	69	168.93421(3)			
Tin	Sn	50	118.710(7)	g		
Titanium	Ti	22	47.88(3)			
Tungsten (Wolfram)	W	74	183.85(3)			
Unnilquadium	Unq	104				A
Unnilpentium	Unp	105				A
Unnihexium	Unh	106				A
Unnilseptium	Uns	107				A
Uranium*	U	92	238.0289(1)	g	m	Z
Vanadium	V	23	50.9415(1)			

TABLE 33.40 *(Continued)*
Standard Atomic Weights (1987)

(Scaled to A_r (^{12}C) = 12)

The atomic weights of many elements are not invariant but depend on the origin and treatment of the material. The footnotes to this table elaborate the types of variation to be expected for individual elements. The values of A_r (E) and uncertainty U_r (E) given here apply to elements as they exist naturally on earth.

Name	Symbol	No.	Atomic Weight		Footnotes
Xenon	Xe	54	131.29(2)	g	m
Ytterbium	Yb	70	173.04(3)	g	
Yttrium	Y	39	88.90585(2)		
Zinc	Zn	30	65.39(2)		
Zirconium	Zr	40	91.224(2)	g	

g = Geological specimens are known in which the element has an isotopic composition outside the limits for normal material. The difference between the atomic weight of the element in such specimens and that given in the table may exceed the implied uncertainty.

m = Modified isotopic compositions may be found in commercially available material because it has been subjected to an undisclosed or inadvertent isotopic separation. Substantial deviations in atomic weight of the element from that given in the table can occur.

r = Range in isotopic composition of normal terrestrial material prevents a more precise A_r(E) being given: the tabulated A_r(E) value should be applicable to any normal material.

A = Radioactive element that lacks a characteristic terrestrial isotopic composition.

Z = An element, without stable nuclide(s), exhibiting a range of characteristic terrestrial compositions of long-lived radionuclide(s) such that a meaningful atomic weight can be given.

* Element has no stable nuclides.

See end of section for source.

D. STATISTICS

Statistical analysis is an integral part of a toxicology study. Advances in computer technology have allowed for more sophisticated statistical analyses to be conducted more easily and quickly on data generated in toxicology studies than would ever have been thought possible just a few decades ago. Figure 33.1 presents a decision tree for choosing the proper statistical tests for analysis of a variety of data. Although other equally valid tests may be used in place of those indicated, the scheme that is shown is a good representation of the statistical approach commonly used for assessing toxicological data. Refer to the referenced texts for a detailed discussion of the various statistical tests and their uses.

The reader should be aware of several important limitations associated with the use of statistics in toxicology: 1) statistics cannot make "poor" data "better"; 2) statistical significance may not imply biological significance; 3) an effect that may have biological significance may not be statistically significant; 4) the lack of statistical significance does not prove safety. The importance and relevance of any effect observed in a study must be assessed within the limitations imposed by the study design and the species being studied.

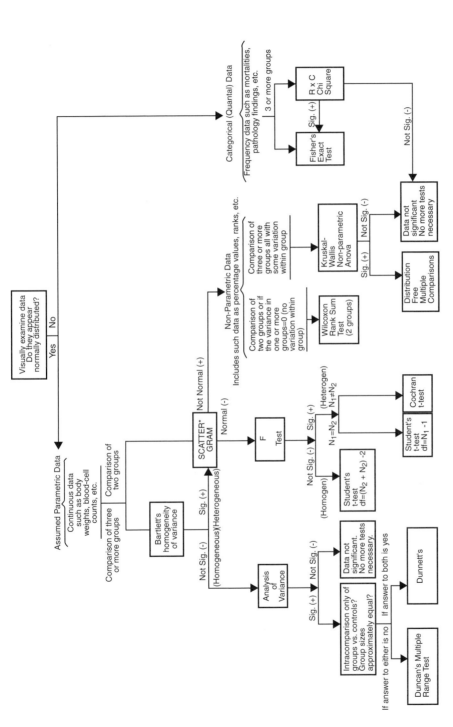

FIGURE 33.1 Decision tree for selecting hypothesis-testing procedures. Dunn's summed rank test is generally performed after the Kruskal-Wallis ANOVA for multiple comparisons of nonparametric data. For trend analysis of parametric data, Jonckheere test for monotonic trend can be used. From Gad, S. and Weil, C.S., in *Statistics and Experimental Design for Toxicologists*, Telford Press, Caldwell, NJ, 1986. With permission.

TABLE 33.41
Transformation of Percentages into Logits

Percentage	0	1	2	3	4	5	6	7	8	9
50	0	0.04	0.08	0.12	0.16	0.20	0.24	0.28	0.32	0.36
60	0.41	0.45	0.49	0.53	0.58	0.62	0.66	0.71	0.75	0.80
70	0.85	0.90	0.94	0.99	1.05	1.10	1.15	1.21	1.27	1.32
80	1.38	1.45	1.52	1.59	1.66	1.73	1.82	1.90	1.99	2.09
90	2.20	2.31	2.44	2.59	2.75	2.94	3.18	3.48	3.89	4.60
99	4.60	4.70	4.82	4.95	5.11	5.29	5.52	5.81	6.21	6.91

See end of section for source.

TABLE 33.42
Transformation of Percentages into Probits

Percentage	0	1	2	3	4	5	6	7	8	9
0	[–]	2.67	2.95	3.12	3.25	3.36	3.45	3.52	3.59	3.66
10	3.72	3.77	3.82	3.87	3.92	3.96	4.01	4.05	4.08	4.12
20	4.16	4.19	4.23	4.26	4.29	4.33	4.36	4.39	4.42	4.45
30	4.48	4.50	4.53	4.56	4.59	4.61	4.64	4.67	4.69	4.72
40	4.75	4.77	4.80	4.82	4.85	4.87	4.90	4.92	4.95	4.97
50	5.00	5.03	5.05	5.08	5.10	5.13	5.15	5.18	5.20	5.23
60	5.25	5.28	5.31	5.33	5.36	5.39	5.41	5.44	5.47	5.50
70	5.52	5.55	5.58	5.61	5.64	5.67	5.71	5.74	5.77	5.81
80	5.84	5.88	5.92	5.95	5.99	6.04	6.08	6.13	6.18	6.23
90	6.28	6.34	6.41	6.48	6.55	6.64	6.75	6.88	7.05	7.33
99	7.33	7.37	7.41	7.46	7.51	7.58	7.65	7.75	7.88	8.07

See end of section for source.

TABLE 33.43
Areas under the Standard Normal Curve

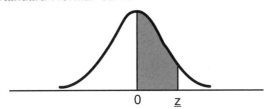

z	0.00	0.01	0.02	0.03	0.04	0.05	0.06	0.07	0.08	0.09
0.0	0.0000	0.0040	0.0080	0.0120	0.0160	0.0199	0.0239	0.0279	0.0319	0.0359
0.1	0.0398	0.0438	0.0478	0.0517	0.0557	0.0596	0.0636	0.0675	0.0714	0.0753
0.2	0.0793	0.0832	0.0871	0.0910	0.0948	0.0987	0.1026	0.1064	0.1103	0.1141
0.3	0.1179	0.1217	0.1255	0.1293	0.1331	0.1368	0.1406	0.1443	0.1480	0.1517
0.4	0.1554	0.1591	0.1628	0.1664	0.1700	0.1736	0.1772	0.1808	0.1844	0.1879
0.5	0.1915	0.1950	0.1985	0.2019	0.2054	0.2088	0.2123	0.2157	0.2190	0.2224
0.6	0.2257	0.2291	0.2324	0.2357	0.2389	0.2422	0.2454	0.2486	0.2517	0.2549
0.7	0.2580	0.2611	0.2642	0.2673	0.2704	0.2734	0.2764	0.2794	0.2823	0.2852
0.8	0.2881	0.2910	0.2939	0.2967	0.2995	0.3023	0.3051	0.3078	0.3106	0.3133
0.9	0.3159	0.3186	0.3212	0.3238	0.3264	0.3289	0.3315	0.3340	0.3365	0.3389
1.0	0.3413	0.3438	0.3461	0.3485	0.3508	0.3531	0.3554	0.3577	0.3599	0.3621
1.1	0.3643	0.3665	0.3686	0.3708	0.3729	0.3749	0.3770	0.3790	0.3810	0.3830
1.2	0.3849	0.3869	0.3888	0.3907	0.3925	0.3944	0.3962	0.3980	0.3997	0.4015
1.3	0.4032	0.4049	0.4066	0.4082	0.4099	0.4115	0.4131	0.4147	0.4162	0.4177
1.4	0.4192	0.4207	0.4222	0.4236	0.4251	0.4265	0.4279	0.4292	0.4306	0.4319
1.5	0.4332	0.4345	0.4357	0.4370	0.4382	0.4394	0.4406	0.4418	0.4429	0.4441
1.6	0.4452	0.4463	0.4474	0.4484	0.4495	0.4505	0.4515	0.4525	0.4535	0.4545
1.7	0.4554	0.4564	0.4573	0.4582	0.4591	0.4599	0.4608	0.4616	0.4625	0.4633
1.8	0.4641	0.4649	0.4656	0.4664	0.4671	0.4678	0.4686	0.4693	0.4699	0.4706
1.9	0.4713	0.4719	0.4726	0.4732	-0.4738	0.4744	0.4750	0.4756	0.4761	0.4767
2.0	0.4772	0.4778	0.4783	0.4788	0.4793	0.4798	0.4803	0.4808	0.4812	0.4817
2.1	0.4821	0.4826	0.4830	0.4834	0.4838	0.4842	0.4846	0.4850	0.4854	0.4857
2.2	0.4861	0.4864	0.4868	0.4871	0.4875	0.4878	0.4881	0.4884	0.4887	0.4890
2.3	0.4893	0.4896	0.4898	0.4901	0.4904	0.4906	0.4909	0.4911	0.4913	0.4916
2.4	0.4918	0.4920	0.4922	0.4925	0.4927	0.4929	0.4931	0.4932	0.4934	0.4936
2.5	0.4938	0.4940	0.4941	0.4943	0.4945	0.4946	0.4948	0.4949	0.4951	0.4952
2.6	0.4953	0.4955	0.4956	0.4957	0.4959	0.4960	0.4961	0.4962	0.4963	0.4964
2.7	0.4965	0.4966	0.4967	0.4968	0.4969	0.4970	0.4971	0.4972	0.4973	0.4974
2.8	0.4974	0.4975	0.4976	0.4977	0.4977	0.4978	0.4979	0.4979	0.4980	0.4981
2.9	0.4981	0.4982	0.4982	0.4983	0.4984	0.4984	0.4985	0.4985	0.4986	0.4986
3.0	0.4987	0.4987	0.4987	0.4988	0.4988	0.4989	0.4989	0.4989	0.4990	0.4990

See end of section for source.

TABLE 33.44
Poisson Distribution

Each number in this table represents the probability of obtaining at least X successes, or the area under the histogram to the right of and including the rectangle whose center is at X.

m	X = 0	X = 1	X = 2	X = 3	X = 4	X = 5	X = 6	X = 7	X = 8	X = 9	X = 10	X = 11	X = 12	X = 13	X = 14
.10	1.000	.095													
.20	1.000	.181	.005												
.30	1.000	.259	.018	.001											
.40	1.000	.330	.037	.004											
.50	1.000	.393	.062	.008	.001										
.60	1.000	.451	.090	.014	.002										
.70	1.000	.503	.122	.023	.003										
.80	1.000	.551	.156	.034	.006	.001									
.90	1.000	.593	.191	.047	.009	.001									
1.00	1.000	.632	.228	.063	.013	.002									
1.1	1.000	.667	.264	.080	.019	.004	.001								
1.2	1.000	.699	.301	.100	.026	.005	.001								
1.3	1.000	.727	.337	.120	.034	.008	.002								
1.4	1.000	.753	.373	.143	.043	.011	.002								
1.5	1.000	.777	.408	.167	.054	.014	.003	.001							
1.6	1.000	.798	.442	.191	.066	.019	.004	.001							
1.7	1.000	.817	.475	.217	.079	.024	.006	.001							
1.8	1.000	.835	.507	.243	.093	.030	.008	.002							
1.9	1.000	.850	.537	.269	.109	.036	.010	.003	.001						
2.0	1.000	.865	.566	.296	.125	.044	.013	.003	.001						
2.2	1.000	.889	.594	.323	.143	.053	.017	.005	.001						
2.4	1.000	.909	.645	.377	.181	.072	.025	.007	.002						
2.6	1.000	.926	.692	.430	.221	.096	.036	.012	.003	.001					
2.8	1.000	.939	.733	.482	.264	.123	.049	.017	.005	.001					
3.0	1.000	.950	.769	.531	.308	.152	.065	.024	.008	.002					
3.2	1.000	.959	.801	.577	.353	.185	.084	.034	.012	.004	.001				
3.4	1.000	.967	.829	.620	.397	.219	.105	.045	.017	.006	.001				
3.6	1.000	.973	.853	.660	.442	.256	.129	.058	.023	.008	.002				
3.8	1.000	.978	.874	.697	.485	.294	.156	.073	.031	.012	.003	.001			
4.0	1.000	.982	.893	.731	.527	.332	.184	.091	.040	.016	.004	.001			
4.2	1.000	.985	.908	.762	.567	.371	.215	.111	.051	.021	.006	.002	.001		
4.4	1.000	.988	.922	.790	.605	.410	.247	.133	.064	.028	.008	.003	.001		
4.6	1.000	.990	.934	.815	.641	.449	.280	.156	.079	.036	.011	.004	.002	.001	
4.8	1.000	.992	.944	.837	.674	.487	.314	.182	.095	.045	.015	.006	.003	.001	
5.0	1.000	.993	.952	.857	.706	.524	.349	.209	.113	.056	.020	.008	.004	.001	
			.960	.875	.735	.560	.384	.238	.133	.068	.025	.010	.005	.001	.001

See end of section for source.

TABLE 33.45
t-Distribution

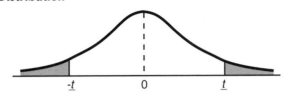

Deg. freedom. *f*	90% (*P* = .1)	95% (*P* = .05)	99% (P = .01)
1	6.314	12.706	63.657
2	2.920	4.303	9.925
3	2.353	3.182	5.841
4	2.132	2.776	4.604
5	2.015	2.571	4.032
6	1.943	2.447	3.707
7	1.895	2.365	3.499
8	1.860	2.306	3.355
9	1.833	2.262	3.250
10	1.812	2.228	3.169
11	1.796	2.201	3.106
12	1.782	2.179	3.055
13	1.771	2.160	3.012
14	1.761	2.145	2.977
15	1.753	2.131	2.947
16	1.746	2.120	2.921
17	1.740	2.110	2.898
18	1.734	2.101	2.878
19	1.729	2.093	2.861
20	1.725	2.086	2.845
21	1.721	2.080	2.831
22	1.717	2.074	2.819
23	1.714	2.069	2.807
24	1.711	2.064	2.797
25	1.708	2.060	2.787
26	1.706	2.056	2.779
27	1.703	2.052	2.771
28	1.701	2.048	2.763
29	1.699	2.045	2.756
inf.	1.645	1.960	2.576

See end of section for source.

TABLE 33.46
χ^2 **Distribution**

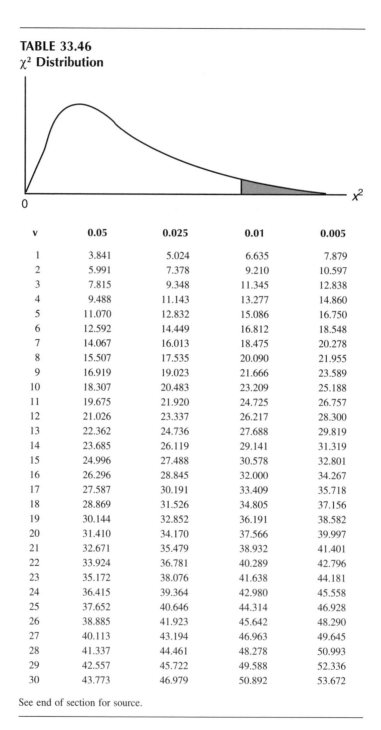

v	0.05	0.025	0.01	0.005
1	3.841	5.024	6.635	7.879
2	5.991	7.378	9.210	10.597
3	7.815	9.348	11.345	12.838
4	9.488	11.143	13.277	14.860
5	11.070	12.832	15.086	16.750
6	12.592	14.449	16.812	18.548
7	14.067	16.013	18.475	20.278
8	15.507	17.535	20.090	21.955
9	16.919	19.023	21.666	23.589
10	18.307	20.483	23.209	25.188
11	19.675	21.920	24.725	26.757
12	21.026	23.337	26.217	28.300
13	22.362	24.736	27.688	29.819
14	23.685	26.119	29.141	31.319
15	24.996	27.488	30.578	32.801
16	26.296	28.845	32.000	34.267
17	27.587	30.191	33.409	35.718
18	28.869	31.526	34.805	37.156
19	30.144	32.852	36.191	38.582
20	31.410	34.170	37.566	39.997
21	32.671	35.479	38.932	41.401
22	33.924	36.781	40.289	42.796
23	35.172	38.076	41.638	44.181
24	36.415	39.364	42.980	45.558
25	37.652	40.646	44.314	46.928
26	38.885	41.923	45.642	48.290
27	40.113	43.194	46.963	49.645
28	41.337	44.461	48.278	50.993
29	42.557	45.722	49.588	52.336
30	43.773	46.979	50.892	53.672

See end of section for source.

TABLE 33.47
Variance Ratio

					F (95%)					
					n_1					
n_2	**1**	**2**	**3**	**4**	**5**	**6**	**8**	**12**	**24**	**∞**
1	161.4	199.5	215.7	224.6	230.2	234.0	238.9	243.9	249.0	254.3
2	18.51	19.00	19.16	19.25	19.30	19.33	19.37	19.41	19.45	19.50
3	10.13	9.55	9.28	9.12	9.01	8.94	8.84	8.74	8.64	8.53
4	7.71	6.94	6.59	6.39	6.26	6.16	6.04	5.91	5.77	5.63
5	6.61	5.79	5.41	5.19	5.05	4.95	4.82	4.68	4.53	4.36
6	5.99	5.14	4.76	4.53	4.39	4.28	4.15	4.00	3.84	3.67
7	5.59	4.74	4.35	4.12	3.97	3.87	3.73	3.57	3.41	3.23
8	5.32	4.46	4.07	3.84	3.69	3.58	3.44	3.28	3.12	2.93
9	5.12	4.26	3.86	3.63	3.48	3.37	3.23	3.07	2.90	2.71
10	4.96	4.10	3.71	3.48	3.33	3.22	3.07	2.91	2.74	2.54
11	4.84	3.98	3.59	3.36	3.20	3.09	2.95	2.79	2.61	2.40
12	4.75	3.88	3.49	3.26	3.11	3.00	2.85	2.69	2.50	2.30
13	4.67	3.80	3.41	3.18	3.02	2.92	2.77	2.60	2.42	2.21
14	4.60	3.74	3.34	3.11	2.96	2.85	2.70	2.53	2.35	2.13
15	4.54	3.68	3.29	3.06	2.90	2.79	2.64	2.48	2.29	2.07
16	4.49	3.63	3.24	3.01	2.85	2.74	2.59	2.42	2.24	2.01
17	4.45	3.59	3.20	2.96	2.81	2.70	2.55	2.38	2.19	1.96
18	4.41	3.55	3.16	2.93	2.77	2.66	2.51	2.34	2.15	1.92
19	4.38	3.52	3.13	2.90	2.74	2.63	2.48	2.31	2.11	1.88
20	4.35	3.49	3.10	2.87	2.71	2.60	2.45	2.28	2.08	1.84
21	4.32	3.47	3.07	2.84	2.68	2.57	2.42	2.25	2.05	1.81
22	4.30	3.44	3.05	2.82	2.66	2.55	2.40	2.23	2.03	1.78
23	4.28	3.42	3.03	2.80	2.64	2.53	2.38	2.20	2.00	1.76
24	4.26	3.40	3.01	2.78	2.62	2.51	2.36	2.18	1.98	1.73
25	4.24	3.38	2.99	2.76	2.60	2.49	2.34	2.16	1.96	1.71
26	4.22	3.37	2.98	2.74	2.59	2.47	2.32	2.15	1.95	1.69
27	4.21	3.35	2.96	2.73	2.57	2.46	2.30	2.13	1.93	1.67
28	4.20	3.34	2.95	2.71	2.56	2.44	2.29	2.12	1.91	1.65
29	4.18	3.33	2.93	2.70	2.54	2.43	2.28	2.10	1.90	1.64
30	4.17	3.32	2.92	2.69	2.53	2.42	2.27	2.09	1.89	1.62
40	4.08	3.23	2.84	2.61	2.45	2.34	2.18	2.00	1.79	1.51
60	4.00	3.15	2.76	2.52	2.37	2.25	2.10	1.92	1.70	1.39
120	3.92	3.07	2.68	2.45	2.29	2.17	2.02	1.83	1.61	1.25
∞	3.84	2.99	2.60	2.37	2.21	2.10	1.94	1.75	1.52	1.00
					F (99%)					
1	4,052	4,999	5,403	5,625	5,764	5,859	5,982	6,106	6,234	6,366
2	98.50	99.00	99.17	99.25	99.30	99.33	99.37	99.42	99.46	99.50
3	34.12	30.82	29.46	28.71	28.24	27.91	27.49	27.05	26.60	26.12
4	21.20	18.00	16.69	15.98	15.52	15.21	14.80	14.37	13.93	13.46
5	16.26	13.27	12.06	11.39	10.97	10.67	10.29	9.89	9.47	9.02
6	13.74	10.92	9.78	9.15	8.75	8.47	8.10	7.72	7.31	6.88
7	12.25	9.55	8.45	7.85	7.46	7.19	6.84	6.47	6.07	5.65
8	11.26	8.65	7.59	7.01	6.63	6.37	6.03	5.67	5.28	4.86
9	10.56	8.02	6.99	6.42	6.06	5.80	5.47	5.11	4.73	4.31
10	10.04	7.56	6.55	5.99	5.64	5.39	5.06	4.71	4.33	3.91
11	9.65	7.20	6.22	5.67	5.32	5.07	4.74	4.40	4.02	3.60
12	9.33	6.93	5.95	5.41	5.06	4.82	4.50	4.16	3.78	3.36
13	9.07	6.70	5.74	5.20	4.86	4.62	4.30	3.96	3.59	3.16
14	8.86	6.51	5.56	5.03	4.69	4.46	4.14	3.80	3.43	3.00
15	8.68	6.36	5.42	4.89	4.56	4.32	4.00	3.67	3.29	2.87
16	8.53	6.23	5.29	4.77	4.44	4.20	3.89	3.55	3.18	2.75
17	8.40	6.11	5.18	4.67	4.34	4.10	3.79	3.45	3.08	2.65

TABLE 33.47 *(Continued)*
Variance Ratio

	F (99%)									
	n_1									
n_2	1	2	3	4	5	6	8	12	24	∞
18	8.28	6.01	5.09	4.58	4.25	4.01	3.71	3.37	3.00	2.57
19	8.18	5.93	5.01	4.50	4.17	3.94	3.63	3.30	2.92	2.49
20	8.10	5.85	4.94	4.43	4.10	3.87	3.56	3.23	2.86	2.42
21	8.02	5.78	4.87	4.37	4.04	3.81	3.51	3.17	2.80	2.36
22	7.94	5.72	4.82	4.31	3.99	3.76	3.45	3.12	2.75	2.31
23	7.88	5.66	4.76	4.26	3.94	3.71	3.41	3.07	2.70	2.26
24	7.82	5.61	4.72	4.22	3.90	3.67	3.36	3.03	2.66	2.21
25	7.77	5.57	4.68	4.18	3.86	3.63	3.32	2.99	2.62	2.17
26	7.72	5.53	4.64	4.14	3.82	3.59	3.29	2.96	2.58	2.13
27	7.68	5.49	4.60	4.11	3.78	3.56	3.26	2.93	2.55	2.10
28	7.64	5.45	4.57	4.07	3.75	3.53	3.23	2.90	2.52	2.06
29	7.60	5.42	4.54	4.04	3.73	3.50	3.20	2.87	2.49	2.03
30	7.56	5.39	4.51	4.02	3.70	3.47	3.17	2.84	2.47	2.01
40	7.31	5.18	4.31	3.83	3.51	3.29	2.99	2.66	2.29	1.80
60	7.08	4.98	4.13	3.65	3.34	3.12	2.82	2.50	2.12	1.60
120	6.85	4.79	3.95	3.48	3.17	2.96	2.66	2.34	1.95	1.38
∞	6.64	4.60	3.78	3.32	3.02	2.80	2.51	2.18	1.79	1.00

See end of section for source.

GENERAL STATISTICAL REFERENCES

Adler, H. L. and Roessler, E. B., *Introduction to Probability and Statistics*, 6th ed., H. Freeman, New York, 1977.
Gad, S. and Weil, C. S., *Statistics and Experimental Design for Toxicologists*, Telford Press, NJ, 1986.
Hollander, M. and Wolfe, D. A., *Nonparametric Statistical Methods*, John Wiley & Sons, New York, 1973.
Snedecor, G. W. and Cochran, W. G., *Statistical Methods*, 6th ed., Iowa State University Press, Ames, IA, 1967.
Tallarida, R. J. and Murray, R. B., *Manual of Pharmacologic Calculations with Computer Programs*, 2nd ed., Springer-Verlag, New York, 1987.

E. KINETICS

TABLE 33.48
Table of Equations and their Uses

$$k = \frac{0.693}{t_{1/2}} \tag{1}$$

Equation 1 is useful for determining the value of the rate constant when the half-time is known or for determining the half-time when the rate constant is known. Rate constants and half-times are measured in dynamic binding experiments. The ratio of the dissociation rate constant to the association rate constant is an alternative way to determine the equilibrium dissociation constant. This relationship is only valid for first order processes or pseudo first order processes where all but one component is constant over time. Plotting the log of the concentration of the substance of interest vs. time will give a straight line if the process is first order.

$$\Delta G^0 = -RT \ln K_D \tag{2}$$

TABLE 33.48 *(Continued)*
Table of Equations and their Uses

Equation 2 is useful for determining the free energy difference between reactants and products at equilibrium when the equilibrium constant for the reaction is known. Alternatively, if the energy difference between reactants and products at equilibrium is known, Equation 2 can be used to determine the equilibrium constant. Calorimetric measurements can be used to measure ΔG^0 values associated with binding interactions.

$$B_L = \frac{B_{Lmax}[L]}{K_D + [L]} \tag{3}$$

The Langmuir binding isotherm[1] describes the characteristics of binding of molecules to other molecules or surfaces. We are concerned here with the binding of ligands to receptors. The useful parameters are the maximum binding capacity of the receptors (B_{max}) and their affinity for binding the ligand (K_D). Nonlinear fitting to Equation is the best way of evaluating these parameters.

$$Y = \frac{[L]}{K_D + [L]} \tag{4}$$

An alternative means of expressing the Langmuir binding isotherm is in terms of fractional receptor occupancy (Y). This has the effect of confining the dependent variable to a scale from 0 to 1. This allows direct graphic comparisons (Y vs. log $[L]$) of the affinity of the interactions of different receptor-ligand systems. The ordinate scale is the same for each receptor-ligand interaction regardless of the magnitude of B_{max}. The only difference is the position of the curve, right or left, which is a measure of the affinity.

$$\frac{1}{B_L} = \frac{1}{[L]} \frac{K_D}{B_{Lmax}} + \frac{1}{B_{Lmax}} \tag{5}$$

The double-reciprocal or Lineweaver-Burk equation is the most widely used and understood of the linear transformations of Equation 3. For this reason it is useful as a means of displaying data for graphic presentation. With the wide availability of computer programs for nonlinear fitting, Equation 5 is now of only limited value for evaluating binding parameters.

$$\frac{B_L}{[L]} = -\frac{B_L}{K_D} + \frac{B_{Lmax}}{K_D} \tag{6}$$

The Rosenthal-Scatchard equation is particularly sensitive to the presence of heterogeneity of binding and for the presence of multiple binding sites for the same ligand on a single receptor. Either of these phenomena have the potential to produce nonlinearity. Multiple binding sites for the same ligand on a single receptor will produce convex curvature while binding site heterogeneity can produce convex, concave, or no curvature. The value of this transformation of Equation is in graphic analysis for nonlinearity.

$$B_L = -\frac{B_L}{[L]} K_D + B_{Lmax} \tag{7}$$

The Eadie-Hofstee equation is essentially the same equation as the Rosenthal-Scatchard equation. The major difference between the two equations is that the axes are reversed. Equation 7 is useful for the same analyses as the Rosenthal-Scatchard equation and it has the additional advantage of providing the values of the binding parameters directly rather than as reciprocals or in combinations.

$$\frac{[L]}{B_L} = -\frac{[L]}{B_{Lmax}} + \frac{K_D}{B_{Lmax}} \tag{8}$$

The Woolf equation is the least used of the linear transformations of the Langmuir binding isotherm. It is the best one for minimizing the effect of weighting errors. However, since nonlinear fitting to the Langmuir binding isotherm, as a means of evaluating binding parameters, is now widely available this feature of the equation is of diminished importance.

$$pL = pK_D + \log\left(\frac{[R]}{[RL]}\right) \tag{9}$$

Equation 9 is the ligand binding equivalent of the Henderson Hasselbalch pH equation. This equation can be used like the Henderson-Hasselbalch equation, for example, to calculate the fractional receptor occupancy for any given ligand concentration when the K_D is known.

$$\frac{E_L}{E_{max}} = \frac{\alpha}{\dfrac{K_D}{[L]} + 1} \tag{10}$$

Equation 10 is a rearrangement that incorporates terms for relative intrinsic activity due to the phenomenon of partial agonism. When the maximum physiological effect for a receptor system is known, Equation 10 can be employed to evaluate the relative intrinsic activity (α) of any given agonist.

$$\log\left(\frac{Y}{1-Y}\right) = n\log[L] - \log K_D \tag{11}$$

The Hill equation is useful for evaluating the presence of interacting binding sites on a receptor (cooperativity). The Hill equation also detects multiple noninteracting binding sites for the same ligand with different affinities on the same receptor. It is incapable of distinguishing between these two mechanisms. A Hill coefficient (n) greater than 1 is an indication of either cooperativity of binding or multiple noninteracting binding sites on the same receptor. The deficiency of the Hill equation is that the K_D value is a composite of multiple values and the Hill coefficient determined from experimental data, which is supposed to represent the number of different or interacting binding sites, is rarely a simple integer value.

$$\frac{B_L}{[L]^n} = -\frac{B_L}{K_D} + \frac{B_{L\,max}}{K_D} \tag{12}$$

Equation 12 is a form of the Scatchard equation that takes into consideration the possibility of multiple binding sites for the same ligand on the receptor. The n in this equation is the same as the Hill coefficient. When n is greater than 1 the Scatchard plot will exhibit pronounced convex curvature. This equation has the same deficiency as the Hill equation.

$$\log\left(\frac{Y}{1-Y}\right) = \log[L] - \log K_{D_2} - \log\left(1 + \frac{K_D}{[L]}\right) \tag{13}$$

Equation 13 is a modification of the Hill equation that takes into consideration the individual affinity constants for a receptor with two binding sites for the ligand where only the RLL complex is capable of producing a physiological effect. When these sites interact, or when they have different affinities, they will produce a downward curving Hill plot. When such behavior is noted, this equation can be used to evaluate the relative contributions of the two binding sites to the overall binding and effect.

$$\log\left(\frac{Y}{1-Y}\right) = 2\log[L] - \log(K_{D_1}K_{D_2}) + \log\left(1 + k\frac{K_{D_2}}{[L]}\right) \tag{14}$$

Equation 14 is a modified version of the Hill equation that takes into consideration the individual affinity constants for a receptor with two binding sites when both RL and RLL are capable of producing a physiological effect. This mechanism will produce Hill plots with an upward curvature. This equation, like Equation 13, is useful for evaluation of the relative contributions of the two binding sites to the overal binding and effect.

$$B_L = \frac{B_{L\,max}[L]}{K_D\left(1 + \dfrac{[I]}{K_I}\right) + [L]} \tag{15}$$

TABLE 33.48 *(Continued)*
Table of Equations and their Uses

Equation 15 is a modified version of the Langmuir binding isotherm which takes into consideration the contribution of a competitive inhibitor. This equation, in combination with Equation 3, is useful for the evaluation of the inhibition constant employing nonlinear fitting methods.

$$\frac{1}{B_L} = \frac{1}{[L]}\frac{K_D}{B_{L\max}}\left(1+\frac{[I]}{K_I}\right)+\frac{1}{B_{L\max}} \tag{16}$$

Equation 16 is a modified version of the double-reciprocal transformation of the Langmuir binding isotherm that takes into consideration the contribution of a competitive inhibitor. This equation is useful for the graphic analysis of competitive inhibition. If the inhibitor changes only the slope, and not the abscissal intercept, this indicates that the inhibition is competitive.

$$\log\left(\frac{[L']}{[L]}-1\right) = \log[I] + pK_I \tag{17}$$

The Schild equation is useful for calculating the concentration of agonist needed to restore the same level of effect when a known concentration of competitive inhibitor is added. Alternatively, it is useful for calculating the competitive inhibitor concentration when a known increase in agonist concentration is necessary to maintain the same level of effect.

$$E_L = \frac{E_{L\max}[L]}{K_D\left(1+\frac{[I]}{K_I}\right)+[L]\left(1+\frac{[I]}{K_I}\right)} \tag{18}$$

Equation 18 is a modified version of the Langmuir binding isotherm which takes into consideration the contribution of a simple noncompetitive inhibitor. This equation is useful for the evaluation of the inhibition constant employing nonlinear fitting methods.

$$\frac{1}{E_L} = \frac{1}{[L]}\frac{K_D}{E_{L\max}}\left(1+\frac{[I]}{K_I}\right)+\frac{1}{E_{L\max}}\left(1+\frac{[I]}{K_I}\right) \tag{19}$$

Equation 19 is a modified version of the double-reciprocal transformation of the Langmuir binding isotherm that takes into consideration the contribution of a simple noncompetitive inhibitor. This equation is useful for the graphic analysis of simple noncompetitive inhibition. If the inhibitor changes both the slope and the abscissal intercept, this indicates that the inhibition is noncompetitive.

$$\frac{E_L}{E_{L\max}} = \frac{[L]}{K_{D_I}\left(1+\frac{[I]}{K_{I_1}}\right)+[L]\left(1+\frac{[I]}{K_{I_2}}\right)} \tag{20}$$

Equation 20 is a modified version of the Langmuir binding isotherm which takes into consideration the contribution of a heterotropic-cooperative noncompetitive inhibitor. This equation is useful for the evaluation of the effect of agonist binding on the inhibition constant employing nonlinear fitting methods.

$$\frac{1}{E_L} = \frac{1}{[L]}\frac{K_{D_1}}{E_{L\max}}\left(1+\frac{[I]}{K_{I_1}}\right)+\frac{1}{E_{L\max}}\left(1+\frac{[I]}{K_{I_2}}\right) \tag{21}$$

Equation 21 is a modified version of the double-reciprocal transformation of the Langmuir binding isotherm that takes into consideration the contribution of a heterotropic-cooperative noncompetitive inhibitor. This equation is useful for the graphic analysis of heterotropic-cooperative noncompetitive inhibition. If the inhibitor changes both the slope and the abscissal intercept, this indicates that the inhibition is noncompetitive. If the intersection of the lines is above or below the ordinate, this indicates that the binding of substrate influences the binding of inhibitor and the binding of inhibitor influences the binding of substrate. When this is true, the mechanism is heterotropic-cooperative noncompetitive inhibition.

TABLE 33.48 *(Continued)*
Table of Equations and their Uses

$$Y = \cfrac{1}{\cfrac{K_{D_1}\left(1 + \cfrac{[I]}{K_{I_1}}\right)}{[L]\left(1 + \cfrac{[I]}{K_{I_2}}\right)} + 1} \tag{22}$$

Equation 22 is a modified version of the Langmuir binding isotherm which takes into consideration the contribution of a heterotropic-cooperative noncompetitive inhibitor that reduces the affinity of the receptor for the agonist without preventing the physiological effect. This is allosteric competitive inhibition. This equation is useful by virtue of the fact that it predicts that, at very high inhibitor concentration, there will be a decrease in the B_{Lmax}. Thus, allosteric competitive inhibition can be distinguished from simple competitive inhibition by employing very high inhibitor concentrations.

$$Y = \cfrac{1}{\cfrac{K_{D_2}}{[L]}\left(1 + \cfrac{K_{S_1}}{[S]}\right) + \left(1 + \cfrac{K_{S_2}}{[S]}\right)} \tag{23}$$

Equation 23 is a modified version of the Langmuir binding isotherm which takes into consideration the contribution of a simple noncompetitive stimulator. This equation is useful for the evaluation of the stimulation constant employing nonlinear fitting methods. An alternative way to think about a stimulator is that it can also represent, under some circumstances, a second agonist at the receptor where both agonists must bind before a physiological effect can be produced.

$$\frac{1}{E_L} = \frac{1}{[L]}\frac{K_{D_2}}{E_{Lmax}}\left(1 + \frac{K_{S_1}}{[S]}\right) + \frac{1}{E_{Lmax}}\left(1 + \frac{K_{S_2}}{[S]}\right) \tag{24}$$

Equation 24 is a modified version of the double-reciprocal transformation of the Langmuir binding isotherm that takes into consideration the contribution of a simple noncompetitive stimulator. This equation is useful for the graphic analysis of simple noncompetitive stimulation. If the stimulator changes both the slope and the abscissal intercept, this indicates that the stimulation is noncompetitive.

$$\frac{E_L}{E_{Lmax}} = \cfrac{1}{\cfrac{K_D}{[L]} + \left(1 + \cfrac{[I]}{K_I}\right)} \tag{25}$$

Equation 25 is a modified version of the Langmuir binding isotherm which takes into consideration the contribution of an uncompetitive inhibitor. This equation is useful for the evaluation of the inhibition constant using nonlinear fitting methods.

$$\frac{1}{E_L} = \frac{1}{[L]}\frac{K_D}{E_{Lmax}} + \frac{1}{E_{Lmax}}\left(1 + \frac{[I]}{K_I}\right) \tag{26}$$

Equation 26 is a modified version of the double-reciprocal transformation of the Langmuir binding isotherm that takes into consideration the contribution of an uncompetitive inhibitor. This equation is useful for the graphic analysis of uncompetitive inhibition. If the inhibitor changes the abscissal intercept without affecting the slope, this indicates that the inhibition is uncompetitive. Uncompetitive inhibition can, under some circumstances, represent a special case of heterotropic-cooperative noncompetitive inhibition where binding of substrate increases the affinity of binding of the inhibitor from near zero to its final value.

$$V = \frac{V_{max}[S]}{K_M + [S]} \tag{27}$$

TABLE 33.48 *(Continued)*
Table of Equations and their Uses

The Michaelis-Menten equation for enzyme kinetics is equivalent in form to the Langmuir binding isotherm. A number of special conditions and assumptions are involved in the derivation of the Michaelis-Menten equation which are not necessary for the Langmuir binding isotherm. If these conditions and assumptions are not met, the Michaelis-Menten equation is not valid for the analysis of enyme kinetic data. This equation is useful for the evaluation of the K_M and V_{max} parameters of enzyme reactions using nonlinear fitting methods.

$$V = \frac{V_{max}[S_1][S_2]}{K_{D_1}K_{M_2} + K_{M_1}[S_2] + K_{M_2}[S_1] + [S_1][S_2]} \tag{28}$$

Equation 28 is a modified version of the Michaelis-Menten equation for enzyme reactions that require two substrates to add to the enzyme before any product formation can occur. Normally, one substrate is present at saturating concentration. When this is true, the equation simplifies to Equation 27. This equation is useful for analyzing kinetic parameters when it is not feasible to hold one substrate at saturation.

$$V = \frac{V_{max}[S_1][S_2]}{K_{M_1}[S_2] + K_{M_2}[S_1] + [S_1][S_2]} \tag{29}$$

Equation 29 is a modified version of the Michaelis-Menten equation for enzyme reactions that exhibit a ping-pong mechanism. These enzymes have two substrates and two products. The first substrate combines with the enzyme and is converted to product. This reaction alters the enzyme such that it can then combine with the second substrate and convert it to product. The second reaction converts the enzyme back to its original form. Normally one of the substrates is present at saturating concentration. When this is true, the equation simplifies to Equation 27. This equation is useful for analyzing kinetic parameters when it is not feasible to hold one substrate at saturation.

Source: Matthews, J. C., *Fundamentals of Receptor, Enzyme, and Transport Kinetics*, CRC Press, Boca Raton, FL, 1993. With permission.

MATHEMATICS, SYMBOLS, PHYSICAL CONSTANTS, CONVERSIONS, AND STATISTICS

Materials in this section were reprinted from the following sources:

Lide, D. R., Ed., *CRC Handbook of Chemistry and Physics*, 73rd ed., CRC Press, Boca Raton, FL, 1992: International System of Units (SI), conversion constants and multipliers (conversion of temperatures), symbols and terminology for physical and chemical quantities, fundamental physical constants, classification of electromagnetic radiation, electrical resistivity (pure metals, selected alloys), dielectric constants, properties of semiconductors, properties of magnetic alloys, resistance of wires.

Beyer, W. H., Ed., *CRC Standard Mathematical Tables and Formulae*, 29th ed., CRC Press, Boca Raton, FL, 1991: Greek alphabet, conversion constants and multipliers (recommended decimal multiples and submultiples, metric to English, English to metric, general, temperature factors), physical constants, series expansion, integrals, the Fourier transforms, numerical methods, probability, positional notation.

Tallarida, R. J., *Pocket Book of Integrals and Mathematical Formulas*, 2nd ed., CRC Press, Boca Raton, FL, 1992: Elementary algebra and geometry; determinants, matrices, and linear systems of equations; trigonometry; analytic geometry; series; differential calculus; integral calculus; vector analysis; special functions; statistics; tables of probability and statistics; table of derivatives.

Pankow, J. F., *Aquatic Chemistry Concepts*, Chelsea, MI, Lewis Publishers, 1991: Periodic table of the elements.

Shackelford, J. and Alexander, W. Eds., *CRC Materials Science and Engineering Handbook*, CRC Press, Boca Raton, FL, 1992: Electrical resistivity of selected alloy cast irons, resistivity of selected ceramics.

SECTION 4. CALCULATIONS, PREPARATION, AND PROPERTIES OF VARIOUS TYPES OF SUBSTANCES COMMONLY USED IN TOXICOLOGY

A. MOLARITY, MOLALITY, NORMALITY, OSMOLARITY CALCULATIONS

1. Molarity (M) $= \dfrac{\text{Number of moles of solute}}{\text{Liter of solution}}$

   Where: Number of moles $= \dfrac{\text{Grams of chemical}}{\text{Molecular weight}}$

2. Molality (m) $= \dfrac{\text{Number of moles of solute}}{\text{Kilogram of solution}}$

3. Normality (N) $= \dfrac{\text{Number of equivalents of solute}}{\text{Liter of solution}}$

   Where: Number of equivalents $= \dfrac{\text{Grams of chemical}}{\text{Equivalent weight}}$

   Equivalent weight $= \dfrac{\text{Molecular weight}}{n}$

   For acids and bases, $n =$ The number of replaceable H^+ or OH^- ions per molecule

4. Normality $= n$ Molarity
   Where $n:$ = Number of replaceable H^+ or OH^- ions per molecule.

5. Osmolarity $= n$ Molarity
   Where $n:$ = Number of dissociable ions per molecule.

B. SOLUTION CALCULATIONS

6. Volume percent (% v / v) $= \dfrac{\text{Volume of solute}}{\text{Volume of solution}} \times 100$

7. Weight percent (% w / w) $= \dfrac{\text{Weight of solute}}{\text{Weight of solution}} \times 100$

8. Weight / volume percent (% w / v) $= \dfrac{\text{Weight of solute (g)}}{\text{Volume of solution (ml)}} \times 100$

9. Milligram percent (mg%) $= \dfrac{\text{Weight of solute (mg)}}{100 \text{ mL of solution}} \times 100$

10. Parts per million (ppm) $= \dfrac{\text{Weight of solute}}{\text{Weight of solution}} \times 10^6$

11. Parts per million (for gases)

    ppm $= \dfrac{(mg / m^3)\,(R)}{\text{Molecular weight}}$

    Where: $R = 24.5$ at 25°C.

12. $(\text{volume}_C)\,(\text{concentration}_C) = (\text{volume}_D)\,(\text{concentration}_D)$
    Where: C = Concentrated solution
    D = Dilute solution

The above relationship is useful in preparing dilute solutions from concentrated solutions.

C. pH Calculations

13. $pH = -\log [H^+] = \log \dfrac{1}{[H^+]}$

14. $pH = pKa + \log \dfrac{[A^-]}{[HA]}$

Where: $HA \Leftrightarrow H^+ + A^-$
(weak acid) (conjugate base)
$pK_a = -\log Ka$
(equilibrium constant)

D. Glossary of Terms Associated with Solutions

Dispersion Two-phase system that consists of finely divided particles distributed throughout a bulk substance. Examples include gas:liquid (foam); solid:gas (aerosol); gas:solid (foamed plastic); liquid:gas (fog); liquid:liquid (emulsion); solid:liquid (paint); solid:solid (carbon black in rubber).

Emulsion A system containing two or more immiscible liquids in which one is dispersed in the form of very small globules throughout the other.

Miscible Capable of being mixed and remaining so after the mixing process ceases. Materials that do not mix at all are said to be immiscible (e.g., oil and water).

Mixture A mutual incorporation of two or more substances without chemical union, the physical characteristics of each of the components being retained. The components may or may not be uniformly dispersed and can usually be separated by mechanical means. Mixtures can be broadly grouped into two classes: *mechanical mixtures* which consist of a mixture of particles or masses distinguishable as such under a microscope or by other methods; *physical mixtures* consisting of a more intimate mixture of molecules such as with gases and many solutions.

Solubility The ability or tendency of one substance to blend uniformly with another. Examples include solid in liquid, liquid in liquid, gas in liquid, gas in gas. Usually, liquids and gases are said to be miscible in other liquids and gases rather than soluble.

Soluble Capable of being dissolved.

Solution A uniformly dispersed mixture at the molecular or ionic level of one or more substances (the solute) in one or more other substances (the solvent).

Suspension The dispersion through a liquid of very small particles (solid, semisolid, or liquid) of a size large enough to be detected by optical means. If the particles are small enough to pass through filter membranes but still large enough to scatter light, they will generally remain dispersed indefinitely and the system is called a colloidal suspension.

REFERENCES
(SUBSECTIONS A.→D.)

1. Segel, I. H., *Biochemical Calculations,* 2nd ed., John Wiley & Sons, New York, 1976.
2. Skoog, D. A. and West, D. M., *Fundamentals of Analytical Chemistry,* 2nd ed., Holt, Rinehart and Winston, New York, 1969.
3. Sax, N. I. and Lewis, R. J. Sr., *Hawley's Condensed Chemical Dictionary,* 11th ed., Van Nostrand Reinhold Company, New York, 1987.
4. *Stedman's Medical Dictionary,* 22nd ed., Williams & Wilkins Company, Baltimore, 1972.

TABLE 33.49
Strengths of Concentrated Solutions of Acids and Bases

Acid or Base	Specific Gravity	% by Weight	Weight (g/l)	Approximate Molarity
Hydrochloric acid (HCl)	1.19	37	440	12.1
Sulfuric acid (H_2SO_4)	1.84	96	1,730	18
Nitric acid (HNO_3)	1.42	70	990	15.7
Acetic acid (CH_3COOH)	1.06	99.5	1,060	17.4
Ammonium hydroxide (NH_4OH)	0.880	29	250	15–17
Sodium hydroxide (saturated solution) (NaOH)	1.50–1.53	about 50	600–700	15–18
Potassium hydroxide (saturated solution) (KOH)	1.55	about 50	800	14

TABLE 33.50
Physiological Solutions (g/l)

	NaCl	KCl	$CaCl_2$	$MgCl_2$	$NaHCO_3$	NaH_2PO_4	KH_2PO_4	$MgSO_4$	Glucose
Saline (mammal)	9.00	—	—	—	—	—	—	—	—
Ringer (mammal)	9.00	0.42	0.24	—	0.50	—	—	—	1.00
Ringer (by Cattell)	9.00	0.42	0.12	—	—	—	0.100	—	1.00
Ringer (by Dresel)	6.00	0.531	0.35	—	2.10	—	0.081	0.147	0.90
Ringer (by Evans)	—	0.42	0.12	0.200	—	—	—	—	1.00[a,b]
Ringer (by Genell)	8.00	0.42	0.24	0.005	1.00	—	—	—	0.50
Ringer (by Moran)	7.00	0.42	0.24	0.200	2.10	—	—	—	1.80
Ringer-Dale (by Stewart)	9.00	0.42	2.015	0.003	0.50	—	—	—	0.50
Ringer-Locke (same as Locke's)	9.00	0.42	.024	—	0.15	—	—	—	1.75
Ringer-Locke (by Feldberg)	9.00	0.20	0.20	—	0.30	—	—	—	1.00
Ringer-Locke (by Gaddum)	9.00	0.42	0.06	—	0.50	—	—	—	0.50
Ringer-Locke (by Hukovic)	9.00	0.42	0.24	—	0.50	—	—	—	2.00
Locke's (by Burn)	9.00	0.42	0.24	0.005	0.50	—	—	—	0.50
Krebs-Henseleit	6.87	0.40	0.28	—	2.10	0.140	—	0.140	2.00
Krebs-Henseleit- Ringer	6.90	0.354	0.280	—	2.10	—	0.162	0.294	—
Krebs-Henseleit (by Furchgott)	6.90	0.354	0.282	—	2.10	—	0.162	0.294	1.80
Krebs (by Hukovic)	6.60	0.350	0.280	—	2.10	—	0.162	0.294	2.08
Beauvilain's	9.00	0.42	0.06	0.005	0.50	—	—	—	0.50
McEwan's	7.60	0.42	0.24	—	2.10	0.143	—	—	2.00[c]
Tyrode (isolated gut)	8.00	0.20	0.20	0.100	1.00	0.050	—	—	1.00
Feigen's (isolated heart)	9.00	0.42	0.62	—	0.60	—	—	—	1.00

[a] K_2SO_4 = 22.00.
[b] $KHCO_3$ = 3.60.
[c] Sucrose = 4.50.

TABLE 33.51
Composition of a Typical Organ Perfusion Medium

	Component	Concentration
Electrolytes	NaCl	115 mM
	KCl	5.4 mM
	$MgSO_4$	2.4 mM
	$CaCl_2$	3.0 mM
Buffer	NaH_2PO_4	1.5 mM
	$NaHCO_3$	25 mM
Source of energy	Glucose	5 mM
	Glutamine	2 mM
Oncotic agent	Bovine serum albumin	60 g l^{-1}
Other additions	Alanine	2 mM
	Glutathione	2 mM

TABLE 33.52
Properties of Carrier Gases for Gas Chromatography

Carrier Gas	Density (kg/m³)	Thermal Conductivity × 10⁻² (W/[m · K])	Thermal Conductivity Differences			Viscosity × 10⁻³ (Pa · s)	Heat Capacity (J/[kg · K])	Relative Molecular Mass
			δλ (He)	δλ (N₂)	δλ (Al)			
Hydrogen	0.08988	19.71	3.97	16.96	17.81	0.876 (20.7°C)	14,112.7	2.016
						1.086 (129.4°C)		
						1.381 (299.0°C)		
Helium	0.17847	15.74	—	12.99	13.84	1.941 (20.0°C)	5,330.6	4.003
						2.281 (100.0°C)		
						2.672 (200.0°C)		
Methane	0.71680	3.74	−12.00	0.99	1.84	1.087 (20.0°C)	2,217.2	16.04
						1.331 (100.0°C)		
						1.605 (200.5°C)		
Oxygen	1.42904	2.85	−12.89	0.10	0.95	2.018 (19.1°C)	915.3	32.00
						2.568 (127.7°C)		
						3.017 (227.0°C)		
Nitrogen	1.25055	2.75	−12.99	—	0.85	1.781 (27.4°C)	1,030.5	28.016
						2.191 (127.2°C)		
						2.559 (226.7°C)		
Carbon monoxide	1.25040	2.67	−13.07	−0.08	0.77	1.753 (21.7°C)	1,030.7	28.01
						2.183 (126.7°C)		
						2.548 (227.0°C)		
Ethane	1.35660	2.44	−13.30	−0.31	0.54	0.901 (17.2°C)	1,614.0	30.07
						1.143 (100.4°C)		
						1.409 (200.3°C)		
Ethene	1.26040	2.30	−13.44	−0.45	0.40	1.008 (20.0°C)	—	28.05
						1.257 (100.0°C)		
						1.541 (200.0°C)		
Propane	2.00960	2.03	−13.71	−0.72	0.13	0.795 (17.9°C)	—	44.09
						1.009 (100.4°C)		
						1.253 (199.3°C)		
Argon	1.78370	1.90	−13.84	−0.85	—	2.217 (20.0°C)	523.7	39.94
						2.695 (100.0°C)		
						3.223 (200.0°C)		
Carbon dioxide	1.97690	1.83	−13.91	−0.92	−0.07	1.480 (20.0°C)	836.6	44.01
						1.861 (99.1°C)		
						2.221 (182.4°C)		
n-Butane	2.51900	1.82	−13.92	−0.93	−0.08	0.840 (14.7°C)	—	58.12
Sulfur hexafluoride	6.50 (20°C)	1.63	−14.11	−1.12	−0.27	1.450 (21.1°C)	647.0	146.05

Note: Values refer to a pressure of 101 kPa (760 torr). Density values are given at 0°C (120°F).

Reprinted from Bruno, T. J. and Svoronos, P. D. N., *CRC Handbook of Basic Tables for Chemical Analysis*, CRC Press, Boca Raton, FL, 1989, p. 4. With permission.

TABLE 33.53
Solvents for Ultraviolet Spectrophotometry

Solvent	Wavelength Cutoff (nm)	Dielectric Constant (20°C)	
Acetic acid	260	6.15	
Acetone	330	20.7	(25°C)
Acetonitrile	190	37.5	
Benzene	280	2.284	
2-Butanol	260	15.8	(25°C)
n-Butyl acetate	254		
Carbon disulfide	380	2.641	
Carbon tetrachloride	265	2.238	
1-Chlorobutane	220	7.39	(25°C)
Chloroform[a]	245	4.806	
Cyclohexane	210	2.023	
1,2-Dichloroethane	226	10.19	(25°C)
1,2-Dimethoxyethane	240		
N,N-Dimethylacetamide	268	59	(83°C)
N,N-Dimethylformamide	270	36.7	
Dimethylsulfoxide	265	4.7	
1,4-Dioxane	215	2.209	(25°C)
Diethyl ether	218	4.335	
Ethanol	210	24.30	(25°C)
2-Ethoxyethanol	210		
Ethyl acetate	255	6.02	(25°C)
Glycerol	207	42.5	(25°C)
n-Hexadecane	200	2.06	(25°C)
n-Hexane	210	1.890	
Methanol	210	32.63	(25°C)
2-Methoxyethanol	210	16.9	
Methyl cyclohexane	210	2.02	(25°C)
Methyl ethyl ketone	330	18.5	
Methyl isobutyl ketone	335		
2-Methyl-1-propanol	230	1	
N-Methyl-2-pyrrolidone	285	32.0	
Pentane	210	1.844	
n-Pentyl acetate	212		
1-Propanol	210	20.1	(25°C)
2-Propanol	210	18.3	(25°C)
Pyridine	330	12.3	(25°C)
Tetrachloroethylene[b]	290		
Tetrahydrofuran	220	7.6	
Toluene	286	2.379	(25°C)
1,1,2-Trichloro-1,2,2-trifluoroethane	231		
2,2,4-Trimethylpentane	215	1.936	(25°C)
o-Xylene	290	2.568	
m-Xylene	290	2.374	
p-Xylene	290	2.270	
Water		78.54	(25°C)

[a] Stabilized with ethanol to avoid phosgene formation.

[b] Stabilized with thymol (isopropyl meta-cresol).

Reprinted from Bruno, T. J. and Svoronos, P. D. N., *CRC Handbook of Basic Tables for Chemical Analysis*, CRC Press, Boca Raton, FL, 1989, p. 212. With permission.

TABLE 33.54
[13]C Chemical Shifts of Useful NMR Solvents

Solvent	Formula	Chemical Shift (npm)
Acetone-d_6	$(CD_3)_2C=O$	29.2 (CD_3) 204.1 ($>C=O$)
Acetonitrile-d_3	$CD_3C\equiv N$	1.3 (CD_3) 117.1 ($C\equiv N$)
Benzene-d_6	C_6D_6	128.4
Carbon disulfide	CS_2	192.3
Carbon tetrachloride	CCl_4	96.0
Chloroform-d_3	$CDCl_3$	77.05
Cyclohexane-d_{12}	C_6D_{12}	27.5
Dichloromethane-d_2	CD_2Cl_2	53.6
Dimethylformamide-d_7	$(CD_3)_2NCOD$	31 (CD_3) 36 (CD_3) 162.4 ($DC=O$)
Dimethylsulfoxide-d_6	$(CD_3)_2S=O$	39.6
Dioxane-d_8	$C_6D_8O_2$	67.4
Methanol-d_4	CD_3OD	49.3
Nitromethane-d_3	$CD_3.NO_2.$	57.3
Pyridine-d_5	C_5D_5N	123.9 (C-3) 135.9 (C-4) 150.2 (C-2)
1, 1,2,2-Tetrachloroethane-d_2	$CDCl_2.CDCl_2$	75.5
Tetrahydrofuran-d_8	C_4D_8O	25.8 (C-2) 67.9 (C-1)
Trichlorofluoromethane	$CFCl_3$	117.6
Water (heavy)	D_2O	—

Reprinted from Bruno, T. J. and Svoronos, P. D. N., *CRC Handbook of Basic Tables for Chemical Analysis*, CRC Press, Boca Raton, FL, 1989, p. 330. With permission.

TABLE 33.55
Important Peaks in the Mass Spectra of Common Solvents

Solvents	Formula	M[+]	Important Peaks (*m/e*)
Water	H_2O	18(100%)	17
Methanol	CH_3OH	32	31 (100%), 29, 15
Acetonitrile	CH_3CN	41(100%)	40, 39, 38, 28, 15
Ethanol	CH_3CH_2OH	46	45, 31 (100%), 27, 15
Dimetyl ether	CH_3OCH_3	46(100%)	45,29, 15
Acetone	CH_3COCH_3	58	43 (100%), 42, 39, 27, 15
Acetic acid	CH_3CO_2H	60	45, 43, 18, 15
Ethylene glycol	$HOCH_2CH_2OH$	62	43, 33, 31 (100%), 29, 18, 15
Furan	C_4H_4O	68(100%)	42, 39, 38, 37, 29, 18
Tetrahydrofuran	C_4H_8O	72	71, 43, 42 (100%), 41, 40, 39, 27, 18, 15
n-Pentane	C_5H_{12}	72	57, 43 (100%), 42, 41, 39, 29, 28, 27, 15
Dimethylformamide (DMF)	$HCON(CH_3)_2$	73(100%)	58, 44, 42, 30, 29, 28, 18, 15
Diethylether	$(C_2H_5)_2O$	74	59, 45, 41, 31 (100%), 29, 27, 15
Methylacetate	$CH_3CO_2CH_3$	74	59, 43 (100%), 42, 32, 29, 28, 15
Carbon disulfide	CS_2	76(100%)	64, 44, 38, 32
Benzene	C_6H_6	78(100%)	77, 52, 51, 50, 39, 28
Pyridine	C_5H_5N	79(100%)	80, 78, 53, 52, 51, 50, 39, 26
Dichloromethane	CH_2Cl_2	84	86, 51, 49 (100%), 48, 47, 35, 28
Cyclohexane	C_6H_{12}	84	69, 56, 55, 43, 42, 41, 39, 27
n-Hexane	C_6H_{14}	86	85, 71, 69, 57, (100%), 43, 42, 41, 39, 29, 28, 27
p-Dioxane	$C_4H_8O_2$	88(100%)	87, 58, 57, 45, 43, 31, 30, 29, 28
Tetramethylsilane (TMS)	$(CH_3)_4Si$	88	74, 73, 55, 45, 43, 29

TABLE 33.55 *(Continued)*
Important Peaks in the Mass Spectra of Common Solvents

Solvents	Formula	M+	Important Peaks (*m/e*)
1,2-Dimethoxy ethane	$(CH_3OCH_2)_2$	90	60, 58, 45 (100%), 31, 29
Toluene	$C_6H_5CH_3$	92	91 (100%), 65, 51, 39, 28
Chloroform	$CHCl_3$	118	120, 83, 81 (100%), 47, 35, 28
Chloroform-d_1	$CDCl_3$	119	121, 84, 82 (100%), 48, 47, 35, 28
Carbon tetrachloride	CCl_4	152 (not seen)	121, 119, 117 (100%), 84, 82, 58.5, 47, 35, 28
Tetrachloroethene	$CCl_2 = CCl_2$	164 (not seen)	168, 166 (100%), 165, 164, 131, 128, 129, 95, 94, 82, 69, 59, 47, 31, 24

Reprinted from Bruno, T. J. and Svoronos, P. D. N., *CRC Handbook of Basic Tables for Chemical Analysis*, CRC Press, Boca Raton, FL, 1989, p. 357. With permission.

TABLE 33.56
Solvents for Liquid Chromatography

Solvent	Viscosity (mPa . s; 20°C)	UV Cutoff (nm)	Refractive Index (20°C)	Normal Boiling Point (°C)	Dielectric Constant (20°C)
Acetic acid	1.31(15)		1.372	117.9	6.15
Acetone	0.30(25)	330	1.359	56.3	20.7(25)
Acetonitrile	0.34(25)	190	1.344	81.6	37.5
Benzene	0.65	278	1.501	80.1	2.284
1-Butanol	2.95	215	1.399	117.7	17.8
2-Butanol	4.21	260	1.397	99.6	15.8(25)
n-Butyl acetate	0.73	254	1.394	126.1	
n-Butyl chloride	0.47(15)	220	1.402	78.4	
Carbon tetrachloride	0.97	263	1.460	76.8	2.238
Chlorobenzene	0.80	287	1.525	131.7	2.708
Chloroform	0.58	245	1.446	61.2	4.806
Cyclohexane	0.98	200	1.426	80.7	2.023
Cyclopentane	0.44	200	1.406	49.3	1.965
o-Dichlorobenzene	1.32(25)	295	1.551	180.5	9.93(25)
N,N-Dimethylacetamide	2.14	268	1.438	166.1	37.8
Dimethylformamide	0.92	268	1.430	153.0	36.7
Dimethyl sulfoxide	2.20	286	1.478	189.0	4.7
Dioxane	1.44(15)	215	1.422	101.3	2.209(25)
2-Ethoxyethanol	2.05	210	1.408	135.6	
Ethyl acetate	0.46	256	1.372	77.1	6.02(25)
Ethyl ether	0.24	218	1.352	34.6	4.335
Glyme (ethylene glycol dimethyl ether)	0.46(25)	220	1.380	93.0	
Heptane	0.42	200	1.388	98.4	1.92
Hexadecane	3.34	200	1.434	287.0	
Hexane	0.31	200	1.375	68.7	1.890
Isobutyl alcohol	4.70(15)	200	1.396	107.7	15.8(25)
Methanol	0.55	205	1.328	64.7	32.63(25)
2-Methoxyethanol	1.72	210	1.402	124.6	16.9
2-Methoxyethyl acetate		254	1.402	144.5	
Methylene chloride	0.45(15)	233	1.424	39.8	9.08

TABLE 33.56 *(Continued)*
Solvents for Liquid Chromatography

Solvent	Viscosity (mPa . s; 20°C)	UV Cutoff (nm)	Refractive Index (20°C)	Normal Boiling Point (°C)	Dielectric Constant (20°C)
Methylethylketone	0.42(15)	329	1.379	79.6	18.5
Methylisoamylketone		330	1.406	−144.0	
Methylisobutylketone	0.54(25)	334	1.396	116.5	
N-Methyl-2-pyrrolidone	1.67(25)	285	1.488	202.0	32.0
Nonane	0.72	200	1.405	150.8	1.972
Pentane	0.24	200	1.357	36.1	1.84
Petroleum ether	0.30	226		30–60	
β–Phenethylamine		285	1.529(25)	197–198	
1-Propanol	2.26	210	1.386	97.2	20.1(25)
2-Propanol	2.86(15)	205	1.377	82.3	18.3(25)
Propylene carbonate			1.419	240.0	
Pyridine	0.95	330	1.510	115.3	12.3(25)
Tetrachloroethylene	0.93(15)	295	1.506	121.2	
Tetrahydrofuran	0.55	212	1.407	66.0	7.6
Tetramethyl urea		265	1.449(25)	175.2	23.0
Toluene	0.59	284	1.497	110.6	2.379(25)
Trichloroethylene	0.57	273	1.477	87.2	3.4(16)
1,2,2-Trichloro- 1,2,2-trifluoroethane	0.71	231	1.356(25)	47.6	
2,2,4-Trimethylpentane	0.50	215	1.391	99.2	1.94
Water	1.00	<190	1.333	100.0	78.54
o-Xylene	0.81	288	1.505	144.4	2.568
p-Xylene		290	1.496	138.5	2.270

Reprinted from Bruno, T. J. and Svoronos, P. D. N., *CRC Handbook of Basic Tables for Chemical Analysis*, CRC Press, Boca Raton, FL, 1989, p. 89. With permission.

SECTION 5. NATIONAL STANDARDS

Table 33.57 gives threshold limits for selected airborne contaminants in the workplace. The limits are set by:

> American Conference of Governmental Industrial Hygienists
> 1330 Kemper Meadow Drive
> Cincinnati, OH 45240-1634
> www.acgih.org

Threshold limit values are airborne concentrations under which it is believed that nearly all workers may be repeatedly exposed day after day without adverse effect. However, it should be noted that a small percentage of individuals may be affected at concentrations at or below these limits because of unusual susceptibility or preexisting conditions. Publications by the organization cited above should be consulted for full details.

In Table 33.57, the threshold limit valve (TLV) is given in parts per million (ppm) by volume in air at 25°C and 760 torr (101.325 kPa). For most substances, the quantity tabulated is the time-weighted average (TWA) for a normal 8-h workday and 40-h workweek. However, a C following a TLV entry indicates a ceiling value which should not be exceeded even for short periods.

The abbreviations used in the table are as follows: *asphy*, compound that may not have significant physiological effects but is an asphyxiant when present in high concentrations (fire and explosion hazards may also exist for these compounds); *CAS RN*, Chemical Abstracts Service Registry Number.

Compounds are listed by molecular formula in the modified Hill order.

TABLE 33.57
Threshold Limit Values for Airborne Contaminants[a]

Molecular Formula	Compound	CAS RN	TLV-TWA (ppm)	
AsH_3	Arsine	7784-42-1	0.05	
BBr_3	Boron tribromide	10294-33-4	1	C
BF_3	Boron trifluoride	7637-07-2	1	C
B_2H_6	Diborane	19287-45-7	0.1	
B_5H_{11}	Pentaborane	19624-22-7	0.005	
BrH	Hydrogen bromide	10035-10-6	3	C
Br_2	Bromine	7726-95-6	0.1	
$ClFO_3$	Perchloryl fluoride	7616-94-6	3	
ClF_3	Chlorine trifluoride	7790-91-2	0.1	C
ClH	Hydrogen chloride	7647-01-0	5	C
ClO_2	Chlorine dioxide	10049-04-4	0.1	
Cl_2	Chlorine	7782-50-5	0.5	
Cl_2CrO_2	Chromyl chloride	14977-61-8	0.025	
Cl_2OS	Thionyl chloride	7719-09-7	1	C
Cl_3OP	Phosphorous oxychloride	10025-87-3	0.1	
Cl_3P	Phosphorous trichloride	7719-12-2	0.2	
Cl_5P	Phosphorous pentachloride	10026-13-8	0.1	
FH	Hydrogen fluoride	7664-39-3	3	C
F_2	Fluorine	7782-41-4	1	
F_2O	Oxygen difluoride	7783-41-7	0.05	C
F_2O_2S	Sufuryl fluoride	2699-79-8	5	
F_3N	Nitrogen trifluoride	7783-54-2	10	
F_4S	Sulfur tetrafluoride	7783-60-0	0.1	C
F_5S	Sulfur pentafluoride	5714-22-7	0.01	C
F_6S	Sulfur hexafluoride	2551-62-4	1000	
F_6Se	Selenium hexafluoride	7783-79-1	0.05	
HNO_3	Nitric acid	7697-37-2	2	
H_2O_2	Hydrogen peroxide	7722-84-1	1	
H_2S	Hydrogen sulfide	7783-06-4	5	
H_2Se	Hydrogen selenide	7783-07-5	0.05	
H_3N	Ammonia	7664-41-7	25	
H_3P	Phosphine	7803-51-2	0.3	
H_3Sb	Stibine	7803-52-3	0.1	
H_4N_2	Hydrazine	302-01-2	0.1	
H_4Si	Silane	7803-62-5	5	
I_2	Iodine	7553-56-2	0.1	C
NO	Nitric oxide	10102-43-9	25	
NO_2	Nitrogen dioxide	10102-44-0	3	
O_2S	Sulfur dioxide	7446-09-5	2	
CBr_2F_2	Dibromodifluoromethane	75-61-6	100	
CClN	Cyanogen chloride	506-77-4	0.3	C

TABLE 33.57 *(Continued)*
Threshold Limit Values for Airborne Contaminants[a]

Molecular Formula	Compound	CAS RN	TLV-TWA (ppm)	
CCl_2F_2	Dichlorodifluoromethane	75-71-8	1000	
CCl_2O	Phosgene	75-44-5	0.1	
CCl_3F	Trichlorofluoromethane	75-69-4	1000	C
CBr_4	Carbon tetrabromide	558-13-4	0.1	
CCl_4	Carbon tetrachloride	56-23-5	5	
CF_2O	Carbonyl fluoride	353-50-4	2	
CO	Carbon monoxide	630-08-0	25	
CO_2	Carbon dioxide	124-38-9	5000	
CS_2	Carbon disulfide	75-15-0	10	
$CHBr_3$	Tribromomethane (Bromoform)	75-25-2	0.5	
$CHClF_2$	Chlorodifluoromethane	75-45-6	1000	
$CHCl_2F$	Dichlorofluoromethane	75-43-4	10	
$CHCl_3$	Chloroform	67-66-3	10	
CHI_3	Triiodomethane (Iodoform)	75-47-8	0.6	
CHN	Hydrogen Cyanide	74-90-8	4.7	C
CH_2BrCl	Bromochloromethane	74-97-5	200	
CH_2Cl_2	Dichloromethane	75-09-2	50	
CH_2N_2	Diazomethane	334-88-3	0.2	
CH_2O	Formaldehyde	50-00-0	0.3	
CH_2O_2	Formic acid	64-18-6	5	
CH_2Br	Methyl bromide	74-83-9	1	
CH_3Cl	Methyl chloride	74-87-3	50	
CH_3I	Methyl iodide	74-88-4	2	
CH_3NO	Formamide	75-12-7	10	
CH_3NO_2	Nitromethane	75-52-5	20	
CH_4	Methane	74-82-8	asphy.	
CH_4O	Methanol	67-56-1	200	
CH_4S	Methyl mercaptan	74-93-1	0.5	
CH_5N	Methylamine	74-89-5	5	
CH_6N_2	Methylhydrazine	60-34-4	0.01	C
C_2ClF_5	Chloropentafluoroethane	76-15-3	1000	
C_2Cl_2	Dichloroacetylene	7572-29-4	0.1	C
C_2Cl_4	Tetrachloroethylene	127-18-4	25	
C_2Cl_6	Hexachloroethane	67-72-1	1	
C_2N_2	Cyanogen	460-19-5	10	
C_2HCl_3	Trichloroethylene	79-01-6	50	
$C_2HCl_3O_2$	Trichloroacetic acid	76-03-9	1	
C_2H_2	Acetylene	74-86-2	asphy.	
$C_2H_2Cl_2$	1,1-Dichloroethylene	75-35-4	5	
$C_2H_2Cl_2O$	Chloroacetyl chloride	79-04-9	0.05	
$C_2H_2Cl_4$	1,1,2,2-Tetrachloroethane	79-34-5	1	
C_2H_2O	Ketene	463-51-4	0.5	
C_2H_3Br	Vinyl bromide	593-60-2	0.5	
C_2H_3Cl	Vinyl chloride	75-01-4	1	C
C_2H_3ClO	Chloroacetaldehyde	107-20-0	1	C
$C_2H_3Cl_3$	1,1,1-Trichloroethane	71-55-6	350	C
$C_2H_3Cl_3$	1,1,2-Trichloroethane	79-00-5	10	
C_2H_3N	Acetonitrile	75-05-8	40	

TABLE 33.57 *(Continued)*
Threshold Limit Values for Airborne Contaminants[a]

Molecular Formula	Compound	CAS RN	TLV-TWA (ppm)	
C$_2$H$_3$NO	Methylisocyanate	624-83-9	0.02	
C$_2$H$_4$	Ethylene	74-85-1	asphy.	
C$_2$H$_4$Cl$_2$	1,2-Dichloroethane	107-06-2	10	
C$_2$H$_4$Cl$_2$O	*Bis*-(chloromethyl)ether	542-88-1	0.001	
C$_2$H$_4$O	Acetaldehyde	75-07-0	25	C
C$_2$H$_4$O$_2$	Acetic acid	64-19-7	10	
C$_2$H$_4$O	Ethylene oxide	75-21-8	1	
C$_2$H$_4$O$_2$	Methyl formate	107-31-3	100	
C$_2$H$_5$Br	Bromoethane (Ethyl bromide)	74-96-4	5	
C$_2$H$_5$Cl	Chloroethane (Ethyl chloride)	75-00-3	100	
C$_2$H$_5$ClO	2-Chloroethanol	107-07-3	1	C
C$_2$H$_5$N	Ethyleneimine	151-56-4	0.5	
C$_2$H$_5$NO$_2$	Nitroethane	79-24-3	100	
C$_2$H$_6$	Ethane	74-84-0	asphy.	
C$_2$H$_6$O	Ethanol	64-17-5	1000	
C$_2$H$_6$O$_2$	Ethylene glycol	107-21-1	100 mg/m^3	C
C$_2$H$_6$S	Ethyl mercaptan	75-08-1	0.5	
C$_2$H$_7$N	Dimethylamine	124-40-3	5	
C$_2$H$_7$N	Ethylamine	75-04-7	5	
C$_2$H$_7$NO	Ethanolamine	141-43-5	3	
C$_2$H$_8$N$_2$	1,1-Dimethylhydrazine	57-14-7	0.01	
C$_2$H$_8$N$_2$	Ethylenediamine	107-15-3	10	
C$_3$F$_6$O	Hexafluoroacetone	684-16-2	0.1	
C$_3$H$_3$N	Acrylonitrile	107-13-1	2	
C$_3$H$_4$	Methylacetylene	74-99-7	1000	
C$_3$H$_4$O	Acrolein	107-02-8	0.1	C
C$_3$H$_4$O	Propargyl alcohol	107-19-7	1	
C$_3$H$_4$O$_2$	Acrylic acid	79-10-7	2	
C$_3$H$_4$O$_2$	*p*-Propiolactone	57-57-8	0.5	
C$_3$H$_5$Cl	Allyl chloride	107-05-1	1	
C$_3$H$_5$ClO	Epichlorohydrin	106-89-8	0.5	
C$_3$H$_5$NO	Acrylamide	79-06-1	0.03 mg/m^3	
C$_3$H$_6$O	Acetone	67-64-1	500	
C$_3$H$_6$O	Allyl alcohol	107-18-6	0.5	
C$_3$H$_6$O$_2$	Ethyl formate	109-94-4	100	
C$_3$H$_6$O$_2$	Methyl acetate	79-20-9	200	
C$_3$H$_6$O$_2$	Propionic acid	79-09-4	10	
C$_3$H$_6$O	1,2-Propylene oxide	75-56-9	2	
C$_3$H$_7$N	Propyleneimine	75-55-8	2	
C$_3$H$_7$NO	*N,N*-Dimethylformamide	68-12-2	10	
C$_3$H$_8$	Propane	74-98-6	2500	
C$_3$H$_8$O	*n*-Propanol	71-23-8	200	
C$_3$H$_8$O	Isopropanol	67-63-0	200	
C$_3$H$_9$N	Isopropylamine	75-31-0	5	
C$_3$H$_9$N	Trimethylamine	75-50-3	5	
C$_4$Cl$_6$	Hexachlorobutadiene	87-68-3	0.02	
C$_4$NiO$_4$	Nickel carbonyl	13463-39-3	0.05	
C$_4$H$_2$O$_3$	Maleic anhydride	108-31-6	0.1	

TABLE 33.57 (Continued)
Threshold Limit Values for Airborne Contaminants[a]

Molecular Formula	Compound	CAS RN	TLV-TWA (ppm)	
C_4H_5N	Methylacrylonitrile	126-98-7	1	
C_4H_6	1,3-Butadiene	106-99-0	2	
C_4H_6O	*trans*-Crotonaldehyde	4170-30-3	0.3	C
$C_4H_6O_2$	Methacrylic acid	79-41-4	20	
$C_4H_6O_2$	Methyl acrylate	96-33-3	2	
$C_4H_6O_2$	Vinyl acetate	108-05-4	10	
$C_4H_6O_3$	Acetic anhydride	108-24-7	5	C
C_4H_8O	Methyl ethyl ketone	78-93-3	200	
C_4H_8O	Tetrahydrofuran	109-99-9	200	
$C_4H_8O_2$	1,4-Dioxane	123-91-1	20	
$C_4H_8O_2$	Ethylacetate	141-78-6	400	
C_4H_9NO	Morpholine	110-91-8	20	
C_4H_{10}	*n*-Butane	106-97-8	800	
$C_4H_{10}O$	*n*-Butanol	71-36-3	20	C
$C_4H_{10}O$	*sec*-Butanol	78-92-2	100	
$C_4H_{10}O$	*tert*-Butanol	75-65-0	100	
$C_4H_{10}O$	Isobutanol	78-83-1	50	
$C_4H_{10}O$	Diethyl ether	60-29-7	400	
$C_4H_{10}S$	*n*-Butyl mercaptan	109-79-5	0.5	
$C_4H_{11}N$	Diethylamine	109-89-7	5	
$C_4H_{11}NO_2$	Diethanolamine	111-42-2	2 mg/m³	
$C_5H_4O_2$	Furfural	98-01-1	2	
C_5H_5N	Pyridine	110-86-1	5	
C_5H_6	Cyclopentadiene	542-92-7	75	
$C_5H_8O_2$	Ethyl acrylate	140-88-5	5	
$C_5H_8O_2$	Methyl methacrylate	80-62-6	50	
C_5H_{10}	Cyclopentane	287-92-3	600	
$C_5H_{10}O$	Cyclohexanone	108-94-1	25	
$C_5H_{10}O$	Diethyl ketone	96-22-0	200	
$C_5H_{10}O$	Mesityl oxide	141-79-7	15	
$C_5H_{10}O$	*n*-Valeraldehyde	110-62-3	50	
$C_5H_{10}O_2$	Isopropyl acetate	108-21-4	100	
$C_5H_{10}O_2$	*n*-Propyl acetate	109-60-4	200	
C_5H_{12}	*n*-Pentane	109-66-0	600	
$C_4H_3Cl_2$	1,2,4-Trichlorobenzene	120-82-1	5	C
$C_6H_4Cl_2$	*o*-Dichlorobenzene	95-50-1	25	
$C_6H_4Cl_2$	*p*-Dichlorobenzene	106-46-7	10	
$C_6H_4O_2$	*p*-Benzoquinone	106-51-4	0.1	
C_6H_5Cl	Chlorobenzene	108-90-7	10	
$C_6H_5NO_2$	Nitrobenzene	98-95-3	1	
C_6H_6	Benzene	71-43-2	0.5	
C_6H_6O	Phenol	108-95-2	5	
C_6H_6S	Phenyl mercaptan	108-98-5	0.5	
C_6H_7N	Aniline	62-53-3	2	
C_6H_{10}	Cyclohexene	110-83-8	300	
$C_6H_{11}NO$	Caprolactam	105-60-2	5 mg/m³	
C_6H_{12}	Cyclohexane	110-82-7	200	
$C_6H_{12}O$	Cyclohexanol	108-93-0	50	

TABLE 33.57 *(Continued)*
Threshold Limit Values for Airborne Contaminants[a]

Molecular Formula	Compound	CAS RN	TLV-TWA (ppm)
$C_6H_{12}O$	Methyl isobutyl ketone	108-10-1	50
$C_6H_{12}O_2$	*n*-Butyl acetate	123-86-4	150
$C_6H_{12}O_2$	Isobutyl acetate	110-19-0	150
$C_6H_{13}N$	Cyclohexylamine	108-91-8	10
$C_6H_{12}O_2$	Diacetone alcohol	123-42-2	50
$C_6H_{15}N$	Diisopropylamine	108-18-9	5
C_6H_{14}	*n*-Hexane	110-54-3	50
C_7H_7Cl	*o*-Chlorotoluene	95-49-8	50
C_7H_7Cl	Chloromethylbenzene	100-44-7	1
$C_7H_7NO_2$	*o*-Nitrotoluene	88-72-2	2
$C_7H_7NO_2$	*m*-Nitrotoluene	99-08-1	2
$C_7H_7NO_2$	*p*-Nitrotoluene	99-99-0	2
C_7H_8	Toluene	108-88-3	50
C_7H_8O	*o*-Cresol	95-48-7	5
C_7H_8O	*m*-Cresol	108-39-4	5
C_7H_8O	*p*-Cresol	106-44-5	5
C_7H_9N	*o*-Toluidine	95-53-4	2
C_7H_9N	*m*-Toluidine	108-44-1	2
C_7H_9N	*p*-Toluidine	106-49-0	2
C_7H_9NO	*p*-Anisidine	104-94-9	0.1
$C_7H_{14}O_2$	*n*-Pentyl acetate	628-63-7	50
C_7H_{16}	*n*-Heptane	142-82-5	400
$C_8H_4O_3$	Phthalic anhydride	85-44-9	1
C_8H_8	Styrene	100-42-5	20
$C_8H_8N_2$	Phenylhydrazine	100-63-0	0.1
C_8H_{10}	Ethylbenzene	100-41-4	100
C_8H_{10}	*o*-Xylene	95-47-6	100
C_8H_{10}	*m*-Xylene	108-38-3	100
C_8H_{10}	*p*-Xylene	106-42-3	100
$C_8H_{11}N$	*N*,*N*-Dimethylaniline	121-69-7	5
C_8H_{18}	*n*-Octane	111-65-9	300
$C_9H_6N_2O_2$	Toluene-2,4-diisocyanate	584-84-9	0.005
C_9H_8	Indene	95-13-6	10
C_9H_{10}	Vinyl toluene	25013-15-4	50
C_9H_2O	*n*-Nonane	111-84-2	200
$C_{10}H_8$	Naphthalene	91-20-3	10
$C_{10}H_{16}O$	Camphor	76-22-2	2
$C_{12}H_{10}$	Biphenyl	92-52-4	0.2
$C_{12}H_{12}N_2$	*p*-Benzidine	92-87-5	
$C_{20}H_{12}$	Benzo(a)pyrene	50-32-8	

[a] Based on values as of year 2000.

Some values may have changed since 2000.

TABLE 33.58
U.S. National Primary Drinking Water Standards
for selected contaminants (as of 7/2000)

Chemical Contaminants	Maximum Contaminant Level (mg/l)
Arsenic	0.05
Barium	2.0
Cadmium	0.005
Chromium	0.1
Lead	0.015 (action level)
Mercury	0.002
Nitrate (as nitrogen)	10
Selenium	0.05
Silver	0.10
Fluoride	4.0
Endrin	0.002
Lindane	0.0002
Methoxychlor	0.04
Toxaphene	0.003
2,4-D	0.07
2,4,5-TP	0.05
Trihalomethanes	0.10

Source: www.EPA.gov.

SECTION 6. DESIGN AND PERFORMANCE OF
TOXICOLOGY STUDIES

A. ACCEPTABLE TOXICOLOGY STUDY REQUIREMENTS

Table 33.59 lists the minimum requirements which must be met for a toxicology study to be acceptable under present day standards.[1] Some of these are addressed in detail in the referenced Good Laboratory Practices Standards (GLP).[2–4] Generally, United States GLP satisfy similar regulatory requirements of other countries. Additional acceptability requirements may be associated with specific study designs (e.g., neurotoxicity, reprotoxicity, etc.) and need to be addressed on a case-by-case basis.

TABLE 33.59
Minimum Requirements for an Acceptable Toxicology Study

1. The study should be conducted at a laboratory recognized by accreditation and/or reputation as having the scientific capability, expertise, and experience to conduct the study of interest.
2. The study should be conducted according to Good Laboratory Practices (GLP).
3. The objectives and design of the study should be specified in a study-specific protocol approved by the study director and the sponsor (if applicable).
4. The chemical nature of the tested material should be precisely defined and documented including chemical identity, stability, and degree of purity with any impurities clearly defined.
5. The specificity of any methodology used should be adequate for the degree of detection of the endpoints to be evaluated. Such methods must be validated. Positive controls and standards should be used as necessary.
6. The number of test and control animals should be sufficient to allow the detection of biological variability in response to exposure, to allow trends to be appreciated and to be sufficient for statistical analyses.

TABLE 33.59 *(Continued)*
Minimum Requirements for an Acceptable Toxicology Study

7. Ideally, doses or exposure levels should be sufficient to detect toxicity, define thresholds, and establish no-effect levels.
8. Statistical procedures used should be appropriate for the type of data analyzed.
9. The study should be reported in a clear and unambiguous manner with all necessary detail to allow the reader to understand the study design, interpret the results and draw conclusions. All deviations from the protocol which have occurred should be clearly stated and the potential impact on the study assessed.
10. The report should be signed by the study director to indicate agreement with the results and conclusions. In addition, the study director should sign the GLP compliance statement which states whether the study was conducted in full GLP compliance and if not, the areas of noncompliance. The report should also contain the signed Quality Assurance statement providing dates of inspection and reporting to management.

REFERENCES

1. Ballantyne, B. B. and Sullivan, J. B., Basic principles of toxicology, in *Hazardous Materials Toxicology: Clinical Principles of Environmental Health*, Sullivan, J. B., and Krieger, G. R., Eds., Williams and Wilkens, Baltimore, 1992, chap. 2.
2. Toxic Substances Control Act (TSCA); Good Laboratory Practice Standards; Final Rule. Code of Federal Regulations (CFR) 40, Part 792, United States Environmental Protection Agency, 1989.
3. Federal Insecticide, Fungicide and Rodenticide Act (FIFRA); Good Laboratory Practice Regulations; Final Rule, Code of Federal Regulations (CFR) 40, Part 160, United Stated Environmental Protection Agency, 1989.
4. Food and Drug Administration; Good Laboratory Practice Regulations; Final Rule, Code of Federal Regulations (CFR) 21, Part 58, 1991 (revision), United States Department of Health and Human Services.

B. Estimated Costs and Test Sample Requirements for Standard Toxicology Tests

The following tables provide estimated costs and test sample requirements for standard toxicology tests. The costs indicated are based on year 2000 estimates. For later years, add for inflation at a minimum. Test sample requirements, especially for longer term studies by inhalation, can vary considerably and depend on the toxic potency of the material and the physical nature of the test substance (for inhalation studies). For example, an inhalation study of a minimally toxic dust will require orders of magnitude, more test material, than an equivalent study of a highly toxic gas.

When comparing costs, attention should be paid to the design of the study being offered. The cost of mammalian studies, particularly acute studies, can be influenced by several factors including the use of vehicle control groups, degree of gross and microscopic pathology required, use of positive controls, requirements for dedicated animal rooms, need for dose range-finding studies, type and number of observations required, cost of animals (particularly rabbits), and the degree of statistical analyses and report format required. Analytical method development can add considerable costs to inhalation and aquatic studies. The requirement for a flow-through design can increase the costs of aquatic studies. Factors affecting the cost of genetic studies include the number of bacterial strains and method of exposure to liver enzymes utilized, the number of harvest times, the type and degree of endpoint analyses performed and the need for range-finding studies and confirmatory tests.

Test costs do not necessarily correlate with quality. The most expensive labs may not always represent the best choice. Conversely, a lab should not be ruled out of consideration on the basis of low prices.

TABLE 33.60
Mammalian Toxicology Tests — Cost and Material Requirements

Study Type	Typical Costs	Estimated Material Requirements
Acute Oral Toxicity in Rats, Limit Test[a]	$1,900	50 g
Acute Oral Toxicity in Rats, LD_{50} (4 Levels)[b]	$4,200	50 g
Acute Dermal Toxicity in Rabbits, Limit Test[a]	$2,900	50 g
Acute Dermal Toxicity in Rabbits, LD_{50} (4 Levels)[b]	$6,500	100 g
Acute Inhalation Toxicity in Rats (4 hr. exp.) Limit Test[a]	$5,000	100–5,000 g
Acute Inhalation Toxicity in Rats (4 hr. exp.) LC_{50} (4 Levels)[b,c]	$16,000	500–50,000 g
Primary Eye Irritation in Rabbits[d]	$1,800	10 g
Primary Skin Irritation in Rabbits[d]	$1,800	10 g
Dermal Sensitization in Guinea Pigs, Maximization[e]	$6,000	80 g
Dermal Sensitization in Guinea Pigs, Buehler Type[e,f]	$5,500	80 g
1-Month Oral Toxicity in Rats-Gavage	$60,000	100–200 g
1-Month Inhalation in Rats	$130,000	1–200 kg
1-Month Intravenous Toxicity in Rats	$65,000	100–150 g
1-Month Intravenous Toxicity in Dogs	$100,000	2–3 kg
1-Month Dermal Toxicity in Rats	$60,000	100–300 g
1-Month Oral Toxicity in Dogs-Capsule	$90,000	2–3 kg
3-Month Oral Toxicity in Rats-Gavage	$95,000	600–1200 g
3-Month Inhalation in Rats[c]	$205,000	3–600 kg
3-Month Inhalation in Primates[c]	$300,000	3–600 kg
3-Month Dermal Toxicity in Rats	$120,000	300–900 g
3-Month Oral Toxicity in Dogs-Capsule	$130,000	7–10 kg
6-Month Oral Toxicity in Rats-Gavage	$150,000	6–12 kg
1-Year Oral Toxicity in Dogs-Capsule	$350,000	30–40 kg
18-Month Oncogenicity in Mice-Gavage	$600,000	1–2 kg
24-Month Oncogenicity in Rats-Gavage	$700,000	12–24 kg
24-Month Inhalation in Rats[c]	$1,400,000	20–4,000 kg
3-Month Dietary Study in Rats	$100,000	150–200 g
3-Month Dietary Study in Dogs	$140,000	12–16 kg
General Fertility and Reproductive Performance (Segment I) in Rats	$95,000	500–2,000 g
Range Finding Teratology Study in Rats	$20,000	50–100 g
Teratology (Segment II) Study in Rats	$50,000	50–500 g
Range Finding Teratology Study in Rabbits	$25,000	100–500 g
Teratology (Segment II) Study in Rabbits	$62,000	100–1000 g
Perinatal and Postnatal Study (Segment III) in Rats	$150,000	100–750 g
2-Generation Reproduction Study in Rats	$300,000	3–12 kg
Human Repeat Insult Patch Test (RIPT), 100 Subjects, Nondedicated Panel[g]	$2,800 per sample	300–400 g
Human RIPT, 200 Subjects, Nondedicated Panel[g]	$5,400 per sample	600–800 g
Human RIPT, 100 Subjects, Dedicated Panel[h]	$26,000 (max 8–12 samples)	300–400 g

[a] Lower cost design may not include control groups, bodyweight measurements, or gross necropsy.

[b] Costs may be higher depending on histopathology and performance of dose range finding study.

[c] Costs will be higher if analytical method development and/or extraordinary analytical methods are required.

[d] Additional cost if extended observation periods are required.

[e] Additional cost for positive control.

[f] Number of induction times may vary.

[g] Panel may be shared with other sponsors (8–12 samples per subject).

[h] Panel dedicated to one sponsor.

TABLE 33.61
Genetic Toxicology Tests — Cost and Material Requirements

Study Type	Typical Costs[a]	Estimated Material Requirements
Ames Assay [b,c]	$3,500	20 g
Mouse Lymphoma Assay	$16,000	5–10 g
in vitro Chromosome Aberrations (CHO cells)	$18,000	5 g
in vitro Chromosome Aberrations (Human Lymphocytes)	$20,000	5 g
in vitro Chromosome Aberrations (Rat Lymphocytes)	$22,000	5 g
in vivo Chromosome Aberrations (Mouse Bone Marrow)	$28,000	25–50 g
in vivo Chromosome Aberration (Rat Bone Marrow)	$30,000	50–100 g
in vitro Unscheduled DNA Synthesis (UDS)	$11,000	5 g
in vivo/in vitro UDS	$32,000	25–50 g
in vitro Cell Transformation (Syrian Hamsters)	$20,000	5 g
Drosophilia Sex-Linked Recessive Lethal	$45,000	50 g
Dominant Lethal (Mouse)	$30,000	25–50 g
Dominant Lethal (Rat)	$32,000	100 g
Mouse Micronucleus	$12,000	50 g
in vitro SCE (CHO cells)	$8,000	5 g
in vivo SCE (Mouse)	$22,000	25–50 g

[a] Costs will be higher if confirmatory studies are required.
[b] Costs will vary depending on method of liver enzyme exposure.
[c] Costs will be higher if additional bacterial strains are required.

TABLE 33.62
Aquatic/Ecotoxicology Tests — Cost and Material Requirements

Study Type	Estimated Cost[a]	Estimated Material Requirements
Fish Static Acute (Freshwater) (96 h)[b]	$3,000	10 g
Fish 35-Day Embryo/Larval	$25,000	150 g[c]
Fish 90-Day Embryo/Larval	$38,000	350 g[c]
Daphnid Static Acute (48 h)[b]	$2,500	5 g
Daphnid 21-Day Chronic Reproduction	$16,000	100 g[c]
Algal Static Acute[b] (96 h)	$5,000	5 g
Algal Static 14-Day[b]	$12,000	5 g
28-Day Bioconcentration with Depuration Phase	$39,000	200 g[c]
Earthworm (48 h — Filter Paper)	$4,800	5 g
Earthworm (14 Day — Soil)	$6,000	30 g

[a] Costs will be higher if analytical method development and/or extraordinary analytical methods are required.
[b] Additional cost if flow-through design required.
[c] Assumes highest test concentration of 10 mg/l.

C. CONTRACT LABORATORIES

The following table (Table 33.63) provides a directory of commercial contract laboratories. This listing is intended as a general reference source that allows for the quick identification of laboratories offering general mammalian, genetic, ecotoxicological/aquatic and clinical (Human) testing. The reader should consult the referenced sources or contact the laboratories directly for more detailed information about staff, facilities, and specific tests offered. Directories of laboratories providing ancillary testing related to toxicology such as physiochemical analysis, microbiological screening, environmental fate analysis, etc. are published elsewhere and are beyond the scope of this book.

The information provided in this directory was reasonably accurate at the time of its preparation. Changes to the information supplied in the referenced sources were made when updated information was known. Much effort was made to include all commercial laboratories offering the listed services but it is possible that some were missed unintentionally. Inclusion in this directory does not represent an endorsement of the laboratory; likewise, absence from this list does not indicate a lack of endorsement.

TABLE 33.63
Directory of Contract Toxicology Laboratories[a]

Laboratory	Mammalian	Genetic	Ecotoxicological Aquatic	Clinical
ABEL Scientific-Aquatic Biological Evaluation Laboratory 1551 Jennings Mill Road, Suite 3200-B Bogart, GA 30622 (706) 549-9443			X	
ABC Laboratories 7200 East ABC Lane Columbia, MO 65205 (573) 443-9033 and 38 Castle Roe Road Coleraine, N. Ireland BT51 3RL (44) 2870 320639			X	X
Applied Preclinical Services 161 Janes Chapel Road Oxford, NJ 07863 (908) 637- 4427	X			
Aqua Survey, Inc. 499 Point Breeze Road Flemington, NJ 08822 (908) 788-8700			X	
Battelle 505 King Avenue Columbus, OH 43201-2693 (614) 424-5295	X	X	X	
Battelle Pacific Northwest National Laboratory PO Box 999 Richland, WA 99352 (509) 373-6218		X	X	
BIBRA International Woodmansterne Road Carshalton, Surrey SM5 4DS UNITED KINGDOM (44) 20 8652 1024	X	X		X

TABLE 33.63 *(Continued)*
Directory of Contract Toxicology Laboratories[a]

Laboratory	Mammalian	Genetic	Ecotoxicological Aquatic	Clinical
Biodevelopment Laboratories, Inc. 30 Memorial Drive Cambridge, MA 02142 (617) 441-1088	X	X		
Biocon, Inc. 15801 Crabbs Branch Way Rockville, MD 20855 (301) 762-3202	X			
BioDynamics Walton Manor Walton Milton Keynes, MK7 7AJ United Kingdom (44) 1908 201653	X			X
Bio-Life Associates, Ltd. N6230 County Road G Neillsville, WI 54456 (715) 743-4557	X		X	
Biology and Zoology Research Center, Inc. 36-7 Oyama-Cho, Shibuya-ku Tokyo, 151 Japan (3) 5453 8101	X			
Biological Test Center 2525 McGraw Avenue Irvine, CA 92714 (949) 660-3185	X	X		
Biologic Safety Research, Inc. 510 West Hackley Avenue Muskegon, MI 49444 (616) 739-5511	X			
BioReliance 14920 Broschart Drive Rockville, MD 20850 301 738-1000	X	X		
Braton Biotech, Inc. 1 Taft Court Rockville, MD 20850 (301) 762-5301	X	X		
California Primate Research Center University of California/Davis Davis, CA 95616 (503) 752-8091	X			

TABLE 33.63 *(Continued)*
Directory of Contract Toxicology Laboratories[a]

Laboratory	Mammalian	Genetic	Ecotoxicological Aquatic	Clinical
Central Toxicology Laboratory/ AstraZeneca (CTL) Alderley Park Macclesfield, Cheshire SK 10 4TJ United Kingdom (44) 16255 14534	X	X		
Centre International de Toxicologie (CIT) BP 585 Miserey 27005 Evreux Cedex France (33) 2 32 29 2626	X	X	X	X
CIRION 230 Bernard-Belleau, Suite 169 Laval, QC H7V 4A9 Canada (450) 688-6445		X		X
ClinTrials BioResearch Ltd. (CTBR) 87 Senneville Road Senneville (Montreal) Quebec, Canada H9X 3R3 (514) 630-8200	X	X		
Comparative Biosciences, Inc. 2672 Bayshore Parkway Mountain View, CA 94043 (650) 404-0940	X			
Comparative Toxicology Laboratories VSC, Kansas State University Manhattan, KS 66506 (913) 532-5679	X			X
Consumer Product Testing Co. 70 New Dutch Lane Fairfield, NJ 07004 (973) 808-7111	X	X		X
Covance Laboratories 3301 Kinsman Blvd. Madison, WI 53707-7545 (888) 268-2623 (USA) (44) 1 423 500888(Europe) (65) 56 77333 (Asia) (61) 2 8879 2000 (Australia)	X	X	X	X
DermTech International 15222B Avenue of Science San Diego, CA (858) 618-1328				X

TABLE 33.63 *(Continued)*
Directory of Contract Toxicology Laboratories[a]

Laboratory	Mammalian	Genetic	Ecotoxicological Aquatic	Clinical
Earthnet Labs 414 West California Ruston, LA 71270 (318) 255-0060			X	
Ecology & Environment, Inc. 368 Pleasant View Drive Lancaster, NY 14086 (716) 684-8060			X	
Environmental Health Research & Testing Inc. 3235 Omni Drive Cincinnati, OH (513) 752-2950	X	X		
Environmental Science & Engineering, Inc. (ESE) PO Box 1703 Gainesville, FL 32602 (904) 332-2626			X	
Fraunhofer Institute Nikolai-Fuchs-Strasse 1 30625 Hannover Germany (49) 511 5350 402	X	X		X
Genesis Laboratories 10122 N.E. Frontage Road Wellington, CO 80549 (303) 568-7059	X		X	
Genesys Research, Inc. 2300 Englert Drive PO Box 14165 Research Triangle Park, NC 27709-4165 (919) 544-9500		X		
Gentest Corporation 6 Henshaw Street Woburn, MA 01801 (781) 935-5115	X	X		
Gibraltar Biological Laboratories 122 Fairfield Road Fairfield, NJ 07004 (973) 227-6882	X	X		
Harris Laboratories, Inc. 624 Peach Street, Box 80837 Lincoln, NE 68501 (402) 476-2811			X	

TABLE 33.63 *(Continued)*
Directory of Contract Toxicology Laboratories[a]

Laboratory	Mammalian	Genetic	Ecotoxicological Aquatic	Clinical
Heartland BioTechnologies 125 West 76th Street Davenport, Iowa 52806 (319) 388-6422		X		
Hill Top Research PO Box 420501 Cincinnati, OH 45242 (513) 831-2240				X
H.T.I. Bio-Services, Inc. 26578 Old Julian Highway Santa Ysabel, CA 92070 (619) 788-9691	X			
Huntigdon Life Sciences Alconbury Wooley Road Huntingdon, Cambridgeshire PE175HS ENGLAND (44) 1480 892000 and 100 Mettlers Road East Millstone, NJ 08875-2360 (732) 873-2550	X	X	X	X
IIT Research Institute 10 West 35th Street Chicago, IL 60616 (312) 567-4357	X	X		X
Ina Research Inc. Taguchi Bldg. 7F 1-52-16 Akabane, Kita-ku, Tokyo 115-0045, Japan 03 3902 2377	X	X	X	
Integrated Laboratory Systems 801 Capitola Drive Durham, NC 27713 (919) 544-4589	X	X	X	
Inveresk Research Tranent, Scotland EH33 2NE United Kingdom (44) 1875-614545	X	X	X	X
ITR Laboratories Canada, Inc. 19601 Boul. Clark Graham Montreal, Quebec Canada H9X 27I (514) 457-7400	X			

TABLE 33.63 *(Continued)*
Directory of Contract Toxicology Laboratories[a]

Laboratory	Mammalian	Genetic	Ecotoxicological Aquatic	Clinical
Jai Research Foundation (JRF)/ **JRF International (JRFI)** 3268 Allison Court Carmel, IN 46033 (317) 573-9395	X	X	X	
Kemic Bioresearch Laboratories, Ltd. Valley Professional Centre 70 Exhibition Street PO Box 878 Kentville, Nova Scotia Canada B4N 4H8 (902) 678-8195	X			X
LabCorp 1904 Alexander Drive Research Triangle Park, NC (919) 572-6900				X
LAB Pre-Clinical Research International 560 Cartier Boulevard Laval, Quebec H7V 3P6 Canada (450) 973-2240	X			
Laboratory of Pharmacology & Toxicology P.O. Box 920461 D-21134 Hamburg Germany +49 40 702 020	X	X		X
Laboratory Research Enterprises, Inc. 6321 South 6th Street Kalamazoo, MI 49009 (616) 375-0482	X			
LCG Bioscience Bourn Hall Clinic Bourn Cambridge, CB3 7TR United Kingdom (44) 1954 717 271	X	X	X	X
Life Science Research Israel, Ltd. PO Box 139 Nessziona 70 451 Israel (08) 472599, 472777	X			
Lovelace Respiratory Research Institute 2425 Ridgecrest Drive, S.E. Albuquerque, NM 108-5127 (505) 845-1075	X	X		X

TABLE 33.63 *(Continued)*
Directory of Contract Toxicology Laboratories[a]

Laboratory	Mammalian	Genetic	Ecotoxicological Aquatic	Clinical
MB Research Labs, Inc. PO Box 178 Steinsburg & Wentz Roads Spinnerstown, PA 18968 (215) 536-4110	X			
McWill Research Laboratories, Inc. 564 Lee Street, SW PO Box 10916 Atlanta, GA 30310-0916 (404) 753-1226 or 753-1227	X			X
medcon Kontraktlabor GmbH Sudkampen NR.31 D-29664 Walsrode Germany (49) 5166 590	X			
Medtox Via Trinacria 34 Tremestieri Etneo 92125 Catania, Italy 095 223027 (609) 730 8568 (USA)	X			
Midwest Research Institute 425 Volker Boulevard Kansas City, MO 64110 (816) 753-7600	X	X	X	X
Mitsubishi Chemical Safety Institute Ltd. (MSI) 1-30 Shiba, 2-Chome Minato-Ku Tokyo, 105-0014 Japan (81) 3 3454 7571	X	X	X	
MPI Research 54943 North Main Street Mattawan, MI 49071 (616) 668-3336	X			
Next Century Inc. Delaware Technology Park 1 Innovation Way, Suite 301 Newark, DE 19711 (302) 453-4460 and 18-5 CITIC Building No.9 Jian Wai Da Jie street Beijing, China		X		

TABLE 33.63 *(Continued)*
Directory of Contract Toxicology Laboratories[a]

Laboratory	Mammalian	Genetic	Ecotoxicological Aquatic	Clinical
NM RPRL/Primate Research Laboratory PO Box 1027 Holloman Airforce Base New Mexico 88330-1027 (505) 479-6101	X			
North American Science Associates, Inc. 2261 Tracy Road Toledo, OH 43619 (419) 666-9455	X	X		X
Northview Biosciences 2800 7th Street Berkeley, CA 94710 (510) 548-8440	X			
Notox BV PO Box 3476 5203 DL's-Hertogenbosch The Netherlands (31) 73641 9575	X	X	X	X
OMNI Research, Inc. El Retiro Industrial Zone PO Box 325 San German, PR 00753 (809) 892-2680	X			
Oxford Biomedical Ltd. The Spendlove Research Center Enstone Road Charlbury, Oxfordshire ENGLAND (44) 608 81128	X			X
Pharmakon Research International, Inc. PO Box 609 Waverly, PA 18471 (717) 586-2411	X	X		
Pharmatox Beratung und Forschung GmbH Vogtel-Ruthe-Strasse 26 3163 Sehndel 13 (Wirringen) Germany 05138/20 85-20 86	X			X
Phoenix International Life Sciences, Inc. 2350 Cohen Street Saint-Laurant (Montreal), Quebec H4R 2N6 (514) 333-0033	X			

TABLE 33.63 *(Continued)*
Directory of Contract Toxicology Laboratories[a]

Laboratory	Mammalian	Genetic	Ecotoxicological Aquatic	Clinical
Primate Research Institute Box 1027 Holloman Air Force Base New Mexico 88330 (505) 479-6101	X			
Primedica Corporation (Argus, Mason and Redfield Labs) 57 Union Street Worcester, MA 01608 (508) 890-0100	X			
Product Investigations, Inc. 151 East 10th Avenue Conshohocken, PA 19428 (610) 825-5855				X
Product Safety Labs 725 Cranbury Road East Brunswick, NJ 08816 (732) 545-9200	X	X		
Protox Aventis Pharma Deutschland GmbH Mainser Landstrasse 500 65795 Hattersheim Germany (49) 6190 807 361	X			
PTRL East, Inc. 3945 Simpson Lane Richmond, KY 40475 (859) 624-8111	X		X	
Quintiles Bromyard Road Ledbury, Herefordshire HR8 1LH United Kingdom (44) 153 613 4121 and 10245 Hickman Mills Drive Kansas City, MO 64134 (816) 767-3900	X			
RCC, LTD. ZELGLIWEG 1 4452 Itingen Switzerland (41) 61 975 1107	X	X	X	X

TABLE 33.63 *(Continued)*
Directory of Contract Toxicology Laboratories[a]

Laboratory	Mammalian	Genetic	Ecotoxicological Aquatic	Clinical
Research Triangle Institute 3040 Cornwallis Road PO Box 12194 Research Triangle Park, NC 27709-2194 (919) 541-7103	X	X		
Ricerca, Inc. 7528 Auburn Road Painsville, OH 44077-1000 (440) 357-3300	X		X	
Roy F. Weston, Inc. 1 Wall Street Manchester, NH 03101 (603) 656-5400			X	
Safepharm Laboratories Ltd. PO Box 45 Derby DE1 2BT Derbyshire, England (44) 1 332 792896	X	X	X	
Scantox HesteHaueves 36A EJBY DK-4623, Lille Skensved Denmark (45) 56 82 1500	X	X		
Scientific Associates, Inc. 6200 South Lindbergh Blvd. St. Louis, MO 63123 (314) 487-6776	X			
Serquest 2000 Ninth Avenue, South Birmingham, AL 35205 (205) 581-2830	X			
Sierra Biomedical-a Charles River Company 587 Dunn Circle Sparks, NV 89431 (775) 331-2289	X			
Sitek Research Laboratories 15235 Shady Grove Road Rockville, MD 20850 Suite 303 (301) 926- 4900	X	X		

TABLE 33.63 *(Continued)*
Directory of Contract Toxicology Laboratories[a]

Laboratory	Mammalian	Genetic	Ecotoxicological Aquatic	Clinical
SkeleTech, Inc 22002 26th Avenue, SE Suite 104 Bothell, WA 98021 (425) 424-2663	X			
SNBL USA, Ltd. 6605 Merril Creek Parkway Everett, Washington (425) 407-0121 and 2438 Miyanoura, Yoshida Kagoshima, 891-1394, Japan (81) 992 94 2600	X	X		
Southern Research Institute 2000 9th Avenue, South Birmingham, AL 35205 (205) 581-2689	X	X		
Southwest Research Institute 6220 Culebra Road San Antonio, TX 78284-2900 (210) 522-2658	X		X	
Springborn Laboratories, Inc. Ohio Research Center 640 N. Elizabeth Avenue Spencerville, OH 45887 (419) 647-4196 and Massachusetts Research Center 790 Main Street Wareham, MA 02543 (508) 295-2550 and Swiss Research Center Seestrasse 21 Horn, CH-9326 Switzerland (41) 71 844 6970	X		X	
Spring Valley Laboratories, Inc. P.O. Box 242 Woodbine, MD 21797 (410) 795-2242	X			
SRI International 333 Ravenswood Avenue Menlo Park, CA 94025 (650) 859-6459	X	X	X	

TABLE 33.63 *(Continued)*
Directory of Contract Toxicology Laboratories[a]

Laboratory	Mammalian	Genetic	Ecotoxicological Aquatic	Clinical
Stillmeadow, Inc. 12852 Park One Drive Sugarland, TX 77478 (281) 240-8828	X		X	
Syracuse Research Corporation Environmental Science Center 6225 Running Ridge Road North Syracuse, NY 13212 (315) 426-3200			X	
TherImmune Research Corporation 555 Quince Orchard Road, Suite 460 Gaithersburg, MD 20878 (301) 330-3733	X			
TKL Research, Inc. 4 Forest Avenue Paramus, NJ 07652 (201) 587-0500				X
TNO Toxicology Utrechtseweg 48 PO Box 360 3700 A7 Zeist The Netherlands (31) 306 944449	X	X	X	
Toxicology Pathology Services, Inc. PO Box 333 Mt. Vernon, IN 47620 (812) 985-5900		X		
ToxLabs Bioscience GmbH Suedkampen 31 D-29664 Walsrode (49) 5166 98 85 00	X			
Tox Monitor Laboratories/BSR, Inc. 33 West Chicago Avenue Oak Park, IL 60302 (708) 345-6970	X			
Toxicol Laboratories, Ltd. Bromyard Road Ledbury, Herefordshire HR8 1LH UNITED KINGDOM (44) 01531-634121	X	X		X

TABLE 33.63 *(Continued)*
Directory of Contract Toxicology Laboratories[a]

Laboratory	Mammalian	Genetic	Ecotoxicological Aquatic	Clinical
Toxicology Research Laboratory 1940 West Taylor Street Room 312 Chicago, IL 60612 (312) 996-9185	X			
Toxikon Corporation 15 Wiggins Ave. Bedford, MA 01730 (781) 275-3330	X	X	X	
TPS, Inc. 10424 Middle Mt. Vernon Road Mt. Vernon, IN 47620 (812) 985-5900	X			
T.R. Wilbury Laboratories, Inc. 40 Doaks Lane Marblehead, MA 01945 (617) 631-2923			X	
United States Testing Corporation Biological Services Division 1415 Park Avenue Hoboken, NJ 07030 (201) 792-2400	X	X	X	
ViroMED Laboratories, Inc. 2540 Executive Drive St. Paul, MN 55120 (612) 931-0077	X	X		
White Eagle Laboratories, Inc. 2003 Lower State Road Doylestown, PA 18901 (215) 348-3868	X			
Wildlife International, Ltd. 8598 Commerce Drive Easton, MD 21601 (410) 822-8600			X	
WIL Research Laboratories, Inc. 1407 George Road Ashland, OH 44805 (419) 289-8700 or (800) 221-9610	X			
Xenobiotic Laboratories, Inc. 107 Morgan Lane Plainsboro, NJ 08536 (609) 799-2295	X		X	

[a] Area codes in the U.S. are subject to change.

REFERENCES

1. Regulatory Assistance Corporation, *Directory of Toxicological and Related Testing Laboratories,* Hemisphere Publishing, Washington, D.C., 1991.
2. Jackson, E. M., Ed., Special issue: International directory of contract laboratories, *J. Toxicol. Cutaneous Occul. Toxicol.,* 7, 1, 1988.
3. Society of Toxicology Exhibitor Directory, 2000.
4. Freudenthal, R. I., *Directory of Toxicology Laboratories Offering Contract Services,* Aribet Books, West Palm Beach, FL, 2000.

SECTION 7. ORGANIZATIONS AND AGENCIES

Table 33.64 contains a listing of organizations and agencies associated with toxicology and/or toxicological issues. Contacts have been listed where a main address or phone number for a central office were not available. The contacts listed in the referenced sources as office holders, administrators, or in some other way involved in the organization listed, may or may not currently hold the same position. However, because it would be impossible to maintain a current listing in a publication of this type, especially because office holders often change every year, the editors believe that the contacts listed would be willing to supply updated information to an inquirer. We ask for the contacts understanding and apologize for any inconvenience that this might create.

TABLE 33.64
Organizations and Agencies Associated with Toxicology and/or Toxicological Issues[a]

Academy of Toxicological Sciences (ATS)
Contact: Mildred S. Christian
905 Sheehy Drive
Horsham, PA 19044
(215) 443-8710

Agency for Toxic Substances and Disease Registry (ATSDR)
1600 Clinton Road N.E.
Atlanta, GA 30333
1-888-422-8737

American Academy of Clinical Toxicology
777 East Park Drive
P.O. Box 8820
Harrisburg, PA 17105
(717) 558-7847

American Academy of Veterinary and Comparative Toxicology (AAVCT)
Contact: H. Dwight Mercer, DVM, Ph.D.
Drawer V
Mississippi State, MS 39762
(601) 325-3432

American Association of Poison Control Centers (AAPCC)
3201 New Mexico Avenue
Suite 310
Washington, D.C. 20016
(202) 362-7217

TABLE 33.64 *(Continued)*
Organizations and Agencies Associated with Toxicology and/or Toxicological Issues[a]

American Board of Medical Toxicology (ABMT)
Contact: Lewis Goldfrank, M.D.
Bellevue Hospital Center
27th St and First Avenue
New York, NY 10016
(212) 562-4317

American Board of Toxicology (ABT)
PO Box 30054
Raleigh, NC 27662-0054
(919) 847-8720

American Chemical Society (ACS)
1155 16th Street, NW
Washington, D.C. 20036
(202) 872-4600

American Chemistry Council (ACC)
(Formerly Chemical Manufacturers Association (CMA))
1300 Wilson Boulevard
Arlington, VA 22209
(703) 741-5131

American College of Toxicology (ACT)
9650 Rockville Pike
Bethesda, MD 20814
(301) 571-1840

American Conference of Governmental Industrial Hygienists (ACGIH)
1330 Kemper Meadow Drive
Suite 600
Cincinnati, OH 45240
(513) 742-2020

American Industrial Hygiene Association (AIHA)
1700 Prosperity Avenue, Suite 250
Fairfax, VA 22031
(703) 849-8888

American Society for Pharmacology and Experimental Therapeutics (ASPET)
9650 Rockville Pike
Bethesda, MD 20814
(301) 530-7060

Board on Environmental Studies and Toxicology
Commission of Life Sciences
National Research Council
2101 Constitution Avenue, NW
Washington, D.C. 20418
(202) 334-2318

TABLE 33.64 *(Continued)*
Organizations and Agencies Associated with Toxicology and/or Toxicological Issues[a]

Centers for Disease Control
1600 Clifton Road, NE
Atlanta, GA 30333
(404) 639-3311

Chemical Emergency Preparedness
 Program (CEPP) Hotline
(800) 535-0202

CIIT Centers for Health Research
6 Davis Drive
PO Box 12137
Research Triangle Park, NC 27709
(919) 558-1200

Consumer Product Safety Commission (CPSC)
4330 East-West Highway
Bethesda, MD 20814-4408
(301) 504-0990

Cosmetic Toiletry and Fragrance Association (CTFA)
1101 17th Street, NW
Suite 300
Washington, D.C. 20036-4072
(202) 331-1770

Council on Environmental Quality (CEQ)
722 Jackson Place, NW
Washington, D.C. 20006
(202) 395-5750

Department of Agriculture (USDA)
Fourteenth St and Independence Ave, SW
Washington, D.C. 20250
(202) 447-2791

Department of Energy (DOE)
1000 Independence Avenue SW
Washington, D.C. 20585
(202) 586-5000

Department of the Interior
Fish and Wildlife Service
Washington, D.C. 20240
(202) 208-4131

Department of Transportation (DOT)
Research and Special Programs Administration
Office of Hazardous Material Technology
400 Seventh Street, SW
Washington, D.C. 20590
(202) 366-4545

TABLE 33.64 *(Continued)*
Organizations and Agencies Associated with Toxicology and/or Toxicological Issues[a]

Drinking Water Hotline
Environmental Protection Agency
Washington, D.C.
(800) 426-4791

Environmental Defense Fund (EDF)
257 Park Avenue South
New York, NY 10010
(212) 505-2100

Environmental Law Institute (ELI)
1616 P Street, NW
Suite 200
Washington, D.C. 20036
(202) 939-3800

Environmental Mutagen Society (EMS)
11250 Roger Bacon Drive
Suite 8
Reston, VA 20190-5202
(703) 437-4377

Environmental Protection Agency (EPA)
(headquarters)
Ariel Rios Building
1200 Pennsylvania Avenue, NW
Washington, D.C. 20460
(202) 260-2090

Environmental Protection Agency
Region I
1 Congress Street, Suite 1100
Boston, MA 02114-2023
(617) 918-1111

Environmental Protection Agency
Region 2
290 Broadway
New York, NY 10007-1866
(212) 637-3000

Environmental Protection Agency
Region 3
1650 Arch Street
Philadelphia, PA 19103-2029
(215)- 814-5000

Environmental Protection Agency
Region 4
Atlanta Federal Center
61 Forsyth Street, SW
Atlanta, GA 30303-3104
(404) 562-9900

TABLE 33.64 *(Continued)*
Organizations and Agencies Associated with Toxicology and/or Toxicological Issues[a]

Environmental Protection Agency
Region 5
77 West Jackson Boulevard
Chicago, IL 60604-3507
(312) 353-2000

Environmental Protection Agency
Region 6
Fountain Place, 12th Floor, Suite 1200
1445 Ross Avenue
Dallas, TX 75202-2733
(214) 665-2200

Environmental Protection Agency
Region 7
901 North 5th Street
Kansas City, KS 66101
(913) 551-7003

Environmental Protection Agency
Region 8
999 18th Street, Suite 500
Denver, CO 80202-2405
(303) 312-6312

Environmental Protection Agency
Region 9
75 Hawthorne Street
San Francisco, CA 94105
(415) 744-1305

Environmental Protection Agency
Region 10
1200 Sixth Avenue
Seattle, WA 98101
(206) 553-1200

European Society of Toxicology (EUROTOX)
Contact: Professor Eino Hietanen
University of Turku
Dept. of Clinical Physiology
Fin-20520 Turku, Finland
+358-2-261-2664

Federal Bureau of Investigation
Law Enforcement Services
FBI Laboratory
Scientific Analysis Section
Chemistry-Toxicology Unit
J. Edgar Hoover Building
935 Pennsylvania Ave, NW
Washington, D.C. 20535
(202) 324-3000

TABLE 33.64 *(Continued)*
Organizations and Agencies Associated with Toxicology and/or Toxicological Issues[a]

Food and Drug Administration (FDA)
5600 Fishers Lane
Rockville, MD 20857
(888) 463-6332

Genetic Toxicology Association (GTA)
Contact: Andrea Ham
PMB 311
4142 Ogletown-Stanton Road
Newark, DE 19713-4169
(302) 366-6322

International Life Sciences Institute (ILSI)
1126 Sixteenth Street, NW Suite 300
Washington, D.C. 20036-4804
(202) 659-0074

International Society of Regulatory Toxicology and Pharmacology (ISRTP)
6546 Belleview Drive
Columbia, MD 21046
(410) 992-9083

International Society on Toxicology (IST)
Contact: Dr. Philip Rosenberg
Department of Pharmacology and Toxicology
University of Connecticut School of Pharmacy, U-92
Storrs, CT 06268
(203) 486-2213

Inhalation Toxicology Research Institute (ITRI)
Office of Energy Research
Department of Energy
P.O. Box 5890
Albuquerque, NM 87185
(505) 845-1037

International Union of Toxicology (IUTOX)
Contact: Meryl H. Karol
University of Pittsburgh
260 Kappa Drive
Pittsburgh, PA
(412) 967-6530

(*Note:* IUTOX has over 40 international toxicology societies as members. Contacts for member societies can be obtained from the IUTOX web site www.toxicology.org/iutox)

National Cancer Institute (NCI)
Public Inquiries Office
31 Center Drive
Bethesda, MD 20892
(301) 435-3848

TABLE 33.64 *(Continued)*
Organizations and Agencies Associated with Toxicology and/or Toxicological Issues[a]

National Center for Toxicological Research (NCTR)
Contact: Daniel Casciano, Director
Jefferson, AK 72079
(870) 543-7517

National Eye Institute (NEI)
9000 Rockville Pike
Bethesda, MD 20892
(301) 496-1776

National Heart, Lung and Blood Institute
9000 Rockville Pike
Bethesda, MD 20892
(301) 496-1776

National Institute of Environmental Sciences (NIEHS)
111 Alexander Drive
P.O. Box 12233
Research Triangle Park, NC 27709
(919) 541-3345

National Institutes of Health
9000 Rockville Pike
Bethesda, MD 20892
(301) 496-1766

National Institute for Occupational Safety and Health (NIOSH)
1600 Clifton Road NE
Atlanta, GA 30333
(800) 356-4674
outside U.S.A. (513) 533-8328

National Library of Medicine (NLM)
Toxicology Information Program (TIP)
8600 Rockville Pike
Bethesda, MD 20894
(888) 346-3656
outside U.S.A. (301) 594-5983

National Toxicology Program
Public Information Office
P.O. Box 12233
Research Triangle Park, NC 27709
(919) 541-3419

National Toxicological Information Service
P.O. Box 1133
Washington, D.C. 20013-1133
(800) 336-4700

NIOSH Publications
4676 Columbia Parkway
Cincinnati, OH 45226
(800) 356-4674

TABLE 33.64 *(Continued)*
Organizations and Agencies Associated with Toxicology and/or Toxicological Issues[a]

Occupational Safety and Health Administration (OSHA)
200 Constitution Avenue, NW
Washington, D.C. 20210
(202) 693-1999

Oak Ridge National laboratory
P.O. Box 2008
One Bethel Valley Road
Oak Ridge, TN 37831
Life Sciences Division (865) 574-5845
Environmental Sciences (865) 574-7374

Organization for Economic Cooperation and Development (OECD)
2 rue Andre Pascal
75775 Paris CEDEX 16, France
+33-(0)-1-45-24-82-00

Society of Environmental Toxicology and Chemistry (SETAC)
1010 North 12th Avenue
Pensacola, FL 32501
(850) 469-1500
and
Avenue E. Mounier 83, Box 3
1200 Brussels, Belgium
32-2-772-7281

Society of Forensic Toxicologists (SOFT)
P.O. Box 5543
Mesa, AZ 85211-5543
(480) 839-9106

Society of Toxicologic Pathologists
19 Mantua Road
Mount Royal, NJ 08061
(856) 423-3610

Society of Toxicology (SOT)
Suite 302
1767 Business Center Drive
Reston, VA 20190
(703) 438-3115

Synthetic Organic Chemical Manufacturers Association (SOCMA)
1850 M Street, NW, Suite 700
Washington, D.C. 20036
(202) 721-4100

Teratology Society
1767 Business Center Drive
Suite 302
Reston, VA 20190
(703) 438-3104

TABLE 33.64 *(Continued)*
Organizations and Agencies Associated with Toxicology and/or Toxicological Issues[a]

Toxicology Forum
1575 Eye Street, NW, Suite 325
Washington, D.C. 20005
(202) 659-0030

Toxicology Information Center (TIC)
National Research Council
National Academy Press
2101 Constitution Avenue, NW
Washington, D.C. 20055
(202) 624-8373

Toxicology Information Response Center (TIRC)
Oak Ridge National Laboratory
1060 Commerce Park, MS 6480
Oak Ridge, TN 37830
(423) 576- 1746

TSCA Information Service
Environmental Protection Agency
Toxic Assistance Office
401 M Street, SW
Washington, D.C. 20460
(202) 554-1404

UN Environmental Program (UNEP)
1818 H. Street, NW
Washington, D.C. 20433
(202) 458-9695

Women's Occupational Health Resource Center
Contact: Jeanne M. Stellman
School of Public Health
Columbia University
600 West 168th Street
New York, NY 10032
(212) 305-1164

World Health Organization
Avenue Appia 20
1211 Geneva 27, Switzerland
41-22-791-21-11

[a] Area codes in the U.S. are subject to change.
Note: For additional information on U.S. government agencies and direct links to Web sites, refer to http://www.netserveint.com/resources/usgovsites.html.

SECTION 8. INTERNET/WEB SITES

TABLE 33.65
Useful Internet Sites

Internet Site	URL
ACS Chemcenter	www.chemcenter.org
Agency for Toxic Substances and Disease Registry	www.atsdr.cdc.gov/atsdrhome.html
American Academy of Clinical Toxicology	www.clintox.org
American Association of Poison Control Centers	www.aapcc.org
American Chemical Society (ACS)	www.acs.org
American Chemistry Council	www.AmericanChemistry.com
American Conference of Governmental Industrial hygienists	www.acgih.org
American Industrial Hygiene Association	www.aiha.org
American Society for Pharmacology and Experimental Therapeutics	www.faseb.org/aspet/
BELLE	www.belleonline.com
Centers for Disease Control and Prevention	www.cdc.gov
Chem-Dex (global list of chemistry sites)	www.chempex.org
Chemical Abstract Services	www.cas.org
Chemical Accident Risk Assessment Thesarus (OECD)	www.oecd.org/ehs/carat
Chemical Safety and Hazard Investigation Board	www.chemsafety.gov
ChemWeb (UK)	www.chemweb.com
CIIT Centers for Health Research	www.ciit.org
Consumer Products Safety Commission	www.cpsc.gov
Conversion Tool Site	www.onlineconversion.com
Department of Agriculture	www.usda.gov
Department of Transportation	www.dot.gov
Endocrine/Estrogen Letter Links page	www.eeletter.com/links.htm
Environmental Defense Fund	www.edf.org
Environmental Organization Web Directory	www.webdirectory.com
Environmental RouteNet (encyclopedic resource)	www.csa.com/routenet
EUROTOX	www.uta.fi/eurotox/index.htm
EXTOXNET (University Network)	www.ace.orst.edu/info/extoxnet
Genetic Terms Glossary	www.nhgri.nih.gov/DIR/VIP/Glossary
Harvard University Center for Risk Analysis	www.hcra.harvard.edu
Health Effects Institute	www.healtheffects.org
International Agency for Research on Cancer	www.iarc.fr
International Society for Exposure Analysis	www.ISEAweb.org
International Union of Toxicology (IUTOX)	www.toxicology.org/iutox/
Mid-Atlantic Chapter Society of Toxicology	www.masot.org
National Academy of Science	www.nas.edu
National Cancer Institute	www.nci.nih.gov
National Center for Biotechnology Information Resources Center (NCBI Genbank)	www.ncbi.nlm.nih.gov
National Environmental Information Resources Center	www.gwis.circ.gwu.edu/~greenu
National Institute for Occupational Safety and Health	www.cdc.gov/niosh/homepage.html
National Institute of Environmental Health Sciences (NIEHS)	www.niehs.nih.gov
National Institutes of Health	www.nih.gov
National Library for the Environment	www.cnie.org/nle
National Library of Medicine	www.nlm.nih.gov/
National Research Council	www.nas.edu/nrc/
National Science Foundation	www.nsf.gov
National Toxicology Program	www.ntp-server.niehs.gov

TABLE 33.65 *(Continued)*
Useful Internet Sites

Internet Site	URL
Occupational Safety and Health Administration	www.osha.gov/index.html
PathIT (pathology links)	www.pathit.com
Research Triangle Foundation	www.rtp.org
Risk Assessment Information System	www.risk.lsd.ornl.gov/rap-hp.shtml
Royal Society of Chemistry	www.rsc.org
Society for Environmental Toxicology and Chemistry	www.setac.org
Society for Risk Analysis	www.sra.org
Society of Toxicology	www.toxicology.org
The Chemical Industry Home Page	www.neis.com
The Endocrine Society	www.endo-society.org
TOXNET (toxicology data network)	www.toxnet.nlm.nih.gov/
United States Environmental Protection Agency	www.epa.gov
United States Food and Drug Administration	www.fda.gov
WebElements (periodic table)	www.shef.ac.uk/~chem/web- elements
World Health Organization	www.who.int/

Note: For additional sites see Tables 26.15, 30.12, 32.1, and Section 9 of Chapter 8.

SECTION 9. ACRONYMS

TABLE 33.66
Frequently Encountered Acronyms

AAALAC	American Association for Accreditation of Laboratory Animal Care
AADA	Abbreviated Antibiotic Drug Application
AALAS	American Association for Laboratory Animal Science
AAPCO	Association of American Pesticide Control Officials
ACB	Analytical Chemistry Branch (re: OPP)
ACC	American Chemistry Council
ACP	Associates of Clinical Pharmacology
ACS	American Chemical Society
ACT	American College of Toxicology
ACUP	Animal Care and Use Procedure
ADE	Adverse Drug Experience/Effect/Event
ADI	Acceptable Daily Intake (see also RfD)
ADME	Absorption Distribution, Metabolism, Excretion
ADR	Adverse Drug Reaction
AE	Adverse Experience/Event
AERS	Adverse Event Reporting System
AHI	Animal Health Institute
ai/A	Active Ingredient per Acre
AI	Active Ingredient
ALISS	"A — List" Inventory Support System (re: SRRD)
ALJ	Administrative Law Judge
ANADA	Abbrieviated New Animal Drug Application
ANDA	Abbreviated New Drug Application
ANSI	American National Standards Institute
AOAC	Association of Official Analytical Chemists

TABLE 33.66 *(Continued)*
Frequently Encountered Acronyms

ARAR	Applicable, Relevant and Appropriate Requirements (re: Superfund)
APB	Antimicrobial Program Branch
ARB	Accelerated Reregistration Branch (re: SRRD of OPP)
ARS	Agricultural Research Service (re: USDA)
ARTS	Accelerated Reregistration Tracking System (re: SRRD of OPP)
ASAP	Administrative System Automations Project
ASQC	American Society of Quality Control
ASR	Analytical Summary Report
ASTHO	Association of State and Territorial Health Officials
ASTM	Association of Standard Test Methods
AWA	Animal Welfare Act
BAB	Biological Analysis Branch (re: BEAD of OPP)
BARQA	The British Association of Research Quality Assurance
BDAT	Best Demonstrated Available Technology
BEAD	Biological and Economic Analysis Division (re: OPP)
CANADAs	Computer Assisted New Drug Applications
CANADA	Computer Assisted New Animal Drug Application
CAP	Compliance Audit Program
CAPER	Computer Assisted Preclinical Electronic Review
CAPLA	Computer Assisted Product License Application (Re: Biologics)
CB	Communications Branch (re: OPP)
CB I & II	Chemistry Branch I and II (re: OPP)
CBER	Center for Biologics Evaluation and Research (re: FDA)
CBI	Confidential Business Information
CDC	Centers for Disease Control (see also USCDC)
CDER	Center for Drug Evaluation and Research (re: FDA)
CDRH	Center for Devices and Radiological Health (re: FDA)
CEO	Council on Environmental Quality
CERCLA	Comprehensive, Environmental, Response, Compensation, and Liability Act
CFD	Call For Data
CFR	Code of Federal Regulations
CGMP	Current Good Manufacturing Practices (see also GMP)
CLIA	Clinical Laboratory Improvement Act
CMA	Chemical Manufacturers Association
CMC	Chemistry Manufacturing and Controls
CNAEL	Committee on National Accreditation for Environmental Laboratories
CORT	toxicology studies set: Chronic feeding; Oncogenicity; Reproduction; Teratology
CPDA	Chemical Producers and Distributors Association
CPG	Compliance Policy Guide
CPGM	Compliance Program Guidance Manuals (re: Bioresearch Monitoring Program)
CPSC	Consumer Product Safety Commission
CRA	Clinical Research Associate
CRADA	Cooperative Research and Development Agreement
CRF	Case Report Form
CRO	Contract Research Organization
CRP	Child-Resistant Packaging
CSA	Clinical & Scientific Affairs
CSF	Confidential Statement of Formula
CSMA	Chemical Specialities Manufacturers Association
CSO	Consumer Safety Officer (re: FDA)
CSRS	Cooperative State Research Service

TABLE 33.66 *(Continued)*
Frequently Encountered Acronyms

CTB	Certification and Training Branch (re: FOD of OPP)
CV	Curriculum Vitae
CVM	Center for Veterinary Medicine (re: FDA)
CWA	Clean Water Act
DAMOS	Drug Application Methodology with Optical Storage (re: EC)
DCI	Data Call-In notice (re: RD or SRRD of OPP)
DEA	Drug Enforcement Agency
DEB	Dietary Exposure Branch (see also CB I and II)
DFE	Design for the Environment
DI	Department of Interior (see also USDI)
DIA	Drug Information Association
DIS	Drug information System
DISLODG	Dislodgeable Foliar Residue (re: EPA)
DMF	Drug Master File
DOE	Department of Energy (see also USDOE)
DOT	Department of Transportation
DQOs	Data Quality Objectives (re: EPA work)
DRES	Dietary Risk Evaluation System (re: OPP)
EAB	Economic Analysis Branch (re: OPP)
EC	Emulsifiable Concentrate
EC	European Community (see also EEC)
EDF	Environmental Defense Fund
EEB	Ecological Effects Branch (re: OPP)
EEC	European Economic Community (see also EC)
EFED	Environmental Fate and Effects Division (re: OPP)
EFGWB	Environmental Fate and Groundwater Branch (re: OPP)
EIR	Establishment Inspection Report
ELA	Establishment License Report (re: Biologics)
ELGIN	Environmental Liaison Group International
ELI	Environmental Law Institute
EMO	Experimental Manufacturing Order
EP	End-Use Product
EPA	Environmental Protection Agency (see also USEPA)
EPCRA	Emergency Planning and Community Right to Know Act
EPRS	Establishment/Product Registration System
ESA	Entomological Society of America
EUP	Experimental Use Permit (re: EPA FIFRA)
FACTS	Field Accomplishments and Compliance Tracking System
FDA	Food and Drug Administration (see also USFDA)
FDB	Field Data Book
FD&C	Federal Food, Drug and Cosmetic Act (see also FFDCA, FDCL)
FDCL	Food, Drug Cosmetic Law (see also FD&C, FFDCA)
FDLI	Food & Drug Law Institute
FFDCA	Federal Food, Drug and Cosmetic Act (see also FD&C, FDCL)
FHB	Fungicide-Herbicide Branch (re: RD of OPP)
FHSA	Federal Health and Safety Act
FIFRA	Federal Insecticide, Fungicide and Rodenticide Act
FOD	Field Operations Division (re: OPP)
FOI	Freedom of Information (see also FOIA)
FOIA	Freedom of Information Act (see also FOI)
FPLA	Fair Packaging & Labeling Act

TABLE 33.66 *(Continued)*
Frequently Encountered Acronyms

FR	Federal Register
FRD	Field Research Director
FTC	Federal Trade Commission
FWS	Fish and Wildlife Service (see also USFWS)
GALP	Good Automated Laboratory Practices
GARPs	Good Academic Research Practices (draft 1992)
GAO	General Accounting Office
GATT	General Agreement on Tariffs and Trade
GCP	Good Clinical Practices
GLP	Good Laboratory Practices
GLPS	Good Laboratory Practice Standards
GMP	Good Manufacturing Practices
GH_2O	Groundwater Studies (re: EPA)
GRAE	Generally Recognized As Effective
GRAS	Generally Recognized As Safe
HDT	Highest Dose Tested (re: EPA)
HED	Health Effects Division (re: OPP)
HEI	Health Effects Institute
HES	Health and Environmental Safety
HHS	Health and Human Services
HIMA	Health Industry Manufacturers Association
HPB	Health Protection Branch (re: Canada)
HPV-SIDS	High Production Volume-Screening Info Data Set (re: OECD)
HRS	Hazard Ranking System (re: Superfund)
IACUC	Institutional Animal Care and Use Committee
IB	Investigator's Brochure
ICH	International Conference on Harmonization
ICR	Information Collection Request
IDB	Investigational Drug Brochure
IDE	Investigational Device Exemption
IG	Inspector General (see also OIG)
INAD	Investigational New Animal Drug
IND	Investigational New Drug
IPM	Integrated Pest Management (re: OPP)
IR-4	Interregional Research Project #4 for Minor Crops (re: USDA)
IRB	Insecticide and Rodenticide Branch (re: RD of OPP)
IRB	Institutional Review Board
IS	Information Standards
ISA	Information Systems Architecture
ISB	Information Services Branch (re: PMSD of OPP)
ISQA	International Society of Quality Assurance
ITC	Interagency Testing Committee (re: TSCA)
LAC	Laboratory Accreditation Committee
LADD	Lifetime Average Daily Dose (re: OPP)
LADD	Lowest Acceptable Daily Dose (re: OPP)
LC_{50}	Lethal Concentration for 50% of test population
LD_{50}	Lethal Dose for 50% of test population
LDT	Lowest Dose Tested
LEL	Lowest Effective Level
LRD	Laboratory Research Director
LUIS	Label Use information System (re: OPP)

TABLE 33.66 *(Continued)*
Frequently Encountered Acronyms

MARSQA	Mid-Atlantic Region Society of Quality Assurance
MCA	Medicines Control Agency (UK equivalent to FDA)
MCL	Maximum Contaminant Level
MCLG	Maximum Contaminant Level Goal
MDDI	Medical Devices, Diagnostics and Instrumentation
MNVP	Medically Necessary Veterinary Product (re: FDA-CVM)
MOE	Margin of Exposure
MOS	Margin of Safety
MOU	Memorandum of Understanding
MP	Manufacturing Use Product (re: OPP, see also MUP)
MPI	Maximum Permitted Intake
MRID #	Master Record Identification Number
MS	Master Schedule
MSS	Master Schedule Sheet
MSDS	Material Safety Data Sheet
MTL	Master Testing List
MUP	Manufacturing Use Product (re: OPP, see also MP)
MURS	Multi-User Regulatory Submission (International Multi-Agency Project)
NACA	National Agricultural Chemical Association
NADA	New Animal Drug Application
NADE	New Animal Drug Evaluation, office of (re: FDA-CVM)
NAF	Notice of Adverse Findings
NAI	No Action Indicated
NAICC	National Alliance of Independent Crop Consultants
NARA	National Agrichemical Retailers Association
NAS	National Academy of Sciences
NASDA	National Association of State Departments of Agriculture
NCAMP	National Coalition Against the Misuse of Pesticides
NCE	New Chemical Entity
NCP	National Contingency Plan (re: Superfund)
NBS	National Bureau of Standards (now called NIST)
NDA	New Drug Application
NDS	New Drug Submission
NEIC	National Enforcement Investigation Center (re: USEPA)
NIEHS	National Institute of Environmental Health Sciences
NIH	National Institutes of Health
NIOSH	National Institute for Occupational Safety and Health
NIST	National Institute of Standards and Technology (formerly NBS)
NPCA	National Pest Control Association
NPDES	National Pollutant Discharge Elimination System
NPIRS	National Pesticide Information Retrieval System
NPL	National Priority List (re: Superfund)
NPTN	National Pesticide Telecommunications Network
NRDC	Natural Resources Defense Council
NTIS	National Technical Information Service
OAI	Official Action Indicated
OASIS	Operational and Administrative System for Import Support
ODW	Office of Drinking Water
OECD	Organization for Economic Cooperation and Development
OECA	Office of Enforcement and Compliance Assurance
OES	Office of Endangered Species (re: FWS of DI)

TABLE 33.66 *(Continued)*
Frequently Encountered Acronyms

OGD	Office of Generic Drugs (re: FDA)
OIG	Office of the Inspector General (see also IG)
OLTS	On-Line Tracking System
OMB	Office of Management and Budget
OPM	Office of Personnel Management
OPP	Office of Pesticide Programs (re: EPA)
OPPT	Office of Pollution Prevention and Toxics (formerly OTS; re. TSCA)
OPPTS	Office of Prevention, Pesticides and Toxic Substances
OREB	Occupational and Residential Exposure Branch (re: HED of OPP)
OSB	Occupational Safety Branch (re: FOD of OPP)
OSHA	Occupational Safety and Health Administration
OSW	Office of Solid Waste (re: EPA)
OSWER	Office of Solid Waste and Emergency Response
OTA	Office of Technology Assessment (re: Congress)
OTC	Over the Counter
OTS	Office of Toxic Substances (now called OPPT)
OWPE	Office of Waste Programs Enforcement
PAG	Pesticide Assessment Guidelines
PAI	Pure Active Ingredient
PBA	Preliminary Benefit Analysis
PCO	Pest Control Operator
PDA	Parenteral Drug Association
PDMS	Pesticide Document Management System
PDR	Physician's Desk Reference
PDUFA	Prescription Drug User Fee Act
PES	Planning and Evaluation Staff
PHED	Pesticide Handlers Exposure Database (re: EPA)
PHI	Pre-Harvest Interval
PHI	Post-Harvest Interval
PIMS	Pesticide Incident Monitoring System
PLA	Product License Application (re: Biologics)
PM	Product Manager
PMA	Pharmaceutical Manufacturers Association
PMN	Premanufacturers Notification (re: TSCA)
PMSD	Program Management and Support Division (re: OPP)
P&P guide	Policy and Procedures guide (re: FDA-CVM)
PPIS	Pesticide Product Information Systems
PR#	Pesticide Clearance Request Number
PR notice	Pesticide Registration notice
PRATS	Pesticide Registration Activity Tracking System
PRCSQA	Pacific Regional Chapter of the Society of Quality Assurance
PRP	Potentially Responsible Party (re: Superfund)
PSA	Product Safety Assurance
QA	Quality Assurance
QAAS	Quality Assurance Advisory Subcommittee
QAO	Quality Assurance Officer
QAP	Quality Assurance Project Plan
QAU	Quality Assurance Unit
QC	Quality Control
QMP	Quality Management Plan
QUA	Qualitative Use Assessment

TABLE 33.66 *(Continued)*
Frequently Encountered Acronyms

R&D	Research and Development
R&E	Research and Experimental
RAC	Raw Agricultural Commodity (see also RAC-PC)
RAC	Risk Assessment Council
RAC-PC	Raw Agricultural Commodity Processing (re: EPA)
RAF	Risk Assessment Forum
RAPS	Regulatory Affairs Professional Society
RB	Reregistration Branch
RCFs	Refractory Ceramic Fibers
RCRA	Resource Conservation and Recovery Act
RD	Registration Division (re: OPP)
RDRA	Remedial Design/Remedial Action (re: Superfund)
RED	Reregistration Eligibility Document
REI	Reentry Interval (re: OPP)
RFC	Regional Field Coordinator
RfD	Reference Dose
RFD	Recommended for Development
RI/FS	Remedial Investigation/Feasibility Study (re: Superfund)
RLC	Regional Laboratory Coordinator
RM	Review Manager (re: OPP)
RM-1	Risk Management–1 (re: EPA)
RM-2	Risk Management–2 (re: EPA)
RMEB	Resource Management and Evaluation Branch (re: PMSD of OPP)
ROD	Record of Decision (re: Superfund)
RPAR	Rebuttable Presumption Against Registration (re: OPP; see also SR)
RRC	Regulatory Review Committee of the Society of Quality Assurance
RRD	Residue Research Director
RS	Registration Standard (re: OPP)
RSB	Registration Support Branch
RTECS	Registry of Toxic Effects of Chemical Substances
RUP	Restricted Use Pesticide
SAB	Scientific Advisory Board (re: EPA)
SACB	Science Analysis and Coordination Branch (re: HED of OPP)
SACS	Science Analysis and Coordination Staff (re: EFED of OPP)
SAES	State Agricultural Experiment Stations
SAP	Scientific Advisory Panel (re: FIFRA)
SARA	Superfund Amendments and Reauthorization Act
SB	Systems Branch (re: PMSD of OPP)
SD	Study Director
SDLC	Software Development Life Cycles
SDWA	Safe Drinking Water Act
SETAC	Society of Environmental Toxicology & Chemistry
SFIREG	State FIFRA Issues, Research and Evaluation Group
SGML	Standard General Mark-up Language (Computer Language)
SITE	Superfund Innovative Technology Evaluation Program
SMART	Submission Management and Review Tracking
SMARTS	Simple Maintenance of ARTS (see also ARTS)
SOP	Standard Operating Procedure
SOT	Society of Toxicology
SPI	Standard Practice Instructions
SQA	Society of Quality Assurance

TABLE 33.66 *(Continued)*
Frequently Encountered Acronyms

SR	Special Review (re: OPP; formerly RPAR)
SRB	Special Review Branch (re: SRRD of OPP)
SRRD	Special Review and Reregistration Division (re: OPP)
STARS	Submission Tracking And Reporting System
STP	Society of Toxicologic Pathologists
TCLP	Toxicity Characteristic Leaching Procedure, RCRA
TEP	Typical End-use Product
TFM	Testing Facility Management
TGAI	Technical Grade Active Ingredient
TMRC	Theoretical Maximum Residue Contribution (re: OPP)
TOSCA	Toxic Substances Control Act (see also TSCA)
TQ	Total Quality
TQM	Total Quality Management
TQSS	Total Quality Specialty Section of the Society of Quality Assurance
TRI	Toxics Release Inventory (re: EPCRA)
TSCA	Toxic Substances Control Act (see also TOSCA)
TSCATS	TSCA Test Submissions
TVOCs	Total Volatile Organic Compounds
UN	United Nations
USC	United States Code
USCDC	United States Centers for Disease Control (see also CDC)
USDA	United States Department of Agriculture
USDOE	United States Department of Energy (see also DOE)
USDI	United States Department of Interior (see also DI)
USEPA	United States Environmental Protection Agency (see also EPA)
USFDA	United States Food and Drug Administration (see also FDA)
USFWS	United States Fish and Wildlife Service (see also FWS)
VAI	Voluntary Action Indicated
WEX-WPS	Worker Exposure Studies — Worker Protection Standards (re: EPA)
WHO	World Health Organization
WP	Wettable Powders
WSS	Weed Science Society

From Society of Quality Assurance, with permission.

SECTION 10. ACADEMIC PROGRAMS IN TOXICOLOGY

Table 33.67 presents an overview of academic degree programs in Toxicology offered by United States and Canadian institutions.[1] All the schools that appeared in this listing in the first edition of this book have been retained. Additional schools have been added for this edition. Inclusion in this list does not represent an endorsement; likewise, absence from this list does not indicate a lack of endorsement. A more detailed description of the programs and degree requirements can be found in the reference sources or obtained by contacting the academic institution listed.

TABLE 33.67
Academic Programs in Toxicology: United Stated and Canada

Institution	Bachelors	Masters	Doctoral
Albany Medical College Dept. Pharmacology and Toxicology Albany, NY 12208		×	×
Ashland University Department of Toxicology 401 College Avenue Ashland, OH 44805	×		
Auburn University Interdisciplinary Toxicology Program Auburn University, AL 36849-5122		×	×
Brown University Dept. of Pathology and Laboratory Medicine Biomedical Center Providence, RI 02912			×
Case Western Reserve University Dept. of Environmental Health Sciences Cleveland, OH 44106		×	×
Clemson University The Institute of Wildlife & Environmental Toxicology Clemson, SC 29634		×	×
Colorado State University Department of Environmental Health Environmental Health Building Fort Collins, CO 80523-167		×	×
Dartmouth College Dartmouth Medical School Dept. of Pharmacology and Toxicology Hanover, NH 03756			×
Duke University Medical Center and School of the Environment Durham, NC 27710			×
Duquesne University Dept. of Pharmacology and Toxicology Pittsburgh, PA 15282		×	

TABLE 33.67 *(Continued)*
Academic Programs in Toxicology: United Stated and Canada

Institution	Bachelors	Masters	Doctoral
Eastern Michigan University Dept. of Chemistry Program in Toxicology-Biochemistry Ypsilanti, MI 48105	×		
Florida A&M University College of Pharmacy and Pharmaceutical Sciences Tallahassee, FL 32307			×
Harvard University Laboratory of Toxicology and Dept. of Biological Chemistry and Molecular Pharmacology: Joint Program in Toxicology Boston, MA 02115			×
Indiana University Pharmacology and Toxicology 635 Barnhill Drive Medical Science Building MS 1021 Indianapolis, IN 46202		×	×
Iowa State University Interdepartmental Toxicology Major Ames, IA 50011		×	×
The John Hopkins University Division of Toxicological Sciences School of Hygiene and Public Health Baltimore, MD 21205		×	×
Kansas State University Comparative Toxicology Laboratories Manhattan, KS 66506		×	×
Long Island University Arnold and Marie Schwartz College of Pharmacy and Health Sciences Brooklyn, NY 11202		×	
Louisiana State University Medical Center — Shreveport Dept. of Pharmacology and Therapeutics Section of Toxicology Shreveport, LA 71130		×	×
Massachusetts Institute of Technology Division of Bioengineering and Environmental Health Cambridge, MA 02139		×	×
Medical College of Ohio Toxicology Program Toledo, OH 43614		×	×

TABLE 33.67 *(Continued)*
Academic Programs in Toxicology: United Stated and Canada

Institution	Bachelors	Masters	Doctoral
Michigan State University Institute for Environmental Toxicology East Lansing, MI 48824			×
Mississippi State University Center for Environmental Health Sciences Mississippi State, MS 39762		×	×
Montclair State University Toxicology Program Upper Montclair, NJ 07043	×		
New Mexico State University Interdisciplinary Toxicology Program Las Cruces, NM 88003		×	×
New York Medical College Graduate School of Health Sciences Environmental Health Sciences Program Valhalla, NY 10595		×	×
New York University Institute of Environmental Medicine Program in Environmental Health Sciences New York, NY 10016			×
North Carolina State University College of Agriculture and Life Sciences Raleigh, NC 27695		×	×
Northeast Louisiana University Division of Pharmacology and Toxicology School of Pharmacy Monroe, LA 71209-0470	×	×	×
Northeastern University Toxicology Program Boston, MA 02115	×	×	×
Oklahoma State University Dept. of Physiological Sciences Graduate Program in Toxicology/Pharmacology Stillwater, OK 74078-0353		×	×
Oregon State University Toxicology Program Corvallis, OR 97331		×	×
Philadelphia College of Pharmacy and Science Dept. of Pharmacology and Toxicology Philadelphia, PA 19104	×	×	×
Purdue University School of Health Sciences West Lafayette, IN 47907		×	×

TABLE 33.67 *(Continued)*
Academic Programs in Toxicology: United Stated and Canada

Institution	Bachelors	Masters	Doctoral
Rutgers, The State University of NJ University of Medicine and Dentistry of NJ Dept. of Pharmacology and Toxicology School of Pharmacy Piscataway, NJ 08855-0789		×	×
San Diego State University Graduate School of Public Health Division of Occupational and Environmental Health San Diego, CA 92182		×	×
State University of New York at Albany Environmental Health and Toxicology Wadsworth Center, C-236 Albany, NY 12201		×	×
State University of New York at Buffalo School of Medicine and Biomedical Sciences Dept. of Pharmacology and Therapeutics Buffalo, NY 14214		×	×
St. John's University Pharmaceutical Sciences Jamaica, NY 11439	×	×	×
Texas A&M University Dept. of Veterinary Physiology and Pharmacology College Station, TX 77843		×	×
Texas Tech University The Institute of Environmental and Human Health Box 41163 Lubbock, TX 79409-1163		×	×
Thomas Jefferson University Daniel Baugh Institute Anatomy Department Philadelphia, PA 19107			×
University of Alabama at Birmingham Dept of Environmental Health Services Birmingham, AL 35294		×	×
University of Arizona College of Pharmacy Tucson, AZ 85721		×	×
University of Arkansas for Medical Sciences Dept. of Pharmacology and Toxicology College of Medicine Little Rock, AR 72205		×	×
The University of British Columbia Faculty of Pharmaceutical Sciences Vancouver, BC Canada V6T 1W5		×	×

TABLE 33.67 *(Continued)*
Academic Programs in Toxicology: United Stated and Canada

Institution	Bachelors	Masters	Doctoral
University of California at Berkeley Environmental Health Sciences Program Berkeley, CA 94720		×	×
University of California, Davis Graduate Group in Pharmacology & Toxicology Davis, CA 95616		×	×
University of California, Irvine Dept. of Community and Environmental Medicine College of Medicine 370 Medical Surge II Irvine, CA 92697-1820		×	×
University of California, Riverside College of Natural and Agricultural Sciences Riverside, CA 92521		×	×
University of California at San Francisco Division of Toxicology San Francisco, CA 94143-0446			×
University of Cincinnati College of Medicine Dept. of Environmental Health Cincinnati, OH 45267-0056		×	×
University of Colorado Health Sciences Center Pharmaceutical Sciences, School of Pharmacy Box C238, 4200 East Ninth Avenue Denver, CO 80262			×
University of Connecticut Dept. of Pharmaceutical Sciences Storrs, CT 06269-2092		×	×
University of Florida Center for Environmental and Human Toxicology Box 110885 Gainesville, FL 110885			×
University of Georgia College of Pharmacy Athens, GA 30602		×	×
University of Guelph Collaborative Interdepartmental Program in Toxicology Guelph, Ontario Canada		×	×
University of Illinois at Urbana-Champaign College of Veterinary Medicine Department Veterinary Biosciences Urbana, IL 61801		×	×

TABLE 33.67 *(Continued)*
Academic Programs in Toxicology: United Stated and Canada

Institution	Bachelors	Masters	Doctoral
University of Kansas Medical Center Department of Pharmacology, Toxicology, and Therapeutics 3901 Rainbow Boulevard Kansas City, KS 66160-7417			×
University of Kentucky Graduate Center for Toxicology 306 Health Sciences Research Building Lexington, KY 40536-0305		×	×
University of Louisville Dept. of Pharmacology and Toxicology Louisville, KY 40292		×	×
University of Maryland Program in Toxicology Baltimore, MD 21201		×	×
Univ. of Medicine and Dentistry of NJ at Newark Dept. of Pharmacology and Toxicology Newark, NJ 07103			×
University of Michigan School of Public Health Ann Arbor, MI 48109		×	×
University of Minnesota Dept. of Pharmacology Program in Toxicology Minneapolis, MN 55455			×
University of Mississippi Medical Center Dept. of Pharmacology and Toxicology Jackson, MS 39216-4505		×	×
Universite de Montreal Dept. of Environmental Health Department of Pharmacology Montreal, Quebec Canada H3C 3I7		×	×
University of Nebraska Center for Environmental Toxicology Program 986805 Nebraska Medical Center Omaha, NE 68198-6805		×	×
University of North Carolina at Chapel Hill Curriculum in Toxicology Chapel Hill, NC 27599			×
The University of Oklahoma College of Pharmacy Graduate Program in Toxicology Oklahoma City, OK 73190			×

TABLE 33.67 *(Continued)*
Academic Programs in Toxicology: United Stated and Canada

Institution	Bachelors	Masters	Doctoral
University of Pittsburgh Dept. of Industrial Environmental Health Sciences Toxicology Program Pittsburgh, PA 15261			×
The University of Rhode Island Dept. of Pharmacology and Toxicology Kingston, RI 02881		×	×
University of Rochester School of Medicine and Dentistry Environmental Health Sciences Center Rochester, NY 14642		×	×
University of Saskatchewan Saskatoon Saskatchewan Graduate Training Programs in Toxicology Postgraduate Diploma Saskatoon, Saskatchewan Canada S7N 0W0		×	×
University of South Carolina School of Public Health Dept. of Environmental Health Sciences Columbia, SC 29208		×	×
University of South Florida College of Public Health Dept. of Environmental and Occupational Health Tampa, FL 33612		×	×
The University of Southern California Institute for Toxicology Los Angeles, CA 90033		×	×
University of Texas at Austin College of Pharmacy Division of Pharmacology and Toxicology Austin, TX 78712		×	×
The University of Texas Health Science Center at Houston School of Public Health Houston, TX 77225		×	×
University of Texas Medical Branch Graduate School of Biomedical Sciences Galveston, TX 77550			×
University of the Sciences in Philadelphia Pharmaceutical Sciences 600 S. 43rd Street Philadelphia, PA 19104		×	×

TABLE 33.67 *(Continued)*
Academic Programs in Toxicology: United Stated and Canada

Institution	Bachelors	Masters	Doctoral
University of Toronto Toxicology Graduate Program Toronto, Ontario M5S 1A4 Canada		×	×
University of Utah Dept. of Pharmacology and Toxicology Salt Lake City, UT 84112			×
University of Washington Dept. of Environmental Health Seattle, WA 98195		×	×
University of Wisconsin — Madison Graduate Program in Environmental Toxicology Madison, WI 53706		×	×
Utah State University Graduate Program in Toxicology Logan, UT 84322-5600		×	×
Vanderbilt University Graduate Study in Toxicology & Carcinogenesis Nashville, TN 37232			×
Virginia Maryland Regional College of Veterinary Medicine Blacksburg, VA 24061		×	×
Washington State University Graduate Program in Pharmacology/Toxicology Pullman, WA 99164-1030		×	×
Wayne State University Institute of Chemical Toxicology 2727 Second Avenue Detroit, MI 48201			×
West Virginia University Dept of Pharmacology and Toxicology Morgantown, WV 26506			×
Wright State University Biomedical Sciences Doctoral Program Toxicology and Environmental Chemistry Dayton, OH 45435			×

REFERENCES

1. *Resource Guide to Careers in Toxicology,* Society of Toxicology, Washington, D.C., 1989.
2. *Resource Guide to Careers in Toxicology,* 4th ed., Society of Toxicology Web site (*www. toxicology.org*), 2000.

SECTION 11. MISCELLANEOUS

A. RADIOACTIVITY

1. SI Units of Radioactivity

The unit of radioactivity in the International System of Units (SI) is the becquerel, which is equal to one nuclear transformation per second.

Conversion factors are:

1 becquerel, (Bq)	= 1 nuclear transformation/second
1 curie (Ci)	= 3.7 × 10^10 becquerels (exactly)
	= 37 gigabecquerels (GBq)
1 millicurie (mCi)	= 3.7 × 10^7 becquerels
	= 37 megabecquerels (MBq)
1 microcurie (μCi)	= 3.7 × 10^4 becquerels
	= 37 kilobecquerels (kBq)
1 gigabecquerel (GBq)	= 27.027 millicuries (mCi)
1 megabecquerel (MBq)	= 27.027 microcuries (μCi)
1 kilobecquerel (kBq)	= 27.027 nanocuries (nCi)

TABLE 33.68
Decay Constants and Modes for Selected Radionuclides

Nuclide	Half-life	Decay Mode[a]
Carbon- 11	20.3 min	β+
Carbon- 14	5730 yr	β−
Cesium-137	30.0 yr	β−
Chromium-51	27.8 day	E.C.
Cobalt-57	270 day	E.C.
Cobalt-60	5.26 yr	β−
Gallium-67	78 h	E.C.
Gold- 198	2.7 day	β−
Hydrogen-3 (tritium)	12.4 yr	β−
Indium- 111	2.8 day	E.C.
Indium-113m	100 min	I.T.
Iodine-123	13.3 h	E.C.
Iodine- 125	60 day	E.C.
Iodine- 131	8.05 day	β−
Iron-59	45 day	β−
Mercury- 197	65 h	E.C.
Nitrogen- 13	10.0 min	β+
Phosphorus-32	14.3 day	β−
Oxygen- 15	124 sec	β+
Selenium-75	120 day	E.C.
Sulphur-35	87.4 day	β−
Technetium-99m	6.0 h	I.T.
Thallium-201	73 h	E.C.
Xenon- 133	5.3 day	β−
Ytterbium-169	31.8 day	E.C.

[a] Decay modes include: β−, beta decay; β+, positron emission; E.C., electron capture; I.T., isomeric transition.

B. IONIZATION

TABLE 33.69
pK$_a$ Values of Common Drugs

Drug	pK$_a$	Drug	pK$_a$
Acetanilid	0.3	Methamphetamine	9.9
Acetazolamide	7.2	Metoprolol	9.6
N-Acetylaminoantipyrine	0.5	Morphine	8.2
α-Acetylmethadol	8.3	Nortriptyline	9.7
Acetylsalicylic acid	3.5	Orphenadrine	8.4
Aminopyrine	5.0	Oxyphenbutazone	4.7
Amitriptyline	9.4	Papaverine	6.4
Amphetamine	9.9	Pentobarbital	8.1
Amylobarbital	7.9	Pentazocine	8.8
Aniline	4.6	Phencyclidine	8.5
Antipyrine	1.4	Phenobarbital	7.2
Ascorbic acid	4.1, 11.8	Phenylbutazone	4.5
Atropine	10.0	Phenylpropanolamine	9.1
Barbital	7.5	Physostigmine	8.5
Barbituric acid	4.0	Pilocarpine	6.9
Caffeine	0.8	Probenecid	3.4
Chlorpheniramine	9.0	Propoxyphene	6.3
Chlorpromazine	8.2	Propranolol	9.5
Cocaine	8.5	Pseudoephedrine	9.7
Cycloserine	4.5, 7.4	Quinine	4.1, 8.5
Desipramine	10.2	Reserpine	6.1
Dextromethorphan	8.3	Salicylic acid	3.0
Dicumarol	5.7	Secobarbital	7.9
Diphenhydramine	8.3	Strychnine	8.3
Doxepin	8.0	Sulfadiazine	6.5
Ephedrine	9.9	Sulfaguanidine	> 10.00
Ethylbiscoumacetate	3.1	Sulfanilamide	10.4
Glutethimide	11.2	Sulfapyridine	8.4
Hexachlorophene	5.4, 10.9	Sulfathiazole	7.1
Hydrocodone	8.9	Sulfinpyrazone	2.8
Hydromorphone	8.2	Theophylline	0.7
Imipramine	9.5	Thiopental	7.6
Levorphanol	9.2	Tolazoline	10.3
Lidocaine	7.9	Triamterene	6.2
Loxapine	6.6	Trimethobenzamide	8.3
Mecamylamine	11.2	Trimethoprim	7.2
Meperidine	8.7	Vinblastine	5.4, 7.4
Methadone	8.3	Vincristine	5.0, 7.4

The following table gives approximate pH values for a number of substances of biological importance. All values are rounded off to the nearest tenth and are based on measurements made at 25°C.

TABLE 33.70
Approximate pH Values of Biological Materials and Foods

Biological Materials

Blood, plasma, human	7.3–7.5	Gastric contents, human	1.0–3.0	Milk, human	6.6–7.6
Spinal fluid, human	7.3–7.5	Duodenal contents, human	4.8–8.2	Bile, human	6.8–7.0
Blood, whole, dog	6.9–7.2	Feces, human	4.6–8.4		
Saliva, human	6.5–7.5	Urine, human	4.8–8.4		

Foods

Apples	2.9–3.3	Gooseberries	2.8–3.0	Potatoes	5.6–6.0
Apricots	3.6–4.0	Grapefruit	3.0–3.3	Pumpkin	4.8–5.2
Asparagus	5.4–5.8	Grapes	3.5–4.5	Raspberries	3.2–3.6
Bananas	4.5–4.7	Hominy (lye)	6.8–8.0	Rhubarb	3.1–3.2
Beans	5.0–6.0	Jams, fruit	3.5–4.0	Salmon	6.1–6.3
Beer	4.0–5.0	Jellies, fruit	2.8–3.4	Sauerkraut	3.4–3.6
Beets	4.9–5.5	Lemons	2.2–2.4	Shrimp	6.8–7.0
Blackberries	3.2–3.6	Limes	1.8–2.0	Soft drinks	2.0–4.0
Bread, white	5.0–6.0	Maple syrup	6.5–7.0	Spinach	5.1–5.7
Butter	6.1–6.4	Milk, cows	6.3–6.6	Squash	5.0–5.4
Cabbage	5.2–5.4	Olives	3.6–3.8	Strawberries	3.0–3.5
Carrots	4.9–5.3	Oranges	3.0–4.0	Sweet potatoes	5.3–5.6
Cheese	4.8–6.4	Oysters	6.1–6.6	Tomatoes	4.0–4.4
Cherries	3.2–4.0	Peaches	3.4–3.6	Tuna	5.9–6.1
Cider	2.9–3.3	Pears	3.6–4.0	Turnips	5.2–5.6
Corn	6.0–6.5	Peas	5.8–6.4	Vinegar	2.4–3.4
Crackers	6.5–8.5	Pickles, dill	3.2–3.6	Water, drinking	6.5–8.0
Dates	6.2–6.4	Pickles, sour	3.0–3.4	Wine	2.8–3.8
Eggs, fresh white	7.6–8.0	Pimento	4.6–5.2		
Flour, wheat	5.5–6.5	Plums	2.8–3.0		

Source: Handbook of Chemistry and Physics, Lide, D. R., Ed., CRC Press, Boca Raton, FL, 1990. With permission.

C. CHEMICAL FUNCTIONAL GROUPS

Table 33.71 presents the chemical structure of functional groups frequently encountered in toxicology.

TABLE 33.71
Chemical Functional Groups

Acetamido (acetylamino)	CH_3CONH-
Acetimido (acetylimino)	$CH_3C(=NH)-$
Acetoacetamido	CH_3COCH_2CONH-
Acetoacetyl	CH_3COCH_2CO-
Acetonyl	CH_3COCH_2-
Acetonylidene	$CH_3COCH=$
Acetyl	CH_3CO-
Acrylyl	$CH_2=CHCO-$

TABLE 33.71 *(Continued)*
Chemical Functional Groups

Adipyl (from adipic acid)	$-OC(CH_2)_4CO-$
Alanyl (from alanine)	$CH_3CH(NH_2)CO-$
β-alanyl	$HN(CH_2)_2CO-$
Allophanoyl	$H_2NCONHCO-$
Allyl (2-propenyl)	$CH_2=CHCH_2-$
Allylidene (2-propenylidene)	$CH_2=CHCH=$
Amidino (aminoiminomethyl)	$H_2NC(=NH)-$
Amino	H_2N-
Amyl (pentyl)	$CH_3(CH_2)_4-$
Anilino (phenylamino)	C_6H_5NH-
Anisidino	$CH_3OC_6H_4NH-$
Anisyl (from anisic acid)	$CH_3OC_6H_4CO-$
Anthranoyl (2-aminobenzoyl)	$2-H_2NC_6H_4CO-$
Arsino	AsH_2-
Azelaoyl (from azelaic acid)	$-OC(CH_2)_7CO-$
Azido	N_3-
Azino	$=NN=$
Azo	$-N=N-$
Azoxy	$-N(O)N-$
Benzal	$C_6H_5CH=$
Benzamido (benzylamino)	C_6H_5CONH-
Benzhydryl (diphenylmethyl)	$(C_6H_5)_2CH-$
Benzimido (benzylimino)	C_6H_5COO-
Benzoxy (benzoyloxy)	C_6H_5COO-
Benzoyl	C_6H_5CO-
Benzyl	$C_6H_5CH_2-$
Benzylidine	$C_6H_5CH=$
Benzyldyne	$C_6H_5C\equiv$
Biphenylyl	$C_6H_5C_6H_5-$
Biphenylene	$-C_6H_4C_6H_4-$
Butoxy	C_4H_9O-
Sec-butoxy	$C_2H_5CH(CH_3)O-$
Tert-butoxy	$(CH_3)_3CO-$
Butyl	$CH_3(CH_2)_3-$
Iso-butyl (3-methylpropyl)	$(CH_3)_2(CH_2)_2-$
sec-butyl (1-methylpropyl)	$C_2H_5CH(CH_3)-$
Tert-butyl (1,1, dimethylethyl)	$(CH_3)_3C-$
Butyryl	C_3H_7CO-
Caproyl (from caproic acid)	$CH_3(CH_2)_4CO-$
Capryl (from capric acid)	$CH_3(CH_2)_6CO-$
Caprylyl (from caprylic acid)	$CH_3(CH_2)_6CO-$
Carbamido	$H_2NCONH-$
Carbamoyl (aminocarbonyl)	H_2NCO-
Carbamyl (aminocarbonyl)	H_2NCO-
Carbazoyl (hydrazinocarbonyl)	$H_2NNHCO-$
Carbethoxy	$C_2H_5O_2C-$
Carbobenzoxy	$C_6H_5CH_2O_2C-$
Carbonyl	$-C=O-$
Carboxy	$HOOC-$
Cetyl	$CH_3(CH_2)_{15}-$
Chloroformyl (chlorocarbonyl)	$ClCO-$

TABLE 33.71 *(Continued)*
Chemical Functional Groups

Cinnamyl (3-phenyl-2-propenyl)	$C_6H_5CH{=}CHCH_2{-}$
Cinnamoyl	$C_6H_5CH{=}CHCO{-}$
Cinnamylidene	$C_6H_5CH{=}CHCH{=}$
Cresyl (hydroxymethylphenyl)	$HO(CH_3)C_6H_4{-}$
Crotoxyl	$CH_3CH{=}CHCO{-}$
Crotyl (2-butenyl)	$CH_3CH{=}CHCH_2{-}$
Cyanamido (cyanoamino)	$NCNH{-}$
Cyanato	$NCO{-}$
Cyano	$NC{-}$
Decanedioyl	$-OC(CH_2)_6CO{-}$
Decanoly	$CH_3(CH_2)_6CO{-}$
Diazo	$N_2{=}$
Diazoamino	$-NHN{=}N{-}$
Disilanyl	$H_2SiSiH_2{-}$
Disiloxanoxy	$H_3SiOSiH_2O{-}$
Disulfinyl	$-S(O)S(O){-}$
Dithio	$-SS{-}$
Enanthyl	$CH_3(CH_2)_5CO{-}$
Epoxy	$-O{-}$
Ethenyl (vinyl)	$CH_2{=}CH{-}$
Ethinyl	$HC{\equiv}C{-}$
Ethoxy	$C_2H_5O{-}$
Ethyl	$CH_3CH_2{-}$
Ethylthio	$C_2H_5S{-}$
Formamido (formylamino)	$HCONH{-}$
Formyl	$HCO{-}$
Fumaroyl (from fumaric acid)	$-OCCH{=}CHCO{-}$
Furfuryl (2-furanylmethyl)	$OC_4H_3CH_2{-}$
Furfurylidene (2-furanylmethylene)	$OC_4H_3CH{=}$
Furyl (furanyl)	$OC_4H_3{-}$
Glutamyl (from glutamic acid)	$-OC(CH_2)_2CH(NH_2)CO{-}$
Glutaryl (from glutaric acid)	$-OC(CH_2)CO{-}$
Glycidyl (oxiranylmethyl)	$CH_2CHCH_2{-}$
Glycinamido	$H_2NCH_2CONH{-}$
Glycolyl (hydroxyacetyl)	$HOCH_2CO{-}$
Glycyl (aminoacetyl)	$H_2NCH_2CO{-}$
Glyoxylyl (oxoacetyl)	$HCOCO{-}$
Guanidino	$H_2NC({=}NH)NH{-}$
Guanyl	$H_2NC({=}NH){-}$
Heptadecanoyl	$CH_3(CH_2)_{15}CO{-}$
Heptanamido	$CH_3(CH_2)_{15}CONH{-}$
Heptanedioyl	$-OC(CH_2)_5CO{-}$
Heptanoyl	$CH_3(CH_2)_5CO{-}$
Hexadecanoyl	$CH_3(CH_2)_4CO{-}$
Hexamethylene	$-(CH_2)_6{-}$
Hexanedioyl	$-OC(CH_2)_4CO{-}$
Hippuryl (N-benzoylglycyl)	$C_6H_5CONHCH_2CO{-}$
Hydantoyl	$H_2NCONHCH_2CO{-}$
Hydrazino	$N_2NNH{-}$
Hydrazo	$-HNNH{-}$
Hydrocinnamoyl	$C_6H_5(CH_2)_2CO{-}$

TABLE 33.71 *(Continued)*
Chemical Functional Groups

Hydroperoxy	HOO–
Hydroxamino	HONH–
Hydroxy	HO–
Imino	HN=
Lodoso	OI–
Isoamyl (isopentyl)	$(CH_3)_2CH(CH_2)_2$–
Isobutenyl (2-methyl-1-propenyl)	$(CH_3)_2C=CH$–
Isobutoxy	$(CH_3)_2CHCH\ O$–
Isobutyl	$(CH_3)_2CHCH_2$–
Isobutylidene	$(CH_3)_2CHCH=$
Isobutyryl	$(CH_3)_2CHCO$–
Isocyanato	OCN–
Isocyano	CN–
Isohexyl	$(CH_3)_2CH(CH_2)_3$–
Isoleucyl (from isoleucine)	$C_2H_3CH(CH_3)CH(NH_4)CO$–
Isonitroso	HON=
Isopentyl	$(CH_3)_2CH(CH_2)_2$–
Isopentylidene	$(CH_3)_2CHCH_2CH=$
Isopropenyl	$H_2C=C(CH_3)$–
Isopropoxy	$(CH_3)_2CHO$–
Isopropyl	$(CH_3)_2CH$–
Isopropylidene	$(CH_3)_2C=$
Isothiocyanato (isothiocyano)	SCN–
Isovaleryl (from isovaleric acid)	$(CH_3)_2CHCH_2CO$–
Keto (oxo)	O=
Lactyl (from lactic acid)	$CH_3CH(OH)CO$–
Lauroyl (from lauric acid)	$CH_3(CH_2)_{10}CO$–
Leucyl (from leucine)	$(CH_3)_2CHCH_2CH(NH_2)CO$–
Levulinyl (From levulinic acid)	$CH_3CO(CH_2)_2CO$–
Malonyl (from malonic acid)	$–OCCH_2CO$–
Mandelyl (from mandelic acid)	$C_6H_5CH(OH)CO$–
Mercapto	HS–
Methacrylyl (from methacrylic acid)	$CH_2=C(CH_3)CO$–
Methallyl	$CH_2=C(CH_3)CH_2$–
Methionyl (from methionine)	$CH_3SCH_2CH_2CH(NH_2)CO_2$–
Methoxy	CH_3O–
Methyl	H_3C–
Methylene	$H_2C=$
Methylenedioxy	$–OCH_2O$–
Methylenedisulfonyl	$–O_2SCH_2SO_2$–
Methylol	$HOCH_2$–
Methylthio	CH_2S–
Myristyl (from myristic acid)	$CH_3(CH_2)_{12}CO$–
Naphthal	$(C_{10}H_7)CH=$
Naphthobenzyl	$(C_{10}H_7)CH_2$–
Naphthoxy	$(C_{10}H_7)O$–
Naphthyl	$(C_{10}H_7)$–
Naphthylidene	$(C_{10}H_6)=$
Neopentyl	$(CH_3)_3CCH_2$–
Nitramino	O_2NNH–
Nitro	O_2N–

TABLE 33.71 *(Continued)*
Chemical Functional Groups

Nitrosamino	ONNH–
Nitrosimino	ONN=
Nitroso	ON–
Nonanoyl (from nonanoic acid)	$CH_3(CH_2)_7CO–$
Oleyl (from oleic acid)	$CH_3(CH_2)_7CH=CH(CH_2)_7CO–$
Oxalyl (from oxalic acid)	–OCCO–
Oxamido	$H_2NCOCONH–$
Oxo (keto)	O=
Palmityl (from palmitic acid)	$CH_3(CH_2)_{14}CO–$
Pelargonyl (from pelargonic acid)	$CH_3(CH_2)_7CO–$
Pentamethylene	$–(CH_2)_5–$
Pentyl	$CH_3(CH_2)_4–$
Phenacyl	$C_6H_5COCH_2–$
Phenacylidene	$C_6H_5COCH=$
Phenanthryl	$(C_{14}H_9)–$
Phenethyl	$C_6H_5CH_2CH_2–$
Phenoxy	$C_6H_5O–$
Phenyl	$C_6H_5–$
Phenylene	$–C_6H_4–$
Phenylenedioxy	$–OC_6H_4O–$
Phosphino	$H_2P–$
Phosphinyl	$H_2P(O)–$
Phospho	$O_2P–$
Phosphono	$(HO)_2P(O)–$
Phthalyl (from phthalic acid)	$1,2-C_6H_4(CO–)_2$
Picryl (2,4,6-trinitrophenyl)	$2,4,6–(NO_2)_2C_6H_2–$
Pimelyl (from pimelic acid)	$–OC(CH_2)_5CO–$
Piperidino	$C_5H_{10}N–$
Piperidyl (piperidinyl)	$(C_5H_{10}N)–$
Piperonyl	$3,4-(CH_2O_2)C_6H_3CH_2–$
Pivalyl (from pivalic acid)	$(CH_3)_3CCO–$
Prenyl (3-methyl-2-butenyl)	$(CH_3)_2C=CHCH_2–$
Propargyl (2-propynyl)	$HC≡CCH_2–$
Propenyl	$CH_2=CHCH_2–$
iso-propenyl	$(CH_3)_2C=$
Propionyl	$CH_3CH_2CO–$
Propoxy	$CH_3CH_2CH_2O–$
Propyl	$CH_3CH_2CH_2–$
iso-propyl	$(CH_3)_2CH–$
Propylidene	$CH_3CH_2CH=$
Pyridino	$C_5H_5N–$
Pyridyl (pyridinyl)	$(C_5H_4N)–$
Pyrryl (pyrrolyl)	$(C_3H_4N)–$
Salicyl (2-hydroxybenzoyl)	$2-HOC_6H_4CO–$
Selenyl	HSe–
Seryl (from serine)	$HOCH_2CH(NH_2)CO–$
Siloxy	$H_3SiO–$
Silyl	$H_3Si–$
Silylene	$H_2Si=$
Sorbyl (from sorbic acid)	$CH_3CH=CHCH=CHCO–$

TABLE 33.71 *(Continued)*
Chemical Functional Groups

Stearyl (from stearic acid)	$CH_3(CH_2)_{16}CO-$
Styryl	$C_6H_5CH=CH-$
Suberyl (from suberic acid)	$-OC(CH_2)_6CO-$
Succinamyl	$H_2NCOCH_2CH_2CO-$
Succinyl (from succinic acid)	$-OCCH_2CH_2CO-$
Sulfamino	$HOSO_2NH-$
Sulfamyl	H_2NSO-
Sulfanilyl	$4-H_2NC_6H_4SO_2-$
Sulfeno	$HOS-$
Sulfhydryl (mercapto)	$HS-$
Sulfinyl	$OS=$
Sulfo	HO_3S-
Sulfonyl	$-SO_2-$
Terephthalyl	$1,4-C_6H_4(CO-)_2$
Tetramethylene	$-(CH_2)_4-$
Thenyl	$(C_4H_3S)CH-$
Thienyl	$(C_4H_3S)-$
Thiobenzoyl	C_6H_5CS-
Thiocarbamyl	H_2NCS-
Thiocarbonyl	$-CS-$
Thiocarboxy	$HOSC-$
Thiocyanato	$NCS-$
Thionyl (sulfinyl)	$-SO-$
Thiophenacyl	$C_6H_5CSCH_2-$
Thiurain(aminothioxomethyl)	H_2NCS-
Threonyl (from threonine)	$CH_3CH(OH)CH(NH_2)CO-$
Toluidino	$CH_3C_6H_4NH-$
Toluyl	$CH_3C_6H_4CO-$
Tolyl (methylphenyl)	$CH_3C_6H_4-$
α-tolyl	$C_6H_5CH_2-$
Tolylene (methylphenylene)	$(CH_3C_6H_3)=$
α-tolylene	$C_6H_5CH=$
Tosyl [(4-methylphenyl) sulfonyl)]	$4-CH_3C_6H_4SO_2-$
Triazano	$H_2NNHNH-$
Trimethylene	$-(CH_2)_3-$
Triphenylmethyl (trityl)	$(C_6H_5)_3C-$
Tyrosyl (from tyrosine)	$4-HOC_6H_4CH_2CH(NH_2)CO-$
Ureido	$H_2NCONH-$
Valeryl (from valeric acid)	C_4H_9CO
Valyl (from valine)	$(CH_3)_2CHCH(NH_2)CO-$
Vinyl	$CH_2=CH-$
Vinylidene	$CH_2=C=$
Xenyl (biphenylyl)	$C_6H_5C_6H_4-$
Xylidino	$(CH_3)_2C_6H_3NH-$
Xylyl (dimethylphenyl)	$(CH_3)_2C_6H_3-$
Xylylene	$-CH_2C_6H_4CH_2-$

From *CRC Handbook of Chemistry and Physics,* 73rd ed., Lide, D. R., Ed., CRC Press, Boca Raton, FL, 1992–1993. With permission.

Table 33.72 gives selected properties of 20-α-amino acids commonly found in proteins. The compounds are listed in alphabetical order by the three-letter symbols. Dissociation constants refer to aqueous solutions at 25°C. M_r = molecular weight; T_m = melting point; pK_a = negative of the logarithm of the dissociation constant for the α-COOH group; pK_b = negative of the logarithm of the dissociation constant for the $\alpha - NH_3^+$ group; pK_x = negative of the logarithm of the dissociation constant for any other group present in the molecule; pI = pH at the isoelectronic point; S = solubility in water at 25°C in units of grams per kilogram of water.

TABLE 33.72
Properties of Common Amino Acids

Symbol	Name	Mol. form.	M_r	$t_m/°C$	pK_a	pK_b	pK_x	pI	S/g kg⁻¹
Ala	Alanine	$C_3H_7NO_2$	89.09	297	2.33	9.71		6.00	165.0
Arg	Arginine	$C_6H_{14}N_4O_2$	174.20	244	2.03	9.00	12.10	10.76	182.6
Asn	Asparagine	$C_4H_8N_2O_3$	132.12	235	2.16	8.73		5.41	25.1
Asp	Aspartic acid	$C_4H_7NO_4$	133.10	270	1.95	9.66	3.71	2.77	4.95
Cys	Cysteine	$C_3H_7NO_2S$	121.16	240	1.91	10.28	8.14	5.07	v.s.
Glu	Glutamic acid	$C_5H_9NO_4$	147.13	160	2.16	9.58	4.15	3.22	8.61
Gln	Glutamine	$C_5H_{10}N_2O_3$	146.15	185	2.18	9.00		5.65	42
Gly	Glycine	$C_2H_5NO_2$	75.07	290	2.34	9.58		5.97	250.9
His	Histidine	$C_6H_9N_3O_2$	155.16	287	1.70	9.09	6.04	7.59	43.5
Ile	Isoleucine	$C_6H_{13}NO_2$	131.17	284	2.26	9.60		6.02	34.2
Leu	Leucine	$C_6H_{13}NO_2$	131.17	293	2.32	9.58		5.98	22.0
Lys	Lysine	$C_6H_{14}N_2O_2$	146.19	224	2.15	9.16	10.67	9.74	5.8
Met	Methionine	$C_5H_{11}NO_2S$	149.21	281	2.16	9.08		5.74	56
Phe	Phenylalanine	$C_9H_{11}NO_2$	165.19	283	2.18	9.09		5.48	27.9
Pro	Proline	$C_5H_9NO_2$	115.13	221	1.95	10.47		6.30	1623
Ser	Serine	$C_3H_7NO_3$	105.09	228	2.13	9.05		5.68	421.7
Thr	Threonine	$C_4H_9NO_3$	119.12	256	2.20	8.96		5.60	98.1
Trp	Tryptophan	$C_{11}H_{12}N_2O_2$	204.23	289	2.38	9.34		5.89	13.2
Try	Tyrosine	$C_9H_{11}NO_3$	181.19	343	2.24	9.04	10.10	5.66	0.46
Val	Valine	$C_5H_{11}NO_2$	117.15	315	2.27	9.52		5.96	88.5

M_r — Molecular weight

T_m — Melting point

pK_a, pK_b, pK_c, pK_d — Negative of the logarithm of the acid dissociation constants for the COOH and NH_2 groups (and, in some cases, other groups) in the molecule (at 25°C)

pI — pH at the isoelectric point

S — Solubility in water at 25°C in units of grams of compound per kilogram of water; when quantitative data are not available, the notations sl.s. (for slightly soluble and v.s. (for very soluble) are used.

D. MATERIAL SAFETY DATA SHEETS

TABLE 33.73
Information Disclosed on a Material Safety Data Sheet (MSDS)

SECTION 1.   **Chemical Product and Company Identification**
Product Name
Generic Names/Synonyms
Product Use
Manufacturer's Name and Address
Name and Phone Number of the Person/Group Who Prepared the MSDS
Date MSDS was Prepared
Emergency Phone Number

SECTION 2.   **Composition/Information on Ingredients**
Ingredient Name(s)
CAS Number(s)
Percent by Weight

SECTION 3.   **Hazards Identification**
Potential Human Health Hazards:
    To Skin (irritancy, sensitization)
    To Eyes (irritancy)
    via Inhalation (acute effects)
    via Ingestion (acute effects)
    Delayed Effects (chronic effects)
    Carcinogenicity, reproductive and developmental effects, mutagenicity, other

SECTION 4.   **First Aid Measures**
Specific First Aid Measures for Various Routes of Exposure
Notes to Physician Including Antidotes and Medical Conditions Affected by the
    Product

SECTION 5.   **Fire Fighting Measures**
Flammable Properties (flashpoint, autoignition temperature, etc.)
Extinguishing Media
Hazardous Combustion Products
Explosion Hazards
Firefighting Precautions and Instructions

SECTION 6.   **Accidental Release Measures**
Procedures to be Followed in Case of Spill or Other Release

SECTION 7.   **Handling and Storage**
Normal Handling Procedures
Storage Recommendations

SECTION 8.   **Exposure Controls/Personal Protection**
Engineering Controls
Personal Protective Equipment
Exposure Guidelines (TLV, PEL, other)

SECTION 9.   **Physical and Chemical Properties**
Appearance Boiling Point
Physical State   Melting Point
Odor Vapor   Pressure
Specific Gravity   Vapor Density
Solubility   Evaporation Rate
pH   % Volatiles

TABLE 33.73 *(Continued)*
Information Disclosed on a Material Safety Data Sheet (MSDS)

SECTION 10.	**Stability and Reactivity**	
	Stability Conditions	
	Incompatibilities	
	Hazardous Decomposition Products	
	Hazardous Polymerization	
SECTION 11.	**Toxicity Information**	
	Acute Effects (LD_{50}, LC_{50})	
	Subchronic and Chronic Effects	
	Irritancy	
	Sensitization	
	Neurotoxicity	
	Reprotoxicity	
	Developmental Toxicity	
	Mutagenicity	
SECTION 12.	**Ecological Information**	
	Aquatic Toxicity	
	Terrestrial Toxicity	
	Bioaccumulation Potential	
	Biodegradability	
	Microbial Toxicity	
SECTION 13.	**Disposal Information**	
SECTION 14.	**Shipping Information**	
	D.O.T. Hazard Class	
	D.O.T. I.D. Number	
SECTION 15.	**Regulatory Information**	
	TSCA Inventory Status	
	Other Federal, State, Local	
	Foreign Regulatory Information	
SECTION 16.	**Information not covered in the other 15 sections**	

REFERENCES

Fasman, G. D., Ed., *Practical Handbook of Biochemistry and Molecular Biology*, CRC Press, Boca Raton, FL, 1989.

Hinz, H. J., Ed., *Thermodynamic Datafor Biochemistry and Biotechnology*, Springer-Verlag, Heidelberg, 1986.

Smith, E. L. et al., *Principles of Biochemistry,* 7th ed., McGraw Hill, New York, 1983.

Index

A